Nurse's Manual of Laboratory and Diagnostic Tests

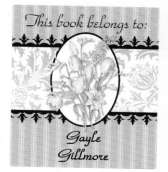

Nurse's Manual of Laboratory and Diagnostic Tests
3rd Edition

Bonita Morrow Cavanaugh, RN, PhD
Assistant Professor and
Baccalaureate Program Director
University of Colorado
Health Sciences Center
School of Nursing
Denver, Colorado

 F. A. DAVIS COMPANY • Philadelphia

F. A. Davis Company
1915 Arch Street
Philadelphia, PA 19103

Printed in the United States of America

Last digit indicates print number: 10 9 8 7 6 5 4 3 2 1

Acquisitions Editor: Lisa Biello
Developmental Editor: Diane Blodgett
Production Editor: Jessica Howie Martin
Cover Designer: Louis J. Forgione

As new scientific information becomes available through basic and clinical research, recommended treatments and drug therapies undergo changes. The author and publisher have done everything possible to make this book accurate, up to date, and in accord with accepted standards at the time of publication. The author, editors, and publisher are not responsible for errors or omissions or for consequences from application of the book, and make no warranty, expressed or implied, in regard to the contents of the book. Any practice described in this book should be applied by the reader in accordance with professional standards of care used in regard to the unique circumstances that may apply in each situation. The reader is advised always to check product information (package inserts) for changes and new information regarding dose and contraindications before administering any drug. Caution is especially urged when using new or infrequently ordered drugs.

Library of Congress Cataloging-in-Publication Data

Cavanaugh, Bonita Morrow, 1952–
    Nurse's manual of laboratory and diagnostic tests. -- 3rd ed. /
Bonita Morrow Cavanaugh.
       p.   cm.
    Rev. ed. of: Nurse's manual of laboratory and diagnostic tests /
Juanita Watson. 2nd. ed. c1995.
    Includes bibliographical references and index.
    ISBN 0-8036-0363-0 (pbk.)
    1. Diagnosis, Laboratory --Handbooks, manuals, etc. 2. Nursing-
-Handbook, manuals, etc. I. Watson, Juanita, 1946–   Nurse's
manual of laboratory and diagnostic tests.   II. Title.
    [DNLM: 1.   Laboratory Techniques and Procedures nurses' instruction
handbooks.   QY 39 C377n 1999]
RT48.5.W38   1999
616.07′5--dc21
DNLM/DLC
for Library of Congress
                                     98-50920
                                       CIP

To Laurie O'Neil Good, the finest nurse I have ever known.

Love,
Bonnie

Preface

➤ This book is designed to provide both students and practitioners of nursing with the information they need to care for individuals undergoing laboratory and diagnostic tests and procedures. The content is presented as a guiding reference for planning care, providing specific interventions, and evaluating outcomes of nursing care.

The major difference in the third edition is the reorganization of the text. The background information and description of the test or procedure are now followed directly by the clinical applications data, starting with reference values, for each test or group of tests. In addition, a nursing care plan appendix and critical thinking exercises in the form of case studies have been developed.

The introductory sections (formerly called Background Information) include the anatomic, physiological, and pathophysiological content necessary for a thorough understanding of the purpose of and indications for specific tests and procedures. The inclusion of this information makes this book unlike many other references on this subject matter. This feature enhances the integration of basic science knowledge with understanding of and application to diagnostic testing. This is extremely helpful for nursing students in developing critical thinking and clinical judgment.

For each test or study within the respective sections, reference values, including variations related to age or gender, are provided. Critical values, where appropriate, are highlighted. Both conventional units and international units are provided. Readers are encouraged to be aware of some variation in laboratory values from agency to agency.

For all tests, interfering factors are noted where appropriate. Contraindications and Nursing Alerts are included to provide information crucial to safe and reliable testing and nursing care.

Other features of this manual that contribute to its practical use are presentation of detailed content in tabular format when appropriate and the use of appendices to provide essential information applicable to most, if not all, tests and procedures.

Every effort has been made to include tests and procedures currently in use in practice settings. It is recognized that newer tests and procedures may have become available after this manuscript was prepared. Readers are encouraged to keep abreast of current literature and consult with laboratories and agencies in their area for new developments in the field of diagnostic tests.

Bonita Morrow Cavanaugh

Acknowledgments

➤ This book would not have been possible without the help, support, and encouragement of a number of people. Special appreciation is due to the staff of the F. A. Davis Company. I am particularly indebted to Lisa Biello, Nursing Editor, for her major contribution in developing the unique format of this text, for her encouragement, and for always being available for help when I needed it. I would also like to acknowledge Robert Martone, Nursing Publisher, who encouraged me to pursue this project, and Robert H. Craven, Jr., President, for his support and patience as the book evolved. Special thanks are also due to Ruth De George, Editorial Assistant and Michele Reese, Editorial Aide, for their invaluable assistance. Many other individuals at the F. A. Davis Company contributed to the production of this book, and I wish to extend to all of them my sincere appreciation for their expertise and dedication to the high standards necessary to produce a good book. Special recognition in this regard is due to Jessica Howie Martin, Production Editor, and Bob Butler, Director of Production.

I thank the consultants who served as reviewers of the manuscript for their thoroughness and generosity in sharing their ideas and suggestions. Your comments proved invaluable! Finally, a special thanks to those family members, friends, and associates who offered and gave their support, patience, and encouragement.

B.M.C.

Consultants

Janice Brownlee, BScN, MAEd
Professor
Canadore College of Applied Arts
    and Technology
North Bay, Ontario, Canada

Marie Colucci, BS, MS, EdD
Associate Professor
Riverside Community College
Riverside, California

Mary Jo Goolsby, MSN, ARNP, EdD
Instructor
Florida State University
Tallahassee, Florida

Shelby Hawk, RN, MSN
Instructor
Mid Michigan Community College
Harrison, Michigan

Priscilla Innocent, RN, MSN
Associate Professor
Indiana Wesleyan University
Marion, Indiana

Dr. Fran Keen, RN, DNSc
Associate Professor
University of Miami
Coral Gables, Florida

Dolores Philpot, BSMT, AND, MSN
Instructor
University of Tennessee
Knoxville, Tennessee

Sylvan L. Settle, RN
Vocational Teacher
Tennessee Technology Center
Memphis, Tennessee

Joyce Taylor, RN, MSN, DSN, BA
Associate Professor
Henderson State University
Arkadelphia, Arkansas

Shelley M. Tiffin, ART (CSMLS), BMLSc
Bachelor of Medical Laboratory
    Science Program
Department of Pathology and
    Laboratory Medicine
University of British Columbia
Vancouver, British Columbia, Canada

Donna Yancey, BSN, MSN, DNS
Assistant Professor
Purdue University
West Lafayette, Indiana

Contents

➤ **SECTION ONE:** Laboratory Tests, **1**

1. Hematology and Tests of Hematopoietic Function, 3
2. Hemostasis and Tests of Hemostatic Function, 49
3. Immunology and Immunologic Testing, 81
4. Immunohematology and Blood Banking, 129
5. Blood Chemistry, 141
6. Studies of Urine, 309
7. Sputum Analysis, 379
8. Cerebrospinal Fluid Analysis, 389
9. Analysis of Effusions, 403
10. Amniotic Fluid Analysis, 423
11. Semen Analysis, 435
12. Analysis of Gastric and Duodenal Secretions, 445
13. Fecal Analysis, 461
14. Analysis of Cells and Tissues, 477
15. Culture and Sensitivity Tests, 511

➤ **SECTION TWO:** Diagnostic Tests and Procedures, **525**

16. Endoscopic Studies, 527
17. Radiologic Studies, 585
18. Radiologic Angiography Studies, 651
19. Ultrasound Studies, 685
20. Nuclear Scan and Laboratory Studies, 727
21. Non-Nuclear Scan Studies, 799
22. Manometric Studies, 829
23. Electrophysiologic Studies, 851
24. Studies of Specific Organs or Systems, 885
25. Skin Tests, 947

Appendices

   I. Obtaining Various Types of Blood Specimens, **967**

  II. Obtaining Various Types of Urine Specimens, **977**

 III. Guidelines for Isolation Precautions in Hospitals, **981**

  IV. Units of Measurement (Including SI Units), **983**

   V. Profile or Panel Groupings and Laboratory Tests, **991**

  VI. Nursing Care Plan for Individuals Experiencing Laboratory and Diagnostic Testing, **999**

 VII. Discussion and Answers to Case Studies and Critical Thinking Exercises, **1001**

General Index, **1007**

Index of Tests and Procedures Covered, **1029**

Laboratory Tests

1

Hematology and Tests of Hematopoietic Function

> ### TESTS COVERED

Bone Marrow Examination, *8*
Reticulocyte Count, *11*
Iron Studies, *13*
Vitamin B$_{12}$ and Folic Acid
   Studies, *16*
Complete Blood Count (CBC), *18*
Erythrocyte (RBC) Count, *22*
Hematocrit (Hct), *24*
Hemoglobin (Hgb), *25*
Red Blood Cell (RBC) Indices, *27*
Stained Red Blood Cell (RBC)
   Examination, *28*

Hemoglobin (Hgb)
   Electrophoresis, *29*
Osmotic Fragility, *34*
Red Blood Cell (RBC) Enzymes, *35*
Erythrocyte Sedimentation Rate
   (ESR, Sed Rate), *37*
White Blood Cell (WBC) Count, *40*
Differential White Blood Cell (WBC)
   Count, *41*
White Blood Cell (WBC)
   Enzymes, *42*

INTRODUCTION

Blood constitutes 6 to 8 percent of total body weight. In terms of volume, women have 4.5 to 5.5 L of blood and men 5 to 6 L. The principal functions of blood are the transport of oxygen, nutrients, and hormones to all tissues and the removal of metabolic wastes to the organs of excretion. Additional functions of blood are (1) regulation of temperature by transfer of heat to the skin for dissipation by radiation and convection, (2) regulation of the pH of body fluids through the buffer systems and facilitation of excretion of acids and bases, and (3) defense against infection by transportation of antibodies and other substances as needed.

Blood consists of a fluid portion, called plasma, and a solid portion that includes red blood cells (erythrocytes), white blood cells (leukocytes), and platelets (thrombocytes). Plasma makes up 45 to 60 percent of blood volume and is composed of water (90 percent), amino acids, proteins, carbohydrates, lipids, vitamins, hormones, electrolytes, and cellular wastes.[1] Of the "solid" or cellular portion of the blood, more than 99 percent consists of red blood cells. Leukocytes and thrombocytes, although functionally essential, occupy a relatively small portion of the total blood cell mass.[2]

Erythrocytes remain within the blood throughout their normal life span of 120 days, transporting oxygen in the hemoglobin component and carrying away carbon dioxide. Leukocytes, while they are in the blood, are merely in transit,

3

because they perform their functions in body tissue. Platelets exert their effects at the walls of blood vessels, performing no known function in the bloodstream itself.[3]

Hematology traditionally limits itself to the study of the cellular elements of the blood, the production of these elements, and the physiologic derangements that affect their functions. Hematologists also are concerned with blood volume, the flow properties of blood, and the physical relationships of red cells and plasma. The numerous substances dissolved or suspended in plasma fall within the province of other laboratory disciplines.[4]

HEMATOPOIESIS

Hematopoiesis is the process of blood cell formation. In normal, healthy adults, blood cells are manufactured in the red marrow of relatively few bones, notably the sternum, ribs, vertebral bodies, pelvic bones, and proximal portions of the humerus and the femur. This production is in contrast to that taking place in the embryo, in which blood cells are derived from the yolk sac mesenchyme. As the fetus develops, the liver, the spleen, and the marrow cavities of nearly all bones become active hematopoietic sites (Fig. 1–1). In the newborn, hematopoiesis occurs primarily in the red marrow, which is found in most

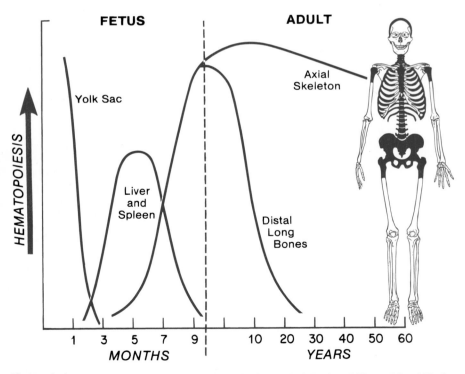

Figure 1–1   Location of active marrow growth in the fetus and adult. (from Hillman, RS and Finch, CA: Red Cell Manual, ed 7. FA Davis, Philadelphia, 1996, p 2, with permission.)

bones at that stage of development. Beginning at about age 5 years, the red marrow is gradually replaced by yellowish fat-storage cells (yellow marrow), which are inactive in the hematopoietic process. By adulthood, blood cell production normally occurs in only those bones that retain red marrow activity.[5]

Adult reticuloendothelial cells retain the potential for hematopoiesis, although in the healthy state reserve sites are not activated. Under conditions of hematopoietic stress in later life, the liver, the spleen, and an expanded bone marrow may resume the production of blood cells.

All blood cells are believed to be derived from the "pluripotential stem cell,"[6] an immature cell with the capability of becoming an erythrocyte, a leukocyte, or a thrombocyte. In the adult, stem cells in hematopoietic sites undergo a series of divisions and maturational changes to form the mature cells found in the blood (Fig. 1–2). As they achieve the "blast" stage, stem cells are committed to becoming a specific type of blood cell. This theory also explains the origin of the several types of white blood cells (neutrophils, monocytes, eosinophils, basophils, and lymphocytes). As the cells mature, they lose their ability to reproduce and cannot further divide to replace themselves. Thus, there is a need for continuous hematopoietic activity to replenish worn-out or damaged blood cells.

Erythropoiesis, the production of red blood cells (RBCs), and *leukopoiesis,* the production of white blood cells (WBCs), are components of the hematopoietic process. Erythropoiesis maintains a population of approximately 25×10^{12} circulating RBCs, or an average of 5 million erythrocytes per cubic millimeter of blood. The production rate is about 2 million cells per second, or 35 trillion cells per day. With maximum stimulation, this rate can be increased sixfold to eightfold, or one volume per day equivalent to the cells contained in 0.5 pt of whole blood.

The level of tissue oxygenation regulates the production of RBCs; that is, erythropoiesis occurs in response to tissue hypoxia. Hypoxia does not, however, directly stimulate the bone marrow. Instead, RBC production occurs in response to *erythropoietin,* precursors of which are found primarily in the kidney and to a lesser extent in the liver. When the renal oxygen level falls, an enzyme, renal erythropoietic factor, is secreted. This enzyme reacts with a plasma protein to form erythropoietin, which subsequently stimulates the bone marrow to produce more RBCs. Specifically, erythropoietin (1) accelerates production, differentiation, and maturation of erythrocytes; (2) reduces the time required for cells to enter the circulation, thereby increasing the number of circulating immature erythrocytes such as reticulocytes (Fig. 1–2); and (3) facilitates the incorporation of iron into RBCs. When the number of produced erythrocytes meets the body's tissue oxygenation needs, erythropoietin release and RBC production are reduced. Table 1–1 lists causes of tissue hypoxia that may stimulate the release of erythropoietin.

Threats to normal erythropoiesis occur if sufficient amounts of erythropoietin cannot be produced or if the bone marrow is unable to respond to erythropoietic stimulation. People without kidneys or with severe impairment of renal function are unable to produce adequate amounts of renal erythropoietic factor. In these individuals, the liver is the source of erythropoietic factor. The quantity produced, however, is sufficient to maintain only a fairly stable state of severe anemia that responds minimally to hypoxemia.

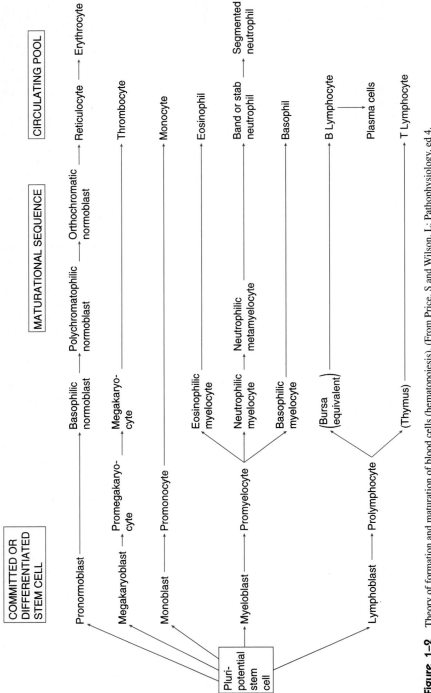

Figure 1–2   Theory of formation and maturation of blood cells (hematopoiesis). (From Price, S and Wilson, L: Pathophysiology, ed 4. Mosby Year-Book, St Louis, 1992, p 176, with permission.)

Table 1–1 ➤ CAUSES OF TISSUE HYPOXIA THAT MAY STIMULATE ERYTHROPOIETIN RELEASE
Acute blood loss
Impaired oxygen–carbon dioxide exchange in the lungs
Low hemoglobin levels
Impaired binding of oxygen to hemoglobin
Impaired release of oxygen from hemoglobin
Excessive hemolysis of erythrocytes due to hypersplenism or hemolytic disorders of antibody, bacterial, or chemical origin
Certain anemias in which abnormal red blood cells are produced (e.g., hereditary spherocytosis)
Compromised blood flow to the kidneys

Inadequate erythropoiesis may occur also if the bone marrow is depressed because of drugs, toxic chemicals, ionizing radiation, malignancies, or other disorders such as hypothyroidism. Also, in certain anemias and hemoglobinopathies, the bone marrow is unable to produce sufficient normal erythrocytes.

Other substances needed for erythropoiesis are vitamin B_{12}, folic acid, and iron. Vitamin B_{12} and folic acid are required for DNA synthesis and are needed by all cells for growth and reproduction; because cellular reproduction occurs at such a high rate in erythropoietic tissue, formation of RBCs is particularly affected by a deficiency of either of these substances. Iron is needed for hemoglobin synthesis and normal RBC production. In addition to dietary sources, iron from worn-out or damaged RBCs is available for reuse in erythropoiesis.[7]

Leukopoiesis, the production of WBCs, maintains a population of 5,000 to 10,000 leukocytes per cubic millimeter of blood, with the capability for rapid and dramatic change in response to a variety of stimuli. No leukopoietic substance comparable to erythropoietic factor has been identified, but many factors are known to influence WBC production, with a resultant excess (leukocytosis) or deficiency (leukopenia) in leukocytes (Table 1–2).

It should be noted that WBC levels vary in relation to diurnal rhythms; thus, the time at which the sample is obtained may influence the results. Overall, leukocytes may increase by as many as 2000 cells per milliliter from morning to evening, with a corresponding overnight decrease. Eosinophils decrease until about noon and then rise to peak between midnight and 3 AM. This variation may be related to adrenocortical hormone levels, which peak between 4 and 8 AM, because an increase in these hormones can cause circulating lymphocytes and eosinophils to disappear in a few hours.

Evaluation of Hematopoiesis

Abnormal results of studies such as a complete blood count (CBC) (p. 18) and WBC count (p. 40) and differential (p. 41) indicate the need to determine the individual's hematopoietic function. Evaluation of hematopoiesis begins with the examination of a bone marrow sample and may subsequently require other studies and a sample of peripheral blood, either venous or capillary.

Although the collection of blood specimens is usually the responsibility of the laboratory technician or phlebotomist, it is often the responsibility of the nurse in emergency departments, critical care units, and community and home

Table 1–2 ➤ CAUSES OF ALTERED LEUKOPOIESIS		
	Physiological	**Pathological**
Leukocytosis	Pregnancy	All types of infection
	Early infancy	Anemias
	Emotional stress	Cushing's disease
	Strenuous exercise	Erythroblastosis fetalis
	Menstruation	Leukemias
	Exposure to cold	Polycythemia vera
	Ultraviolet light	Transfusion reactions
	Increased epinephrine	Inflammatory disorders
	secretion	Parasitic infestations
Leukopenia	Diurnal rhythms	Bone marrow depression
		Toxic and antineoplastic drugs
		Radiation
		Severe infection
		Viral infections
		Myxedema
		Lupus erythematosus and other autoimmune disorders
		Peptic ulcers
		Uremia
		Allergies
		Malignancies
		Metabolic disorders
		Malnutrition

care settings. A detailed description of procedures for obtaining peripheral blood samples is provided in Appendix I.

BONE MARROW EXAMINATION

Bone marrow examination (aspiration, biopsy) requires removal of a small sample of bone marrow by aspiration, needle biopsy, or open surgical biopsy. Cells normally present in hematopoietic marrow include erythrocytes and granulocytes (neutrophils, basophils, and eosinophils) in all stages of maturation; megakaryocytes (from which platelets develop); small numbers of lymphocytes; and occasional plasma cells (Fig. 1–2, p. 6). Nucleated WBCs in the bone marrow normally outnumber nucleated (immature) RBCs by about 3:1. This is called the myeloid to erythroid (M:E) ratio.[8] Causes of increased and decreased values on bone marrow examination are presented in Table 1–3.

Various stains followed by microscopic examination can be performed on bone marrow aspirate to diagnose and differentiate among the different types of leukemia. A Sudan B stain differentiates between acute granulocytic and lymphocytic leukemia. A periodic acid–Schiff (PAS) stain assists in the diagnosis of acute lymphocytic leukemia and erythroleukemia. A terminal deoxynucleotidyl transferase test differentiates between lymphoblastic leukemia and lymphoma.[9]

Because bone marrow examination involves an invasive procedure with risks of infection, trauma, and bleeding, a signed consent is required.

Reference Values

Cell Type (%)	Adults	Infants	Children
Undifferentiated	0–1.0	—	—
Reticulocytes	0.5–2.5	—	—
Neutrophils (total)	56.5	32.4	57.1
Myeloblasts	0.3–5.0	0.62	1.2
Promyelocytes	1.4–8.0	0.76	1.4
Myelocytes	4.2–15.0	2.5	18.4
Neutrophilic	5.0–19.0	—	—
Eosinophilic	0.5–3.0	—	—
Basophilic	0–0.5	—	—
Bands (stabs)	13.0–34.0	14.1	0
Lymphocytes	14.0–16.0	49.0	16.0
Monocytes	0.3–6.0	—	—
Plasma cells	0.3–3.9	0.02	0.4
Megakaryocytes	0.1–3.0	0.05	0.1
M:E ratio	2.3–3.5:1	4.4:1	2.9:1
Pronormoblasts	0.2–1.3	0.1	0.5
Normoblasts	25.6	8.0	23.1
Basophilic	1.4–4.0	0.34	1.7
Polychromatophilic	6.0–29.0	6.9	18.2
Orthochromic	1.0–4.6	0.54	2.7
Eosinophils	0.5–3.0	2.6	3.6
Basophils	0–0.2	0.07	0.06

Note: There may be differences in normal values among individuals and in values obtained by different laboratory techniques.

Indications for Bone Marrow Examination

➤ Evaluation of abnormal results of CBC (e.g., anemia), of WBC count with differential (e.g., increased numbers of leukocyte precursors), or of both tests

➤ Monitoring of effects of exposure to bone marrow depressants

➤ Monitoring of bone marrow response to antineoplastic or radiation therapy for malignancies

➤ Evaluation of hepatomegaly (enlarged liver) or splenomegaly (enlarged spleen)

➤ Identification of bone marrow hyperplasia or hypoplasia, although the study may not indicate the cause of the quantitative abnormality

➤ Determination of marrow differential (proportion of the various types of cells present in the marrow) and M:E ratio

➤ Diagnosis of various disorders associated with abnormal hematopoiesis
 • Multiple myeloma
 • Most leukemias, both acute and chronic
 • Disseminated infections (granulomatous, bacterial, fungal)
 • Lipid or glycogen storage diseases
 • Hypoplastic anemia (which may be caused by chronic infection, hypothyroidism, chronic renal failure, advanced liver disease, and a number of "idiopathic" conditions)

Table 1–3 ➤ **CAUSES OF ALTERATIONS IN BONE MARROW CELLS**

Cell Type	Increased Values	Decreased Values
Reticulocytes	Compensated RBC loss	Aplastic crisis of sickle cell disease or hereditary spherocytosis
	Response to vitamin B_{12} therapy	Aplastic anemia
Neutrophils (total)	Myeloid (chronic) leukemias	Leukemias (monocytic and lymphoblastic)
	Acute myeloblastic leukemia	
Lymphocytes	Lymphatic leukemia	
	Lymphosarcoma	
	Lymphomas	
	Mononucleosis	
	Aplastic anemia	
Plasma cells	Myeloma	
Normoblasts	Polycythemia vera	Deficiency of folic acid or vitamin B_{12}
		Aplastic anemia
		Hemolytic anemia
Eosinophils	Bone marrow carcinoma	
	Lymphadenoma	
	Myeloid leukemia	

- Erythropoietic hyperplasia (which may be caused by iron deficiency, thalassemias, hemoglobinopathies, disorders of folate and vitamin B_{12} metabolism, hypersplenism, glucose-6-phosphate dehydrogenase (G-6-PD) deficiency, hereditary spherocytosis, and antibody-mediated bacterial or chemical hemolysis)
- Lupus erythematosus
- Porphyria erythropoietica
- Parasitic infestations
- Amyloidosis
- Polycythemia vera
- Aplastic anemia (which may be caused by drug toxicity, idiopathic marrow failure, or infection)

Contraindications

➤ Known coagulation defects, although the test may be performed if the importance of the information to be obtained outweighs the risks involved in carrying out the test

Nursing Care Before the Procedure

Explain to the client:

➤ The purpose of the study

➤ That it will be done at the bedside by a physician and requires about 20 minutes

➤ The general procedure, including the sensations to be expected (momentary pain as the skin is injected with local anesthetic and again as the needle penetrates the periosteum, the "pulling" sensation as the specimen is withdrawn)

➤ That discomfort will be minimized with local anesthetics or systemic analgesics

➤ That the site may remain tender for several weeks

Ensure that a signed consent has been obtained. Then:

➤ Take and record vital signs.

➤ Provide a hospital gown if necessary to provide access to the biopsy site or to prevent soiling of the client's clothes with the solution used for skin preparation.

➤ Administer premedication prescribed for pain or anxiety.

The Procedure

The client is assisted to the desired position depending on the site to be used. In young children, the most frequently chosen site is the proximal tibia; in older children, vertebral bodies T10 to L4 are preferred. In adults, the sternum or iliac crests are the preferred sites.

The prone or side-lying position is used if the spinous processes are the sites to be used. (These sites are preferred if more than one specimen is to be obtained.) The client may also be sitting, supported by a pillow on an overbed table for a spinous process site. The side-lying position is used if the iliac crest or tibia is the site. For sternal punctures, the supine position is used.

The skin is prepared with an antiseptic solution, draped, and anesthetized, preferably with procaine, which is painless when injected. Asepsis must be meticulous to prevent systemic infection.

For aspiration, a large needle with stylet is advanced into the marrow cavity. Penetration of the periosteum is painful. The stylet is removed and a syringe is attached to the needle. An aliquot of 0.5 mL of marrow is withdrawn. At this time, the discomfort is a "pulling" sensation rather than pain. The needle is removed and pressure applied to the site. The aspirate is immediately smeared on slides and, when dry, sprayed with a fixative.

For needle biopsy, the local anesthetic is introduced deeply enough to include the periosteum. A special cutting biopsy needle is introduced through a small skin incision and bored into the marrow cavity. A core needle is introduced through the cutting needle and a plug of marrow is removed. The needles are withdrawn and the specimen placed in a preservative solution. Pressure is applied to the site for 5 to 10 minutes and a dressing applied.

Nursing Care After the Procedure

➤ Care and assessment after the procedure include assisting the client to lie on the biopsied side, if the iliac crest was entered, or supine, if the vertebral bodies were used, to maintain pressure on the site for 10 to 15 minutes.

➤ For sternal punctures, place the client in the supine position or other position of comfort.

➤ Provide bed rest for at least 30 minutes after the procedure.

➤ Assess puncture site every 10 to 15 minutes for bleeding. Apply an ice bag to the puncture site to alleviate discomfort and prevent bleeding.

➤ Assess for infection at the site; note any redness, swelling, or drainage.

➤ Administer analgesics to alleviate discomfort.

RETICULOCYTE COUNT

Reticulocytes are immature RBCs. As RBC precursors mature (see Fig. 1–2, p. 6), the cell nucleus decreases in size and eventually becomes a dense, structureless mass.[10] At the same time, the hemoglobin content of the cell increases. Reticulocytes are cells that have lost their nuclei but still retain fragments of mitochondria and other organelles. They also are slightly larger than mature RBCs.[11] RBCs normally enter the circulation as reticulocytes and attain the mature form (erythrocytes) in 1 to 2 days.

Under the stress of anemia or hypoxia, an increased output of erythropoietin may lead to an increased number of circulating reticulocytes (see Table 1-1, p. 7). The extent of such an increase depends on the functional integrity of the bone marrow, the severity and duration of anemia or hypoxia, the adequacy of the erythropoietin response, and the amount of available iron.[12] For example, a normal reticulocyte count in the presence of a normal hemoglobin level indicates normal marrow activity, whereas a normal reticulocyte count in the presence of a low hemoglobin level indicates an inadequate response to anemia. This may be a result of defective erythropoietin production, bone marrow function, or hemoglobin formation. After blood loss or effective therapy for certain kinds of anemia, an elevated reticulocyte count (reticulocytosis) indicates that the bone marrow is normally responsive and is attempting to replace cells lost or destroyed. Individuals with defects of RBC maturation and hemoglobin production may show a low reticulocyte count (reticulocytopenia) because the cells never mature sufficiently to enter the peripheral circulation.

Performing a reticulocyte count involves examining a stained smear of peripheral blood to determine the percentage of reticulocytes in relation to the number of RBCs present.

Reference Values

Newborns	3.2% of RBCs, declining by 2 mo
Infants	2–5%
Children	0.5–4%
Adults	0.5–2% of RBCs; can be higher in pregnant women
Reticulocyte index	1.0
Critical Values	**>20% increase**

Indications for Reticulocyte Count

➤ Evaluation of the adequacy of bone marrow response to stressors such as anemia or hypoxia
  • A normal response is indicated by an increase in the reticulocyte count.
  • Failure of the reticulocyte count to increase may indicate depressed bone marrow functioning, defective erythropoietin production, or defective hemoglobin production.
➤ Evaluation of anemia of unknown etiology to determine the type of anemia
  • Elevated reticulocyte counts are found in hemolytic anemias and sickle cell disease.
  • Decreased counts are seen in pernicious anemia, thalassemia, aplastic anemia, and severe iron-deficiency anemia.
➤ Monitoring response to therapy for anemia
  • In iron-deficiency anemia, therapeutic administration of iron should produce reticulocytosis within 3 days and the count should remain elevated until normal hemoglobin levels are achieved.

- Vitamin B$_{12}$ therapy for pernicious anemia should cause a prompt, continuing reticulocytosis.
➤ Monitoring physiologic response to blood loss
  - After a single hemorrhagic episode, reticulocytosis should begin in 24 to 48 hours and peak in 4 to 7 days.
  - Persistent reticulocytosis or a second rise in the count indicates continuing blood loss.
➤ Confirmation of aplastic crisis in clients with known aplastic anemia as evidenced by a drop in the usually high level of reticulocytes, indicating that RBC production has stopped despite continuing RBC destruction[13]

Nursing Care Before the Procedure

Client preparation is the same as that for any study involving the collection of a peripheral blood sample (see Appendix I).

The Procedure

If the client is an adult, a venipuncture is performed and the sample is collected in a lavender-topped tube. A capillary sample may be obtained in infants and children as well as in adults for whom venipuncture may not be feasible.

Nursing Care After the Procedure

Care and assessment after the procedure are the same as for any study involving the collection of a peripheral blood sample (see Appendix I).
➤ *Abnormal values:* Note and report fatigue, weakness, and color changes associated with a decrease in counts and pain, changes in mental state and visual perception associated with an increase in counts. Increased counts in 4 to 7 days indicate that the therapy to treat loss of RBCs is effective, whereas decreased counts indicate an ineffective production of RBCs, and further testing and evaluation are needed to determine the cause. Assess for continuing blood loss (pulse, blood pressure, skin color, weakness, dizziness).
➤ **Critical values:** Polycythemia with reticulocyte increases of greater than 20 percent requires immediate communication to the physician. Prepare the client for possible phlebotomy to reduce volume of blood and intravenous fluids to reduce viscosity of blood. Administer ordered myelosuppressive drugs.

IRON STUDIES

Iron plays a principal role in erythropoiesis, as it is necessary for proliferation and maturation of RBCs and for hemoglobin synthesis. Of the body's normal 4 g of iron (somewhat less in women), about 65 percent resides in hemoglobin and about 3 percent in myoglobin. A tiny but vital amount of iron is found in cellular enzymes, which catalyze the oxidation and reduction of iron. The remainder is stored in the liver, bone marrow, and spleen as ferritin or hemosiderin.[14]

Except for blood transfusions, the only way iron enters the body is orally. Normally, only about 10 percent of ingested iron is absorbed, but up to 20 percent or more can be absorbed in cases of iron-deficiency anemia. It is never possible to absorb all ingested iron, no matter how great the body's need. In addition to dietary sources, iron from worn-out or damaged RBCs is available for reuse in erythropoiesis.[15]

Serum Iron, Transferrin, and Total Iron-Binding Capacity (TIBC)

Any iron present in the serum is in transit among the alimentary tract, bone marrow, and available iron storage forms. Iron travels in the bloodstream bound to transferrin, a protein (β-globulin) manufactured by the liver. Unbound iron is highly toxic to the body, but generally much more transferrin is available than that needed for iron transport. Usually, transferrin is only 30 to 35 percent saturated, with a normal range of 20 to 55 percent. If excess transferrin is available in relation to body iron, the percentage saturation is low. Conversely, in situations of iron excess, both serum iron and percentage saturation are high.

Measurement of serum iron is accomplished by using a specific color reagent to quantitate iron after it is freed from transferrin. Transferrin may be measured directly through immunoelectrophoretic techniques or indirectly by exposure of the serum to sufficient excess iron such that all the transferrin present can combine with the added iron. The latter result is expressed as total iron-binding capacity (TIBC). The percentage saturation is calculated by dividing the serum iron value by the TIBC value.

Ferritin

Iron is stored in the body as ferritin or hemosiderin. Many individuals who are not anemic and who can adequately synthesize hemoglobin may still have decreased iron stores. For example, menstruating women, especially those who have borne children, usually have less storage iron. In contrast, persons with disorders of excess iron storage such as hemochromatosis or hemosiderosis have extremely high serum ferritin levels.[16]

Serum ferritin levels are used to measure iron storage status and are obtained by either radioimmunoassay or enzyme-linked immunoassay. The amount of ferritin in the circulation usually is proportional to the amount of storage iron (ferritin and hemosiderin) in body tissues. It should be noted that serum ferritin levels vary according to age and gender (Fig. 1-3).

Reference Values

	Conventional Units	SI Units
Serum Iron		
Newborns	350–500 μg/dL	62.7–89.5 μmol/L
Children	40–200 μg/dL	7.2–35.8 μmol/L
Adults		
Men	60–170 μg/dL	10.7–30.4 μmol/L
Women	50–130 μg/dL	9.0–23.3 μmol/L
Elderly Persons	40–80 μg/dL	7.2–14.3 μmol/L
Transferrin		
Newborns	60–170 mg/dL	0.6–1.7 g/L
Adults	250–450 mg/dL	2.5–4.5 g/L
% Saturation (of Transferrin)		
Newborns	65% saturation	0.65
Adults	20–55% saturation	0.20–0.55

TIBC		
Children	100–350 μg/dL	18–63 μmol/L
Adults	300–360 μg/dL	54–64 μmol/L
Elderly Persons	200–310 μg/dL	36–56 μmol/L
Ferritin		
Children	20–40 μg/dL	20–40 μg/L
Adults		
Men	50–200 μg/dL	50–200 μg/L
	(average 100 μg/dL)	(avg 100 μg/L)
Women (menstruating)	12–100 μg/dL	12–100 μg/L
	(average 30 μg/dL)	(avg 30 μg/L)

Indications for Iron Studies

➤ Anemia of unknown etiology to determine cause and type of anemia
  - Decreased serum iron with increased transferrin levels is seen in iron-deficiency anemia and blood loss.
  - Decreased serum iron and decreased transferrin levels may be seen in disorders involving diminished protein synthesis or defects in iron absorption (e.g., chronic diseases, infections, widespread malignancy, malabsorption syndromes, malnutrition, nephrotic syndrome). Percentage saturation of transferrin may be normal if serum iron and transferrin levels are proportionately decreased; if the problem is solely one of protein homeostasis (with normal iron stores), percentage saturation will be high.

➤ Support for diagnosing hemochromatosis or other disorders of iron metabolism and storage

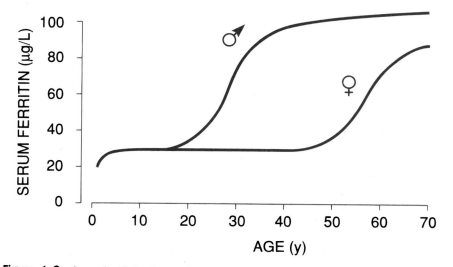

Figure 1–3   Serum ferritin levels according to sex and age. (From Hillman, RS and Finch, CA: Red Cell Manual, ed 7. FA Davis, Philadelphia, 1996, p 64, with permission.)

- Serum iron and ferritin levels may be elevated in hemochromatosis and hemosiderosis; percentage saturation of transferrin is elevated, whereas TIBC is decreased.
- Serum iron levels can be elevated in lead poisoning, after multiple blood transfusions, and in severe hemolytic disorders that cause release of iron from damaged RBCs.

➤ Monitoring hematologic responses during pregnancy, when serum iron is usually decreased, transferrin levels are increased (in the third trimester), percentage saturation is low, TIBC may be increased, and ferritin may be decreased (*Note:* Transferrin levels may be increased in women taking oral contraceptives, whereas ferritin levels may be decreased in women who are menstruating or who have borne children.)

Nursing Care Before the Procedure

Client preparation is the same as that for any study involving the collection of a peripheral blood sample (see Appendix I).

➤ Blood for serum iron and TIBC should be drawn in the morning, in the fasting state, and 24 hours or more after discontinuing iron-containing medications.[17]

The Procedure

A venipuncture is performed and the sample collected in a red-topped tube. A capillary sample may be obtained in infants and children as well as in adults for whom venipuncture may not be feasible.

Nursing Care After the Procedure

Care and assessment after the procedure are the same as for any study involving the collection of a peripheral blood sample (see Appendix I).

➤ Food, fluids, and medications withheld before the test may be resumed after the sample is obtained.

➤ *Complications and precautions:* Note and report signs and symptoms of anemia: decreases in test levels, fatigue and weakness, increased pulse, exertional dyspnea, and dizziness. If anemia is caused by blood loss, prepare to administer a transfusion of blood products. If anemia is caused by iron deficiency, administer ordered oral or parenteral (intramuscular) iron supplement and instruct client in dietary inclusion of foods high in iron content. After 4 to 7 days check iron studies, RBC count, reticulocyte count, and hemoglobin levels to see whether iron stores have been replenished.

VITAMIN B_{12} AND FOLIC ACID STUDIES

Vitamin B_{12} (cyanocobalamin) and folic acid (pteroylglutamic acid) are essential for the production and maturation of erythrocytes. Both must be present for normal DNA replication and cell division. In humans, vitamin B_{12} is obtained only by eating animal proteins, milk, and eggs, which places strict vegetarians at risk for developing cobalamin deficiency; hydrochloric acid (HCl) and intrinsic factor are required for absorption. Folic acid (or folate) is present in liver and in many foods of vegetable origin such as lima beans, kidney beans, and dark-green leafy vegetables. It should be noted that canning and prolonged cooking destroy folate. Normally functioning intestinal mucosa is necessary for absorption of both vitamin B_{12} and folic acid.

Vitamin B_{12} is normally stored in the liver in sufficient quantity to withstand 1 year of zero intake. In contrast, most of the folic acid absorbed goes directly to the tissues, with a smaller amount stored in the liver. Folate stores are adequate for only 2 to 4 months.

Reference Values

		Conventional Units	**SI Units**
Vitamin B_{12}	Serum	200–900 pg/mL	148–664 pmol/L
Folic acid	Serum	1.8–9 ng/mL	4–20 nmol/L
	RBCs	95–500 ng/mL	215–1133 nmol/L

Indications for Vitamin B_{12} and Folic Acid Studies

➤ Determination of the cause of megaloblastic anemia
  • Diagnosis of pernicious anemia, a megaloblastic anemia characterized by vitamin B_{12} deficiency despite normal dietary intake
  • Diagnosis of megaloblastic anemia caused by deficient folic acid intake or increased folate requirements (e.g., in pregnancy and hemolytic anemias) or both, as indicated by decreased serum levels of folic acid
➤ Monitoring response to disorders that may lead to vitamin B_{12} deficiency (e.g., gastric surgery, age-related atrophy of the gastric mucosa, surgical resection of the ileum, intestinal parasites, overgrowth of intestinal bacteria)
➤ Monitoring response to disorders that may lead to folate deficiency (e.g., disease of the small intestine, sprue, cirrhosis, chronic alcoholism, uremia, some malignancies)[18]
➤ Monitoring effects of drugs that are folic acid antagonists (e.g., alcohol, anticonvulsants, antimalarials, and certain drugs used to treat leukemia)[19]
➤ Monitoring effects of prolonged parenteral nutrition

Nursing Care Before the Procedure

Client preparation is the same as that for any study involving the collection of a peripheral blood sample (see Appendix I).
➤ Samples should be drawn after the client has fasted for 8 hours and before injections of vitamin B_{12} have been given.
➤ Alcohol also should be avoided for 24 hours before the test.

The Procedure

A venipuncture is performed and the sample collected in a red-topped tube. A capillary sample may be obtained in infants and children as well as in adults for whom venipuncture may not be feasible.

Nursing Care After the Procedure

Care and assessment after the procedure are the same as for any study involving the collection of a peripheral blood sample (see Appendix I).
➤ Foods and drugs withheld before the test may be resumed after the sample is obtained.

➤ *Complications and precautions (anemia):* Note and report folic acid levels of less than 4 ng and a normal level of vitamin B_{12}, indicating folic acid anemia. Prepare to administer ordered oral replacement therapy of folic acid; dosage and duration depend on the cause of the deficiency. Perform nursing activities for vitamin B_{12} deficiency as in pernicious anemia diagnosed by the Schilling test (see Chap. 20).

COMPLETE BLOOD COUNT (CBC)

A CBC includes (1) enumeration of the cellular elements of the blood, (2) evaluation of RBC indices, and (3) determination of cell morphology by means of stained smears. Counting is performed by automated electronic devices capable of rapid analysis of blood samples with a measurement error of less than 2 percent.[20]

Reference values for the CBC vary across the life cycle and between the genders. In the neonate, when oxygen demand is high, the number of erythrocytes also is high. As demand decreases, destruction of the excess cells results in decreased erythrocyte, hemoglobin, and hematocrit levels. During childhood, RBC levels again rise, although hemoglobin levels may decrease slightly.

In prepubertal children, normal erythrocyte and hemoglobin levels are the same for boys and girls. During puberty, however, values for boys rise, whereas values for girls decrease. In men, these higher values persist to age 40 or 50, decline slowly to age 70, and then decrease rapidly thereafter. In women, the drop in hemoglobin and hematocrit that begins with puberty reverses at about age 50 but never rises to prepubertal levels or to that of men of the same age.

The difference between men and women results partly from menstrual blood loss in women and partly from the effects of androgens in men. Castration of men usually causes hemoglobin and hematocrit to decline to nearly the same levels as those of women. It should be noted that there is a decline in erythrocytes for both genders in old age.[21]

More detailed discussions of the RBC and WBC components of the CBC are included in succeeding sections of this chapter. Platelets are discussed in Chapter 2.

Reference Values

The components of the CBC and their reference values across the life cycle are shown in Table 1–4.

Indications for a Complete Blood Count (CBC)

Because the CBC provides much information about the overall health of the individual, it is an essential component of a complete physical examination, especially when performed upon admission to a health-care facility or before surgery. Other indications for a CBC are as follows:

➤ Suspected hematologic disorder, neoplasm, or immunologic abnormality
➤ History of hereditary hematologic abnormality
➤ Suspected infection (local or systemic, acute or chronic)
➤ Monitoring effects of physical or emotional stress
➤ Monitoring desired responses to drug therapy and undesired reactions to drugs that may cause blood dyscrasias (Table 1–5)

Table 1–4 ▶ REFERENCE VALUES FOR COMPLETE BLOOD COUNT

CBC Component	Newborn	1 Mo	6 Mo	1–10 Yr	ADULT Male	ADULT Female
Red blood cells (RBCs)	4.8–7.1 million/mm^3 4.8–7.1 × 10^{12}/L (SI units)	4.1–6.4 million/mm^3	3.8–5.5 million/mm^3	4.5–4.8 million/mm^3	4.6–6.2 million/mm^3	4.2–5.4 million/mm^3
Hematocrit (Hct)	4.4–64%	35–49%	30–40%	35–41%	40–54%	38–47%
Hemoglobin (Hgb)	14–24 g/dL (SI units) 140–240 g/L (SI units)	11–20 g/dL 110–200 g/L	10–15 g/dL 100–150 g/L	11–16 g/dL 110–160 g/L	13.5–18 g/dL 135–180 g/L	12–16 g/dL 120–160 g/L
RBC indices						
MCV*	96–108 μm^3 96–108 fL (SI units)	82–91 μm^3 82–91 fL (SI units)	—	—	80–94 μm^3 80–94 fL	81–99 μm^3 81–99 fL
MCH†	32–34 pg	27–31 pg	—	—		27–31 pg
MCHC‡	32–33% 320–330 S/L (SI units)	32–36% 320–360 S/L	—	—		32–36% 320–360 S/L
Stained RBC examination	Normochromic and normocytic for all age groups and both sexes (see p. 27)					
White blood cells (WBCs)	9,000–30,000/mm^3 9,000–30,000 × 10^9/L (SI units)	6,000–18,000/mm^3	6,000–16,000/mm^3	5,000–13,000/mm^3	5,000–10,000/mm^3	
Differential WBC						
Neutrophils	≤45% by 1 wk	≤40% by 4 wk	32%	60% after age 2 yr	—	54–75% (3000–7500/mm^3)
Bands	—	—	—	—	—	3–8% (150–700/mm^3)
Eosinophils	—	—	—	0–3%	—	1–4% (50–400/mm^3)
Basophils	—	—	—	1–3%	—	0–1% (25–100/mm^3)
Monocytes	—	—	—	4–9%	—	2–8% (100–500/mm^3)
Lymphocytes	≥41% by 1 wk	56% by 4 wk	61%	59% after age 2 yr	—	25–40% (1500–4500/mm^3)
T lymphocytes	—	—	—	—	—	60–80% of lymphocytes
B lymphocytes	—	—	—	—	—	10–20% of lymphocytes
Platelets	140,000–300,000/mm^3 140–300 × 10^9/L (SI units)	150,000–390,000/mm^3 150–390 × 10^9/L	200,000–473,000/mm^3 200–473 × 10^9/L	150,000–450,000/mm^3 150–450 × 10^9/L	150,000–450,000/mm^3 150–450 × 10^9/L	

*Mean corpuscular volume.
†Mean corpuscular hemoglobin.
‡Mean corpuscular hemoglobin concentration.

Table 1–5 ➤ DRUGS THAT MAY CAUSE BLOOD DYSCRASIAS

Generic Name or Class	Trade Names
Acetaminophen and acetaminophen compounds	Bancap, Capital, Colrex, Comtrex, Darvocet-N, Datril, Dolene, Duradrin, Duradyne, Esgic, Excedrin, Liquiprin, Midrin, Neopap Supprettes, NyQuil, Ornex, Panadol, Parafon Forte, Percogesic, Phrenilin, Sedapap, Sinarest, Sinutab, Supac, Tylenol, Tempra, Tylenol with Codeine, Valadol, Vanquish, Wygesic
Acetophenazine maleate	Tindal
Aminosalicylic acid	Pamisyl, PAS, Rezipas
Amphotericin B	Fungizone, Mysteclin F
Antineoplastic agents	
Arsenicals	
Carbamazepine	Tegretol
Chloramphenicol	Chloromycetin
Chloroquine	Aralen
Ethosuximide (methsuximide, phensuximide)	Zarontin
Furazolidone	Furoxone
Haloperidol	Haldol
Hydantoin derivatives	
Ethotoin	Peganone
Mephenytoin	Mesantoin
Phenytoin	Dilantin, Diphenylan
Hydralazine	Apresazide, Apresoline, Bolazine, Ser-Ap-Es, Serpasil-Apresoline
Hydroxychloroquine sulfate	Plaquenil
Indomethacin	Indocin
Isoniazid	INH, Nydrazid, Rifamate
MAO inhibitors	Eutonyl, Nardil, Parnate
Mefenamic acid	Ponstel
Mepacrine	Atabrine
Mephenoxalone	Lenetron
Mercurial diuretics	Thiomerin
Metaxalone	Skelaxin
Methaqualone	Quaalude, Sopor
Methyldopa	Aldoclor, Aldomet, Aldoril
Nitrites	
Nitrofurantoin	Cyantin, Furadantin, Macrodantin
Novobiocin	Albamycin
Oleandomycin	Matromycin
Oxyphenbutazone	Oxalid, Tandearil
Paramethadione	Paradione
Pencillamine	Cuprimine, Depen
Penicillins	
Phenacemide	Phenurone
Phenobarbital	
Phenylbutazone	Azolid, Butazolidin
Phytonadione	AquaMEPHYTON, Konakion
Primaquine	
Primidone	Mysoline
Pyrazolone derivatives	Butazolidin, Tandearil, Oxalid
Pyrimethamine	Daraprim
Rifampin	Rifadin, Rifamate, Rimactane
Radioisotopes	
Spectinomycin	Trobicin

(Continued on page 21)

Table 1–5 ➤ DRUGS THAT MAY CAUSE BLOOD DYSCRASIAS *(Continued)*

Generic Name or Class	Trade Names
Sulfonamides	
Mafenide	Sulfamylon cream
Phthalylsulfathiazole	Sulfathalidine
Sulfabenzamide	Sultrin vaginal cream
Sulfacetamide	Bleph-10, Cetamide ointment, Isopto Cetamide, Sulamyd, Sultrin vaginal cream
Sulfachlorpyridazine	Sonilyn
Sulfacytine	Renoquid
Sulfadiazine	Silvadene
Sulfameter	Sulla
Sulfamethiozole	Thiosulfil Forte
Sulfamethoxazole	Azo Gantanol, Bactrim, Gantanol, Septra
Sulfamethoxypyridazine	Midicel
Sulfanilamide	AVC vaginal cream
Sulfasalazine	Azulfidine,
Sulfathiazole	Sultrin vaginal cream, Triple Sulfa cream
Sulfinpyrazone	Anturane
Sulfisoxazole	Azo Gantrisin, Gantrisin
Sulfones	
Dapsone	
DDS	
Sulfoxone	
Sulfonylureas	
Acetohexamide	Dymelor
Chlorpropamide	Diabinese
Tolazamide	Tolinase
Tolbutamide	Orinase
Tetracyclines	Achromycin
Chlortetracycline	Aureomycin
Demeclocycline	Declomycin
Doxycycline	Doxychel, Doxy, Vibramycin, Vibra-Tabs
Meclocycline	Meclan
Methacycline	Rondomycin
Minocycline	Minocin
Oxytetracycline	Oxlopar, Terramycin
Thiazide diuretics (rare hematologic side effects)	Ademol, Diuril, Enduron, Exna, Naturetin, Naqua, Renese, Saluron
Thiocyanates	
Trimethadione	Tridione
Tripelennamine	Pyribenzamine, PBZ
Troleandomycin	Cyclamycin, Tao capsules and suspension
Valproic acid	
Valproate	
Vitamin A	Aquasol A, Alphalin

➤ Monitoring progression of nonhematologic disorders such as chronic obstructive pulmonary disease, malabsorption syndromes, malignancies, and renal disease

Nursing Care Before the Procedure

Client preparation is the same as that for any study involving the collection of a peripheral blood sample (see Appendix I).

The Procedure

A venipuncture is performed and the sample collected in a lavender-topped tube. A capillary sample may be obtained in infants and children, as well as in adults for whom venipuncture may not be feasible.

Nursing Care After the Procedure

Care and assessment after the procedure are the same as for any study involving the collection of a peripheral blood sample (see Appendix I).

➤ *Abnormal range of values:* Note and report decreases in individual or entire CBC (pancytopenia) panel. Prepare to administer drugs and treatments, or both, that have been ordered to manage anemia (RBC, hematocrit [Hct], hemoglobin [Hgb], RBC indices), clotting process (platelet), or infectious process (WBC, differential).

ERYTHROCYTE STUDIES

The mature RBC (erythrocyte) is a biconcave disk with an average life span of 120 days. Because it lacks a nucleus and mitochondria, it is unable to synthesize protein, and its limited metabolism is barely enough to sustain it. Erythrocytes function primarily as containers for Hgb. As such, they transport oxygen from the lungs to all body cells and transfer carbon dioxide from the cells to the organs of excretion. The RBC is resilient and capable of extreme changes in shape. It is admirably designed to survive its many trips through the circulation.[22]

Old, damaged, and abnormal erythrocytes are removed mainly by the spleen and also by the liver and the red bone marrow. The iron is returned to plasma transferrin (see p. 14) and is transported back to the erythroid marrow or stored within the liver and spleen as ferritin and hemosiderin (see p. 14). The bilirubin component of Hgb is carried by plasma albumin to the liver, where it is conjugated and excreted into the bile. Most of this conjugated bilirubin is ultimately excreted in the stool, although some appears in the urine or is returned to bile.

The hematologist determines the numbers, structure, color, size, and shape of erythrocytes; the types and amount of Hgb they contain; their fragility; and any abnormal components.

ERYTHROCYTE (RBC) COUNT

The erythrocyte (RBC) count, a component of the CBC, is the determination of the number of RBCs per cubic millimeter. In international units, this is expressed as the number of RBCs per liter of blood. The test is less significant by itself than it is in computing Hgb, Hct, and RBC indices.

Many factors influence the level of circulating erythrocytes. Decreased numbers are seen in disorders involving impaired erythropoiesis (see p. 10), excessive blood cell destruction (e.g., hemolytic anemia), and blood loss, and in chronic inflammatory diseases. A relative decrease also may be seen in situations with increased body fluid in the presence of a normal number of RBCs (e.g., pregnancy). Increases in the RBC count are most commonly seen in poly-

cythemia vera, chronic pulmonary disease with hypoxia and secondary polycythemia, and dehydration with hemoconcentration. Excessive exercise, anxiety, and pain also produce higher RBC counts. Many drugs may cause a decrease in circulating RBCs (Table 1–5), whereas a few drugs, such as
methyldopa and gentamicin, may cause an increase.[23]

Reference Values

	Conventional Units	**SI Units**
Newborns	4.8–7.1 million/mm^3	4.8–7.1 × 10^{12}/L
1 mo	4.1–6.4 million/mm^3	4.1–6.4 × 10^{12}/L
6 mo	3.8–5.5 million/mm^3	3.8–5.5 × 10^{12}/L
1–10 yr	4.5–4.8 million/mm^3	4.5–4.8 × 10^{12}/L
Adults		
Men	4.6–6.2 million/mm^3	4.6–6.2 × 10^{12}/L
Women	4.2–5.4 million/mm^3	4.2–5.4 × 10^{12}/L

Interfering Factors

➤ Excessive exercise, anxiety, pain, and dehydration may lead to false elevations.
➤ Hemodilution in the presence of a normal number of RBCs may lead to
false decreases (e.g., excessive administration of intravenous fluids, normal
pregnancy).
➤ Many drugs may cause a decrease in circulating RBCs (see Table 1–5,
pp. 20–21).
➤ Drugs such as methyldopa and gentamicin may cause an elevated RBC
count.

Indications for an Erythrocyte (RBC) Count

➤ Routine screening as part of a CBC (see p. 18)
➤ Suspected hematologic disorder involving RBC destruction (e.g., hemolytic
anemia)
➤ Monitoring effects of acute or chronic blood loss
➤ Monitoring response to drug therapy that may alter the RBC count (see
Table 1–5, pp. 20–21)
➤ Monitoring clients with disorders associated with elevated RBC counts
(e.g., polycythemia vera, chronic obstructive pulmonary disease)
➤ Monitoring clients with disorders associated with decreased RBC counts
(e.g., malabsorption syndromes, malnutrition, liver disease, renal disease,
hypothyroidism, adrenal dysfunction, bone marrow failure)

Nursing Care Before the Procedure

Client preparation is the same as that for any study involving the collection of a
peripheral blood sample (see Appendix I).

The Procedure

A venipuncture is performed and the sample collected in a lavender-topped
tube. A capillary sample may be obtained in infants and children as well as in
adults for whom venipuncture may not be feasible.

Nursing Care After the Procedure

Care and assessment after the procedure are the same as for any study involving the collection of a peripheral blood sample (see Appendix I).

➤ *Anemia:* Note and report signs and symptoms of anemia associated with decreased counts in combination with Hgb and Hct decreases. Prepare to administer ordered oral or parenteral iron preparation or a transfusion of whole blood or packed RBCs. Prepare for phlebotomy if levels are increased in polycythemia vera or secondary polycythemia.

HEMATOCRIT (HCT)

Blood consists of a fluid portion (plasma) and a solid portion that includes RBCs, WBCs, and platelets. More than 99 percent of the total blood cell mass is composed of RBCs. The Hct or packed RBC volume measures the proportion of RBCs in a volume of whole blood and is expressed as a percentage.

Several methods may be used to perform the test. In the classic method, anticoagulated venous blood is pipetted into a tube 100 mm long and then centrifuged for 30 minutes so that the plasma and blood cells separate. The volumes of packed RBCs and plasma are read directly from the millimeter marks along the side of the tube. In the micro method, venous or capillary blood is used to fill a small capillary tube, which is then centrifuged for 4 to 5 minutes. The proportions of plasma and RBCs are determined by means of a calibrated reading device. Both techniques allow visual estimation of the volume of WBCs and platelets.[24]

With the newer, automated methods of cell counting, Hct is calculated indirectly as the product of the RBC count and mean cell volume. Although this method is generally quite accurate, certain clinical situations may cause errors in interpreting the Hct. Abnormalities in RBC size and extremely elevated WBC counts may produce false Hct values. Elevated blood glucose and sodium may produce elevated Hct because of the resultant swelling of the erythrocyte.[25]

Normally, the Hct parallels the RBC count. Thus, factors influencing the RBC count also affect the results of the Hct (see p. 10).

Reference Values

	Conventional Units	**SI Units**
Newborns	44–64%	0.44–64
1 mo	35–49%	0.35–0.49
6 mo	30–40%	0.30–0.40
1–10 yr	35–41%	0.35–0.41
Adults		
Men	40–54%	0.40–0.54
Women	38–47%	0.38–0.47
Critical Values	**<14% or >60%**	**<0.14– >0.60**

Note: Values vary across the life cycle and between genders.

Interfering Factors

➤ Abnormalities in RBC size and extremely elevated WBC counts may alter Hct values.

➤ Elevated blood glucose and sodium may produce elevated Hct because of swelling of the erythrocyte.

➤ Factors that alter the RBC count such as hemodilution and dehydration also influence the Hct (see p. 10).

Indications for a Hematocrit (Hct) Test

➤ Routine screening as part of a CBC (see p. 18)

➤ Along with an Hgb (i.e., an "H and H"), to monitor blood loss and response to blood replacement

➤ Along with an Hgb, to evaluate known or suspected anemia and related treatment

➤ Along with an Hgb, to monitor hematologic status during pregnancy

➤ Monitoring responses to fluid imbalances or to therapy for fluid imbalances
* A decreased Hct may indicate hemodilution.
* An increased Hct may indicate dehydration.

Nursing Care Before the Procedure

Client preparation is the same as that for any study involving the collection of a peripheral blood sample (see Appendix I).

The Procedure

The volume of the sample needed depends on the method used to determine the Hct. With the exception of the classic method of Hct determination, a capillary sample is usually sufficient to perform the test. If a venipuncture is performed, the sample is collected in a lavender-topped tube.

Nursing Care After the Procedure

Care and assessment after the procedure are the same as for any study involving the collection of a peripheral blood sample (see Appendix I).

➤ **Critical values:** Notify the physician at once if the Hct is greater than 60 percent or less than 14 percent. Prepare the client for possible transfusion of blood products or infusion of intravenous fluids and for further procedures to evaluate the cause or source of the blood loss or hemoconcentration.

HEMOGLOBIN (HGB)

Hgb is the main intracellular protein of the RBC. Its primary function is to transport oxygen to the cells and to remove carbon dioxide from them for excretion by the lungs. The Hgb molecule consists of two main components: heme and globin. Heme is composed of the red pigment porphyrin and iron, which is capable of combining loosely with oxygen. Globin is a protein that consists of nearly 600 amino acids organized into four polypeptide chains. Each chain of globin is associated with a heme group.

Each RBC contains approximately 250 million molecules of hemoglobin, with some erythrocytes containing more hemoglobin than others. The oxygen-binding, -carrying, and -releasing capacity of Hgb depends on the ability of the globin chains to shift position normally during the oxygenation-deoxygenation process. Structurally abnormal chains that are unable to shift normally have decreased oxygen-carrying ability. This decreased oxygen transport capacity is characteristic of anemia.

Hgb also functions as a buffer in the maintenance of acid-base balance. During transport, carbon dioxide (CO_2) reacts with water (H_2O) to form carbonic acid (H_2CO_3). This reaction is speeded by carbonic anhydrase, an enzyme contained in RBCs. The carbonic acid rapidly dissociates to form hydrogen ions (H^+) and bicarbonate ions (HCO_3^-). The hydrogen ions combine with the Hgb molecule, thus preventing a buildup of hydrogen ions in the blood. The bicarbonate ions diffuse into the plasma and play a role in the bicarbonate buffer system. As bicarbonate ions enter the bloodstream, chloride ions (Cl^+) are repelled and move back into the erythrocyte. This "chloride shift" maintains the electrical balance between RBCs and plasma.[26]

Hgb determinations are of greatest use in the evaluation of anemia, because the oxygen-carrying capacity of the blood is directly related to the Hgb level rather than to the number of erythrocytes. To interpret results accurately, the Hgb level must be determined in combination with the Hct level (see p. 24). Normally, Hgb and Hct levels parallel each other and are commonly used together to express the degree of anemia. The combined values are also useful in evaluating situations involving blood loss and related treatment. The Hct level is normally three times the Hgb level. If erythrocytes are abnormal in shape or size or if Hgb manufacture is defective, the relationship between Hgb and Hct is disproportionate.[27,28]

Reference Values

	Conventional Units	SI Units
Newborns	14–24 g/dL	140–240 g/L
1 mo	11–20 g/dL	110–200 g/L
6 mo	10–15 g/dL	100–150 g/L
1–10 yr	11–16 g/dL	110–160 g/L
Adults		
Men	13.5–18 g/dL	135–180 g/L
Women	12–16 g/dL	120–160 g/L
Critical Values	**<6.0 g/dL**	**<60 g/L**
	>200 g/dL	**>200 g/L**

Ratio of hemoglobin to hematocrit = 3 : 1.

Interfering Factors

Factors that alter the RBC count may also influence Hgb levels (see p. 23).

Indications for Hemoglobin (Hgb) Determination

➤ Routine screening as part of a CBC (see p. 18)
➤ Along with an Hct (i.e., an "H and H"), to evaluate known or suspected anemia and related treatment
➤ Along with an Hct, to monitor blood loss and response to blood replacement
➤ Along with an Hct, to monitor hematologic status during pregnancy

Nursing Care Before the Procedure

Client preparation is the same as that for any study involving the collection of a peripheral blood sample (see Appendix I).

The Procedure

A venipuncture is performed and the sample collected in a lavender-topped tube. A capillary sample may be obtained in infants and children as well as in adults for whom venipuncture may not be feasible.

Nursing Care After the Procedure

Care and assessment after the procedure are the same as for any study involving the collection of a peripheral blood sample (see Appendix I).

➤ **Critical values:** Notify the physician at once if the Hgb is less than 6.0 g/dL. Prepare the client for possible transfusion of blood products and for further procedures to evaluate cause or source of blood loss.

RED BLOOD CELL (RBC) INDICES

RBC indices are calculated mean values that reflect the size, weight, and Hgb content of individual erythrocytes. They consist of the mean corpuscular volume (MCV), the mean corpuscular hemoglobin (MCH), and the mean corpuscular hemoglobin concentration (MCHC). MCV indicates the *volume* of the Hgb in each RBC, MCH is the *weight* of the Hgb in each RBC, and MCHC is the *proportion* of Hgb contained in each RBC. MCHC is a valuable indicator of Hgb deficiency and of the oxygen-carrying capacity of the individual erythrocyte. A cell of abnormal size, abnormal shape, or both may contain an inadequate proportion of Hgb.

RBC indices are used mainly in identifying and classifying types of anemias. Anemias are generally classified according to RBC size and Hgb content. *Cell size* is indicated by the terms normocytic, microcytic, and macrocytic. *Hgb content* is indicated by the terms normochromic, hypochromic, and hyperchromic. Table 1–6 shows anemias classified according to these terms and in relation to the results of RBC indices.

To calculate the RBC indices, the results of an RBC count, Hct, and Hgb are necessary. Thus, factors that may influence these three determinations (e.g., abnormalities of RBC size or extremely elevated WBC counts) may also result in misleading RBC indices. For this reason, a stained blood smear may be used to compare appearance with calculated values and to determine the etiology of identified abnormalities.

Reference Values

	Men	Women	Newborns	SI Units
MCV	80–94 μm^3	81–99 μm^3	96–108 μm^3	81–99 fL (women)
				96–108 fL (newborns)
MCH	27–31 pg	27–31 pg	32–34 pg	32–34 pg (women)
				32–34 pg (newborns)
MCHC	32–36%	32–36%	32–33%	320–360 g/L (women)
				320–330 g/L (newborns)

Normal values for RBC indices are shown in Table 1–4 (p. 19) in relation to the CBC and also are repeated above for adults. Values in newborn infants are slightly different, but adult levels are achieved within approximately 1 month of age.

Table 1-6 ➤ CLASSIFICATION OF ANEMIAS

Anemia	Examples of Causes	MCV* (μm³)	MCH† (pg)	MCHC‡ (%)
Normocytic, normochromic	Sepsis, hemorrhage, hemolysis, drug-induced aplastic anemia, radiation, hereditary spherocytosis	82–92	25–30	32–36
Microcytic, normochromic	Renal disease, infection, liver disease, malignancies	<80	20–25	27
Microcytic, hypochromic	Iron deficiency, lead poisoning, thalassemia, rheumatoid arthritis	50–80	12–25	25–30
Macrocytic, normochromic	Vitamin B₁₂ and folic acid deficiency, some drugs, pernicious anemia	95–150	30–50	32–36

*Mean corpuscular volume.
†Mean corpuscular hemoglobin.
‡Mean corpuscular hemoglobin concentration.

Interfering Factors

Because RBC indices are calculated from the results of the RBC count, Hgb, and Hct, factors that influence the latter three tests (e.g., abnormalities of RBC size, extremely elevated WBC counts) also influence RBC indices.

Indications for Red Blood Cell Indices

➤ Routine screening as part of a CBC (see p. 18)
➤ Identification and classification of anemias (see Table 1–6)

Nursing Care Before the Procedure

Client preparation is the same as that for any study involving the collection of a peripheral blood sample (see Appendix I).

The Procedure

A venipuncture is performed and the sample collected in a lavender-topped tube. A capillary sample may be obtained in infants and children as well as in adults for whom venipuncture may not be feasible.

Nursing Care After the Procedure

Care and assessment after the procedure are the same as for any study involving the collection of a peripheral blood sample (see Appendix I).

STAINED RED BLOOD CELL (RBC) EXAMINATION

The stained RBC examination (RBC morphology) involves examination of RBCs under a microscope. It is usually performed to compare the actual appearance of the cells with the calculated values for RBC indices. Cells are examined for abnormalities in color, size, shape, and contents. The test is performed by spreading a drop of fresh anticoagulated blood on a glass slide. The addition of stain to the specimen is used to enhance RBC characteristics.

As with RBC indices, RBC color is described as normochromic, hypochromic, or hyperchromic, indicating, respectively, normal, reduced, or elevated amounts of Hgb. Cell size may be described as normocytic, microcytic, or macrocytic, depending on whether cell size is normal, small, or abnormally large, respectively. Cell shape is described using terms such as poikilocyte, anisocyte, leptocyte, and spherocyte (Table 1–7). The cells are examined also for inclusions or abnormal cell contents; for example, Heinz bodies, Howell-Jolly bodies, Cabot's rings, and siderotic granules (Table 1–8).

Reference Values

In a normal smear, all cells are uniform in color, size, and shape and are free of abnormal contents. A normal RBC may be described as a normochromic, normocytic cell.

Indications for a Stained Red Blood Cell (RBC) Examination

➤ Abnormal calculated values for RBC indices
➤ Evaluation of anemia and related disorders involving RBCs (see Tables 1–6, p. 28; 1–7, p. 30; and 1–8, p. 31)

Nursing Care Before the Procedure

Client preparation is the same as that for any study involving the collection of a peripheral blood sample (see Appendix I).

The Procedure

A venipuncture is performed and the sample collected in a lavender-topped tube. A capillary sample may be obtained in infants and children as well as in adults for whom venipuncture may not be feasible.

Nursing Care After the Procedure

Care and assessment after the procedure are the same as for any study involving the collection of a peripheral blood sample (see Appendix I).

HEMOGLOBIN (HGB) ELECTROPHORESIS

The Hgb molecule consists of four polypeptide globin chains and four heme components containing iron and the red pigment porphyrin. Hgb formation is genetically determined, and the types of globin chains normally formed are termed alpha (α), beta (β), gamma (γ), and delta (δ). Combinations of these chains form various types of Hgb. Disorders of synthesis and production of globin chains result in the formation of abnormal Hgb.

Hgb electrophoresis is a technique for identifying the types of Hgb present and for determining the percentage of each type. Exposed to an electrical current, the several types of Hgb migrate toward the positive pole at different rates. The patterns created are compared with standard patterns.

At birth, most RBCs contain fetal hemoglobin (Hgb F), which is made up of two α chains and two γ chains. Within a few months, through sequential suppression and activation of individual genes, Hgb F largely disappears and is replaced by adult hemoglobin (Hgb A). Hgb A, composed of two α chains and two β chains, makes up more than 95 percent of Hgb in adults. A minor type of Hgb, Hgb A_2, consisting of two α chains and two δ chains, also is found in

Table 1–7 ➤ RED BLOOD CELL ABNORMALITIES SEEN ON STAINED SMEAR

Descriptive Term	Observation	Significance
Macrocytosis	Cell diameter >8 μm MCV* >95 μm³	Megaloblastic anemias Severe liver disease Hypothyroidism
Microcytosis	Cell diameter <6 μm MCV <80 μm³ MCHC† <27	Iron-deficiency anemia Thalassemias Anemia of chronic disease
Hypochromia	Increased zone of central pallor	Diminished Hgb content
Hyperchromia	Microcytic, hyperchromic cells Increased bone marrow stores of iron	Chronic inflammation Defect in ability to use iron for Hgb synthesis
Polychromatophilia	Presence of red cells not fully hemoglobinized	Reticulocytosis
Poikilocytosis	Variability of cell shape	Sickle cell disease Microangiopathic hemolysis Leukemias Extramedullary hematopoiesis Marrow stress of any cause
Anisocytosis	Variability of cell size	Reticulocytosis Transfusing normal blood into microcytic or macrocytic cell population
Leptocytosis	Hypochromic cells with small central zone of Hgb ("target cells")	Thalassemias Obstructive jaundice
Spherocytosis	Cells with no central pallor, loss of biconcave shape MCHC high	Loss of membrane relative to cell volume Hereditary spherocytosis Accelerated red blood cell destruction by reticuloendothelial system
Schistocytosis	Presence of cell fragments in circulation	Increased intravascular mechanical trauma Microangiopathic hemolysis
Acanthocytosis	Irregularly spiculated surface	Irreversibly abnormal membrane lipid content Liver disease Abetalipoproteinemia
Echinocytosis	Regularly spiculated cell surface	Reversible abnormalities of membrane lipids High plasma-free fatty acids Bile acid abnormalities Effects of barbituates, salicylates, and so on
Stomatocytosis	Elongated, slitlike zone of central pallor	Hereditary defect in membrane sodium metabolism Severe liver disease
Elliptocytosis	Oval cells	Hereditary anomaly, usually harmless

Adapted from Sacher, RA, and McPherson, RA: Widmann's Clinical Interpretation of Laboratory Tests, ed 10. FA Davis, Philadelphia, 1991, p 49.
*Mean corpuscular volume.
†Mean corpuscular hemoglobin concentration.

Table 1–8 ➤ TYPES OF ABNORMAL RED BLOOD CELL INCLUSIONS AND THEIR CAUSES	
Type (Composition)	**Causes of Inclusions**
Heinz bodies (denatured Hgb)	α-Thalassemia
	G-6-PD deficiency
	Hemolytic anemias
	Methemoglobinemia
	Splenectomy
	Drugs: analgesics, antimalarials, antipyretics, nitrofurantoin (Furadantin), nitrofurazone (Furacin), phenylhydrazine, sulfonamides, tolbutamide, vitamin K (large doses)
Basophilic stippling (residual cytoplasmic RNA)	Anemia caused by liver disease
	Lead poisoning
	Thalassemia
Howell-Jolly bodies (fragments of residual DNA)	Splenectomy
	Intense or abnormal RBC production resulting from hemolysis or inefficient erythropoiesis
Cabot's rings (composition unknown)	Same as for Howell-Jolly bodies
Siderotic granules (iron-containing granules)	Abnormal iron metabolism
	Abnormal hemoglobin manufacture

small amounts (2 to 3 percent) in adults. Traces of Hgb F persist throughout life (Fig. 1–4).[29]

More than 150 genetic abnormalities in the Hgb molecule have been identified. These are termed thalassemias and hemoglobinopathies. Thalassemias are genetic disorders in globin chain synthesis that result in decreased production rates of α or β globin chains. Hemoglobinopathies refer to disorders involving abnormal amino acid sequence in the globin chains.

In α-thalassemia, for example, there is decreased production of α chains and Hgb A. The oversupply of β chains results in the formation of hemoglobin H (Hgb H), which consists of four β chains (Fig. 1–5). Complete absence of α chain production (homozygous thalassemia A) is incompatible with life and generally results in stillbirth during the second trimester of pregnancy. The cord blood of such fetuses shows high levels of hemoglobin Barts, a type of Hgb that evolves from unpaired γ chains. Hemoglobin Barts itself has such a high affinity for oxygen that it releases none to the tissues.

In β-thalassemia minor, there is a decrease in β chain production and, therefore, a reduction in the amount of Hgb A formed. In β-thalassemia major, all β chain production is lost and no Hgb A is formed. The α chains are then used to form Hgb F and Hgb A_2.

Among the most common Hgb abnormalities are the sickle cell disorders, in which there is a double β gene defect that results in the production of hemoglobin S (Hgb S). In Hgb S, the amino acid valine is substituted for glutamine at a critical position on the globin chain, which causes the β chains to "lock" when deoxygenated, deforming the erythrocyte into the sickled shape. Repeated sickling damages RBC membranes and shortens the cells' life spans. The abnormally shaped cells pass more sluggishly through the circulation, leading to impaired tissue oxygenation.

Chromosomes

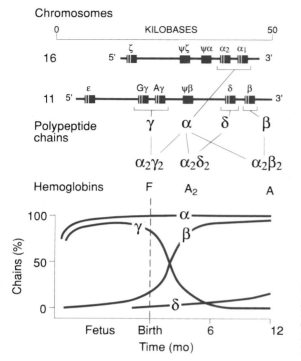

Polypeptide chains

Hemoglobins

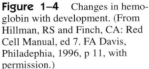

Figure 1–4 Changes in hemoglobin with development. (From Hillman, RS and Finch, CA: Red Cell Manual, ed 7. FA Davis, Philadelphia, 1996, p 11, with permission.)

The gene for Hgb S is most prevalent in black populations and may be present as either sickle cell trait (having one recessive gene for Hgb S) or sickle cell disease (having both recessive genes for Hgb S). The Sickledex test, a screening test for sickle cell disorders, detects sickled erythrocytes under conditions of oxygen deprivation. Hgb electrophoresis is necessary, however, to differentiate sickle cell trait (20 to 40 percent Hgb S) from sickle cell disease (70 percent Hgb S).

Many other types of abnormal Hgb are caused by defects in globin chain synthesis. Hemoglobin C (Hgb C), for example, has an abnormal amino acid substitution on the β chain and may lead to a form of mild hemolytic anemia. Other examples of abnormal Hgb resulting from rearrangement or substitution of the amino acids on the globin chains include hemoglobin E (Hgb E), hemoglobin Lepore (β chain abnormalities), and hemoglobin Constant Spring (α chain abnormality).[30]

Other disorders involving Hgb pertain to the oxygen-combining ability of the heme portion of the molecule. Examples of types of Hgb associated with such disorders are methemoglobin (Hgb M), sulfhemoglobin, and carboxyhemoglobin. Hgb M is formed when the iron contained in the heme portion of the Hgb molecule is oxidized to a ferric instead of a ferrous form, thus impairing its oxygen-combining ability. Methemoglobinemia may be hereditary or acquired. The acquired form may be caused by excessive radiation or by the toxic effects of chemicals and drugs (e.g., nitrates, phenacetin, lidocaine). It should be noted that Hgb F is more easily converted to Hgb M than is Hgb A.

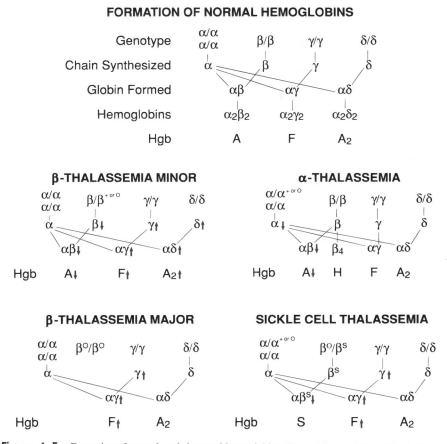

Figure 1–5 Formation of normal, and abnormal hemoglobins. (From Hillman, RS and Finch, CA: Red Cell Manual, ed 6. FA Davis, Philadephia, 1992, p 84, with permission.)

Sulfhemoglobin is a pigment that results from Hgb combining with inorganic sulfides. It occurs in those who take sulfonamides or acetanilid.

Carboxyhemoglobin results when Hgb is exposed to carbon monoxide. Although this type of Hgb is most commonly seen in individuals with excessive exposure to automobile exhaust fumes, it may also occur in heavy smokers.[31] Tests other than Hgb electrophoresis are used to determine the presence of Hgb M and carboxyhemoglobin.

Reference Values

The normal values shown for Hgb electrophoresis are for adults. In newborn infants, 60 to 90 percent of Hgb may consist of Hgb F. This amount decreases to 10 to 20 percent by 6 months of age and to 2 to 4 percent by 1 year. Abnormal forms of Hgb (e.g., Hgb S, Hgb H) are not normally present.

	Conventional Units	**SI Units**
Hgb A	95–97%	>0.95
Hgb A$_2$	2–3%	0.02–0.03
Hgb F	>1%	>0.01
Methemoglobin (Hgb M)	2% or 0.06–0.24 g/dL	
Sulfhemoglobin	Minute amounts	
Carboxyhemoglobin	0–2.3%	
	4–5% in smokers	

Indications for Hemoglobin (Hgb) Electrophoresis

- Suspected thalassemia, especially in individuals with positive family history for the disorder
- Differentiation among the types of thalassemias
- Evaluation of a positive Sickledex test (see p. 32) to differentiate sickle cell trait (20 to 40 percent Hgb S) from sickle cell disease (70 percent Hgb S)
- Evaluation of hemolytic anemia of unknown etiology
- Diagnosis of Hgb C anemia
- Identification of the numerous types of abnormal Hgb, most of which do not produce clinical disease

Nursing Care Before the Procedure

Client preparation is the same as that for any study involving the collection of a peripheral blood sample (see Appendix I).

The Procedure

A venipuncture is performed and the sample collected in a lavender-topped tube. A capillary sample may be obtained in infants and children as well as in adults for whom venipuncture may not be feasible.

Nursing Care After the Procedure

Care and assessment after the procedure are the same as for any study involving the collection of a peripheral blood sample (see Appendix I).

- *Complications and precautions:* Note and report signs and symptoms associated with the specific type of anemia identified by electrophoresis. Prepare to instruct in therapy and prevention of complications. Offer information about genetic factors and counseling or both, if appropriate.

Osmotic Fragility

The osmotic fragility test determines the ability of the RCB membrane to resist rupturing in a hypotonic saline solution. Normal disk-shaped cells can imbibe water and swell significantly before membrane capacity is exceeded, but spherocytes (RBCs that lack the normal biconcave shape) and cells with damaged membranes burst in saline solutions only slightly less concentrated than normal saline. Conversely, in thalassemia, sickle cell disease, and other disorders, RBCs are more than normally resistant to osmotic damage (Table 1–9).

The test is performed by exposing RBCs to increasingly dilute saline solutions. The percentage of the solution at which the cells swell and rupture is then noted.

Table 1-9 ➤ CAUSES OF ALTERED ERYTHROCYTE OSMOTIC FRAGILITY

Decreased Fragility	Increased Fragility
Iron-deficiency anemias	Hereditary spherocytosis
Hereditary anemias (sickle cell, hemoglobin C, thalassemias)	Hemolytic anemias
	Autoimmune anemias
Liver diseases	Burns
Polycythemia vera	Toxins (bacterial, chemical)
Splenectomy	Hypotonic infusions
Obstructive jaundice	Transfusion with incompatible blood
	Mechanical trauma to RBCs (prosthetic heart valves, disseminated intravascular clotting, parasites)
	Enzyme deficiencies (PK, G-6-PD)

Reference Values

Normal erythrocytes rupture in saline solutions of 0.30 to 0.45 percent. RBC rupture in solutions of greater than 0.50 percent saline indicates increased fragility. Lack of rupture in solutions of less than 0.30 percent saline indicates decreased RBC fragility.

Indications for Osmotic Fragility Test

➤ Confirmation of disorders that alter RBC fragility, including hereditary anemias (see Table 1-9)
➤ Evaluation of the extent of extrinsic damage to RBCs from burns, inadvertent instillation of hypotonic intravenous fluids, microorganisms, and excessive exercise

Nursing Care Before the Procedure

Client preparation is the same as that for any study involving the collection of a peripheral blood sample (see Appendix I).

The Procedure

A venipuncture is performed and the sample collected in a green-topped tube. A capillary sample may be obtained in infants and children as well as in adults for whom a venipuncture may not be feasible.

Nursing Care After the Procedure

Care and assessment after the procedure are the same as for any study involving the collection of a peripheral blood sample (see Appendix I).

➤ *Abnormal test results, complications, and precautions:* Respond as for any laboratory analysis to determine RBC abnormalities leading to anemia (see p. 28).

RED BLOOD CELL (RBC) ENZYMES

To maintain normal shape and flexibility as well as to combine with and release oxygen, RBCs must generate energy. The needed energy is produced almost exclusively through the breakdown of glucose, a process that is catalyzed by a number of enzymes. Deficiencies of these enzymes are associated with hemolytic anemia. Two of the most common deficiencies, both hereditary, involve the RBC enzymes glucose-6-phosphate dehydrogenase and pyruvate kinase.

Glucose-6-Phosphate Dehydrogenase (G-6-PD)

Glucose-6-phosphate dehydrogenase (G-6-PD) is an enzyme pivotal in generating the reduced form of nicotinamide adenine dinucleotide phosphate (NADPH) through the pentose pathway in glucose metabolism. More than 100 structural and functional variants of the normal G-6-PD molecule (called type B) have been identified, most of which are clinically insignificant. One variant form (called type A) does, however, produce clinical disease. The type A variant is caused by a sex-linked genetic defect. The abnormal gene is carried by women and is transmitted to men who inherit the disorder.

Persons with the type A enzyme (15 percent of blacks) experience no difficulty until challenged by an oxidative stressor, which induces rapid intravascular hemolysis of susceptible cells. Among these stressors are systemic infections, septicemia, metabolic acidosis, and exposure to oxidant drugs (aspirin, chloramphenicol [Chloromycetin], nitrofurantoin [Furadantin], phenacetin, primaquine, probenecid [Benemid], quinidine, quinine, sulfonamides, thiazide diuretics, and tolbutamide [Orinase]).

A Mediterranean variant also may occur, especially in individuals of Greek and Italian descent and in some small, inbred Jewish populations. This variant severely reduces enzymatic activity and leads to more severe hemolytic episodes, which are triggered by a greater variety of stimuli and are less likely to be self-limited than in persons with the type A variant. In addition to the oxidative stressors just listed, ingestion of fava beans is known to precipitate hemolytic events in individuals with Mediterranean-type G-6-PD deficiency.[32]

Pyruvate Kinase (PK)

Pyruvate kinase (PK) functions in the formation of pyruvate and adenosine diphosphate (ADP) in glycolysis. The pyruvate thus formed is subsequently converted to lactate. RBCs that lack PK have a low affinity for oxygen. Episodes of hemolysis in individuals lacking this enzyme are severe and chronic and are exacerbated by stressors such as infection.

The inherited form of this disorder is transmitted as an autosomal recessive trait; both parents must carry the abnormal gene for the child to be affected. The acquired form of PK deficiency is usually caused by either drug ingestion or metabolic liver disease.

Reference Values

	Conventional Units	**SI Units**
G-6-PD	4.3–11.8 IU/g Hgb	0.28–0.76 mμ/mol Hgb
	125–281 U/dL packed RBCs (PRBCs)	1.25–2.81 kU/L RBC
	251–511 U/10^6 cells	0.25–0.51 nU/L RBC
	1211–2111 IU/mL PRBCs	
PK	2.0–8.8 U/g Hgb	
	0.3–0.91 mg/dL	

Interfering Factors

Young RBCs have higher enzyme levels than do older ones; thus, if the tests are performed within 10 days of a hemolytic episode (when the body is actively replacing lost cells through increased erythropoiesis) or after a recent blood transfusion, the results may be falsely normal.

Indications for Red Blood Cell (RBC) Enzymes Study

➤ Hemolytic anemia of uncertain etiology, especially when it occurs in infancy or early childhood

➤ Suspected G-6-PD or PK deficiency, especially in individuals with positive family history or with jaundice occurring in response to stressors, oxidant drugs, or foods such as fava beans

Nursing Care Before the Procedure

Client preparation is the same as that for any study involving the collection of a peripheral blood sample (see Appendix I).

The Procedure

A venipuncture is performed and the sample collected in a lavender-topped tube. A capillary sample may be collected in infants and children as well as in adults for whom venipuncture may not be feasible.

Nursing Care After the Procedure

Care and assessment after the procedure are the same as for any study involving the collection of a peripheral blood sample (see Appendix I).

➤ *Abnormal test results, complications, and precautions:* Respond as for any laboratory analysis to determine RBC abnormalities leading to anemia (see p. 28).

ERYTHROCYTE SEDIMENTATION RATE (ESR, SED RATE)

The erythrocyte sedimentation rate (ESR, sed rate) measures the rate at which RBCs in anticoagulated blood settle to the bottom of a calibrated tube. In normal blood, relatively little settling occurs because the gravitational pull on the RBCs is almost balanced by the upward force exerted by the plasma. If plasma is extremely viscous or if cholesterol levels are very high, the upward trend may virtually neutralize the downward pull on the RBCs. In contrast, anything that encourages RBCs to aggregate or stick together increases the rate of settling. Inflammatory and necrotic processes, for example, cause an alteration in blood proteins that results in clumping together of RBCs because of surface attraction. These clumps are called *rouleaux.* If the proportion of globin to albumin increases or if fibrinogen 3 levels are especially high, rouleaux formation is enhanced and the sed rate increases.[33] Specific causes of altered ESRs are presented in Table 1–10.

Reference Values

Normal values for the ESR follow. Note that several laboratory methods may be used to determine the ESR. Values vary according to the method used.

	Wintrobe (mm/hr)	Westergren (mm/hr)	Cutler (mm/hr)
Men			0–8
<50 yr	0–7	0–15	
>50 yr	5–7	0–20	
Women			0–10
<50 yr	0–15	0–20	
>50 yr	25–30	0–30	

	Landau Micro Method	Smith Micro Method
Children		
Newborn–2 yr	1–6	0–1 (newborns)
4–14 yr	1–9	3–13

Interfering Factors

Delays in performing the test after the sample is collected may retard the ESR and cause abnormally low results; the test should be performed within 3 hours of collecting the sample.

Indications for Erythrocyte Sedimentation Rate (ESR, Sed Rate) Test

➤ Suspected organic disease when symptoms are vague and clinical findings uncertain

➤ Identification of the presence of an inflammatory or necrotic process

➤ Monitoring response to treatment for various inflammatory disorders (e.g., rheumatoid arthritis, systemic lupus erythematosus)

➤ Support for diagnosing disorders associated with altered ESRs (see Table 1–10)

Table 1–10 ➤ CAUSES OF ALTERED ERYTHROCYTE SEDIMENTATION RATES

Increased Rate	Decreased Rate
Pregnancy (uterine and ectopic)	Polycythemia vera
Toxemia of pregnancy	Congestive heart failure
Collagen disorders (immune disorders of connective tissue)	Sickle cell, Hgb C disease
	Degenerative joint disease
Inflammatory disorders	Cryoglobulinemia
Infections	Drug toxicity (salicylates, quinine derivatives,
Acute myocardial infarction	adrenal corticosteroids)
Most malignancies	
Drugs (oral contraceptives, dextran, penicillamine, methyldopa, procainamide, theophylline, vitamin A)	
Severe anemias	
Myeloproliferative disorders	
Renal disease (nephritis)	
Hepatic cirrhosis	
Thyroid disorders	
Acute heavy metal poisoning	

Nursing Care Before the Procedure

Client preparation is the same as that for any study involving the collection of a peripheral blood sample (see Appendix I).

The Procedure

A venipuncture is performed and the sample collected in a lavender-topped tube. A capillary sample may be obtained in infants and children as well as in adults for whom venipuncture may not be feasible.

The sample should be transported promptly to the laboratory, as the test must be performed within 3 hours of collecting the sample. Delays may retard the ESR and cause abnormally low results.

Nursing Care After the Procedure

Care and assessment after the procedure are the same as for any study involving the collection of a peripheral blood sample (see Appendix I).

➤ *Abnormal values:* Note and report increases or decreases in the rate in relation to other test results used to determine the presence of or to monitor the progress of a disease. As the rate increases, note signs of infection or inflammation (pain, temperature) and activity intolerance (fatigue, weakness), and perform activities that conserve the client's energy. Administer ordered anti-inflammatory or antibiotic therapy. As the rate decreases, evaluate for improvement in condition and possible increases in client activity.

LEUKOCYTE STUDIES

Leukocytes (white blood cells, WBCs) constitute the body's primary defense against "foreignness"; that is, leukocytes protect the body from foreign organisms, substances, and tissues. The main types of leukocytes are neutrophils, monocytes, eosinophils, basophils, and lymphocytes. All of these cells are produced in the bone marrow. Lymphocytes may be produced in additional sites, however. Each of these types of leukocytes has different functions, and each behaves as a related but different system.[34]

Neutrophils and monocytes, the most mobile and active phagocytic leukocytes, are capable of breaking down various proteins and lipids such as those in bacterial cell membranes. The function of eosinophils is uncertain, although they are believed to detoxify foreign proteins that enter the body through the lungs or intestinal tract. The function of basophils also is not clearly understood, but the cells themselves are known to contain heparin, histamine, and serotonin. Basophils are believed to cause increased blood flow to injured tissues while preventing excessive intravascular clotting. Lymphocytes play an important role in immunity and may be divided into two main categories, B lymphocytes and T lymphocytes. B lymphocytes are responsible for humoral immunity and antibody production. It is B lymphocytes that ultimately develop into the antibody-producing plasma cells (see Fig. 1–2, p. 6). T lymphocytes are responsible for cellular immunity and they interact directly with the antigen.[35,36] Lymphocytes and related studies are discussed in greater detail in Chapter 3.

It should be noted that leukocytes perform their functions outside the vascular bed. Thus, WBCs are merely in transit while in the blood. Because of the many leukocyte functions, alterations in the number and types of cells may be indicative of numerous pathophysiologic problems.

WHITE BLOOD CELL (WBC) COUNT

The WBC count determines the number of leukocytes per cubic millimeter of whole blood. The counting is performed very rapidly by electronic devices. The WBC may be performed as part of a CBC, alone, or with differential WBC count. An elevated WBC count is termed *leukocytosis;* a decreased count, *leukopenia.* In addition to the normal physiologic variations in WBC count, many pathologic problems may result in an abnormal WBC count (see Table 1–2, p. 8).

If the WBC count is low, a buffy coat smear can be performed to identify leukemia or solid tumor cells in the blood. An alteration in total WBC count indicates the degree of response to a pathologic process but is not specifically diagnostic for any one disorder. A more complete evaluation is obtained through the differential WBC count.

Reference Values

The normal range of WBCs for adults is 5,000 to 10,000. Variations in the WBC count across the life cycle are shown in Table 1–4 (p. 19). Abnormal results may be classified by degree of severity as indicated.

	Elevations		Decreases	
	Conventional Units	**SI Units**	**Conventional Units**	**SI Units**
Slight	11,000–20,000	$11.0–20.0 \times 10^9$ L	3000–4500	$3.4–4.5 \times 10^9$ L
Moderate	20,000–30,000	$20.0–30.0 \times 10^9$ L	1500–3000	$1.5–3.0 \times 10^9$ L
Severe	>50,000	$>50.0 \times 10^9$ L	<1500	$<1.5 \times 10^9$ L

Indications for a White Blood Cell (WBC) Count

➤ Routine screening as part of a CBC (see p. 8)
➤ Suspected inflammatory or infectious process (see Table 1–2, p. 8)
➤ Suspected leukemia, autoimmune disorder, or allergy
➤ Suspected bone marrow depression
➤ Monitoring response to stress, malnutrition, and therapy for infectious or malignant processes

Nursing Care Before the Procedure

Client preparation is the same as that for any study involving the collection of a peripheral blood sample (see Appendix I).

The Procedure

A venipuncture is performed and the sample collected in a lavender-topped tube. A capillary sample may be obtained in infants and children as well as in adults for whom venipuncture may not be feasible.

Because of the normal diurnal variation of WBC levels, it is important to note the time the sample was obtained.

Nursing Care After the Procedure

Care and assessment after the procedure are the same as for any study involving the collection of a peripheral blood sample (see Appendix I).

➤ *Abnormal test results:* Provide support when diagnostic findings are revealed, especially if malignancy is a possibility or is confirmed. Reinforce information given by the physician, and answer questions or direct them to the appropriate professionals.

➤ *Abnormal values:* Note and report signs and symptoms of infection or inflammation associated with an increased count (temperature, chills), including those reflective of the site affected (pain, edema, redness, drainage). Carry out appropriate standard precautions to prevent spread to other sites. Collect a specimen for culture and sensitivities. Administer ordered antipyretic and antibiotic therapy to treat infection. Administer chemotherapeutic agents for malignancy identified and monitored by WBC and differential counts. Note and report decreased count and carry out reverse isolation procedures to protect immunosuppressed client from infection.

➤ **Critical values:** Notify the physician at once if a new client has a WBC count of less than 2000 per microliter or greater than 50,000 per microliter or if a client whose WBC count was less than 4000 per microliter has a change of 1000 per microliter. Take precautions to protect the client from infection. Prepare for further diagnostic procedures to identify the cause or source of increases or decreases in the count.

DIFFERENTIAL WHITE BLOOD CELL (WBC) COUNT

The differential WBC count indicates the percentage of each type of leukocyte present per cubic millimeter of whole blood. If necessary for further evaluation of results, the percentage for each cell type can be multiplied by the total WBC count to obtain the absolute number of each cell type present.

Causes of alterations in the differential WBC count according to type of leukocyte are presented in Table 1–11. An increase in immature neutrophils (i.e., bands, stabs) indicates the body's attempt to produce more neutrophils in response to the pathologic process. A decreased neutrophil count is fairly common in children during viral infections. An increase in bands is sometimes referred to as a "shift to the left." This terminology derives from the traditional headings used on laboratory slips to report WBC differential results, which are the following: Bands, Neutrophils, Eosinophils, Basophils, Monocytes, and Lymphocytes.

In contrast, the meaning of a "shift to the right" is less well defined. This may refer to an increase in neutrophils or other granulocytes or to an increase in lymphocytes or monocytes.

Reference Values

The normal percentage of each WBC type in adults is shown next. Variations across the life cycle are listed in Table 1–4 (p. 19).

	Conventional Units	SI Units
Bands	3–8%	0.03–0.08
Neutrophils	54–75%	0.54–0.75
Eosinophils	1–4%	0.01–0.04
Basophils	0–1%	0–0.01
Monocytes	2–8%	0.02–0.08
Lymphocytes	25–40%	0.25–0.40

Indications for Differential White Blood Cell (WBC) Count

➤ Routine screening as part of a CBC (see p. 18)
➤ Abnormal total WBC count to determine the source of the elevation
➤ Confirmation of the presence of various disorders associated with increases and decreases in the several types of WBCs (see Table 1–11, p. 43)
➤ Monitoring of response to treatment for acute infections, with a therapeutic response indicated by a decreasing number of bands and a stabilizing number of neutrophils
➤ Monitoring of physiologic responses to chemotherapy

Nursing Care Before the Procedure

Client preparation is the same as that for any study involving the collection of a peripheral blood sample (see Appendix I).

The Procedure

A venipuncture is performed and the sample collected in a lavender-topped tube. A capillary sample may be obtained in infants and children as well as in adults for whom venipuncture may not be feasible.

Nursing Care After the Procedure

Care and assessment after the procedure are the same as for any study involving the collection of a peripheral blood sample (see Appendix I).

WHITE BLOOD CELL (WBC) ENZYMES

WBCs in peripheral blood samples retain enzymatic activity and can alter substrates added in the laboratory. The presence of enzymatic activity is useful in studying cells that are so morphologically abnormal on stained smear that it is difficult to determine their cell line of origin (see Fig. 1–2, p. 6). The two most common WBC enzyme tests are the test for leukocyte alkaline phosphatase, an enzyme found in neutrophils; and the periodic acid–Schiff stain, which tests for enzymes found in granulocytes and erythrocytes. Both tests are used to diagnose hematologic disorders, especially leukemias. Specific causes of alterations in WBC enzymes are presented in Table 1–12. Another WBC enzyme test, tartrate-resistant acid phosphatase, is performed to diagnose hairy cell leukemia, as this enzyme activity is present in the lymphocytic cells of this type of leukemia. Additional details of each test are briefly discussed subsequently.

Table 1–11 ➤ CAUSES OF ALTERED WHITE BLOOD CELL DIFFERENTIAL BY CELL TYPE

Cell Type	Increased Levels	Decreased Levels
Neutrophils	Stress (allergies, exercise, childbirth, surgery) Extremes of temperature Acute hemorrhage or hemolysis Infectious diseases Inflammatory disorders (rheumatic fever, gout, rheumatoid arthritis, drug reactions, vasculitis, myositis) Tissue necrosis (burns, crushing injuries, abscesses Malignancies Metabolic disorders (uremia, eclampsia, diabetic ketoacidosis, thyroid crisis, Cushing's syndrome) Drugs (epinephrine, histamine, lithium, heavy metals, heparin, digitalis, ACTH) Toxins and venoms (turpentine, benzene) Leukemia (myelocytic)	Bone marrow depression (viruses, toxic chemicals, overwhelming infection, Felty's syndrome, Gaucher's disease, myelofibrosis, hypersplenism, pernicious anemia, radiation) Anorexia nervosa, starvation, malnutrition Folic acid deficiency Vitamin B_{12} deficiency Acromegaly Addison's disease Thyrotoxicosis Anaphylaxis Disseminated lupus erythematosus Drugs (alcohol, phenylbutazone [Butazolidin], phenacetin, penicillin, chloramphenicol, streptomycin, phenytoin [Dilantin], mephenytoin [Mesantoin], phenacemide [Phenurone], tripelennamine [PBZ], aminophylline, quinine, chlorpromazine, barbiturates, dinitrophenols, sulfonamides, antineoplastics)
Bands (immature neutrophils)	Infections Antineoplastic drugs Any condition that causes neutrophilia	None, as bands should be absent or present only in only small numbers
Basophils	Leukemia Hodgkin's disease Polycythemia vera Ulcerative colitis Nephrosis Chronic hypersensitivity states	None, as normal value is 0–1%
Eosinophils	Sickle cell disease Asthma Chorea Hypersensitivity reactions Parasitic infestations Autoimmune diseases Addison's disease Malignancies Sarcoidosis Chronic inflammatory diseases and dermatoses Leprosy Hodgkin's disease Polycythemias Ulcerative colitis Autoallergies Pernicious anemia	Disseminated lupus erythematosus Acromegaly Elevated steroid levels Stress Infectious mononucleosis Hypersplenism Cushing's syndrome Congestive heart failure Hyperplastic anemia Hormones (ACTH, thyroxine, epinephrine)

(Continued on page 44)

Table 1–11 ➤ CAUSES OF ALTERED WHITE BLOOD CELL DIFFERENTIAL BY CELL TYPE *(Continued)*

Cell Type	Increased Levels	Decreased Levels
Monocytes	Splenectomy Infections (bacterial, viral, mycotic, rickettsial, amebic) Cirrhosis Collagen diseases Ulcerative colitis Regional enteritis Gaucher's disease Hodgkin's disease Lymphomas Carcinomas Monocytic leukemia Radiation Polycythemia vera Sarcoidosis Weil's disease Systemic lupus erythematosus Hemolytic anemias Thrombocytopenic purpura	Not characteristic of specific disorders
Lymphocytes	Infections (bacterial, viral) Lymphosarcoma Ulcerative colitis Banti's disease Felty's syndrome Myeloma Lymphomas Addison's disease Thyrotoxicosis Malnutrition Rickets Waldenström's macroglobulinemia Lymphocytic leukemia	Immune deficiency diseases Hodgkin's disease Rheumatic fever Aplastic anemia Bone marrow failure Gaucher's disease Hemolytic disease of the newborn Hypersplenism Thrombocytopenic purpura Transfusion reaction Massive transfusions Pernicious anemia Septicemia Pneumonia Burns Radiation Toxic chemicals (benzene, bismuth, DDT) Antineoplastic agents Adrenal corticosteroids (high doses)

Leukocyte Alkaline Phosphatase (LAP)

Leukocyte alkaline phosphatase (LAP) is an enzyme found in neutrophils. This enzyme is completely independent of serum alkaline phosphatase, which reflects osteoblastic activity and hepatic function. The LAP content of neutrophils increases as the cells mature; therefore, the LAP study is useful in assessing cellular maturation and in evaluating departures from normal differentiation.

The LAP study is used to distinguish among various hematologic disorders. For example, LAP increases in polycythemia vera, myelofibrosis, and

Table 1–12 ➤ CAUSES OF ALTERATIONS IN WHITE BLOOD CELL ENZYMES		
	CAUSES OF ALTERATIONS	
Enzyme	**Elevated Levels**	**Decreased Levels**
Leukocyte alkaline phosphatase (LAP)	Chronic myelocytic leukemia Polycythemia vera Myelofibrosis Leukemoid reactions Oral contraceptives Pregnancy Adrenocorticotropic hormone (ACTH) excess Cushing's syndrome Down syndrome Multiple myeloma Lymphomas	Acute myelocytic leukemia Acute monocytic leukemia Chronic granulocytic leukemia Anemias (aplastic, pernicious) Thrombocytopenia Infectious mononucleosis Paroxysmal nocturnal hemoglobinuria Hereditary hypophosphatasia Collagen diseases
	Positive	**Negative**
Periodic acid–Schiff (PAS) stain	Acute granulocytic leukemia Acute lymphoblastic leukemia Erythroleukemia Amyloidosis Thalassemia Lymphomas	Early granulocyte precursors Severe iron-deficiency anemia Normal erythrocyte precursors Mature RBCs

leukemoid reactions to infections but decreases in chronic granulocytic leukemia. Because all of these conditions have increased numbers of immature circulating neutrophils, LAP scores can be helpful in differentiating among them.

Periodic Acid–Schiff (PAS) Stain

In the periodic acid–Schiff (PAS) stain, compounds that can be oxidized to aldehydes are localized by brilliant fuschia staining. Many elements in many tissues are PAS-positive, but in blood cells the PAS-positive material of diagnostic importance is cytoplasmic glycogen. Early granulocytic precursors and normal erythrocytic precursors are PAS-negative. Mature RBCs remain PAS-negative, but granulocytes acquire increasing PAS positivity as they mature.[37]

Reference Values

Leukocyte alkaline phosphatase (LAP)	13–130 U
Periodic acid–Schiff (PAS) stain	Granulocytes—positive
	Agranulocytes—negative
	Granulocytic precursors—negative
	Erythrocytes—negative
	Erythrocytic precursors—negative
Tartrate-resistant acid phosphatase (TRAP)	Activity absent

Indications for White Blood Cell (WBC) Enzymes Study

> ➤ Identification of morphologically abnormal WBCs on stained smear
> ➤ Suspected leukemia or other hematologic disorders (see Table 1–12, p. 45)

Nursing Care Before the Procedure

Client preparation is the same as that for any study involving the collection of a peripheral blood sample (see Appendix I).

The Procedure

A capillary sample is generally preferred for these tests. The sample is spread on a slide, fixed, and stained.

Nursing Care After the Procedure

Care and assessment after the procedure are the same as for any study involving the collection of a peripheral blood sample (see Appendix I).

Student Name _____ Class _____

Instructor _____ Date _____

CASE STUDY AND CRITICAL THINKING EXERCISE

1. Ms. White, age 25, is admitted to the clinic. She complains of fatigue that has lasted for 3 months. Physical exam reveals VS: T 99°F (37.2°C), P 102, R 22, BP 110/60. Lab values are Hct 47%, MCV 130 μm^3, and MCH 30 pg.

   a. What is the probable diagnosis?

   b. Interpret the lab values relative to the diagnosis.

   c. A Schilling test is ordered. Explain purpose, procedure, and expected findings.

2. Jim, age 9 years, is brought to the clinic for a checkup. His mother reports that he has recently shown less interest in participating on his soccer team and complains of fatigue. Physical exam reveals VS: T 99.2°F (37.5°C), P 88, R 16, BP 98/60. His skin is pale, with ecchymotic areas on his trunk and lower extremities. Liver and spleen are not palpable. CBC reveals Hgb 9.2g/dl, Hct 30%, RBC 3 × 10/mm³, WBC 16 × 10/mm³, lymphocytes 4500/mm³, blasts much higher than normal, platelets 30 × 10/mm³.

   a. What is the probable diagnosis?

   b. Interpret the lab data relative to this diagnosis.

   c. Describe treatment considerations.

References

1. Hole, JW: Human Anatomy and Physiology, ed 4. Wm C Brown, Dubuque, Iowa, 1987, p 614.
2. Sacher, RA, and McPherson, RA: Widmann's Clinical Interpretation of Laboratory Tests, ed 10. FA Davis, Philadelphia, 1991, p 21.
3. Ibid, p 21.
4. Ibid, p 21.
5. Hillman, RS, and Finch, CA: Red Cell Manual, ed 6. FA Davis, Philadelphia, 1992, p 2.
6. Price, S, and Wilson, L: Pathophysiology, ed 3. McGraw-Hill, New York, 1986, p 180.
7. Hole, op cit, p 619.
8. Sacher and McPherson, op cit, p 30.
9. Fischbach, FT: A Manual of Laboratory and Diagnostic Tests, ed 4. JB Lippincott, Philadelphia, 1992, pp 89–91.
10. Hillman and Finch, op cit, pp 4–5.
11. Sacher and McPherson, op cit, p 32.
12. Hillman and Finch, op cit, pp 6–7.
13. Sacher and McPherson, op cit, p 32.
14. Ibid, p 41.
15. Ibid, p 41.
16. Ibid, p 43.
17. Ibid, p 32.
18. Hillman and Finch, op cit, pp 95-96.
19. Fischbach, op cit, p 88.
20. Hillman and Finch, op cit, p 42.
21. Sacher and McPherson, op cit, p 45.
22. Hillman and Finch, op cit, p 12.
23. Fischbach, op cit, p 43.
24. Sacher and McPherson, op cit, p 46.
25. Hillman and Finch, op cit, p 43.
26. Hole, op cit, p 603.
27. Hillman and Finch, op cit, p 43.
28. Sacher and McPherson, op cit, p 44.
29. Hillman and Finch, op cit, pp 10–11.
30. Ibid, pp 87, 110.
31. Fischbach, op cit, p 82.
32. Sacher and McPherson, op cit, pp 99–100.
33. Ibid, pp 67–68.
34. Boggs, DR, and Winkelstein, A: White Cell Manual, ed 4. FA Davis, Philadelphia, 1983, p 1.
35. Hole, op cit, pp 625–627.
36. Boggs and Winkelstein, op cit, pp 63–65.
37. Sacher and McPherson, op cit, pp 70–71.

Bibliography

Bunn, HF, and Forget, BG: Hemoglobin: Molecular, Genetic and Clinical Aspects. WB Saunders, Philadelphia, 1986.

Byrne, CJ, et al: Laboratory Tests: Implications for Nursing Care, ed 2. Addison-Wesley, Menlo Park, Calif, 1986.

Chernecky, CC, and Berger, BJ; Cullen, BN (ed): Laboratory Tests and Diagnostic Procedures, ed 2. WB Saunders, Philadelphia, 1996.

Clinical Laboratory Tests: Values and Implications, ed 2. Springhouse Corporation, Springhouse, Pa, 1995.

Corbett, JV: Laboratory Tests and Diagnostic Procedures with Nursing Diagnoses, ed 4. Appleton & Lange, Norwalk, Conn, 1995.

Deglin, JH, and Vallerand, AH: Davis's Drug Guide for Nurses, ed 6. FA Davis, Philadelphia, 1999.

Delamore, IW, and Yin, JAL: Haematological Aspects of Systemic Disease. WB Saunders, Philadelphia, 1990.

Hayhoe, FGJ, and Flemans, RJ: Color Atlas of Hematological Cystology, ed 3. Mosby–Year Book, St Louis, 1992.

Henry, JB: Clinical Diagnosis and Management by Laboratory Methods, ed 19. WB Saunders, Philadelphia, 1996.

Kee, JL: Handbook of Laboratory and Diagnostic Tests with Nursing Implications, ed 3. Appleton & Lange, Norwalk, Conn, 1997.

Kuhn, M: Pharmacotherapeutics: A Nursing Process Approach, ed 4. FA Davis, Philadelphia, 1997.

Lewis, SM, et al (eds): Medical-Surgical Nursing: Assessment and Management of Clinical Problems, ed 4. Mosby–Year Book, St Louis, 1995.

Pagana, KD, and Pagana, TJ: Diagnostic and Laboratory Test Reference, ed 3. Mosby–Year Book, St Louis, 1996.

Porth, CM: Pathophysiology: Concepts of Altered Health States, ed 4. JB Lippincott, Philadelphia, 1993.

Powers, LW: Diagnostic Hematology: Clinical and Technical Principles. Mosby–Year Book, St Louis, 1989.

Ravel, R: Clinical Laboratory Medicine: Clinical Application of Laboratory Data, ed 6. Mosby–Year Book, St Louis, 1994.

Springhouse Corporation: Nurse's Reference Library, Diagnostic Tests, ed 3. Springhouse, Springhouse, Pa, 1991.

Tietz, NW (ed): Clinical Guide to Laboratory Tests, ed 3. WB Saunders, Philadelphia, 1997.

Whaley, LF: Nursing Care of Infants and Children, ed 4. Mosby–Year Book, St Louis, 1991.

2

Hemostasis and Tests of Hemostatic Functions

➤ **TESTS COVERED**

Platelet Count, *54*
Bleeding Time, *56*
Platelet Aggregation Test, *59*
Clot Retraction Test, *60*
Rumple-Leeds Capillary Fragility Test
  (Tourniquet Test), *61*
Prothrombin Time (PT, Pro Time), *63*
Partial Thromboplastin Time
  (PTT)/Activated Partial
  Thromboplastin Time (aPTT), *66*

Whole Blood Clotting Time
  (Coagulation, CT, Lee-White
  Coagulation Time), *68*
Thrombin Clotting Time (TCT, Plasma
  Thrombin Time), *69*
Prothrombin Consumption Time (PCT,
  Serum Prothrombin Time), *70*
Factor Assays, *71*
Plasma Fibrinogen, *74*
Fibrin Split Products (FSP), *75*
Euglobulin Lysis Time, *76*

INTRODUCTION

Hemostasis is the collective term for all the mechanisms the body uses to protect itself from blood loss. In other words, failure of hemostasis leads to hemorrhage. Hemostatic mechanisms are organized into three categories: (1) vascular activity, (2) platelet function, and (3) coagulation.

VASCULAR ACTIVITY

Vascular activity consists of constriction of muscles within the walls of the blood vessels in response to vascular damage. This vasoconstriction narrows the path through which the blood flows and may sometimes entirely halt blood flow. The vascular phase of hemostasis affects only arterioles and their dependent capillaries; large vessels cannot constrict sufficiently to prevent blood loss. Even in small vessels, vasoconstriction provides only a brief hemostasis.

PLATELET FUNCTION

Platelets serve two main functions: (1) to protect intact blood vessels from endothelial damage provoked by the countless microtraumas of day-to-day existence and (2) to initiate repair through the formation of platelet plugs when blood vessel walls are damaged.

When overt trauma or microtrauma damages blood vessels, platelets adhere to the altered surface. Adherence requires the presence of ionized calcium

49

(coagulation factor IV), fibrinogen (coagulation factor I), and a protein associated with coagulation factor VIII, called von Willebrand's factor (vWF). The process of adherence involves reversible changes in platelet shape and, usually, the release of adenosine diphosphate (ADP), adenosine triphosphate (ATP), calcium, and serotonin. With a strong enough stimulus, the next phase of platelet activity, platelet aggregation, occurs and results in the formation of a loose plug in the damaged endothelium. The platelet plug aids in controlling bleeding until a blood clot has had time to form.[1]

Platelets generate prostaglandins that ultimately promote platelet adherence, whereas the endothelial cells lining the blood vessels produce a different prostaglandin that inhibits platelet aggregation. Ingestion of aspirin inhibits the actions of the prostaglandins released by platelets, an effect that may persist for many days after a person takes even a small amount of aspirin. Aspirin also may affect the actions of the prostaglandins produced by endothelial cells, but not to the extent that it affects platelet prostaglandins.[2] Thus, the net effect of aspirin is to inhibit hemostasis.

Thrombin, which is generated by the coagulation sequence (see the next section), independently promotes the release of substances from the platelets. Release of platelet factor 3 enhances coagulation mechanisms, thereby increasing thrombin generation. Platelet factor 4, also released by platelets, reinforces the interactions between coagulation and platelet aggregation by neutralizing the naturally generated anticoagulant, endogenous heparin.[3]

COAGULATION

Coagulation is a complex process by which plasma proteins interact to form a stable fibrin gel.[4] The fibrin strands thus formed create a meshwork that cements blood components together, a process known as syneresis. Ultimately, a blood clot is formed.[5,6] Normal coagulation depends on the presence of all clotting factors and follows specific sequences known as pathways or cascades.

At least 30 substances are believed to be involved in the clotting process. The most significant ones are shown in Table 2–1. Note that clotting factors are

Table 2–1 ➤ CLOTTING FACTORS

I	Fibrinogen
Ia	Fibrin
II	Prothrombin
IIa	Thrombin
III	Thromboplastin, tissue thromboplastin
IV	Calcium, ionized calcium
V	Accelerator globulin (AcG), proaccelerin, labile factor
VII	Proconvertin, autoprothrombin I, serum prothrombin conversion accelerator (SPCA)
VIIa	Convertin
VIII	Antihemophilic factor (AHF), antihemophilic globulin (AHG)
IX	Christmas factor, antihemophilic factor B, plasma thromboplastin component (PTC), autoprothrombin II
X	Stuart factor, Stuart-Prower factor, autoprothrombin III
XI	Plasma thromboplastin antecedent (PTA)
XII	Hageman factor
XIII	Fibrin-stabilizing factor

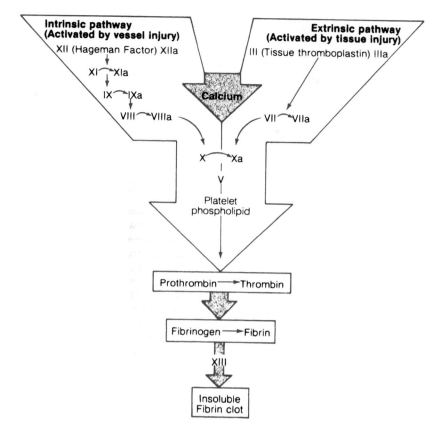

Figure 2–1   Schematic diagram of the intrinsic, extrinsic, and common final coagulation pathways. (From Porth, C: Pathophysiology: Concepts of Altered Health States, ed 4. JB Lippincott, Philadelphia, 1994, p 313, with permission.)

now designated by Roman numerals. The "a" indicates an activated clotting factor.[7] There is no factor VI because that number was originally assigned to what is now known to be activated factor V.[8]

Each of the clotting factors is involved at a specific step in the coagulation process, with one clotting factor leading to activation of the next factor in the sequence. Three major clotting sequences have been identified: (1) the intrinsic pathway, (2) the extrinsic pathway, and (3) the common final pathway.

The intrinsic pathway is activated when blood comes in contact with the injured vessel wall; the extrinsic pathway is activated when blood is exposed to damaged tissues. Both pathways are needed for normal hemostasis, and both lead to the common final pathway.[9] A schematic representation of the intrinsic, extrinsic, and common pathways is shown in Figure 2–1.

The common final pathway is initiated with the activation of factor X. Factors X and V, along with platelet phospholipid and calcium, combine to form prothrombin activator, which converts prothrombin to thrombin. Thrombin subsequently converts fibrinogen to fibrin gel. Thrombin also enhances platelet release reactions, augments the activation of factors V and VIII, and activates factor XIII.[10] Stable (insoluble) fibrin is formed in the presence of activated factor XIII.

Calcium plays an important role throughout the coagulation process. It is necessary for the activation of factors VII, IX, X, and XI; for the conversion of prothrombin (factor II) to thrombin; and for the formation of fibrin. Hypocalcemia usually does not cause bleeding difficulties, however, because cardiac arrest occurs before levels are low enough to precipitate abnormal hemostasis. Citrate, oxalate, and ethylenediaminetetraacetic acid (EDTA) are anticoagulants because they bind calcium and prevent it from participating in the clotting process. Any one of these substances may be added to the vacuum tubes used to collect peripheral blood samples when an uncoagulated specimen is needed (see Appendix I, Table A–1).[11]

ANTAGONISTS TO HEMOSTASIS

Both platelet activation and coagulation are self-perpetuating processes that could potentially continue until an injured vessel is completely occluded. Coagulation inhibitors are present to prevent excessive clotting and to dissolve the clot as tissue repair occurs.

Maintaining adequate blood flow aids in diluting and removing clotting factors and in dispersing aggregated platelets. Partially activated coagulation factors are carried to the liver and the reticuloendothelial system, where they are degraded.[12] Two specific anticoagulation mechanisms also help to prevent excessive clotting: (1) the fibrinolytic system and (2) the antithrombin system.

In the fibrinolytic system, fibrin strands are broken down into progressively smaller fragments by a proteolytic enzyme, *plasmin.* Although plasmin does not circulate in active form, its precursor, *plasminogen,* does. Plasminogen is converted into plasmin by several plasminogen activators, among them factor XII, urokinase, and streptokinase. Once activated, plasmin digests fibrin, splits fibrinogen into peptide fragments (fibrin split products [FSP]), and degrades factors V, VIII, and XIII. In addition, the FSP interfere with platelet aggregation, reduce prothrombin, and interfere with conversion of soluble fibrin to insoluble fibrin. Plasma also contains agents that neutralize plasmin itself. Among these are antiplasmin and alpha$_1$-antitrypsin. A balance between proplasmin and antiplasmin substances aids in maintaining normal coagulation.[13]

The antithrombin system protects the body from excessive clotting by neutralizing the clotting capability of thrombin.[14] Although various substances inhibit thrombin, the most important one is antithrombin III (AT III), a substance that abolishes the activity of thrombin (activated factor II); activated factors X, XI, and XII; and plasmin. Another name for AT III is heparin cofactor. Heparin augments by approximately 100 times the affinity of AT III and the activated clotting factors on which it acts. A deficiency of AT III, which can be congenital or acquired, makes an individual prone to excessive clotting. Platelet factor 4, which is released when platelets are broken down, inhibits AT III activity.[15]

PLATELET STUDIES

Circulating platelets (thrombocytes) are anuclear, cytoplasmic disks that bud off from megakaryocytes, large multinucleated cells found in the bone marrow[16,17] (see Fig. 1–2, p. 6). Platelets survive in the circulation for about 10 days.

Regulation of platelet production is ascribed to *thrombopoietin* by analogy to erythropoietin (see p. 5, Chap. 1), although no single substance has been specifically identified. With pronounced hemostatic stress or marrow stimulation, platelet production can increase to seven to eight times that of normal. Newly generated platelets are larger and have greater hemostatic capacity than mature circulating platelets.[18]

Two thirds of the total number of platelets are in the systemic circulation, and the remaining third exists as a pool of platelets in the spleen. The pool exchanges freely with the general circulation.[19] The spleen also aids in removing old or damaged platelets from the circulation. In disorders involving exaggerated splenic activity (hypersplenism), 90 percent of the body's platelets may be trapped in the enlarged spleen, and the client is predisposed to excessive bleeding. Hypersplenism is seen in certain acute infections (e.g., infectious mononucleosis, miliary tuberculosis), connective tissue diseases (e.g., rheumatoid arthritis, lupus erythematosus), myeloproliferative diseases (e.g., leukemias, lymphomas, hemolytic anemias), and chronic liver diseases (e.g., cirrhosis).[20]

The functions of platelets are discussed in the introduction to this chapter. In general, individuals with too few platelets or with platelets that function poorly experience numerous pinpoint-sized hemorrhages (petechiae) and multiple small, superficial bruises (ecchymoses). Frequently, there is generalized oozing from mucosal surfaces and from venipuncture sites or other small, localized injuries. Large, deep hematomas and bleeding into joints are not characteristic of platelet deficiency (thrombocytopenia).[21]

Platelet studies involve evaluating the number and function of circulating platelets. Platelet numbers are assessed by the platelet count (see the next section). Disorders of platelet function (thrombopathies) are less common than disorders of platelet number. An overview of the causes of altered platelet function is provided in Table 2–2.

Table 2–2 ➤ **OVERVIEW OF CAUSES OF ALTERED PLATELET FUNCTION**

Increased Function	Decreased Function
Trauma	Severe liver disease
Surgery	Uremia
Fractures	Myeloproliferative disorders
Strenuous exercise	Dysproteinemias
	Glanzman's thrombasthenia
Pregnancy	Bernard-Soulier syndrome (hereditary giant platelet syndrome)
	Idiopathic thrombocytopenic purpura
	Infectious mononucleosis
	von Willebrand's disease
	Drugs such as aspirin and other anti-inflammatory agents, antihistamines, antidepressants, alcohol, methylxanthines

PLATELET COUNT

Platelets may be counted manually or with electronic counting devices. Although larger numbers of platelets are capable of being examined with electronic counting, the procedure is subject to error if (1) the white blood cell (WBC) count is greater than 10,000 cells per cubic millimeter, (2) there is severe red blood cell fragmentation, (3) the diluting fluid contains extraneous particles, (4) the plasma sample settles too long during processing, or (5) platelets adhere to one another.

Causes of increased numbers of platelets (thrombocytosis, thrombocythemia) and decreased numbers of platelets (thrombocytopenia) are presented in Table 2–3.

Mean platelet volume can also be determined by the electronic automated method. The test reveals the size of platelets important in the diagnosis of disorders affecting the hematologic system. An increased volume of platelets that are larger than normal in diameter is found in lupus erythematosus, thrombocytopenic purpura, B_{12}-deficiency anemia, hyperthyroidism, and myelogenic and other myeloproliferative diseases. A decreased volume of the larger-sized platelets is found in Wiskott-Aldrich syndrome.[22]

Table 2–3 ➤ CAUSES OF ALTERED PLATELET LEVELS

Increased Levels (Thrombocytosis)	DECREASED LEVELS (THROMBOCYTOPENIA)	
	Decreased Production	Increased Destruction
Leukemias (chronic)	Vitamin B_{12}/folic acid deficiencies	Idiopathic thrombocytopenic purpura
Polycythemia vera	Radiation	Splenomegaly caused by liver disease
Anemias (posthemorrhagic and iron-deficiency)	Viral infections	Lymphomas
Splenectomy	Leukemias (acute)	Hemolytic anemias
Tuberculosis and other acute infections	Histiocytosis	Rocky Mountain spotted fever
Hemorrhage	Bone marrow malignancies	Sarcoidosis
Carcinomatosis	Fanconi's syndrome	Meningococcemia
Trauma	Wiskott-Aldrich syndrome	Antibody/HLA-antigen reactions
Surgery	Uremia	Hemolytic disease of the newborn
Chronic heart disease	Drugs such as anticancer drugs, anticonvulsants, alcohol,	Congenital infections (cytomegalovirus [CMV],
Cirrhosis	carbamates, chloramphenicol,	herpes, syphilis,
Chronic pancreatitis	chlorothiazides, isoniazid,	toxoplasmosis)
Childbirth	pyrazolones, streptomycin,	Disseminated intravascular
Drugs such as epinephrine	sulfonamides, sulfonylureas	coagulation (DIC)
		Immune complex formation
		Chronic cor pulmonale
		Miliary tuberculosis
		Burns
		Drugs and chemicals such as aspirin, benzenes, DDT, digitoxin, gold salts, heparin, quinidine, quinine, thiazides

Reference Values

Values vary slightly across the life cycle, with lower platelet counts seen in newborns (see Table 1–4, p. 19).

➤ 150,000 to 450,000 per mm³ (average = 250,000 per mm³)
➤ Mean platelet volume = 25 μm diameter
➤ **Critical Values <20,000 U/L or >1,000,000 U/L**

Interfering Factors

➤ Altered test results may occur if:
  • The WBC count is greater than 100,000 per cubic millimeter.
  • There is severe red blood cell fragmentation.
  • The fluid used to dilute the sample contains extraneous particles.
  • The plasma sample settles too long during processing.
  • Platelets adhere to one another.
  • The client is receiving drugs that alter platelet functions and numbers (see Tables 2–2, p. 53, and 2–3, p. 54).
➤ Traumatic venipunctures may lead to erroneous results as a result of activation of the coagulation sequence.
➤ Excessive agitation of the sample may cause the platelets to clump together and adhere to the walls of the test tube, thus altering test results.

Indications for Platelet Count

➤ Family history of bleeding disorder
➤ Signs of abnormal bleeding such as epistaxis, easy bruising, bleeding gums, hematuria, and menorrhagia
➤ Determination of effects of diseases and drugs known to alter platelet levels (see Table 2–3, p. 54)
➤ Identification of individuals who may be prone to bleeding during surgical, obstetric, dental, or invasive diagnostic procedures, as indicated by a platelet count of approximately 50,000 to 100,000 per cubic millimeter
➤ Identification of individuals who may be prone to spontaneous bleeding, as indicated by a platelet count of less than 15,000 to 20,000 per cubic millimeter
➤ Differentiation between decreased platelet production and decreased platelet function
  • Platelet dysfunction is defined as a long bleeding time (see p. 56) with a platelet count of greater than 100,000 per cubic millimeter.[23]

Nursing Care Before the Procedure

Client preparation is the same as that for any study involving the collection of a peripheral blood sample (see Appendix I).

The Procedure

A venipuncture is performed and the sample collected in a lavender-topped tube. A capillary sample may be obtained in infants and children as well as in adults for whom venipuncture may not be feasible.

Nursing Care After the Procedure

Care and assessment after the procedure are essentially the same as for any study involving the collection of a peripheral blood sample. Because the client may have a platelet deficiency, maintain digital pressure directly on the puncture site for 3 to 5 minutes after the needle is withdrawn. Also, inspect the site for excessive bruising after the procedure.

➤ *Abnormal increase (thrombocytosis):* Note and report signs of dehydration and input and output (I&O) ratio that can contribute to venous stasis, possible thrombosis, or bleeding tendency if the coagulation process is affected. Administer ordered aspirin and antacid, and observe for bleeding tendency if prothrombin time is increased.

➤ *Abnormal decrease (thrombocytopenia):* Note and report petechiae, bruising, or hematoma. Administer ordered corticosteroids. Protect children from trauma and advise adults to use soft toothbrushes and electric razors, and prevent other trauma by padding side rails and avoiding intramuscular and subcutaneous injections. Assess bleeding from skin and mucous membranes (petechiae, ecchymoses, epistaxis, feces, urine, emesis, sputum). Administer platelet transfusion and assess for any allergic responses, sepsis, or hypervolemia.

➤ **Critical values:** Notify the physician immediately if the platelet count is less than 20,000/mL or greater than 1 million/mL. Prepare for transfusion of platelets by intravenous drip or bolus infusion.

BLEEDING TIME

One of the best indicators of platelet deficiency is prolonged bleeding after a controlled superficial injury; that is, capillaries subjected to a small, clean incision bleed until the defect is plugged by aggregating platelets (see p. 49). When platelets are inadequate in number or if their function is impaired, bleeding time is prolonged.

If the platelet count falls below 10,000 per cubic millimeter, bleeding time is prolonged. Prolonged bleeding time with a platelet count of greater than 100,000 per cubic millimeter indicates platelet dysfunction. Bleeding time is prolonged in von Willebrand's disease, an inherited deficiency of vWF, a protein associated with clotting factor VIII that is necessary for normal platelet adherence. Aspirin ingestion also prevents platelet aggregation and may prolong bleeding time for as long as 5 days after a single 300-mg dose.[24] Other causes of prolonged bleeding times are listed in Table 2–4.

Reference Values

Method	Normal Values
Duke	1–3 min
Ivy	3–6 min
Template	3–6 min

Values vary according to the method used to perform the test (see the section on procedure).

Table 2-4 ➤ CAUSES OF PROLONGED BLEEDING TIME	
Drugs	**Diseases**
Alcohol	Aplastic anemia
Anticoagulants	Bernard-Soulier syndrome (hereditary giant plate syndrome)
Aspirin and other salicylates	Connective tissue diseases
(OTC cold remedies, analgesics)	Disseminated intravascular coagulation (DIC)
Chlorothiazides	Glanzmann's thrombasthenia
High-molecular-weight dextran	Hepatic cirrhosis
Mithramycin	Hypersplenism
Streptokinase	Hypothyroidism
Sulfonamides	Leukemias
Thiazide diuretics	Malignancies such as Hodgkin's disease and multiple myeloma
	Measles
	Mumps
	Scurvy
	von Willebrand's disease

When the platelet count is low, bleeding time may be calculated from platelet numbers using the following formula. The result should be evaluated in relation to the normal values for the Ivy and template methods.

$$\text{Bleeding time} = 30.5 - \frac{\text{platelet count/mm}^3}{3850}$$

The calculated value also may be compared with the actual results of bleeding time obtained by the Ivy and template methods. An actual bleeding time longer than the calculated result suggests defective platelet function in addition to reduced numbers. It is also possible to detect above-normal hemostatic capacity in cases in which active young platelets compose the entire population of circulating platelets, because young platelets have enhanced hemostatic capabilities.[25] This phenomenon may be seen in disorders involving increased platelet destruction (see Table 2-3, p. 54).

Interfering Factors

➤ Ingestion of aspirin and aspirin-containing medications within 5 days of the test may prolong the bleeding time. Other drugs that may prolong bleeding time are listed in Table 2-4.

Indications for Bleeding Time Test

➤ Family history of bleeding disorders, especially von Willebrand's disease (Tests of platelet adhesiveness and levels of factor VIII also are necessary to confirm the diagnosis of von Willebrand's disease.)
➤ Signs of abnormal bleeding such as epistaxis, easy bruising, bleeding gums, hematuria, and menorrhagia
➤ Thrombocytopenia as indicated by platelet count
➤ Identification of individuals who may be prone to bleeding during surgical, obstetric, dental, or invasive diagnostic procedures

➤ Determination of platelet dysfunction as indicated by a prolonged bleeding time with a platelet count of greater than 100,000 per cubic millimeter
➤ Determination of effects of diseases and drugs known to affect bleeding time (see Table 2–4, p. 57)

Nursing Care Before the Procedure

Explain to the client:
➤ That the test will be performed by a laboratory technician and requires approximately 15 minutes
➤ The procedure, including the momentary discomfort to be expected when the skin is incised

Aspirin and aspirin-containing medications should be withheld for at least 5 days before the test. Other drugs that may prolong bleeding time (see Table 2–4, p. 57) should also be withheld.

The Procedure

The test may be performed using the Duke, Ivy, or template method. All three methods involve piercing the skin and observing the duration of bleeding time from the puncture site. Welling blood must be removed, but gently so as not to disrupt the fragile platelet plug. After the skin is pierced, oozing blood is removed at 15-second intervals by touching filter paper to the drop of blood without touching the wound itself. As platelets accumulate, bleeding slows and the oozing drop of blood gets smaller. The end point occurs when there is no fluid blood left to produce a spot on the filter paper.[26] The test is timed with a stopwatch.

For all methods, the site to be used is cleansed with antiseptic and allowed to dry. In the Duke method, the earlobe is incised 3 mm deep with a sterile lancet. For the Ivy and template methods, the volar surface of the forearm is used. A blood pressure cuff is applied above the elbow and inflated to 40 mm Hg; the pressure is maintained throughout the test. In the Ivy method, two incisions 3 mm deep are made freehand with sterile lancets. In the template method, two incisions, each 1 mm deep and 9 mm long, are made with a standardized template. The advantage of the template method is the ability to achieve a reproducible, precise incision every time.

The elapsed time at the point when bleeding ceases is recorded. If bleeding persists beyond 10 minutes, the test is discontinued and a pressure dressing is applied to the puncture site(s).

Nursing Care After the Procedure

When the test is completed, a sterile dressing or Band-Aid is applied to the site. For persistent bleeding, ice may be applied to the site in addition to the pressure dressing.
➤ Observe the puncture site(s) every 5 minutes for bleeding. Clients with clotting factor disorders may rebleed after initial bleeding has stopped. This may occur approximately 20 to 30 minutes after the initial procedure.
➤ Check the puncture site(s) at least twice daily for infection or failure to heal.
➤ For Ivy and template methods, assess for excessive bruising at the blood pressure cuff application site.

PLATELET AGGREGATION TEST

Platelet aggregation can be measured by bringing platelet-rich plasma into contact with known inducers of platelet aggregation. Most inducers, such as collagen, epinephrine, and thrombin, act through the effects of ADP, which is released by the platelets themselves (see p. 50). Adding exogenous ADP causes platelet aggregation directly. Ristocetin, an antibiotic, may also be used for this test.[27]

Platelet aggregation is quantitated by determining whether platelet-rich plasma becomes clear as evenly suspended platelets aggregate and fall to the bottom of a test tube. Normally, platelet aggregates should be visible in less than 5 minutes.

Platelet aggregation in response to specific inducing agents is diagnostic for specific disorders. Aspirin, other anti-inflammatory agents, and many phenothiazines markedly inhibit the aggregating effect of collagen and epinephrine but do not interfere with the direct action of added ADP. Also, conditions that depress the release-inducing effects of collagen and epinephrine and of directly added ADP affect platelet aggregation.

Individuals with von Willebrand's disease have platelets that respond normally to epinephrine, collagen, and ADP. Without vWF in their plasma, however, the platelets will not be aggregated by ristocetin.[28]

Other disorders that may impair platelet aggregation include Glanzmann's thrombasthenia, Bernard-Soulier syndrome (hereditary giant platelet syndrome), idiopathic thrombocytopenic purpura, and infectious mononucleosis. Drugs that interfere with platelet aggregation are listed in Table 2–5.

Reference Values

Platelet aggregates should be visible in less than 5 minutes.

Interfering Factors

➤ Ingestion of aspirin and other drugs known to interfere with platelet aggregation within 5 to 7 days of the test (see Table 2–5).

➤ Delay in processing the sample or excessive agitation of the sample may alter test results.

Indications for Platelet Aggregation Test

➤ Suspected von Willebrand's disease or other inherited platelet disorder

➤ Evaluation of platelet aggregation in clients with disorders known to cause alterations (e.g., uremia, severe liver disease, myeloproliferative disorders, dysproteinemias)

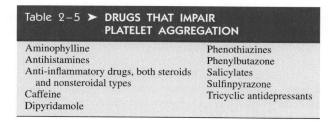

Table 2–5 ➤ DRUGS THAT IMPAIR PLATELET AGGREGATION	
Aminophylline	Phenothiazines
Antihistamines	Phenylbutazone
Anti-inflammatory drugs, both steroids and nonsteroidal types	Salicylates
Caffeine	Sulfinpyrazone
Dipyridamole	Tricyclic antidepressants

➤ Therapy with drugs known to alter platelet aggregation (see Table 2–5, p. 59)

Nursing Care Before the Procedure

Client preparation is essentially the same as that for any study involving the collection of a peripheral blood sample (see Appendix I). It is generally recommended that the person abstain from food for 8 hours before the test and, if possible, from drugs that may impair platelet aggregation for 5 to 7 days before the test.

The Procedure

A venipuncture is performed and the sample collected in a light-blue-topped tube.

Nursing Care After the Procedure

Care and assessment after the procedure are essentially the same as for any study involving the collection of a peripheral blood sample. Because the client may have platelet deficiency, maintain digital pressure directly on the puncture site for 3 to 5 minutes after the needle is withdrawn. Also, inspect the site for excessive bruising after the procedure.

➤ *Complications and precautions:* Note and report drugs that alter platelet aggregation and discontinue if test results indicate prolonged aggregation. Report any abnormal test results to the physician.

CLOT RETRACTION TEST

When blood collected in a test tube first clots, the entire column of blood solidifies. As time passes, the clot diminishes in size. Serum (the fluid remaining after blood coagulates) is expressed, and only the red blood cells remain in the shrunken fibrin clot. Because platelets are necessary for this process, the speed and extent of clot retraction roughly reflect the adequacy of platelet function. Individuals with thrombocytopenia or platelet dysfunction, for example, have samples with scant serum and a soft, plump, poorly demarcated clot.

The results of the clot retraction test should be evaluated in relation to other hematologic, platelet, and coagulation studies. If the client has a low hematocrit, for example, the clot is small and the volume of serum is great. In contrast, individuals with polycythemia or hemoconcentration have poor clot retraction because the numerous red blood cells contained in the clot separate the fibrin strands and interfere with normal retraction.

If fibrinogen levels are low, the initial clot is so fragile that the fibrin strands rupture and red blood cells spill into serum when retraction begins. If there is excessive fibrinolysis, as often happens with reduced fibrinogen levels, the incubated tube may contain only cells and fibrin with no fibrin clot at all. Low fibrinogen levels and excessive fibrinolysis are seen in disseminated intravascular coagulation (DIC).[29]

The clot retraction test also can be modified to demonstrate the inhibitory effect of antiplatelet antibodies, especially those associated with drugs. Clot retraction is abolished if more than 90 percent of platelet activity is neutralized. Serum suspected of containing antibodies can be added to normal blood to see if retraction is inhibited.[30]

Reference Values

A normal clot, gently separated from the side of the test tube and incubated at 37°C (98.6°F), shrinks to about half its original size within 1 hour. The result is a firm, cylindrical fibrin clot that contains all the red blood cells and is sharply demarcated from the clear serum.

Interfering Factors

➤ Rough handling of the sample alters clot formation.

Indications for Clot Retraction Test

➤ Evaluation of adequacy of platelet function
➤ Evaluation of thrombocytopenia of unknown etiology
➤ Suspected antiplatelet antibodies resulting from immune disorders or drug-antibody reactions
➤ Suspected abnormalities of fibrinogen or fibrinolytic activity
➤ Monitoring of response to conditions that predispose to DIC

Nursing Care Before the Procedure

Client preparation is the same as that for any study involving the collection of a peripheral blood sample (see Appendix I).

The Procedure

A venipuncture is performed and approximately 5 mL of blood is collected in a red-topped tube. The sample is sent promptly to the laboratory.

Nursing Care After the Procedure

Care and assessment after the procedure are essentially the same as for any study involving the collection of a peripheral blood sample.
➤ Because the client may have platelet dysfunction or deficiency, maintain digital pressure directly on the puncture site for 3 to 5 minutes after the needle is withdrawn.
➤ Inspect the site for excessive bruising after the procedure.

RUMPLE-LEEDS CAPILLARY FRAGILITY TEST (TOURNIQUET TEST)

The capillary fragility test indicates the ability of capillaries to resist rupturing under pressure. Excessive capillary fragility may be caused by either abnormalities of capillary walls or thrombocytopenia. The causes of positive test results are listed in Table 2–6.

The test is performed by applying a blood pressure cuff inflated to 100 mm Hg to the client's arm for 5 minutes. The resulting petechiae in a circumscribed area are then counted.

This test is unnecessary in the presence of obvious petechiae or large ecchymoses. It also should not be performed on clients known to have or suspected of having DIC.

Reference Values

Fewer than 10 petechiae (excluding those that may have been present before the test) in a 2-inch circle is considered normal. Results may also be reported ac-

Table 2–6 ➤ CAUSES OF POSITIVE RUMPLE-LEEDS CAPILLARY FRAGILITY TEST	
Strongly positive (grade 4)	Aplastic anemia
	Chronic renal disease
	Glanzmann's thrombasthenia
	Idiopathic thrombocytopenic purpura (ITP)
	Leukemia
	Thrombocytopenia caused by acute infectious disease (measles, influenza, scarlet fever)
Moderately positive (grade 3)	Hepatic cirrhosis
Slightly positive (grade 2)	Allergic and senile purpuras
	Decreased estrogen levels
	Deficiency of vitamin K, factor VII, fibrinogen, or prothrombin
	Dysproteinemia
	Polycythemia vera
	von Willebrand's disease

cording to the following scale, with grade 1 indicating a normal or negative result. Causes of positive results are listed in Table 2–6.

Grade	Petechiae per 2-Inch Circle
1	0–10
2	10–20
3	20–50
4	50

Interfering Factors

➤ Repetition of the test on the same extremity within 1 week will yield inaccurate results.

Indications for Rumple-Leeds Capillary Fragility Test (Tourniquet Test)

➤ History of "easy bruising" or production of petechiae by the application of a tourniquet for venipuncture
➤ Verification of increased capillary fragility, although the test itself is not specific for any particular bleeding disorder (see Table 2–6)

Nursing Care Before the Procedure

Explain to the client:
➤ The procedure, including the degree of discomfort to be expected from the inflated blood pressure cuff

Inspect the client's forearms and select a site that is as free as possible of petechiae. Measure an area 2 inches in diameter; the site may be circled lightly with a felt-tipped marker if necessary for reference. If petechiae are present in the site to be measured, note and record the number.

The Procedure

A blood pressure cuff is applied to the arm and inflated to 100 mm Hg. The pressure is maintained for 5 minutes. The blood pressure cuff is then removed and the petechiae counted and the number recorded.

Nursing Care After the Procedure

➤ There is no specific aftercare. If the arm feels "tense" or "full," it may be elevated for a few minutes to hasten venous drainage.

➤ *Complications and precautions:* Note and report tendency for easy bruising or presence of petechiae. Take measures to prevent trauma to the skin and mucous membranes if results are above the normal values.

COAGULATION STUDIES

Coagulation studies are performed to evaluate the components and pathways of the coagulation sequence (see pp. 50–51). Innumerable tests have been devised to diagnose inherited, acquired, and iatrogenic deficiencies of coagulation. Some of these require specialized techniques or rare reagents available only in laboratories that perform many such tests. Other tests are less precisely diagnostic but more available and more readily applicable to immediate clinical situations. The tests included here are widely available.

Screening tests of hemostatic function include the platelet count, bleeding time, prothrombin time (PT), and partial thromboplastin time (PTT). When a "coagulation profile" or "coagulogram" is ordered, it includes the four screening tests plus clotting time and activated partial thromboplastin time (aPTT).

PROTHROMBIN TIME (PT, PRO TIME)

The prothrombin time (PT, pro time) test is used to evaluate the extrinsic pathway of the coagulation sequence. It represents the time required for a firm fibrin clot to form after tissue thromboplastin (coagulation factor III) and calcium are added to the sample. These added substances directly activate factor X, the key factor in all three coagulation pathways (see Fig. 2–1, p. 51). Neither platelets nor the factors involved in the intrinsic pathway are necessary for the clot to form.

To give a normal PT result, plasma must have at least 100 mg/dL of fibrinogen (normal: 150 to 400 mg/dL) and adequate levels of factors X, VII, V, and II (prothrombin). Because the test bypasses the clotting factors of the intrinsic pathway, the PT cannot detect the two most common congenital coagulation disorders: (1) deficiency of factor VIII (hemophilia A, or "classic" hemophilia) and (2) deficiency of factor IX (hemophilia B, or Christmas disease). Also, thrombocytopenia does not prolong the PT.

PT measurements are reported as time in seconds or as a percentage of normal activity, or both. Time in seconds indicates the length of time for the blood to clot when chemicals are added in comparison to normal blood with the same chemicals added (control value). A value that is higher than the control sample is considered to be deficient in prothrombin. Some laboratories report the results in percentages that are derived from a plotted graph based on dilutions of the control samples and the time in seconds it takes for the sample to clot; the seconds are then converted to percentages. The time then reflects the percentage of normal clotting time by comparing the client's clotting time to its intersection point with the percentage on the graph. Usually an increase in time for clotting equals a decrease in the percentage of activity, although different laboratories can obtain different results when determining the percentages. This difference is because of the different thromboplastins used as reagents in the testing procedure.

Because the variability in responsiveness to the different thromboplastins has resulted in dosing differences, a thromboplastin has been developed by the first International Reference Preparation (IRP). This reagent is used to monitor the therapeutic levels for coagulation during coumarin-type therapy. A standardization of reporting the PT assay test results developed by the World Health Organization (WHO) has been adopted for this reagent. It is known as the International Normalized Ratio (INR). The INR is calculated with the use of a nomogram developed to demonstrate the relationship between the INR and the prothrombin ratios with the International Sensitivity Index (ISI) range (values associated with the available thromboplastin reagents from the various companies that develop them). PT evaluation can now be based on the INR and both are reported as PT and its equivalent INR for evaluation and decisions in oral anticoagulation therapy as endorsed by the Committee on Antithrombotic Therapy of the American College of Chest Physicians (ACCP), the Committee for Thrombosis and Hemostasis, and the International Committee for Standardization in Hematology. The recommended INR therapeutic range for oral anticoagulant therapy is 2.0 to 3.0 in the treatment of venous thrombosis, pulmonary embolism, and the prevention or treatment of systemic embolism. A pro time test system is now available to perform immediate measurement of PT at the bedside using a fresh whole blood sample, reagent cartridges, and a monitor that operates on rechargeable batteries.

Prothrombin is a vitamin K–dependent protein produced by the liver. Thus, any disorder that impairs the liver's ability to use vitamin K or to form proteins (e.g., the various types of cirrhosis) prolongs the PT. Anticoagulants of the coumarin family act by inhibiting hepatic synthesis of the vitamin K–dependent factors II, VII, IX, and X. A natural anticoagulant system dependent on the action of vitamin K on the proteins C and S is different from the activity of this vitamin on coagulation factors II, VII, IX, and X. Protein C acts to neutralize the activity of factors VIIIa and Va, and protein S increases the inactivation of VIIIa and Va by the protein C. Any deficiency of the various factors can alter the balance between the two proteins and result in thrombotic disorders. The tests are performed to determine their functional activity and reveal a tendency toward hypercoagulation and thrombosis or to diagnose a hereditary deficiency.

Reference Values

	Conventional Units	**SI Units**
Newborns	12–21 sec	12–21 s
Adults		
Men	9.6–11.8 sec	9.6–11.8 s
Women	9.5–11.3 sec	9.5–11.3 s
INR	2.0–3.0 sec for anticoagulation, higher (3.0–4.5 sec) for recurrent systemic embolization	2.0–3.0 s 3.0–4.5 s for recurrent systemic embolism
Critical Values	**8–9 sec below control or >40 sec**	**8–9 s below control or >40 s**

Because values may vary according to the source of the substances added to the sample and the type of laboratory equipment used, the result is usually evaluated in relation to a control sample obtained from an individual with normal hemostatic function.

Test results are sometimes given as a percentage of normal activity, comparing the client's results against a curve that shows the normal clotting rate of diluted plasma. The normal value in this case is 100 percent; however, the method itself is thought to be inaccurate because dilution affects the clotting process.

Interfering Factors

Numerous drugs may alter the PT results, including:
➤ Drugs that prolong the PT, such as coumarin derivatives, quinidine, quinine, thyroid hormones, adrenocorticotropic hormone (ACTH), steroids, alcohol, phenytoin, indomethacin, and salicylates
➤ Drugs that may shorten the PT, such as barbiturates (especially chloral hydrate), oral contraceptives, and vitamin K[31]
  • Traumatic venipuncture may lead to erroneous results because of activation of the coagulation sequence.
  • Excessive agitation of the sample may erroneously prolong the PT.
  • A fibrinogen level of less than 100 mg/dL (SI units, 1.00 g/L) (normal: 150 to 400 mg/dL [SI units, 1.50–4.00 g/L]) may prolong the PT.

Indications for Prothrombin Time (PT)

➤ Signs of abnormal bleeding such as epistaxis, easy bruising, bleeding gums, hematuria, and menorrhagia
➤ Identification of individuals who may be prone to bleeding during surgical, obstetric, dental, or invasive diagnostic procedures
➤ Evaluation of response to anticoagulant therapy with coumarin derivatives and determination of dosage required to achieve therapeutic results
➤ Differentiation of clotting factor deficiencies of V, VII, and X, which prolong the PT, from congenital coagulation disorders such as hemophilia A (factor VIII) and hemophilia B (factor IX), which do not alter the PT
➤ Monitoring of effects on hemostasis of conditions such as liver disease, protein deficiency, and fat malabsorption

Nursing Care Before the Procedure

In general, client preparation is the same as that for any study involving the collection of a peripheral blood sample (see Appendix I).
➤ Because many drugs may affect the PT result, all medications taken by the client should be noted.
➤ If the individual is receiving anticoagulant therapy, the time and the amount of the last dose should be noted.

The Procedure

A venipuncture is performed and the sample collected in a light-blue-topped tube. Traumatic venipunctures and excessive agitation of the sample should be avoided.

Nursing Care After the Procedure

Care and assessment after the procedure are essentially the same as for any study involving the collection of a peripheral blood sample.

➤ Because the client may have a coagulation deficiency, maintain digital pressure directly on the puncture site for 3 to 5 minutes after the needle is withdrawn.

➤ Inspect the site for excessive bruising after the procedure.

• *Bleeding episode:* Note and report increase in PT, medications taken that affect the PT and expected test values, symptoms such as bleeding from any area (blood in sputum, feces, urine; bleeding from nose, skin), headache, increased pulse, or pain in the abdomen or back. Report changes related to administration of coumarin-type medication and adjust drug dosage as ordered until desired INR is reached. Protect skin, mucous membranes, and organs from trauma (shaving, brushing teeth, suctioning, intramuscular [IM], subcutaneous [SC], and intravenous [IV] injections, falls, activities that are strenuous, straining). Test for occult blood in body secretions and excretions. Inform client to avoid drugs that potentiate the effect of coumarin-type drugs. Instruct client in importance and frequency of PT laboratory testing.

• *Venous thrombosis:* Note and report decreases in PT or other factors predisposing to formation of venous thrombi. Provide leg exercises and adequate fluid intake. Advise client to avoid crossing legs, wearing constrictive clothing, or participating in other activities that impair circulation. Inform client of importance and frequency of PT testing.

• **Critical values:** Notify the physician immediately of an increase of greater than 40 seconds or 15 seconds above the control time. Prepare the client for administration of IM vitamin K or IV frozen plasma. Notify the physician immediately of an increase of greater than 24 seconds in individuals with a liver disease if they are experiencing hypoprothrombinemia from vitamin K deficiency. Notify the physician immediately if there is a decrease of less than than 8 to 9 seconds or 11 to 12 seconds below the control time. Prepare the client for possible SC administrations of heparin.

PARTIAL THROMBOPLASTIN TIME (PTT)/ACTIVATED PARTIAL THROMBOPLASTIN TIME (aPTT)

The partial thromboplastin time (PTT) test is used to evaluate the intrinsic and common pathways of the coagulation sequence. It represents the time required for a firm fibrin clot to form after phospholipid reagents similar to thromboplastin reagent are added to the specimen. Because coagulation factor VII is not required for the PTT, the test bypasses the extrinsic pathway (see Fig. 2–1, p. 51).

To give a normal PTT result, factors XII, XI, IX, VIII, X, V, II (prothrombin), and I (fibrinogen) must be present in the plasma. The PTT is more sensitive than the PT in detecting minor deficiencies of clotting factors because factor levels below 30 percent of normal prolong the PTT.

The activated partial thromboplastin time (aPTT) is essentially the same as the PTT but is faster and more reliably reproducible. In this test, the thromboplastin reagent may be kaolin, celite, or ellagic acid, all of which more rapidly activate factor XII.

It is possible to infer which factors are deficient by comparing the results of the PTT with those of the PT. A prolonged PTT with a normal PT points to a deficiency of factors XII, XI, IX, and VIII and to von Willebrand's disease. In contrast, a normal PTT with a prolonged PT occurs only in factor VII deficiency.[32]

In addition to heparin therapy and coagulation factor deficiencies, the following also prolong the PTT: circulating products of fibrin and fibrinogen degradation, polycythemia, severe liver disease, vitamin K deficiency, DIC, and established therapy with coumarin anticoagulants.

Reference Values

Newborns	Time in sec is higher up to 3 mo of age than for adults
Adults	
PTT	30–45 sec
aPTT	35–45 sec*
Critical Values	**>20 sec more than control if not receiving heparin therapy**
	<53 sec or >2.5 times control if receiving heparin therapy

*Values can vary among laboratories.

Interfering Factors

➤ Heparin and established therapy with coumarin derivatives alter the PTT.
➤ Traumatic venipunctures may lead to erroneous results because of activation of the coagulation sequence.
➤ Excessive agitation of the sample may prolong the PTT.

Indications for PTT/aPTT Test

➤ Signs of abnormal bleeding such as epistaxis, easy bruising, bleeding gums, hematuria, and menorrhagia
➤ Identification of individuals who may be prone to bleeding during surgical, obstetric, dental, or invasive diagnostic procedures
➤ Evaluation of responses to anticoagulant therapy with heparin or established therapy, or both, with coumarin derivatives and determination of dosage required to achieve therapeutic results
➤ Detection of congenital deficiencies in clotting factors such as hemophilia A (factor VIII) and hemophilia B (factor IX), which alter the PTT
➤ Monitoring of effects on hemostasis of conditions such as liver disease, protein deficiency, and fat malabsorption

Nursing Care Before the Procedure

In general, client preparation is the same as that for any study involving the collection of a peripheral blood sample (see Appendix I).
➤ If the individual is receiving anticoagulant therapy, the time and the amount of the last dose should be noted.

The Procedure

A venipuncture is performed and the sample collected in a light-blue-topped tube. Traumatic venipunctures and excessive agitation of the sample should be avoided.

Nursing Care After the Procedure

Care and assessment after the procedure are essentially the same as for any study involving the collection of a peripheral blood sample.

➤ Because the client may have a coagulation deficiency, maintain digital pressure directly on the puncture site for 3 to 5 minutes after the needle is withdrawn.

➤ Inspect the site for excessive bruising after the procedure.

- *Bleeding episode:* Report increase in PTT or aPTT during heparin therapy; note that a therapeutic range is maintained (usually 1.5 to 2.5 times the control). Note also (1) drugs taken that can interfere with the action of heparin therapy, (2) the administration of prophylactic low-dose heparin that does not require PTT testing, and (3) symptoms such as bleeding from any area (blood in sputum, urine, feces; bleeding from nose, skin, mucous membranes). Adjust dosage according to physician order. Protect from trauma to skin, mucous membranes, organs, joints (falls; rough handling of extremities; shaving; brushing teeth; IM, SC, and IV injections; suctioning). Test for occult blood in body secretions and excretions. Inform client to avoid drugs that affect the PTT. Provide special considerations to allay anxiety related to possible bleeding tendencies.

- **Critical values:** Notify the physician at once of an increase of greater than 20 seconds above the control if the individual is not receiving heparin therapy. If heparin therapy is administered, a PTT level of less than 53 seconds indicates an inadequate anticoagulation effect; the physician should be told immediately if a level is greater than 2.5 times the control time level.

WHOLE BLOOD CLOTTING TIME (COAGULATION TIME, CT, LEE-WHITE COAGULATION TIME)

Whole blood clotting time, also known as coagulation time (CT) or Lee-White coagulation time, is the oldest but least accurate of the coagulation tests. It measures the time it takes blood to clot in a test tube. Because the sensitivity of the test is low, coagulation problems of mild to moderate severity are not apparent. Heparin prolongs clotting time; therefore, the test was once used to monitor heparin therapy. Partial thromboplastin time or activated partial thromboplastin time (PTT or aPTT) is currently used to evaluate such therapy.

Reference Values

4 to 8 minutes

Because this test is relatively insensitive and difficult to standardize, a normal result does not rule out a coagulation defect.

Interfering Factors

➤ Heparin prolongs the whole blood clotting time.
➤ Traumatic venipuncture may lead to erroneous results.

Indications for Whole Blood Clotting Time Test

➤ Evaluation of response to heparin therapy
- Adequate anticoagulation is indicated by a clotting time of about 20 minutes.

➤ Signs of abnormal bleeding such as epistaxis, easy bruising, bleeding gums, hematuria, and menorrhagia

➤ Suspected congenital coagulation defect that involves the intrinsic coagulation pathway (e.g., deficiencies of factors VIII, IX, XI, and XII)

Nursing Care Before the Procedure

In general, client preparation is the same as that for any study involving the collection of a peripheral blood sample (see Appendix I).

➤ If the individual is receiving heparin anticoagulant therapy, the time and the amount of the last dose should be noted.

The Procedure

A venipuncture is performed and 3 mL of blood collected in a syringe and then discarded. A new syringe, glass or plastic, is attached to the venipuncture needle, and an additional 3 mL of blood is withdrawn. Traumatic venipunctures and excessive movement of the needle in the vein must be avoided if accurate results are to be obtained.

As the second sample is withdrawn, timing is begun with a stopwatch. The sample is immediately and gently transferred into three glass tubes (1 mL in each). The test tubes are placed in a water bath at 98.6°F (37°C) and are tilted gently every 30 seconds until a firm clot has formed in each tube.

Timing is completed when all tubes contain firm clots, and the interval is recorded as the clotting time.

Nursing Care After the Procedure

Care and assessment after the procedure are essentially the same as for any study involving the collection of a peripheral blood sample. Because the client may have a coagulation deficiency, maintain digital pressure directly on the puncture site for 3 to 5 minutes after the needle is withdrawn. Also, inspect the site for excessive bleeding after the procedure.

➤ *Bleeding tendency:* If anticoagulant therapy is administered, note and report bleeding from any area (skin, nose, mucous membranes; blood in urine, feces; excessive menses). Note results of coagulation factor screen for deficiencies. Protect the skin, mucous membranes, and other organs from trauma. Test for occult blood in body secretions and excretions.

THROMBIN CLOTTING TIME (TCT, PLASMA THROMBIN TIME)

The thrombin clotting time (TCT, plasma thrombin time) is used to evaluate the common final pathway of the coagulation sequence. Preformed thrombin (coagulation factor IIa), usually of bovine origin, can be added to the blood sample to convert fibrinogen (factor I) directly to a fibrin clot. Because the test bypasses the intrinsic and extrinsic pathways, deficiencies in either one do not affect the TCT (see Fig. 2–1, p. 51).

Thrombin-induced clotting is very rapid, and the test result can be standardized to any desired normal value (usually 10 to 15 seconds). The TCT is prolonged if fibrinogen levels are below 100 mg/dL (normal: 150 to 400 mg/dL), if the fibrinogen present is functioning abnormally, or if fibrinogen inhibitors (e.g., streptokinase, urokinase) are present (see below). In all of these conditions, the PT and PTT also are prolonged.[33]

Reference Values

10 to 15 seconds (Values vary among laboratories.)

Interfering Factors

➤ A fibrinogen level of less than 100 mg/dL (SI units, 1.00 g/L) (normal: 150 to 400 mg/dL[SI units, 1.50–4.00 g/L) prolongs the TCT.
➤ Abnormally functioning fibrinogen prolongs the TCT.
➤ Fibrinogen inhibitors such as streptokinase and urokinase prolong the TCT.
➤ Traumatic venipunctures and excessive agitation of the sample may alter results.

Indications for Thrombin Clotting Time Test

➤ Confirmation of suspected DIC as indicated by a prolonged TCT
➤ Detection of hypofibrinogenemia or defective fibrinogen
➤ Monitoring of effects of heparin or fibrinolytic therapy (e.g., with streptokinase)

Nursing Care Before the Procedure

In general, client preparation is the same as that for any study involving the collection of a peripheral blood sample (see Appendix I).
➤ If the individual is receiving anticoagulant therapy, the time and the amount of the last dose should be noted.

The Procedure

A venipuncture is performed and the sample collected in a light-blue-topped tube. Traumatic venipunctures and excessive agitation of the sample should be avoided.

Nursing Care After the Procedure

Care and assessment after the procedure are essentially the same as for any study involving the collection of a peripheral blood sample.
➤ Because the client may have a coagulation deficiency, maintain digital pressure directly on the puncture site for 3 to 5 minutes after the needle is withdrawn.
➤ Inspect the site for excessive bruising after the procedure.

PROTHROMBIN CONSUMPTION TIME (PCT, SERUM PROTHROMBIN TIME)

The prothrombin consumption time (PCT, serum prothrombin time) test measures utilization of prothrombin when a blood clot forms. Normally, the formation of a clot "consumes" prothrombin by converting it to thrombin. Individuals with deficiencies in platelets, platelet factor 3, or factors involved in the intrinsic coagulation pathway (see pp. 50–51 and Fig. 2–1, p. 51) are not able to convert as much prothrombin to thrombin. In such cases, excess prothrombin remains in the serum after the clot is formed, thus shortening the PCT. The PCT also may be shortened in persons receiving anticoagulant therapy or in those with DIC, hypoprothrombinemia, and cirrhosis.

Abnormal PCT results must be evaluated in relation to coagulation studies such as PT, PTT, and factor assays, to differentiate platelet factor deficiencies from clotting factor deficiencies.

Reference Values

15 to 20 seconds with more than 80 percent of the prothrombin consumed

Interfering Factors

➤ Traumatic venipunctures and excessive agitation of the sample may alter test results.
➤ Therapy with anticoagulants may shorten the PCT.

Indications for Prothrombin Consumption Time Test

➤ Suspected deficiency of platelet factor 3 or of the clotting factors involved in the intrinsic coagulation pathway (i.e., factors VIII, IX, XI, and XII), as indicated by a shortened PCT
➤ Suspected DIC, as indicated by a shortened PCT
➤ Monitoring of effects on hemostasis of conditions such as liver disease and protein deficiency

Nursing Care Before the Procedure

In general, client preparation is the same as that for any study involving the collection of a peripheral blood sample (see Appendix I).
➤ If the client is receiving anticoagulant therapy, the time and the amount of the last dose should be noted.

The Procedure

A venipuncture is performed and the sample collected in a red-topped tube. As with other coagulation studies, traumatic venipunctures and excessive agitation of the sample should be avoided.

Nursing Care After the Procedure

Care and assessment after the procedure are essentially the same as for any study involving the collection of a peripheral blood sample.
➤ Because the client may have a coagulation deficiency, maintain digital pressure directly on the puncture site for 3 to 5 minutes after the needle is withdrawn.
➤ Inspect the site for excessive bruising after the procedure.

FACTOR ASSAYS

If the PT or PTT/aPTT is abnormal but the nature of the factor deficiency unknown, specific coagulation factors may be measured. Factor assays require specialized techniques not available in many laboratories. Factor assays are used to discriminate among mild, moderate, and severe deficiencies and to follow the course of acquired factor inhibitors. States associated with particular factor deficiencies are presented in Table 2–7.

Factors of the extrinsic (II, V, VII, X) and intrinsic (VIII, IX, XI, XII) co-agulation pathways are usually measured separately. The factor XIII assay is a separate test in which a blood clot is observed for 24 hours. Clot dissolution within this time indicates severe factor XIII deficiency. The test for fibrinogen (factor I) is discussed later.

Reference Values

	Conventional Units	SI Units
Extrinsic Pathway		
Factor II	70–130 mg/100 mL	0.7–1.3 U
Factor V	70–130 mg/100 mL	0.7–1.3 U
Factor VII	70–150 mg/100 mL	0.7–1.5 U
Factor X	70–130 mg/100 mL	0.7–1.3 U
Intrinsic Pathway		
Factor VIII	50–200 mg/100 mL	0.5–2.0 U
Factor IX	70–130 mg/100 mL	0.7–1.3 U
Factor XI	70–130 mg/100 mL	0.7–1.3 U
Factor XII	30–225 mg/100 mL	0.3–2.2 U
Common Pathway		
Factor XIII	Dissolution of a formed clot within 24 hr	

Normal values vary among laboratories.

Interfering Factors

➤ Therapy with anticoagulants and other drugs known to alter hemostasis.
➤ Traumatic venipunctures and excessive agitation of the sample may alter test results.

Indications for Factor Assays

➤ Prolonged PT or PTT of unknown etiology
  • If the PT is prolonged but the PTT is normal, factors of the extrinsic pathway are evaluated (i.e., factors, II, V, VII, and X).
  • If the PTT is prolonged but the PT is normal, factors of the intrinsic pathway are evaluated (i.e., factors VIII, IX, XI, XII).
➤ Monitoring of effects of disorders and drugs known to lead to deficiencies in clotting factors (see Table 2–7, p. 73)

Nursing Care Before the Procedure

Client preparation is the same as that for any study involving the collection of a peripheral blood sample (see Appendix I).
➤ If the individual is receiving anticoagulant therapy, the time and the amount of the last dose should be noted.

The Procedure

For assays of the factors involved in the intrinsic and extrinsic coagulation pathways, a venipuncture is performed and the sample collected in a light-blue-

Table 2–7 ➤ STATES ASSOCIATED WITH COAGULATION FACTOR DEFICIENCIES

| Factor | Synonym(s) | STATES ASSOCIATED WITH DEFICIENCY | |
		Congenital	Acquired
Extrinsic Pathway			
II	Prothrombin	Hypoprothrombinemia	Vitamin K deficiency Liver disease
V	Accelerator globulin (AcG), proaccelerin, labile factor	Parahemophilia	Liver disease Acute leukemia Surgery
VII	Proconvertin, autoprothrombin I, serum prothrombin conversion accelerator (SPCA)	Factor VII deficiency	Liver disease Vitamin K deficiency Antibiotic therapy
X	Stuart factor, Stuart-Prower factor, autoprothrombin III	Stuart factor deficiency	Liver disease Vitamin K deficiency Anticoagulants Normal pregnancy Disseminated intravascular coagulation (DIC) Hemorrhagic disease of the newborn
Intrinsic Pathway			
VIII*	Antihemophilic factor (AHF), antihemophilic globulin (AHG)	Hemophilia A (classic hemophilia) von Willebrand's disease	Disseminated intravascular coagulation (DIC) Fibrinolysis
IX	Christmas factor, antihemophilic factor B, plasma thromboplastin component (PTC), autoprothrombin II	Hemophilia B (Christmas disease)	Liver disease Vitamin K deficiency Anticoagulants Nephrotic syndrome
XI	Plasma thromboplastin antecedent (PTA)	Factor XI deficiency	Liver disease Vitamin K deficiency Anticoagulants Congenital heart disease
XII	Hageman factor	Hageman trait	Normal pregnancy Nephrotic syndrome
Common Pathway			
XIII	Fibrin-stabilizing factor	Factor XIII deficiency	Liver disease Lead poisoning Multiple myeloma Agammaglobulinemia Elevated fibronogen levels Postoperatively

*Factor VIII is increased in normal pregnancy (as is factor X) and in states of inflammation and other physiologic stress.

topped tube. For factor XIII assays, the sample is collected in a red-topped tube. As with other coagulation studies, traumatic venipunctures and excessive agitation of the sample should be avoided. The samples should be sent to the laboratory immediately.

Nursing Care After the Procedure

Care and assessment after the procedure are essentially the same as for any study involving the collection of a peripheral blood sample.

➤ Because the client may have a coagulation deficiency, maintain digital pressure directly on the puncture site for 3 to 5 minutes after the needle is withdrawn.

➤ Inspect the site for excessive bruising after the procedure.

PLASMA FIBRINOGEN

In the common final pathway, fibrinogen (factor I) is converted to fibrin by thrombin (see Fig. 2–1, p. 51). Plasma fibrinogen studies are based on the fact that, in normal healthy individuals, the serum should contain no residual fibrinogen after clotting has occurred.

Three different techniques may be used to perform the test: (1) standard assay (classical procedure), (2) immunologic technique, and (3) heat-precipitation tests. In the standard assay, thrombin is added to the blood sample to induce clotting. Because fibrinogen is a plasma protein, the amount of protein in the resulting clot is measured. The quantity of precursor fibrinogen present is then extrapolated from this value. In the immunologic technique, the degree of reactivity between the plasma sample and antifibrinogen antibodies is measured. The assumption underlying this method is that any plasma constituent that reacts with antifibrinogen antibodies is, indeed, fibrinogen. Heat-precipitation tests are based on a similar assumption that all of the material responsive to the precipitation technique is really fibrinogen.[34]

Reference Values

150–450 mg/dL

Interfering Factors

➤ Transfusions of whole blood, plasma, or fractions within 4 weeks of the test may lead to erroneous results.

➤ Traumatic venipuncture and excessive agitation of the sample may alter test results.

Indications for Plasma Fibrinogen Test

➤ Confirmation of suspected DIC, as indicated by decreased fibrinogen levels

➤ Evaluation of congenital or acquired dysfibrinogenemias

➤ Monitoring of hemostasis in disorders associated with low fibrinogen levels (e.g., severe liver diseases and cancer of the prostate, lung, or pancreas)

➤ Detection of elevated fibrinogen levels, which may predispose to excessive thrombosis in various situations (e.g., immune disorders of connective tissue; glomerulonephritis; oral contraceptive use; cancer of the breast, stomach, or kidney)

Nursing Care Before the Procedure

Client preparation is the same as that for any study involving the collection of a peripheral blood sample (see Appendix I).
➤ If the individual is receiving anticoagulant therapy, the time and amount of the last dose should be noted.

The Procedure

A venipuncture is performed and the sample collected in a light-blue-topped tube. As with other coagulation studies, traumatic venipunctures and excessive agitation of the sample should be avoided. The sample should be sent to the laboratory immediately.

Nursing Care After the Procedure

Care and assessment after the procedure are essentially the same as for any study involving the collection of a peripheral blood sample.
➤ Because the client may have a coagulation deficiency, maintain digital pressure directly on the puncture site for 3 to 5 minutes after the needle is withdrawn.
➤ Inspect the site for excessive bruising after the procedure.

FIBRIN SPLIT PRODUCTS (FSP)

After a fibrin clot has formed, the fibrinolytic system acts to prevent excessive clotting (see p. 51). In this system, plasmin digests fibrin. Fibrinogen also may be degraded if there is a disproportion among plasmin, fibrin, and fibrinogen. The substances that result from this degradation—fibrin split products (FSP) or fibrinogen degradation products (FDP)—interfere with normal coagulation and with formation of the hemostatic platelet plug.

Normally, FSP are removed from the circulation by the liver and the reticuloendothelial system. In situations such as widespread bleeding or DIC, however, FSP are found in the serum.

Tests for FSP are performed on serum using immunologic techniques. Because FSP do not coagulate, they remain in the serum after fibrinogen is removed through clot formation. Antifibrinogen antibodies are added to the serum to detect the presence of FSP. Because normal serum contains neither FSP nor fibrinogen, there should be nothing present to react with the antibodies. If a reaction occurs, FSP are present.[35]

Reference Values

2 to 10 μg/mL

Interfering Factors

> ➤ Heparin, fibrinolytic drugs such as streptokinase and urokinase, and large doses of barbiturates may produce elevated levels of FSP.
> ➤ Traumatic venipunctures and excessive agitation of the sample may alter test results.

Indications for Fibrin Split Products (FSP) Test

> ➤ Confirmation of suspected DIC, as indicated by elevated FSP levels
> ➤ Evaluation of response to therapy with fibrinolytic drugs
> ➤ Monitoring of effects on hemostasis of trauma, extensive surgery, obstetric complications, and disorders such as liver disease

Nursing Care Before the Procedure

Client preparation is the same as that for any study involving the collection of a peripheral blood sample (see Appendix I).

> ➤ If the individual is receiving anticoagulant therapy, the time and the amount of the last dose should be noted.

The Procedure

A venipuncture is performed and the sample collected in a red-topped tube or in a special tube provided for the FSP test by the laboratory. As with other coagulation studies, traumatic venipunctures and excessive agitation of the sample should be avoided. The sample should be sent to the laboratory promptly.

Nursing Care After the Procedure

Care and assessment after the procedure are essentially the same as for any study involving the collection of a peripheral blood sample.

> ➤ Because the client may have a coagulation deficiency, maintain digital pressure directly on the puncture site for 3 to 5 minutes after the needle is withdrawn.
> ➤ Inspect the site for excessive bruising after the procedure.

EUGLOBULIN LYSIS TIME

The euglobulin lysis time test is used to document excessive fibrinolytic activity (see p. 52). Euglobulins are proteins that precipitate from acidified dilute plasma; these include fibrinogen, plasminogen, and plasminogen activator but very little antiplasmin activity. In euglobulins prepared from normal blood, the initial clot dissolves in 2 to 6 hours. With excessive fibrinolytic activity, a clot forms if thrombin is added to the sample.

Shortened euglobulin lysis times are seen in fibrinolytic therapy with streptokinase or urokinase, prostatic cancer, severe liver disease, extensive vascular trauma or surgery, and shock.

Reference Values

Lysis in 2 to 6 hours

Interfering Factors

➤ Decreased fibrinogen levels may lead to falsely shortened lysis time because of the reduced amount of fibrin to be lysed.[36]
➤ Traumatic venipunctures and excessive agitation of the sample may alter results.

Indications for Euglobulin Lysis Time Test

➤ Suspected abnormal fibrinolytic activity as indicated by lysis of the clot within about 1 hour[37]
➤ Differentiation of primary fibrinolysis from DIC, which usually presents with a normal euglobulin lysis time
➤ Monitoring of effects of fibrinolytic therapy on normal coagulation

Nursing Care Before the Procedure

Client preparation is the same as that for any study involving the collection of a peripheral blood sample (see Appendix I).

➤ If the individual is receiving anticoagulant therapy, the time and the amount of the last dose should be noted.

The Procedure

A venipuncture is performed and the sample collected in a light-blue-topped tube. As with other coagulation studies, traumatic venipuncture and excessive agitation of the sample should be avoided. The sample should be sent to the laboratory promptly.

Nursing Care After the Procedure

Care and assessment after the procedure are essentially the same as for any study involving the collection of a peripheral blood sample.

➤ Because the client may have a coagulation deficiency, maintain digital pressure directly on the puncture site for 3 to 5 minutes after the needle is withdrawn.
➤ Inspect the site for excessive bruising after the procedure.
➤ *Clot lysis:* Note and report decreases in lysis level during fibrinolytic therapy. Monitor client response and effect of therapy on coagulation.

Case Study and Critical Thinking Exercise appears on page 78.

Student Name _____ Class _____

Instructor _____ Date _____

CASE STUDY AND CRITICAL THINKING EXERCISE

Mr. Brown, age 54, comes to the health clinic complaining of "tiny red spots" covering his trunk and limbs. He also states that he has noticed that his gums bleed when he brushes his teeth. VS: T 98.6°F (37°C), P 82, R 16, and BP 148/86. His lab values reveal the following: platelets 30,000 per mm^3 and bleeding time 6 min by the Duke method.

a. What is the probable diagnosis?

b. What nursing measures are indicated relative to this diagnosis?

References

1. Sacher, RA, and McPherson, RA: Widmann's Clinical Interpretation of Laboratory Tests, ed 10. FA Davis, Philadelphia, 1991, pp 182–183.
2. Ibid, p 185.
3. Ibid, p 185.
4. Ibid, p 190.
5. Porth, CM: Pathophysiology: Concepts of Altered Health States, ed 4. JB Lippincott, Philadelphia, 1993, p 168.
6. Fischbach, FT: A Manual of Laboratory and Diagnostic Tests, ed 4. JB Lippincott, Philadelphia, 1992, p 95.
7. Ibid, p 118.
8. Porth, op cit, p 169.
9. Ibid, p 121.
10. Sacher and McPherson, op cit, pp 192–193.
11. Ibid, p 195.
12. Ibid, p 195.
13. Ibid, p 196.
14. Fischbach, op cit, p 98.
15. Sacher and McPherson, op cit, p 197.
16. Thompson, AR, and Harker, LA: Manual of Hemostasis and Thrombosis. FA Davis, Philadelphia, 1983, p 9.
17. Sacher and McPherson, op cit, p 182.
18. Ibid, p 182.
19. Thompson and Harker, op cit, p 18.
20. Springhouse Corporation: Professional Guide to Diseases, ed 2. Springhouse, Springhouse, Pa, 1987, pp 1026–1027.
21. Sacher and McPherson, op cit, p 187.
22. Fischbach, op cit, pp 125–126.
23. Thompson and Harker, op cit, p 61.
24. Sacher and McPherson, op cit, p 190.
25. Ibid, p 190.
26. Ibid, p 190.
27. Ibid, pp 188–189.
28. Ibid, p 189.
29. Ibid, p 187.
30. Ibid, pp 187–188.
31. Ibid, p 193.
32. Ibid, p 201.
33. Ibid, p 200.
34. Ibid, p 200.
35. Ibid, pp 139–140.
36. Ibid, p 203.
37. Thompson and Harker, op cit, pp 140–141.

Bibliography

Byrne, CJ, et al: Laboratory Tests: Implications for Nursing Care. Addison-Wesley, Menlo Park, Calif, 1986.

Chernecky, CC, and Berger, BJ; Cullen, BN (ed): Laboratory Tests and Diagnostic Procedures, ed 2. WB Saunders, Philadelphia, 1996.

Collier, BS: Progress in Hemostasis and Thrombosis, vol 10. WB Saunders, Philadelphia, 1991.

Corbett, JV: Laboratory Tests and Diagnostic Procedures with Nursing Diagnoses, ed 4. Appleton & Lange, Norwalk, Conn, 1995.

Hann, IM (ed): Fetal and Neonatal Haematology. WB Saunders, Philadelphia, 1991.

Henry, JB: Clinical Diagnosis and Management by Laboratory Methods, ed 19. WB Saunders, Philadelphia, 1996.

Kee, JL: Handbook of Laboratory and Diagnostic Tests with Nursing Implications, ed 3. Appleton & Lange, Norwalk, Conn, 1997.

Laposata, M, et al: The Clinical Hemostasis Handbook. Mosby–Year Book, St Louis, 1989.

Lewis, SM, et al (eds): Medical-Surgical Nursing: Assessment and Management of Clinical Problems, ed 4. Mosby–Year Book, St Louis, 1995.

Pagana, KD, and Pagana, TJ: Diagnostic and Laboratory Test Reference, ed 3. Mosby–Year Book, St Louis, 1996.

Ratnoff, OD, and Forbes, CD: Disorders of Hemostasis, ed 3. WB Saunders, Philadelphia, 1996.

Springhouse Corporation: Nurse's Reference Library, Diagnostic Tests, ed 3. Springhouse, Springhouse, Pa, 1991.

Tietz, NW (ed): Clinical Guide to Laboratory Tests, ed 3. WB Saunders, Philadelphia, 1997.

Whaley, LF: Nursing Care of Infants and Children, ed 4. Mosby–Year Book, St Louis, 1991.

Wu, KK, and Rossi, EC: Pathophysiology and Management of Thromboembolic Disorders. Mosby–Year Book, St Louis, 1984.

3

Immunology and Immunologic Testing

➤ **TESTS COVERED**

T- and B-Lymphocyte Assays, *84*
Immunoblast Transformation
  Tests, *88*
Immunoglobulin Assays, *90*
Serum Complement Assays, *95*
Immune Complex Assays, *96*
Radioallergosorbent Test (RAST)
  for IgE, *97*
Autoantibody Tests, *98*
Fungal Infection Antibody Tests, *102*
Staphylococcal Tests, *104*
Streptococcal Tests, *106*
Febrile/Cold Agglutinin Tests, *107*
Fluorescent Treponemal Antibody-
  Absorption (FTA-ABS) Test, *109*

Venereal Disease Research
  Laboratory (VDRL) and Rapid
  Plasma Reagin (RPR) Tests, *110*
Viral Infection Antibody Tests, *112*
Infectious Mononucleosis Tests, *113*
Hepatitis Tests, *115*
Acquired Immunodeficiency
  Syndrome (AIDS) Tests, *117*
Serum α-Fetoprotein (AFP) Test, *120*
Carcinoembryonic Antigen (CEA)
  Test, *122*
CA 15-3, CA 19-9, CA 50, and
  CA 125 Antigen Tests, *123*

INTRODUCTION

The immune system protects the body from invasion by foreign elements ranging from microorganisms and pollens to transplanted organs and subtly altered autologous proteins. An *antigen* is any substance that elicits an immune response in an immunocompetent host to whom that substance is foreign.

The cells responsible for immune reactivity are lymphocytes and macrophages. The primary function of the lymphocytes is to react with antigens and thus initiate immune responses. There are two main categories of immune response: (1) the cell-mediated response, produced by locally active T lymphocytes present at the same time and place as the specific antigen, and (2) the humoral response, the manufacture by B lymphocytes of antibody proteins that enter body fluids for widespread distribution throughout the body.[1]

The immune system also removes damaged or worn-out cells and destroys abnormal cells as they develop in the body. The cells responsible for these functions are the macrophages, which engulf particulate debris (phagocytosis) and also secrete a vast array of enzymes, enzyme inhibitors, oxidizing agents, chemotactic agents, bioactive lipids (prostaglandins and related substances), complement components, and products that stimulate or inhibit multiplication of other cells. These phagocytic and secretory activities help mediate responses to immune stimulation. Macrophages also are critically important in the induction of immunity. Only after macrophages process antigen and present it to lymphocytes can immunologic reactivity develop.

Laboratory tests can demonstrate with remarkable sensitivity many of the body's immune activities. In general, quantification of cellular components, presence and activities of antibodies and antigens, and measurement of biologically active secretions constitute the laboratory tests of immune functions.

TESTS OF LYMPHOCYTE FUNCTIONS

Lymphocytes, the second most numerous of the several types of white cells in the peripheral blood (see Table 1–4, p. 19), are essential components of the immune system. Diseases affecting lymphocytes frequently manifest as an inability to protect the individual against environmental pathogens (immune deficiency disorders) or as the development of immune reactions to the individual's own cells.[2]

The lymphocytes in the circulation represent only a small fraction of the total body pool of these cells. The majority are located in the spleen, lymph nodes, and other organized lymphatic tissues. The lymphocytes in the blood are able to enter and leave the circulation freely. Thus, there is continuous movement of cells from one area or compartment to another. Despite this process, the number of lymphocytes in the blood and tissues is kept quite constant. Lymphocytes have been divided into two major categories based on their immunologic activity: T lymphocytes and B lymphocytes. There also is a third group of lymphocytes that lack the characteristics of either T or B cells; they are called *null cells.*[3]

T lymphocytes are primarily responsible for cell-mediated immunity, which requires direct cell contact between the antigen and the lymphocyte. This immune reaction occurs at the local site and generally develops slowly. Examples of cell-mediated immune responses include reactions against intracellular pathogens such as bacteria, viruses, fungi, and protozoa; positive tuberculin skin test results; contact dermatitis; transplant rejection (acute and chronic reactions); and tumor immunity.

As with other blood cells, T lymphocytes develop from stem cells (see Fig. 1–2, p. 6) and then migrate to the thymus, where they proliferate and mature. Thymopoiesis is, however, an ineffective process, and many T lymphocytes die either within the thymus or shortly after leaving it. Only a small portion of the T lymphocytes reach the peripheral tissues as mature T cells capable of effecting cell-mediated immunity.[4]

It should be noted that the thymus functions primarily during fetal life. The peripheral T-lymphoid system is fully developed at birth and normally does not require a constant input of new cells for maintenance after birth. Thus, it is possible to surgically remove the thymus (e.g., as is done to treat myasthenia gravis) without impairing the individual's cell-mediated immune system. In contrast, failure of the thymus to develop during fetal life leads to a severe de-

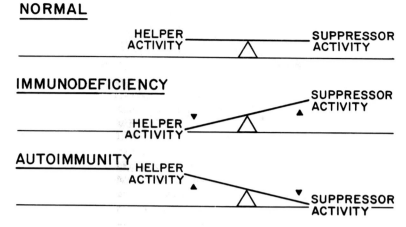

Figure 3–1   In normal, healthy individuals, there is a balance between helper and suppressor activities. Many immunodeficiency syndromes appear to be caused by a disturbance of this balance such that a state of unresponsiveness is created. This could result from either a lack of helper activity or an excess of suppressor activity. Conversely, autoimmunity, which results from aberrant responses directed at the host's own antigens, could result from abnormal immunoregulation from either excessive helper or reduced suppressor activities. (From Boggs, DR and Winkelstein, A: White Cell Manual, ed 4. FA Davis, Philadelphia, 1983, p 71, with permission.)

fect in cellular immunity (Di George's syndrome), usually resulting in death during infancy as a consequence of repeated infections.[5]

Two subsets of T lymphocytes have been identified: helper T cells and suppressor T cells. Helper T cells promote the proliferation of T lymphocytes, stimulate B-lymphocyte reactivity, and activate macrophages, thereby increasing their bactericidal and cytotoxic functions. Suppressor T cells limit the magnitude of the immune response. In normal individuals, there is a balance between helper and suppressor activities. Many immune diseases are associated with deficiencies or excesses of the T-lymphocyte subtypes (Fig. 3–1).[6]

The B lymphocytes are responsible for humoral immunity through the production of circulating antibodies. Examples of humoral immunity include elimination of encapsulated bacteria, neutralization of soluble toxins, protection against viruses, transplant rejection (hyperacute reaction), and possible tumor immunity. Pathologic alterations in antibody production are responsible for disorders such as autoimmune hemolytic anemia, immune thrombocytopenia, allergic responses, some forms of glomerulonephritis and vasculitis, and transfusion reactions.[7]

Actual production of antibodies (immunoglobulins) occurs in plasma cells, the most differentiated form of B lymphocyte. All B lymphocytes have immunoglobulins (Ig) on their surfaces. These serve as receptors for specific antibodies. Five classes of immunoglobulins are currently identified (IgG, IgM, IgA, IgD, and IgE). Immune activation requires interaction not only of surface Ig with the specific antigen but also of B lymphocytes with the helper T cells. The activated B lymphocytes undergo transformation into immunoblasts that

CENTRAL LYMPHOID
TISSUES   PERIPHERAL LYMPHOID
                                                          TISSUES

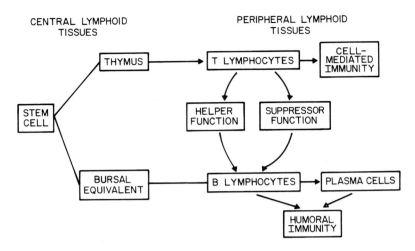

Figure 3–2   The relationship between the T-lymphocyte and B-lymphocyte systems. (From Boggs, DR and Winkelstein, A: White Cell Manual, ed 4. FA Davis, Philadelphia, 1983, p 64, with permission.)

replicate and then differentiate into either plasma cells, which produce antibodies, or memory cells ("small lymphocytes"), which retain the ability to recognize the antigen. Similar memory cells have been found in the T-lymphocyte system.[8]

The relationships between the T-lymphocyte and B-lymphocyte systems are diagrammed in Figure 3–2. In both cellular and humoral immune responses, initial exposure to specific antigens initiates the primary immune response. Depending on the nature and quantity of the antigen, it may take days, weeks, or months for the cells to recognize and respond to the antigen. Subsequent exposure to the same antigen, however, elicits the secondary (anamnestic) response much more rapidly than the primary response.[9]

Tests of lymphocyte functions include T- and B-lymphocyte assays, immunoblast transformation tests, and immunoglobulin assays.

T- AND B-LYMPHOCYTE ASSAYS

T- and B-lymphocyte assays are used to diagnose a number of immunologic disorders (Tables 3–1 and 3–2). A variety of methods are used. The most common way to assess T-cell activity is to measure the individual's response to delayed hypersensitivity skin tests. This involves intradermal injection of minute amounts of several antigens to which the individual has previously been sensitized (e.g., tuberculin, mumps, *Candida*). Erythema and induration should occur at the site within 24 to 48 hours. Absence of response is termed *anergy* and, thus, the test is frequently called an *anergy panel*. Anergy to skin tests reflects either a temporary or a permanent failure of cell-mediated immunity.[10]

Other measures of T and B lymphocytes involve determination of the number of cell types present. T lymphocytes are recognized by their ability to

Table 3-1 ➤ CAUSES OF ALTERED LEVELS OF T AND B LYMPHOCYTES	
Increased Levels	**Decreased Levels**
	T Lymphocytes
Acute lymphocytic leukemia	Di George's syndrome
Multiple myeloma	Chronic lymphocytic leukemia
Infectious mononucleosis	Acquired immunodeficiency syndrome (AIDS)
Graves' disease	Hodgkin's disease
	Nezelof syndrome
	Wiskott-Aldrich syndrome
	Waldenström's macroglobulinemia
	Severe combined immunodeficiency disease (SCID)
	Long-term therapy with immunosuppressive drugs
	B Lymphocytes
Chronic lymphocytic leukemia	Acute lymphocytic leukemia
Multiple myeloma	X-linked agammaglobulinemia
Di George's syndrome	SCID
Waldenström's macroglobulinemia	
Acute lupus erythematosus	

form rosettes with sheep erythrocytes (i.e., the sheep red cells surround the T lymphocyte). Although the sheep erythrocytes adhere to the cell membrane of the T lymphocytes, they react to neither B lymphocytes nor null cells.[11]

T lymphocytes and their subsets also may be distinguished by their ability to react with various monoclonal antibodies. Monoclonal antibodies constitute a single species of immunoglobulins with specificity for a single antigen and are produced by immunizing mice with specific antigens. The most commonly used monoclonal antibodies to T lymphocytes are designated T3, T4, and T8.

Table 3-2 ➤ DISORDERS ASSOCIATED WITH ABNORMAL T-CELL SUBSETS
Immune Deficiency Diseases (Helper and/or Suppressor Activity)
Common variable hypogammaglobulinemia
Acute viral infections (infectious mononucleosis, cytomegalic inclusion disease)
Chronic graft-versus-host disease
Multiple myeloma
Chronic lymphomocytic leukemia
Primary biliary cirrhosis
Sarcoidosis
Immunosuppressive drugs (azathioprine, corticosteroids, cyclosporin A)
Acquired immunodeficiency syndrome (AIDS)
Autoimmunity (Helper and/or Suppressor Activity)
Connective tissue diseases (e.g., systemic lupus erythematosus)
Acute graft-versus-host disease
Autoimmune hemolytic anemia
Multiple sclerosis
Myasthenia gravis
Inflammatory bowel diseases
Atopic eczema

Adapted from Boggs, DR, and Winkelstein, A: White Cell Manual, ed 4. FA Davis, Philadelphia, 1983, p 72.

T3 is a pan-T-cell antibody that reacts with a determinant that is present on all mature peripheral T lymphocytes and can, therefore, be used to enumerate the total number of T cells present. T4 antibodies identify helper T cells, and T8 antibodies identify suppressor T cells.[12]

Other monoclonal antibodies include T10, T9, and T6. T10 and T9 antibodies react with very immature T lymphocytes (thymocytes) that are found in the thymus gland but not in the peripheral circulation. T10 antigen also is seen in mature thymocytes that are localized primarily in the medullary regions of the thymus. T6 antibodies also react with certain immature thymocytes. As T lymphocytes mature, reactivity to T6 antibodies is lost. Tests involving reactivity to immature T lymphocytes are useful in diagnosing T-cell leukemias and lymphomas.[13]

B lymphocytes are detected by immunofluorescent techniques, accomplished by mixing lymphocyte suspensions with heterologous antisera to immunoglobulins that have been labeled with a dye such as fluorescein. The antisera combine with B lymphocytes and when the suspension is examined by fluorescent microscopy, only B lymphocytes appear.[14]

T and B lymphocytes can be differentiated by electron microscopy, as T cells are smooth and B cells have surface projections. This technique is not, however, available in many laboratories.

Reference Values

T lymphocytes	60–80% of circulating lymphocytes*
B lymphocytes	10–20% of circulating lymphocytes
Null cells	5–20% of circulating lymphocytes
Helper T lymphocytes	50–65% of circulating T lymphocytes
Suppressor T lymphocytes	20–35% of circulating T lymphocytes
Ratio of helper to suppressor T lymphocytes 2 : 1	

*A decreased lymphocyte count (lymphopenia) usually indicates a decrease in the number of circulating T lymphocytes.

Indications for T- and B-Lymphocyte Assays

➤ Diagnosis of disorders associated with abnormal levels of T and B lymphocytes (see Table 3–1, p. 85)
➤ Diagnosis of disorders associated with abnormal T-cell subtypes (see Table 3–2, p. 85)
➤ Support for diagnosing acquired immunodeficiency syndrome (AIDS), as indicated by decreased helper T cells, normal or increased suppressor T cells, and a decreased ratio of helper to suppressor T cells
➤ Diagnosis of severe combined immunodeficiency disease (SCID), an inherited disorder characterized by failure of the stem cell to differentiate into T and B lymphocytes (Fig. 3–3)
➤ Diagnosis of Di George's syndrome, characterized by failure of the thymus (and parathyroids) to develop, with a resulting decrease in T lymphocytes (Fig. 3–3)
➤ Diagnosis of X-linked agammaglobulinemia, characterized by severe B-lymphocyte deficiency (Fig. 3–3)

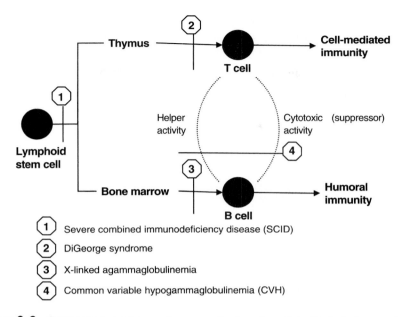

1. Severe combined immunodeficiency disease (SCID)
2. DiGeorge syndrome
3. X-linked agammaglobulinemia
4. Common variable hypogammaglobulinemia (CVH)

Figure 3–3 Several immunodeficiency diseases can be viewed as cellular blocks in the normal maturation of lymphocytes. (From Winkelstein, A et al: White Cell Manual, ed 5. FA Davis, Philadelphia, 1998, p 103, with permission.)

➤ Diagnosis of common variable hypogammaglobulinemia (CVH), characterized by absent, decreased, or defective B cells and most commonly caused by either lack of helper T lymphocytes or abnormal suppressor T cells (Fig. 3–3)

Nursing Care Before the Procedure

Client preparation is the same as that for any study involving the collection of a peripheral blood sample (see Appendix I).

The Procedure

A venipuncture is performed and the sample collected in a green-topped tube or other type of blood collection tube, depending on laboratory preference.

Nursing Care After the Procedure

Care and assessment after the procedure are the same as for any study involving the collection of a peripheral blood sample.

➤ Because the client may be immunosuppressed, assess the site for signs of infection.

➤ *Complications and precautions for compromised immune status:* Note and report helper T-cell level and relation to suppressor T-cell level or decreased B cells. Administer chemotherapy or other ordered medications. Provide reverse protective precautions to prevent infection.

Cell-Mediated Immunity

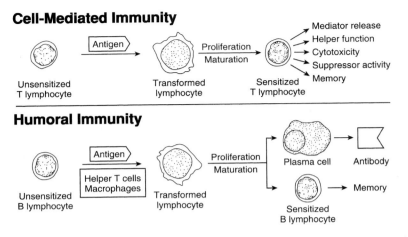

Figure 3–4   Responses of mature lymphocytes to antigens. In both the T- and B-cell systems, stimulated cells undergo a redifferentiation process leading to immature-appearing lymphoblasts. (From Winkelstein, A, et al: White Cell Manual, ed 5. FA Davis, Philadelphia, 1998, p 83, with permission.)

IMMUNOBLAST TRANSFORMATION TESTS

When responding to a specific antigen, mature lymphocytes undergo a series of morphologic and biochemical changes that enable them to become actively proliferating cells (immunoblasts). The lymphocytes enlarge, synthesize new nucleic acids and proteins, and undergo a series of mitoses. This proliferative expansion increases the pool of antigen-responsive cells (Fig. 3–4).[15] Immunoblast transformation tests evaluate the capability of lymphocytes to change to proliferative cells and, thus, to respond normally to antigenic challenge.

Several methods of performing immunoblast transformation tests may be used. Nonimmune transformation tests involve exposing a sample of the client's lymphocytes to mitogens, agents that cause normally responsive lymphocytes to become immunoblasts independent of any antigenic effect. Effective mitogens include plant extracts such as phytohemagglutinin (PHA), concanavalin A (conA), and pokeweed mitogen. PHA and conA stimulate primarily T lymphocytes; pokeweed stimulates both T and B lymphocytes, although the effect on B lymphocytes is greater. Approximately 72 hours after the lymphocytes have been incubated with the mitogens, radiolabeled thymidine is added and then incorporated into the deoxyribonucleic acid (DNA) of the proliferating cells. The rate of uptake of radioactive thymidine indicates the extent of lymphocyte proliferation.[16]

After immune capability has been established, antigen-specific transformation tests can demonstrate whether the person's T cells have encountered specific antigens; that is, an individual's cell-mediated immunities can be documented by observing the way T cells respond to a battery of known antigens (e.g., soluble viral or bacterial antigens or tissue antigens of human white cells from organ donors).

The mixed lymphocyte culture (MLC) technique is widely used in testing before organ transplantation. This test is based on the fact that cultured lymphocytes can recognize and respond to foreign antigens that have not previously sensitized the host. Immunologically responsive lymphocytes cultured together with cells possessing unfamiliar or unknown surface antigens gradually develop sensitivity; after a lag period of 48 to 72 hours, the responding cells undergo immunoblast transformation if the stimulating cells possess antigens different from those of the host.[17]

Reference Values

Nonimmune transformation tests	A stimulation index of greater than 10 indicates immunocompetence.
Antigen-specific transformation tests	A stimulation index of greater than 3 indicates prior exposure to the antigen.
Mixed lymphocyte culture	Nonresponsiveness indicates good histocompatibility.

Interfering Factors

➤ Radioisotope studies performed within 1 week of the test may alter test results.
➤ Pregnancy or oral contraceptive use may lead to a decreased response to PHA in nonimmune transformation tests (see p. 88).

Indications for Immunoblast Transformation Tests

➤ Support for diagnosing immunodeficiency disorders as indicated by a decreased response to nonimmune transformation tests
➤ Identification of microorganisms to which the individual was previously exposed as indicated by an increased response to antigen-specific transformation tests
➤ Support for identifying compatible organ donors and recipients as indicated by nonresponsiveness on mixed lymphocyte culture

Nursing Care Before the Procedure

Client preparation is the same as that for any study involving the collection of a peripheral blood sample (see Appendix I).
➤ All clients should be interviewed to determine whether they have undergone any radioisotope tests within the past week; if the client is a woman, it should be determined whether she is pregnant or using oral contraceptives.

The Procedure

A venipuncture is performed and the sample collected in a green-topped tube or other type of blood collection tube, depending on laboratory preference. The sample should be transported to the laboratory promptly.

Nursing Care After the Procedure

Care and assessment after the procedure are the same as for any study involving the collection of a peripheral blood sample.

➤ Because the client may be immunosuppressed, assess the site for signs of infection.

• *Complications and precautions:* Note and report the lymphocyte response to an antigenic challenge in relation to signs and symptoms of tissue rejection or allergic condition.

IMMUNOGLOBULIN ASSAYS

Immunoglobulins are serum antibodies produced by the plasma cells of the B lymphocytes. Immunoglobulins (Ig) have been subdivided into the five classes, IgG, IgA, IgM, IgD, and IgE; their functions are listed in Table 3–3. IgG, IgA, and IgM have been further divided into subclasses (e.g., IgG_1, IgG_2, IgG_3, and IgG_4).

Four techniques may be used to assess Ig: (1) serum protein electrophoresis, (2) immunoelectrophoresis, (3) radial immunodiffusion, and (4) radioimmunoassay. Serum protein electrophoresis, although not specific to the immunoglobulins, may indicate the presence of immunologic disorders such that additional testing may not be needed. Electrophoresis separates the serum proteins into albumin and globulin components, with the latter being further broken down into α_1, α_2, β, and γ fractions. Most of the γ fraction derives from IgG molecules, whereas IgM contributes to the β portion.[18]

Three types of alterations in immunoglobulins can be identified by serum protein electrophoresis: (1) hypogammaglobulinemia, a reduction in the total quantity of immunoglobulins; (2) monoclonal gammopathy, excessive amounts of single immunoglobulins or proteins related to immunoglobulins (seen in multiple myeloma and macroglobulinemia); and (3) polyclonal gammopathy, excessive amounts of several different immunoglobulins (seen in many infections and diffuse inflammatory conditions).[19,20] Examples of these serum protein electrophoretic patterns are diagrammed in Figure 3–5. Additional examples of disorders associated with monoclonal and polyclonal gammopathies are listed in Table 3–4.

Immunoelectrophoresis is not a quantitative technique, but it provides such detailed separation of the individual immunoglobulins that modest deficiencies are readily detected. It identifies the presence of monoclonal protein and its type. Radial immunodiffusion allows measurement of the quantity of individual immunoglobulins to concentrations as low as 10 to 20 mg/dL. Radioimmunoassay provides better results when immunoglobulin levels are below 20 mg/dL. Serum IgD and IgE are normally well below this level, as are immunoglobulin levels in most body fluids other than serum.

Cryoglobulin is an immunoglobulin that precipitates in the cold and, in those who develop high concentrations, causes the blockage of small capillaries in fingers, ears, and toes exposed to cold temperatures. The test is performed by first cooling the blood serum in a refrigerator to note whether a precipitate forms in 2 to 7 days and then measuring the volume in relation to the percentage of the total serum to obtain a numerical value analogous to a hematocrit. Three positive types of cryoglobulins can be identified by immunoelectrophore-

Table 3–3 ▶ IMMUNOGLOBULINS

Class	Locations	Functions	Increased	Decreased
			CAUSES OF ALTERED LEVELS	
IgG	Plasma Interstitial fluid Placenta	Produces antibodies against bacteria, viruses, and toxins Protects neonate Activates the complement system Is a major factor in secondary (anamnestic) response	Infections—all types, acute and chronic Starvation Liver disease Rheumatic fever Sarcoidosis IgG myelomas	Lymphocytic leukemia Agammaglobulinemia Amyloidosis Toxemia of pregnancy
IgA	Respiratory tract Gastrointestinal tract Genitourinary tract Tears Saliva Milk, colostrum Exocrine secretions	Protects mucous membranes from viruses and bacteria Includes antitoxins, antibacterial agglutinins, antinuclear antibodies, and allergic reagins Activates complement through the alternative pathway	Autoimmune diseases Chronic infections Liver disease Wiskott-Aldrich syndrome IgA myeloma	Lymphocytic leukemia Agammaglobulinemia Malignancies Hereditary ataxia-telangiectasia Hypogammaglobulinemia Malabsorption syndromes
IgM	—	Primary responder to antigens Produces antibody against rheumatoid factors, gram-negative organisms, and the ABO blood group Activates the complement system	Lymphosarcoma Brucellosis, actinomycosis Trypanosomiasis Relapsing fever Malaria Infectious mononucleosis Rubella virus in newborn Waldenström's macroglobulinemia Chronic infections	Lymphocytic leukemia Agammaglobulinemia Amyloidosis IgG and IgA myeloma Dysgammaglobulinemia
IgD	Serum Cord blood	Unknown	IgD myelomas	—
IgE	Serum Interstitial fluid	Allergic reactions Anaphylaxis Protects against parasitic worm infestations	Atopic skin disorders Hay fever Asthma Anaphylaxis IgE myeloma	Congenital agammaglobulinemia

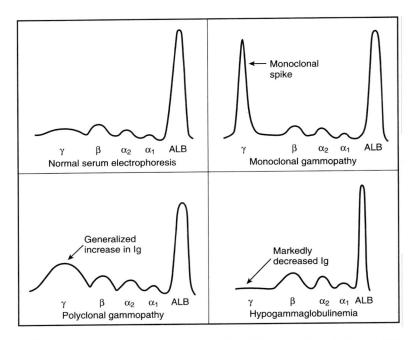

Figure 3–5 Serum protein electrophoretic patterns. (From Winkelstein, A, et al: White Cell Manual, ed 5. FA Davis, Philadelphia, 1998, p 95, with permission.)

sis. Pyroglobulin is a protein identified by heating the blood serum to obtain a precipitate, indicating an abnormality. The test is performed to determine cold sensitivity as well as to assist in the diagnosis of collagen disorders, malignancies, or infections.[21]

Table 3–4 ➤ CONDITIONS CAUSING EXCESSIVE GLOBULIN LEVELS

Monoclonal Gammopathies	
Usually found	Multiple myeloma, Waldenström's macroglobulinemia, heavy chain disease, essential cryoglobulinemia
Sometimes found	Chronic lymphocytic leukemia, lymphomas, "benign" monoclonal gammopathy, age >80
Rarely found	Amyloidosis, autoimmune disorders, chronic active hepatitis, biliary cirrhosis
Polyclonal Gammopathies	
Usually found	Advanced cirrhosis, chronic active hepatitis, biliary cirrhosis, sarcoidosis, narcotics addiction, systemic lupus erythematosus, congenital infections, many parasitic diseases
Sometimes found	Chronic infections, infectious mononucleosis, pulmonary hypersensitivity diseases, rheumatoid arthritis, amyloidosis, scleroderma
Rarely found	Down syndrome, berylliosis, immunoglobulin A disorders

Adapted from Sacher, RA, and McPherson, RA: Widmann's Clinical Interpretation of Laboratory Tests, ed 10. FA Davis, Philadelphia, 1991, p 169, with permission.

Reference Values

Serum Protein Electrophoresis	*Percentage of Total Protein*	
	Conventional Units	**SI Units**
Constituent		
Albumin	52–68	0.520–0.680
Globulin	32–48	0.320–0.480
α_1-Globulin	2.4–5.3	0.024–0.053
α_2-Globulin	6.6–13.5	0.066–0.135
β-Globulin	8.5–14.5	0.085–0.145
γ-Globulin	10.7–21.0	0.107–0.210

Immunoglobulins	IgG, mg/dL	IgA, mg/dL	IgM, mg/dL	IgD, mg/dL	IgE, mg/dL
Neonates	650–1250	0–12	5–30	—	—
SI Units	6.5–12.5 g/L	0.00–0.12 g/L	0.05–0.30 g/L		
6 mo	200–1100	10–90	10–80	—	—
SI Units	2.0–11.0 g/L	0.10–0.90 g/L	0.10–0.80 g/L		
1 yr	300–1400	20–150	20–100	—	—
SI Units	3.0–14.0 g/L	0.20–1.50 g/L	0.20–1.0 g/L		
6 yr	550–1500	50–175	22–100	—	—
SI Units	5.50–15.0 g/L	0.50–1.75 g/L	0.22–1.0 g/L		
12 yr	660–1450	50–200	30–120	—	—
SI Units	6.60–14.5 g/L	0.50–2.0 g/L	0.30–1.20 g/L		
16 yr	700–1050	7–225	35–75	—	—
SI Units	7.0–10.5 g/L	0.70–2.25 g/L	0.35–0.75 g/L		
Adults	800–1800	100–400	55–150	0.5–3	0.01–0.04
SI Units	8.0–18.0 g/L	1.0–4.0 g/L	0.55–1.50 g/L	0.005–0.03 g/L	0–430 μg/L
Percentage of total immunoglobulins in adults	75–80%	15%	10%	0.2%	0.0002%

Interfering Factors

➤ Immunizations within 6 months before the test may alter test results.
➤ Transfusions of either whole blood or fractions within 2 months may alter test results.

Indications for Immunoglobulin Assays

➤ Suspected immunodeficiency, either congenital or acquired
➤ Suspected immunoproliferative disorders such as multiple myeloma or Waldenström's macroglobulinemia
➤ Suspected autoimmune disorder
➤ Suspected malignancy involving the lymphoreticular system
➤ Monitoring of effects of chemotherapy or radiation therapy, or both, which may suppress the immune system
➤ Identification of hypogammaglobulinemia, monoclonal gammopathy, and polyclonal gammopathy by serum protein electrophoresis (see Fig. 3–5, p. 92, and Table 3–4, p. 92)
➤ Support for diagnosing a variety of disorders associated with altered immunoglobulin levels (see Table 3–3, p. 91)

Nursing Care Before the Procedure

Client preparation is the same as that for any study involving the collection of a peripheral blood sample (see Appendix I).

➤ The client should be interviewed to determine whether he or she has received immunizations within 6 months before the test or transfusions of whole blood or fractions within 2 months before the test.

The Procedure

A venipuncture is performed and the sample collected in a red-topped tube or other type of blood collection tube, depending on laboratory preference. The sample should be transported to the laboratory promptly.

Nursing Care After the Procedure

Care and assessment after the procedure are the same as for any study involving the collection of a peripheral blood sample.

➤ Because the client may be immunosuppressed, assess the site for signs of infection.

 • *Complications and precautions:* Note and report abnormal levels in relation to immunodeficiency, malignant, or autoimmune disorders.

TESTS OF THE COMPLEMENT SYSTEM

Complement is a system of protein molecules, the sequential interactions of which produce biologic effects on surface membranes, on cellular behavior, and on the interactions of other proteins. Each of the proteins of the complement system is inactive by itself. Activation occurs through a cascadelike sequence after contact with substances such as IgG or IgM antigen-antibody complexes, aggregated IgA, certain naturally occurring polysaccharides and lipopolysaccharides, activation products of the coagulation system, and bacterial endotoxins. Activation of the complement system results in an inflammatory response that destroys or damages cells.

Complement proteins are identified by letters and numbers and are listed here in order of activation in the "classical pathway" of the complement cascade: $C1_q$, $C1_r$, $C1_s$, C4, C2, C3, and then C5 through C9. The "alternate pathway" bypasses C1, C4, and C2 activation and begins directly with C3. The key step in the alternate pathway is activation of properdin, a serum protein without biologic effects in its inactive form. Contact with aggregated IgA, with bacterial endotoxins, or with complex molecules such as dextran, agar, and zymosan alters properdin and initiates the sequence at C3.[22]

Complete activation to C9 leads to membrane disruption and irreversible cell damage. Along the way to complete activation, the following activities occur: C2 releases a low-molecular-weight peptide with kinin activity. Activation of products of C3 and C5 affects mast cells, smooth muscle, and leukocytes to produce an anaphylactic effect; other elements of C3 and C5 bind to cell membranes and render them more susceptible to phagocytosis, a process called opsonization. Fragments of C3 and C4 cause immune adherence, in which complement-coated particles bind to cells with surface membranes that have complement receptors; activated C3 and C4 are also capable of virus neutralization. C3 and C5 exert chemotactic activity on neutrophils, and the C5 to C9 complex influences the procoagulant activity of platelets. Conversely, procoagulant factor XII can initiate C1 activation, and plasmin (the substance that dissolves fibrin) and thrombin (which converts fibrinogen to fibrin) can cleave C3 into its active form.[23]

SERUM COMPLEMENT ASSAYS

Radioimmunoassay and immunodiffusion techniques have made it possible to quantify each of the complement components. For clinical purposes, however, only total complement, C3, and C4 are measured. Total complement (CH_{50}), also known as a *hemolytic assay,* is measured by exposing a sample of human serum to sheep red cells coated with complement-requiring antibody. Results are expressed as CH_{50} units, reflecting the dilution at which adequate complement exists to lyse one half of the test cells. C3 and C4 levels are measured individually by radial immunodiffusion. These latter tests take 24 to 36 hours to complete, and results are easily affected by improper handling of the specimen.[24]

The causes of alterations in C3 and C4 levels are presented in Table 3–5.

Reference Values

		Conventional Units	**SI Units**
Total complement (CH_{50})		40–90 U/mL	0.4–0.9 g/L
C3	Men	80–180 mg/dL	0.80–1.80 g/L
	Women	76–120 mg/dL	0.76–1.20 g/L
C4	Men	15–60 mg/dL	0.15–0.60 g/L
	Women	15–52 mg/dL	0.15–0.52 g/L

Values for total complement, C3, and C4 may vary according to laboratory methods and the reference range established by the laboratory performing the test.

Table 3–5 ➤ CAUSES OF ALTERATIONS IN C3 AND C4 LEVELS

Component	Increased Levels	Decreased Levels
C3	Acute rheumatic fever Rheumatoid arthritis Early SLE Most cancers	Advanced systemic lupus erythematosus (SLE) Glomerulonephritis Renal transplant rejection Chronic active hepatitis Cirrhosis Multiple sclerosis Anemias Gram-negative septicemia Subacute bacterial endocarditis Inborn C3 deficiency Serum sickness Immune complex disease
C4	Rheumatoid spondylitis Juvenile rheumatoid arthritis Most cancers	SLE Lupus nephritis Acute poststreptococcal glomerulonephritis Chronic active hepatitis Cirrhosis Subacute bacterial endocarditis Inborn C4 deficiency Serum sickness Immune complex disease

Interfering Factors

➤ Failure to transport the sample to the laboratory immediately may alter test results because complement deteriorates rapidly at room temperature.

➤ Hemolysis of the sample may alter test results.

Indications for Serum Complement Assays

➤ Suspected acute inflammatory disorder as generally indicated by elevated total complement levels

➤ Suspected immune or infectious disorder (e.g., acute glomerulonephritis, systemic lupus erythematosus [SLE], rheumatoid arthritis, hepatitis, sub-acute bacterial endocarditis, gram-negative sepsis) or both, as indicated by decreased total complement levels

➤ Support for diagnosing hereditary deficiencies of complement components as indicated by decreased levels of total complement or of specific components such as C3 and C4, or of both (see Table 3–5, p. 95)

➤ Support for diagnosing cancer, especially that of the breast, lung, digestive system, cervix, ovary, and bladder, as indicated by increased levels of C3 and C4 (see Table 3–5, p. 95)

➤ Monitoring for the progression of malignant disease as indicated by declining complement levels as the disease progresses

➤ Support for diagnosing a variety of immune and inflammatory disorders as indicated by altered C3 and C4 levels (see Table 3–5, p. 95)

➤ Monitoring of progress after various immune and inflammatory disorders as indicated by levels approaching or within the reference ranges

Nursing Care Before the Procedure

Client preparation is the same as that for any study involving the collection of a peripheral blood sample (see Appendix I).

The Procedure

A venipuncture is performed and the sample collected in a red-topped tube or other type of blood collection tube, depending on laboratory preference. The sample must be handled gently to avoid hemolysis and transported to the laboratory immediately.

Nursing Care After the Procedure

Care and assessment after the procedure are the same as for any study involving the collection of a peripheral blood sample.

➤ *Complications and precautions:* Note and report types and deficiencies of complement components and their relation to an inflammatory or infectious disorder.

IMMUNE COMPLEX ASSAYS

Immune complexes are combinations of antigen and antibody that are capable of activating the complement cascade. Although the activated agent is directed against the immune complex, tissues that are "innocent bystanders" may also be severely damaged, especially when immune complexes are produced too rapidly for adequate clearance by the body. Immune complexes are commonly present in autoimmune disorders and also are found in immune hypersensitivities that do not involve autoimmunity.

Two methods can be used to determine the circulating immune complexes (CIC) in the blood in the diagnosis of autoimmune and infectious diseases. One involves screening for large amounts of precipitate in serum that has been refrigerated. The other is the Raji cell assay, in which these specially prepared cells that bind complement (C3) are combined with the serum sample and then incubated. Further incubation with a radiolabeled antihuman immunoglobulin allows for binding of the CIC on the surface of the Raji cells. This is followed by washing of the cells and measurement of the radioactivity to determine the CIC in the blood.[25]

Reference Values

Immune complexes are not normally found in the serum.

Interfering Factors

➤ Rough handling of the sample and failure to transport the sample promptly to the laboratory may cause deterioration of any immune complexes present.

Indications for Immune Complex Assays

➤ Suspected immune disorders such as SLE, scleroderma, dermatomyositis, polymyositis, glomerulonephritis, and rheumatic fever as indicated by the presence of immune complexes
➤ Monitoring of the effects of therapy for various immune disorders
➤ Suspected serum sickness or allergic reactions to drugs as indicated by the presence of immune complexes

Nursing Care Before the Procedure

Client preparation is the same as that for any study involving the collection of a peripheral blood sample (see Appendix I).

The Procedure

A venipuncture is performed and the sample collected in a red-topped tube or other type of blood collection tube, depending on laboratory preference. The sample must be handled gently and transported to the laboratory promptly.

Nursing Care After the Procedure

Care and assessment after the procedure are the same as for any study involving the collection of a peripheral blood sample.
➤ *Complications and precautions:* Note and report the presence of complexes in relation to signs and symptoms of an existing or suspected autoimmune disease.

RADIOALLERGOSORBENT TEST (RAST) FOR IGE

IgE antibodies are responsible for hypersensitivity reactions described as atopic (allergic) or anaphylactic. Examples of IgE-mediated diseases include hay fever, asthma, certain types of eczema, and idiosyncratic, potentially fatal reactions to insect venoms, penicillin, and other drugs or chemicals.

Almost all of the body's active IgE is bound to tissue cells, with only small amounts in the blood. Thus, IgE antibodies cannot circulate in search of antigen but must wait for antigens to appear in their area. Once this happens, the interaction of IgE antibodies with specific antigens causes mast cells (tissue basophils) to release histamine and other substances that promote vascular permeability.[26]

The radioallergosorbent test (RAST) for IgE measures the quantity of IgE antibodies in the serum after exposure to specific antigens selected on the basis of the person's history. RAST has replaced skin tests and provocation procedures, which were inconvenient, painful, and hazardous to the client.

Reference Values

If the client is not allergic to the antigen, IgE antibody is not detected. A positive test result in relation to a specific antigen is more than 400 percent of control. Results of the test may vary depending on the reference serum used for the control.

Interfering Factors

➤ Radioisotope tests within 1 week before the test may alter results.

Indications for Radioallergosorbent Test (RAST) for IgE

➤ Onset of asthma, hay fever, dermatitis
➤ Systemic reaction to insect venom, drugs, or chemicals
➤ Identification of the specific antigen(s) to which the client reacts
➤ Monitoring of response to desensitization procedures

Nursing Care Before the Procedure

Client preparation is the same as that for any study involving the collection of a peripheral blood sample (see Appendix I).

➤ All clients should be interviewed to determine whether they have undergone any radioisotope tests within the past week.

The Procedure

A venipuncture is performed and the sample collected in a red-topped tube or other type of blood collection tube, depending on laboratory preference. The allergy panel desired should be indicated on the laboratory request form. Each panel usually consists of six antigens.

Nursing Care After the Procedure

Care and assessment after the procedure are the same as for any study involving the collection of a peripheral blood sample.

➤ *Complications and precautions:* Instruct client to avoid contact with substances, ingestion of drugs, or exposure to insects that cause reactions.

AUTOANTIBODY TESTS

Antibodies directed against "self" components are believed to be responsible for the pathogenesis of many diseases. Some show widespread systemic involvement (Table 3–6), whereas others are confined to a specific organ system (Table 3–7).

Table 3–6 ► SUMMARY OF AUTOANTIBODY-RELATED DISORDERS AND TESTS USED IN DIAGNOSIS

| | INCIDENCE | | |
Antibody	Present in 90% or More of Cases	Present in 50–90% of Cases	Present in <50% of Cases
C-reactive protein (CRP)	Rheumatic fever Rheumatoid arthritis Acute bacterial infections Viral hepatitis	Active tuberculosis Gout Advanced cancers Leprosy Cirrhosis Burns Peritonitis	Multiple sclerosis Guillain-Barré syndrome Scarlet fever Varicella Surgery Intrauterine contraceptive devices
Rheumatoid factor (RF)	Rheumatoid arthritis	Early rheumatoid arthritis SLE Scleroderma Dermatomyositis	Advanced age Juvenile rheumatoid arthritis (20%) Infectious diseases Healthy adults (<5%)
Antinuclear antibodies (ANA)	Systemic lupus erythematosus (SLE)	Sjögren's syndrome Scleroderma Drug-induced SLE-like syndrome Chronic active hepatitis Heart disease, with long-term procainamide therapy	Burns Asbestosis Juvenile chronic polyarthritis Rheumatoid arthritis Rheumatic fever Myasthenia gravis Advanced age Dermatomyositis Polyarteritis nodosa Primary biliary cirrhosis Juvenile rheumatoid arthritis Progressive systemic sclerosis Drug-induced SLE-like syndrome Uveitis
Anti-DNA	Active SLE	SLE in remission	
Cold agglutinins	Atypical pneumonia Influenza Pulmonary embolus	Viral infections Infectious mononucleosis Lymphoreticular malignancy	Congenital syphilis Malaria Anemia Cirrhosis
Lupus erythematosus (LE) cell preparation	SLE	—	—
Cryoglobulins	Raynaud's syndrome Cryoglobulinemia	—	—

Reference Values

	Conventional Units	SI Units
C-reactive protein (CRP)	Negative to trace	
Antinuclear antibodies (ANA)	Negative	
Rheumatoid factor (RF)	Negative (<1:20)	
Anti-DNA antibodies	<1 μg/mL	<2.0 kU/L
Antimitochondrial antibodies	Negative	
Antiskin antibodies	Negative	
Antiadrenal cortex antibodies	Negative	
Antithyroglobulin, antithyroid microsome antibodies	<1:100	
Antismooth muscle antibodies	Negative	
Antiparietal cell, anti-intrinsic factor antibodies	Negative	
Antistriated muscle antibodies	Negative	
Antimyocardial antibodies	Negative	
Antiglomerular basement membrane antibodies	Negative	
Anti-insulin antibodies	Negative	
Acetylcholine receptor antibodies	Negative	
Anti-SS-A and anti-SS-B antibodies	Negative	
Lupus erythematosus cell test (LE prep)	Negative	
Cold agglutinins	<1:16	
Cryoglobulins	Negative	
Antiglobulin tests (Coombs' tests)*		
Direct	Negative	
Indirect	Negative	

*See also Chapter 4.

Interfering Factors

➤ Many drugs may cause false-positive results in certain autoantibody tests (Table 3–8).

Indications for Autoantibody Tests

➤ Signs and symptoms of the disorder for which each test is pathognomonic or for which the test provides confirming data (see Tables 3–6, p. 99, and 3–7, p. 101)
➤ Monitoring of response to treatment for autoimmune disorders

Nursing Care Before the Procedure

Client preparation is the same as that for any study involving the collection of a peripheral blood sample (see Appendix I).
➤ Food and fluids are not restricted, except for the cryoglobulin test, which requires a 4-hour fast from food.

The Procedure

The procedure is the same for all autoantibody tests, except cryoglobulins. A venipuncture is performed and the sample collected in a red-topped tube. For cryoglobulins, the sample is collected in a prewarmed red-topped tube. The sample must be handled gently to avoid hemolysis and sent promptly to the laboratory.

Table 3–7 ➤ **CELL- AND TISSUE-SPECIFIC ANTIBODIES**

Antibody Target Cell/Tissue	Diseases for Which the Test Is Usually Diagnostic	Other Diseases in Which This Antibody May Also Be Present
Skeletal muscle	Myasthenia gravis	
Cardiac muscle	Myocardial infarction	Acute rheumatic fever
Smooth muscle	Chronic active hepatitis	Biliary cirrhosis
		Viral hepatitis
		Infectious mononucleosis
		Systemic lupus erythematosus (SLE) (10%)
Mitochondria	Primary biliary cirrhosis	Chronic active hepatitis
	Drug-induced jaundice	Viral hepatitis
		SLE (20%)
Skin	Pemphigus	—
Altered IgG	Rheumatoid arthritis	—
Adrenal cells	Addison's disease	—
Intrinsic factor, parietal cells	Pernicious anemia	SLE (5%)
Long-acting thyroid stimulator	Graves' disease	—
	Hashimoto's thyroiditis	
Long-acting thyroid microsomes	Primary myxedema	SLE (5%)
	Juvenile lymphocytic thyroiditis	Pernicious anemia (25%)
	Graves' disease	Allergies
		Healthy adults
Thyroglobulin	Hashimoto's thyroiditis	Pernicious anemia
	Primary myxedema	Allergies
	Graves' disease	Healthy adults (5–10%)
Salivary ducts	Sjögren's syndrome	Rheumatoid arthritis
Red blood cell membrane	Autoimmune hemolytic anemia	Transfusion reaction
Platelet cell membrane	Idiopathic thrombocytopenic purpura	—
Basement membranes of lungs, renal glomeruli	Goodpasture's syndrome Glomerulonephritis	—

Nursing Care After the Procedure

Care and assessment after the procedure are the same as for any study involving the collection of a peripheral blood sample. Resume food withheld before the test.

➤ *Complications and precautions:* Note and report the presence of cell-specific or tissue-specific antibodies in relation to a suspected disease and the presenting signs and symptoms.

IMMUNOLOGIC ANTIBODY TESTS

Exposure to bacteria, fungi, viruses, and parasites induces production of antibodies that either can be identified only during acute disease or can remain identifiable for many years. Exposure can be through immunization, from previous infection so minimal that it passed unrecognized, or from current symptomatic or prepathogenic infection. Detection and identification of specific antibodies in the blood by assays performed in the serology laboratory are preferred for obtaining diagnostic information. This is especially true when the antigen assays or culture techniques performed in the microbiology laboratory

Table 3–8 ➤ DRUGS THAT MAY CAUSE FALSE-POSITIVE REACTIONS IN AUTOANTIBODY TESTS*	
Antibiotics	Para-aminosalicylic acid
Anti-DNA	Penicillin
Chlorpromazine	Phenylbutazone
Clofibrate	Phenytoin
Ethosuximide	Procainamide
Griseofulvin	Propylthiouracil
Hydralazine	Quinidine
Isoniazid	Radioactive diagnostics
Mephenytoin	Streptomycin
Methyldopa	Sulfonamides
Methysergide	Tetracyclines
Oral contraceptives	Trimethadione

*The drugs listed here may cause false-positive reactions in the following tests: antinuclear antibodies, lupus erythematosus (LE) prep, and antiglobulin (Coombs') tests.

are ineffective in producing a causative agent or in clients who cannot tolerate an invasive procedure necessary to collect a specimen for culture.

Various methods for detection of antibodies are used. They include immunoprecipitation, complement fixation, neutralization assay, particle agglutination/agglutination inhibition, immunofluorescence assay, enzyme immunoassay, and radioimmunoassay. The concentrations of antibody are referred to as the *titer,* and their predictable patterns are useful in both diagnosing a disease and monitoring its course.

Fungal Infection Antibody Tests

Most pathogenic fungi elicit antibodies in immunocompetent hosts. Assays for fungal antibodies are used to diagnose invasive deep-seated recent or current infections. Serologic testing for parasitic organisms or antibodies in the blood sample is also used in the diagnosis of infections. Depending on the antibody to be identified, testing uses the various assay techniques mentioned in the introduction of this chapter. Table 3–9 indicates the fungal and parasitic infections for which tests are available and the causes of alteration in the test results.

Reference Values

Organism	Complement Fixation Titers	Immunodiffusion Test	Agglutination	Other Tests
Fungi				
Histoplasma capsulatum	<1:8	Negative	—	—

(Continued on page 103)

Blastomyces dermatitidis	<1:8	Negative	—	—
Coccidioides immitis	<1:2	Negative	—	—
Aspergillus fumigatus	<1:8	Negative	—	—
Cryptococcus neoformans	—	—	Negative	—
Sporotrichum schenckii	—	—	1:40	—
Candida albicans	—	—	—	Latex agglutination (LA) test <1:8
Parasite				
Toxoplasma gondii	—	—	—	Indirect fluorescent antibody tests <1:16
Entamoeba histolytica	—	—	—	Indirect hemagglutination test <1:32

Interfering Factors

➤ Recent fungal skin tests may alter results.
➤ Obtaining the sample near fungal skin lesions may contaminate the specimen and alter test results.

Indications for Fungal Infection Antibody Tests

➤ Suspected infection with the fungus for which the test is performed
➤ Persistent pulmonary symptoms after pneumonia
➤ Acute meningitis of unknown etiology
➤ Identification of the state of infection by rising or falling titers
➤ Confirmation of previous exposure to the fungus despite absence of clinical signs of illness

Table 3–9 ➤ FUNGAL AND PARASITIC IMMUNOLOGIC TESTS

Organism	Tests Available	Causes of Alterations
Fungi		
Histoplasma capsulatum	CF, I, LA	Prior exposure to organism or cross-reactive agent, recent skin test
Blastomyces dermatitidis	EIA	Blastomycosis
Coccidioides immitis	CF, I, LA	Acute or chronic infection, repeated skin testing with coccidioidin
Aspergillus fumigatus	CF, I	Pulmonary aspergillosis, aspergillosis allergy
Cryptococcus neoformans	A	Test demonstrates antigen, not antibodies, in infection
Sporotrichum schenckii	A	Deep tissue infection
Candida albicans	LA	Systemic infection, vaginal infection
Parasites		
Toxoplasma gondii	IFA, EIA	Acute or chronic toxoplasmosis
Entamoeba histolytica	A, IFA	Amebic dysentary

A = agglutination, CF = complement fixation, I = immunodiffusion, IFA = indirect fluorescent antibody tests, LA = latex agglutination, EIA = enzyme immunoassary.

Nursing Care Before the Procedure

Client preparation is the same as that for any study involving the collection of a peripheral blood sample (see Appendix I).

➤ The client should be interviewed to determine if he or she has undergone any recent fungal skin tests that may alter test results.

The Procedure

A venipuncture is performed and the sample collected in a red-topped tube. Venipuncture should not be performed on or near any fungal skin lesions. The sample must be handled gently and transported promptly to the laboratory.

Nursing Care After the Procedure

Care and assessment after the procedure are the same as for any study involving the collection of a peripheral blood sample.

➤ *Complications and precautions:* Note and report signs and symptoms of fungal infection, superficial or deep-seated presence, and rise of serum antibodies to a specific fungal or parasitic microorganism or culture identification of the microorganism. Assess factors that can cause infection such as travel or residence in areas where infection is endemic; antibiotic or corticosteroid therapy; chemotherapy; presence of an intravenous (IV) line to administer fluids, medications, or parenteral nutrition; or invasive procedures such as surgery. Note symptoms of vaginitis such as itching and foul-smelling, white, cheeselike secretion. Administer ordered antifungals via oral, IV, or vaginal routes. Monitor respiratory status for changes in rate, ease, depth, and breath sounds and place on respiratory precautions according to universal standards, if appropriate. Prepare client for skin tests if ordered.

Bacterial Infection Antibody Tests

Although most bacterial infections are successfully diagnosed by culture, serologic testing is performed for antibodies to screen for past, recent, or existing infection in those with negative cultures. Clients in whom these tests are performed usually have sustained a fever of unknown origin or have been treated with antimicrobials. Table 3–10 indicates the commonly performed tests for recent bacterial infections for identification and titers that are suggestive of recent infection. Also, specific individual serologic tests that have special applications in bacterial antibody detection of recent or existing infectious diseases are individually outlined and discussed. They include staphylococcal, streptococcal, and febrile/cold agglutinin tests.

STAPHYLOCOCCAL TESTS

The teichoic acid antibody is measured to diagnose infections caused by *Staphylococcus aureus.* Teichoic acid attaches to the organism's cell wall. High titers are associated with invasive infections such as bacterial endocarditis and osteomyelitis.

Table 3–10 ➤ COMMONLY PERFORMED SEROLOGIC TESTS FOR DIAGNOSIS OF RECENT BACTERIAL INFECTIONS

Organism	Test	Clinically Significant Result*
Staphylococcus aureus	Immunodiffusion for teichoic acid antibodies	≥1:4
Streptococcus pyogenes	Antistreptolysin O (ASO)	≥1:240
	Anti-DNAase B	≥1:240
	Antihyaluronidase	≥4× titer rise
Salmonella typhi (typhoid fever)	Widal test	≥4× titer rise
Legionella pneumophila (legionnaires' disease)	Indirect immunofluorescence	≥1:256
Treponema pallidum	Rapid plasma reagin (RPR)	≥1:8
	Venereal Disease Research Laboratory (VDRL)	≥1:8
	Fluorescent treponemal antibody-absorption (FTA-ABS) (IgM)	Positive
Borrelia burgdorferi (Lyme disease)	Indirect immunofluorescence	≥1:128
Mycoplasma pneumoniae (atypical pneumonia)	Cold agglutinins	≥1:128
	Complement fixation	≥1:32
Rickettsia rickettsii (spotted and typhus fevers)	Weil-Felix (OX-19)	≥1:320

*Titers greater than or equal to those displayed in the table or fourfold or greater rises in titer between acute and convalescent sera are only suggestive of recent infection by all of the agents listed. Titers less than those displayed in the table do not rule out infection.

Adapted from Sacher, RA, and McPherson, RA: Widmann's Clinical Interpretation of Laboratory Tests, ed 10. FA Davis, Philadelphia, 1991, p 528.

Reference Values

Teichoic acid antibody titer <1:2

Interfering Factors

➤ Improper technique in testing

Indications for Staphylococcal Tests

➤ Suspected infection caused by *Staphylococcus aureus*
➤ Diagnosis of osteomyelitis or endocarditis caused by a bacterial infection
➤ Monitoring of ongoing therapy administered for gram-positive bacterial infections

Nursing Care Before the Procedure

Client preparation is the same as for any study involving the collection of a peripheral blood sample (see Appendix I).
➤ Inform the client that repeat or serial blood sampling and testing can be performed.

The Procedure

A venipuncture is performed and the sample collected in a red-topped tube. The tube should be labeled as an acute or convalescent sample, whichever applies.

Nursing Care After the Procedure

Care and assessment after the procedure are the same as for any study involving the collection of a peripheral blood sample.

➤ Inform the client of the time to return for a repeat test, usually in 2 weeks, to determine the change in titers between the acute and convalescent stages.

• *Abnormal values:* Note and report increases in titers. Assess for signs and symptoms associated with staphylococcal infections such as temperature elevation, bone pain in osteomyelitis, and changes in heart sounds in endocarditis. Administer ordered analgesic and antibiotic therapy and instruct in preventive antibiotic therapy in those at risk.

STREPTOCOCCAL TESTS

Group A β-hemolytic streptococci produce a variety of extracellular products capable of stimulating antibody production. Such antibodies do not act on the bacteria and have no protective effect, but their existence indicates recent active streptococci. Antibody production is most reliably noted in response to streptolysin O, and the test for this antibody is termed an *antistreptolysin O (ASO) titer.* Antibodies in response to hyaluronidase (AH), streptokinase (anti-SK), deoxyribonuclease B (ADN-B), and nicotinamide (anti-NADase) also can be produced. When ASO titers are low, tests for these latter antibodies can be produced to substantiate the diagnosis, as they are more sensitive tests.

Elevated antistreptococcal antibody titers can occur in healthy carriers of β-hemolytic streptococci. Elevated levels also are seen in those with rheumatic fever, glomerulonephritis, bacterial endocarditis, scarlet fever, otitis media, and streptococcal pharyngitis.

Reference Values

Antistreptolysin O (ASO) Titer	
Preschool children	<85 Todd units/mL
School-age children	<170 Todd units/mL
Adults	<85 Todd units/mL
Antideoxyribonuclease B (ADN-B) Titer	
Preschool children	<60 Todd units/mL
School-age children	<170 Todd units/mL
Adults	<85 Todd units/mL
Antihyaluronidase (AH) Titer	<128 Todd units/mL
Antistreptokinase (anti-SK) Titer	<128 Todd units/mL

Interfering Factors

➤ Therapy with antibiotics and adrenal corticosteroids may result in falsely decreased levels.

➤ Elevated blood β-lipoproteins may result in falsely elevated levels.

Indications for Streptococcal Tests

➤ Suspected streptococcal infection, to confirm the diagnosis
➤ Detection and monitoring of response to therapy for poststreptococcal illnesses such as rheumatic fever and glomerulonephritis
➤ Differentiation of rheumatic fever from rheumatoid arthritis, with the former indicated by elevated levels

Nursing Care Before the Procedure

Client preparation is the same as that for any study involving the collection of a peripheral blood sample (see Appendix I).

➤ Medications that the client is currently taking or has recently taken should be noted, because therapy with antibiotics and adrenal corticosteroids may alter test results.

The Procedure

A venipuncture is performed and the sample collected in a red-topped tube. A capillary sample may be obtained in infants and children as well as in adults for whom a venipuncture may not be feasible. The sample must be handled gently and sent promptly to the laboratory.

Nursing Care After the Procedure

Care and assessment after the procedure are the same as for any study involving the collection of a peripheral blood sample.

➤ *Abnormal values:* Note and report increased levels of specific tests in relation to signs and symptoms of joint or renal disease. Assess for joint pain, elevated temperature, sore throat, and history of a recent infection. Administer ordered antipyretics, analgesics, and antibiotic therapy. Prepare for additional tests if more specificity is needed.

FEBRILE/COLD AGGLUTININ TESTS

Febrile agglutinin tests are performed concurrently with blood culture for microorganism identification to diagnose the infectious cause of a febrile condition. The test is performed with the use of antigens to specific organisms and their reaction (agglutination) with antibodies in the client's blood serum. Diseases that can be diagnosed using these tests, along with the type of febrile agglutinin test used, are listed in Table 3–11.

The cold agglutinin test is performed to identify cold agglutinins, antibodies that result from *Mycoplasma pneumoniae* infection. This infection is caused by a nonbacterial agent, but it still manifests a febrile condition. The antibodies cause agglutination of red blood cells at temperature ranges of 35.6 to 46.4°F (2 to 8°C), with a positive titer resulting in those with atypical pneumonia or cold agglutination disorders, depending on the severity of the disease.

Table 3–11 ➤ **FEBRILE AGGLUTININ TESTS**	
Diseases	**Test**
Rickettsial Infections Rocky Mountain spotted fever, typhus (murine, scrub, epidemic, and recrudescent)	Weil-Felix reaction (*Proteus* antigen test)
Salmonella Infections Typhoid and paratyphoid fevers	Widal's test (O and H antigen tests)
Brucella Infections Cattle, hog, goat (Hosts may transmit infections to humans.)	*Brucella* agglutination test (slide agglutination test)
Tularemia Rabbit fever and deer fly fever	Tularemia agglutination test (tube dilution test)

Reference Values

Weil-Felix reaction (*Proteus* antigen test)	<1:80
Widal's test (O and H antigen tests)	<1:160
Brucella agglutination test (slide agglutination test)	<1:80
Tularemia agglutination test (tube dilution test)	<1:40
Mycoplasma pneumoniae (cold agglutinin test)	<1:32

Interfering Factors

➤ Vaccination, chronic exposure to infected animals, and cross-reactions with other antibodies may result in falsely elevated titers.

➤ Individuals who are immunosuppressed or are receiving antibiotic therapy may have false-negative results.

Indications for Febrile/Cold Agglutinin Tests

➤ Determination of possible cause of fever of unknown origin (FUO)

➤ Suspected typhus, Rocky Mountain spotted fever, or other disorder for which selected tests are specific

➤ Suspected "carrier" state for typhoid

➤ Positive blood or stool culture for *Salmonella*

Nursing Care Before the Procedure

Client preparation is the same as that for any study involving the collection of a peripheral blood sample (see Appendix I).

The Procedure

A venipuncture is performed and the sample collected in a red-topped tube. The sample must be handled gently to avoid hemolysis and transported immediately to the laboratory.

Nursing Care After the Procedure

Care and assessment after the procedure are the same as for any study involving the collection of a peripheral blood sample.

➤ *Abnormal values:* Note and report increased titers in cold agglutinin test in relation to specific signs and symptoms of the disease such as fever, change in respiratory status, and nonproductive cough; also note increased titers in febrile disorders in relation to specific infectious processes. Assess for culture results or need to obtain culture for organism identification; place on enteric precautions as appropriate. Administer ordered antimicrobial therapy. Inform client of the need for serial testing during acute and convalescent stages.

Syphilis Tests

Infection with *Treponema pallidum* provides two distinct categories of antibodies: (1) reagin (a nonspecific antibacterial antibody) and (2) antitreponemal antibody. Reagin tests, by their nature nonspecific, include the Wassermann and Reiter complement fixation tests, now seldom used. Reagin tests currently used for screening are the Venereal Disease Research Laboratory (VDRL) and rapid plasma reagin (RPR) flocculation tests. Because reagin screening tests often yield false-positive reactions (Table 3–12), positive test results are confirmed by means of treponemal antibody tests. The best of these is the fluorescent treponemal antibody-absorption (FTA-ABS) test with absorbed serum.[27]

FLUORESCENT TREPONEMAL ANTIBODY-ABSORPTION (FTA-ABS) TEST

The fluorescent treponemal antibody-absorption (FTA-ABS) test is conducted on a sample of the client's serum that is layered onto a slide fixed with *Treponema*

Table 3–12 ➤ CAUSES OF FALSE-POSITIVE REACTIONS TO REAGIN TESTS	
Transiently Positive	**Persistently Positive**
Occurring in >10% of Clients with the Following:	
Infectious mononucleosus	Systemic lupus erythematosus
Malaria	Rheumatoid arthritis
Brucellosis	Illicit drug use
Typhus	Hepatitis
Lymphogranuloma venereum	Leprosy
Subacute bacterial endocarditis	Malaria
	Advanced age
	Nonsyphilitic treponemal disease (pints, yaws, bejel)
Occurring Rarely in Clients with the Following:	
Hepatitis	Tuberculosis
Measles	Scleroderma
Chickenpox	
Mycoplasma pneumonia	
After smallpox vaccination	

pallidum organisms. If the antibody is present, it will attach to the organisms and can subsequently be demonstrated by its reaction with fluorescein-labeled antiglobulin serum.

The FTA-ABS test rarely gives false-positive results, except sporadically in clients with SLE; the pattern of fluorescence may have an atypical beaded appearance in these cases. Elderly individuals and clients with immune complex diseases (see p. 97) occasionally also have false-positive results.[28]

Reference Values

Negative

Interfering Factors

➤ False-positive results may occasionally occur in elderly individuals and in clients with SLE or other immune complex diseases.

Indications for Fluorescent Treponemal Antibody-Absorption (FTA-ABS) Test

➤ Confirmation of the presence of treponemal antibodies in the serum (*Note:* the test also may be applied to cerebrospinal fluid [CSF] to diagnose tertiary syphilis.)
➤ Verification of syphilis as the cause of positive VDRL and RPR test results (see p. 109)

Nursing Care Before the Procedure

Client preparation is the same as that for any study involving the collection of a peripheral blood sample (see Appendix I).
➤ The client's history should be reviewed for possible sources of false-positive results.

The Procedure

A venipuncture is performed and the sample collected in a red-topped tube. The sample must be handled gently to avoid hemolysis and must be transported promptly to the laboratory.

Nursing Care After the Procedure

Care and assessment after the procedure are the same as for any study involving the collection of a peripheral blood sample.

VENEREAL DISEASE RESEARCH LABORATORY (VDRL) AND RAPID PLASMA REAGIN (RPR) TESTS

The venereal disease research laboratory (VDRL) and rapid plasma reagin (RPR) tests are flocculation tests for reagin and are used in screening for syphilis. The VDRL test uses heat-inactivated serum and can be made on slides or in tubes. The RPR test uses unheated serum or plasma, which is added to a reagent-treated plasma card. Automated procedures have been adapted for multichannel analyzers.[29]

It is noted that these tests are not specific for antibodies to *Treponema pallidum,* and many factors, including laboratory procedures, may cause false-positive results (see Table 3–12, p. 109).

Reference Values

Results are reported qualitatively as strongly reactive, reactive, weakly reactive, or negative. A degree of quantification is possible by diluting the serum and reporting the highest titer that remains positive. Positive results must be further evaluated either by repeat testing or with tests specific for antitreponemal antibodies.[30]

Interfering Factors

➤ Many factors, including laboratory procedures, may cause false-positive results (see Table 3–12, p. 109).

Indications for Venereal Disease Research Laboratory (VDRL) and Rapid Plasma Reagin (RPR) Tests

➤ Routine screening for possible syphilis
➤ Known or suspected exposure to syphilis, including congenital syphilis
➤ Verification of an antigen-antibody reaction to reagin, although a positive result is not necessarily diagnostic for syphilis
➤ Monitoring of response to treatment for syphilis, with effective treatment indicated by decreasing titers

Nursing Care Before the Procedure

Client preparation is the same as that for any study involving the collection of a peripheral blood sample (see Appendix I).

➤ A thorough history should be obtained to identify possible causes of false-positive results (see Table 3–12, p. 109).
➤ It is recommended that alcohol ingestion be avoided for 24 hours before the test.

The Procedure

A venipuncture is performed and the sample collected in a red-topped tube. The sample must be handled gently to avoid hemolysis and transported promptly to the laboratory.

➤ For neonates, a sample of cord blood may be obtained at delivery. Subsequent samples of venous blood from the infant may be required if the mother's titer is lower than that of the infant, indicating active syphilis in the infant despite successful treatment of the mother.

Nursing Care After the Procedure

Care and assessment after the procedure are the same as for any study involving the collection of a peripheral blood sample.

➤ *Abnormal values:* Note and report positive result and degree of reactivity. Assess for pregnancy and sexual contacts. Ensure that positive results are reported to the health department for follow-up and treatment of sexual contacts. Administer ordered antibiotic medication regimen. Instruct in importance of preventive measures to take during sexual activity, especially if pregnant, and the screening and treatment of sexual partner. Inform that the test should be repeated every 3 months for at least 1 year or until the reaction becomes negative. Provide a sensitive, nonjudgmental environment for the client.

Viral Infection Antibody Tests

Viral cultures either are not available or can be disproportionately expensive in relation to the potential benefit, because effective antiviral treatment is not available for most organisms. For these reasons, viral antibody tests are used to determine exposure to and existing infections with certain viruses that are difficult to culture, or they are used to screen donors before blood donation or organ transplantation (Table 3–13).

Because many types of tests can be performed, requests for viral antibody tests must be specific and include enough clinical information to permit selection of the appropriate study. A request for "viral studies" is meaningless. Antibody assays for detection of some specific disease entities, although in-

Table 3–13 ➤ TESTS FOR VIRAL DISEASE

Virus/Disease	Serologic Tests
Respiratory syndromes	
Influenza	CF, HI
Parainfluenza	
Adenoviruses	CF, HI, NT
Chlamydia	CF, IFA
Respiratory syncytial virus	
Arbovirus	CF, HI, NT
Colorado tick fever	
Yellow fever	
Meningoencephalitis	Antibodies to echo, herpes, polio, and coxsackie viruses by neutralization tests
Herpes viruses	Fluorescein-tagged antibodies in cells, EIA,
Herpes simplex*	Indirect HI
Varicella zoster	
Cytomegalovirus*	
Epstein-Barr virus	Heterophile antibody (Monotest), agglutination test, IFA
Rubella*	IgM titers, CF, HI
Mumps	
Measles	
Infectious hepatitis	IgM titers, IgG titers, hepatitis A virus antibodies (anti-Ha), CF, RIA
Serum hepatitis	Antibodies to hepatitis B virus surface antigen (HBsAb) (HBsAg)
Cytomegalic inclusion disease	CF, HI, EIA
Acquired immunodeficiency syndrome (AIDS)	Human immunodeficiency virus (HIV-1) antibodies, IFA, EIA, WIB
Leukemia and tropical spastic paraparesis	HTLV-1 and HTLV-II antibodies, ETA, WIB

Note: In the TORCH test, antibodies to *Toxoplasma gondii* (see Table 3–9, p.103), rubella virus, cytomegalovirus, and herpesvirus are measured.

CF = complement fixation, EIA = enzyme immunoassay, HI = hemagglutination inhibition, IFA = immunofluorescent antibody, NT = neutralization test, RIA = radioimmunoassay, WIB = Western immunoblot assay.

cluded in Table 3–13 (see p. 109), are outlined and discussed in the next section. They include infectious mononucleosis, hepatitis, and AIDS tests.

Reference Values

In general, lack of exposure to the virus yields a negative test result. Reference values vary with the type of viral antibody test. The laboratory performing the test should be consulted.

Indications for Viral Infection Antibody Tests

➤ Suspected AIDS or exposure to human immunodeficiency virus (HIV)
➤ Retrospective confirmation of viral infection
➤ Determination of immunity to rubella in women of childbearing age
➤ Confirmation of exposure to rubella in early pregnancy
➤ Suspected herpes encephalitis
➤ Determination of immunity to chickenpox in children with leukemia, as this infection may be fatal in such children
➤ Identification of asymptomatic carriers of cytomegalovirus (CMV)
➤ Monitoring of the course of prolonged viral disease
➤ Monitoring of mothers and neonates for exposure to viral infections that may cause congenital disease in the newborn infant (usually done by the toxoplasmosis, other infections, rubella, cytomegalovirus infection, and herpes simplex [TORCH] test—see Table 3–13, p. 112)

Nursing Care Before the Procedure

Client preparation is the same as that for any study involving the collection of a peripheral blood sample (see Appendix I).

The Procedure

A venipuncture is performed and the sample collected in a red-topped tube. The sample must be handled gently to avoid hemolysis and transported promptly to the laboratory.

Nursing Care After the Procedure

Care and assessment after the procedure are the same as for any study involving the collection of a peripheral blood sample.
➤ Women of childbearing age with low rubella titers should be appropriately immunized.
  • *Abnormal test results, complications, and precautions:* Response is dependent on the type of viral antibody test and the specific infectious process identified in Table 3–13 (see p. 109). See the specific tests that follow for nursing implications related to aftercare and observations.

INFECTIOUS MONONUCLEOSIS TESTS

Diagnosis of infectious mononucleosis, caused by Epstein-Barr virus (EBV), depends on serologic (antigen-antibody) confirmation of clinical manifestations of the disease that include fever, sore throat, and lymphadenopathy. EBV stimulates the formation of new antigens that, in turn, stimulate a humoral and cellular immune response. The humoral response is characterized by an increased titer of the antibodies IgG and IgM early in the disease. The cellular response is characterized by the activation of T cells later in the illness in response to the EBV-induced infection.

The hallmark of EBV infection is the heterophil antibody, also called the Paul-Bunnell antibody, the formation of which is stimulated by the virus. The heterophil antibody is an IgM that agglutinates sheep or horse red cells. Forssman antibody, which can be present in the serum of normal people as well as in that of individuals with serum sickness, also agglutinates with sheep erythrocytes. The Davidsohn differential absorption test can be used to distinguish between the Paul-Bunnell antibody and the Forssman antibody. Currently, more rapid and sensitive tests are available that use red blood cells from horses in a single-step agglutination test.[31] These tests (e.g., Monospot, Monoscreen) are used as screening tests for infectious mononucleosis and are gradually replacing the more traditional techniques.

Reference Values

Negative, or a titer of less than 1:56 heterophile antibodies

Interfering Factors

➤ False-positive results may occur in the presence of narcotic addiction, serum sickness, lymphomas, hepatitis, leukemia, cancer of the pancreas, and phenytoin therapy.

Indication for Infectious Mononucleosis Tests

➤ Suspected infectious mononucleosis. (Of individuals with EBV infectious mononucleosis, 95 percent will have a positive result, 86 percent in the first week of illness.)

Nursing Care Before the Procedure

Client preparation is the same as that for any study involving the collection of a peripheral blood sample (see Appendix I).

➤ A thorough history should be obtained to identify possible sources of false-positive results.

The Procedure

A venipuncture is performed and the sample collected in a red-topped tube. For screening tests, the directions accompanying the test kit are followed. For traditional tests, the sample should be sent to the laboratory promptly.

Nursing Care After the Procedure

Care and assessment after the procedure are the same as for any study involving the collection of a peripheral blood sample.

➤ *Abnormal values:* Note and report increased heterophile titer or titers against EBV. Assess signs and symptoms of infection such as fever, chills, malaise, sore throat, anorexia, enlarged lymph nodes, and fatigue. Provide rest, adequate nutritional and fluid intake, and activities that do not cause fatigue or stress.

HEPATITIS TESTS

Hepatitis tests include measurements of serologic markers that appear during the course of the disease caused by the hepatitis A virus (HAV), hepatitis B virus (HBV), hepatitis C virus (HCV), hepatitis D virus (HDV), and hepatitis E virus. Laboratory methods used in the detection of specific antigens or antibodies include radioimmunoassay (RIA) and enzyme immunoassay (EIA).

Hepatitis A is a self-limiting disease that does not usually cause liver damage or chronic infectious state. It occurs as the result of oral ingestion of the virus and is characterized by malaise, anorexia, fever, and nausea. The virus is present in the feces, but diagnosis is based on serologic markers (anti-HAV, IgM, IgG) identified in the laboratory. The diagnosis is made for hepatitis A if anti-HAV antibodies can be demonstrated in the early acute stage of the disease or if there is a high level of IgM anti-HAV compared to the level of the IgG antibody to HAV. IgM antibodies appear in the early stages, and IgG antibodies indicate past infection and immunity to reinfection.

Hepatitis B, also known as the Australian antigen, is a more serious, prolonged disease that can result in liver damage and chronic active hepatitis. HBV virus can be found in the blood, feces, saliva, semen, sweat, urine, or any body fluid of infected individuals and can be transmitted by exposure to blood products or parenteral contact with articles contaminated with material containing the virus. Diagnosis is made by identification of the hepatitis B surface antigen (HBsAg) circulating in the blood before and during the acute early stage before enzyme elevations or in chronic carriers after an acute illness. It is the first indicator of acute hepatitis infection. The recovery from and immunity to HBV as late as 6 to 10 months after an active infection are identified by the detection of anti-HBs. The presence of hepatitis B antibody (anti-HBe, HBeAB) indicates the resolution of acute infection or, along with positive HBsAg, indicates an asymptomatic, healthy carrier. The presence of hepatitis Be antigen (HBeAg) is an early indicator of hepatitis B infection. If HBeAg persists for more than 3 months, it is indicative of chronic infection. Delta hepatitis coinfects with HBV, and diagnosis is made by detection of the antibodies (anti-D) in the blood.

Hepatitis C is a parenterally acquired disease usually caused by blood transfusion but also by IV drug abuse. The disease can lead to chronic hepatitis and cirrhosis of the liver. The test is performed to detect the antibodies to HCV in the blood of those at risk for the infection and transmission of the virus as a blood donor. Antibody formation can take as long as a year after exposure to the virus.

Hepatitis D is caused by a "defective" virus that can produce infection only when HBV is present. HDV antigens do not circulate and are found only in hepatocytes. Hepatitis D occurs with HBV and can result in more serious disease in individuals with chronic HBV infection. Hepatitis D is also known as *delta agent hepatitis.*

Hepatitis E is similar in presentation and disease course to hepatitis A. It occurs primarily in Asia, Africa, and South America.[32]

Reference Values

Hepatitis A	
Anti-HAV	Negative
IgM	Negative
IgG	Negative
Hepatitis B	
Surface antigen (HBsAg)	Negative
Surface antibody (HBsAb)	Negative
B antigen (HBeAg)	Negative
B antibody (HBeAb)	Negative
Core antibody (anti-HBcAb)	Negative
Hepatitis C	
C antibody (anti-HCV)	Negative
Hepatitis D	
Delta antibody (anti-HDV)	Negative

Interfering Factors

➤ The administration of radionuclides within 1 week of testing using RIA technique can cause inaccurate results.
➤ Rheumatoid factor and competing IgG-specific antibody can cause inaccurate positive and negative results.

Indications for Hepatitis Tests

➤ Detection of the presence of antigen or antibody to a specific type of hepatitis depending on symptoms and stage of the disease in the diagnosis of the condition
➤ Determination of possible hepatitis carrier status
➤ Determination of past exposure or immunity status in those with a history of hepatitis
➤ Screening of pretransfusion donors for a history or presence of hepatitis, especially if asymptomatic and information source questionable
➤ Determination of progression to chronic hepatitis or persistent signs and symptoms of liver dysfunction

Nursing Care Before the Procedure

Client preparation is the same as for any study involving the collection of a peripheral blood sample (see Appendix I).
➤ Obtain a thorough history regarding possible ingestion of contaminated water or foods, environmental sanitation factors conducive to occurrence, recent blood transfusion, parenteral exposure to materials contaminated by blood or body fluids, personal contact through sexual activity, or presence of pregnancy (the infection could be transmitted to the infant).[33]

The Procedure

A venipuncture is performed and the sample collected in a red-topped tube. For screening tests, the directions accompanying the test kit are followed. For traditional testing, the sample should be sent to the laboratory promptly, with the test performed within 7 days or frozen for future analysis.

Nursing Care After the Procedure

Care and assessment after the procedure are the same as for any study involving the collection of a peripheral blood sample.

➤ *Abnormal values:* Note and report presence of antigen or antibody to a specific type of hepatitis. Provide rest and energy-saving assistance as needed, skin care for jaundice and pruritus, and adequate nutritional and fluid intake.

➤ *Disease transmission:* Note and report type of hepatitis. If hepatitis A, place client on enteric precautions. If hepatitis B, C, or D, observe standard precautions for blood-borne pathogens (see Appendix III for hand protection, personal protection, and needles and sharps), and instruct in precautions against transmission via sharing of needles by IV drug abusers and sexual contact.

➤ *Disease prevention:* Hepatitis A and B vaccines for active immunity. Instruct client to avoid donating blood for 6 months if a transfusion has been received and to never donate blood if diagnosis of hepatitis B has been made.

ACQUIRED IMMUNODEFICIENCY SYNDROME (AIDS) TESTS

AIDS and the early stages of HIV infection are diseases of the immune system caused by the human immunodeficiency virus or HIV-2. This virus is responsible for infecting and destroying the T-helper lymphocytes (CD4 cells). This destruction, in turn, affects the ability of the body to produce antibodies and suppresses cellular immune responses, leading to disorders and infections by many opportunistic infectious agents. The average time from HIV infection to full-blown AIDS is approximately 10 years. The clinical manifestations of the infection also can vary from an initially mild illness to an acute state. Those at high risk for the disease include male homosexuals, hemophiliacs, recipients of blood or blood products before 1985, and IV drug users who share needles. Heterosexual transmission of the virus is on the rise.[34]

After the virus has been acquired, antigens are detectable in the blood serum as early as 2 weeks, and they remain for 2 to 4 months. At this time, antibodies appear. Late in the disease, antigens reappear and antibodies decrease, indicating a poor prognosis. The most common tests to screen for HIV-1 virus antibodies are the EIA, also known as the enzyme-linked immunosorbent assay (ELISA), and the immunofluorescence assay. The test is repeated if the results are positive or borderline. Repeat testing after a positive value requires confirmation by the Western immunoblot (WIB) assay, which has the ability to identify antibodies to at least nine different epitopes of HIV-1. Antigen testing in the early stages of HIV-1 infections before antibodies are detected can be undertaken to monitor clients for progression of the disease and response to therapy. It is also useful to diagnose HIV-1 infection in infants when maternal antibodies are passively transferred and diagnosis based on serologic testing is difficult.[35]

Reference Values

➤ Negative for HIV antigen by antigen capture assay during initial infectious state and in advanced state of the disease

➤ Negative for HIV antibodies by antibody detection methods, EIA, and immunofluorescence assay

➤ Negative for confirmation test for HIV antibodies by WIB

Interfering Factors

➤ Negative results can occur in infected individuals because of lack of anti-body formation early in the disease and in late stages because of loss of ability to produce antibodies.

➤ Inaccurate results can occur with the use of test kits that contain proteins if an individual has been exposed to the media used in the kits.

➤ Cross-reactive antibodies directed to antigenic determinants found in non-pathogenic retroviruses can result in inaccurate positive results.[36]

➤ Children who become infected before birth through an infected mother can have inaccurate negative results.

➤ Corticosteroids can affect lymphocyte subset test results.

➤ Protease inhibitors can inhibit replication of infected cells and cell-to-cell spread of HIV.

Indications for Acquired Immunodeficiency Syndrome (AIDS) Tests

➤ Detection of the core p24 protein and antibodies to the identified protein in the diagnosis and staging or progression of infections in AIDS

➤ Confirmation of positive test results obtained by EIA to ensure accurate results

➤ Determination of the extent of CD4 (T-helper lymphocytes) cell decreases in relation to normal or increased levels of CD8 (T-suppressor) cells to pre-dict immunodeficiency state

➤ Prediction of exacerbation of the disease by increased protein β_2-microglob-ulin, indicating destruction of lymphocytes and macrophages

➤ Assistance in the diagnosis of AIDS in the presence of opportunistic infec-tions determined by culture and microorganism identification

➤ Screening of those in high-risk groups for the development of AIDS

➤ Screening of blood donors by blood banks before obtaining blood donations

➤ Screening of blood before using for transfusion or preparation of blood products

Nursing Care Before the Procedure

Client preparation is the same as for any study involving the collection of a pe-ripheral blood sample (see Appendix I).

➤ Obtain a history regarding possible contact with the virus such as sexual practices, drug abuse with needle sharing, transfusion with contaminated blood products, or presence of pregnancy (virus could be transmitted to the infant). Inform the client of confidentiality and legal requirements regarding the test performance and test results.

The Procedure

A venipuncture is performed and the sample collected in a red- (antigen or anti-body) or lavender-topped (lymphocyte or microglobulin) tube, depending on the tests to be performed. Appropriate apparel (gloves and mask) and precau-tions for blood-borne pathogens are carried out when obtaining and caring for the blood samples (see Appendix III).

Nursing Care After the Procedure

Care and assessment after the procedure are the same as for any study involving the collection of a peripheral blood sample.

➤ *Abnormal values:* Note and report positive test results. Inform client of the most current information regarding medications, economic and social assistance, and possible psychological counseling services. Instruct client in adequate nutritional and fluid intake. Provide a sensitive, nonjudgmental, and caring environment for the client.

➤ *Disease transmission:* Instruct client in precautions to take during sexual activity; advise to avoid sharing needles during drug use and to avoid donating blood. Provide care using standard precautions and observing transmission-based isolation procedures for blood-borne pathogens.

➤ *Medicolegal aspects:* Observe regulations for confidentiality in reporting test results, such as use of computer or telephone. Maintain confidentiality of records containing test results. Carry out state regulation regarding the reporting of positive results. Provide a form for physician to sign regarding any risks associated with testing and obtain a signed informed permission request before the test.

IMMUNOLOGIC TESTS RELATED TO CANCER

Tumor markers are defined as a substance produced by malignant or benign cells in response to the presence of cancer. They are detected by the examination of body fluids and tissue specimens. Their use includes tumor prediction, detection, and identification; monitoring of the course and prognosis; and evaluation of therapy protocols. The most desirable markers are those that can detect malignancy in a remote area by the analysis of body fluids (serum, urine, fluid from effusion, and CSF) rather than by invasive procedures to obtain a tissue sample. The markers are classified as endocrine (hormones), metabolic consequences associated with tumor (albumin, blood cells, lipids), enzymes and isozymes, oncofetal antigens or glycoproteins, and gene alteration or oncogenes. Current tumor markers and some clinical associations in use at this time are listed in Table 3–14.[37,38] Panels of tumor markers to assist in the identification or confirmation of a malignancy in relation to tissue site and to assist in monitoring the course and prognosis of the malignancy are also performed.

Malignancies or cancer can invade organ tissue, access vascular channels, and metastasize to other body sites. They are characterized by an abnormal number of cells that grow without the normal control and immune abilities of the body. There is no single molecular or morphologic characteristic specific to malignancies.[39] This allows for the presence of abnormal reference values associated with benign cells and conditions other than cancer. Complete specific test information regarding the blood cells, enzyme, hormone, endocrine, and metabolic markers listed in Table 3–14 (see p. 120) is included in the respective chapters. These tests are commonly performed to obtain information about many other disorders, and differentiation is made when analyzing the results in the diagnosis of malignancy. Antigens and globulins, used in the diagnosis and treatment of cancer and commonly found in fetal life, are considered individually in this section. These substances are considered abnormal in adults if present in excessive amounts.

Table 3-14 ➤ CANCER TESTS AND TUMOR MARKERS

Marker	Clinical Association
Alkaline phosphatase (ALP) (enzyme isozyme)	Osteogenic sarcoma, osteoblastic carcinoma metastasis
α-Fetoprotein (AFP) (oncofetal antigen)	Testicular, hepatic carcinoma
CA 15-3 antigen (oncofetal antigen)	Breast malignancy
CA 19-9 antigen (oncofetal antigen)	Stomach, colon, pancreatic carcinoma
CA 50 antigen (oncofetal antigen)	Stomach, colon, pancreatic carcinoma
CA 125 antigen (oncofetal antigen)	Ovarian, fallopian tube carcinoma
Calcitonin (polypeptide hormone)	Thyroid medullary carcinoma
Carcinoembryonic antigen (CEA) (oncofetal antigen)	Breast, colon, lung carcinoma
Catecholamines (vanillylmandelic acid metabolite)	Neuroblastoma and pheochromocytoma
Creatine kinase isoenzyme (CK-BB) (enzyme isoenzyme)	Breast, pulmonary carcinoma
DU-PAN-2 (glycoprotein antigen)	Pancreatic carcinoma
Galactosyltransferase (GT II) (enzyme isoenzyme)	Pancreatic carcinoma
Genetic mutation (DNA, oncogenes)	Predisposition to development of carcinoma, leukemia, lymphoma
Human chorionic gonadotropin (hCG) (glycoprotein hormone)	Testicular carcinoma
5-Hydroxyindoleacetic acid (5-HIAA) (serotonin metabolite)	Carcinoid tumor
Immunoglobulins produced by B lymphocytes	Multiple myeloma, lymphomas
Lactate dehydrogenase (LD) (enzyme isoenzyme LD_1)	Renal carcinoma, leukemia, lymphoma
Lymphocyte B- and T-cell surface antigens (blood cell)	Lymphomas, lymphoblastic leukemia
Neuron-specific enolase (NSE) (enolase isoenzyme)	Neuroblastoma, lung carcinoma
Prostate-specific antigen (PSA) (serine protease)	Prostatic carcinoma
Prostatic acid phosphatase (PAP) (enzyme isozyme)	Prostatic carcinoma
Tissue polypeptide antigen (TPA) (oncofetal antigen)	Breast, lung, liver, pancreas, colorectal, stomach, ovary, prostate, bladder, head and neck, thyroid carcinoma
Squamous cell carcinoma (SCC) antigen (protein antigen)	Cervical, lung, esophageal, head and neck carcinoma
Vasoactive intestinal peptide (VIP)	Intestinal tumor

SERUM α-FETOPROTEIN (AFP) TEST

During the first 10 weeks of life, the major serum protein is not albumin, but α-fetoprotein (AFP). Fetal liver synthesizes huge quantities of AFP until about the 32nd week of gestation. Thereafter, synthesis declines until, at 1 year of age, the serum normally contains no more than 30 ng/mL.

Resting liver cells (hepatocytes) normally manufacture very little AFP, but rapidly multiplying hepatocytes resume synthesis of large amounts.[40] Thus, the test's greatest usefulness is in monitoring for recurrence of hepatic carcinoma or metastatic lesions involving the liver. It should be noted that 30 to 50 percent of Americans with liver cancer do not have elevated AFP levels. More consistent elevations are seen in those Asian and African populations with a very high incidence of hepatocellular carcinoma.[41]

Measurement of AFP levels in maternal blood and amniotic fluid is used to detect certain fetal abnormalities, especially neural tube defects such as anencephaly, spina bifida, and myelomeningocele (see Chap. 10). Routine prenatal screening includes determination of the mother's serum AFP level at 13 to 16 weeks of pregnancy. If maternal blood levels are elevated on two samples obtained 1 week apart, an ultrasound may be performed, and AFP levels in amniotic fluid may be analyzed. Other possible causes of elevated AFP levels during pregnancy include multiple pregnancy and fetal demise.

Reference Values

	Conventional Units	**SI Units**
Neonates	600,000 ng/mL	600,000 µg/L
1 yr old to adults	<30 ng/mL	<30 µg/L

Indications for Serum α-Fetoprotein (AFP) Tes

➤ Monitoring for hepatic carcinoma or metastatic lesions involving the liver, as indicated by highly elevated levels (e.g., 10,000 to 100,000 ng/mL)
➤ Monitoring for response to treatment for hepatic carcinoma, with successful treatment indicated by an immediate drop in levels
➤ Monitoring for recurrence of hepatic carcinoma, with elevated levels occurring 1 to 6 months before the client becomes symptomatic
➤ Suspected hepatitis or cirrhosis, as indicated by slightly to moderately elevated levels (e.g., 500 ng/mL)
➤ Routine prenatal screening for fetal neural tube defects and other disorders, as indicated by elevated levels
➤ Suspected intrauterine fetal death, as indicated by elevated levels
➤ Support for diagnosing embryonal gonadal teratoblastoma, hepatoblastoma, and ataxia-telangiectasia

Nursing Care Before the Procedure

For serum studies, client preparation is the same as that for any study involving the collection of a peripheral blood sample (see Appendix I).

For amniotic fluid studies, the client is prepared for amniocentesis, as described in Chapter 10.

The Procedure

For serum studies, a venipuncture is performed and the sample collected in a red-topped tube. The sample must be handled gently to avoid hemolysis and transported promptly to the laboratory. For amniotic fluid studies, amniocentesis is performed (see Chap. 10).

Nursing Care After the Procedure

Care and assessment after the procedures are the same as for any study involving collection of a peripheral blood sample or amniocentesis (see Chap. 10).

➤ *Abnormal adult values:* Note and report increased levels and relate to tissue healing or regeneration. Assess history for presence and/or treatment of malignancy; assist in coping with need for additional treatments.
➤ *Abnormal fetal values:* Note and report increased levels in amniotic fluid analysis results or pregnant woman's serum test results. Assess for fear and

anxiety levels while waiting for test results. Provide information about genetic counseling or termination of pregnancy, or both.

CARCINOEMBRYONIC ANTIGEN (CEA) TEST

Carcinoembryonic antigen (CEA) is a glycoprotein normally produced only during early fetal life and during rapid multiplication of epithelial cells, especially those of the digestive system. Elevations of CEA occur with many cancers, primary and recurrent, as well as with a number of nonmalignant diseases and in smokers (Table 3–15). Although the test is not diagnostic for any specific disease, it is used primarily when various types of carcinomas are suspected.

Reference Values

Less than 2.5 ng/mL

Interfering Factors

➤ Levels may be elevated in smokers who do not have malignancies.

Indications for Carcinoembryonic Antigen (CEA) Test

➤ Monitoring of clients with inflammatory intestinal disorders with a high risk of malignancy
➤ Suspected carcinoma of the colon, pancreas, or lung, as these cancers produce the highest CEA levels

Table 3–15 ➤ CAUSES OF ALTERATIONS IN CEA LEVELS

Cause of Alteration	PERCENTAGE WITH CEA LEVELS, NG/ML			
	<2.5	2.6–5	5.1–10	>10
Nonsmokers	97	3	0	0
Smokers	81	15	3	1
Ex-smokers	93	5	1	1
Carcinomas				
Colorectal	28	23	14	34
Pulmonary	24	25	25	25
Gastric	39	32	10	19
Pancreatic	9	31	26	35
Breast	53	21	13	14
Head/neck	48	32	14	5
Other	53	27	12	9
Leukemias	63	25	8	5
Lymphoma	65	24	11	0
Sarcoma	68	26	5	0
Benign tumors	82	12	6	1
Benign breast disease	85	11	4	0
Pulmonary emphysema	43	37	16	4
Alcoholic cirrhosis	29	44	24	2
Ulcerative colitis	69	18	8	5
Regional ileitis	60	27	11	2
Gastric ulcer	55	29	15	1
Colorectal polyps	81	14	3	1
Diverticulitis	73	20	5	2

➤ Monitoring of response to therapy for cancer, with effective treatment indicated by normal levels within 4 to 6 weeks
➤ Monitoring for recurrence of carcinoma, with elevated levels occurring several months before the client becomes symptomatic
➤ Suspected leukemia, gammopathy, or other disorder associated with elevated CEA levels (Table 3–15, p. 122)

Nursing Care Before the Procedure

Client preparation is the same as that for any study involving the collection of a peripheral blood sample (see Appendix I).

The Procedure

A venipuncture is performed and the sample collected in a red-topped tube. The sample must be handled gently to avoid hemolysis and transported promptly to the laboratory.

Nursing Care After the Procedure

Care and assessment after the procedure are the same as for any study involving collection of a peripheral blood sample.
➤ *Abnormal values:* Note and report increased values or return of increased values. Assess history for presence of malignancy and site or treatment of malignancy. Assist client and family in coping with need for additional treatments or poor prognosis.

CA 15-3, CA 19-9, CA 50, AND CA 125
ANTIGEN TESTS

Cancer antigens are substances detected in serum or tissue and are defined by one or two monoclonal antibodies. Immunologic methods are used to detect the substances in serum and immunohistochemical methods in tissue. Assay kits for these markers are available to ensure consistent values among agencies performing the tests. These tumor markers are not used for screening malignancy in asymptomatic populations.

CA 15-3 is a serum antigen defined by two monoclonal antibodies found in breast cancer and breast cancer metastasis to the liver as well as in benign diseases of the breast. CA 19-9 is a serum antigen defined by a monoclonal antibody found in malignancies of the pancreas, gallbladder, salivary glands, and endocervix as well as in benign disorders such as acute pancreatitis, inflammatory bowel disease, and hepatobiliary disease. The test is commonly performed to monitor the course of a malignancy that is known to produce the antigen. CA 50 is a serum antigen defined by a monoclonal antibody found in pancreatic, colorectal, and gastrointestinal malignancies. Besides its diagnostic value, CA 50 is used to monitor the course of a tumor that produces the antigen. CA 125 is a serum antigen defined by a monoclonal antibody found in ovarian and pelvic organ malignancies as well as in breast and pancreatic malignancies. Nonmalignant conditions such as ascites of benign cause, pregnancy, menstruation, endometriosis, and pelvic inflammatory disease also cause increases in this antigen. The test is undertaken to monitor surgical removal of malignant ovarian tumor for recurrence and metastasis. Another test, tissue polypeptide antigen (TPA), is a marker identified in serum and tissue in those with a variety of malignancies in relation to the extent of the disease and subsequent recurrence or regression after surgical removal of the tumor.[42]

Reference Values

	Conventional Units	SI Units
CA 15-3	<35 U/ml	<35 kU/L
CA 19-9	<37 U/ml	<37 kU/L
CA 50	<37 U/ml	<37 kU/L
CA 125	<35 U/ml	<35 kU/L

Interfering Factors

➤ Chemotherapeutic agents administered to treat tumor.
➤ Levels can be increased in the absence of disease or in benign disorders and can affect diagnostic findings for malignancy.

Indications for CA 15-3, CA 19-9, CA 50, and CA 125 Antigen Tests

➤ Diagnosis and confirmation of presence of local and metastatic malignancy, suggested by an increased level or a gradual rise in levels of the specific cancer antigen
➤ Determination of residual tumor after surgical intervention to remove the malignancy
➤ Monitoring of course of the malignancy and effectiveness of therapeutic regimen to determine progression, prognosis, or recurrence
➤ Differentiation between malignant and benign disorders of specific organ tissues

Nursing Care Before the Procedure

Client preparation is the same as for any study involving the collection of a peripheral blood sample (see Appendix I).
➤ Obtain a history regarding the presence of other acute or chronic diseases and the assessment data that support the diagnoses.
➤ Ensure that neoplastic medication protocols are administered.

The Procedure

A venipuncture is performed and the sample collected in a red-topped tube. The sample should be transported promptly to the laboratory for analysis by immunoassay methods.

Nursing Care After the Procedure

Care and assessment after the procedure are the same as for any study involving the collection of a peripheral blood sample.
➤ *Abnormal values:* Note and report increased values or return of increased values. Assess for presence of malignancy site or metastasis or both, past or ongoing treatments, and procedures for malignancy. Assist client and family to reduce anxiety and to cope with need for additional treatments or poor prognosis.

Student Name _____ Class _____

Instructor _____ Date _____

CASE STUDY AND CRITICAL THINKING EXERCISE

Mr. Good, a 36-year-old man, comes to the clinic with a 3-month history of night sweats, bouts of diarrhea, and increasing fatigue. He has hepato-splenomegaly and generalized lymphadenopathy. His WBC is 1600. An ELISA test indicates a positive result.

a. What do you suspect Mr. Good's diagnosis to be?

b. What specific manifestations did you consider in identifying this diagnosis?

c. What is an ELISA test?

d. What is Pneumocystis carinii pneumonia (PCP)? How does it relate to this diagnosis?

References

1. Sacher, RA, and McPherson, RA: Widmann's Clinical Interpretation of Laboratory Tests, ed 10. FA Davis, Philadelphia, 1991, p 63.
2. Boggs, DR, and Winkelstein, A: White Cell Manual, ed 4. FA Davis, Philadelphia, 1983, p 61.
3. Ibid, pp 61–62.
4. Ibid, p 63.
5. Ibid, pp 63–64.
6. Ibid, pp 68–71.
7. Ibid, p 74.
8. Sacher and McPherson, op cit, pp 242–243.
9. Ibid, p 244.
10. Boggs and Winkelstein, op cit, p 69.
11. Ibid, p 69.
12. Ibid, pp 69–73.
13. Ibid, pp 72–73.
14. Ibid, p 74.
15. Ibid, p 65.
16. Sacher and McPherson, op cit, p 256.
17. Ibid, p 256.
18. Ibid, pp 252–253.
19. Ibid, pp 252–254.
20. Boggs and Winkelstein, op cit, pp 83–84.
21. Sacher and McPherson, op cit, p 253.
22. Ibid, p 246.
23. Ibid, p 246.
24. Ibid, pp 254–255.
25. Ibid, p 255.
26. Ibid, p 262.
27. Ibid, pp 531–532.
28. Ibid, p 531.
29. Ibid, p 531.
30. Ibid, p 532.
31. Ibid, p 542.
32. Centers for Disease Control and Prevention, Hepatitis Branch: Epidemiology and prevention of viral hepatitis A to E: An overview. CDC, 1998.
33. Sacher and McPherson, op cit, pp 441–442.
34. Ray, CG, and Minnich, LL: Viruses, rickettsia, and chlamydia. In James, JB: Clinical Diagnosis and Management by Laboratory Methods, ed 18. WB Saunders, Philadelphia, 1991, p 1249.
35. Ibid, pp 1249–1250.
36. Stevens, RW, and McQuillan, GM: Serodiagnosis of human immunodeficiency virus (HIV) and hepatitis B virus (HBV) infections. In James, JB: Clinical Diagnosis and Management by Laboratory Methods, ed 18. WB Saunders, Philadelphia, 1991, pp 913–914.
37. Rooney, MT, and Henry, JB: Molecular markers of malignant neoplasms. In James, JB: Clinical Diagnosis and Management by Laboratory Methods, ed 18. WB Saunders, Philadelphia, 1991, pp 285–286.
38. Sacher and McPherson, op cit, p 779.
39. Rooney and Henry, op cit, p 286.
40. Sacher and McPherson, op cit, pp 437–438.
41. Ibid, p 438.
42. Rooney and Henry, op cit, pp 297–298.

Bibliography

Bellanti, JA: Immunology: Basic Processes, ed 2. WB Saunders, Philadelphia, 1985.

Bryant, NJ: Laboratory Immunology and Serology, ed 3. WB Saunders, Philadelphia, 1992.

Byrne, CJ, et al: Laboratory Tests: Implications for Nursing Care. Addison-Wesley, Menlo Park, Calif, 1986.

Chernecky, CC, and Berger, BJ; Cullen, BN (ed): Laboratory Tests and Diagnostic Procedures, ed 2. WB Saunders, Philadelphia, 1996.

Corbett, JV: Laboratory Tests and Diagnostic Procedures with Nursing Diagnoses, ed 4. Appleton & Lange, Norwalk, Conn, 1995.

Deglin, JH, and Vallerand, AH: Davis's Drug Guide for Nurses, ed 6. FA Davis, Philadelphia, 1999.

Fischbach, FT: A Manual of Laboratory and Diagnostic Tests, ed 5. Lippincott-Raven, Philadelphia, 1995.

Henry, JB: Clinical Diagnosis and Management by Laboratory Methods, ed 19. WB Saunders, Philadelphia, 1996.

Kee, JL: Handbook of Laboratory and Diagnostic Tests with Nursing Implications, ed 3. Appleton & Lange, Norwalk, Conn, 1997.

Lewis, SM, et al (eds): Medical-Surgical Nursing: Assessment and Management of Clinical Problems, ed 4. Mosby–Year Book, St Louis, 1995.

Miller, LE, et al: Manual of Laboratory Immunology, ed 2. Williams & Wilkins, Baltimore, 1990.

Pagana, KD, and Pagana, TJ: Diagnostic and Laboratory Test Reference, ed 3. Mosby–Year Book, St Louis, 1996.

Porth, CM: Pathophysiology: Concepts of Altered Health States, ed 4. JB Lippincott, Philadelphia, 1993.

Sheehan, C: Clinical Immunology: Principles and Laboratory Diagnosis, ed 2. Lippincott-Raven, Philadelphia, 1997.

Springhouse Corporation: Clinical Laboratory Tests: Values and Implications, ed 2. Springhouse, Springhouse, Pa, 1995.

Springhouse Corporation: Nurse's Reference Library, Diagnostic Tests, ed 3. Springhouse, Springhouse, Pa, 1991.

Tietz, NW: Clinical Guide to Diagnostic Tests, ed 3. WB Saunders, Philadelphia, 1997.

Turgeon, ML: Immunology and Serology in Laboratory Medicine, ed 2. Mosby – Year Book, St Louis, 1996.

Whaley, LF: Nursing Care of Infants and Children, ed 4. Mosby – Year Book, St Louis, 1991.

Wallach, J: Interpretation of Diagnostic Tests: A Synopsis of Laboratory Medicine, ed 6. Little, Brown & Co, Boston, 1996.

4

Immunohematology and Blood Banking

➤ **TESTS COVERED**

ABO Blood Typing, *129*
Rh Typing, *132*
Direct Antiglobulin Test (DAT, Direct Coombs'), *134*

Indirect Antiglobulin Test (IAT, Indirect Coombs', Antibody Screening Test), *135*
Human Leukocyte Antigens (HLA), *136*

INTRODUCTION

Immunohematology is the study of the antigens present on blood cell membranes and the antibodies stimulated by their presence. For red cells, more than 300 antigenic configurations have been discovered and classified. A specific biologic role has been identified for only a few of these (e.g., ABO and Rh typing for blood transfusions). One commonality is that blood cell antigens are inherited, and the genes that determine them follow the laws of mendelian genetics.[1] Thus, the greatest usefulness of many of the blood cell antigens that have been identified to date is in genetic studies.

The focus of this chapter is on tests of blood cell antigens and related antibodies that are used in determining the compatibility of blood and blood products for transfusions.

ABO BLOOD TYPING

The major antigens in the ABO system are A and B. An individual with A antigens has type A blood; an individual with B antigens has type B blood. A person with both A and B antigens has type AB blood, and one having neither A nor B antigens has type O blood. The genes determining the presence or absence of A or B antigens reside on chromosome number 9.[2] Immunologically competent individuals more than 6 months of age have serum antibodies that react with the A and B antigens absent from their own red cells (Table 4–1). Thus, a person with type A blood has anti-B antibodies, whereas one with type B blood has anti-A antibodies. Individuals with type AB blood have neither of these antibodies, whereas those with type O blood have both. These antibodies are not inherited, but develop after exposure to environmental antigens that are chemically similar to red cell antigens (e.g., pollens and bacteria). Individuals do not, however, develop antibodies to their own red cell antigens.[3,4]

Table 4–1 ➤ ANTIGENS AND ANTIBODIES IN ABO BLOOD GROUPS

Blood Group	Antigens on Red Cells	Antibodies in Serum	FREQUENCY, % IN US POPULATIONS			
			Whites	American Blacks	Native Americans	Asians
A	A	Anti-B	40	27	16	28
B	B	Anti-A	11	20	4	27
O	Neither	Anti-A Anti-B	45	49	79	40
AB	A and B	Neither	4	4	<1	5

From Sacher, RA, and McPherson, RA: Widmann's Clinical Interpretation of Laboratory Tests, ed 10. FA Davis, Philadelphia, 1991, p. 268, with permission.

Anti-A and anti-B antibodies are strong agglutinins and cause rapid, complement-mediated destruction (see Chap. 3) of any incompatible cells encountered. Although most of the anti-A and anti-B activity resides in the IgM class of immunoglobulins (see Chap. 3), some activity rests with IgG. Anti-A and anti-B antibodies of the IgG class coat the red cells without immediately affecting their viability and can readily cross the placenta, resulting in hemolytic disease of the newborn. Persons with type O blood frequently have more IgG anti-A and anti-B antibodies than do individuals with type A or B blood. Thus, ABO hemolytic disease of the newborn (erythroblastosis fetalis) affects infants of type O mothers almost exclusively.[5]

When blood transfusions are required, the client is normally given blood of his or her own type to prevent adverse antigen-antibody reactions. In emergency situations, however, some individuals may be given blood of other ABO types. For example, because type O blood has neither A nor B antigens, it may be given to individuals with types A, B, and AB blood. Thus, a person with type O blood is called a *universal donor.* With the advent of colloid expanders (e.g., dextran), untyped blood is not given even in cases of hemorrhage. Further, because persons with type O blood have both anti-A and anti-B antibodies, they can receive only type O blood.

The situation is reversed for those with type AB blood. Because these individuals lack anti-A and anti-B antibodies, they may receive transfusions of types A, B, and O blood in emergencies when type AB blood is not available. Thus, a person with type AB blood is called a *universal recipient.*

ABO blood typing is an agglutination test in which the client's red cells are mixed with anti-A and anti-B sera, a process known as *forward grouping.* The procedure is then reversed, and the person's serum is mixed with known type A and type B cells (i.e., *reverse grouping*). When a transfusion is to be administered, cross-matching blood from the donor and the recipient is performed along with typing. Cross-matching detects antibodies in the sera of the donor and the recipient, which may lead to a transfusion reaction as a result of red cell destruction.

Other pretransfusion or post-transfusion tests can be performed to determine the cause of transfusion reactions. The leukoagglutinins are antibodies in the donor blood that react with white blood cells in the recipient's blood, producing fever, cough, dyspnea, and other lung complications, depending on the severity of the reaction after the transfusion. It requires that leukocyte-poor blood be used to transfuse these clients. Platelet antibody tests are performed to detect specific antibodies that cause post-transfusion purpuric reactions. Assays as well as platelet typing can be performed to support a diagnosis of post-transfusion purpura and thrombocytopenic purpura.[6]

Reference Values

The normal distribution of the four ABO blood groups in the United States is shown in Table 4–1 (p. 130). Discrepancies in the results of forward and reverse grouping may occur in infants, elderly persons, and persons who are immunosuppressed or who have a variety of immunologic disorders.[7]

Indications for ABO Typing

➤ Identification of the client's ABO blood type, especially before surgery or other procedures in which blood loss is a threat or for which replacement may be needed, or both
➤ Identification of donor ABO blood type for stored blood
➤ Determination of ABO compatibility of donor's and recipient's bloods
➤ Identification of maternal and infant ABO blood types to predict potential hemolytic disease of the newborn

Nursing Care Before the Procedure

Client preparation is the same as that for any study involving the collection of a peripheral blood sample (see Appendix I).
➤ Immunosuppressive drugs taken by the client or the presence of immunologic disorder should be noted.

The Procedure

A venipuncture is performed and the sample collected in a red-topped tube or other type of blood collection tube, depending on laboratory preference. The sample must be handled gently to avoid hemolysis and sent promptly to the laboratory.

Although correct client identification is important for all laboratory and diagnostic procedures, it is crucial when blood is collected for ABO typing. One of the most common sources of error in ABO typing is incorrect identification of the client and the specimens.[8]

Nursing Care After the Procedure

Care and assessment after the procedure are the same as for any study involving the collection of a peripheral blood sample.
➤ The client should be informed of his or her blood type, and the information should be recorded on a card or other document (e.g., driver's license) that the client normally carries in the event of an emergency requiring a blood transfusion.
➤ *Circulatory overload:* Report increased blood pressure; bounding pulse; and signs of pulmonary edema such as dyspnea, rapid and labored breathing, cough producing blood-stained sputum, and cyanosis.

➤ *Blood transfusion reaction:* Note and report reduced blood pressure, elevated temperature, chills, palpitations, substernal or flank pain, warmth at the infusion site, or anxiety. Discontinue transfusion and infuse saline. Send the leftover unit of blood and a blood and urine specimen to the laboratory.

➤ **Critical values:** Notify physician immediately if there is an incompatible cross-match.

RH TYPING

After the ABO system, the Rh system is the group of red cell antigens with the greatest importance.[9] The antigen was called the Rh factor because it was produced by immunizing guinea pigs and rabbits with red cells of rhesus monkeys. Researchers found that the serum from the immunized animals agglutinated not only the rhesus monkey red cells but also the red cells of approximately 85 percent of humans. Thus, human red cells could be classified into two new blood types: Rh-positive and Rh-negative. This discovery was a great breakthrough in explaining transfusion reactions to blood that had been tested for ABO compatibility as well as in explaining hemolytic disease of the newborn not caused by ABO incompatibility between mother and fetus.[10]

It is now known that the Rh system includes many different antigens. The major antigen is termed Rh_o or D. Persons whose red cells possess D are called Rh-positive; those who lack D are called Rh-negative, no matter what other Rh antigens are present, because the D antigen is more likely to provoke an antibody response than any other red cell antigen, including those of the ABO system. The other major antigens of the Rh system are C, E, c, and e.[11] Among blacks, there are many quantitative and qualitative variants of the Rh antigens that do not always fit into the generally accepted classifications.[12]

Rh-negative individuals may produce anti-D antibodies if exposed to Rh-positive cells through either blood transfusions or pregnancy. Although 50 to 70 percent of Rh-negative individuals develop antibodies if transfused with Rh-positive blood, only 20 percent of Rh-negative mothers develop anti-D antibodies after carrying an Rh-positive fetus. This difference occurs because a greater number of cells are involved in a blood transfusion than are involved in pregnancy.

When Rh antibodies develop, they are predominantly IgG. Thus, they coat the red cells and set them up for destruction in the reticuloendothelial system. The antibodies seldom activate the complement system (see Chap. 3). Anti-D antibodies readily cross the placenta from mother to fetus and are the most common cause of severe hemolytic disease of the newborn. Immunosuppressive therapy (e.g., with Rh_o [D] immune globulin [RhoGAM]) successfully prevents antibody formation when given to an unimmunized Rh-negative mother just after delivery or abortion of an Rh-positive fetus.[13]

Rh typing involves an agglutination test in which the client's red cells are mixed with serum containing anti-D antibodies. Agglutination indicates that the D antigen is present, and the person is termed Rh-positive.

Reference Values

The D antigen is present on the red cells of 85 percent of whites and a higher percentage of blacks, Native Americans, and Asians.

Indications for Rh Typing

➤ Identification of the client's Rh type, especially before surgery or other procedures in which blood loss is a threat or for which replacement may be needed, or for both
➤ Identification of donor Rh type for stored blood
➤ Determination of Rh compatibility of donor's and recipient's blood
➤ Identification of maternal and infant Rh types to predict potential hemolytic disease of the newborn
➤ Determination of anti-D antibody titer after sensitization by pregnancy with an Rh-positive fetus
➤ Determination of the need for immunosuppressive therapy (e.g., with RhoGAM) when an Rh-negative woman has delivered or aborted an Rh-positive fetus

Nursing Care Before the Procedure

Client preparation is the same as that for any study involving the collection of a peripheral blood sample (see Appendix I).

The Procedure

A venipuncture is performed and the sample collected in a red-topped tube or other type of blood collection tube, depending on laboratory preference. The sample must be handled gently to avoid hemolysis and sent promptly to the laboratory.

As with ABO typing, correct client and sample identifications are crucial in avoiding erroneous results.

Nursing Care After the Procedure

Care and assessment after the procedure are the same as that for any study involving the collection of a peripheral blood sample.
➤ As with ABO typing, the client should be informed of his or her Rh type.
➤ Women of childbearing age who are Rh-negative should be informed of the need for follow-up should pregnancy occur.
  • *Rh incompatibility:* Note and report Rh factors of mother and father, number of pregnancies, and past transfusions of Rh-positive blood given to an Rh-negative mother. Communicate incompatible test results to the physician. Inform client and prepare client for administration of Rh immunoglobulins (RhoGAM).

ANTIGLOBULIN TESTS (COOMBS' TESTS)

Antiglobulin (Coombs') tests are used to detect nonagglutinating antibodies or complement molecules on red cell surfaces. They are used most commonly in immunohematology laboratories and blood banks for routine cross-matching, antibody screening tests, and preliminary investigations of hemolytic anemias.[14,15]

The tests are based on the principle that immunoglobulins (i.e., antibodies) act as antigens when injected into a nonhuman host. This principle was originally published by Moreschi in 1908, but his findings drew little notice. In 1945, Coombs independently rediscovered the principle when he prepared antihuman serum by injecting human serum into rabbits. The rabbit antibody produced against the human globulin was then collected and purified. This antihuman globulin was used to demonstrate incomplete human antibodies that were adsorbed to red cells and did not cause visually apparent agglutination unless Coombs' rabbit serum was used. The two applications of the test currently used are (1) the direct antiglobulin test (direct Coombs') and (2) the indirect antiglobulin test (indirect Coombs').[16]

DIRECT ANTIGLOBULIN TEST (DAT, DIRECT COOMBS')

It is never normal for circulating red cells to be coated with antibody. The direct antiglobulin test (DAT, direct Coombs') is used to detect abnormal in vivo coating of red cells with antibody globulin (IgG) or complement, or both.

When this test is performed, the red cells are taken directly from the sample, washed with saline (to remove residual globulins left in the client's serum surrounding the red cells but not actually attached to them), and mixed with antihuman globulin (AHG). If the AHG causes agglutination of the client's red cells, specific antiglobulins may be used to determine if the red cells are coated with IgG, complement, or both.

The most common cause of a positive DAT is autoimmune hemolytic anemia, in which affected individuals have antibodies against their own red cells. Other causes of positive results include hemolytic disease of the newborn, transfusion of incompatible blood, and red cell–sensitizing reactions caused by drugs. In the latter, the red cells may be coated with the drug or with immune complexes composed of drugs and antibodies that activate the complement system.[17,18] Drugs associated with such reactions are listed in Table 4–2. Positive DAT results may also be seen in individuals with *Mycoplasma* pneumonia, leukemias, lymphomas, infectious mononucleosis, lupus erythematosus and other immune disorders of connective tissue, and metastatic carcinoma. Other conditions, such as the aftermath of cardiac vascular surgery, are associated with production of autoantibodies.

Reference Values

Negative (no agglutination)

Interfering Factors

➤ Many drugs may cause positive reactions (Table 4–2).

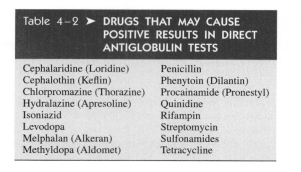

Table 4–2 ➤ DRUGS THAT MAY CAUSE POSITIVE RESULTS IN DIRECT ANTIGLOBULIN TESTS

Cephalaridine (Loridine)	Penicillin
Cephalothin (Keflin)	Phenytoin (Dilantin)
Chlorpromazine (Thorazine)	Procainamide (Pronestyl)
Hydralazine (Apresoline)	Quinidine
Isoniazid	Rifampin
Levodopa	Streptomycin
Melphalan (Alkeran)	Sulfonamides
Methyldopa (Aldomet)	Tetracycline

Indications for Direct Antiglobulin Test

➤ Suspected hemolytic anemia or hemolytic disease of the newborn as indicated by a positive reaction
➤ Suspected transfusion reaction as indicated by a positive result
➤ Suspected drug sensitivity reaction as indicated by a positive result

Nursing Care Before the Procedure

For samples collected by venipuncture, client preparation is the same as that for any study involving the collection of a peripheral or cord blood sample (see Appendix I).

➤ Drugs currently taken by the client should be noted.
➤ If the test is to be performed on the newborn, the parent(s) should be informed that a sample of umbilical cord blood will be obtained at delivery and will not result in blood loss to the infant.

The Procedure

A venipuncture is performed and the sample collected in a red-topped tube or other type of blood collection tube, depending on laboratory preference. For cord blood, the sample is collected in a red- or lavender-topped tube (depending on the laboratory) from the maternal segment of the cord after it has been cut and before the placenta has been delivered.

Nursing Care After the Procedure

For venipunctures, care and assessment after the procedure are the same as for any study involving the collection of a peripheral blood sample.

➤ *Complications and precautions:* Note and report a positive value in cord blood of a neonate with possible erythroblastosis fetalis for direct Coombs' because this test result indicates that antibodies are attached to the circulating erythrocytes. Assess associated bilirubin and hemoglobin levels. Prepare the infant for exchange transfusion of fresh whole blood that has been typed and cross-matched with the mother's serum.

INDIRECT ANTIGLOBULIN TEST (IAT, INDIRECT COOMBS', ANTIBODY SCREENING TEST)

The indirect antiglobulin test (IAT, indirect Coombs', antibody screening test) is used primarily to screen blood samples for unexpected circulating antibodies that may be reactive against transfused red blood cells.

In this test, the client's serum serves as the source of antibody, and the red cells to be transfused serve as the antigen. The test is performed by incubating the serum and red cells in the laboratory (in vitro) to allow any present antibodies every opportunity to attach to the red cells. The cells are then washed with saline to remove any unattached serum globulins, and AHG is added. If the client's serum contains an antibody that reacts with and attaches to the donor red cells, the AHG will cause the antibody-coated cells to agglutinate.

If there is no agglutination after addition of AHG, it means that no antigen-antibody reaction has occurred. The serum may contain an antibody, but the red cells against which it is tested do not have the relevant antigen. Thus, the reaction is negative.[19]

Reference Values

Negative (no agglutination)

Interfering Factors

➤ Recent administration of dextran, whole blood or fractions, or intravenous contrast media may result in a false-positive reaction.

➤ Drugs that may cause false-positive reactions are cephalosporins, insulin, isoniazid, levodopa, mefenamic acid, methyldopa, methyldopa hydrochloride, penicillins, procainamide hydrochloride, quinidine, rifampin, sulfonamides, and tetracyclines.

Indications for Indirect Antiglobulin Test (IAT, Indirect Coombs', Antibody Screening Test)

➤ Antibody screening and cross-matching before blood transfusions, especially to detect antibodies whose presence may not be elicited by other methods such as ABO and Rh typing

➤ Determination of antibody titers in Rh-negative women sensitized by an Rh-positive fetus

➤ Testing for the weak Rh variant antigen D^u

➤ Detection of other antibodies in maternal blood that may be potentially harmful to the fetus

Nursing Care Before the Procedure

Client preparation is the same as that for any study involving the collection of a peripheral blood sample (see Appendix I).

➤ Exposure to substances that may cause false-positive reactions should be noted. The medication history should also be noted.

The Procedure

A venipuncture is performed and the sample collected in a red-topped tube or other blood collection tube, depending on laboratory preference. The sample must be handled gently to avoid hemolysis and sent promptly to the laboratory.

Nursing Care After the Procedure

Care and assessment after the procedure are the same as for any study involving the collection of a peripheral blood sample.

➤ *Complications and precautions:* Note and report positive value for antibody detection, especially in a pregnant woman. Inform the client that further testing will be undertaken to identify the antibodies.

HUMAN LEUKOCYTE ANTIGENS (HLA)

All nucleated cells have human leukocyte antigens (HLA) on their surface membranes. Although sometimes described as "white cell antigens," HLA characterize virtually all cell types except red blood cells. HLA consist of a glycoprotein chain and a globulin chain. They are classified into five series designated A, B, C, D, and DR (D-related), each series containing 10 to 20 distinct antigens. A, B, C, and D antigens characterize the membranes of virtually all cells except mature red blood cells; DR antigens seem to reside only on B lymphocytes and macrophages (see Chap. 3).

Some antigens have been identified with specific diseases (Table 4–3). Arthritic disorders, for example, have been closely linked to HLA-B27. In addition, HLA typing is valuable in determining parentage. If the HLA phenotypes of a child and one parent are known, it is possible to assess fairly accurately whether a given individual is the other parent.[20]

Reference Values

HLA combinations vary according to certain races and populations. The most common B antigens in American whites, for example, are B7, B8, and B12. In American blacks, the most common of the B series are Bw17, Bw35, and a specificity characterized as 1AG. This combination is in contrast to that of African blacks, whose most common B antigens are B7, Bw17, and 1AG. Similar variations among the A antigens also have been found among various races and populations.

Indications for HLA Tests

➤ Determination of donor and recipient compatibility for tissue transplantation, especially when they are blood relatives[21]
➤ Determination of compatibility of donor platelets in individuals who will receive multiple transfusions over a long period of time
➤ Support for diagnosing HLA-associated diseases (see Table 4–3), especially when signs and symptoms are inconclusive
➤ Determination of biologic parentage

Nursing Care Before the Procedure

Client preparation is the same as that for any study involving the collection of a peripheral blood sample (see Appendix I).

Table 4–3 ➤ DISEASES ASSOCIATED WITH HUMAN LEUKOCYTE ANTIGENS	
Disease	**Associated Antigen**
Ankylosing spondylitis	B27
Reiter's syndrome	B27
Diabetes mellitus (juvenile, or insulin-dependent)	B8, Bw15
Multiple sclerosis	A3, B7, B18
Acute anterior uveitis	B27
Graves' disease	B8
Juvenile rheumatoid arthritis	B27
Celiac disease	B8
Psoriasis vulgaris	B13, Bw17
Myasthenia gravis	B8
Dermatitis herpetiformis	B8
Autoimmune chronic active hepatitis	B8

The Procedure

A venipuncture is performed and the sample collected in a green-topped tube or other blood collection device, depending on laboratory preference. The sample is sent promptly to the laboratory performing the test (not all laboratories are equipped to do so).

Nursing Care After the Procedure

Care and assessment after the procedure are the same as for any study involving the collection of a peripheral blood sample.

➤ *Medicolegal implications:* HLA testing results for biologic parentage exclusion are not allowed as evidence in all jurisdictions.

Student Name _____ Class _____

Instructor _____ Date _____

CASE STUDY AND CRITICAL THINKING EXERCISE

A client (para 2 gravida 2) is admitted to the delivery room. Her blood type is B−. Her first child was born 2 years ago and has a blood type of AB+.

a. What possible serious complication might her second child experience if the mother was exposed to her first child's blood type?

b. Is the same complication a consideration if a mother is B+ and the baby AB−?

References

1. Sacher, RA, and McPherson, RA: Widmann's Clinical Interpretation of Laboratory Tests, ed 10. FA Davis, Philadelphia, 1991, p 265.
2. Ibid, p 266.
3. Harmening, D: Modern Blood Banking and Transfusion Practices, ed 2. FA Davis, Philadelphia, 1992, p 79.
4. Sacher and McPherson, op cit, pp 268–269.
5. Ibid, p 269.
6. Fischbach, FT: A Manual of Laboratory and Diagnostic Tests, ed 4. JB Lippincott, Philadelphia, 1992, pp 556–558.
7. Harmening, op cit, p 89.
8. Ibid, p 80.
9. Sacher and McPherson, op cit, p 269.
10. Harmening, op cit, p 105.
11. Sacher and McPherson, op cit, p 271.
12. Harmening, op cit, p 110.
13. Sacher and McPherson, op cit, pp 272–273.
14. Ibid, p 275.
15. Harmening, op cit, pp 65–66.
16. Ibid, pp 65–66.
17. Ibid, p 66.
18. Sacher and McPherson, op cit, p 276.
19. Ibid, p 279.
20. Harmening, op cit, p 374.
21. Ibid, p 369.

Bibliography

Byrne, CJ, et al: Laboratory Tests: Implications for Nursing Care. Addison-Wesley, Menlo Park, Calif, 1986.

Chernecky, CC, and Berger, BJ; Cullen, BN (ed): Laboratory Tests and Diagnostic Procedures, ed 2. WB Saunders, Philadelphia, 1996.

Corbett, JV: Laboratory Tests and Diagnostic Procedures with Nursing Diagnoses, ed 4. Appleton & Lange, Norwalk, Conn, 1995.

Henry, JB: Clinical Diagnosis and Management by Laboratory Methods, ed 19. WB Saunders, Philadelphia, 1996.

Kee, JL: Handbook of Laboratory and Diagnostic Tests with Nursing Implications, ed 3. Appleton & Lange, Norwalk, Conn, 1997.

Lewis, SM, et al (eds): Medical-Surgical Nursing: Assessment and Management of Clinical Problems, ed 4. Mosby–Year Book, St Louis, 1995.

Pagana, KD, and Pagana, TJ: Diagnostic and Laboratory Test Reference, ed 3. Mosby–Year Book, St Louis, 1996.

Porth, CM: Pathophysiology: Concepts of Altered Health States, ed 4. JB Lippincott, Philadelphia, 1993.

Salmon, C: Blood Groups and Other Red Cell Surface Markers in Health and Disease. Mosby–Year Book, St Louis, 1984.

Springhouse Corporation: Nurse's Reference Library: Diagnostic Testing, ed 3. Springhouse, Springhouse, Pa, 1991.

Tietz, NW (ed): Clinical Guide to Laboratory Tests, ed 3. WB Saunders, Philadelphia, 1997.

Whaley, LF: Nursing Care of Infants and Children, ed 4. Mosby–Year Book, St Louis, 1991.

Blood Chemistry

> **TESTS COVERED**

Blood Glucose (Serum Glucose, Plasma Glucose), *144*

Two-Hour Postprandial Blood Glucose (Postprandial Blood Sugar, PPBS), *146*

Oral Glucose Tolerance Test (OGTT), *148*

Intravenous Glucose Tolerance Test (IVGTT), *151*

Cortisone Glucose Tolerance Test (Cortisone GTT), *152*

Glycosylated Hemoglobin, *153*

Tolbutamide Tolerance Test, *154*

Serum Proteins, *156*

α_1-Antitrypsin (α_1-AT), *160*

Haptoglobin, *161*

Ceruloplasmin (Cp), *162*

Urea Nitrogen, *164*

Serum Creatinine, *166*

Ammonia, *168*

Serum Creatine, *169*

Uric Acid, *170*

Free Fatty Acids (FFA), *173*

Triglycerides, *175*

Total Cholesterol, *177*

Phospholipids, *179*

Lipoprotein and Cholesterol Fractionation, *181*

Lipoprotein Phenotyping, *184*

Bilirubin, *186*

Alanine Aminotransferase (ALT, SGPT), *191*

Aspartate Aminotransferase (AST, SGOT), *192*

Alkaline Phosphatase (ALP), *194*

5'-Nucleotidase (5'-N), *196*

Leucine Aminopeptidase (LAP), *197*

γ-Glutamyl Transpeptidase (GGT), *198*

Isocitrate Dehydrogenase (ICD), *199*

Ornithine Carbamoyltransferase (OCT), *200*

Serum Amylase, *201*

Serum Lipase, *203*

Acid Phosphatase (ACP), *204*

Prostate-Specific Antigen (PSA), *206*

Aldolase (ALS), *207*

Creatine Phosphokinase (CPK) and Isoenzymes, *208*

Lactic Dehydrogenase (LDH) and Isoenzymes, *211*

Hexosaminidase, *213*

α-Hydroxybutyric Dehydrogenase (α-HBD, HBD), *214*

Cholinesterases, *215*

Renin, *217*

Growth Hormone (GH, STH, SH), *221*

Growth Hormone (GH) Stimulation Tests, *223*

Growth Hormone (GH) Suppression Test, *224*

Prolactin (hPRL, LTH), *225*

Adrenocorticotropic Hormone (ACTH), *226*

Thyroid-Stimulating Hormone (TSH), *228*

TSH Stimulation Test, *230*

Follicle-Stimulating Hormone (FSH), *231*

FSH/LH Challenge Tests, *232*

Luteinizing Hormone (LH, ICSH), *234*

Antidiuretic Hormone (ADH), *235*

Thyroxine (T_4), *238*

Triiodothyronine (T_3), *240*

T_3 Uptake ($RT_3 U$), *241*

Thyroxine-Binding Globulin (TBG), *243*

Thyroid-Stimulating
Immunoglobulins (TSI, TSIg), *243*
Calcitonin, *244*
Parathyroid Hormone (PTH), *245*
Cortisol/ACTH Challenge Tests, *248*
Aldosterone Challenge Tests, *250*
Catecholamines, *252*
Estrogens, *254*
Progesterone, *256*
Testosterone, *258*
Human Chorionic Gonadotropin
(hCG), *259*
Human Placental Lactogen (hPL),
261
Insulin, *263*
C-Peptide, *264*
Glucagon, *265*

Gastrin, *267*
Serum Sodium (Na), *268*
Serum Potassium (K), *271*
Serum Chloride (Cl), *274*
Serum Bicarbonate (HCO$_3$,
HCO$_3^-$), *276*
Serum Calcium (Ca, Ca^{++}), *279*
Serum Phosphorus/Phosphate
(P), *282*
Serum Magnesium (Mg, Mg^{++}), *284*
Serum Osmolality, *286*
Arterial Blood Gases (ABGs), *288*
Vitamin A, *292*
Vitamin C, *293*
Vitamin D, *295*
Trace Minerals, *296*
Drugs and Toxic Substances, *297*

INTRODUCTION

The blood transports innumerable substances that participate in and reflect ongoing metabolic processes. Relatively few of these substances are routinely measured. Some materials are analyzed to provide information about specific organs and processes; other substances reflect the summed effects of numerous metabolic events.[1] "Chemistry" includes measurement of glucose, proteins, lipids, enzymes, electrolytes, hormones, vitamins, toxins, and other substances that may indicate derangement of normal physiological processes. In recent years, the diagnosis of many disorders associated with abnormal blood chemistries has become more rapid and accurate with the use of automated analyzers that can measure multiple chemistry components in a single blood sample.

CARBOHYDRATES

The body acquires most of its energy from oxidative metabolism of glucose. Glucose, a simple six-carbon sugar, enters the diet as part of the sugars called sucrose, lactose, and maltose and as the major constituent of the complex polysaccharides called dietary starch. Complete oxidation of glucose yields carbon dioxide (CO_2), water, and energy that is stored as adenosine triphosphate (ATP).

If glucose is not immediately metabolized, it can be stored in the liver or muscle as glycogen. Unused glucose may also be converted by the liver into fatty acids, which are stored as triglycerides, or into amino acids, which can be used for protein synthesis. The liver is pivotal in distributing glucose as needed for immediate fuel or as indicated for storage or for structural purposes. If available glucose or glycogen is insufficient for energy needs, the liver can synthesize glucose from fatty acids or even from protein-derived amino acids.[2]

Glucose fuels most cell and tissue functions. Thus, adequate glucose is a critical requirement for homeostasis. Many cells can derive some energy from burning fatty acids, but this energy pathway is less efficient than burning glucose and generates acid metabolites (e.g., ketones) that are harmful if they ac-

Table 5–1 ➤ HORMONES THAT INFLUENCE BLOOD GLUCOSE LEVELS

Hormone	Tissue of Origin	Metabolic Effect	Effect on Blood Glucose
Insulin	Pancreatic beta cells	1. Enhances entry of glucose into cells 2. Enhances storage of glucose as glycogen, or conversion to fatty acids 3. Enhances synthesis of proteins and fatty acids 4. Suppresses breakdown of protein into amino acids; of adipose tissue, into free fatty acids	Lowers
Somatostatin	Pancreatic D cells	1. Suppresses glucagon release from alpha cells (acts locally) 2. Suppresses release of insulin, pituitary tropic hormones, gastrin, and secretin	Lowers
Glucagon	Pancreatic alpha cells	1. Enhances release of glucose from glycogen 2. Enhances synthesis of glucose from amino acids or fatty acids	Raises
Epinephrine	Adrenal medulla	1. Enhances release of glucose from glycogen 2. Enhances release of fatty acids from adipose tissue	Raises
Cortisol	Adrenal cortex	1. Enhances synthesis of glucose from amino acids or fatty acids 2. Antagonizes insulin	Raises
Adrenocorticotropic hormone (ACTH)	Anterior pituitary	1. Enhances release of cortisol 2. Enhances release of fatty acids from adipose tissue	Raises
Growth hormone	Anterior pituitary	1. Antagonizes insulin	Raises
Thyroxine	Thyroid	1. Enhances release of glucose from glycogen 2. Enhances absorption of sugars from intestine	Raises

Note: From Sacher, RA, and McPherson, RA: Widmann's Clinical Interpretation of Laboratory Tests, ed 10. FA Davis, Philadelphia, 1991, p 324, with permission.

cumulate in the body. Many hormones (Table 5–1) participate in maintaining blood glucose levels in steady-state conditions or in response to stress. Measuring blood glucose indicates whether the regulation is successful. Pronounced departure from normal, either too high or too low, indicates abnormal homeostasis and should initiate a search for the etiology.[3] The causes of abnormal blood glucose levels are summarized in Table 5–2.

Two major methods are used to measure blood glucose: chemical and enzymatic. Chemical methods use the nonspecific reducing properties of the glucose molecule. In enzymatic methods, glucose oxidase reacts with its specific substrate, glucose, liberating hydrogen peroxide, the effects of which are then measured. Values are 5 to 15 mg/dL higher for the reducing (chemical) methods than for enzymatic techniques because blood contains other reducing substances in addition to glucose. Urea, for example, can contribute up to 10 mg/dL in normal serum and even more when uremia exists. Several different indicator systems are used for automated enzymatic methods, yielding somewhat different normal values.[4]

It should also be noted that, in the past, blood glucose values were given in terms of whole blood. Today, most laboratories measure serum or plasma glu-

Table 5-2 ➤ CAUSES OF ALTERED BLOOD GLUCOSE LEVELS

Hyperglycemia	Hypoglycemia
PERSISTENT CAUSES	
Diabetes mellitus	Insulinoma
Hemochromatosis	Addison's disease
Cushing's syndrome	Hypopituitarism
Hyperthyroidism	Galactosemia
Acromegaly, gigantism	Ectopic insulin production from tumors (adrenal
Obesity	carcinoma, retroperitoneal sarcomas, pleural
Chronic pancreatitis	fibrous mesotheliomas)
Pancreatic adenoma	Starvation
TRANSIENT CAUSES	
Pheochromocytoma	Acute alcohol ingestion
Pregnancy (gestational diabetes)	Severe liver disease
Severe liver disease	Severe glycogen storage diseases
Acute stress reaction	Stress-related catecholamine excess ("functional"
Shock, trauma	hypoglycemia)
Convulsions, eclampsia	Hereditary fructose intolerance
Malabsorption syndrome	Myxedema
Postgastrectomy "dumping syndrome"	
DRUGS	
Glucagon	Clonidine
Adrenocorticosteroids	Dextrothyroxine
Oral contraceptives	Niacin
Estrogens	Salicylates
Thyroid hormones	Antituberculosis agents
Anabolic steroids	Sulfonylureas
Thiazide diuretics	Sulfonamides
Loop diuretics	Insulin
Propranolol	Ethanol
Antipsychotic drugs	Clofibrate
Hydantoins	MAO inhibitors

cose levels. Because of its higher water content, serum contains more dissolved glucose, and the resultant values are 1.15 times higher than are those for whole blood. Serum or plasma should be separated promptly because red and white blood cells continue to metabolize glucose. In blood with very high white blood cell levels, excessive glycolysis may actually lower glucose results. Arterial, capillary, and venous blood samples have comparable glucose levels in a fasting individual. After meals, venous levels are lower than those in arterial or capillary blood.[5]

Blood Glucose (Serum Glucose, Plasma Glucose)

Blood glucose (serum glucose, plasma glucose) is measured in a variety of situations. In the fasting state, the serum glucose level gives the best indication of overall glucose homeostasis.[6]

Blood glucose levels also may be measured at regular intervals throughout the day to monitor responses to diet and medications in persons with a diagnosis of abnormalities of glucose metabolism. Such monitoring may take place in a hospital setting or in the home with kits specially designed for self-monitoring of blood glucose. Serial blood glucose levels also are used to determine insulin requirements in clients with uncontrolled diabetes mellitus and for individuals receiving total parenteral or enteral nutritional support.

In addition to situations characterized by actual or potential elevations in blood sugar, glucose levels are evaluated in individuals suspected or known to have hypoglycemia.

Reference Values

	Newborns		Children		Adults	
	Conventional Units	**SI Units**	**Conventional Units**	**SI Units**	**Conventional Units**	**SI Units**
Whole blood	25–51 mg/dL	1.4–2.8 mmol/L	50–90 mg/dL	2.8–5.0 mmol/L	60–100 mg/dL	3.3–5.6 mmol/L
Serum/plasma	30–60 mg/dL	1.7–3.3 mmol/L	60–105 mg/dL	3.3–5.8 mmol/L	70–110 mg/dL	3.9–6.1 mmol/L
Critical Values	**<30 mg/dL or >300 mg/dL**	**<1.6 mmol/L or >16.5 mmol/L**	**<40 mg/dL or >700 mg/dL**	**<2.2 mmol/L or >38.6 mmol/L**	**<40 mg/dL or >700 mg/dL**	**<2.2 mmol/L or >38.6 mmol/L**

Values may vary depending on the laboratory method used (see pp. 143 to 144).

Interfering Factors

➤ Elevated urea levels and uremia may lead to falsely elevated levels.

➤ Extremely elevated white blood cell counts may lead to falsely decreased values.

➤ Failure to follow dietary restrictions before a fasting blood glucose may lead to falsely elevated values.

➤ Administration of insulin or oral hypoglycemic agents within 8 hours of a fasting blood glucose may lead to falsely decreased values.

Indications for Blood Glucose Test

➤ Routine screening for diabetes mellitus
  • Fasting blood glucose levels greater than 140 to 150 mg/dL on two or more occasions may be considered diagnostic of diabetes mellitus if other possible causes of hyperglycemia are eliminated as sources of elevation (see Table 5–2).
  • Random (nonfasting) blood glucose levels of greater than 200 mg/dL may be pathognomonic of diabetes mellitus.[7]

➤ Clinical symptoms of hypoglycemia or hyperglycemia

➤ Known or suspected disorder associated with abnormal glucose metabolism (see Table 5–2).

➤ Identification of abnormal hypoglycemia as indicated by a fasting blood sugar as low as 50 mg/dL in men or 35 mg/dL in women[8]

➤ Monitoring of response to therapy for abnormal glucose metabolism

➤ Determination of insulin requirements (i.e., "insulin coverage")

➤ Monitoring of metabolic response to drugs known to alter blood glucose levels (see Table 5–2).

> Monitoring of metabolic response to parenteral or enteral nutritional support to determine insulin requirements

Nursing Care Before the Procedure

Client preparation is essentially the same as that for any study involving the collection of a peripheral blood sample (see Appendix I).

> If a fasting sample is to be drawn, food and insulin or any oral hypo-glycemic agent should be withheld for approximately 8 hours before the test (i.e., the client usually takes only water from midnight until the sample is drawn in the morning).

> For home glucose monitoring, the client should be instructed in the correct use of the testing equipment and in the method used to obtain the blood sample.

The Procedure

A venipuncture is performed and the sample is obtained in either a gray- or a red-topped tube, depending on the laboratory performing the test. The sample should be handled gently to avoid hemolysis and transported promptly to the laboratory.

A capillary sample may be obtained in infants and children as well as in adults for whom venipuncture may not be feasible. Capillary samples also are used for self-monitoring of blood glucose.

Nursing Care After the Procedure

Care and assessment after the procedure are the same as for any study involving collection of a peripheral blood sample.

> Resume food and medications withheld before the test after the sample is drawn.

> *Abnormal values:* Note and report increased levels. Assess for symptoms associated with hyperglycemia such as polyuria and possible dehydration, polydipsia, or weight loss. Prepare for additional glucose tests for diabetes mellitus. Monitor intake and output (I&O). Prepare to administer ordered medications (insulin or oral hypoglycemic) to treat known diabetic condi-tion. Instruct client on diabetic diet in relation to medications, activities, and blood and urine test results. Note and report decreased levels. Assess for symptoms associated with hypoglycemia such as weakness, sweating, ner-vousness, hunger, confusion, or palpitations. Prepare to administer sucrose or glucose orally or intravenously (IV). Instruct client to keep readily ab-sorbed carbohydrates on hand. Instruct client on diet and its relation to med-ications, activities, and blood and urine test results.

> **Critical values:** Notify the physician immediately of a blood glucose level of less than 30 mg/dL in infants or less than 40 mg/dL in adults or a blood glucose level of greater than 300 mg/dL in infants or greater than 700 mg/dL in adults.

Two-Hour Postprandial Blood Glucose (Postprandial Blood Sugar, PPBS)

The 2-hour postprandial blood glucose (postprandial blood sugar, PPBS) test reflects the metabolic response to a carbohydrate challenge.[9] In normal individ-uals, the blood sugar returns to the fasting level within 2 hours.

In contrast, postprandial hypoglycemia appears to result from delayed or exaggerated response to the insulin secreted in relation to dietary blood sugar rise. It may occur as an early event in individuals with non–insulin-dependent diabetes mellitus (NIDDM, type II diabetes mellitus) or in individuals with gastrointestinal malfunction. Frequently, no cause is demonstrated and the hypoglycemia is considered "functional." Postprandial hypoglycemia differs from fasting hypoglycemia (i.e., hypoglycemia that occurs after 10 or more hours without food) in that the latter nearly always has pathological significance. It results from either overproduction of insulin or undermobilization of glucose and is most commonly seen in clients with tumors of the pancreatic beta cells (insulinoma), liver disease, and chronic alcohol ingestion.[10]

Reference Values

	Children		Adults		Elderly Persons	
	Conventional Units	SI Units	Conventional Units	SI Units	Conventional Units	SI Units
Blood	120 mg/dL	6.6 mmol/L	≤120 mg/dL	6.6 mmol/L	≤140 mg/dL	7.7 mmol/L
Serum/plasma	150 mg/dL	8.3 mmol/L	≤140 mg/dL	7.7 mmol/L	≤160 mg/dL	8.8 mmol/L

Values may vary, depending on the laboratory method used.

With advancing age, the speed of glucose clearance declines. Two-hour levels in persons who do not have diabetes and in those with negative family histories may increase an average of 6 mg/dL for each decade over age 30.[11]

Interfering Factors

➤ Failing to follow dietary instructions may alter test results.
➤ Smoking and drinking coffee during the 2-hour test period may lead to falsely elevated values.
➤ Strenuous exercising during the 2-hour test period may lead to falsely decreased values.

Indications for 2-Hour Postprandial Blood Glucose (Postprandial Blood Sugar, PPBS) Test

➤ Abnormal fasting blood sugar
➤ Routine screening for diabetes mellitus, as indicated by a blood glucose level greater than the fasting level and especially by a 2-hour level greater than 200 mg/mL
➤ Identification of postprandial hypoglycemia and differentiation of this state from fasting hypoglycemia, with fasting hypoglycemia almost always indicative of a pathological state (see p. 144)
➤ Known or suspected disorder associated with abnormal glucose metabolism (see Table 5–2, p. 144)
➤ Monitoring of metabolic response to drugs known to alter blood glucose levels (see Table 5–2, p. 144)

Nursing Care Before the Procedure

General client preparation is the same as that for any test involving collection of a peripheral blood sample.

➤ Specific preparation includes ingesting a meal (usually breakfast) containing at least 100 g of carbohydrate 2 hours before the test.

➤ The American Diabetes Association recommends a 300-g carbohydrate diet for 2 to 3 days before the test, but this recommendation is not universally followed.

➤ The time of the last meal before the test should be noted.

➤ The client should then fast from food and avoid coffee, smoking, and strenuous exercise until the sample is obtained.

➤ Although medications are not withheld for this test, those taken should be noted.

The Procedure

Two hours after the carbohydrate challenge is ingested, a venipuncture is performed and the sample is collected in either a gray- or a red-topped tube, depending on the laboratory performing the test. A capillary sample may be obtained in children and in adults for whom venipuncture may not be feasible. Capillary samples are also used when the test is performed for mass screenings. It should be noted that in some instances a fasting blood sugar level may be obtained before the carbohydrate challenge.

Nursing Care After the Procedure

Care and assessment after the procedure are the same as for any study involving collection of a peripheral blood sample. Resume usual diet and activities.

➤ *Complications and precautions:* Abnormal increased or decreased values are treated in the same way as for blood glucose testing. If the glucose level does not return to a fasting state in 2 hours, an additional glucose tolerance test is required, and there are no critical values to report (see p. 147).

Glucose Tolerance Tests (GTTs)

Glucose tolerance tests (GTTs) are used to evaluate the response to a carbohydrate challenge throughout a 3- to 5-hour period. When a glucose load is presented, the normal individual's blood insulin level rises in response to it, with peak levels occurring 30 to 60 minutes after the carbohydrate challenge. Blood glucose levels, although elevated immediately after the carbohydrate challenge, return to normal fasting levels 2 to 3 hours later. For individuals in whom abnormal hypoglycemia or gastrointestinal malabsorption is suspected, the test may be extended to a 5-hour period.[12–14]

Several methods may be used to perform a glucose tolerance test. The oral, IV, and cortisone glucose tolerance tests are discussed in this section. Tolerance tests also may be performed for pentose, lactose, galactose, and D-xylose.

ORAL GLUCOSE TOLERANCE TEST (OGTT)

The oral glucose tolerance test (OGTT) is used for individuals who are able to eat and who are not known to have problems with gastrointestinal malabsorption. The client should be in a normal nutritional state and should be capable of normal physical activity (i.e., not immobilized or on bed rest), because carbohydrate depletion and inactivity may impair glucose tolerance. In addition, drugs that affect blood glucose levels (see Table 5–2, p. 144) should not be taken for several days before the test. Because oral glucose tolerance testing is affected by so many variables, the results are subject to many diagnostic interpretations.[15]

The OGTT may be performed using blood samples only or using urine samples as well. The urine is normally negative for sugar throughout the test; that is, because the average renal threshold for glucose is 180 mg/dL, the plasma glucose level must be approximately 180 mg/dL before sugar appears in the urine. Renal threshold levels vary, however, and urine testing during an OGTT may show how much glucose the individual spills, if any, at various blood glucose levels. As long as the renal threshold is not surpassed by the blood glucose levels, all of the glucose presented to the kidneys is reabsorbed from the glomerular filtrate by the renal tubules, provided that renal function is normal.

Reference Values

| | \multicolumn{8}{c}{Time After Carbohydrate Challenge} | | | | | | | |
| | \multicolumn{2}{c}{30 min} | | \multicolumn{2}{c}{1 Hr} | | \multicolumn{2}{c}{2 Hr} | | \multicolumn{2}{c}{3 Hr} | |
	Conventional Units	SI Units	Conventional Units	SI Units	Conventional Units	SI Units	Conventional Units	SI Units
Whole blood glucose	<150 mg/dL	≥8.3 mmol/L	<160 mg/dL	≥8.8 mmol/L	<115 mg/dL	≥6.6 mmol/L	Same as fasting	Same as fasting
Serum/ plasma	<160 mg/dL	>8.8 mmol/L	<170 mg/dL	>9.4 mmol/L	<125 mg/dL	>7.1 mmol/L	Same as fasting	Same as fasting
Urine glucose	Negative throughout test							

Values for children over age 6 years are the same as those for adults. Values for elderly individuals are 10 to 30 mg/dL higher at each interval because of the age-related decline in glucose clearance.

Interfering Factors

➤ Failure to ingest a diet with sufficient carbohydrate content (e.g., 150 g/day) for at least 3 days before the test may result in falsely decreased values.

➤ Impaired physical activity may lead to falsely increased values.

➤ Excessive physical activity before or during the test may lead to falsely decreased values.

➤ Smoking before or during the test may lead to falsely increased values.

➤ Ingestion of drugs known to alter blood glucose levels may lead to falsely increased or decreased values (see Table 5–2, p. 144).

Indications for Oral Glucose Tolerance Test (OGTT)

➤ Abnormal fasting or postprandial blood glucose levels that are not clearly indicative of diabetes mellitus

➤ Identification of impaired glucose metabolism without overt diabetes mellitus, which is characterized by a modest elevation in blood glucose after 2 hours and a normal level after 3 hours

➤ Evaluation of glucose metabolism in women of childbearing age, especially those who are pregnant and have a history of previous fetal loss, birth of babies weighing 9 pounds or more, or positive family history for diabetes mellitus

➤ Support for diagnosing hyperthyroidism and alcoholic liver disease, which are characterized by a sharp rise in blood glucose followed by a decline to subnormal levels

➤ Identification of true postprandial hypoglycemia (5-hour GTT) caused by excessive insulin response to a glucose load

➤ Support for diagnosing gastrointestinal malabsorption, which is characterized by peak glucose levels lower than that normally expected and hypoglycemia in the latter hours of the test (5-hour GTT)

➤ Identification of abnormal renal tubular function, if glycosuria occurs without hyperglycemia

---

➤➤ Nursing Alert

- Individuals with fasting blood sugars of greater than 150 mg/dL or postprandial blood glucose levels greater than 200 mg/dL should not receive the glucose load required for this test.
- If the client vomits the oral glucose preparation, notify the laboratory and physician immediately, and implement any treatment ordered.
- If signs and symptoms of hypoglycemia are observed or reported, obtain a blood sugar immediately and administer orange juice with 1 tsp of sugar or other beverage containing sugar; notify the physician that the test has been terminated.

Nursing Care Before the Procedure

Explain to the client:

➤ The general procedure for the test, including the administration of glucose and the frequency of collection of blood and urine samples

➤ The importance of eating a diet containing at least 150 g carbohydrate per day for 3 days before the test (Provide sample menus or lists of foods that demonstrate how this may be accomplished.)

➤ Which medications, if any, are to be withheld before the test

➤ That no food may be eaten after midnight before the test but that water is not restricted

➤ The importance of not smoking or performing strenuous exercise after midnight before the test and until the test is completed

➤ The symptoms of hypoglycemia and the necessity of reporting such symptoms immediately

Provide containers for collection of urine samples.

The Procedure

A venipuncture is performed and a sample is obtained for a fasting blood sugar. At the same time, a second voided (double-voided) urine sample is collected and tested for glucose. To collect a second-voided specimen, have the client void 30 minutes before the required specimen is due. Discard this urine, then collect the second voided specimen at the designated time.

The glucose load is administered orally. This is a calculated dose, either 1.75 g/kg body weight or 50 g/m² body surface. Several commercial preparations are available that are flavored for palatability. Blood and urine samples are obtained at ½-hour, 1-hour, 2-hour, and 3-hour intervals. The second voided urine specimen is necessary only at the beginning of the test. The client should drink one glass of water each time a urine sample is collected to ensure adequate urinary output for remaining specimens. If the test is extended to 5 hours, additional samples are collected at 4- and 5-hour intervals.

The test may be performed with blood samples only, depending on the desired information to be obtained from the test.

Nursing Care After the Procedure

Care and assessment after the procedure are essentially the same as those for any test involving the collection of peripheral blood samples.

➤ Resume food and medications withheld before the test, as well as usual activities.

➤ *Complications and precautions:* Same as for blood glucose. Closely monitor those clients whose pretest levels are greater than 200 mg/dL for possible reactions to the additional glucose intake required for the test (see p. 150).

INTRAVENOUS GLUCOSE TOLERANCE TEST (IVGTT)

The intravenous glucose tolerance test (IVGTT) is essentially the same as the OGTT, except that the carbohydrate challenge is administered IV instead of orally. Because the results are somewhat difficult to interpret, the IVGTT is used only in certain clinical situations or for research purposes.

Reference Values

The reference values are the same as those for the OGTT, except that the blood glucose level at the ½-hour interval may be 300 to 400 mg/dL because of the direct IV administration of the glucose load.

Interfering Factors

➤ Those factors that may alter results of an OGTT may also alter the results of an IVGTT (see p. 149).

➤ Infusions of total parenteral nutrition (TPN, hyperalimentation) during the test may lead to falsely elevated values; alternative solutions with less glucose should be infused for at least 3 hours before and during the test.

Indications for Intravenous Glucose Tolerance Test (IVGTT)

➤ Inability to take or tolerate oral glucose preparations used for the OGTT

➤ Suspected gastrointestinal malabsorption problems that interfere with accurate performance of the OGTT

➤ Evaluation of blood glucose control without the effects of gastrin, secretin, cholecystokinin, and gastric inhibitory peptide, all of which stimulate insulin production after oral ingestion of glucose

Nursing Care Before the Procedure

Client preparation is essentially the same as that for the OGTT.

➤ If the person is receiving TPN, an alternative solution with less glucose should be prescribed and infused for at least 3 hours before and during the test.

The Procedure

The procedure is essentially the same as that for the OGTT except that an intermittent venous access device (e.g., heparin lock) may be inserted to administer the glucose load and to obtain blood samples. Existing IV lines also may be used to administer the carbohydrate challenge, which is usually 50 percent glucose, with the amount to be given determined by the client's weight or body surface.

Nursing Care After the Procedure

Care and assessment after the procedure are the same as those for the OGTT.

➤ If an intermittent venous access device was inserted for the procedure, remove it after completion of the test and apply a pressure bandage to the site.

➤ Resume food and medications withheld before the test, as well as usual activities.

➤ Resume infusions of TPN as ordered.

CORTISONE GLUCOSE TOLERANCE TEST (CORTISONE GTT)

The cortisone glucose tolerance test (cortisone GTT) combines administration of a carbohydrate challenge with a cortisone challenge. Cortisone enhances the synthesis of glucose from amino acids and fatty acids (gluconeogenesis) and, when administered with a glucose load, may produce an abnormal GTT that would not be otherwise evident. The cortisone GTT is used only in certain clinical situations and for research purposes.

Reference Values

The reference values are similar to those for the OGTT except that the blood glucose level at the 2-hour interval may be 20 mg/dL higher than the client's fasting level.

Interfering Factors

➤ Those factors that may alter results of an OGTT may also alter the results of a cortisone GTT (see p. 149).

➤ Failure to administer or take the oral cortisone as prescribed for the test will alter results.

Indications for Cortisone Glucose Tolerance Test (Cortisone GTT)

➤ Inconclusive results of OGTT when prediabetes or "borderline" diabetes is suspected, with a 2-hour level of greater than 165 mg/dL considered indicative of diabetes

Nursing Care Before the Procedure

Client preparation is essentially the same as that for the OGTT.

➤ In addition, the client should be instructed on the purpose and administration of the oral cortisone acetate.

The Procedure

The procedure is the same as that for the OGTT except that cortisone acetate is administered orally 8 hours and again 2 hours before the standard GTT is begun.

Nursing Care After the Procedure

Care and assessment after the procedure are the same as for the OGTT.

Glycosylated Hemoglobin

Throughout the red blood cell's life span, the hemoglobin molecule incorporates glucose onto its beta chain. Glycosylation is irreversible and occurs at a stable rate. The amount of glucose permanently bound to hemoglobin depends on the blood sugar level. Thus, the level of glycosylated hemoglobin, designated Hgb A_{1c}, reflects the average blood sugar over a period of several weeks.

The test is used to evaluate the overall adequacy of diabetic control and provides information that may be missed by individual blood and urine glucose tests. Insulin-dependent diabetics, for example, may have undetected periods of hyperglycemia alternating with postinsulin periods of normoglycemia or even hypoglycemia. High Hgb A_{1c} levels reflect inadequate diabetic control in the preceding 3 to 5 weeks.

In addition to providing a more accurate assessment of overall blood glucose control, the test is more convenient for diabetic clients because it is performed only every 5 to 6 weeks and because there are no dietary or medication restrictions before the test.

Reference Values

Hgb A_{1c} is 3 to 6 percent of hemoglobin.

Hgb A_{1c} is 7 to 11 percent in diabetes under control.

Interfering Factors

➤ Individuals with hemolytic anemia and high levels of young red blood cells may have spuriously low levels.

➤ Individuals with elevated hemoglobin levels or on heparin therapy may have falsely elevated levels.

Indications for Glycosylated Hemoglobin Test

➤ Monitoring overall blood glucose control in clients with known diabetes, as the test aids in assessing blood glucose levels over a period of several weeks and provides data that may be missed by random blood or urine glucose tests

  • With prolonged hyperglycemia, levels of Hgb A_{1c} may rise to as high as 18 to 20 percent.

  • After normoglycemic levels are stabilized, Hgb A_{1c} levels return to normal in about 3 weeks.[16]

➤ Monitoring adequacy of insulin dosage for blood glucose control, especially that administered by automatic insulin pumps

➤ Evaluating the diabetic client's degree of compliance with the prescribed therapeutic regimen, as fasting or adjusting medications shortly before the test will not significantly alter results

Nursing Care Before the Procedure

Client preparation is the same as that for any test involving collection of a peripheral blood sample (see Appendix I).

➤ The client should be informed that fasting or adjusting medications for diabetes shortly before the test will not significantly alter results.

The Procedure

A venipuncture is performed and the sample obtained in a lavender-topped tube. The sample must be mixed adequately with the anticoagulant contained in the tube and transported promptly to the laboratory.

Nursing Care After the Procedure

Care and assessment after the procedure are the same as for any study involving collection of a peripheral blood sample.

➤ *Complications and precautions:* A value of greater than 15 percent of total Hgb A_{1c} indicates that the diabetes is out of control. Notify the physician at once.

Tolbutamide Tolerance Test

Tolbutamide (Orinase) is a hypoglycemic agent that produces hypoglycemia by stimulating the beta cells of the pancreas to secrete and release insulin. An IV infusion of tolbutamide raises the serum insulin and causes a rapid decrease in the blood glucose level. Thus, the test demonstrates the pancreatic beta-cell response to drug-induced stimulation. It should be noted that the test may be performed with glucagon or leucine instead of tolbutamide for clients who are sensitive to sulfonylureas or sulfonamides.

Reference Values

A decrease in serum glucose levels is evident within 5 to 10 minutes of administration of the drug. The lowest glucose levels occur in about 20 to 30 minutes and are generally about half of the client's usual fasting level. The glucose level returns to pretest values in 1 to 3 hours.

Interfering Factors

➤ The factors that may alter results of an OGTT may also alter the results of a tolbutamide tolerance test (see p. 149).

Indications for Tolbutamide Tolerance Test

➤ Evaluation of fasting or postprandial hypoglycemia by assessing the degree of pancreatic beta-cell response to drug-induced stimulation

➤ Suspected insulinoma (insulin-producing tumor of the pancreatic beta cells) as indicated by glucose levels that drop markedly in response to tolbutamide and take 3 or more hours to return to normal levels

➤ Suspected prediabetic state that may be characterized by excessive insulin release, as indicated by glucose levels that are lower than expected but that follow the overall pattern of a normal response to the test

---

➤➤ Nursing Alert

- Because of the expected drop in blood sugar levels, the test should be performed with extreme caution, if at all, on individuals with fasting blood sugars of 50 mg/dL or less.
- If the client is allergic to sulfonylureas or sulfonamides, the test should be performed using glucagon or leucine instead of tolbutamide.

Nursing Care Before the Procedure

Client preparation is essentially the same as that for an OGTT (see p. 146).
➤ The individual should be informed that venous access will be established with either a continuous infusion or an intermittent device and that a medication that lowers blood sugar will be administered.
➤ The client should be questioned regarding allergies to sulfonylureas or sulfonamides.
➤ Clients with a history of abnormal hypoglycemia will need reassurance that they will be monitored closely during the test.

The Procedure

Venous access is established and a sample is obtained for a fasting blood sugar (FBS). The IV catheter is then connected to an intermittent device (e.g., heparin lock) or to a continuous IV infusion of normal saline at a keep-vein-open (KVO) rate. Tolbutamide 1.0 g mixed in 20 mL sterile water is administered IV. Blood glucose samples are obtained via the IV catheter at 15-minute intervals for the first hour and then at 1½-, 2-, and 3-hour intervals. Observe the client closely for signs and symptoms of hypoglycemia. If hypoglycemia occurs, obtain a stat fasting blood sugar, notify the physician, and initiate an IV infusion of 5 percent glucose and water, if ordered.

Note any signs or symptoms of sensitivity reaction to tolbutamide. If a reaction occurs, notify the physician and administer drugs as ordered. Maintain an open IV line until there is no further danger of adverse drug reaction.

Nursing Care After the Procedure

The venous access device is left in place until any danger of hypoglycemia is past. It is then removed and a pressure bandage applied to the site. Food and medications withheld before the test, as well as usual activities, should be resumed on its completion.
➤ Continue to observe for signs and symptoms of hypoglycemia for 2 hours or more, depending on results of the 3-hour interval blood sugar.
➤ Assess the venipuncture site for signs of hematoma or phlebitis.
➤ Observe for adequate intake when foods are resumed.

PROTEINS

Proteins, also called polypeptides, consist of amino acids linked together by peptide bonds. Although all human proteins are constructed from a mere 20 amino acids, variations in chain length, amino acid sequence, and incorporated constituents combine to make possible an almost infinite number of protein molecules. All cells manufacture proteins, with different proteins characterizing different cell types. The amino acids needed for these processes enter the body from dietary sources. These amino acids are rapidly distributed to tissue cells, which promptly incorporate them into proteins.

Three fourths of the body's solid matter is protein and, except for hemoglobin, relatively little circulates in whole blood. The major plasma proteins are albumin, the globulins, and fibrinogen. Fibrinogen evolves into insoluble fibrin when blood coagulates. The fluid that remains after coagulation is called serum. Serum and plasma have the same protein composition except that serum lacks fibrinogen and several other coagulation factors (prothrombin, factor VIII, factor V, and factor XIII).

The proteins in circulating blood transport amino acids from one site to another, providing raw materials for synthesis, degradation, and metabolic interconversion. Circulating proteins also function as buffers in acid-base balance, contribute to the maintenance of colloidal osmotic pressure, and aid in transporting lipids, enzymes, hormones, vitamins, and certain minerals.

Most plasma proteins originate in the liver. Hepatocytes synthesize fibrinogen, albumin, and 60 to 80 percent of the globulins. The remaining globulins are immunoglobulins (antibodies), which are manufactured by the lymphoreticular system. Immunoglobulins are studied as part of the immune system (see Chap. 3), whereas fibrinogen is usually studied as part of a coagulation work-up (see Chap. 2). The focus of this section is on the major serum proteins (albumin and nonantibody globulins), binding proteins, and protein metabolites.[17]

Serum Proteins

General assessment of the serum proteins includes measurement of total protein, albumin, globulin, and the albumin-globulin (A-G) ratio. Although these tests are being replaced by serum protein electrophoresis (see Chap. 3), they may still be ordered for screening purposes or as components of multitest chemistry profiles, because they provide an overall picture of protein homeostasis.

Several disorders can cause alterations in serum proteins. Those affecting total protein levels are listed in Table 5–3. Albumin levels show less variation. Except for dehydration, exercise, and effects of certain drugs (e.g., gallamine triethiodide [Flaxedil]), elevated albumin levels do not occur. Albumin may be decreased in a number of situations caused, in general, by (1) decreased hepatic synthesis, (2) excessive renal excretion, (3) increased metabolic degradation, and (4) complex combined disorders. Specific problems associated with hypoalbuminemia are listed in Table 5–4.

Globulin levels show more variation than do albumin levels, probably because of the multiple production sites for this protein. Causes of altered globulin levels are listed in Table 5–5 according to the type of globulin affected.

Table 5-3 ➤ CAUSES OF ALTERED TOTAL SERUM PROTEINS

Increased Levels	Decreased Levels
Kala-azar	Renal disease
Dehydration	Ulcerative colitis
Macroglobulinemias	Water intoxication
Sarcoidosis	Cirrhosis
	Severe burns
Drugs	Scleroderma
Adrenocorticotropic hormone (ACTH), corticosteroids	Malnutrition
Clofibrate	Hodgkin's disease
Dextran	Hemorrhage
Growth hormone	
Heparin	*Drugs*
Insulin	Ammonium ion
Sulfobromophthalein (Bromsulphalein, BSP)	Dextran
Thyroid preparations	Oral contraceptives
Tolbutamide	Pyrazinamide
X-ray contrast media	Salicylates

The A-G ratio indicates the balance between total albumin and total globulin and is usually evaluated in relation to the total protein level. A low protein level and a reversed A-G ratio (i.e., decreased albumin and elevated globulins) suggest chronic liver disease. A normal total protein level with a reversed A-G ratio suggests myeloproliferative disease (e.g., leukemia, Hodgkin's disease) or certain chronic infectious diseases (e.g., tuberculosis, chronic hepatitis).

Reference Values

The reference values for total protein, albumin, and globulin vary slightly across the life cycle and are listed accordingly. Values for γ-globulins are provided for comparison purposes.

Age	Total Protein Conventional Units	SI Units	Albumin Conventional Units	SI Units	Globulins Conventional Units	SI Units	γ-Globulins Conventional Units	SI Units
Newborns	5.0–7.1 g/dL	50–70 g/L	2.5–5.0 g/dL	25–50 g/L	1.2–4.0 g/dL	12–40 g/L	0.7–0.9 g/dL	7–9 g/L
3 mo	4.7–7.4 g/dL	47–74 g/L	3.0–4.2 g/dL	30–42 g/L	1.0–3.3 g/dL	10–33 g/L	0.1–0.5 g/dL	1–5 g/L
1 yr	5.0–7.5 g/dL	50–75 g/L	2.7–5.0 g/dL	27–50 g/L	2.0–3.8 g/dL	20–38 g/L	0.4–1.2 g/dL	4–12 g/L
15 yr	6.5–8.6 g/dL	65–86 g/L	3.2–5.0 g/dL	32–50 g/L	2.0–4.0 g/dL	20–40 g/L	0.6–1.2 g/dL	6–12 g/L
Adults	6.6–7.9 g/dL	66–79 g/L	3.3–4.5 g/dL	33–45 g/L	2.0–4.2 g/dL	20–42 g/L	0.5–1.6 g/dL	5–16 g/L

Albumin-globulin (A-G) ratio 1.5 : 1–2.5 : 1.

Although discussed in Chapter 3, the normal values for serum protein electrophoresis are repeated next for reference purposes. Values are reported as percentage of total proteins.

Total Globulins		Albumin		α_1		α_2		β		γ	
Conven-tional Units	SI Units	Conven-tional Units	SI Units	Conven-tional Units	SI Units	Conven-tional Units	SI Units	Conven-tional Units	SI Units	Conven-tional Units	SI Units
52– 68	0.520– 0.680	32– 48	0.320– 0.480	10.7– 21.0	0.107– 0.210	8.5– 14.5	0.085– 0.145	6.6– 13.5	0.066– 0.135	2.4– 5.3	0.024– 0.053

Interfering Factors

➤ High serum lipid levels may interfere with accurate testing.
➤ Numerous drugs may alter protein levels (see Tables 5–3 and 5–4).

Table 5–4 ➤ CAUSES OF HYPOALBUMINEMIA

Decreased Synthesis of Albumin
Malnutrition (starvation, malabsorption iron deficiency)
Chronic diseases (tuberculosis)
Acute infections (hepatitis, brucellosis)
Chronic liver disease
Collagen disorders (scleroderma, systemic lupus erythematosus [SLE])

Drugs
Acetaminophen (Tylenol)
Azathioprine (Imuran)
Conjugated estrogens (Premarin)
Cyclophosphamide (Cytoxan)
Dextran
Ethinyl estradiol (Estinyl)
Heroin
Mestranol/norethynodrel (Enovid)
Niacin
Nicotinyl alcohol (Roniacol)

Increased Loss of Albumin
Ascites
Burns (severe)
Nephrotic syndrome
Chronic renal failure

Increased Catabolism of Albumin
Malignancies (leukemias, advanced tumors)
Trauma

Multifactorial Causes
Cirrhosis
Congestive heart failure (CHF)
Pregnancy
Toxemia of pregnancy
Diabetes mellitus
Myxedema
Rheumatic fever
Rheumatoid arthritis
Hypocalcemia

Table 5–5 ➤ CAUSES OF ALTERED SERUM GLOBULIN LEVELS

Globulin	Increased Levels	Decreased Levels
α_1 (Alpha$_1$)	Pregnancy Malignancies Acute infections Tissue necrosis	Genetic deficiency of α_1-antitrypsin
α_2 (Alpha$_2$)	Acute infections Trauma, burns Advanced malignancies Rheumatic fever Rheumatoid arthritis Acute myocardial infarction Nephrotic syndrome	Hemolytic anemia Severe liver disease
β (Beta)	Hypothyroidism Biliary cirrhosis Nephrotic syndrome Diabetes mellitus Cushing's syndrome Malignant hypertension	Hypocholesterolemia
γ (Gamma)	Connective tissue diseases (such as systemic lupus erythematosus [SLE] and rheumatoid arthritis) Hodgkin's disease Chronic active liver disease Drugs Tolazamide (Tolinase) Tubocurarine Anticonvulsants	Nephrotic syndrome Lymphocytic leukemia Lymphosarcoma Drugs Bacille Calmette-Guérin (BCG) vaccine Methotrexate

Indications for Serum Proteins Test

➤ Routine screening as part of a complete physical examination, with normal results indicating satisfactory overall protein homeostasis

➤ Clinical signs of diseases associated with altered serum proteins (see Tables 5–3, 5–4, and 5–5)

➤ Monitoring of response to therapy with drugs that may alter serum protein levels

Nursing Care Before the Procedure

Client preparation is the same as that for any test involving collection of a peripheral blood sample (see Appendix I).

➤ Some laboratories require an 8-hour fast before the test, as well as a low-fat diet for several days before the test, because high serum lipid levels may interfere with accurate testing.

The Procedure

A venipuncture is performed and the sample collected in a red-topped tube. The sample should be handled gently and sent promptly to the laboratory.

Nursing Care After the Procedure

Care and assessment after the procedure are the same as for any study involving collection of a peripheral blood sample. Resume any foods withheld before the test.

➤ *Abnormal values:* Note and report increased levels. Assess for symptoms of dehydration that can cause hyperproteinemia such as thirst, dry skin and mucous membranes, or poor skin turgor. Assess fluid loss resulting from vomiting, diarrhea, or renal dysfunction. Note and report decreased levels. Assess in relation to hypoalbuminuria and for edema in serum albumin levels as low as 2.0 to 2.5 g/dL. Assess for causes of hypoalbuminemia such as acute or chronic liver disease or renal dysfunction. Assess for stress, injury, or infection that requires increased protein intake. Prepare for IV administration of albumin replacement in severe conditions. Monitor I&O. Encourage and instruct in increased dietary protein intake.

α_1-Antitrypsin (α_1-AT)

α_1-Antitrypsin (α_1-AT) is an α_1-globulin produced by the liver. Its function is inhibition of the proteolytic enzymes trypsin and plasmin, which are released by alveolar macrophages and by bacteria in the lungs. As with many other proteins, the α_1-AT molecule has several structural variants. Some of these variant molecules have different electrophoretic mobility and reduced ability to inhibit proteolytic enzymes.

Inherited deficiencies in normal α_1-AT activity are associated with the development, early in life, of lung and liver disorders in which functional tissue is destroyed and replaced with excessive connective tissue; that is, emphysema and cirrhosis may develop in children and young adults who are deficient in α_1-AT, without the usual predisposing factors associated with onset of these disorders. Such deficiencies are seen on serum protein electrophoresis as a flat area where the normal α_1-globulin hump should be. More detailed physiochemical analysis can demonstrate which variant form is present. Decreased levels of α_1-AT also are seen in nephrotic syndrome and malnutrition.

Reference Values

80 to 213 mg/dL

Interfering Factors

➤ Pregnancy
➤ Oral contraceptive and steroid administration
➤ Extreme physical stress caused by trauma or surgery

Indications for α_1-Antitrypsin (α_1-AT) Test

➤ Genetic absence or deficiency of α_1-AT, indicated by decreased levels of the protease
➤ Suspected inflammation, infection, and necrosis processes, indicated by increased levels of the protease
➤ Family history of α_1-AT deficiency

Nursing Care Before the Procedure

Client preparation is the same as that for any test involving collection of a peripheral blood sample (see Appendix I).
➤ The client should fast for 8 hours before the test.
➤ Water is not restricted.

➤ Oral contraceptives and steroids should be withheld 24 hours before the study, although this practice should be confirmed with the person ordering the test.

The Procedure

A venipuncture is performed and the sample collected in a red-topped tube. The sample should be handled gently to avoid hemolysis and frozen if not tested immediately.

Nursing Care After the Procedure

Care and assessment after the procedure are the same as for any study involving the collection of a peripheral blood sample.

➤ Resume meals or medications withheld before the test.

➤ *Abnormal values:* Note and report decreased levels. Assess for pulmonary or liver disorders and associated signs and symptoms, smoking history, and pollution in the home or work environment. Inform client of stop-smoking clinics and resources for genetic counseling. Instruct client in ways to protect pulmonary system from irritants. Inform client of the importance of medical follow-up. Suggest ongoing support resources to assist client in coping with illness and possible early death.

Binding Proteins

HAPTOGLOBIN

Haptoglobin, an α_2-globulin produced in the liver, binds free hemoglobin released by the hemolysis of red blood cells in the bloodstream. Most red blood cells are normally removed in the reticuloendothelial system (e.g., liver, spleen) by a process known as extravascular destruction. Approximately 10 percent of red blood cells are, however, broken down in the circulation (intravascular destruction). This percentage may increase in situations caused by excessive red blood cell hemolysis (e.g., transfusion reaction, hemolytic anemia).

The free hemoglobin released from intravascular red blood cell destruction is unstable in plasma and dissociates into components (α-β dimers) that are quickly bound to haptoglobin. Formation of the haptoglobin-hemoglobin complex prevents the renal excretion of plasma hemoglobin and stabilizes the heme-globin bond. The haptoglobin-hemoglobin complex is removed from the circulation by the liver.

There is a limit to the capacity of the haptoglobin-binding mechanism, and a sudden intravascular release of several grams of hemoglobin can exceed binding capacity. Furthermore, because haptoglobin itself is removed from the circulation as a haptoglobin-hemoglobin complex and is catabolized by the liver, a decrease in or absence of haptoglobin may be used to indicate increased intravascular red blood cell hemolysis.

Because haptoglobin is formed in the liver, chronic liver disease with impaired protein synthesis also may result in decreased haptoglobin levels. Although haptoglobin is absent in most newborns, congenital absence of haptoglobin (congenital ahaptoglobinemia) also may occur in a very small percentage of the population.

If haptoglobin is deficient or its binding capacity overwhelmed, unbound hemoglobin dimers are free to be filtered by the renal glomerulus, after which they are reabsorbed by the renal tubules and converted into hemosiderin (a storage form of iron). If renal tubular uptake capacity is exceeded, either free hemoglobin or methemoglobin (a type of hemoglobin with iron in the ferric, instead of the ferrous, form) is excreted in the urine. It should be noted that reabsorption of free hemoglobin may damage the renal tubules because of excessive deposition of hemosiderin.[18]

Elevated haptoglobin levels are seen in inflammatory diseases (e.g., ulcerative colitis, arthritis, pyelonephritis) and in disorders involving tissue destruction (e.g., malignancies, burns, acute myocardial infarction). Steroid therapy may also elevate haptoglobin levels. Elevated levels are not of major clinical significance except to indicate that additional testing may be necessary to determine the source of the elevation.

Reference Values

	Conventional Units	SI Units
Newborns	0–10 mg/dL	0–0.1 g/L
Adults	30–160 mg/dL	0.3–1.6 g/L

Interfering Factors

➤ Steroid therapy may result in elevated levels.

Indications for Haptoglobin Test

➤ Known or suspected disorder characterized by excessive red blood cell hemolysis, as indicated by decreased levels
➤ Known or suspected chronic liver disease, as indicated by decreased levels
➤ Suspected congenital ahaptoglobinemia, as indicated by decreased levels
➤ Known or suspected disorders involving a diffuse inflammatory process or tissue destruction, as indicated by elevated levels

Nursing Care Before the Procedure

Client preparation is the same as that for any test involving collection of a peripheral blood sample (see Appendix I).

The Procedure

A venipuncture is performed and the sample collected in a red-topped tube. Some laboratories require that the sample be placed in ice immediately upon collection. The sample should be handled gently to avoid hemolysis, which may alter test results, and sent promptly to the laboratory.

Nursing Care After the Procedure

Care and assessment after the procedure are the same as for any study involving the collection of a peripheral blood sample.

CERULOPLASMIN (CP)

Ceruloplasmin (Cp) is an α_2-globulin that binds copper for transport within the circulation after it is absorbed from the gastrointestinal tract. Among the disorders associated with abnormal ceruloplasmin levels is Wilson's disease (hepato-lenticular degeneration), an inherited disorder characterized by excessive absorption of copper from the gastrointestinal tract, decreased ceruloplasmin, and deposition of copper in the liver, brain, corneas (Kayser-Fleischer rings), and kidneys. In addition to low ceruloplasmin levels, serum copper levels are decreased because of excessive excretion of unbound copper in the kidneys and deposition of copper in the body tissues. The disorder manifests during the first three decades of life and is fatal unless treatment is instituted.

Other causes of abnormal ceruloplasmin levels are listed in Table 5–6.

Reference Values

	Conventional Units	**SI Units**
Newborns	2–13 mg/dL	20–130 μmol/L
Adults	23–50 mg/dL	230–500 μmol/L

Indications for Ceruloplasmin (Cp) Test

➤ Family history of Wilson's disease (hepatolenticular degeneration)
➤ Signs of liver disease combined with neurological changes, especially in a young person, with Wilson's disease indicated by decreased levels
➤ Monitoring of ceruloplasmin levels in disorders associated with abnormal values (see Table 5–6)
➤ Monitoring of response to total parenteral nutrition (hyperalimentation), which may lead to decreased levels

Nursing Care Before the Procedure

Client preparation is the same as that for any test involving collection of a peripheral blood sample (see Appendix I).

The Procedure

A venipuncture is performed and the sample collected in a red-topped tube. Some laboratories require that the sample be placed in ice immediately on col-

Table 5–6 ➤ CAUSES OF ALTERED LEVELS OF CERULOPLASMIN	
Increased Levels	**Decreased Levels**
Acute infections	Wilson's disease
Hepatitis	Malabsorption syndromes
Hodgkin's disease	Long-term total parenteral nutrition (TPN)
Hyperthyroidism	Menkes' kinky hair syndrome
Pregnancy	Nephrosis
Malignancies of bone, lung, stomach	Severe liver disease
Myocardial infarction	Early infancy
Rheumatoid arthritis	
Drugs	
Oral contraceptives	
Estrogens	
Methadone	
Phenytoin (Dilantin)	

lection. The sample should be handled gently to avoid hemolysis and sent promptly to the laboratory.

Nursing Care After the Procedure

Care and assessment after the procedure are the same as for any study involving the collection of a peripheral blood sample.

➤ *Abnormal values:* Note and report decreased levels. Assess for hepatic or neurological or psychiatric manifestations of Wilson's disease. Assess for history of ceruloplasmin deficiency by Kayser-Fleischer rings determined by slit-lamp examination. Inform of need for follow-up medical care and genetic counseling.

Protein Metabolites

Most nitrogen in the blood resides in proteins, and the amount of nitrogen contained in proteins is high in relation to amino acid content. When proteins are metabolized, the nitrogen-containing components are removed from the amino acids, a process known as deamination. The resulting protein metabolites include urea, creatinine, ammonia, creatine, and uric acid. Levels of these nonprotein nitrogenous compounds reflect various aspects of protein balance and metabolism.

UREA NITROGEN

Urea is a nonprotein nitrogenous compound that is formed in the liver from ammonia. Although urea diffuses freely into both extracellular and intracellular fluid, it is ultimately excreted by the kidneys. Blood urea levels reflect the balance between production and excretion of urea. Changes in protein intake, fluid balance, liver function, and renal excretion affect blood urea levels. Specific causes of alterations are listed in Table 5–7.

Blood urea analysis involves measurement of nitrogen; the result is expressed as urea nitrogen. Nitrogen contributes 46.7 percent of the total weight of urea. The concentration of urea can be calculated by multiplying the urea nitrogen result by 2.14.[19]

Reference Values

	Conventional Units [Urea Nitrogen]	**SI Units [Urea]**
Newborns	4–18 mg/dL	1.4–6.4 mmol/L
Children	7–18 mg/dL	2.5–6.4 mmol/L
Adults	5–20 mg/dL	1.8–7.1 mmol/L
Critical Values	**>100 mg/dL**	**>35.7 mmol/L**

Interfering Factors

➤ Therapy with drugs known to alter urea nitrogen levels (see Table 5–7)

Indications for Urea Nitrogen Test

➤ Known or suspected disorder associated with impaired renal function, as indicated by increased levels

Table 5-7 ➤ CAUSES OF ALTERED UREA LEVELS

Increased Levels	Decreased Levels
Congestive heart failure (CHF)	Inadequate dietary protein
Shock	Severe liver disease
Hypovolemia	Water overload
Urinary tract obstruction	Nephrotic syndrome
Renal diseases	Pregnancy
Starvation	Amyloidosis
Infection	Malabsorption syndromes
Myocardial infarction	
Diabetes mellitus	*Drugs*
Burns	IV dextrose
Gastrointestinal bleeding	Phenothiazines
Advanced pregnancy	Thymol
Nephrotoxic agents	
Excessive protein ingestion	
Malignancies	
Addison's disease	
Gout	
Pancreatitis	
Tissue necrosis	
Advanced age	
Drugs	
Aspirin	
Acetaminophen	
Cancer chemotherapeutic agents	
Antibiotics (amphotericin B, cephalosporins, aminoglycosides)	
Thiazide diuretics	
Indomethacin (Indocin)	
Morphine	
Codeine	
Sulfonamides	
Methyldopa (Aldomet)	
Propranolol (Inderal)	
Guanethidine (Ismelin)	
Pargyline (Eutonyl)	
Lithium carbonate	
Dextran	
Sulfonylureas	

- Obstructive, inflammatory, or toxic damage to the kidneys, nephron loss caused by aging, or extrarenal conditions that reduce the glomerular filtration rate (GFR) increase retention of urea.
- ➤ Monitoring for the effects of disorders associated with altered fluid balance
  - Dehydration or hypovolemia caused by vomiting, diarrhea, hemorrhage, or inadequate fluid intake raises the urea nitrogen.
  - Fluid overload decreases the urea nitrogen if renal function is adequate.
- ➤ Known or suspected liver disease as indicated by decreased levels caused by the liver's inability to convert ammonia to urea (80 percent of liver function may be lost before this is evident)
- ➤ Monitoring for effects of drugs known to be nephrotoxic or hepatotoxic

➤ Monitoring of response to various disorders known to result in altered urea nitrogen levels (see Table 5–7, p. 165)

Nursing Care Before the Procedure

Client preparation is the same as that for any test involving collection of a peripheral blood sample (see Appendix I).

➤ Some laboratories require an 8-hour fast before the test.

The Procedure

A venipuncture is performed and the sample is obtained in either a gray-topped or red-topped tube, depending on the laboratory performing the test. The sample should be handled gently to avoid hemolysis and transported promptly to the laboratory.

Nursing Care After the Procedure

Care and assessment after the procedure are the same as for any study involving the collection of a peripheral blood sample.

➤ If the client's diet has been restricted before the test, the usual diet may be resumed.

➤ *Abnormal levels:* Note and report decreased levels. Assess hydration status for overhydration, I&O, osmolality, and sodium levels. Note and report increased levels and assess in relation to creatinine level. Assess electrolyte panel and for signs and symptoms of anemia, gastrointestinal bleeding, oliguria, confusion, level of consciousness if urea nitrogen rises to greater than 20 to 50 mg/dL. Monitor urinary output every hour. Provide safety measures if consciousness is altered. Instruct as to restriction in fluid and dietary intake of protein (meat, fish, poultry).

➤ *Critical values:* Notify the physician immediately if levels are greater than 100 mg/dL.

SERUM CREATININE

Creatinine is the end product of creatine metabolism. Creatine, although synthesized largely in the liver, resides almost exclusively in skeletal muscle, where it reversibly combines with phosphate to form the energy storage compound phosphocreatine. This reaction (creatine + phosphate ⇌ phosphocreatine) repeats as energy is released and regenerated, but in the process small amounts of creatine are irreversibly converted to creatinine, which serves no useful function and circulates only for transportation to the kidneys. The amount of creatinine generated in an individual is proportional to the mass of skeletal muscle present; level of muscular activity is not a critical determinant.

Daily generation of creatinine remains fairly constant unless crushing injury or degenerative diseases cause massive muscle damage. The kidneys excrete creatinine very efficiently. Levels of blood and urine flow affect creatinine excretion much less than they influence urea excretion because temporary alterations in renal blood flow and glomerular function can be compensated by increased tubular secretion of creatinine. Thus, serum creatinine is a more sensitive indicator of renal function than is urea nitrogen.[20]

Reference Values

	Conventional Units	SI Units
Children <6 yr	0.3–0.6 mg/dL	24–54 μmol/L
Children 6–18 yr	0.4–1.2 mg/dL	36–106 μmol/L
Adults		
Men	0.6–1.3 mg/dL	53–115 μmol/L
Women	0.5–1.0 mg/dL	44–88 μmol/L
Critical Values	**>10 mg/dL**	**>880 μmol/L**

Indications for Serum Creatinine Test

➤ Known or suspected impairment of renal function, including therapy with nephrotoxic drugs
  • In the absence of disorders affecting muscle mass, elevated creatinine levels indicate decreased renal function.
  • Creatinine levels may be normal in situations in which a slow decline in renal function occurs simultaneously with a slow decline in muscle mass, as may occur in elderly individuals (in such situations, a 24-hour urine collection yields lower than normal excretion levels).
➤ Along with a urea nitrogen, to provide additional client information
  • An elevated urea nitrogen with a normal creatinine usually indicates a nonrenal cause for the excessive urea.
  • The urea nitrogen rises more steeply than creatinine as renal function declines, and it falls more rapidly with dialysis.
  • With severe, permanent renal impairment, urea levels continue to climb, but creatinine values tend to plateau (at very high circulating creatinine levels, some is excreted through the gastrointestinal tract).
➤ Known or suspected disorder involving muscles, including crushing injury to muscles
  • In the absence of renal disease, elevated serum creatinine levels are associated with trauma or disorders causing excessive muscle mass (gigantism, acromegaly).
  • Decreased levels are associated with muscular dystrophy.

Nursing Care Before the Procedure

Client preparation is the same as that for any test involving collection of a peripheral blood sample (see Appendix I).
➤ Some laboratories require an 8-hour fast before the test.

The Procedure

A venipuncture is performed and the sample collected in a red-topped tube. The sample should be sent promptly to the laboratory.

Nursing Care After the Procedure

Care and assessment after the procedure are the same as for any study involving the collection of a peripheral blood sample.
➤ *Complications and precautions:* Increased levels should be assessed in relation to the urea nitrogen; notify the physician immediately if levels are greater than 10 mg/dL unless the client is on dialysis.

AMMONIA

Blood ammonia comes from two sources: (1) deamination of amino acids during protein metabolism and (2) degradation of proteins by colon bacteria. The liver converts ammonia to urea, generating glutamine as an intermediary. The kidneys then use glutamine as a source for synthesizing ammonia for renal regulation of electrolyte and acid-base balance. Serum ammonia levels have little effect on renal excretion of ammonia.

Circulating blood normally contains very little ammonia because the liver converts ammonia in the portal blood to urea. When liver function is severely compromised, especially in situations when decreased hepatocellular function is combined with impaired portal blood flow, ammonia levels rise. Both elevated serum ammonia and abnormal glutamine metabolism have been implicated as etiologic factors in hepatic encephalopathy (hepatic coma).[21] Additional causes of altered serum ammonia levels are listed in Table 5–8.

Reference Values

	Conventional Units	**SI Units**
Newborns	90–150 μg/dL	64–107 μmol/L
Children	40–80 μg/dL	23–47 μmol/L
Adults	15–45 μg/dL	11–32 μmol/L

Table 5–8 ➤ CAUSES OF ALTERED BLOOD AMMONIA LEVELS

Increased Levels	**Decreased Levels**
Liver failure, late cirrhosis	Renal failure
GI hemorrhage	Hypertension
Late congestive heart failure (CHF)	
Azotemia	*Drugs*
Hemolytic disease of the newborn	Arginine (R-Gene)
Chronic obstructive pulmonary disease (COPD)	Benadryl
Leukemias	Sodium salts
Reye's syndrome	Glutamic acid (Acidulin)
Inborn enzyme deficiency	MAO inhibitors
Excessive protein ingestion	Antibiotics (tetracycline
Alkalosis	[Achromycin], kanamycin
	[Kantrex], neomycin)
Drugs	Potassium salts
Acetazolamide (Diamox)	
Ammonium salts	
Barbiturates	
Colistin (Coly-Mycin S)	
Diuretics	
Ethanol	
Heparin	
Isoniazid	
Methicillin	
Morphine	
Tetracycline	

Indications for Serum Ammonia Test

➤ Evaluation of advanced liver disease or other disorders associated with altered serum ammonia levels (see Table 5–8)
➤ Identification of impending hepatic encephalopathy in clients with known liver diseases (e.g., after bleeding from esophageal varices or other gastrointestinal sources, or after excessive ingestion of protein) as indicated by rising levels
➤ Monitoring for the effectiveness of treatment for hepatic encephalopathy as indicated by declining levels

Nursing Care Before the Procedure

Client preparation is essentially the same as that for any study involving the collection of a peripheral blood sample (see Appendix I). An 8-hour fast from food is required before the test.

The Procedure

A venipuncture is performed and the sample collected in a green-topped tube. Some laboratories require that the sample be placed in ice immediately on collection. The sample should be handled gently to avoid hemolysis and sent promptly to the laboratory.

Nursing Care After the Procedure

Care and assessment after the procedure are the same as for any study involving the collection of a peripheral blood sample. Resume foods withheld before the test.

SERUM CREATINE

Creatine is a nitrogen-containing compound found largely in skeletal muscle, where it functions as an energy source. Its use by muscles results in loss proportionate to the muscle mass and level of muscular activity. Measurement of serum creatine reflects this loss, which is fairly constant under normal conditions.

Reference Values

	Conventional Units	SI Units
Men	0.1–0.4 mg/dL	9–35 μmol/L
Women	0.2–0.7 mg/dL	18–62 μmol/L

Interfering Factors

➤ Failure to follow dietary restrictions and vigorous exercise within 8 hours of the test may alter results.

Indications for Serum Creatine Test

➤ Signs and symptoms of muscular disease (e.g., muscle injury, muscular dystrophies, dermatomyositis), as indicated by elevated levels
➤ Monitoring for the progression of muscle-wasting diseases with serial measurements indicating the rate of muscle deterioration

➤ Evaluation of the effects of hyperthyroidism and rheumatoid arthritis on muscle tissue

Nursing Care Before the Procedure

Client preparation is essentially the same as that for any study involving the collection of a peripheral blood sample (see Appendix I).

➤ Food, fluids, and vigorous exercise are not permitted for at least 8 hours before the test.

The Procedure

A venipuncture is performed and the sample collected in a red-topped tube. The sample should be handled gently to avoid hemolysis and sent promptly to the laboratory.

Nursing Care After the Procedure

Care and assessment after the procedure are the same as for any test involving the collection of a peripheral blood sample.

➤ Resume foods and fluids withheld before the test, as well as usual activities.

URIC ACID

Uric acid (urate) is the end product of purine metabolism. Purines are important constituents of nucleic acids; purine turnover occurs continuously in the body, producing substantial amounts of uric acid even in the absence of dietary purine (e.g., meats, legumes, yeasts) intake. Most uric acid is synthesized in the liver and excreted by the kidneys. Serum urate levels are affected by the amount of uric acid produced as well as by the efficiency of renal excretion.

Both gout and urate renal calculi (kidney stones) are associated with elevated uric acid levels. Other disorders and drugs associated with altered uric acid levels are listed in Table 5–9.

Reference Values

	Conventional Units	**SI Units**
Children	2.5–5.5 mg/dL	0.15–0.33 mmol/L
Men	4.0–8.5 mg/dL	0.24–0.51 mmol/L
Women	2.7–7.3 mg/dL	0.16–0.43 mmol/L
Critical Values	**>12 mg/dL**	**0.71 mmol/L**

Interfering Factors

➤ Therapy with drugs known to alter uric acid levels (see Table 5–9), unless the test is being conducted to monitor such drug effects

Indications for Uric Acid Test

➤ Family history of gout (autosomal dominant genetic disorder) or signs and symptoms of gout, or both, with the disorder indicated by elevated levels

➤ Known or suspected renal calculi, to determine the cause

➤ Signs and symptoms of disorders associated with altered uric acid levels (see Table 5–9)

Table 5–9 ➤ **CAUSES OF ALTERED URIC ACID LEVELS**

Increased Levels	**Decreased Levels**
Excessive dietary purines	Fanconi's syndrome
Polycythemia	Wilson's disease
Gout	Yellow atrophy of the liver
Psoriasis	
Type III hyperlipidemia	***Drugs***
Chemotherapy, radiation therapy for malignancies	Probenecid
von Gierke's disease	Sulfinpyrazone
Sickle cell anemia	Aspirin (>4 g/day)
Pernicious anemia	Adrenocorticotropic hormone (ACTH),
Acute tissue destruction (infection, starvation, exercise)	corticosteroids
Eclampsia, hypertension	Coumarin
Hyperparathyroidism	Estrogens
Decreased excretion from lactic acidosis, ketoacidosis,	Allopurinol
renal failure, congestive heart failure (CHF)	Acetohexamide (Dymelor)
	Azathioprine (Imuran)
Drugs	Clofibrate
Alcohol	2-Phenylcinchoninic acid (Cinchophen)
Aspirin (<2 g/day)	Chlorprothixene (Taractan)
Thiazide diuretics	Mannitol
Diazoxide (Hyperstat)	Marijuana
Epinephrine	
Ethacrynic acid (Edecrin)	
Furosemide	
Phenothiazines	
Dextran	
Methyldopa	
Ascorbic acid	
Aminophylline	
Antibiotics (gentamicin)	
Griseofulvin	
Rifampin	
Triamterene (Dyrenium)	

➤ Monitoring for the effects of drugs known to alter uric acid levels (see Table 5–9), either as a side effect or as a therapeutic effect

➤ Evaluation of the extent of tissue destruction in infection, starvation, excessive exercise, malignancies, chemotherapy, or radiation therapy

➤ Evaluation of possible liver damage in eclampsia, as indicated by elevated levels

Nursing Care Before the Procedure

Client preparation is the same as that for any study involving the collection of a peripheral blood sample (see Appendix I).

➤ Some laboratories require an 8-hour fast from food before the test.

The Procedure

A venipuncture is performed and the sample collected in a red-topped tube. The sample should be handled gently to avoid hemolysis and sent promptly to the laboratory.

Nursing Care After the Procedure

Care and assessment after the procedure are the same as for any study involving the collection of a peripheral blood sample.

➤ Resume foods withheld before the test.

➤ *Abnormal values:* Note and report increased level. Assess for symptoms associated with renal stones and joint pain. Prepare to administer ordered medications (allopurinol, probenecid, nonsteroidal anti-inflammatory analgesics). Increase fluid intake. Instruct client to avoid high-purine fluids and foods (sardines, organ meats, legumes, alcohol, caffeine-containing beverages).

➤ **Critical values:** Notify the physician immediately if levels are greater than 12 mg/dL.

LIPIDS

Lipids are carbon- and hydrogen-containing compounds that are insoluble in water but soluble in organic solvents. Biologically important categories of lipids are the neutral fats (e.g., triglycerides), the conjugated lipids (e.g., phospholipids), and the sterols (e.g., cholesterol). Lipids function in the body as sources of energy for various metabolic processes. Other functions include contributing to the formation of cell membranes, bile acids, and various hormones.

Lipids are derived from both dietary sources and internal body processes. Almost the entire fat portion of the diet consists of triglycerides, which are combinations of three fatty acids and one glycerol molecule. Triglycerides are found in foods of both animal and plant origin. The usual diet also includes small quantities of phospholipids, cholesterol, and cholesterol esters. Phospholipids and cholesterol esters contain fatty acids. In contrast, cholesterol does not contain fatty acids, but its sterol nucleus is synthesized from their degradation products. Because cholesterol has many of the physical and chemical properties of other lipids, it is included as a dietary fat. It should be noted that cholesterol occurs only in foods of animal origin, including eggs and cheese.

Nearly all dietary fats are absorbed into the lymph. Ingested triglycerides are emulsified by bile and then broken down into fatty acids and glycerol by pancreatic and enteric lipases. The fatty acids and glycerol then pass through the intestinal mucosa and are resynthesized into triglycerides that aggregate and enter the lymph as minute droplets called chylomicrons. Although chylomicrons are composed primarily of triglycerides, cholesterol and phospholipids absorbed from the gastrointestinal tract also contribute to their composition (Table 5–10).

In addition to dietary sources of lipids, the body itself is able to produce various fats. Unused glucose and amino acids, for example, may be converted into fatty acids by the liver. Similarly, nearly all body cells are capable of forming phospholipids and cholesterol, although most of the endogenous production of these lipids occurs in the liver or intestinal mucosa.

Because lipids are insoluble in water, special transport mechanisms are required for circulation in the blood. Free fatty acids travel through blood combined with albumin and in this form are called nonesterified fatty acids. Very little free fatty acid is normally present in the blood; therefore, the major lipid components found in serum are triglycerides, cholesterol, and phospholipids.

Table 5–10 ➤ LIPOPROTEIN COMPOSITION					
	Triglyceride %	**Cholesterol %**	**Phospholipid %**	**Protein %**	**Electrophoretic Mobility**
Chylomicrons	85–95	3–5	5–10	1–2	Remain at origin
Very-low-density lipoproteins	60–70	10–15	10–15	10	α_2-Lipoprotein, pre-β-lipoprotein
Low-density lipoproteins	5–10	45	20–30	15–25	β-Lipoprotein
High-density lipoproteins	Very little	20	30	50	α_1-Lipoprotein

Note: From Sacher, RA, and McPherson, RA: Widmann's Clinical Interpretation of Laboratory Tests, ed 10. FA Davis, Philadelphia, 1991, p 343, with permission.

These lipids exist in blood as macromolecules complexed with specialized proteins (apoproteins) to form lipoproteins.

Lipoproteins are classified according to their density, which results from the amounts of the various lipids they contain (see Table 5–10). The least dense lipoproteins are those with the highest triglyceride levels. Lipoprotein densities also are reflected in the electrophoretic mobility of the various types. As with the formation of other endogenous lipids, most lipoproteins are formed in the liver.[22,23]

FREE FATTY ACIDS (FFA)

Free fatty acids (FFA) travel through the blood combined with albumin and in this form are called nonesterified fatty acids (NEFA). Normally, approximately three fatty acid molecules are combined with each molecule of albumin. If, however, the need for fatty acid transport is great (e.g., when needed carbohydrates are not available or cannot be used for energy), as many as 30 fatty acids can combine with one albumin molecule. Thus, although blood levels of FFA are never very high, they rise impressively after stimuli to release fat. The same stimuli that elevate FFA will, in most cases, also elevate serum triglycerides and may produce alterations in lipoprotein levels. Specific causes of both elevated and decreased FFA, including drugs, are listed in Table 5–11.

Reference Values

	Conventional Units	**SI Units**
Free fatty acids	8–25 mg/dL	0.30–0.90 mmol/L

Interfering Factors

➤ Ingestion of alcohol within 24 hours before the test may result in falsely elevated values.

➤ Failure to follow dietary restrictions before the test may alter values.

➤ Drugs known to alter FFA levels should not be ingested unless the test is being performed to evaluate such effects (see Table 5–11).

Table 5–11 ➤ FACTORS ASSOCIATED WITH ALTERED FREE FATTY ACID LEVELS

Increased Levels	Decreased Levels
Diabetes mellitus	*Drugs*
Starvation	Aspirin
Pheochromocytoma	Clofibrate
Acute alcohol intoxication	Glucose
Chronic hepatitis	Insulin
Acute renal failure	Neomycin
Glycogen storage disease	Streptozocin
Hypoglycemia	
Hypothermia	
Hormones	
Adrenocorticotropic hormone (ACTH)	
Cortisone	
Epinephrine, norepinephrine	
Growth hormone (GH)	
Thyroid-stimulating hormone (TSH)	
Thyroxine	
Drugs	
Amphetamines	
Caffeine	
Chlorpromazine	
Isoproterenol	
Nicotine	
Reserpine	
Tolbutamide	

Indication for Free Fatty Acids (FFA) Test

➤ Support for diagnosing uncontrolled or untreated diabetes mellitus, as indicated by elevated levels
➤ Evaluation of response to treatment for diabetes, as indicated by declining levels
➤ Suspected malnutrition, as indicated by elevated levels
➤ Known or suspected disorder associated with excessive hormone production (see Table 5–11), as indicated by elevated levels
➤ Evaluation of response to therapy with drugs known to alter FFA levels (see Table 5–11)

Nursing Care Before the Procedure

Client preparation is essentially the same as that for any study involving the collection of a peripheral blood sample (see Appendix I).
➤ The client should abstain from alcohol for 24 hours and from food for at least 8 hours before the test; water is not restricted.
➤ Drugs known to affect FFA levels (see Table 5–11) may be withheld before the test, although this may not always be done if the therapeutic effect on FFA levels is being evaluated.

The Procedure

A venipuncture is performed and the sample collected in a red-topped tube. The sample should be sent immediately to the laboratory.

Nursing Care After the Procedure

Care and assessment after the procedure are the same as for any study involving the collection of a peripheral blood sample.

➤ Resume foods and any drugs withheld before the test.

➤ *Abnormal values:* Note and report any increased level. Assess in relation to glucose and ketone and to lipid and lipoprotein electrophoresis levels. Assess for recent weight gain or loss. Instruct in appropriate fat and carbohydrate intake in the diet.

TRIGLYCERIDES

Triglycerides, which are combinations of three fatty acids and one glycerol molecule, are used in the body to provide energy for various metabolic processes, with excess amounts stored in adipose tissue. Fatty acids readily enter and leave the triglycerides of adipose tissue, providing raw materials needed for conversion to glucose (gluconeogenesis) or for direct combustion as an energy source. Although fatty acids originate in the diet, many also derive from unused glucose and amino acids that the liver and, to a smaller extent, the adipose tissue convert into storage energy.

Altered triglyceride levels are associated with a variety of disorders and also are affected by hormones and certain drugs, including alcohol (Table 5–12). Diets high in calories, fats, or carbohydrates will elevate serum triglyceride levels, which is considered a risk factor for atherosclerotic cardiovascular disease.

Reference Values

	Conventional Units	SI Units
<2 yr	5–40 mg/dL	0.06–0.45 mmol/L
2–20 yr	10–140 mg/dL	0.11–1.58 mmol/L
20–40 yr		
Men	10–140 mg/dL	0.11–1.58 mmol/L
Women	10–150 mg/dL	0.11–1.68 mmol/L
40–60 yr		
Men	10–180 mg/dL	0.11–2.01 mmol/L
Women	10–190 mg/dL	0.11–2.21 mmol/L

Values for serum triglycerides may vary according to the laboratory performing the test. In addition, values have been found to vary in relation to race, income level, level of physical activity, dietary habits, and geographic location as well as in relation to age and gender, as shown here.

Interfering Factors

➤ Failure to follow the usual diet for 2 weeks before the test may yield results that do not accurately reflect client status.

Table 5–12 ➤ DISORDERS AND DRUGS ASSOCIATED WITH ALTERED TRIGLYCERIDE LEVELS

Elevated Levels	Decreased Levels
DISORDERS	
Primary hyperlipoproteinemia	Acanthocytosis
Atherosclerosis	Cirrhosis
Hypertension	Inadequate dietary protein
Myocardial infarction	Hyperthyroidism
Diabetes mellitus	Hyperparathyroidism
Obstructive jaundice	
Hypothyroidism (primary)	
Hypoparathyroidism	
Nephrotic syndrome	
Chronic obstructive pulmonary disease (COPD)	
Down syndrome	
von Gierke's disease	
DRUGS	
Alcohol	Clofibrate
Cholestyramine	Dextrothyroxine
Corticosteroids	Heparin
Colestipol	Menotropins (Pergonal)
Oral contraceptives	Sulfonylureas
Thyroid preparations	Norethindrone
Estrogen	Androgens
Furosemide	Niacin
Miconazole	Anabolic steroids
	Ascorbic acid

➤ Ingestion of alcohol 24 hours before and food 12 hours before the test may falsely elevate levels.

➤ Drugs known to alter triglyceride levels shold not be ingested within 24 hours before the test unless the test is being conducted to evaluate such effects (see Table 5–12).

Indications for Serum Triglycerides Test

➤ As a component of a complete physical examination, especially for individuals over age 40 or who are obese, or both, to estimate the degree of risk for atherosclerotic cardiovascular disease

➤ Family history of hyperlipoproteinemia (hyperlipidemia)

➤ Known or suspected disorders associated with altered triglyceride levels (see Table 5–12)

➤ Monitoring of response to drugs known to alter triglyceride levels or lipid-lowering agents

Nursing Care Before the Procedure

General client preparation is the same as that for any procedure involving collection of a peripheral blood sample (see Appendix I).

➤ For this test, the client should ingest a normal diet, so that no weight gain or loss will occur for 2 weeks before the study, and should abstain from alcohol for 24 hours and from food for 12 hours before the test.

➤ Water is not restricted.
➤ It is also recommended that drugs that may alter triglyceride levels be withheld for 24 hours before the test, although this practice should be confirmed with the person ordering the study.

The Procedure

A venipuncture is performed and the sample collected in a red-topped tube. The sample should be sent promptly to the laboratory.

Nursing Care After the Procedure

Care and assessment after the procedure are the same as for any study involving the collection of a peripheral blood sample.
➤ Resume foods and any drugs withheld before the test.
➤ *Abnormal values:* Note and report increased level. Assess in relation to cholesterol and lipoprotein electrophoresis. Instruct in low-fat diet and weight reduction caloric intake as appropriate.

TOTAL CHOLESTEROL

Cholesterol is necessary for the formation of cell membranes and is a component of the materials that render the skin waterproof. Cholesterol also contributes to the formation of bile salts, adrenocorticosteroids, estrogens, and androgens.

Cholesterol has two sources: (1) that obtained from the diet (exogenous cholesterol) and (2) that which is synthesized in the body (endogenous cholesterol). Although most body cells can form some cholesterol, most is produced by the liver and the intestinal mucosa. Because cholesterol is continuously synthesized, degraded, and recycled, it is probable that very little dietary cholesterol enters directly into metabolic reactions. Altered cholesterol levels are associated with a variety of disorders and also are affected by hormones and certain drugs (Table 5–13).

Reference Values

	Conventional Units	**SI Units**
<25 yr	125–200 mg/dL	3.27–5.20 mmol/L
25–40 yr	140–225 mg/dL	3.69–5.85 mmol/L
40–50 yr	160–245 mg/dL	4.37–6.35 mmol/L
50–65 yr	170–265 mg/dL	4.71–6.85 mmol/L
>65 yr	175–265 mg/dL	4.71–6.85 mmol/L

Values for total cholesterol may vary according to the laboratory performing the test. In addition, values have been found to vary according to gender, race, income level, level of physical activity, dietary habits, and geographic location as well as in relation to age, as shown here.

Interfering Factors

➤ Ingestion of alcohol 24 hours before and food 12 hours before the test may falsely elevate levels.
➤ Ingestion of drugs known to alter cholesterol levels within 12 hours of the test may alter results, unless the test is being conducted to evaluate such effects (see Table 5–13).

Table 5–13 ➤ DISORDERS AND DRUGS ASSOCIATED WITH ALTERED CHOLESTEROL LEVELS	
Elevated Levels	**Decreased Levels**
DISORDERS	
Familial hyperlipoproteinemia	Malabsorption syndromes
Atherosclerosis	Liver disease
Hypertension	Hyperthyroidism
Myocardial infarction	Cushing's syndrome
Obstructive jaundice	Pernicious anemia
Hypothyroidism (primary)	Carcinomatosis
Nephrosis	
Xanthomatosis	
Pregnancy	
Oophorectomy	
DRUGS	
Adrenocorticotropic hormone (ACTH)	Antidiabetic agents
Androgens	Cholestyramine
Bile salts	Clofibrate
Catecholamines	Colchicine
Corticosteroids	Colestipol
Oral contraceptives	Dextrothyroxine
Phenothiazines	Estrogen
Salicylates	Glucagon
Thiouracils	Haloperidol (Haldol)
Vitamins A and D (excessive)	Heparin
	Kanamycin
	Neomycin
	Nitrates, nitrites
	Para aminosalicylate (PAS)
	Phenytoin (Dilantin)

Indications for Total Cholesterol Test

➤ As a component of a complete physical examination, especially for individuals over age 40 or those who are obese, or both, to estimate the degree of risk for atherosclerotic cardiovascular disease
  * In general, the desirable blood cholesterol level is less than 200 mg/dL.
  * Cholesterol levels of 200 to 240 mg/dL are considered borderline, and the person is considered at high risk if other factors such as obesity and smoking are present; for the latter individuals, additional tests such as lipoprotein and cholesterol fractionation (see p. 181) should be performed.
  * Cholesterol levels of greater than 250 mg/dL place the person at definite high risk for cardiovascular disease and require treatment; additional tests such as lipoprotein and cholesterol fractionation should be performed.
➤ Family history of hypercholesterolemia or cardiovascular disease or both
➤ Known or suspected disorders associated with altered cholesterol levels (see Table 5–13)
➤ Monitoring of response to dietary treatment of hypercholesterolemia and support for decisions regarding need for drug therapy (cholesterol levels may fall with diet modification alone over a period of 6 months, only to return gradually to previous levels)

➤ Monitoring for response to drugs known to alter cholesterol levels (see Table 5–13) or lipid-lowering agents

Nursing Care Before the Procedure

General client preparation is the same as that for any procedure involving collection of a peripheral blood sample (see Appendix I).

➤ For this test, the client should abstain from alcohol for 24 hours and from food for 12 hours before the study.

➤ Water is not restricted.

➤ It also is recommended that drugs that may alter cholesterol levels be withheld for 12 hours before the test, although this practice should be confirmed with the person ordering the study.

The Procedure

A venipuncture is performed and the sample collected in a red-topped tube. The sample should be sent promptly to the laboratory.

Nursing Care After the Procedure

Care and assessment after the procedure are the same as for any study involving the collection of a peripheral blood sample.

➤ Resume food and any drugs withheld before the test.

PHOSPHOLIPIDS

Phospholipids consist of one or more fatty acid molecules and one phosphoric acid radical, and they usually have a nitrogenous base. The three major types of body phospholipids are the lecithins, the cephalins, and the sphingomyelins. In addition to diet as a source of phospholipids, nearly all body cells are capable of forming these lipids. Most endogenous phospholipids are formed, however, in the liver and intestinal mucosa. The phospholipids are transported together in circulating blood in the form of lipoproteins.

Phospholipids are important for the formation of cell membranes and for the transportation of fatty acids through the intestinal mucosa into lymph. Phospholipids also serve as donors of phosphate groups for intracellular metabolic processes and may act as carriers in active transport systems. Saturated lecithins are essential for pulmonary gas exchange, whereas the cephalins are major constituents of thromboplastin, which is necessary to initiate the clotting process. Sphingomyelin is present in large quantities in the nervous system and acts as an insulator around nerve fibers.[24]

Phospholipids may be measured as part of an overall lipid evaluation, but the significance of altered levels is not completely understood. A direct relationship between elevated phospholipids and atherosclerotic cardiovascular disease has not been demonstrated.

Alterations in phospholipid levels may be seen in situations similar to those in which serum triglycerides and cholesterol also are abnormal. For example, elevated levels are associated with diabetes mellitus, nephrotic syndrome, chronic pancreatitis, obstructive jaundice, and early starvation. Decreased levels are seen in clients with primary hypolipoproteinemia, severe malnutrition and malabsorption syndromes, and cirrhosis. Antilipemic drugs (e.g., clofibrate) may lower phospholipid levels, and epinephrine, estrogens, and chlorpromazine tend to elevate them.

Another clinical application of phospholipid data is the use of the lecithin : sphingomyelin (L : S) ratio in estimating fetal lung maturity, with adequate lung maturity indicated by lecithin levels greater than those for sphingomyelin by a ratio of 2 : 1 or greater (see Chap. 10).

Reference Values

	Conventional Units	**SI Units**
Infants	100–275 mg/dL	1.00–2.75 g/L
Children	180–295 mg/dL	1.80–2.95 g/L
Adults	150–380 mg/dL	1.50–3.80 g/L

Values may vary, depending on the laboratory performing the test and the age of the client.

Interfering Factors

➤ Ingestion of alcohol 24 hours before and food 12 hours before the test may falsely elevate levels.
➤ Ingestion of drugs known to alter phospholipid levels within 12 hours before the test may alter results unless the test is being conducted to evaluate such effects.
➤ Antilipemic drugs (e.g., clofibrate) may lower phospholipid levels.
➤ Epinephrine, estrogens, and chlorpromazine tend to elevate phospholipid levels.

Indications for Serum Phospholipids Test

➤ Known or suspected disorders that cause or are associated with altered lipid metabolism
  • Altered phospholipid levels are seen in situations similar to those in which serum triglycerides and cholesterol also are altered (see Tables 5–12 and 5–13, pp. 176 and 178).
  • Elevated levels are associated with diabetes mellitus, nephrotic syndrome, chronic pancreatitis, obstructive jaundice, and early starvation.
  • Decreased levels are seen in primary hypolipoproteinemia, severe malnutrition, malabsorption syndromes, and cirrhosis.
➤ Support for identifying problems related to fat metabolism and transport
  • Phospholipid formation parallels deposition of triglycerides in the liver, and severely decreased levels result in low levels of lipoproteins that are essential for fat transport.
➤ Abnormal bleeding of unknown origin, with decreased cephalin (a type of phospholipid), a possible contributor to low levels of thromboplastin
➤ Suspected neurological disorder, which may be associated with decreased levels of sphingomyelin (a type of phospholipid)

Nursing Care Before the Procedure

General client preparation is the same as that for any procedure involving collection of a peripheral blood sample (see Appendix I).

➤ For this test, the client should abstain from alcohol for 24 hours and from food for 12 hours before the study.

➤ Water is not restricted.

➤ It also is recommended that drugs that may alter phospholipid levels be withheld for 12 hours before the test, although this practice should be confirmed with the person ordering the study.

The Procedure

A venipuncture is performed and the sample collected in a red-topped tube. The sample should be sent promptly to the laboratory.

Nursing Care After the Procedure

Care and assessment after the procedure are the same as for any study involving the collection of a peripheral blood sample.

➤ Resume foods and any drugs withheld before the test.

LIPOPROTEIN AND CHOLESTEROL FRACTIONATION

Lipids are transported in the blood as lipoproteins—complex molecules consisting of triglycerides, cholesterol, phospholipids, and proteins. Lipoproteins exist in several forms that reflect the different concentrations of their constituents. These forms, or fractions, are classified according to either their densities or their electrophoretic mobility.

The lipoprotein fractions in relation to density are (1) chylomicrons, (2) very-low-density lipoproteins (VLDL), (3) low-density lipoproteins (LDL), and (4) high-density lipoproteins (HDL). The least dense lipoproteins—chylomicrons and VLDL—contain the highest levels of triglycerides and lower amounts of cholesterol and protein. LDL and HDL contain the lowest amounts of triglycerides and relatively higher amounts of cholesterol and protein (see also Table 5–10, p. 173).

Lipoprotein densities correspond to electrophoretic mobility patterns of the several lipoprotein fractions. The two main fractions of lipoproteins, as identified by electrophoresis, are α and β. α-Lipoproteins, which approximate the HDL (α_1), migrate with the α-globulins. The β-lipoproteins, which reflect the VLDL (pre-β) and the LDL (β), migrate with the β-globulins. Chylomicrons remain at the origin.

The cholesterol content of the HDL and LDL fractions also can be determined by measuring total cholesterol remaining after one fraction has been removed. It should be noted, however, that HDL cholesterol does not correlate well with the total cholesterol concentration, is higher in women than in men, and tends to be inversely proportional to triglyceride levels. High HDL cholesterol and low LDL cholesterol levels are predictive of a lessened risk of cardiovascular disease, whereas high LDL cholesterol and low HDL cholesterol levels are considered risk factors for atherosclerotic cardiovascular disease. Further, many health-care providers believe that an adequate lipid assessment need include only (1) total cholesterol, (2) HDL cholesterol, (3) serum triglycerides, and (4) estimate of chylomicron concentration.

Specific conditions associated with altered levels of lipoprotein fractions are listed in Table 5–14.

Reference Values

	Conventional Units	**SI Units**	
Total lipoproteins	400–800 mg/dL	—	—
Lipoprotein fractions			
Chylomicrons	—	—	—
VLDL or pre-β	3–32 mg/dL	—	—
LDL or β	38–40 mg/dL	0.98–1.04 mmol/L	
HDL or α$_1$	20–48 mg/dL	0.51–1.24 mmol/L	

	LDL Cholesterol		HDL Cholesterol	
Age	**Conventional Units**	**SI Units**	**Conventional Units**	**SI Units**
<25 yr	73–138 mg/dL	1.87–3.53 mmol/L	32–57 mg/dL	0.82–1.46 mmol/L
25–40 yr	90–180 mg/dL	2.30–4.60 mmol/L	32–60 mg/dL	0.82–1.54 mmol/L
40–50 yr	100–185 mg/dL	2.56–4.74 mmol/L	33–60 mg/dL	0.84–1.54 mmol/L
50–65 yr	105–190 mg/dL	2.69–4.96 mmol/L	34–70 mg/dL	0.87–1.79 mmol/L
>65 yr	105–200 mg/dL	2.69–5.12 mmol/L	35–75 mg/dL	0.90–1.92 mmol/L

HDL cholesterol values are normally lower in men than in women, with an average range of 22 to 68 mg/dL.

Interfering Factors

➤ Failure to follow usual diet for 2 weeks before the test may yield results that do not accurately reflect client status.

Table 5–14 ➤ CONDITIONS ASSOCIATED WITH ALTERED LEVELS OF LIPOPROTEIN FRACTIONS		
Lipoprotein	**Increased Level**	**Decreased Level**
Chylomicrons	Ingested fat Ingested alcohol Types I and V hyperlipoproteinemia	Not applicable—normal value is zero
VLDL	Ingested fat Ingested carbohydrate Ingested alcohol All types of hyperlipoproteinemia Exogenous estrogens Diabetes mellitus Hypothyroidism (primary) Nephrotic syndrome Alcoholism Pancreatitis Pregnancy	Abetalipoproteinemia Cirrhosis Hypobetalipoproteinemia
LDL cholesterol	Ingested cholesterol Ingested saturated fatty acids Types II and III hyperlipoproteinemia Hypothyroidism (primary) Biliary obstruction Nephrotic syndrome	Types I and V hyperlipoproteinemia Hypobetalipoproteinemia Abetalipoproteinemia Hyperthyroidism Cirrhosis
HDL cholesterol	Ingested alcohol (moderate amounts) Chronic hepatitis Hypothyroidism (primary) Early biliary cirrhosis Biliary obstruction	All types of hyperlipoproteinemia Exogenous estrogens Hyperthyroidism Cirrhosis Tangier disease

➤ Ingestion of alcohol 24 hours before and food 12 hours before the test may alter results.

➤ Excessive exercise 12 hours before the test may alter results (regular exercise has been found to lower HDL cholesterol levels).

➤ Numerous drugs may alter results, including those that are known to alter lipoprotein components (see Tables 5–12 and 5–13, pp. 176 and 178).

Indications for Lipoprotein and Cholesterol Fractionation

➤ Serum cholesterol levels of greater than 250 mg/dL, which indicate high risk for cardiovascular disease and the need for further evaluation and possible treatment (see p. 178)

➤ Estimation of the degree of risk for cardiovascular disease
  • Individuals with LDL cholesterol levels greater than 160 mg/dL are considered to be at high risk.
  • Individuals at or above the upper reference range for HDL cholesterol have half the average risk, whereas those at or near the bottom have two, three, or more times the average risk.

➤ Known or suspected disorders associated with altered lipoprotein levels (see Table 5–14)

➤ Evaluation of response to treatment for altered levels and support for decisions regarding the need for drug therapy (LDL cholesterol levels may decrease with dietary modification alone; if not, drug treatment is recommended.)

Nursing Care Before the Procedure

General client preparation is the same as that for any procedure involving collection of a peripheral blood sample (see Appendix I).

➤ For this test, the client should ingest a normal diet, such that no weight gain or loss will occur for 2 weeks before the study, and should abstain from alcohol for 24 hours and from food for 12 hours before the test.

➤ Water is not restricted.

➤ The client also should avoid excessive exercise for at least 12 hours before the test.

➤ It also is recommended that drugs that may alter lipoprotein components be withheld for 24 to 48 hours before the test (see Tables 5–12 and 5–13, pp. 176 and 178), although this practice should be confirmed with the person ordering the study.

The Procedure

A venipuncture is performed and the sample collected in a red-topped tube. The sample should be sent promptly to the laboratory.

Nursing Care After the Procedure

Care and assessment after the procedure are the same as for any study involving the collection of a peripheral blood sample.

➤ Resume food and any drugs withheld before the test, as well as usual activities.

➤ *Abnormal values:* Note and report increased or decreased levels indicating atherosclerosis and high risk for heart disease. Administer ordered medications. Provide information for a low-fat, low-cholesterol, and low-calorie diet, if needed.

LIPOPROTEIN PHENOTYPING

Lipoprotein phenotyping is an extension of the information obtained through lipoprotein fractionation (see pp. 181 and 183) and provides another approach to correlating laboratory findings with disease.

Six different lipoprotein distribution patterns (phenotypes) are seen in serums with high levels of cholesterol or triglycerides or both. These phenotypes, which are referred to by their assigned numbers, have been correlated with genetically determined abnormalities (familial or primary hyperlipoproteinemias) and with a variety of acquired conditions (secondary hyperlipoproteinemias).

Phenotype descriptions have proved useful in classifying diagnoses and in evaluating treatment and preventive regimens. Most hyperlipemic serums can be categorized into lipoprotein phenotypes without performing electrophoresis if the following are known: (1) chylomicron status, (2) serum triglyceride level, (3) total cholesterol, and (4) HDL cholesterol.

Table 5–15 shows the clinical significance of each of the lipoprotein phenotypes as primary familial syndromes and as secondary occurrences caused by disorders that alter lipid metabolism.

Reference Values

	Phenotype					
	I	**IIa**	**IIb**	**III**	**IV**	**V**
Frequency	Very rare	Common	Common	Uncommon	Very common	Rare
Chylomicrons	↑ ↑ ↑	Normal	Normal	Normal or ↑	Normal	↑ ↑
Pre-β-lipoproteins (approximates VLDL)	↑	↑ ↑	↑	(these two bands merge)	↑ ↑ ↑	↑ ↑
β-Lipoproteins (approximates LDL)	↓	↑ ↑	↑ ↑		Normal or ↑	Normal or ↓
α₁-Lipoproteins (approximates HDL)	↓	Normal	Normal	Normal	Normal or ↓	Normal or ↓
Total cholesterol	Normal or ↑	↑ ↑	↑ ↑	↑ ↑	Normal or ↑	↑ ↑
Total triglycerides	↑ ↑ ↑	Normal	↑	↑ ↑ or ↑ ↑ ↑	↑ ↑ or ↑ ↑ ↑	↑ ↑ ↑
Refrigerated serum or plasma	"Cream"/ clear or turbid	Clear	+ or + + turbid	+ + + turbid	+ + + turbid	"Cream"/+ + turbid

From Sacher, RA, and McPherson, RA: Widmann's Clinical Interpretation of Laboratory Tests, ed 10. FA Davis, Philadelphia, 1991, p 344, with permission.

Interfering Factors

➤ Failure to follow usual diet for 2 weeks before the test may yield results that do not accurately reflect client status.

➤ Ingestion of alcohol 24 hours before and food 12 hours before the test may alter results.

➤ Excessive exercise 12 hours before the test may alter results.

Table 5–15 ▶ CLINICOPATHOLOGICAL SIGNIFICANCE OF LIPOPROTEIN PHENOTYPES

Phenotype	Familial Syndrome	May Occur Secondary to	Remarks
I	Abdominal pain Eruptive xanthomas Lipemia retinalis Early vascular disease absent	Insulin-dependent diabetes Lupus erythematosus Dysglobulinemias Pancreatitis	Lipoprotein lipase is deficient.
II	Early, severe vascular disease Prominent xanthomas	High-cholesterol diet Nephrotic syndrome Porphyria Hypothyroidism Dysglobulinemias Obstructive liver diseases	Familial trait is autosomal-dominant; homozygotes are especially severely affected.
III	Accelerated vascular disease, onset in adulthood Xanthomas, palmar yellowing Abnormal glucose tolerance Hyperuricemia	Hypothyroidism Dysglobulinemias Uncontrolled diabetes	Diet, lipid-lowering drugs are very effective
IV	Accelerated vascular disease, onset in adulthood Abnormal glucose tolerance Hyperuricemia	Obesity High alcohol intake Oral contraceptives Diabetes Nephrotic syndrome Glycogen storage disease	Weight loss lowers VLDL. High-fat diet may convert to type V.
V	Abdominal pain Pancreatitis Eruptive xanthomas Abnormal glucose tolerance Vascular disease not associated	High alcohol intake Diabetes Nephrotic syndrome Pancreatitis Hypercalcemia	Weight loss does not lower VLDL.

Note: From Sacher, R.A., and McPherson, R.A: Widmann's Clinical Interpretation of Laboratory Tests, ed 10. FA Davis, Philadelphia, 1991, p 345, with permission.

➤ Numerous drugs, including those that are known to alter lipoprotein components (see Tables 5–12, p. 176; 5–13, p. 178; and 5–15, p. 185), may alter
results.

Indications for Lipoprotein Phenotyping

➤ Further evaluation of elevated serum cholesterol levels and results of
lipoprotein and cholesterol fractionation (see p. 183)
➤ Family history of primary hyperlipoproteinemia (hyperlipidemia)
➤ Identification of the client's specific lipoprotein phenotype
➤ Known or suspected disorders associated with the several lipoprotein phe-
notypes (see Table 5–15, p. 185)

Nursing Care Before the Procedure

General client preparation is the same as that for any study involving collection
of a peripheral blood sample (see Appendix I).
➤ For this test, the client should ingest a normal diet, so that no weight gain or
loss will occur for 2 weeks before the study, and should abstain from alcohol for 24 hours and from food for 12 hours before the test.
➤ Water is not restricted.
➤ The client also should avoid excessive exercise for at least 12 hours before
the test.
➤ It also is recommended that drugs that may alter lipoprotein components be
withheld for 24 to 48 hours or longer before the test (see Tables 5–12,
p. 176; 5–13, p. 178, and 5–15, p. 185), although this practice should be
confirmed with the person ordering the study.

The Procedure

A venipuncture is performed and the sample collected in either a red- or
a lavender-topped tube, depending on the laboratory's procedure for determining lipoprotein phenotypes. The sample should be sent to the laboratory
immediately.

Nursing Care After the Procedure

Care and assessment after the procedure are the same as for any study involving
the collection of a peripheral blood sample.
➤ Resume food and any drugs withheld before the test, as well as usual
activities.

BILIRUBIN

Bilirubin is a degradation product of the pigmented heme portion of hemoglobin. Old, damaged, and abnormal erythrocytes are removed from the circulation
by the spleen and to some extent by the liver and bone marrow. The heme component of the red blood cells is oxidized to bilirubin by the reticuloendothelial
cells and released into the blood.

In the blood, the fat-soluble bilirubin binds to albumin as unconjugated
(prehepatic) bilirubin for transport to the liver. In the liver, hepatocytes detach
bilirubin from albumin and conjugate it with glucuronic acid, which renders the

bilirubin water-soluble. Most of the conjugated (posthepatic) bilirubin is excreted into the hepatic ducts and then into bile. Only small amounts of conjugated bilirubin diffuse from the liver back into the blood. Thus, most circulating bilirubin is normally in the unconjugated form.

Bilirubin is an excretory product that serves no physiological function in bile or blood. Once the conjugated bilirubin in bile enters the intestine, most is converted to a series of urobilinogen compounds and excreted into the stool as stercobilinogen after oxidation. A lesser amount is recycled to the liver and either returned to bile or excreted in urine as urobilinogen, which is oxidized to urobilin.

Bilirubin and its degradation products are pigments and provide the yellow tinge in normal serum, the yellow-green hue in bile, the brown in stools, and the yellow in urine. Abnormally elevated serum bilirubin levels produce jaundice; obstruction to biliary excretion of bilirubin may produce light-colored stools and dark urine.

The terms "indirect" and "direct," which are used to describe unconjugated (prehepatic) and conjugated (posthepatic) bilirubin, respectively, derive from the methods of testing for their presence in serum. Conjugated bilirubin is described as direct (direct reacting) because it is water-soluble and can be measured without modification. Unconjugated bilirubin must be rendered soluble with alcohol or other solvents before the test can be performed and is thus referred to as indirect (indirect reacting).

Impaired liver function causes dramatic increases in serum bilirubin levels (hyperbilirubinemia). Bilirubin must be in the conjugated form for normal excretion via bile, stools, and urine. When the liver is unable to conjugate bilirubin adequately, serum levels of unconjugated bilirubin rise. Disorders in which excessive hemolysis of red blood cells is combined with impaired liver function also produce hyperbilirubinemia. An example is physiological jaundice of the newborn, in which the increased destruction of red blood cells, common after birth, is combined with the immature liver's inability to conjugate sufficient bilirubin. Kernicterus, a complication of newborn hyperbilirubinemia, occurs when unconjugated bilirubin is deposited in brain tissue.

Impaired excretion of conjugated (posthepatic, direct) bilirubin from the liver into the bile ducts or from the biliary tract itself causes this form of bilirubin to be reabsorbed from the liver into the blood, with resultant elevated serum levels. Because conjugated bilirubin is water-soluble and readily crosses the renal glomerulus, excessive amounts may be excreted in the urine. The stools, however, are lighter in color because of diminished amounts of conjugated bilirubin in the gut.

Serum bilirubin levels are measured as total bilirubin, indirect bilirubin, and direct bilirubin. Total bilirubin reflects the combination of unconjugated and conjugated bilirubin in the serum and may be used to screen clients for possible disorders involving bilirubin production and excretion. If total bilirubin is normal, the levels of indirect (unconjugated) and direct (conjugated) bilirubin also are assumed to be normal in most cases.

When total bilirubin levels are elevated, indirect and direct bilirubin levels are measured to determine the source of the overall elevation. Specific causes of elevations in indirect and direct bilirubin are shown in Table 5–16. Numerous drugs also may alter bilirubin levels.

Table 5–16 ➤ **CAUSES OF ELEVATIONS IN INDIRECT AND DIRECT BILIRUBIN LEVELS**

Increased Indirect (Unconjugated) Bilirubin	Increased Direct (Conjugated) Bilirubin
Hemolysis: hemoglobinopathies, spherocytosis, G-6-PD deficiency, autoimmunity, transfusion reaction Red blood cell degradation: hemorrhage into soft tissues or body cavities, inefficient erythropoiesis, pernicious anemia Defective hepatocellular uptake or conjugation: viral hepatitis, hereditary enzyme deficiencies (Gilbert, Crigler-Najjar syndromes), hepatic immaturity in newborns	Intrahepatic disruption: viral hepatitis, alcoholic hepatitis, chlorpromazine, cirrhosis Bile duct disease: biliary cirrhosis, cholangitis (idiopathic, infectious), biliary atresia Extrahepatic bile duct obstruction: gallstones; carcinoma of gallbladder, bile ducts, or head of pancreas; bile duct stricture from inflammation or surgical misadventure

Reference Values

	Conventional Units	SI Units
Total Bilirubin		
Newborns	2.0–6.0 mg/dL	34.0–102.0 μmol/L
48 hr	6.0–7.0 mg/dL	102.0–120.0 μmol/L
5 day	4.0–12.0 mg/dL	68.0–205.0 μmol/L
1 mo–adults	0.3–1.2 mg/dL	5.0–20.0 μmol/L
Indirect Bilirubin (unconjugated, prehepatic)		
1 mo–adults	0.3–1.1 mg/dL	5.0–19.0 μmol/L
Direct Bilirubin		
1 mo–adults	0.1–0.4 mg/dL	1.7–6.8 μmol/L

Interfering Factors

➤ Prolonged exposure of the client, as well as of the blood sample, to sunlight and ultraviolet light reduces serum bilirubin levels.
➤ Failure to follow dietary restrictions before the test.
➤ Fasting normally lowers indirect bilirubin levels.
➤ In Gilbert's syndrome, a congenital defect in bilirubin degradation, chronically elevated levels of indirect bilirubin increase dramatically in the fasting state.
➤ Numerous drugs may elevate bilirubin levels (e.g., steroids, sulfonamides, sulfonylureas, barbiturates, antineoplastic agents, propylthiouracil, allopurinol, antibiotics, gallbladder dyes, caffeine, theophylline, indomethacin, and any drugs that are considered hepatotoxic); it is recommended that such drugs be withheld for 24 hours before the test, if possible.

Indications for Bilirubin Test

➤ Known or suspected hemolytic disorders, including transfusion reactions, as indicated by elevated total and indirect bilirubin levels (see also Table 5–16)

- Hemolysis alone rarely causes indirect bilirubin levels higher than 4 or 5 mg/dL.
- If hemolysis is combined with impaired or immature liver function, levels may rise more dramatically.

➤ Confirmation of observed jaundice
- Jaundice manifests when serum levels of indirect or direct bilirubin reach 2 to 4 mg/dL.

➤ Determination of the cause of jaundice (e.g., liver dysfunction, hepatitis, biliary obstruction, carcinoma)

➤ Support for diagnosing liver dysfunction as evidenced by elevated direct and total bilirubin levels or by elevation of all three levels if bile duct drainage also is impaired

➤ Support for diagnosing biliary tract obstruction as evidenced by elevated direct and total bilirubin levels or by elevation of all three levels if liver function is impaired[25]

Nursing Care Before the Procedure

General client preparation is the same as that for any study involving collection of a peripheral blood sample (see Appendix I).

➤ For these tests, the client should fast from foods for at least 4 hours before the test; water is not restricted.

➤ Because many drugs may alter bilirubin levels (see section entitled "Interfering Factors"), a medication history should be obtained.

➤ It is recommended that those drugs that may alter test results be withheld for 24 hours before the test, although this practice should be confirmed with the person ordering the study.

The Procedure

A venipuncture is performed and the sample obtained in a red-topped tube. The sample should be handled gently to avoid hemolysis and sent immediately to the laboratory. The sample should not be exposed for prolonged periods to sunlight (i.e., more than 1 hour), ultraviolet light, or fluorescent lights. In infants, a capillary sample is obtained by heelstick.

Nursing Care After the Procedure

Care and assessment after the procedure are the same as for any study involving the collection of a peripheral blood sample.

➤ Resume food and any drugs withheld before the test.

➤ *Abnormal values:* Note and report increased levels. Assess for associated signs and symptoms of hyperbilirubinemia such as jaundice, pruritus, pain caused by liver disease, biliary obstruction, or food intolerances. Administer phenobarbital if levels are greater than 12 mg/dL in newborns, as this can lead to central nervous system damage. Prepare for exchange transfusion if level is greater than 15 mg/dL.

ENZYMES

Enzymes are catalysts that enhance reactions without directly participating in them. Individual enzymes, each of which has its own substrate and product specificity, exist for nearly all the metabolic reactions that maintain body functions.

Enzymes are normally intracellular molecules. Because certain metabolic reactions occur in many tissues, the involved enzymes exist in many cell types. Enzymes with more restricted metabolic functions are found in only one of several specialized cell types. The presence of enzymes in circulating blood indicates cellular changes that have permitted their escape into extracellular fluid. The continuous synthesis and destruction of the cells of the enzymes' origins, for example, allow small amounts of enzymes to appear in the blood. Cellular disruption caused by damage by disease, toxins, or trauma, as well as increased cell wall permeability, also elevates serum enzyme levels. Additional causes of elevated enzyme levels are an increase in the number or activity of enzyme-containing cells and decreases in normal excretory or degradation mechanisms.

Decreased serum enzyme levels rarely have diagnostic significance because so few enzymes are present in substantial quantity. Enzyme levels may decline if the number of synthesizing cells declines, if generalized or specific restriction in protein synthesis occurs (enzymes are proteins), or if excretion or degradation increases.

Very few enzymes are studied routinely. Although highly specialized enzyme analysis is applied to the study of many genetically determined diseases, most diagnostic enzyme studies involve only those enzymes with changing values in serum, providing inferential or confirmatory evidence of various pathological processes. A major goal of enzyme analysis is to localize disease processes to specific organs, preferably to specific functional subdivisions or even to specific cellular activities. Enzymes unique to a single cell type or found in only a few sites are particularly useful in this regard. The source of elevations of those enzymes with widespread distribution also can be determined by partitioning total activity into isoenzyme fractions. Isoenzymes are different forms of a single enzyme with immunologic, physical, or chemical characteristics distinctive for their tissue of origin.

Efforts to standardize the study of enzymes (enzymology) have led to new terminology for naming and measuring enzymes. The Commission on Enzymes of the International Union of Biochemistry (IUB) has classified enzymes according to their biochemical functions, assigning to each a numerical designation that embodies class, subclass, and specification number. The IUB has also assigned descriptive names according to the specific reaction catalyzed and, in many cases, a practical name useful for common reference. One result of this standardization is that enzymes that have been studied for years have been renamed according to the new terminology. For example, the liver enzyme that was formerly called glutamic-oxaloacetic transaminase (GOT) is now named aspartate aminotransferase (AST).

Another attempt to standardize enzymology is the introduction of international units (IU) for reporting enzyme activity. One IU of an enzyme is the amount that catalyzes transformation of 1 μmol of substrate per minute under defined conditions. The actual amounts vary among enzymes, and the IU is not a single universally applicable value that can be used to compare enzymes of different characteristics.[26]

In this section, enzymes associated with organs and tissues such as the liver, pancreas, bone, heart, and muscle are discussed. Enzymes specific to red and white blood cells are included in Chapter 1.

Alanine Aminotransferase (ALT, SGPT)

Alanine aminotransferase (ALT), formerly known as glutamic-pyruvic transaminase (GPT), catalyzes the reversible transfer of an amino group between the amino acid, alanine, and α-ketoglutamic acid. Hepatocytes are virtually the only cells with high ALT concentrations, although the heart, kidneys, and skeletal muscles contain moderate amounts.

Elevated serum ALT levels are considered a sensitive index of liver damage resulting from a variety of disorders and numerous drugs, including alcohol. Elevations also may be seen in nonhepatic disorders such as muscular dystrophy, extensive muscular trauma, myocardial infarction, congestive heart failure (CHF), and renal failure, although the increase in ALT produced by these disorders is not as great as that produced by conditions affecting the liver.

This test was formerly known as serum glutamic-pyruvic transaminase (SGPT).

Reference Values

Conventional Units	SI Units
10–30 U/L	0.17–0.51 μkat/L
1–36 U/L	0.02–0.61 μkat/L
5–35 U/L	0.08–0.60 μkat/L
5–25 U/L	0.08–0.43 μkat/L
8–50 U/L	0.14–0.85 μkat/L
4–36 U/L	0.07–0.61 μkat/L

Reference values vary among laboratories and according to the method used for reporting results.

Interfering Factors

➤ Numerous drugs, including alcohol, may falsely elevate levels.

Indications for Alanine Aminotransferase (ALT, SGPT) Test

➤ Known liver disease or liver damage caused by hepatotoxic drugs
  • Markedly elevated levels (sometimes as high as 20 times normal) are considered confirmatory of liver disease.
  • A sudden drop in serum ALT levels in the presence of acute illness after extreme elevation of blood levels (e.g., as seen in severe viral or toxic hepatitis) is an ominous sign and indicates that so many cells have been damaged that no additional source of enzyme remains.
➤ Monitoring for response to treatment for liver disease, with tissue repair indicated by gradually declining levels

Nursing Care Before the Procedure

General client preparation is the same as that for any study involving collection of a peripheral blood sample (see Appendix I).
➤ For this test, the client should abstain from alcohol for at least 24 hours before the study.
➤ Because many drugs may alter ALT levels, a medication history should be obtained. It is recommended that drugs that may alter test results be with-

held for 12 hours before the test, although this practice should be confirmed with the person ordering the study.

The Procedure

A venipuncture is performed and the sample is collected in a red-topped tube. The sample should be handled gently to avoid hemolysis and transported promptly to the laboratory.

Nursing Care After the Procedure

Care and assessment after the procedure are the same as for any study involving the collection of a peripheral blood sample.

➤ Resume any drugs withheld before the test.

➤ *Abnormal levels:* Note and report increased levels. Assess symptoms of liver dysfunction associated with increases such as jaundice, anorexia, and fatigue. Relate increases to other liver function tests. Provide rest and interventions to conserve energy. Tell client which drugs to avoid and encourage client to eat a healthy diet.

Aspartate Aminotransferase (AST, SGOT)

Aspartate aminotransferase (AST), formerly known as glutamic-oxaloacetic transaminase (GOT), catalyzes the reversible transfer of an amino between the amino acid, aspartate, and α-ketoglutamic acid. ALT exists in large amounts in both liver and myocardial cells and in smaller but significant amounts in skeletal muscles, kidneys, pancreas, and brain.

Serum AST rises when there is cellular damage to the tissues in which the enzyme is found. When heart muscle suffers ischemic damage, serum AST rises within 6 to 8 hours; peak values occur at 24 to 48 hours and decline to normal within 72 to 96 hours. Elevation of AST occurs midway in the time sequence between that of creatine phosphokinase (CPK), which rises very early and falls within 48 hours, and lactic dehydrogenase (LDH), which begins rising 12 hours or more after infarction and remains elevated for a week or more. Elevation of AST cannot be used as the single enzyme indicator for myocardial infarction, because it also rises in several other conditions included in the differential diagnosis of heart attack. Other disorders associated with elevated AST, and the magnitude of those elevations, are listed in Table 5–17. It should also be noted that numerous drugs, especially those known to be hepatotoxic or nephrotoxic, may elevate AST levels.[27]

The test for AST was formerly known as serum glutamic-oxaloacetic transaminase (SGOT).

Reference Values

	Conventional Units	**SI Units**
Newborns	16–72 U/L	0.27–1.22 μkat/L
6 mo	20–43 U/L	0.34–0.73 μkat/L
1 yr	16–35 U/L	0.27–0.60 μkat/L
5 yr	19–28 U/L	0.32–0.48 μkat/L
Adults		
Men	8–46 U/L	0.14–0.78 μkat/L
Women	7–34 U/L	0.12–0.58 μkat/L

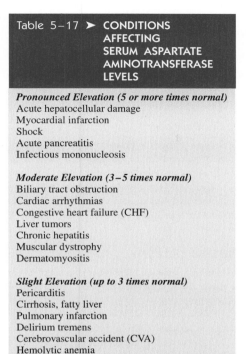

Table 5–17 ➤ CONDITIONS AFFECTING SERUM ASPARTATE AMINOTRANSFERASE LEVELS

Pronounced Elevation (5 or more times normal)
Acute hepatocellular damage
Myocardial infarction
Shock
Acute pancreatitis
Infectious mononucleosis

Moderate Elevation (3–5 times normal)
Biliary tract obstruction
Cardiac arrhythmias
Congestive heart failure (CHF)
Liver tumors
Chronic hepatitis
Muscular dystrophy
Dermatomyositis

Slight Elevation (up to 3 times normal)
Pericarditis
Cirrhosis, fatty liver
Pulmonary infarction
Delirium tremens
Cerebrovascular accident (CVA)
Hemolytic anemia

Note: Adapted from Sacher, RA, and McPherson, RA: Widmann's Clinical Interpretation of Laboratory Tests, ed 10. FA Davis, Philadelphia, 1991, p 403.

Interfering Factors

➤ Numerous drugs may falsely elevate levels.

Indications for Aspartate Aminotransferase (AST, SGOT) Test

➤ Suspected disorders or injuries involving the liver, myocardium, kidneys, pancreas, or brain, with elevated levels indicating cellular damage to tissues in which AST is normally found (see Table 5–17)
  • In myocardial infarction, AST rises within 6 to 8 hours, peaks at 24 to 48 hours, and declines to normal within 72 to 96 hours.
➤ Monitoring of response to therapy with potentially hepatotoxic or nephrotoxic drugs
➤ Monitoring of response to treatment for various disorders in which AST may be elevated, with tissue repair indicated by declining levels

Nursing Care Before the Procedure

General client preparation is the same as that for any study involving collection of a peripheral blood sample (see Appendix I).
➤ Because many drugs alter AST levels, a medication history should be obtained. It is recommended that any drugs that may alter test results be with-

held for 12 hours before the test, although this practice should be confirmed with the person ordering the study.

The Procedure

A venipuncture is performed and the sample is collected in a red-topped tube. The sample should be handled gently to avoid hemolysis and transported promptly to the laboratory.

Nursing Care After the Procedure

Care and assessment after the procedure are the same as for any study involving the collection of a peripheral blood sample.

➤ Resume any drugs withheld before the test, pending test results.

➤ *Complications and precautions:* Increases in this enzyme level in relation to ALT and other assessment data may indicate a cardiac disorder. Monitor vital signs and cardiac activity by electrocardiogram (ECG).

Alkaline Phosphatase (ALP)

Phosphatases are enzymes that cleave phosphate from compounds with a single phosphate group. Those that are optimally active at pH 9 are grouped under the name alkaline phosphatase (ALP).

ALP is elaborated by a number of tissues. Liver, bone, and intestine are the major isoenzyme sources. During pregnancy, the placenta also is an abundant source of ALP, and certain cancers elaborate small amounts of a distinctive form of ALP called the Regan enzyme. Additional sources of ALP are the proximal tubules of the kidneys, the lactating mammary glands, and the granulocytes of circulating blood (see Chap. 1, section entitled "Leukocyte Alkaline Phosphatase").

Bone ALP predominates in normal serum, along with a modest amount of hepatic isoenzyme, which is believed to derive largely from the epithelium of the intrahepatic biliary ducts rather than from the hepatocytes themselves. Levels of intestinal ALP vary; most people have relatively little, but isolated elevations of this enzyme have been observed. Intestinal ALP enters the blood very briefly while fats are being digested and absorbed, but intestinal disease rarely affects serum ALP levels.

Conditions associated with elevated serum ALP levels, and the magnitude of those elevations, are listed in Table 5–18.[28] Numerous drugs also may elevate serum ALP levels.

Decreased levels are seen in cretinism, secondary growth retardation, scurvy, achondroplasia, and, rarely, hypophosphatasia.

Reference Values

	General Reference Levels	Bessey-Lowry Method	Bodansky Method	King-Armstrong Method
Newborns	50–65 U/L	—	—	—
Children	20–150 U/L	3.4–9.0 U/L	5–14 U/L	15–30 U/L
Adults	20–90 U/L	0.8–2.3 U/L	1.5–4.5 U/L	4–13 U/L

Table 5–18 ➤ CONDITIONS ASSOCIATED WITH ELEVATED SERUM ALKALINE PHOSPHATASE LEVELS

Pronounced Elevation (5 or more times normal)
Advanced pregnancy
Biliary obstruction
Biliary atresia
Cirrhosis
Osteitis deformans
Osteogenic sarcoma
Hyperparathyroidism (primary, or secondary to chronic renal disease)
Paget's disease
Infusion of albumin of placental origin

Moderate Elevation (3 to 5 times normal)
Granulomatous or infiltrative liver diseases
Infectious mononucleosis
Metastatic tumors in bone
Metabolic bone diseases (rickets, osteomalacia)
Extrahepatic duct obstruction

Mild Elevation (up to 3 times normal)
Viral hepatitis
Chronic active hepatitis
Cirrhosis (alcoholic)
Healing fractures
Early pregnancy
Growing children
Large doses of vitamin D
Congestive heart failure (CHF)

Interfering Factors

➤ Numerous drugs, including IV albumin, may falsely elevate levels.
➤ Clofibrate, azathioprine (Imuran), and fluorides may falsely decrease levels.

Indications for Serum Alkaline Phosphatase (ALP) Test

➤ Signs and symptoms of disorders associated with elevated ALP levels (e.g., biliary obstruction, hepatobiliary disease, bone disease including malignant processes) (see also Table 5–18)
➤ Differentiation of obstructive biliary disorders from hepatocellular disease, with greater elevations of ALP seen in obstructive biliary disorders
➤ Known renal disease to determine effects on bone metabolism
➤ Signs of growth retardation in children

Nursing Care Before the Procedure

Client preparation is the same as that for any test involving collection of a peripheral blood sample (see Appendix I).

➤ Because many drugs may alter ALP levels, a medication history should be obtained.

The Procedure

A venipuncture is performed and the sample collected in a red-topped tube. The sample should be handled gently to avoid hemolysis and transported promptly to the laboratory.

Nursing Care After the Procedure

Care and assessment after the procedure are the same as for any study involving the collection of a peripheral blood sample.

➤ *Abnormal levels:* Note and report increased levels. Correlate with serum calcium and phosphorus, serum bilirubin, and isoenzymes to determine reason for treatments, progress, and prognosis in diseases of the bone or liver. Assess for jaundice and pathological fracture. If client is pregnant, handle extremities carefully and protect from trauma. Administer ordered vitamin D. Provide comfort measures (soothing bath for pruritus, pain control, support for body image changes) to treat jaundice, if it is present. Advise client to restrict dietary fat.

Alkaline Phosphatase Isoenzymes

If serum alkaline phosphatase (ALP) levels are elevated but the clinical picture does not provide enough information to determine the origin of the excess, ALP isoenzymes are evaluated. The major ALP isoenzymes derive from liver, bone, intestine, and placenta.

ALP isoenzymes may be partitioned by electrophoresis or by exploitation of differences in physical properties on optimal substrates. Electrophoresis has been applied with only modest success. Hepatic and intestinal isoenzymes are easier to differentiate with this method than are hepatic and bone enzymes. Because hepatic ALP is more heat-resistant than bone ALP, the most common way to differentiate between these two isoenzymes is by heating the serum to 132.8°F (56°C).

Evaluation of ALP isoenzymes usually focuses on measuring those of hepatic origin not affected by bone growth or pregnancy. These are 5′-nucleotidase, leucine aminopeptidase, and γ-glutamyl transpeptidase.

5′-NUCLEOTIDASE (5′-N)

5′-Nucleotidase (5′-N), an isoenzyme of ALP, is a specific phosphomonoesterase formed in the hepatobiliary tissues. Elevated serum 5′-N levels are associated with biliary cirrhosis, carcinoma of the liver and biliary structures, and choledocholithiasis or other biliary obstruction.

Reference Values

Conventional Units	SI Units
0–1.6 U	27–233 nmol/s/L
0.3–3.2 U (Bodansky)	

Indications for 5′-Nucleotidase (5′-N) Test

➤ Elevated alkaline phosphatase of uncertain etiology
  • Elevated 5′-N levels support the diagnosis of hepatobiliary disorders as the source of the elevated alkaline phosphatase.

• Normal levels support the diagnosis of bone disease as the source of the elevated alkaline phosphatase.

Nursing Care Before the Procedure

Client preparation is the same as that for any test involving collection of a peripheral blood sample (see Appendix I).

The Procedure

A venipuncture is performed and the sample collected in a red-topped tube. The sample should be handled gently to avoid hemolysis and transported promptly to the laboratory.

Nursing Care After the Procedure

Care and assessment after the procedure are the same as for any study involving the collection of a peripheral blood sample.

LEUCINE AMINOPEPTIDASE (LAP)

Leucine aminopeptidase (LAP), an isoenzyme of alkaline phosphatase, is widely distributed in body tissues, with greatest concentrations found in hepatobiliary tissues, pancreas, and small intestine.

Elevated levels are associated with biliary obstruction resulting from gallstones and tumors, including those of the head of the pancreas, strictures, and atresia. Advanced pregnancy and therapy with drugs containing estrogen and progesterone also may raise LAP levels.

Reference Values

Leucine	Conventional Units	SI Units
Men	0.80–2.00 mg/dL	61.0–152.0 μmol/L
Women	0.75–1.85 mg/dL	57.0–141.0 μmol/L

Values may vary depending on the units of measure used by the laboratory performing the test.

Interfering Factors

➤ Advanced pregnancy and therapy with drugs containing estrogen and progesterone may falsely elevate levels.

Indications for Leucine Aminopeptidase (LAP) Test

➤ Elevated ALP of uncertain etiology
  • Elevated levels support the diagnosis of hepatobiliary or pancreatic disease or both as the source of the elevated ALP.
  • Normal levels support the diagnosis of bone disease as the source of the elevated ALP.

Nursing Care Before the Procedure

Client preparation is the same as that for any test involving the collection of a peripheral blood sample (see Appendix I).

➤ Some laboratories require the client to fast from food for 8 hours before the test.

The Procedure

A venipuncture is performed and the sample collected in a red-topped tube. The sample should be handled gently to avoid hemolysis and transported promptly to the laboratory.

Nursing Care After the Procedure

Care and assessment after the procedure are the same as for any study involving the collection of a peripheral blood sample.
➤ Resume any food withheld before the test.

γ-GLUTAMYL TRANSPEPTIDASE (GGT)

γ-Glutamyl transpeptidase (GGT), an isoenzyme of ALP, catalyzes the transfer of glutamyl groups among peptides and amino acids. Hepatobiliary tissues and renal tubular and pancreatic epithelia contain large amounts of GGT. Other sources include the prostate gland, brain, and heart.

Most GGT in serum derives from hepatobiliary sources, and elevated levels point to hepatobiliary disease.

Reference Values

	Conventional Units	SI Units
Newborns	5 times children's (1–2 yr) values	
Children		
1–2 yr	3–30 U/L	0.05–0.51 μkat/L
5–15 yr	5–27 U/L	0.08–0.46 μkat/L
Adults		
Men	6–37 U/L	0.10–0.63 μkat/L
Women <45 yr	5–27 U/L	0.08–0.46 μkat/L
Women >45 yr	6–37 U/L	0.10–0.63 μkat/L

Interfering Factors

➤ Alcohol, barbiturates, and phenytoin may elevate GGT levels.
➤ Late pregnancy and oral contraceptives may produce lower than normal values.

Indications and Purposes for γ-Glutamyl Transpeptidase (GGT) Test

➤ Elevated alkaline phosphatase of uncertain etiology
  • Pronounced elevations are seen in clients with obstructive disorders of the hepatobiliary tract and hepatocellular carcinoma.
  • Modest elevations occur with hepatocellular degeneration (e.g., cirrhosis) and with pancreatic or renal cell damage or neoplasms.
  • Other disorders associated with elevated GGT levels include CHF, acute myocardial infarction (after 4 to 10 days), hyperlipoproteinemia (type IV), diabetes mellitus with hypertension, and epilepsy.
  • Normal levels in the presence of elevated ALP support the diagnosis of bone disease.

➤ Known or suspected alcohol abuse, including monitoring of individuals participating in alcohol abstinence programs
  • About 60 to 80 percent of individuals considered to have alcohol abuse problems have elevated GGT levels, whether or not other signs of liver damage are present.
  • Moderate increases in GGT levels occur with low alcohol intake.
  • A significant sustained rise occurs with ingestion of six or more drinks per day.
  • Normal levels return within 2 to 6 weeks of abstinence from alcohol.

Nursing Care Before the Procedure

Client preparation is essentially the same as that for any test involving collection of a peripheral blood sample (see Appendix I).
➤ Some laboratories require the client to fast from food for 8 hours before the test.
➤ When the test is conducted to determine whether the liver is the source of elevated ALP, the client should abstain from alcohol for 2 to 3 weeks before the test. This restriction may not apply when the test is used to monitor compliance with alcohol abstinence programs.
➤ The client's reported intake (or nonintake) of alcohol should, however, be noted.

The Procedure

A venipuncture is performed and the sample collected in a red-topped tube. The sample should be handled gently to avoid hemolysis and transported promptly to the laboratory.

Nursing Care After the Procedure

Care and assessment after the procedure are the same as for any study involving the collection of a peripheral blood sample.
➤ Resume any food withheld before the test.

Isocitrate Dehydrogenase (ICD)

Isocitrate dehydrogenase (ICD) catalyzes the decarboxylation of isocitrate in the Krebs cycle. This enzyme is important in controlling the rate of the cycle, which must be precisely adjusted to meet the energy needs of cells. ICD is found in the liver, heart, skeletal muscle, placenta, platelets, and erythrocytes.

Reference Values

	Conventional Units	**SI Units**
Newborns	4.0–28.0 U/L	0.06–0.48 μkat/L
Adults	1.27–7.0 U/L	0.02–0.12 μkat/L

Interfering Factors

➤ Numerous drugs, including those that are hepatotoxic, may cause elevated levels.

Indications for Isocitrate Dehydrogenase (ICD) Test

➤ Elevated serum aspartate aminotransferase (ALT, SGOT) or ALP of uncertain etiology, or both
  • Elevated ICD levels are seen in early viral hepatitis, cancer of the liver, intrahepatic and extrahepatic obstruction, biliary atresia, cirrhosis, and pre-eclampsia.
➤ Therapy with potentially hepatotoxic drugs that may lead to elevated ICD levels early in the course of treatment

Nursing Care Before the Procedure

Client preparation is the same as that for any study involving collection of a peripheral blood sample (see Appendix I).
➤ Because many drugs may alter ICD levels, a medication history should be obtained. It is recommended that any drugs that may alter test results be withheld for 24 hours before the test, although this practice should be confirmed with the person ordering the study.

The Procedure

A venipuncture is performed and the sample collected in a red-topped tube. The sample should be handled gently to avoid hemolysis and transported promptly to the laboratory.

Nursing Care After the Procedure

Care and assessment after the procedure are the same as for any study involving the collection of a peripheral blood sample.
➤ Resume any drugs withheld before the test, pending test results.

Ornithine Carbamoyltransferase (OCT)

Ornithine carbamoyltransferase (OCT), formerly known as ornithine transcarbamoylase, catalyzes ornithine to citrulline in the urea cycle before its link with the citric acid cycle. Its importance stems from its role in the conversion of ammonia to urea by the liver. Decreased levels may be seen in inherited disorders associated with a partial block in the urea cycle.

Reference Values

Conventional Units	SI Units
8–20 mIU/mL	
8–20 U/L	0.02–0.34 µkat/L

Interfering Factors

➤ Hepatotoxic drugs and chemicals may produce elevated levels.

Indications for Ornithine Carbamoyltransferase (OCT) Test

➤ Elevated serum ALP of uncertain etiology
  • Elevated OCT levels are seen in viral hepatitis, cholecystitis, cirrhosis, cancer of the liver, and obstructive jaundice.

➤ Therapy with hepatotoxic drugs or exposure to hepatotoxic chemicals, with early effects indicated by elevated OCT levels

➤ Suspected mushroom poisoning as indicated by elevated levels

Nursing Care Before the Procedure

Client preparation is the same as that for any study involving collection of a peripheral blood sample (see Appendix I).

➤ Because many drugs may alter OCT levels, a medication history should be obtained. It is recommended that any drugs that may alter test results be withheld for 24 hours before the test, although this practice should be confirmed with the person ordering the study.

The Procedure

A venipuncture is performed and the sample collected in a red-topped tube. The sample should be handled gently to avoid hemolysis and transported promptly to the laboratory.

Nursing Care After the Procedure

Care and assessment after the procedure are the same as for any study involving the collection of a peripheral blood sample.

➤ Resume any drugs withheld before the test, pending test results.

Serum Amylase

Amylase is a digestive enzyme that splits starch into disaccharides such as maltose. Although many cells have amylase activity (e.g., liver, small intestine, skeletal muscle, fallopian tubes), amylase circulating in normal serum derives from the parotid glands and the pancreas. Unlike many other enzymes, amylase activity is primarily extracellular; it is secreted into saliva and the duodenum, where it splits large carbohydrate molecules into smaller units for further digestive action by intestinal enzymes.

Elevations in serum amylase are generally seen in pancreatic inflammations, which cause disruption of pancreatic cells and absorption of the extracellular enzyme from the intestine and peritoneal lymphatics. Serum amylase levels also rise sharply after administration of drugs that constrict pancreatic duct sphincters. The most common offender is morphine, and this drug is never indicated for individuals with abdominal pain that could be of pancreatic or biliary tract origin. Other drugs that may produce elevated serum amylase levels are codeine, chlorothiazides, aspirin, pentazocine, corticosteroids, oral contraceptives, pancreozymin, and secretin. Specific causes of elevated serum amylase, and the magnitude of the elevations produced, are listed in Table 5–19.

Reference Values

	Conventional Units	**SI Units**
Children	60–160 U/dL	1.88–5.03 μkat/L
Adults	80–180 U/dL (Somogyi)	1.36–3.0 μkat/L
	45–200 U/dL (dye)	
Values may vary according to the laboratory performing the test.		

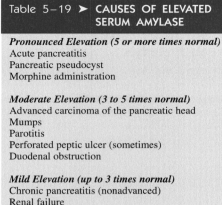

Table 5–19 ➤ CAUSES OF ELEVATED SERUM AMYLASE
Pronounced Elevation (5 or more times normal)   Acute pancreatitis   Pancreatic pseudocyst   Morphine administration
Moderate Elevation (3 to 5 times normal)   Advanced carcinoma of the pancreatic head   Mumps   Parotitis   Perforated peptic ulcer (sometimes)   Duodenal obstruction
Mild Elevation (up to 3 times normal)   Chronic pancreatitis (nonadvanced)   Renal failure   Common bile duct obstruction   Gastric resection

Note: Adapted from Sacher, RA, and McPherson, RA: Widmann's Clinical Interpretation of Laboratory Tests, ed 10. FA Davis, Philadelphia, 1991, p 404.

Interfering Factors

➤ A number of drugs may produce elevated levels (e.g., morphine, codeine, chlorothiazides, aspirin, pentazocine, corticosteroids, oral contraceptives, pancreozymin, and secretin).

➤ High blood glucose levels, which may be a result of diabetes mellitus or IV glucose solutions, may lead to decreased levels.

Indications for Serum Amylase Test

➤ Diagnosis of early acute pancreatitis
- Serum amylase begins rising within 6 to 24 hours after onset and returns to normal in 2 to 7 days.
- Urine amylase levels may remain elevated for several days after serum amylase levels return to normal.

➤ Detection of blunt trauma or inadvertent surgical trauma to the pancreas as indicated by elevated levels

➤ Diagnosis of macroamylasemia, a disorder seen in alcoholism, malabsorption syndrome, and other digestive problems with circulating complexes of amylase and high-molecular-weight dextran (findings include high serum amylase and negative urine amylase)

➤ Support for diagnosing other disorders associated with elevated serum amylase levels (see Table 5–19)

➤ Support for diagnosing disorders associated with decreased amylase levels, such as advanced chronic pancreatitis, advanced cystic fibrosis, liver disease, liver abscess, toxemia of pregnancy, severe burns, and cholecystitis

Nursing Care Before the Procedure

Client preparation is the same as that for any study involving collection of a peripheral blood sample (see Appendix I).

➤ Because many drugs may alter serum amylase levels, a medication history should be obtained. It is recommended that any drugs that may alter test results be withheld for 12 to 24 hours before the test, although this practice should be confirmed with the person ordering the study.

The Procedure

A venipuncture is performed and the sample collected in a red-topped tube. The sample should be handled gently to avoid hemolysis and transported promptly to the laboratory.

Nursing Care After the Procedure

Care and assessment after the procedure are the same as for any study involving the collection of a peripheral blood sample.

➤ Resume any drugs withheld before the test, pending test results.

➤ *Abnormal values:* Note and report increased levels. Correlate with urine amylase, hypocalcemia, hypokalemia, hyperglycemia, and bilirubin in relation to pancreatic diseases. Assess for fluid deficit if pancreatic hemorrhage is present, severity of adominal pain if acute inflammation is present, jaundice if common bile duct is obstructed, and bowel sounds. Maintain nothing by mouth (NPO) status and prepare client for IV fluids, nasogastric tube (NG) insertion, and bowel decompression to decrease pancreatic stimulation. Instruct client to avoid alcohol intake and to reduce carbohydrate intake if absorption problem exists.

Serum Lipase

Lipases split triglycerides into fatty acids and glycerol. Different lipolytic enzymes have different specific substrates, but overall activity is collectively described as lipase. Serum lipase derives primarily from pancreatic lipase, which is secreted into the duodenum and participates in fat digestion. Pancreatic lipase is quite distinct from lipoprotein lipases, which clear the blood of chylomicrons after fats are absorbed.

Viral hepatitis and disorders in which bile salts are decreased may produce low serum lipase levels, as will protamine and IV infusions of saline.

Reference Values

	Conventional Units	**SI Units**
All groups	0–160 U/L	0–2.72 μkat/L

Interfering Factors

➤ Morphine, cholinergic drugs, and heparin may lead to elevated levels.

➤ Protamine and IV infusions of saline may lead to decreased levels.

Indications for Serum Lipase Test

➤ Diagnosis of acute pancreatitis, especially if the client has been ill for more than 3 days
  • Serum amylase levels may return to normal after 3 days, but serum lipase remains elevated for approximately 10 days after onset.
➤ Support for diagnosing pancreatic carcinoma, especially if there is a sustained moderate elevation in serum lipase levels
➤ Support for diagnosing other disorders associated with elevated serum lipase levels (e.g., peptic ulcer, acute cholecystitis, and early renal failure)
➤ Support for diagnosing disorders associated with decreased serum lipase levels (e.g., advanced chronic pancreatitis, cystic fibrosis, advanced carcinoma of the pancreas, and viral hepatitis)

Nursing Care Before the Procedure

Client preparation is the same as that for any test involving collection of a peripheral blood sample (see Appendix I).
➤ The client should fast from food for at least 8 hours before the test.
➤ It is recommended that drugs that may alter test results be withheld for 12 to 24 hours before the test, although this practice should be confirmed with the person ordering the study.

The Procedure

A venipuncture is performed and the sample collected in a red-topped tube. The sample should be handled gently to avoid hemolysis and transported promptly to the laboratory.

Nursing Care After the Procedure

Care and assessment after the procedure are the same as for any study involving the collection of a peripheral blood sample.
➤ Resume food and any drugs withheld before the test.

Acid Phosphatase (ACP)

Phosphatases are enzymes that cleave phosphate from compounds with a single phosphate group. Those that are optimally active at pH 5 are grouped under the name *acid phosphatase (ACP)*.

Many tissues (kidneys, spleen, liver, bone) contain ACP, but the prostate gland, red blood cells (RBCs), and platelets are especially rich in this activity. Two isoenzymes, prostatic fraction and RBC/platelet fraction, are diagnostically significant. These isoenzymes differ from one another in preferred substrate and in the degree to which they are inhibited by various additives during laboratory testing. Normal serum contains more RBC/platelet than prostatic ACP, and small changes in prostatic fraction may be difficult to detect. Tartaric acid inhibits prostatic ACP. Thus, many laboratories report tartrate-inhibitable ACP as well as total ACP in an effort to focus more specifically on the prostatic fraction.

Decreased levels of prostatic ACP are seen after estrogen therapy for prostatic carcinoma and in clients with Down syndrome. Decreased levels are associated with ingestion of alcohol, fluorides, oxalates, and phosphates.

Administration of androgens in women and of clofibrate in both genders produces elevated levels.

Reference Values

	Conventional Units	**SI Units**
Newborns	10.4–16.4 U/L	
1 mo–13 yr	0.5–11.0 U/L (King-Armstrong)	
	6.4–15.2 U/L	108.0–258.0 μkat/L
Adults	0–0.8 U/L	0.0–14.0 μkat/L
	0.1–2.0 U/L (Gutman)	
	0.5–2.0 U/L (Bodansky)	
	0.1–5.0 U/L (King-Armstrong)	
	0.1–0.8 U/L (Bessey-Lowry)	
	0–0.56 U/L (Roy)	

Interfering Factors

➤ Prostatic massage or rectal examination within 48 hours of the test may cause elevated levels.
➤ Administration of androgens in females and of clofibrate in either gender may produce elevated levels.
➤ Ingestion of alcohol, fluorides, oxalates, and phosphates may result in decreased levels.

Indications for Serum Acid Phosphatase (ACP) Test

➤ Enlarged prostate gland, especially if prostatic carcinoma is suspected
  • Prostatic ACP is elevated in 50 to 75 percent of individuals with prostatic carcinoma that has extended beyond the gland.
  • Cancers that remain within the gland cause ACP elevation in only 10 to 25 percent of those affected.
  • Benign hyperplasia, inflammation, or ischemic damage to the prostate rarely causes elevated ACP levels.
➤ Evaluation of the effectiveness of treatment of prostatic carcinoma
  • ACP levels fall to normal within 3 to 4 days of successful estrogen therapy.
  • Recurrent elevation strongly suggests that bone metastases are active.
➤ Support for diagnosing other disorders associated with elevated prostatic ACP levels (e.g., metastatic bone cancer, Paget's disease, osteogenesis imperfecta, hyperparathyroidism, and multiple myeloma)
➤ Known or suspected hematologic disorder
  • Elevated RBC/platelet ACP is seen in hemolytic anemia, sickle cell crisis, thrombocytosis, and acute leukemia.
➤ Support for diagnosing other disorders associated with increased RBC/platelet ACP (e.g., renal insufficiency, liver disease, Gaucher's disease, and Niemann-Pick disease)

Nursing Care Before the Procedure

Client preparation is the same as that for any test involving the collection of a peripheral blood sample (see Appendix I).

➤ It is recommended that any drugs that may alter test results be withheld for 12 to 24 hours before the test, although this practice should be confirmed with the person ordering the study.

The Procedure

A venipuncture is performed and the sample collected in a red-topped tube. The sample should be handled gently to avoid hemolysis and transported promptly to the laboratory. If the test cannot be performed within a few hours, the serum should be frozen.

Nursing Care After the Procedure

Care and assessment after the procedure are the same as for any study involving the collection of a peripheral blood sample.

➤ Resume any drugs withheld before the test.

➤ *Abnormal values:* Note and report increased levels or associated levels of prostate-specific antigen (PSA). Provide support in coping with a life-threatening disease, hormonal therapy, and possible surgical procedure.

Prostate-Specific Antigen (PSA)

Prostate-specific antigen (PSA) is a glycoprotein found in the prostate tissues. Its presence is tested by immunoassay techniques to assist in the detection of prostatic carcinoma. It is considered to be a more specific immunohistochemical marker for metastatic tumor of prostate origin than is ACP. ACP is a test also performed to diagnose prostatic carcinoma, but it is not entirely specific for this disease, as increased values have been noted in bladder as well as in prostatic carcinoma. Increased levels of PSA correlate with the amount of prostatic tissue, both malignant and benign.

Reference Values

	Conventional Units	SI Units
Men <40 yr	<2.0 ng/mL	<2.0 µg/L
Men >40 yr	<2.8 ng/mL	<2.8 µg/L

Interfering Factors

➤ Prostatic massage or rectal examination within 48 hours of the test can cause elevated levels.

Indications for Prostate-Specific Antigen (PSA) Test

➤ Screening for early detection of prostate carcinoma and evaluating those who are at risk for this disease, primarily men over 40 years of age

➤ Diagnosing a malignant tumor of the prostate gland, revealed by increased levels, depending on the volume of the tumor

➤ Determining chemotherapeutic regimen protocol or radiation therapy and monitoring and evaluating the response to therapy, revealed by a decrease in the PSA level

➤ Evaluating progression or recurrence of the tumor, revealed by a rise in the PSA level

Nursing Care Before the Procedure

Client preparation is the same as that for any test involving the collection of a peripheral blood sample (see Appendix I).

The Procedure

A venipuncture is performed and the sample collected in a red-topped tube. The age of the client should be noted on the laboratory form. The sample should be refrigerated if the test is not performed within 24 hours.

Nursing Care After the Procedure

Care and assessment after the procedure are the same as for any study involving the collection of a peripheral blood sample.

Aldolase (ALS)

Aldolase (ALS) is a glycolytic enzyme that catalyzes the breakdown of 1,6-diphosphate into triose phosphate. It is found in many body tissues but is most diagnostically significant in disorders of skeletal and cardiac muscle, liver, and pancreas. Three isoenzymes have been identified: A, originating in skeletal and cardiac muscle; B, originating in liver, kidneys, and white blood cells; and C, originating in brain tissue. Isoenzyme C probably lacks diagnostic capability because it does not cross the blood-brain barrier.

Reference Values

	Conventional Units	SI Units
Newborns	5.2–32.8 U/L (Sibley-Lehninger)	0.09–0.54 μkat/L
Children	2.6–16.4 U/L (Sibley-Lehninger)	0.04–0.27 μkat/L
Adults	1.3–8.2 U/L (Sibley-Lehninger)	0.02–0.14 μkat/L
Men	3.1–7.5 U/L at 98.6°F (37°C)	0.05–0.13 μkat/L
Women	2.7–5.3 U/L at 98.6°F (37°C)	0.04–0.09 μkat/L

Interfering Factors

➤ Hepatotoxic drugs, insecticides, and antihelminthics may cause elevated levels.

➤ Phenothiazines may cause decreased levels.

Indications for Aldolase (ALS) Test

➤ Family history of Duchenne's muscular dystrophy
  • ALS levels rise before clinical signs appear, thus permitting early diagnosis.
➤ Signs and symptoms of neuromuscular disorders, to differentiate muscular disorders from neurological disorders
  • Pronounced elevations are seen in clients having Duchenne's muscular dystrophy, polymyositis, dermatomyositis, trichinosis, and severe crush injuries.
  • Decreased aldolase levels are seen in those with late muscular dystrophy, because of loss of muscle cells, or with use of phenothiazines.
  • ALS is not elevated in those with multiple sclerosis or myasthenia gravis, both of which are of neural origin.

➤ Support for diagnosing other disorders associated with elevated ALS levels
  • Moderate increases are associated with acute hepatitis, neoplasms, and leukemia.
  • Mild elevations are seen in acute myocardial infarction (peak elevation occurs in 24 hours, with gradual return to normal within 1 week).
➤ Evaluation of response to exposure to hepatotoxic drugs or chemicals, with liver damage indicated by elevated levels

Nursing Care Before the Procedure

Client preparation is the same as that for any test involving collection of a peripheral blood sample (see Appendix I).
➤ It is recommended that drugs that may alter test results be withheld for 12 to 24 hours before the test, although this practice should be confirmed with the person ordering the study.

The Procedure

A venipuncture is performed and the sample collected in a red-topped tube. The sample should be handled gently to avoid hemolysis and transported promptly to the laboratory.

Nursing Care After the Procedure

Care and assessment after the procedure are the same as for any study involving the collection of a peripheral blood sample.
➤ Resume any drugs withheld before the test.
➤ *Abnormal values:* Note and report increased levels related to skeletal muscular disorders. Assess for muscle fatigue and strength related to an acute or chronic disorder. Provide energy-saving care to conserve the client's energy while still maintaining as much independence as possible. Instruct in a planned rest and exercise program.

Creatine Phosphokinase (CPK) and Isoenzymes

Creatine phosphokinase (CPK), also called creatine kinase (CK), catalyzes the reversible exchange of phosphate between creatine and adenotriphosphate (ATP). Important in intracellular storage and release of energy, CPK exists almost exclusively in skeletal muscle, heart muscle, and, to a lesser extent, brain. No CPK is found in the liver. Anything that damages skeletal or cardiac muscle elevates serum CPK levels. Brain injury affects serum CPK levels much less, probably because relatively little enzyme crosses the blood-brain barrier.

Spectacular CPK elevations occur in the early phases of muscular dystrophy, but CPK elevation diminishes as the disease progresses and muscle mass decreases. Levels of CPK may be normal to low in late, severe cases. Additional causes of elevated CPK, and the magnitude of those elevations, are listed in Table 5–20.

The CPK molecule consists of two parts, which may be identical or dissimilar. These two constituent chains are called M (muscle) and B (brain). Three diagnostically significant isoenzymes have been identified in relation to the two main components of CPK. Brain CPK (CPK-BB, CPK_1) is almost entirely BB, cardiac CPK (CPK-MB, CPK_2) contains 60 percent MM and 40 percent MB, and skeletal muscle CPK (CPK-MM, CPK_3) contains about 90 percent MM and 10 percent MB. The isoenzyme normally present in serum is almost entirely

Table 5–20 ➤ CAUSES OF ELEVATED CREATINE PHOSPHOKINASE

Pronounced Elevation (5 or more times normal)
Early muscular dystrophy (CPK-MM, CPK$_3$)
Acute myocardial infarction (CPK-MB, CPK$_2$)
Severe angina (CPK-MB, CPK$_2$)
Polymyositis (CPK-MM, CPK$_3$)
Cardiac surgery

Moderate Elevation (2 to 4 times normal)
Vigorous exercise
Deep intramuscular injections
Surgical procedures affecting skeletal muscles
Delirium tremens
Convulsive seizures
Dermatomyositis
Alcoholic myopathy
Hypothyroidism
Pulmonary infarction
Acute agitated psychosis

Mild Elevation (up to 2 times normal)
Late pregnancy
Women heterozygous for the gene causing Duchenne's muscular dystrophy (CPK-MM, CPK$_3$)
Brain injury (CPK-BB, CPK$_1$)

Note: Adapted from Sacher, RA, and McPherson, RA: Widmann's Clinical Interpretation of Laboratory Tests, ed 10. FA Davis, Philadelphia, 1991, p 407.

MM, and only CPK-MM (CPK$_3$) rises when skeletal muscle is damaged. In contrast, serum CPK-MB (CPK$_2$) rises only when heart muscle is damaged.

Drugs that may produce elevated CPK levels include anticoagulants, morphine, alcohol, salicylates in high doses, amphotericin-B, clofibrate, and certain anesthetics. Any medication administered intramuscularly (IM) also elevates CPK. In addition to late muscular dystrophy, decreased levels are seen in early pregnancy.

Reference Values

	Conventional Units	SI Units
Total CPK		
Newborns	30–100 U/L	0.51–1.70 µkat/L
Children	15–50 U/L	0.26–0.85 µkat/L
Adults		
Men	5–55 U/L	—
	55–170 U/L	0.94–2.89 µkat/L
	5–35 µg/mL	—
Women	5–25 U/L	—
	30–135 U/L	0.51–2.30 µkat/L
	5–25 µg/mL	—
Isoenzymes		
CPK-BB (CPK$_1$)	0% of total CK	—
CPK-MB (CPK$_2$)	0–7% of total CK	—
CPK-MM (CPK$_3$)	5–70% of total CK	—

Interfering Factors

➤ Vigorous exercise, deep IM injections, delirium tremens, and surgical procedures in which muscle is transected or compressed may produce elevated levels.

➤ Drugs that may produce elevated CPK levels include anticoagulants, morphine, alcohol, salicylates in high doses, amphotericin-B, clofibrate, and certain anesthetics.

➤ Early pregnancy may produce decreased levels.

Indications for Creatine Phosphokinase (CPK) and Isoenzymes Test

➤ Signs and symptoms of acute myocardial infarction
  * Acute myocardial infarction releases CPK into the serum within the first 48 hours, and values return to normal in about 3 days.
  * CPK levels rise before aspartate aminotransferase (AST, SGOT), and lactic dehydrogenase (LDH) levels rise.
  * The isoenzyme CPK-MB (CPK$_2$) rises only when the heart muscle is damaged; it appears in the first 6 to 24 hours and is usually gone in 72 hours.
  * Both total CPK and MB fraction may rise in severe angina or extensive reversible ischemic damage.[29]
  * Recurrent elevation of CPK suggests reinfarction or extension of ischemic damage.
  * An elevated CPK level helps to differentiate myocardial infarction from CHF and conditions associated with liver damage.

➤ Family history of Duchenne's muscular dystrophy
  * Spectacular CPK elevations occur in the early phases of muscular dystrophy, even before clinical signs or symptoms appear.
  * CPK elevation diminishes as the disease progresses and muscle mass decreases.

➤ Signs and symptoms of other disorders associated with elevated CPK levels (see Table 5–20, p. 209)

Nursing Care Before the Procedure

Client preparation is the same as that for any test involving the collection of a peripheral blood sample (see Appendix I).

➤ It is recommended that any drugs that may alter test results be withheld for 12 to 24 hours before the test, although this practice should be confirmed with the person ordering the study.

➤ Vigorous exercise and IM injections also should be avoided for 24 hours before the test.

The Procedure

A venipuncture is performed and the sample collected in a red-topped tube. The sample should be handled gently to avoid hemolysis and transported promptly to the laboratory.

Nursing Care After the Procedure

Care and assessment after the procedure are the same as those for any study involving the collection of a peripheral blood sample.

➤ Resume any drugs withheld before the test, as well as usual activities.

➤ *Abnormal values:* Note and report increased levels of CPK, CPK-MB, lactic dehydrogenase (in relation to myocardial infarction), and CPK-MM (in relation to muscular dystrophy). Monitor vital signs. Monitor ECG for dysrhythmias. Monitor for fluid overload (distended neck veins, dyspnea, crackles on auscultation). Repeat ordered CPK and lactic dehydrogenase enzyme and isoenzyme tests.

Lactic Dehydrogenase (LDH) and Isoenzymes

Lactic dehydrogenase (LDH) catalyzes the reversible conversion of lactic acid to pyruvic acid within cells. Because many tissues contain LDH, elevated total LDH is considered a nonspecific indication of cellular damage unless other clinical data make the tissue origin obvious. Pronounced elevations in total LDH are seen in clients with megaloblastic anemia, metastatic cancer (especially if the liver is involved), shock, hypoxia, hepatitis, and renal infarction. Moderate elevations occur in those with myocardial and pulmonary infarctions, hemolytic conditions, leukemias, infectious mononucleosis, delirium tremens, and muscular dystrophy. Mild elevations are associated with most liver diseases, nephrotic syndrome, hypothyroidism, and cholangitis.

The most useful diagnostic information is obtained by analyzing the five isoenzymes of LDH through electrophoresis. These isoenzymes are specific to certain tissues. The heart and erythrocytes are rich sources of LDH_1 and LDH_2; however, the brain is a source of LDH_1, LDH_2, and LDH_3. The kidneys contain LDH_3 and LDH_4; the liver and skeletal muscle contain LDH_4 and LDH_5. Certain glands (thyroid, adrenal, and thymus), pancreas, spleen, lungs, lymph nodes, and white blood cells contain LDH_3, whereas the ileum is an additional source of LDH_5.

Situations in which isoenzyme analysis is most useful include distinguishing myocardial infarction from lung or liver problems, diagnosing myocardial infarction in ambiguous settings such as the postoperative period or during severe shock and in hemolysis at a time of bone marrow hypoplasia.

Normally, serum contains more LDH_2 than LDH_1. Damage to tissues rich in LDH_1, however, will cause this ratio to reverse. The reversed ratio (i.e., LDH_1 greater than LDH_2) is an important diagnostic finding that occurs whether or not total LDH is elevated. The reversal is short-lived. In myocardial infarction, for example, the LDH_1 : LDH_2 ratio returns to normal within a week of the infarction even though total LDH may remain elevated.[30] The tissue sources of LDH isoenzymes and common causes of elevations are summarized in Table 5–21.

Numerous drugs may elevate LDH levels: anabolic steroids, anesthetics, aspirin, alcohol, fluorides, narcotics, clofibrate, mithramycin, and procainamide.

Table 5–21 ➤	TISSUE SOURCES AND COMMON CAUSES OF ELEVATED LACTIC DEHYDROGENASE (LDH) ISOENZYMES	
Isoenzyme	**Tissue Sources**	**Causes of Elevated Levels**
LDH₁	Heart Erythrocytes Brain	Acute myocardial infarction Red blood cell hemolysis Cerebrovascular accident (CVA) Renal infarction Muscular dystrophy
LDH₂	Heart Erythrocytes Brain	Acute myocardial infarction Lymphoproliferative disorders Cerebrovascular accident (CVA) Shock Muscular dystrophy
LDH₃	Brain Kidneys Glands (thyroid, adrenal, thymus) Pancreas Spleen Lungs Lymph nodes Leukocytes	Lymphoproliferative disorders Shock Infectious mononucleosis Acute pancreatitis Renal necrosis Pneumonia Pulmonary infarction
LDH₄	Liver Kidneys Skeletal muscles	Pulmonary infarction Pneumonia Shock Hepatitis Cirrhosis Pancreatitis Infectious mononucleosis Muscular dystrophy Acute glomerulonephritis Renal necrosis
LDH₅	Liver Ileum Skeletal muscles	Pulmonary infarction Hepatitis Cirrhosis Liver trauma Shock Infectious mononucleosis Dermatomyositis Muscular dystrophy

Reference Values

	Conventional Units	**SI Units**
Total LDH	80–120 U (Wacker) @ 300°C (636°F) 150–450 U (Wroblewski) 71–207 U/L	1.21–3.52 μkat/L
LDH Isoenzymes	Percentage of Total	Fraction of Total
LDH₁	29–37%	0.29–0.37
LDH₂	42–48%	0.42–0.48
LDH₃	16–20%	0.16–0.20
LDH₄	2–4%	0.02–0.04
LDH₅	0.5–1.5%	0.005–0.015

Values may vary according to the laboratory performing the test.

Interfering Factors

➤ Numerous drugs may produce elevated LDH levels (e.g., anabolic steroids, anesthetics, aspirin, alcohol, fluorides, narcotics, clofibrate, mithramycin, and procainamide).

Indications for Lactic Dehydrogenase (LDH) and Isoenzymes Test

➤ Confirmation of acute myocardial infarction or extension thereof, as indicated by elevation (usually) of total LDH, elevation of LDH_1 and LDH_2, and reversal of the $LDH_1:LDH_2$ ratio within 48 hours of the infarction
➤ Differentiation of acute myocardial infarction from pulmonary infarction and liver problems, which elevate LDH_4 and LDH_5
➤ Confirmation of red blood cell hemolysis or renal infarction, especially as indicated by reversal of the $LDH_1:LDH_2$ ratio
➤ Confirmation of chronicity in liver, lung, and kidney disorders, as evidenced by LDH levels that remain persistently high
➤ Evaluation of the effectiveness of cancer chemotherapy (LDH levels should fall with successful treatment)
➤ Evaluation of the degree of muscle wasting in muscular dystrophy (LDH levels rise early in this disorder and approach normal as muscle mass is reduced by atrophy)
➤ Signs and symptoms of other disorders associated with elevation of the several LDH isoenzymes (see Table 5–21)

Nursing Care Before the Procedure

Client preparation is the same as that for any test involving the collection of a peripheral blood sample (see Appendix I).

➤ It is recommended that drugs that may alter test results be withheld for 12 to 24 hours before the test, although this practice should be confirmed with the person ordering the study.

The Procedure

A venipuncture is performed and the sample collected in a red-topped tube. The sample should be handled gently to avoid hemolysis and transported promptly to the laboratory.

Nursing Care After the Procedure

Care and assessment after the procedure are the same as for any study involving the collection of a peripheral blood sample.

➤ Resume any drugs withheld before the test.

Hexosaminidase

Hexosaminidase A is a test performed to determine the presence of the lysosomal disease known as Tay-Sachs, a genetic autosomal recessive condition characterized by early and progressive retardation in the mental and physical development of the infant, with death resulting by the third or fourth year of life. The deficiency of this enzyme is most common in families of Eastern-European Jewish and French-Canadian origin. Because of this deficiency, gangliosides or complex sphingolipids are not metabolized and accumulate in the brain, causing the paralysis, blindness, dementia, and mental retardation that develop in the children afflicted with this disorder.[31]

Reference Values

56–80 percent of a total normal level (10.4–23.8 U/L)

Interfering Factors

➤ Pregnancy decreases the level of hexosaminidase in relation to the total, resulting in an inaccurate false positive.
➤ Oral contraceptives can decrease the level.

Indications for Hexosaminidase Test

➤ Screening young adults for asymptomatic possession of this gene with or without a family history of Tay-Sachs disease
➤ Identifying carriers in high-risk clients during prenatal examination, revealed by a lowered enzyme activity
➤ Diagnosing Tay-Sachs in infants, revealed by a very low level or absence of enzyme activity
➤ In utero prenatal diagnosis of amniotic fluid or cells obtained from chorionic villi

Nursing Care Before the Procedure

Client preparation is the same as that for any test involving the collection of a peripheral blood sample (see Appendix I).
➤ Food and fluids should be avoided for 8 hours before the test, and oral contraceptives should be withheld.

The Procedure

A venipuncture is performed and the sample collected in a red-topped tube. Refer to the procedures to obtain prenatal samples via chorionic villus biopsy or amniocentesis (see Chaps. 10 and 14).

Nursing Care After the Procedure

Care and assessment after the procedure are the same as for any study involving the collection of a peripheral blood sample.
➤ Resume any drugs withheld before the test.
➤ *Complications and precautions:* Recommend special genetic counseling for those with a family history of the disease or with abnormal test results.

α-Hydroxybutyric Dehydrogenase (α-HBD, HBD)

α-Hydroxybutyric dehydrogenase (α-HBD, HBD) is an enzyme similar to two isoenzymes of lactic dehydrogenase (LDH): LDH_1 and LDH_2. The α-HBD test, however, is cheaper and easier to perform than LDH isoenzyme electrophoresis. Moreover, HBD levels remain elevated for 18 days after acute myocardial infarction, providing a diagnosis when the client has delayed seeking treatment or has not had classic signs and symptoms.

Reference Values

Conventional Units
70–300 U/L
140–350 U/L
Values may vary according to the laboratory performing the test.

Indications for α-Hydroxybutyric Dehydrogenase (α-HBD, HBD) Test

➤ Suspected "silent" myocardial infarction or otherwise atypical myocardial infarction in which the client delayed seeking care
  • HBD levels remain elevated for 18 days after acute myocardial infarction (i.e., when other cardiac enzymes have returned to normal levels).
➤ Support for diagnosing other disorders associated with elevated HBD levels (e.g., megaloblastic and hemolytic anemias, leukemias, lymphomas, melanomas, muscular dystrophy, nephrotic syndrome, and acute hepatocellular disease)

Nursing Care Before the Procedure

Client preparation is the same as that for any test involving the collection of a peripheral blood sample (see Appendix I).

The Procedure

A venipuncture is performed and the sample collected in a red-topped tube. The sample should be handled gently to avoid hemolysis and transported promptly to the laboratory.

Nursing Care After the Procedure

Care and assessment after the procedure are the same as for any study involving the collection of a peripheral blood sample.

Cholinesterases

Cholinesterases hydrolyze concentrated acetylcholine and also cleave other choline esters. Two types of cholinesterase are measured: (1) acetylcholinesterase ("true" cholinesterase) and (2) pseudocholinesterase. Acetylcholinesterase (AcCHS) is found at nerve endings and in erythrocytes; very little is found in serum. Its substrate specificity is limited to acetylcholine, and it is optimally active against very low acetylcholine concentrations. Pseudocholinesterase (PCE) derives from the liver and is normally found in the serum in substantial amounts. It is active against acetylcholine and other choline esters. PCE is unusual in that the diagnostically significant change is depression, not elevation.

An important application of information about PCE is in evaluating individuals for genetic variations of the enzyme before surgery in which succinylcholine, an inhibitor of acetycholine, is to be used to induce anesthesia. Persons homozygous for the abnormal form of PCE have depressed total serum activity and their enzyme does not inactivate succinylcholine; persons who receive the drug during surgery may experience prolonged respiratory depression. Presence of the abnormal form of PCE is determined by exposing the enzyme to dibucaine. Normal PCE is inhibited by dibucaine, whereas abnormal PCE is found to be "dibucaine-resistant."[32]

Reference Values

	Conventional Units	SI Units
Acetylcholinesterase (AcCHS)	0.5 – 1.0 pH units	
Pseudocholinesterase (PCE)	0.5 – 1.3 pH units	
Men	274 – 532 IU/dL	2.74 – 5.32 kU/L
Women	204 – 500 IU/dL	2.04 – 5.00 kU/L

Interfering Factors

➤ Numerous drugs may falsely decrease cholinesterase levels (e.g., caffeine, theophylline, quinidine, quinine, barbiturates, morphine, codeine, atropine, epinephrine, phenothiazines, folic acid, and vitamin K).

Indications for Cholinesterase Determinations

➤ Suspected exposure to organic phosphate insecticides
  • Red blood cell AcCHS levels decline with severe exposure; serum PCE decreases occur earlier.
  • When exposure ceases, serum PCE rises before red blood cell AcCHS returns to normal.
  • Red blood cell AcCHS levels are more useful than are serum PCE levels in determining prior exposure.
➤ Impending use of succinylcholine during anesthesia
  • Persons homozygous for the abnormal form of PCE have depressed total serum activity, and their enzyme does not inactivate succinylcholine, with the abnormal PCE indicated as "dibucaine-resistant."

Nursing Care Before the Procedure

Client preparation is the same as that for any study involving the collection of a peripheral blood sample (see Appendix I).
➤ Because many drugs may alter cholinesterase levels and activity, a medication history should be obtained. It is recommended that those drugs that may alter test results be withheld for 12 to 24 hours before the test, although this practice should be confirmed with the person ordering the study.

The Procedure

A venipuncture is performed and the sample collected in a red-topped tube. The sample should be handled gently to avoid hemolysis and transported promptly to the laboratory.

Nursing Care After the Procedure

Care and assessment after the procedure are the same as for any study involving the collection of a peripheral blood sample.
➤ Resume any medications withheld before the test.

Renin

Renin is an enzyme released by the juxtaglomerular apparatus of the kidney in response to decreased extracellular fluid volume, serum sodium, and renal perfusion pressure. It catalyzes the conversion of angiotensinogen, produced by the liver, to angiotensin I. Angiotensin I is then converted to angiotensin II in the lungs. Angiotensin II elevates systemic blood pressure by causing vasoconstriction and by stimulating the release of aldosterone.

Renin released by the kidneys is found initially in the renal veins. Thus, the output of renin by each kidney may be determined by obtaining samples directly from the right and left renal veins and comparing the results with those obtained from an inferior vena cava sample. This test is indicated when renal artery stenosis is suspected, because the kidney affected by decreased perfusion releases higher amounts of renin. Renal vein assay for renin is performed using fluoroscopy and involves cannulation of the femoral vein and injection of dye to aid in visualizing the renal veins. Because this is an invasive procedure, a signed consent is required.

Reference Values

	Conventional Units	**SI Units**
Peripheral vein	0.4–4.5 (ng/hr)/mL (normal salt intake, standing position)	0.4–4.5 $\mu gh^{-1} L^{-1}$
	1.5–1.6 (ng/hr)/mL or more (normal salt intake, supine position)	1.5–1.6 $\mu gh^{-1} L^{-1}$
Renal vein assay	Difference between each renal sample and the vena cava sample should be <1.4–1.0	

Values for peripheral vein samples should be substantially higher (e.g., 2.9–24 ng/hr/mL) in clients who are sodium-depleted and in the upright position. These values also may vary according to the laboratory performing the test.

Interfering Factors

➤ Failure to follow dietary restrictions, if ordered, before the test.
➤ Failure to take prescribed diuretics, if ordered, before the test.
➤ Failure to maintain required positioning (e.g., upright versus recumbent) for at least 2 hours before the test.
➤ High-dose adrenocorticosteroid therapy, excessive salt intake, and excessive licorice ingestion may produce decreased levels.

Indications for Renin Test

➤ Assessment of renin production by the kidneys when client has hypertension of unknown etiology or when other disorders associated with altered renin levels are suspected
  • Elevated renin levels are seen in renovascular and malignant hypertension, adrenal hypofunction (Addison's disease), salt-wasting disorders, end-stage renal disease, renin-producing renal tumors, and secondary hyperaldosteronism.
  • Decreased levels are associated with primary hyperaldosteronism, hypervolemia, excessive salt ingestion or retention, excessive adrenocortico-

steroid levels resulting from either disease or drug therapy, and excessive licorice ingestion.
- Renin levels may be high, low, or normal in essential hypertension.
- In primary hyperaldosteronism, plasma renin levels are decreased, even with salt depletion before the test (results should be evaluated in relation to the serum aldosterone level, which is elevated in primary hyperaldosteronism).

➤ Suspected renal artery stenosis as the cause of hypertension, as indicated by renal vein output of renin by the affected kidney more than 1.4 times that of the vena cava sample

---

➤➤ Nursing Alert

- The renal vein assay for renin should be performed with extreme caution, if at all, in clients with allergies or previous exposure to radiographic dyes.

Nursing Care Before the Procedure

Client preparation varies according to the method for obtaining the sample and the factors to be controlled (e.g., salt depletion).

1. *Peripheral vein, normal salt intake.* Client preparation is essentially the same as that for any test involving collection of a peripheral blood sample. The client should follow a normal diet with adequate salt and potassium intake. Licorice intake and certain medications may be restricted for 2 weeks or more before the test, although this practice should be confirmed with the person ordering the study. The position relevant to the type of sample (e.g., upright versus recumbent) should be maintained for 2 hours before the test.

2. *Peripheral vein, sodium-depleted.* Client preparation is the same as just described, except that a diuretic is administered for 3 days before the study and dietary sodium is limited to "no added salt" (approximately 3 g/day). Sample menus should be provided. The purpose of the diuretic therapy and sodium restriction should be explained, and client understanding and ability to follow pretest preparation should be ascertained.

Explain to the client:
- ➤ The purpose of the study
- ➤ That a "no added salt" diet must be followed for 3 days before the study
- ➤ That prescribed diuretics must be taken for 3 days before the study
- ➤ Other restrictions in diet (e.g., licorice) or drugs necessary before the study
- ➤ That the test will be performed in the radiology department by a physician and will take about 30 minutes
- ➤ The general procedure, including the sensations to expect (momentary discomfort as the local anesthetic is injected, sensation of warmth as the dye is injected)
- ➤ Whether premedications will be given
- ➤ After-procedure assessment routines (e.g., frequent vital signs) and activity restrictions

Encourage questions and verbalization of concerns appropriate to the client's age and mental status. Then:

➤ Question the client about possible allergies to radiographic dyes.

➤ Ensure that signed consent has been obtained.

➤ To the extent possible, ensure that the dietary and medication regimens and restrictions are followed.

➤ Assist the client in maintaining the upright position (standing or sitting) for 2 hours before the test, if ordered, to stimulate renin secretion.

➤ Take and record vital signs and have the client void; provide a hospital gown.

➤ Administer premedication, if ordered.

➤ Obtain a stretcher for client transport.

The Procedure

The procedure varies with the method for obtaining the sample.

1. *Peripheral vein.* A venipuncture is performed and the sample collected in a chilled lavender-topped tube. The tube should be inverted gently several times to promote adequate mixing with the anticoagulant, placed in ice, and sent to the laboratory immediately.

2. *Renal vein.* The client is assisted to the supine position on the fluoroscopy table, and a site is selected for femoral vein catheterization. The skin may be shaved (if necessary), cleansed with an antiseptic, draped with sterile covers, and injected with a local anesthetic.

   A catheter is inserted into the femoral vein and advanced to the renal veins under fluoroscopic observation. Radiographic dye may be injected into the inferior vena cava at this point to aid in identification of the renal veins. A renal vein is entered and a blood sample obtained. The other renal vein is then entered and a second blood sample obtained. The catheter is then retracted into the inferior vena cava and a third sample obtained.

   The samples are placed in chilled lavender-topped tubes that are labeled to identify collection sites. The tubes should be inverted gently several times to promote adequate mixing with the anticoagulant, placed in ice, and sent to the laboratory immediately.

   The femoral catheter is removed after the third sample is obtained, and pressure is applied to the site for 10 minutes. A pressure dressing is then applied.

Nursing Care After the Procedure

1. *Peripheral vein.* Care and assessment after the procedure are the same as for any study involving the collection of a peripheral blood sample. Pretest diet and medications, which may have been modified or restricted before the study, should be resumed.

2. *Renal vein.* Maintain the client on bed rest for 8 hours after the procedure. Monitor vital signs and record according to the following schedule: every 15 minutes for 1 hour, every 30 minutes for 1 hour, and every hour for 4 hours. Monitor the catheterization site for bleeding or hematoma each time vital signs are checked. Resume previous diet and medications.

   ➤ *Abnormal values:* Note and report results and correlate with urinary sodium, serum, and urinary aldosterone. Monitor blood pressure, especially if antihypertensive medications have been withheld. Monitor I&O for fluid deficit or excess.

➤ *Allergic response (renal vein):* Note and report allergic response to dye injection and assess for rash, urticaria, dyspnea, and tachycardia. Administer ordered antihistamine or steroids and oxygen. Have emergency equipment and supplies on hand.

➤ *Vein thrombosis (renal vein):* Note and report any flank or back pain, hematuria, or abnormal renal test results (blood urea nitrogen, creatinine).

HORMONES

Hormones are chemicals that control the activities of responsive tissues. Some hormones exert their effects in the vicinity of their release; others are released into the extracellular fluids of the body and affect distant tissues. Similarly, some hormones affect only specific tissues (target tissues), whereas others affect nearly all cells of the body. Chemically, hormones are classified as polypeptides, amines, and steroids.

Hormones act on responsive tissues by (1) altering the rate of synthesis and secretion of enzymes or other hormones, (2) affecting the rate of enzymatic catalysis, and (3) altering the permeability of cell membranes. Once the hormone has accomplished its function, its rate of secretion normally decreases. This is known as negative feedback. After sufficient reduction in hormonal effects, negative feedback decreases, and the hormone is again secreted.

Hypophyseal Hormones

The hypophysis, also known as the pituitary gland, lies at the base of the brain in the sella turcica and is connected to the hypothalamus by the hypophyseal stalk. The hypophysis has two distinct portions: (1) the adenohypophysis (anterior pituitary) and (2) the neurohypophysis (posterior pituitary). The adenohypophysis arises from upward growth of pharyngeal epithelium in the embryo, whereas the neurohypophysis arises from the downward growth of the hypothalamus in the embryo.

Almost all hormonal secretion from the hypophysis is controlled by the hypothalamus. Neurohypophyseal hormones are formed in the hypothalamus and travel down nerve fibers to the neurohypophysis, where they are stored and then released into the circulation in response to feedback mechanisms. Adenohypophyseal hormone secretion is controlled by releasing and inhibiting factors that are secreted by the hypothalamus and carried to the adenohypophysis by the hypothalamic-hypophyseal portal vessels. Hypothalamic releasing and inhibiting factors identified thus far include (1) thyrotropin-releasing hormone (TRH); (2) corticotropin-releasing hormone (CRH); (3) gonadotropin-releasing hormone (GnRH), also known as luteinizing hormone–releasing hormone (LHRH) and follicle-stimulating hormone–releasing factor; (4) growth hormone–releasing hormone (GHRH); (5) growth hormone–inhibiting hormone (GHIH); and (6) prolactin inhibitory hormone (PIH). A releasing factor for melanocyte-stimulating hormone also is believed to exist. The releasing factors either stimulate or inhibit the adenohypophysis in the release of its hormones.

The adenohypophysis consists of three major cell types: (1) acidophils, (2) basophils, and (3) chromophobes. The acidophils secrete growth hormone (GH), also called somatotropic hormone (STH, SH) or somatotropin, and prolactin (HPRL), also known as luteotropic hormone (LTH), lactogenic hormone, or lactogen. The basophils secrete adrenocorticotropic hormone (ACTH), also known as adrenocorticotropin and corticotropin; thyroid-stimulating hormone (TSH), also known as thyrotropin; follicle-stimulating hormone (FSH); luteinizing hormone (LH), also known as interstitial cell–stimulating hormone (ICSH); and melanocyte-stimulating hormone (MSH). The chromophobes, which constitute about half of the adenohypophyseal cells, are resting cells capable of transformation to either acidophils or basophils.

The hormones stored and released by the neurohypophysis include antidiuretic hormone (ADH), also known as vasopressin, and oxytocin. Radioimmunoassays are used to determine blood levels of the hypophyseal hormones.

GROWTH HORMONE (GH, STH, SH)

Growth hormone (GH, STH, SH) is secreted in episodic bursts, usually during early sleep. The effects of GH occur throughout the body. GH promotes skeletal growth by stimulating hepatic production of proteins. It also affects lipid and glucose metabolism. Under the influence of growth hormone, free fatty acids enter the circulation for use by muscle; hepatic glucose production (gluconeogenesis) also rises. Growth hormone also increases blood flow to the renal cortex and the glomerular filtration rate; the kidney excretes more calcium and less phosphate than usual. GH is believed to antagonize insulin.

Deficiencies in GH are apparent only in childhood. Children with GH deficiency have very small statures but normal body proportions. The child also may be deficient in other hypophyseal hormones, and this disorder is known as "pituitary dwarfism."

Excessive levels of GH are apparent in all ages. Excess GH in children causes the long bones of the skeleton to enlarge and produces gigantism. In adults, the bones of the skull, hands, and feet thicken to produce the physical appearance of acromegaly. In this disorder, the internal organs, skeletal muscle, and heart muscle hypertrophy. Nerves and cartilage also enlarge and may produce nerve compression and joint disorders.

Reference Values

	Conventional Units	**SI Units**
Newborns	15–40 ng/mL	15–40 μg/L
Children	0–10 ng/mL	0–10 μg/L
Adults	0–10 ng/mL	0–10 μg/L
Values may vary according to the laboratory performing the test.		

Interfering Factors

➤ Hyperglycemia and therapy with drugs such as adrenocorticosteroids and chlorpromazine may cause falsely decreased levels.

➤ Hypoglycemia, physical activity, stress, and a variety of drugs (e.g., amphetamines, arginine, dopamine, levodopa, methyldopa, beta blockers, histamine, nicotinic acid, estrogens) may cause falsely elevated levels.[33]

Indications for Growth Hormone (GH, STH, SH) Test

➤ Growth retardation in children with decreased levels indicative of pituitary etiology
➤ Monitoring for response to treatment of growth retardation caused by GH deficiency
➤ Suspected disorder associated with decreased GH (e.g., pituitary tumors, craniopharyngiomas, tuberculosis meningitis, and pituitary damage or trauma)
➤ Gigantism in children with increased levels indicative of pituitary etiology
➤ Support for diagnosing acromegaly in adults as indicated by elevated levels; acidophil or chromophobe tumors of the adenohypophysis may account for these elevated levels[33]

Nursing Care Before the Procedure

Client preparation is essentially the same as that for any study involving the collection of a peripheral blood sample (see Appendix I).
➤ The client should be informed that the test will be performed on 2 consecutive days, between the hours of 6 and 8 AM.
➤ The client should fast from food and avoid strenuous exercise for 12 hours before each sample is drawn.
➤ Additionally, it is recommended by some that the client be maintained on bed rest for 1 hour before each sample is obtained.
➤ Because many drugs may affect serum GH levels, a medication history should be obtained. It is recommended that those drugs that alter test results be withheld for 12 hours before the study, although this practice should be confirmed with the person ordering the test.

The Procedure

The test is performed on 2 consecutive days, between the hours of 6 and 8 AM. A venipuncture is performed and the sample collected in a red-topped tube. The sample should be handled gently to avoid hemolysis and sent immediately to the laboratory.

Nursing Care After the Procedure

Care and assessment after the procedure are the same as for any study involving the collection of a peripheral blood sample.
➤ Resume food and any medications withheld before the test, as well as usual activities.
➤ *Abnormal values:* Note and report increased levels. Assess for signs and symptoms of hyperglycemia and abnormal (increased) growth pattern. Prepare client for possible surgery or radiation therapy. Note and report decreased levels in association with GH stimulation tests. Assess growth pattern abnormalities for age and gender. Instruct caretaker in availability of replacement therapy and follow-up, if appropriate.

Growth Hormone (GH) Stimulation Tests

Baseline levels of GH are affected by many factors and may be misleading at times. Stimulation tests are performed to determine responsiveness to substances that normally stimulate GH secretion, such as arginine and L-dopa. Insulin also may be given to induce hypoglycemia, which in turn stimulates GH secretion. It has been found that blood sugar levels of less than 50 mg/dL cause GH levels to rise 10 times or more in normal individuals. Idiosyncratic responses to the different stimulants may occur. Thus, it may be necessary to perform two or three different stimulation tests before arriving at diagnostic conclusions.[34]

Reference Values

	Conventional Units	SI Units
Arginine		
Men	>10 ng/mL	>10 µg/L
Women	>15 ng/mL	>15 µg/L
L-Dopa or insulin	>7 ng/mL above baseline level	>7 µg/L

Interfering Factors

➤ Factors that may affect serum GH determinations (see p. 221) also may alter results of GH stimulation tests.

Indications for Growth Hormone (GH) Stimulation Tests

➤ Low or undetectable serum GH levels, with GH deficiency or adult panhypopituitarism confirmed by no increase after administration of the stimulant
➤ Confirmation of the diagnosis of acromegaly as evidenced by reduced GH output after L-dopa is administered as a stimulant (i.e., an idiosyncratic response is seen in acromegaly)

➤➤ Nursing Alert

• If insulin is used as the stimulant, the client should be observed carefully during and after the test for signs and symptoms of extreme hypoglycemia.

Nursing Care Before the Procedure

➤ Initial client preparation is the same as that for serum GH determinations.
➤ The client should be weighed on the day of the test because dosage of the stimulant is determined by weight.
➤ Because several blood samples will be obtained and because certain of the stimulants (i.e., insulin and arginine) are administered IV, the client should be informed that an intermittent venous access device (e.g., heparin lock) will be inserted.

The Procedure

An intermittent venous access device is inserted, usually at about 8 AM, and a venous sample is obtained and placed in a red-topped tube. The sample is handled gently to avoid hemolysis and sent to the laboratory immediately.

The stimulant is then administered. L-Dopa is administered orally; arginine and insulin are administered IV in a saline infusion. If insulin is used to lower blood sugar, an ampule of 50 percent glucose should be on hand in the event that severe hypoglycemia occurs.

After the stimulant is administered, three blood samples are obtained via the venous access device at 30-minute intervals. The samples are placed in red-topped tubes and sent to the laboratory immediately upon collection.

Nursing Care After the Procedure

Care and assessment after the procedure are essentially the same as for serum GH determinations.

➤ If an intermittent venous access device was inserted for the procedure, remove after completion of the test, and apply pressure bandage to the site.

➤ If insulin was used as the stimulant, resume dietary intake as soon as possible after the test is completed, and observe for signs of hypoglycemia.

➤ *Complications and precautions:* If insulin is used, note and report signs and symptoms of hypoglycemia such as sweating, tachycardia, tremors, irritability, or confusion. Prepare client for IV glucose administration.

GROWTH HORMONE (GH) SUPPRESSION TEST

Hyperglycemia suppresses GH secretion in normal individuals. This principle is used in evaluating individuals with abnormally elevated levels and those who are believed to be hypersecreting GH but who show normal levels on routine serum GH determinations. Administration of a glucose load that produces hyperglycemia should decrease serum GH levels within 1 to 2 hours. In individuals who are hypersecreting GH, a decrease in serum GH will not occur in response to hyperglycemia. It should be noted that the test may require repetition to confirm results.

Reference Values

Conventional Units	SI Units
<3 ng/dL	<3 μg/L

Interfering Factors

➤ Factors that may affect serum GH determinations (see p. 221) may also alter results of GH suppression tests.

Indications for Growth Hormone (GH) Suppression Test

➤ Elevated serum GH levels

➤ Signs of GH hypersecretion with serum GH levels within normal limits

➤ Confirmation of GH hypersecretion as indicated by decreased response to GH suppression

Nursing Care Before the Procedure

➤ Initial client preparation is the same as that for serum GH determinations.
➤ The client should be informed that it will be necessary to drink an oral glucose solution and that two blood samples will be obtained.

The Procedure

A venipuncture is performed and a sample collected in a red-topped tube. The sample is handled gently to avoid hemolysis and sent to the laboratory immediately.

The glucose solution (usually 100 g) is administered orally. If the client is unable to drink or retain the glucose solution, the physician is notified. IV glucose may be administered, if necessary, to perform the test.

After 1 to 2 hours, depending on laboratory procedures, a second blood sample is collected in a red-topped tube and sent to the laboratory immediately.

Nursing Care After the Procedure

Care and assessment after the procedure are the same as for serum GH determinations.

➤ *Complications and precautions:* Monitor for hyperglycemia after ingestion of the glucose solution.

PROLACTIN (HPRL, LTH)

Prolactin (hPRL, LTH) is secreted by the acidophil cells of the adenohypophysis. It is unique among hormones in that it responds to inhibition via the hypothalamus rather than to stimulation; that is, prolactin is secreted except when influenced by the hypothalamic inhibiting factor, which is believed to be the neurotransmitter dopamine.

The only known function of hPRL is to induce milk production in a female breast already stimulated by high estrogen levels. Once milk production is established, lactation can continue without elevated prolactin levels. Levels of hPRL rise late in pregnancy, peak with the initiation of lactation, and surge each time a woman breast-feeds. The function of hPRL in men is not known.

Excessive circulating hPRL disturbs sexual function in both men and women. Women experience amenorrhea and anovulation, and they may have inappropriate milk secretion (galactorrhea). Men experience impotence, which occurs even when testosterone levels are normal, and sometimes gynecomastia.[35]

Reference Values

	Conventional Units	SI Units
Children	1–20 ng/mL	1–20 μg/L
Men	1–20 ng/mL	1–20 μg/L
Women		
Nonlactating	1–25 ng/mL	1–25 μg/L
Menopausal	1–20 ng/mL	1–20 μg/L

Interfering Factors

➤ Therapy with drugs such as estrogens, oral contraceptives, reserpine, α-methyldopa, phenothiazines, haloperidol, tricyclic antidepressants, and procainamide derivatives may produce elevated levels.

➤ Episodic elevations may occur in response to sleep, stress, exercise, and hypoglycemia.

➤ Therapy with dopamine, apomorphine, and ergot alkaloids may produce decreased levels.

Indications for Serum Prolactin (hPRL, LTH) Test

➤ Sexual dysfunction of unknown etiology in men and women, because excessive circulating hPRL may indicate the source of the problem (e.g., damage to the hypothalamus, pituitary adenoma)

➤ Failure of lactation in the postpartum period or suspected postpartum hypophyseal infarction (Sheehan's syndrome), or both, as indicated by decreased levels

➤ Suspected tumor involving the lungs or kidneys, with elevated levels indicating ectopic hPRL production

➤ Support for diagnosing primary hypothyroidism as indicated by elevated levels

Nursing Care Before the Procedure

Client preparation is the same as for any study involving the collection of a peripheral blood sample (see Appendix I).

➤ Because many drugs may alter serum hPRL levels, a medication history should be obtained. It is recommended that drugs that may alter test results be withheld for 12 to 24 hours before the test, although this practice should be confirmed with the person ordering the study.

The Procedure

A venipuncture is performed and the sample collected in a red-topped tube. The sample should be handled gently to avoid hemolysis and transported promptly to the laboratory.

Nursing Care After the Procedure

Care and assessment after the procedure are the same as for any study involving the collection of a peripheral blood sample.

➤ Resume any medications withheld before the test.

➤ *Complications and precautions:* Assess for signs and symptoms of pituitary conditions such as mood changes; body image changes; sexual dysfunction in men; and menstrual, milk secretion, and weight gain abnormalities in women.

ADRENOCORTICOTROPIC HORMONE (ACTH)

Adrenocorticotropic hormone (ACTH) is secreted by the basophils of the adenohypophysis. ACTH stimulates the adrenal cortex to secrete (1) glucocorticoids, of which cortisol predominates; (2) adrenal androgens, which are converted by the liver to testosterone; and, to a lesser degree, (3) mineralocorticoids, of which aldosterone predominates. ACTH secretion is closely linked to melanocyte-stimulating hormone; it also is thought to stimulate pancreatic beta cells and the release of GH.

ACTH release, which is stimulated by its corresponding hypothalamic releasing factor, occurs episodically in relation to decreased circulating levels of glucocorticoid, increased stress, and hypoglycemia. ACTH levels also vary diurnally; highest levels occur on awakening, decrease throughout the day, and then begin to rise again a few hours before awakening. Circulating aldosterone levels may influence ACTH secretion to some extent; however, androgens are believed to have no effect on ACTH levels. ACTH assays are expensive to perform and are not universally available.

Reference Values

	Conventional Units	SI Units
BioScience Laboratories	<80 pg/mL at 8 AM	<17.6 pmol/L
Mayo Clinic	<120 pg/mL at 6 to 8 AM	<26.4 pmol/L

Normal values vary according to the laboratory performing the test. Results are usually evaluated in relation to other tests of adrenal-hypophyseal function (e.g., plasma cortisol).

Interfering Factors

> ACTH levels vary diurnally; highest levels occur upon awakening, decrease throughout the day, and then begin to rise again a few hours before awakening.
> Numerous drugs may lead to decreased ACTH levels (e.g., adrenocorticosteroids, estrogens, calcium gluconate, amphetamines, spironolactone, and ethanol).
> Stress, exercise, and blood glucose levels may affect results.

Indications for Plasma Adrenocorticotropic Hormone (ACTH) Test

> Signs and symptoms of adrenocortical dysfunction
>   • Elevated ACTH levels with low cortisol levels indicate adrenocortical hypoactivity (Addison's disease).
>   • Low ACTH levels with high cortisol levels indicate adrenocortical hyperactivity (Cushing's syndrome) caused by benign or malignant adrenal tumors.
>   • High ACTH levels, without diurnal variation, combined with high cortisol levels indicate adrenocortical hyperfunction caused by excessive ACTH production (e.g., resulting from pituitary adenoma and nonendocrine malignant tumors in which there is ectopic ACTH production).
>   • Decreased ACTH levels are associated with panhypopituitarism, hypothalamic dysfunction, and long-term adrenocorticosteroid therapy.

Nursing Care Before the Procedure

General client preparation is the same as that for any study involving the collection of a peripheral blood sample (see Appendix I).

> For this test, the client should follow a low-carbohydrate diet for 48 hours and fast from food for 12 hours before the test.
> In addition, strenuous exercise should be avoided for 12 hours before the test, and 1 hour of bed rest is necessary immediately before the test.

➤ Medications that may alter test results should be withheld for at least 24 to 48 hours or longer before the study, although this practice should be confirmed with the person ordering the test.

➤ The client should be informed that it may be necessary to obtain more than one sample and that samples must be obtained at specific times to detect peak and trough levels of ACTH.

The Procedure

Between 6 and 8 AM (peak ACTH secretion time), a venipuncture is performed and the sample collected in a green-topped tube. The sample must be placed in a container of ice and sent to the laboratory immediately. When ACTH hypersecretion is suspected, a second sample may be obtained between 8 and 10 PM to determine whether diurnal variation in ACTH levels is occurring.

➤ The ACTH stimulation test can be conducted by the timed serial laboratory analysis of blood plasma samples for cortisol levels after the administration of metyrapone. The ACTH suppression test can be conducted by the laboratory analysis of blood plasma samples for cortisol levels after the administration of dexamethasone. The tests are performed to assist in the diagnosis of Addison's disease or Cushing's syndrome.

Nursing Care After the Procedure

Care and assessment after the procedure are the same as for any study involving the collection of a peripheral blood sample.

➤ Resume foods and any medications withheld before the test, as well as usual activities.

➤ *Complications and precautions:* Note cortisol level and its relation to increases in ACTH production by the pituitary gland.

THYROID-STIMULATING HORMONE (TSH)

Thyroid-stimulating hormone (TSH) is produced by the basophil cells of the adenohypophysis in response to stimulation by its hypothalamic releasing factor, thyrotropin-releasing hormone (TRH). TRH responds to decreased circulating levels of thyroid hormones, as well as to intense cold, psychological tension, and increased metabolic need, and it stimulates the adenohypophysis to secrete TSH. TSH accelerates all aspects of hormone production by the thyroid gland and enhances hPRL release. Measuring TSH provides useful information about both hypophyseal and thyroid gland function.

Hypersecretion of TSH by the adenohypophysis (e.g., because of TSH-secreting pituitary tumors) causes hyperthyroidism as a result of excessive stimulation of the thyroid gland. Elevated TSH levels are also seen with prolonged emotional stress and are more common in colder climates. Primary hypothyroidism (i.e., hypothyroidism caused by disorders involving the thyroid gland itself) leads to elevated TSH levels because of normal feedback mechanisms. TSH levels are normally elevated at birth.

It should be noted that increased TSH secretion is associated with excess secretion of exophthalmos-producing substance, which also originates in the adenohypophysis. This substance promotes water storage in the retro-orbital fat pads and causes the eyes to protrude, a common sign of hyperthyroidism.

Exophthalmos sometimes persists after the hyperthyroidism is corrected and also may occur in persons with normal thyroid function.

TSH levels are normal in situations in which the functional ability of the thyroid gland is normal but the thyroid hormone levels are low, a phenomenon that is seen in clients with severe illnesses with protein deficiency (thyroid hormones are proteins) such as neoplastic disease, severe burns, trauma, liver disease, renal failure, and cardiovascular problems. Deficiency of thyroid hormone produces a hypometabolic state. Excess TSH production is not stimulated, however, because circulating thyroid levels are appropriate to the client's metabolic needs (i.e., the person is metabolically euthyroid). Treatment involves correcting the underlying causes. The apparent hypothyroidism is not treated, however, because such treatment could be devastating to a severely debilitated person.

TSH is measured by radioimmunoassay. Immunologic cross-reactivity occurs with glycoprotein hormones such as human chorionic gonadotropin (hCG), follicle-stimulating hormone (FSH), and luteinizing hormone (LH).

Reference Values

	Conventional Units	**SI Units**
Newborns	<25 μIU/mL by day 3	<25 mU/L
Children and adults	<10 μIU/mL	<10 mU/L

Interfering Factors

➤ Aspirin, adrenocorticosteroids, and heparin may produce decreased TSH levels.

➤ Lithium carbonate and potassium iodide may produce elevated TSH levels.

➤ Falsely increased levels may occur in hydatidiform mole, choriocarcinoma, embryonal carcinoma of the testes, pregnancy, and postmenopausal states characterized by high FSH and LH levels.[36]

Indications for Thyroid-Stimulating Hormone (TSH) Test

➤ Signs and symptoms of hypothyroidism, hyperthyroidism, or suspected pituitary or hypothalamic dysfunction, or hypothyroidism or hyperthyroidism combined with suspected pituitary or hypothalamic dysfunction
  • Elevated levels are seen with primary hypothyroidism.
  • Decreased or undetectable levels are associated with secondary hypothyroidism caused by pituitary or hypothalamic hypofunction.
  • Decreased levels are seen with primary hyperthyroidism.
  • Elevated levels may indicate secondary hyperthyroidism resulting from pituitary hyperactivity (e.g., caused by tumor).

➤ Differentiation of functional euthyroidism from true hypothyroidism in debilitated individuals, with the former indicated by normal levels

Nursing Care Before the Procedure

Client preparation is the same as that for any study involving collection of a peripheral blood sample (see Appendix I).

➤ It is recommended that drugs known to alter TSH levels be withheld for 12 to 24 hours before the test, although this practice should be confirmed with the person ordering the study.

The Procedure

A venipuncture is performed and the sample is collected in a red-topped tube. The sample should be handled gently to avoid hemolysis and transported promptly to the laboratory.

➤ The test for TSH is used on newborns to screen for congenital hypothyroidism. It is performed by obtaining a sample of blood from a heelstick and saturating a spot on a special filter paper with the blood. A kit is available for this test; it contains a comparison chart to identify elevations.

Nursing Care After the Procedure

Care and assessment after the procedure are the same as for any study involving the collection of a peripheral blood sample.

➤ Resume any medications withheld before the test.

➤ *Complications and precautions:* Note the relation of TSH to levels of other thyroid tests indicating hypothyroidism as opposed to other thyroid disorders.

TSH STIMULATION TEST

The TSH stimulation test is used to evaluate the thyroid-pituitary-hypothalamic feedback loop. In this test, a purified form of hypothalamic thyrotropin-releasing hormone (TRH) is administered IV. Normally, TRH stimulates the adenohypophysis to release TSH, which, in turn, causes hormonal release from the thyroid gland. A normal response (e.g., elevated TSH levels) indicates that the adenohypophysis is capable of responding to TRH stimulation. If thyroid hormones also are measured as part of the test, elevated levels indicate that the thyroid gland is capable of responding to TSH stimulation.

Reference Values

TSH levels rise within 15 to 30 minutes of thyrotropin-releasing hormone (TRH) administration, peak at 2.5 to 4 times normal, and return to baseline levels within 2 to 4 hours. Thyroid hormone secretion (e.g., T_3 and T_4), which should be increased by 50 to 75 percent, occurs in 1 to 4 hours.

Indications for TSH Stimulation Test

➤ Low or undetectable serum TSH levels, hypothyroidism, or hyperthyroidism of unknown etiology or type, or low serum TSH levels combined with hypothyroidism or hyperthyroidism

• A normal or delayed TSH response in persons with low baseline TSH levels and signs of hypothyroidism indicates hypothalamic dysfunction or disruption of the hypothalamic-hypophyseal portal circulation and confirms the diagnosis of tertiary hypothyroidism.

• A decreased or absent TSH response in persons with low baseline TSH levels and signs of hypothyroidism indicates hypopituitarism and confirms the diagnosis of secondary hypothyroidism.

• A normal or increased TSH response in clients with elevated baseline TSH levels and signs of hypothyroidism, with persistently decreased thyroid gland hormone levels, confirms the diagnosis of primary hypothyroidism.

- A decreased or absent TSH response in persons with low baseline TSH levels and signs of hyperthyroidism, with persistently elevated thyroid gland hormone levels, indicates that thyroid hormone production is occurring autonomously and confirms the diagnosis of primary hyperthyroidism.

Nursing Care Before the Procedure

Initial client preparation is the same as that for serum determinations of TSH.
➤ Because several blood samples will be obtained and because the TRH will be administered IV, the client should be informed that an intermittent venous access device (e.g., heparin lock) may be inserted.

The Procedure

The procedure varies somewhat according to the laboratory performing the test. One example of the procedure is described subsequently.

An intermittent venous access device is inserted and a venous sample is obtained and placed in a red-topped tube. The sample is handled gently to avoid hemolysis and sent promptly to the laboratory. The sample should be labeled either with the time drawn or as the baseline sample.

A bolus of TRH is then administered IV through the access device. Additional blood samples are obtained via the access device ½, 1, 2, 3, and 4 hours after administration of the TRH. Each sample is placed in a red-topped tube, labeled, and sent to the laboratory.

Nursing Care After the Procedure

Care and assessment after the procedure are essentially the same as for serum TSH determinations.
➤ If an intermittent venous access device was inserted for the procedure, remove after completion of the test and apply a pressure bandage to the site.
➤ *Complications and precautions:* Note increased levels in relation to other thyroid tests and prepare client for a nuclear scan laboratory study using the iodine 131 (^{131}I) radionuclide (see Chap. 20).

FOLLICLE-STIMULATING HORMONE (FSH)

Follicle-stimulating hormone (FSH) is secreted by the basophil cells of the adenohypophysis in response to stimulation by hypothalamic gonadotropin-releasing hormone (GnRH), which also is called luteinizing hormone–releasing hormone (LHRH) and follicle-stimulating hormone-releasing factor. FSH affects gonadal function in both men and women. In women, FSH promotes maturation of the graafian (germinal) follicle, causing estrogen secretion and allowing the ovum to mature. In men, FSH partially controls spermatogenesis, but the presence of testosterone also is necessary. GnRH secretion, which in turn stimulates FSH secretion, is stimulated by decreased estrogen and testosterone levels. Isolated FSH elevation also may occur when there is failure to produce spermatozoa, even though testosterone production is normal. FSH production is inhibited by rising estrogen and testosterone levels.

FSH levels are normally low during childhood but begin to rise as puberty approaches. Surges of FSH occur initially during sleep but, as puberty advances, daytime levels also rise. During childbearing years, FSH levels in women vary according to the menstrual cycle. Decreased FSH levels after puberty are associated with male and female infertility. After the reproductive years, estrogen and testosterone levels decline, causing FSH levels to rise in response to normal feedback mechanisms. A 24-hour urine specimen also can be collected and tested for FSH.

FSH/LH CHALLENGE TESTS

The hypothalamic-hypophyseal-gonadal axis can be evaluated by administering drugs and hormones known to affect specfic hormonal interactions. These include clomiphene, GnRH, hCG, and progesterone.

Clomiphene, a drug used to treat infertility, prevents the hypothalamus from recognizing normally inhibitory levels of estrogen and testosterone. Consequently, the hypothalamus continues to secrete GnRH, which, in turn, continues to stimulate the adenohypophysis to secrete FSH and LH. After 5 days of clomiphene, both FSH and LH levels rise, usually 50 to 100 percent above baseline levels. In anovulatory women whose ovaries are normal, clomiphene often enhances FSH and LH levels so that ovulation is induced. If FSH and LH levels do not rise with clomiphene administration, either hypothalamic or hypophyseal dysfunction is indicated. The source of the dysfunction may be identified by administering purified GnRH. If FSH and LH levels rise, the pituitary gland is normal but hypothalamic function is impaired. FSH and LH levels that do not rise indicate hypophyseal dysfunction.

Human chorionic gonadotropin (hCG), a placental hormone with effects similar to those of LH, is used to evaluate testicular activity in men with low testosterone levels. Elevated testosterone levels after hCG administration indicate that testicular function is normal but that hypothalamic-pituitary activity is impaired. Failure of testosterone levels to rise suggests primary testicular dysfunction.

Progesterone, a hormone secreted by the ovary, is used to evaluate amenorrhea. In the normal menstrual cycle, the progesterone surge that follows ovulation inhibits GnRH secretion, and hormonal levels decline. Menstrual bleeding, also called withdrawal bleeding, occurs when the estrogen-stimulated endometrium experiences a drop in hormonal stimulation. This normal situation can be simulated by administering oral or IM progesterone to amenorrheic women already exposed to adequate estrogen levels. If menstrual bleeding occurs, the underlying cause of the amenorrhea is failure to ovulate. Lack of bleeding in response to progesterone administration indicates (1) inadequate estrogen production, resulting from either primary ovarian failure or inadequate pituitary secretion of FSH; (2) hypothalamic dysfunction with defective GnRH secretion; (3) impaired hypophyseal response to GnRH; or (4) abnormal uterine response to hormonal stimulation. These possibilities can be distinguished by administering estrogen to stimulate the endometrium and then repeating the progesterone challenge. If bleeding occurs, then either ovarian failure or inadequately responsive hypothalamic-hypophyseal activity is the underlying cause of the amenorrhea. Measuring FSH, LH, and estrogen levels helps further to diagnose the problem.[37]

Reference Values

	Conventional Units	**SI Units**
Children	5–10 mIU/mL	5–10 IU/L
Men	10–15 mIU/mL	10–15 IU/L
Women (menstruating)		
Early in cycle	5–25 mIU/mL	5–25 IU/L
Midcycle	20–30 mIU/mL	20–30 IU/L
Luteal phase	5–25 mIU/mL	5–25 IU/L
Women (menopausal)	40–250 mIU/mL	40–250 IU/L

Results should be evaluated in relation to other tests of gonadal function.

Interfering Factors

➤ In menstruating women, values vary in relation to the phase of the menstrual cycle.

➤ Values are higher in postmenopausal women.

➤ Administration of the drug clomiphene may result in elevated FSH levels.

➤ Therapy with estrogens, progesterone, and phenothiazines may result in decreased FSH levels.[38]

Indications for Follicle-Stimulating Hormone (FHS) Test

➤ Evaluation of ambiguous sexual differentiation in infants

➤ Evaluation of early sexual development in girls under age 9 or boys under age 10, with precocious puberty associated with elevated levels

➤ Evaluation of failure of sexual maturation in adolescence

➤ Evaluation of sexual dysfunction or changes in secondary sexual characteristics in men and women

   • Elevated levels are associated with ovarian or testicular failure, with polycystic ovary disease, after viral orchitis, and with Turner's syndrome in women and Klinefelter's syndrome in men.

   • Decreased levels may be seen with neoplasms of the testes, ovaries, and adrenal glands, resulting in excessive production of sex hormones.

➤ Suspected pituitary or hypothalamic dysfunction

   • Elevated levels may be seen in pituitary tumors.

   • Decreased levels are associated with hypothalamic lesions and panhypopituitarism.

➤ Suspected early acromegaly as indicated by elevated levels

➤ Suspected disorders associated with decreased FSH levels, such as anorexia nervosa and renal disease

Nursing Care Before the Procedure

Client preparation is the same as that for any study involving the collection of a peripheral blood sample (see Appendix I).

➤ It is recommended that drugs known to alter FSH levels be withheld for 12 to 24 hours before the test, although this practice should be confirmed with the person ordering the study.

➤ In women, the phase of the menstrual cycle should be ascertained, if possible.

The Procedure

A venipuncture is performed and the sample collected in a red-topped tube. The sample should be handled gently to avoid hemolysis and transported to the laboratory immediately.

Nursing Care After the Procedure

Care and assessment after the procedure are the same as for any study involving the collection of a peripheral blood sample.

➤ Resume any medications withheld before the test.

➤ *Complications and precautions:* Note levels in relation to 24-hour urinary FSH and LH results. Prepare client for serial samples for testing.

LUTEINIZING HORMONE (LH, ICSH)

Luteinizing hormone is secreted by the basophil cells of the adenohypophysis in response to stimulation by GnRH, the same hypothalamic releasing factor that stimulates FSH release. LH affects gonadal function in both men and women. In women, a surge of LH occurs at the midpoint of the menstrual cycle and is believed to be induced by high estrogen levels. LH causes the ovum to be expelled from the ovary and stimulates development of the corpus luteum and production of progesterone. As progesterone levels rise, LH production decreases. In men, LH stimulates the interstitial Leydig cells, located in the testes, to produce testosterone.

During childhood, LH levels decrease and are lower than those of FSH. Similarly, LH levels rise after those of FSH as puberty approaches. During the childbearing years, LH levels in women vary according to the menstrual cycle but remain fairly constant in men. Decreased LH levels after puberty are associated with male and female infertility. After the reproductive years, as gonadal hormones decline, LH levels rise in response to normal feedback mechanisms. The rise in LH levels, however, is not as marked as that for FSH levels. A 24-hour urine specimen also can be collected and tested for LH.

Reference Values

	Conventional Units	**SI Units**
Children	5–10 mIU/mL	5–10 IU/L
Men	5–20 mIU/mL	5–20 IU/L
Women (menstruating)		
Early in cycle	5–25 mIU/mL	5–25 IU/L
Midcycle	40–80 mIU/mL	40–80 IU/L
Luteal phase	5–25 mIU/mL	5–25 IU/L
Women (menopausal)	>75 mIU/mL	>75 IU/L

Results should be evaluated in relation to other tests of gonadal function.

Interfering Factors

➤ In menstruating women, values vary in relation to the phase of the menstrual cycle.

➤ Values are higher in postmenopausal women.

➤ Drugs containing estrogen tend to cause elevated LH levels.
➤ Drugs containing progesterone and testosterone may lead to decreased levels.

Indications for Serum Luteinizing Hormone (LH, ICSH) Test

➤ Evaluation of male and female infertility, as indicated by decreased levels
➤ Support for diagnosing infertility caused by anovulation as evidenced by lack of the midcycle LH surge
➤ Evaluation of response to therapy to induce ovulation
➤ Suspected pituitary or hypothalamic dysfunction
  • Elevated levels may be seen in pituitary tumors.
  • Decreased levels are associated with hypothalamic lesions and panhypopituitarism.

Nursing Care Before the Procedure

Client preparation is the same as that for any study involving the collection of a peripheral blood sample (see Appendix I).
➤ It is recommended that any drugs known to alter LH levels be withheld for 12 to 24 hours before the test, although this practice should be confirmed with the person ordering the study.
➤ In women, the phase of the menstrual cycle should be ascertained, if possible.
➤ If the test is being performed to detect ovulation, the client should be informed that it may be necessary to obtain a series of samples over a period of several days to detect peak LH levels.

The Procedure

A venipuncture is performed and the sample collected in a red-topped tube. The sample should be handled gently to avoid hemolysis and transported promptly to the laboratory.

Nursing Care After the Procedure

Care and assessment after the procedure are the same as for any study involving the collection of a peripheral blood sample.
➤ Resume any medications withheld before the test.
➤ *Abnormal test results, complications, and precautions:* Respond as for FSH testing, because LH is usually performed on the same blood sample (see p. 234).

ANTIDIURETIC HORMONE (ADH)

Antidiuretic hormone (ADH) is formed by the hypothalamus but is stored in the neurohypophysis (posterior pituitary gland). ADH is released in response to increased serum osmolality or decreased blood volume. Although as little as a 1 percent change in serum osmolality will stimulate ADH secretion, blood volume must decrease by approximately 10 percent for ADH secretion to be induced. Psychogenic stimuli (e.g., stress, pain, anxiety) also may stimulate ADH release, but the mechanism by which this occurs is unclear.

ADH acts on the epithelial cells of the distal convoluted tubules and the collecting ducts of the kidneys, making them permeable to water. Thus, with

ADH, more water is absorbed from the glomerular filtrate into the bloodstream. Without ADH, water remains in the filtrate and is excreted, producing very dilute urine. In contrast, maximal ADH secretion produces very concentrated urine. ADH also is believed to stimulate mild contractions in the pregnant uterus and to aid in promoting milk ejection in lactation, functions similar to those of oxytocin, which also is secreted by the hypothalamus and released by the neurohypophysis.

Reference Values

Conventional Units	SI Units
2.3 – 3.1 pg/mL	2.3 – 3.1 ng/L

Interfering Factors

➤ Alcohol, phenytoin drugs, β-adrenergic drugs, and morphine antagonists may lead to decreased ADH secretion.

➤ Acetaminophen, barbiturates, cholinergic agents, clofibrate, estrogens, nicotine, oral hypoglycemic agents, cytotoxic agents (e.g., vincristine), tricyclic antidepressants, oxytocin, carbamazepine (Tegretol), and thiazide diuretics may lead to increased ADH secretion.[39]

➤ Pain, stress, and anxiety may lead to increased ADH secretion.

➤ Failure to follow dietary and exercise restrictions before the test may alter results.

Indications for Serum Antidiuretic Hormone (ADH) Test

➤ Polyuria or altered serum osmolality of unknown etiology, or both, to identify possible alterations in ADH secretion as the cause

➤ Central nervous system trauma, surgery, or disease that may lead to impaired secretion of ADH

➤ Differentiation of neurogenic (central) diabetes insipidus from nephrogenic diabetes insipidus
  • Neurogenic diabetes insipidus is characterized by decreased ADH levels.
  • ADH levels may be elevated in nephrogenic diabetes insipidus if normal feedback mechanisms are intact.

➤ Known or suspected malignancy associated with syndrome of inappropriate ADH (SIADH) secretion (e.g., oat cell lung cancer, thymoma, lymphoma, leukemia, and carcinoma of the pancreas, prostate gland, and intestine), with the disorder indicated by elevated ADH levels

➤ Known or suspected pulmonary conditions associated with SIADH secretion (e.g., tuberculosis, pneumonia, and positive pressure mechanical ventilation), with the disorder indicated by elevated ADH levels

Nursing Care Before the Procedure

Client preparation is essentially the same as that for any study involving collection of a peripheral blood sample (see Appendix I).

➤ The client should fast from food and avoid strenuous exercise for 12 hours before the sample is obtained. It is recommended that drugs that may alter

ADH levels be withheld for 12 to 24 hours before the study, although this practice should be confirmed with the person ordering the test.

The Procedure

A venipuncture is performed and the sample collected in a plastic red-topped tube. Plastic is used because contact with glass causes degradation of ADH. The sample should be handled gently to avoid hemolysis and sent to the laboratory immediately.

Nursing Care After the Procedure

Care and assessment after the procedure are the same as for any study involving collection of a peripheral blood sample.

➤ Resume food and any medications withheld before the test, as well as usual activities.

➤ *Abnormal levels:* Note and report increased levels in relation to renin level. Assess for fluid volume excess resulting from sodium and water retention. Monitor I&O, weight gain, edema, and increases in blood pressure. Instruct in diuretic therapy regimen. Note and report decreased levels in relation to sodium level. Assess for fluid volume deficit. Monitor I&O and weight loss. Instruct in long-term fluid, sodium, and corticosteroid therapy regimen.

Thyroid and Parathyroid Hormones

The thyroid gland synthesizes and releases thyroxine (T_4) and triiodothyronine (T_3) in response to stimulation by TSH, which is secreted by the adenohypophysis. The thyroid gland synthesizes its hormones from iodine and the essential amino acid tyrosine. Most of the body's iodine is ingested as iodide through dietary intake and is absorbed into the bloodstream from the gastrointestinal tract. One-third of the absorbed iodide enters the thyroid gland; the remaining two thirds is excreted in the urine. In the thyroid gland, enzymes oxidize iodide to iodine.

The thyroid gland secretes a protein, thyroglobulin, into its follicles. Thyroglobulin has special properties that allow the tyrosine contained in its molecules to react with iodine to form thyroid hormones. The thyroid hormones thus formed are stored in the follicles of the gland as the thyroglobulin-thyroid hormone complex called *colloid.*

When thyroid hormones are released into the bloodstream, they are split from thyroglobulin as a result of the action of proteases, which are secreted by thyroid cells in response to stimulation by TSH. Much more T_4 than T_3 is secreted into the bloodstream. Upon entering the bloodstream, both immediately combine with plasma proteins, mainly thyroxine-binding globulin (TBG), but also with albumin and prealbumin. Although more than 99 percent of both T_4 and T_3 are bound to TBG, physiological activity of both hormones results from only the unbound ("free") molecules. It should also be noted that TBG has greater affinity for T_4 than for T_3, which allows for more rapid release of T_3 from TBG for entry into body cells. T_3 is thought to exert at least 65 to 75 percent of thyroidal hormone effects, and it is believed by some that T_4 has no endocrine activity at all until it is converted to T_3, which occurs when one iodine molecule is removed from T_4.[40]

The main function of thyroid hormones is to increase the metabolic activities of most tissues by increasing the oxidative enzymes in the cells. This increase, in turn, causes increased oxygen consumption and increased utilization of carbohydrates, proteins, fats, and vitamins. Thyroid hormones also mobilize electrolytes and are necessary for the conversion of carotene to vitamin A. Although the mechanism is not known, thyroid hormones are essential for the development of the central nervous system. Thyroid-deficient infants may suffer irreversible brain damage (cretinism). Thyroid deficiency in adults (myxedema) produces diffuse psychomotor retardation, which is reversible with hormone replacement. Thyroid hormones also are thought to increase the rate of parathyroid hormone secretion.

Alterations in thyroid hormone production may be caused by disorders affecting the hypothalamus, which secretes thyrotropin-releasing hormone (TRH) in response to circulating T_4 and T_3 levels; the pituitary gland; or the thyroid gland itself. Such alterations may affect all body systems. *Hypothyroidism* is the general term for the hypometabolic state induced by deficient thyroid hormone secretion, whereas *hyperthyroidism* indicates excessive production of thyroid hormones.

An additional hormone produced by the thyroid gland is calcitonin, which is secreted in response to high serum calcium levels. Calcitonin causes an increase in calcium reabsorption by bone, thus lowering serum calcium.[41]

A number of tests pertaining to thyroid hormones may be performed, some of which may be grouped as a "thyroid screen" (e.g., T_4, T_3, and TSH). A "T_7" is sometimes ordered. This is interpreted as a T_4 plus a T_3, because there is no such substance as T_7. Before it was possible to measure thyroid hormones directly, serum iodine measurements (e.g., protein-bound iodine) were used as indicators of thyroid function. These tests were severely affected by organic and inorganic iodine contaminants and are no longer used to any great extent. Similarly, measurement of thyroidal uptake of radioactive iodine (^{131}I) has been replaced by direct measurements of T_4 and TSH.[42]

THYROXINE (T_4)

Thyroxine (T_4) is measured by competitive protein binding or by radioimmunoassay. In competitive protein binding, the affinity between T_4 and TBG is exploited. Reagent TBG fully saturated with radiolabeled T_4 is incubated with T_4 extracted from the client's serum. The T_4 from the test serum displaces the radiolabeled T_4 in the amount present. This procedure is known as T_4 by displacement (T_4 D), T_4 by competitive binding (T_4 CPB), and T_4 Murphy-Pattee (T_4 MP). T_4 measured by radioimmunoassay (T_4 RIA) is the preferred method to measure T_4 because it is not affected by circulating iodinated substances.

Most T_4 (99.97 percent) in the serum is bound to TBG. The remainder circulates as unbound ("free") T_4 (FT_4) and is responsible for all of the physiological activity of thyroxine. Because FT_4 is not dependent on normal levels of TBG, as is the case with total serum thyroxine, FT_4 levels are considered the most accurate indicator of thyroxine and its thyrometabolic activity. It is difficult, however, to measure FT_4 directly because quantitites are so small and the interference from bound T_4 is great. Free hormone levels are, therefore, usually calculated by multiplying the values for total T_4 by the T_3 uptake ratio (see p. 237). The result is expressed as the free thyroxine index (FT_4 I). The free hormone index varies directly with the amount of circulating hormone and inversely with the amount of unsaturated TBG present in the serum.[43]

Reference Values

	Conventional Units	**SI Units**
T_4D		
Newborns	11.0–23.0 µg/dL	140–230 nmol/L
1–4 mo	7.5–16.5 µg/dL	95–200 nmol/L
4–12 mo	5.5–14.5 µg/dL	70–185 nmol/L
Children	5.0–13.5 µg/dL	65–170 nmol/L
Adults	4.5–13.0 µg/dL	60–165 nmol/L
T_4 RIA	4.0–12.0 µg/dL	50–150 nmol/L
FT_4	0.9–2.3 ng/dL	10–30 nmol/L

Values may vary according to the laboratory performing the test. Results should be evaluated in relation to other tests of thyroid function.

Interfering Factors

➤ Results of T_4D may be altered by circulating iodinated substances; T_4 RIA is not similarly affected.

➤ Pregnancy, estrogen therapy, or estrogen-secreting tumors may produce elevated T_4 levels.

➤ Ingestion of thyroxine will elevate T_4 levels.

➤ Heroin and methadone may produce elevated T_4 levels.

➤ Androgens, glucocorticoids, heparin, salicylates, phenytoin anticonvulsants, sulfonamides, and antithyroid drugs such as propylthiouracil may lead to decreased T_4 levels.

Indications for Thyroxine (T_4) Test

➤ Signs of hypothyroidism, hyperthyroidism, or neonatal screening for congenital hypothyroidism (required in many states), or hypothyroidism or hyperthyroidism combined with neonatal screening
- Decreased T_4 and FT_4 levels indicate hypothyroid states and also may be seen in early thyroiditis.
- Elevated T_4 and FT_4 levels indicate hyperthyroid states.
- Normal T_4 and FT_4 levels in clients with signs of hyperthyroidism may indicate T_3 thyrotoxicosis.
- Normal FT_4 levels are seen in pregnancy, whereas T_4 and TBG are usually elevated.

➤ Monitoring of response to therapy for hypothyroidism or hyperthyroidism
- Elevated T_4 and FT_4 levels indicate response to treatment for hypothyroidism.
- Decreased T_4 and FT_4 levels indicate response to treatment for hyperthyroidism.

➤ Evaluation of thyroid response to protein deficiency associated with severe illnesses (e.g., metastatic cancer, liver disease, renal disease, diabetes mellitus, cardiovascular disorders, burns, and trauma)
- T_4 is decreased in such disorders because of a deficiency of TBG, a protein.
- FT_4 index is normal, if thyroid function is normal, because FT_4 index is not dependent on TBG levels.

Nursing Care Before the Procedure

Client preparation is essentially the same as that for any study involving the collection of a peripheral blood sample (see Appendix I).

➤ It is usually recommended that thyroid medications be withheld for 1 month before the test and that other drugs that may alter thyroxine levels be withheld for at least 24 hours before the study. This practice should be confirmed, however, with the person ordering the test.

➤ For infants, explain to the parent(s) the purpose of the test and that it may require repetition in 3 to 6 weeks because of normal changes in infant thyroid hormone levels.

The Procedure

A venipuncture is performed and the sample collected in a red-topped tube. The sample should be handled gently to avoid hemolysis and transported promptly to the laboratory.

➤ For neonatal screening, the sample is obtained by heelstick. A multiple neonatal screening kit is usually used; the directions provided with the kit must be followed carefully.

Nursing Care After the Procedure

Care and assessment after the procedure are the same as for any study involving the collection of a peripheral blood sample.

➤ Resume any medications withheld before the test.

➤ *Increased levels:* Note and report increased levels and relation to other thyroid tests and procedures performed. Assess for signs and symptoms of hyperthyroidism such as tachycardia, increased appetite, diaphoresis, elevated temperature, exophthalmos, weight loss, insomnia, hyperactivity, or inability to handle stress. Prepare for possible radionuclide therapy or surgical intervention. Administer ordered medications to reduce levels. Instruct in adequate fluid and nutritional dietary intake and eye care for exophthalmos. Instruct client to avoid stressful situations.

➤ *Decreased levels:* Note and report decreased levels and relation to other thyroid tests and procedures. Assess for cold intolerance, weight gain, skin changes, constipation, lethargy, or fatigue. Administer ordered replacement therapy. Instruct client in appropriate fluid and low caloric nutritional dietary intake, long-term thyroid medication regimen, control of environment for relaxation and warmth, and care of skin and hair. Instruct client to avoid sedatives to promote sleep.

TRIIODOTHYRONINE (T_3)

Although produced in smaller quantities than T_4, triiodothyronine (T_3) is physiologically more significant. The competitive protein-binding techniques that are useful in measuring T_4 are not used to measure T_3 because it is present in smaller amounts and has less affinity for TBG than for T_4. Thus, T_3 is measured only by radioimmunoassay (T_3 RIA).

As with T_4, most T_3 (99.7 percent) in the serum is bound to TBG. The remainder circulates as unbound ("free") T_3 (FT_3) and is responsible for all of the physiological activity of T_3. Because FT_3 is not dependent on normal levels of

TBG, as is the case with total T_3, FT_3 levels are the most accurate indicators of thyrometabolic activity. FT_3 levels may be calculated by multiplying total T_3 levels by the T_3 uptake ratio.

Reference Values

	Conventional Units	**SI Units**
T_3 RIA		
Newborns	90–170 ng/dL	1.3–2.6 nmol/L
Adults	80–200 ng/dL	1.2–3.0 nmol/L
FT_3	0.2–0.6 ng/dL	0.003–0.009 nmol/L
Reverse triiodothyronine (rT_3)	38–44 ng/dL	0.58–0.67 nmol/L

Indications for Triiodothyronine (T_4) Test

➤ Support for diagnosing hyperthyroidism in clients with normal T_4 levels, with early hyperthyroidism and T_3 thyrotoxicosis indicated by elevated T_3 levels in the presence of normal T_4 levels

➤ Support for diagnosing "euthyroid sick" syndrome in severely ill clients with protein deficiency, as indicated by low T_3 levels, normal FT_3 levels, and elevated rT_3 levels[44]

Nursing Care Before the Procedure

Client preparation is essentially the same as that for any study involving collection of a peripheral blood sample (see Appendix I).

The Procedure

A venipuncture is performed and the sample collected in a red-topped tube. The sample should be handled gently to avoid hemolysis and transported promptly to the laboratory.

Nursing Care After the Procedure

Care and assessment after the procedure are the same as for any study involving the collection of a peripheral blood sample.

T_3 UPTAKE (RT_3 U)

The T_3 uptake (RT_3 U) test evaluates the quantity of TBG in the serum and the quantity of thyroxine (T_4) bound to it. In the T_3 uptake procedure, a known amount of resin containing radiolabeled T_3 is added to a sample of the client's serum. Normally, TBG in the serum is not fully saturated with thyroid hormones; the saturation level varies in relation to the amounts of TBG and thyroid hormones present. In the T_3 uptake test, the radiolabeled T_3 binds with available TBG sites. Results of the test are determined by measuring the percentage of labeled T_3 that remains bound to the resin after all available sites on TBG have been filled. It should be noted that the percentage of T_3 bound to the resin is inversely proportional to the percentage of TBG saturation in the serum.

Results of the T_3 uptake test are evaluated in relation to serum levels of total T_4 and T_3 and also are used in calculating FT_3 and FT_4 indices. For these calculations, the T_3 uptake ratio (RT_3 UR) is used, a ratio obtained by dividing the client's RT_3 U level by the RT_3 U level determined from a pool of normal serum.

Reference Values

	Conventional Units	**SI Units**
T_3 resin uptake	25–35%	0.25–0.35
T_3 uptake ratio	0.1–1.35	0.1–0.35

Interfering Factors

➤ Drugs that alter TBG levels or that compete for TBG-binding sites may affect test results.

➤ Estrogens may lead to increased TBG levels.

➤ Androgens and glucocorticoids may lead to decreased TBG levels.

➤ Salicylates and phenytoin anticonvulsants compete with T_4 for TBG-binding sites.

➤ Results may vary during pregnancy when TBG levels are usually elevated.

Indications for T_3 Uptake (RT$_3$ U) Test

➤ Signs of hypothyroidism or hyperthyroidism
  • Decreased levels (indicating a low percentage of radiolabeled T_3 remaining) indicate low serum T_4 levels and hypothyroidism.
  • Elevated levels (indicating a high percentage of radiolabeled T_3 remaining) indicate high serum T_4 levels and hyperthyroidism.

➤ Known or suspected problems associated with altered TBG levels (e.g., hereditary abnormality of TBG synthesis, drug therapy, pregnancy, and disorders associated with decreased serum proteins)
  • Elevated levels may indicate low TBG levels.
  • Decreased levels may indicate elevated TBG levels.

➤ Monitoring for response to therapy with drugs that compete with T_4 for TBG-binding sites
  • Elevated levels may indicate that TBG-binding sites are saturated with competing drugs.

➤ Calculation of free T_3 and T_4 indices (see p. 237)

Nursing Care Before the Procedure

Client preparation is essentially the same as that for any study involving the collection of a peripheral blood sample (see Appendix I).

➤ It is recommended that drugs that alter TBG levels or compete for TBG-binding sites be withheld for 12 to 24 hours before the test, although this practice should be confirmed with the person ordering the study.

The Procedure

A venipuncture is performed and the sample collected in a red-topped tube. The sample should be handled gently to avoid hemolysis and transported promptly to the laboratory.

Nursing Care After the Procedure

Care and assessment after the procedure are the same as for any study involving the collection of a peripheral blood sample.

➤ Resume any medications withheld before the test.

THYROXINE-BINDING GLOBULIN (TBG)

Thyroxine-binding globulin (TBG) may be measured directly by radioimmunoassay. Estrogens elevate serum TBG levels; thus, women who are pregnant, who are receiving estrogen therapy or oral contraceptives, or who have estrogen-secreting tumors have higher TBG levels.

Reference Values

Conventional Units	SI Units
16–32 µg/dL	120–180 mg/mL

Interfering Factors

➤ Estrogens elevate serum TBG levels and, thus, women who are pregnant, who are receiving estrogen therapy or oral contraceptives, or who have estrogen-secreting tumors have higher TBG levels.
➤ Androgens and corticosteriods decrease serum TBG levels.

Indications for Thyroxine-Binding Globulin (TBG) Test

➤ Signs and symptoms of hypothyroidism or hyperthyroidism in conditions associated with altered TBG levels (e.g., pregnancy), to differentiate true thyroid disorders from problems related to altered TBG levels
➤ Diagnosis of hereditary abnormality of globulin synthesis, indicated by decreased levels

Nursing Care Before the Procedure

Client preparation is essentially the same as that for any study involving the collection of a peripheral blood sample (see Appendix I).
➤ It is recommended that drugs that may alter TBG levels be withheld for 12 to 24 hours before the test, although this practice should be confirmed with the person ordering the study.

The Procedure

A venipuncture is performed and the sample collected in a red-topped tube. The sample should be handled gently to avoid hemolysis and transported promply to the laboratory.

Nursing Care After the Procedure

Care and assessment after the procedure are the same as for any study involving collection of a peripheral blood sample.
➤ Resume any medications withheld before the test.

THYROID-STIMULATING IMMUNOGLOBULINS (TSI, TSIg)

The globulin formerly known as long-acting thyroid stimulator (LATS) is one of the biologically unique autoantibodies with the effect of stimulating the target cell. Now called thyroid-stimulating immunoglobulins (TSI, TSIg), these antibodies react with the cell surface receptor that usually combines with TSH.

The TSI reacts with the receptors, activates intracellular enzymes, and promotes epithelial cell activity that operates outside the feedback regulation for TSH.

Reference Values

TSI is not normally detected in the serum, although it may be found in the serum of about 5 percent of people without apparent hyperthyroidism or exophthalmos.

Interfering Factors

➤ Administration of radioactive iodine preparations within 24 hours of the test may alter results.

Indications for Thyroid-Stimulating Immunoglobulins (TSI, TSIg) Test

➤ Known or suspected thyrotoxicosis with elevated levels found in 50 to 80 percent of affected individuals
➤ Determination of possible etiology of exophthalmos as indicated by elevated levels
➤ Monitoring of response to treatment for thyrotoxicosis with possible relapse indicated by elevated levels

Nursing Care Before the Procedure

Client preparation is essentially the same as that for any study involving the collection of a peripheral blood sample (see Appendix I).
➤ The client should not have received any radioactive iodine preparations within 24 hours of the test.

The Procedure

A venipuncture is performed and the sample collected in a red-topped tube. The sample should be handled gently to avoid hemolysis and transported promptly to the laboratory.

Nursing Care After the Procedure

Care and assessment after the procedure are the same as for any study involving the collection of a peripheral blood sample.

CALCITONIN

Calcitonin, also called thyrocalcitonin, is secreted by the parafollicular or C cells of the thyroid gland in response to elevated serum calcium levels. Its role is not completely understood, but the following functions are known: (1) It antagonizes the effects of parathormone and vitamin D, (2) it inhibits osteoclasts that reabsorb bone so that calcium continues to be laid down and not reabsorbed into the blood, and (3) it increases renal clearance of magnesium and inhibits tubular reabsorption of phosphates. The net result is that calcitonin decreases serum calcium levels.

Reference Values

	Conventional Units	**SI Units**
Men	<0.155 ng/mL	<0.155 μg/L
Women	<0.105 ng/mL	<0.105 μg/L

Interfering Factors

➤ Failure to fast from food for 8 hours before the test may alter results.

Indications for Calcitonin Test

➤ Support for diagnosing medullary carcinoma of the thyroid gland is indicated by elevated calcitonin levels, when serum calcium levels are normal. (Further verification may require raising the serum calcium level by IV infusion of calcium or pentagastrin and measuring the level to which plasma calcitonin rises in response; a rise of 0.105 to 0.11 ng/mL is to be expected.)

➤ Altered serum calcium levels of unknown etiology may be caused by a disorder associated with altered calcitonin levels.

➤ Elevated calcitonin levels are seen in cancers involving the breast, lung, and pancreas as a result of ectopic calcitonin production by tumor cells.

➤ Elevated calcitonin levels also are seen in primary hyperparathyroidism and in secondary hyperparathyroidism resulting from chronic renal failure.

Nursing Care Before the Procedure

Client preparation is essentially the same as that for any study involving the collection of a peripheral blood sample (see Appendix I).

➤ For this test, the client should fast from food for at least 8 hours before collection of the sample.

The Procedure

A venipuncture is performed and the sample collected in a green-topped tube. The sample should be handled gently to avoid hemolysis and transported promptly to the laboratory.

Nursing Care After the Procedure

Care and assessment after the procedure are the same as for any study involving collection of a peripheral blood sample.

➤ Resume foods withheld before the test.

➤ *Complications and precautions:* Note increased levels. Assess in relation to calcium and parathyroid hormone levels. Prepare the client for subsequent treatment decisions (medication protocol, surgery).

PARATHYROID HORMONE (PTH)

Parathyroid hormone (PTH, parathormone) is secreted by the parathyroid glands in response to decreased levels of circulating calcium. Actions of PTH include (1) mobilizing calcium from bone into the bloodstream, along with phosphates and protein matrix; (2) promoting renal tubular reabsorption of calcium and depression of phosphate reabsorption, thereby reducing calcium excretion and increasing phosphate excretion by the kidneys; (3) decreasing renal secretion of hydrogen ions, which leads to increased renal excretion of bicarbonate and chloride; and (4) enhancing renal production of active vitamin D metabolites, causing increased calcium absorption in the small intestine. The net result of PTH action is maintenance of adequate serum calcium levels.

Reference Values

Conventional Units	SI Units
2.3 – 2.8 pmol/L	
23 – 28 μg/mL	

PTH is measured by radioimmunoassay. As the antibody used for the assay directly affects the results, values vary according to the laboratory performing the test.

Interfering Factors

➤ Failure to fast from food for 8 hours before the test may alter results.

Indications for Parathyroid Hormone (PTH) Test

➤ Suspected hyperparathyroidism
  • Elevated levels occur in primary hyperparathyroidism as a result of hyperplasia or tumor of the parathyroid glands.
  • Elevated levels also may occur in secondary hyperparathyroidism (usually as a result of chronic renal failure, malignant tumors that produce ectopic PTH, and malabsorption syndromes).
➤ Suspected surgical removal of the parathyroid glands or incidental damage to them during thyroid or neck surgery, as indicated by decreased levels
➤ Evaluation of parathyroid response to altered serum calcium levels, with elevated serum calcium levels, especially those resulting from malignant processes, leading to decreased PTH production
➤ Evaluation of parathyroid response to other disorders that may lead to decreased PTH production (e.g., hypomagnesemia, autoimmune destruction of the parathyroid glands)[45]

Nursing Care Before the Procedure

Client preparation is essentially the same as that for any study involving collection of a peripheral blood sample (see Appendix I).
➤ For this test, the client should fast from food for at least 8 hours before collection of the sample.

The Procedure

A venipuncture is performed and the sample collected in a red-topped tube. A sample for serum calcium also may be obtained. The sample(s) should be handled gently to avoid hemolysis and transported promptly to the laboratory.

Nursing Care After the Procedure

Care and assessment after the procedure are the same as for any study involving the collection of a peripheral blood sample.
➤ Resume foods withheld before the test.
➤ *Increased levels:* Note and report increased levels in relation to calcium and phosphate levels. Assess for signs and symptoms of hypercalcemia (greater than 10.5 mg/dL) leading to renal calculi formation, susceptibility to fractures, sluggishness, lethargy, anorexia, and constipation. Instruct in dietary restriction of calcium, medication regimen (corticosteroids, antineoplastics, phos-

phates), or signs and symptoms of hypophosphatemia (less than 3 mg/dL) such as irritability, confusion, and functional deficits. Instruct in dietary intake of foods rich in phosphorus and medication replacement regimen.

➤ *Decreased levels:* Note and report decreased levels in relation to calcium levels. Assess for signs and symptoms of hypocalcemia (less than 8.5 mg/dL), such as muscle cramping and spasms of hands and feet. In mild cases, instruct in dietary intake of calcium and vitamin D supplements; in severe states, prepare for IV administration of calcium.

Adrenal Hormones

Adrenal hormones are secreted by two functionally and embryologically distinct portions of the adrenal gland. The adrenal cortex, which is of mesodermal origin, secretes three types of steroids: (1) glucocorticoids, which affect carbohydrate metabolism; (2) mineralocorticoids, which promote potassium excretion and sodium retention by the kidneys; and (3) adrenal androgens, which the liver converts to testosterone. Cortisol is the predominant glucocorticoid, whereas aldosterone is the predominant mineralocorticoid. Production and secretion of cortisol and adrenal androgens are stimulated by ACTH. Although ACTH also may enhance aldosterone production, the usual stimulants are either increased serum potassium or decreased serum sodium.

The adrenal medulla, which constitutes only about one-tenth of the volume of the adrenal glands, derives from the ectoderm and physiologically belongs to the sympathetic nervous system. The hormones secreted by the adrenal medulla are epinephrine and norepinephrine, which are collectively known as the catecholamines. Epinephrine is secreted in response to sympathetic stimulation, hypoglycemia, or hypotension. Most norepinephrine is manufactured by and secreted from sympathetic nerve endings; only a small amount is normally secreted by the adrenal medulla.[46]

CORTISOL

Cortisol (hydrocortisone), the predominant glucocorticoid, is secreted in response to stimulation by adrenocorticotropic hormone (ACTH). Ninety percent of cortisol is bound to cortisol-binding globulin (CBG) and albumin; the free portion is responsible for its physiological effects. Cortisol stimulates gluconeogenesis, mobilizes fats and proteins, antagonizes insulin, and suppresses inflammation. Cortisol secretion varies diurnally, with the highest levels seen upon awakening and the lowest levels occurring late in the day. Bursts of cortisol excretion also may occur at night.

Elevated cortisol levels occur in Cushing's syndrome, in which there is excessive production of adrenocorticosteroids. Cushing's syndrome may be caused by pituitary adenoma, adrenal hyperplasia, benign or malignant adrenal tumors, and nonendocrine malignant tumors that secrete ectopic ACTH. Therapy with adrenocorticosteroids also may produce cushingoid signs and symptoms. Elevated cortisol levels are additionally associated with stress, hyperthyroidism, obesity, and diabetic ketoacidosis.

Decreased cortisol levels occur with Addison's disease, in which there is deficient production of adrenocorticosteroids. Addison's disease is usually caused by idiopathic adrenal hypofunction, although it may also be seen in pituitary hypofunction, hypothyroidism, tuberculosis, metastatic cancer involving the adrenal glands, amyloidosis, and hemochromatosis. Addison's disease may occur after withdrawal of corticosteroid therapy because of drug-induced atrophy of the adrenal glands.

CORTISOL/ACTH CHALLENGE TESTS

A variety of tests that stimulate or suppress cortisol/ACTH levels may be used further to evaluate individuals with signs and symptoms of adrenal hypofunction or hyperfunction or abnormal cortisol levels.

Dexamethasone is a potent glucocorticoid that suppresses ACTH and cortisol production. In the rapid dexamethasone test, 1 mg of oral dexamethasone is given at midnight; cortisol levels are then measured at 8 AM. Normally, plasma cortisol should be no more than 5 to 10 µg/dL after dexamethasone administration. A 5-hour urine collection test for 17-hydroxycorticoids (17-OHCS), metabolites of glucocorticoids, also may be collected as part of the test. Elevated plasma cortisol levels in response to dexamethasone administration are associated with Cushing's syndrome.

Metyrapone is a drug that inhibits certain enzymes required to convert precursor substances into cortisol. When the drug is administered, plasma cortisol levels decrease and ACTH levels subsequently increase in response. The test involves mainly measurement of urinary excretion of 17-OHCS, which should rise if the adenohypophysis is normally responsive to decreased cortisol levels. Plasma cortisol levels are measured to ensure that sufficient suppression has been induced by the metyrapone such that test results will be valid.

Insulin-induced hypoglycemia (serum glucose of 50 mg/dL or less) also stimulates ACTH production. Adenohypophyseal response to hypoglycemia is usually measured indirectly by plasma cortisol levels because the test is more universally available. A normal response is an increase of 6 µg/dL or more over baseline cortisol levels. Lack of response to hypoglycemic stimulation indicates either pituitary or adrenal hypofunction. They can be differentiated either by directly measuring plasma ACTH levels or by administering ACTH preparations and observing cortisol response.

Purified exogenous ACTH or synthetic ACTH preparations (e.g., cosyntropin) may be used diagnostically to stimulate cortisol secretion. The usual response is an increase in plasma cortisol levels of 7 to 18 µg/dL over baseline levels within 1 hour of ACTH administration. Lack of response indicates adrenal insufficiency.[47]

Reference Values

| | 8 AM | | 4 PM | |
	Conventional Units	SI Units	Conventional Units	SI Units
Children	15–25 µg /dL	410–690 nmol/L	5–10 µg/dL	140–280 nmol/L
Adults	9–24 µg /dL	250–690 nmol/L	3–12 µg/dL	80–330 nmol/L

Interfering Factors

➤ The time of day when the test is performed may alter results because cortisol levels vary diurnally, with highest levels being seen on awakening and lowest levels occurring late in the day.

➤ Stress and excessive physical activity may produce elevated levels.

➤ Pregnancy, therapy with estrogen-containing drugs, lithium carbonate, methadone, and ethyl alcohol may lead to elevated cortisol levels.

➤ Therapy with levodopa, barbiturates, phenytoin (Dilantin), and androgens may produce decreased levels.

➤ Failure to follow dietary restrictions, if ordered, may alter test results.

Indications for Cortisol Assay

➤ Suspected adrenal hyperfunction (Cushing's syndrome) from a variety of causes (see p. 247), as indicated by elevated levels that do not vary diurnally

➤ Evaluation of effects of disorders associated with elevated cortisol levels (e.g., hyperthyroidism, obesity, and diabetic ketoacidosis)

➤ Suspected adrenal hypofunction (Addison's disease) from a variety of causes (see p. 247), as indicated by decreased levels

➤ Monitoring for response to therapy with adrenocorticosteroids

• Elevated levels are seen in clients receiving adrenocorticosteroid therapy.

• Decreased levels may occur for months after therapy is discontinued, resulting from drug-induced atrophy of the adrenal glands.

Nursing Care Before the Procedure

General client preparation is the same as that for any study involving collection of a peripheral blood sample (see Appendix I).

➤ Some laboratories require an 8-hour fast and activity restriction before the test. Medications that may alter cortisol levels should be withheld for 12 to 24 hours before the study, although this practice should be confirmed with the person ordering the test.

➤ The client should be informed that it may be necessary to obtain more than one sample and that samples must be obtained at specific times to detect peak and trough levels of cortisol.

The Procedure

At approximately 8 AM, a venipuncture is performed and the sample is collected in a green-topped tube. The sample should be handled gently to avoid hemolysis and sent promptly to the laboratory. If cortisol hypersecretion is suspected, then a second sample may be obtained at approximately 4 PM to determine whether diurnal variation in cortisol levels is occurring.

Nursing Care After the Procedure

Care and assessment after the procedure are the same as for any study involving the collection of a peripheral blood sample.

➤ Resume food and any medications withheld before the test, as well as usual activities.

➤ *Increased levels:* Note and report increased levels in relation to urinary cortisol, serum glucose, and calcium. Assess potential for infection, fluid volume excess (weight gain, edema, increased blood pressure), hyperglycemia (thirst, polyuria, polydipsia), mood changes (euphoria, psychosis), poor body image (moon face, buffalo hump on the back, acne, hair growth in undesirable areas in women, obese trunk, and thin extremities), and bone or joint pain. Monitor I&O. Provide support for psychophysiological changes. Help client to develop coping skills. Instruct client to increase dietary protein; decrease sodium, calories, and carbohydrates; and avoid infections.

➤ *Decreased levels:* Note and report decreased levels in relation to electrolyte panel (hyponatremia, hyperkalemia) and serum glucose for hypoglycemia. Assess for fluid volume deficit, long-term administration of corticosteroid therapy, and changes in body image (pigmentation of the skin, masculinization in women). Monitor I&O. Administer ordered corticosteroid regimen. Provide support for physical changes affecting body image. Advise client to avoid situations that cause stress or anxiety. Instruct client in long-term supplemental or replacement cortisone regimen.

ALDOSTERONE

Aldosterone, the predominant mineralocorticoid, is secreted by the zona glomerulosa of the adrenal cortex in response to decreased serum sodium, decreased blood volume, and increased serum potassium. It is thought that altered serum sodium and potassium levels directly stimulate the adrenal cortex to release aldosterone. In addition, decreased blood volume and altered sodium and potassium levels stimulate the juxtaglomerular apparatus of the kidney to secrete renin. Renin is subsequently converted to angiotensin II, which then stimulates the adrenal cortex to secrete aldosterone. In normal states, ACTH does not play a major role in aldosterone secretion. In disease or stress states, however, ACTH may also enhance aldosterone secretion.

Aldosterone increases sodium reabsorption in the renal tubules, gastrointestinal tract, salivary glands, and sweat glands. This subsequently results in increased water retention, blood volume, and blood pressure. Aldosterone also increases potassium excretion by the kidneys in exchange for the sodium ions that are retained.

ALDOSTERONE CHALLENGE TESTS

In normal individuals, increased serum sodium levels and blood volume suppress aldosterone secretion. In primary aldosteronism, however, this response is not seen. Serum sodium levels may be elevated through ingestion of a high-sodium diet for approximately 4 days or by infusing 2 L of normal saline intravenously. If there is appropriate control of aldosterone levels through negative feedback systems and the renin-angiotensin system, plasma aldosterone levels will be low normal or decreased in response to the increased sodium load. Fludrocortisone acetate (Florinef), a synthetic mineralocorticoid, produces the same effect after 3 days of administration. Aldosterone challenges are used to differentiate between primary and secondary hyperaldosteronism.[48]

Reference Values

	Conventional Units	**SI Units**
Supine	3–9 ng/dL	0.08–0.30 nmol/L
Standing	5–30 ng/dL	0.14–0.80 nmol/L

Interfering Factors

➤ Upright body posture (see "Nursing Care Before the Procedure"), stress, and late pregnancy may lead to increased levels.

➤ Therapy with diuretics, hydralazine (Apresoline), diazoxide (Hyperstat), and nitroprusside may lead to elevated levels.

➤ Excessive licorice ingestion may produce decreased levels, as may therapy with propranolol and fludrocortisone (Florinef).

➤ Altered serum electrolyte levels affect aldosterone secretion.

➤ Decreased serum sodium and elevated serum potassium increase aldosterone secretion.

➤ Elevated serum sodium and decreased serum potassium suppress aldosterone secretion.

Indications for Plasma Aldosterone Test

➤ Suspected hyperaldosteronism as indicated by elevated levels
  - Primary aldosteronism (e.g., resulting from benign adenomas or bilateral hyperplasia of the aldosterone-secreting zona glomerulosa cells) is indicated by elevated aldosterone and low plasma renin levels (see p. 250).
  - Secondary hyperaldosteronism (e.g., resulting from changes in blood volume and serum electrolytes, CHF, cirrhosis, nephrotic syndrome, chronic obstructive pulmonary disease [COPD], and renal artery stenosis) is indicated by elevated aldosterone and plasma renin levels.

➤ Suspected hypoaldosteronism (e.g., as seen in diabetes mellitus and toxemia of pregnancy) as indicated by decreased levels

➤ Evaluation of hypertension of unknown etiology

Nursing Care Before the Procedure

General client preparation is the same as that for any study involving the collection of a peripheral blood sample (see Appendix I).

➤ The client should not have ingested licorice for 2 weeks before the test. Medications that alter plasma aldosterone levels also may be withheld for up to 2 weeks before the test, although this practice should be confirmed with the person ordering the study.

➤ If hospitalized, the client should be told not to get out of bed in the morning until the sample has been obtained and that it may be necessary to obtain a second sample after he or she has been up for about 2 to 4 hours.

➤ Nonhospitalized individuals should be instructed on when to report to the laboratory in relation to the length of time to be upright before the test.

The Procedure

A venipuncture is performed and the sample is collected in a red-, green-, or lavender-topped tube, depending on laboratory procedures. The client's position and length of time the position was held should be noted on the laboratory request form. The sample(s) should be handled gently to avoid hemolysis and sent to the laboratory immediately. A sample for plasma renin also may be obtained in conjunction with the test.

Nursing Care After the Procedure

Care and assessment after the procedure are the same as for any study involving the collection of a peripheral blood sample.

➤ Resume any medications withheld before the test.

➤ *Increased levels:* Note and report increased levels related to urinary aldosterone levels. Assess for fluid volume excess caused by sodium and fluid retention, and administer ordered diuretics.

➤ *Decreased levels:* Note and report decreased levels related to sodium levels. Assess for fluid volume deficit. Instruct in sodium and corticosteroid replacement regimen.

CATECHOLAMINES

The adrenal medulla, a component of the sympathetic nervous system, secretes epinephrine and norepinephrine, which are collectively known as the catecholamines. A third catecholamine, dopamine, is secreted in the brain, where it functions as a neurotransmitter.

Epinephrine (adrenalin) is secreted in response to generalized sympathetic stimulation, hypoglycemia, or arterial hypotension. It increases the metabolic rate of all cells, heart rate, arterial blood pressure, and levels of blood glucose and free fatty acids, and it decreases peripheral resistance and blood flow to the skin and kidneys.

Norepinephrine is secreted by sympathetic nerve endings, as well as by the adrenal medulla, in response to sympathetic stimulation and the presence of tyramine. It decreases the heart rate, while increasing peripheral vascular resistance and arterial blood pressure. Normally, norepinephrine is the predominant catecholamine.

The only clinically significant disorder involving the adrenal medulla is the catecholamine-secreting tumor, pheochromocytoma. Catecholamine-producing tumors also may originate along sympathetic paraganglia; these tumors are known as functional paragangliomas. Pheochromocytomas may release catecholamines, primarily epinephrine, continuously or intermittently. Because the most common sign of pheochromocytoma is arterial hypertension, measurement of plasma catecholamines (or the urinary metabolites thereof) is indicated in evaluating new-onset hypertension.[49]

Reference Values

	Conventional Units	SI Units
Epinephrine and norepinephrine	100–500 ng/L	
Epinephrine		
Supine	0–110 pg/mL	0–600 pmol/L
Standing	0–140 pg/mL	0–764 pmol/L
Norepinephrine		
Supine	70–750 pg/mL	413–4432 pmol/L
Standing	200–1700 pg/mL	1,182–10,047 pmol/L

Results are usually evaluated in relation to urinary measurements of catecholamine metabolites. Several measurements of plasma levels may also be indicated.

Interfering Factors

➤ Catecholamine levels vary diurnally and with postural changes.
➤ Shock, stress, hyperthyroidism, strenuous exercise, and smoking may produce elevated plasma catecholamines.
➤ Dopamine, norepinephrine (Levophed), sympathomimetic drugs, tricyclic antidepressants, α-methyldopa, hydralazine, quinidine, and isoproterenol (Isuprel) may produce elevated levels.
➤ A diet high in amines (e.g., bananas, nuts, cereal grains, tea, coffee, cocoa, aged cheese, beer, ale, certain wines, avocados, and fava beans) may produce elevated plasma catecholamine levels, although this effect is more likely to be seen in relation to certain urinary metabolites.

Indications for Plasma Catecholamines Test

➤ Hypertension of unknown etiology or suspected pheochromocytoma or paragangliomas or both
➤ Identification of pheochromocytoma as the cause of hypertension as indicated by elevated combined catecholamine and epinephrine levels
➤ Support for diagnosing paragangliomas as indicated by elevated combined catecholamine and norepinephrine levels

Nursing Care Before the Procedure

General client preparation is the same as that for any study involving the collection of a peripheral blood sample (see Appendix I).
➤ For this test, the client should fast for 12 hours and abstain from smoking for 24 hours before the test. Vigorous exercise should be avoided, with provision made for rest in a recumbent position for at least 1 hour before the study.
➤ Medications that may alter test results, especially over-the-counter cold preparations containing sympathomimetics, may be withheld for up to 2 weeks before the test, although this practice should be confirmed with the person ordering the study.
➤ The need for dietary restriction of amine-rich foods for 48 hours before the test should be confirmed with the laboratory performing the test or the person ordering it.

➤ If samples are to be obtained via an intermittent venous access device (e.g., heparin lock), the client should be informed of its purpose and that it may be inserted as long as 24 hours before the test.

The Procedure

If more than one sample is to be obtained, a heparin lock should be inserted 12 to 24 hours before the test; the stress of repeated venipunctures could falsely elevate levels.

➤ For hospitalized individuals, a sample of venous blood should be collected in a chilled lavender-topped tube between 6 and 8 AM. For nonhospitalized clients, the first sample should be obtained after approximately 1 hour of rest in a recumbent position. The sample is handled gently to avoid hemolysis, packed in ice, and sent to the laboratory immediately.

➤ The client should then be helped to stand for 10 minutes, after which a second sample is obtained. The time(s) of collection and the position of the client should be noted on the laboratory request form.

Nursing Care After the Procedure

If an intermittent venous access device was inserted, remove after completion of the test and apply a pressure bandage to the site.

➤ Resume foods and any medications withheld before the test, as well as usual activities.

➤ *Abnormal levels:* Note increased levels in relation to 24-hour urinary vanillylmandelic acid (VMA) and metanephrine levels. Assess for pulse and blood pressure increases, hyperglycemia, shakiness, and palpitations associated with increased values.

Gonadal Hormones

The gonadal hormones, secreted primarily by the ovaries and testes, include estrogens, progesterone, and testosterone. These hormones are essential for normal sexual development and reproductive function in men and women. All gonadal hormones are steroids, and their molecular structures and those of the adrenocorticosteroids are quite similar. Moreover, small amounts of the gonadal hormones or precursors thereof are secreted by the adrenal glands in both men and women.

Secretion of gonadal hormones is regulated via the hypothalamic-hypophyseal system. When blood levels of gonadal hormones decline, the hypothalamus is stimulated to release gonadotropin-releasing hormone (GnRH), which then stimulates the adenohypophysis to release its gonadotropic hormones. These tropic hormones are called, in both men and women, follicle-stimulating hormone (FSH) and luteinizing hormone (LH), even though the ovarian follicle and corpus luteum are unique to women.

ESTROGENS

Estrogens are secreted in large amounts by the ovaries and, during pregnancy, by the placenta. Minute amounts are secreted by the adrenal glands and, possibly, by the testes. Estrogens induce and maintain the female secondary sex characteristics, promote growth and maturation of the female reproductive organs, influence the pattern of fat deposition that characterizes the female form, and cause early epiphyseal closure. They also promote retention of sodium and water by the kidneys and sensitize the myometrium to oxytocin.

Elevated estrogen levels are associated with ovarian and adrenal tumors as well as estrogen-producing tumors of the testes. Decreased levels are associated with primary and secondary ovarian failure, Turner's syndrome, hypopituitarism, adrenogenital syndrome, Stein-Leventhal syndrome, anorexia nervosa, and menopause. Estrogen levels vary in relation to the menstrual cycle.

Many different types of estrogens have been identified, but only three are present in the blood in measurable amounts: estrone, estradiol, and estriol. Estrone (E_1) is the immediate precursor of estradiol (E_2), which is the most biologically potent of the three. In addition to ovarian sources, estriol (E_3) is secreted in large amounts by the placenta during pregnancy from precursors produced by the fetal liver. Through radioimmunoassay, plasma levels of E_2 and E_3 may be determined. Total plasma estrogen levels are difficult to measure and are not routinely performed.

Reference Values

	Conventional Units	SI Units
Estradiol (E_2)		
Children under 6 yr	3–10 pg/mL	10–36 pmol/L
Adults		
Men	12–34 pg/mL	40–125 pmol/L
Women (menstruating)		
Early cycle	24–68 pg/mL	90–250 pmol/L
Midcycle	50–186 pg/mL	200–700 pmol/L
Late cycle	73–149 pg/mL	250–550 pmol/L
Estriol (E_3)		
Weeks of pregnancy		
30–32	2–12 ng/mL	7–40 nmol/L
33–35	3–19 ng/mL	10–65 nmol/L
36–38	5–27 ng/mL	15–95 nmol/L
39–40	10–30 ng/mL	35–105 nmol/L

Interfering Factors

➤ In menstruating women, estrogen levels vary in relation to the menstrual cycle.

➤ Therapy with estrogen-containing drugs and adrenocorticosteroids will elevate levels, whereas clomiphene will decrease them.

Indications for Estrogens Test

➤ Infertility or amenorrhea of unknown etiology, with primary or secondary ovarian failure indicated by low estradiol (E_2) levels

➤ Establishment of the time of ovulation

➤ Evaluation of response to therapy for infertility

➤ Suspected precocious puberty with the disorder indicated by elevated estradiol (E_2) levels

➤ Suspected estrogen-producing tumors, as indicated by consistently high estradiol (E_2) levels without normal cyclic variations

➤ High-risk pregnancy with suspicion of fetal growth retardation, placental dysfunction, or impending fetal jeopardy, as indicated by decreased estriol (E_3) levels relative to the stage of pregnancy

Nursing Care Before the Procedure

Client preparation is the same as that for any study involving collection of a peripheral blood sample (see Appendix I).

➤ It is recommended that drugs known to alter estrogen levels be withheld for 12 to 24 hours before the test, although this practice should be confirmed with the person ordering the study.

➤ In menstruating women, the phase of the menstrual cycle should be ascertained, if possible. If the test is being conducted to detect ovulation, the client should be informed that it may be necessary to obtain a series of samples over a period of several days to detect the normal variation in estrogen levels.

The Procedure

A venipuncture is performed and the sample is collected in a red-topped tube. The sample should be handled gently to avoid hemolysis and transported promptly to the laboratory.

Nursing Care After the Procedure

Care and assessment after the procedure are the same as for any study involving the collection of a peripheral blood sample.

➤ Resume any medications withheld before the test.

➤ *Complications and precautions:* Assess increased or decreased levels in relation to age, gender, pregnancy, and menopausal status and in relation to associated levels of 24-hour urinary analysis and serum estradiol and estriol levels.

PROGESTERONE

Progesterone is secreted in nonpregnant women during the latter half of the menstrual cycle by the corpus luteum and in large amounts by the placenta during pregnancy. It also is secreted in minute amounts by the adrenal cortex in both men and women. Progesterone prepares the endometrium for implantation of the fertilized ovum, decreases myometrial excitability, stimulates proliferation of the vaginal epithelium, and stimulates growth of the breasts during pregnancy. Although progesterone may promote sodium and water retention, its effect is weaker than that of aldosterone, which it directly antagonizes. The net effect is loss of sodium and water from the body.

Reference Values

	Conventional Units	SI Units
Men	<100 ng/dL	<3 nmol/L
Women (menstruating)		
Follicular phase	<150 ng/dL	<5 nmol/L
Luteal phase	300–1200 ng/dL	10–40 nmol/L
Women (pregnant)		
First trimester	1500–5000 ng/dL	50–160 nmol/L
Second and third trimesters	8,000–20,000 ng/dL	250–650 nmol/L
Women (menopausal)	10–22 ng/dL	<2 nmol/L

Interfering Factors

➤ In menstruating women, progesterone levels vary in relation to the menstrual cycle.

➤ Therapy with estrogen, progesterone, or adrenocorticosteroids may produce elevated levels.

Indications for Plasma Progesterone Test

➤ Infertility of unknown etiology with failure to ovulate, indicated by low levels throughout the menstrual cycle

➤ Evaluation of response to therapy for infertility

➤ Support for diagnosing disorders associated with elevated progesterone levels (e.g., precocious puberty, ovarian tumors or cysts, and adrenocortical hyperplasia and tumors)

➤ High-risk pregnancy with suspicion of placental dysfunction, fetal abnormality, impending fetal jeopardy, threatened abortion, or toxemia of pregnancy, as indicated by lower than expected levels for the stage of pregnancy

➤ Support for diagnosing disorders associated with decreased progesterone levels (e.g., panhypopituitarism, Turner's syndrome, adrenogenital syndrome, and Stein-Leventhal syndrome)

Nursing Care Before the Procedure

Client preparation is the same as that for any study involving the collection of a peripheral blood sample (see Appendix I).

➤ It is recommended that any drugs that may alter progesterone levels be withheld for 12 to 24 hours before the test, although this practice should be confirmed with the person ordering the study.

➤ In menstruating women, the phase of the menstrual cycle should be ascertained, if possible. If the test is being performed to detect ovulation, the client should be informed that it may be necessary to obtain a series of samples over a period of several days to detect the normal variation in progesterone levels.

The Procedure

A venipuncture is performed and the sample collected in a green-topped tube. The sample should be handled gently to avoid hemolysis and transported promptly to the laboratory.

Nursing Care After the Procedure

Care and assessment after the procedure are the same as for any study involving the collection of a peripheral blood sample.

➤ Resume any medications withheld before the test.

➤ *Complications and precautions:* Assess increased or decreased levels in relation to age, menstrual or pregnancy status, and 24-hour urinary pregnanediol level.

TESTOSTERONE

Testosterone is produced in men by the Leydig cells of the testes. Minute amounts also are secreted by the adrenal glands in men and women and by the ovaries in women. In the male fetus, testosterone is secreted by the genital ridges and fetal testes.

Testosterone is produced in response to stimulation by luteinizing hormone (LH), which is secreted by the adenohypophysis in response to stimulation by gonadotropin-releasing hormone (GnRH). Testosterone promotes development of the male sex organs and testicular descent in the fetus, induces and maintains secondary sexual characteristics in men, promotes protein anabolism and bone growth, and enhances sodium and water retention to some degree.

Reference Values

	Conventional Units	**SI Units**
Children	0.12–0.16 ng/mL	0.41–0.55 nmol/L
Men		
<60 yr	3.9–7.9 ng/mL	13.59–27.41 nmol/L
>60 yr	1.5–3.1 ng/dL	5.20–10.75 nmol/L
Women		
Menstruating	0.25–0.67 ng/mL	0.87–2.32 nmol/L
Menopausal	0.21–0.37 ng/mL	0.72–1.28 nmol/L

Interfering Factors

➤ Testosterone levels vary diurnally, with highest levels occurring in the early morning.

➤ Administration of testosterone, thyroid and growth hormones, clomiphene, and barbiturates may lead to elevated levels.

➤ Therapy with estrogens and spironolactone (Aldactone) may produce decreased levels.

Indications for Testosterone Test

➤ In men, support for diagnosing precocious puberty, testicular tumors, and benign prostatic hypertrophy, as indicated by elevated levels

➤ In women, support for diagnosing adrenogenital syndrome, adrenal tumors or hyperplasia, Stein-Leventhal syndrome, ovarian tumors or hyperplasia, and luteomas of pregnancy, as indicated by elevated levels

➤ In men and women, support for diagnosing nonendocrine tumors that produce ACTH ectopically, as indicated by elevated levels without diurnal variation

➤ In men, support for diagnosing infertility, with testicular failure indicated by decreased levels

➤ Support for diagnosing other disorders associated with decreased testosterone levels (e.g., hypopituitarism, Klinefelter's syndrome, cryptorchidism [failure of testicular descent], and cirrhosis)

Nursing Care Before the Procedure

Client preparation is the same as that for any study involving the collection of a peripheral blood sample (see Appendix I).

➤ It is recommended that drugs that may alter testosterone levels be withheld for 12 to 24 hours before the test, although this practice should be confirmed with the person ordering the study.

The Procedure

A venipuncture is performed and the sample collected in either a red- or a green-topped tube, depending on the laboratory performing the test. The sample should be handled gently to avoid hemolysis and transported promptly to the laboratory.

Nursing Care After the Procedure

Care and assessment after the procedure are the same as for any study involving the collection of a peripheral blood sample.

➤ Resume any medications withheld before the test.

➤ *Complications and precautions:* Assess increased or decreased levels in relation to age, gender, menstrual or menopausal status, as well as possible sexual dysfunction and medicolegal aspects of the abuse of anabolic steroids related to athletic ability.

Placental Hormones

During pregnancy, the placenta secretes estrogens, progesterone, human chorionic gonadotropin (hCG), and human placental lactogen (hPL). Estrogens and progesterone, which are not specific to pregnancy, are discussed in the preceding sections. In contrast, hCG and hPL are fairly specific to pregnancy, but levels may also be altered in individuals with trophoblastic tumors (e.g., hydatidiform mole, choriocarcinoma) and tumors that ectopically secrete placental hormones.

HUMAN CHORIONIC GONADOTROPIN (HCG)

Human chorionic gonadotropin (hCG) is a glycoprotein that is unique to the developing placenta. Its presence in blood and urine has been used for decades to detect pregnancy. Tests using rabbits, frogs, and rats, however, have now been replaced by immunologic tests that use antibodies to hCG. Earlier immunologic tests were not always reliable, because the antibody used could cross-react with other glycoprotein hormones such as luteinizing hormone (LH). Furthermore, it was sometimes not possible to obtain reliable results until 4 to 8 weeks after the first missed period. Currently, more sensitive and specific tests use antibody that reacts only with the beta subunit of hCG, not with other hormones. The most sensitive of the radioimmunoassays for hCG can detect elevated levels within 8 to 10 days after conception, even before the first missed period.

Because hCG is associated with the developing placenta, it is secreted at increasingly higher levels during the first 2 months of pregnancy, declines during the third and fourth months, and then remains relatively stable until term. Levels return to normal within 1 to 2 weeks of termination of pregnancy. Human chorionic gonadotropin prevents the normal involution of the corpus luteum at the end of the menstrual cycle and stimulates it to double in size and produce large quantities of estrogen and progesterone. It is also thought to stimulate the testes of the male fetus to produce testosterone and to induce descent of the testicles into the scrotum.

Reference Values

	Conventional Units	SI Units
Nonpregnant	<3 mIU/mL	<3 IU/L
Pregnant		
8–10 days	5–40 mIU/mL	5–40 IU/L
1 mo	100 mIU/mL	100 IU/L
2 mo	100,000 mIU/mL	100,000 IU/L
4 mo–term	50,000 mIU/mL	50,000 IU/L

Indications for Human Chorionic Gonadotropin (hCG) Test

➤ Early detection of pregnancy (i.e., within 8 to 10 days of conception), especially in women with a history of infertility or habitual abortion
➤ Prediction of outcome in threatened abortion (levels below 10,000 mIU/mL are highly predictive that abortion will occur)
➤ Suspected intrauterine fetal demise or incomplete abortion as indicated by decreased levels[50]
➤ Suspected hydatidiform mole or choriocarcinoma as indicated by elevated levels
➤ Suspected testicular tumor as indicated by elevated levels
➤ Support for diagnosing nonendocrine tumors that produce hCG ectopically (e.g., carcinoma of the stomach, liver, pancreas, and breast; multiple myeloma; and malignant melanoma), as indicated by elevated levels
➤ Monitoring for the effectiveness of treatment for malignancies associated with ectopic hCG production, as indicated by decreasing levels

Nursing Care Before the Procedure

Client preparation is the same as that for any study involving the collection of a peripheral blood sample (see Appendix I).

The Procedure

A venipuncture is performed and the sample collected in a red-topped tube. The sample should be handled gently to avoid hemolysis and sent promptly to the laboratory.

Nursing Care After the Procedure

Care and assessment after the procedure are the same as for any study involving the collection of a peripheral blood sample.

➤ *Complications and precautions:* Relate age, gender, and time of gestation to the test results.

HUMAN PLACENTAL LACTOGEN (hPL)

Human placental lactogen (hPL), also known as human chorionic somatotropin (hCS), is produced by the placenta but exerts its known effect on the mother. Human placental lactogen causes decreased maternal sensitivity to insulin and causes utilization of glucose, thus increasing the glucose available to the fetus. It also promotes release of maternal free fatty acids for utilization by the fetus. It is also thought that hPL stimulates the action of growth hormone in protein deposition, promotes breast growth and preparation for lactation, and maintains the pregnancy by altering the endometrium.

Human placental lactogen rises steadily through pregnancy, maintaining a high plateau during the last trimester. Blood levels of hPL correlate with placental weight and tend to be high in diabetic mothers. Levels also may be elevated in multiple pregnancy and Rh isoimmunization, as well as in nonendocrine tumors that secrete ectopic hPL.

During pregnancy, hPL levels vary greatly with the individual as well as on a day-to-day basis. Thus, serial determinations may be necessary with the client serving as her own control.[51]

Reference Values

	Conventional Units	SI Units
Men	<0.5 μg/mL	Not detected
Women		
Nonpregnant	<0.5 μg/mL	Not detected
Pregnant		
5–27 weeks	<4.6 μg/mL	<4.6 mg/L
28–31 weeks	2.4–6.1 μg/mL	2.4–6.1 mg/L
32–35 weeks	3.7–7.7 μg/mL	3.7–7.7 mg/L
36 weeks–term	5.0–8.6 μg/mL	5.0–8.6 mg/L
Diabetic at term	10–12 μg/mL	10.0–12.0 mg/L

Interfering Factors

➤ During pregnancy, hPL levels vary greatly with the individual as well as on a day-to-day basis.

➤ Levels tend to be higher in diabetic mothers, multiple gestation, and Rh isoimmunization.

Indications for Human Placental Lactogen (hPL) Test

➤ Detection of placental insufficiency as evidenced by low hPL levels in relation to gestational age

➤ Support for diagnosing intrauterine growth retardation caused by placental insufficiency, as indicated by hPL levels of less than 4 μg/mL, especially when blood estrogen levels are low

➤ Prediction of outcome in threatened abortion as indicated by lower than expected levels for the stage of pregnancy

➤ Support for diagnosing hydatidiform mole and choriocarcinoma as indicated by decreased levels

➤ Support for diagnosing malignancies associated with elevated levels (e.g., nonendocrine tumors that secrete ectopic hPL)

➤ Monitoring for the effectiveness of treatment for malignancies associated with ectopic hPL production as indicated by decreasing levels

Nursing Care Before the Procedure

Client preparation is the same as that for any study involving the collection of a peripheral blood sample (see Appendix I).

➤ The pregnant client should be informed that several determinations may be necessary throughout the pregnancy.

The Procedure

A venipuncture is performed and the sample is collected in a red-topped tube. The sample should be handled gently to avoid hemolysis and sent promptly to the laboratory.

Nursing Care After the Procedure

Care and assessment after the procedure are the same as for any study involving the collection of a peripheral blood sample.

Pancreatic Hormones

The islets of Langerhans, the endocrine cells of the pancreas, produce at least three glucose-related hormones: (1) insulin, which is produced by the beta cells; (2) glucagon, which is produced by the alpha cells; and (3) somatostatin, which is produced by the delta cells.

The overall effect of insulin is to promote glucose utilization and energy storage. It accomplishes this by enhancing glucose and potassium entry into most body cells, stimulating glycogen synthesis in liver and muscle, promoting the conversion of glucose to fatty acids and triglycerides, and enhancing protein synthesis. It exerts its effects by interacting with cell surface receptors.

In contrast to insulin, glucagon increases blood glucose levels by stimulating the breakdown of glycogen and the release of glucose stored in the liver. Somatostatin inhibits secretion of both insulin and glucagon. It also inhibits release of growth hormone, thyroid-stimulating hormone, and adrenocorticotropic hormone by the adenohypophysis and may decrease production of parathormone, calcitonin, and renin. In addition, it is thought to inhibit secretion of gastric acid and gastrin. The exact physiological roles of glucagon and somatostatin are unknown.

Blood levels of insulin are measured by radioimmunoassay and may be determined in most laboratories. Samples for blood glucagon levels require special handling, and tests for its presence may not be routinely available in all laboratories. Somatostatin may be measured but this test is not routinely performed. C-peptide, a metabolically inactive peptide chain formed during the conversion of proinsulin to insulin, may be measured to provide an index of beta cell activity not affected by exogenous insulin.[52]

INSULIN

Insulin is secreted by the beta cells in response to elevated blood glucose, certain amino acids, ketones, fatty acids, cortisol, growth hormone, glucagon, gastrin, secretin, cholecystokinin, gastric inhibitory peptide, estrogen, and progesterone. Because of normal feedback mechanisms, high insulin levels inhibit secretion of insulin. Elevated blood levels of somatostatin, epinephrine, and norepinephrine also inhibit insulin secretion.

Abnormally elevated serum insulin levels are seen with insulin- and proinsulin-secreting tumors (insulinomas), with reactive hypoglycemia in developing diabetes mellitus, and with excessive administration of exogenous insulin.

A blood glucose level is usually obtained with the serum insulin determination. Serum insulin levels may also be measured when glucose tolerance tests are performed (see p. 148).

Reference Values

	Conventional Units	**SI Units**
Fasting	8.0–15.0 µU/mL or 0.3–0.6 ng/mL	55–104 pmol/L
After 100 g glucose		
½ hr	25–231 µU/mL	173–1604 pmol/L
1 hr	18–276 µU/mL	125–1916 pmol/L
2 hr	16–166 µU/mL	111–1152 pmol/L
3 hr	4–38 µU/mL	27–263 pmol/L
Insulin-to-glucose ratio	<0.3 : 1	

Interfering Factors

➤ Administration of insulin or oral hypoglycemic agents within 8 hours of the test may lead to falsely elevated levels.
➤ Failure to follow dietary restrictions before the test may lead to falsely elevated levels.
➤ Therapy with drugs containing estrogen and progesterone may produce elevated levels.

Indications for Serum Insulin Test

➤ Evaluation of postprandial ("reactive") hypoglycemia of unknown etiology
➤ Support for diagnosing early or developing non–insulin-dependent diabetes mellitus as indicated by excessive production of insulin in relation to blood glucose levels (best demonstrated with glucose tolerance tests or 2-hour postprandial tests)

➤ Confirmation of functional hypoglycemia (i.e., no known physiological cause for the hypoglycemia) as indicated by circulating insulin levels appropriate to changing blood glucose levels

➤ Evaluation of fasting hypoglycemia of unknown etiology

➤ Support for diagnosing insulinoma as indicated by sustained high levels of insulin and absence of blood glucose-related variations

➤ Evaluation of uncontrolled insulin-dependent diabetes mellitus

➤ Differentiation between insulin-resistant diabetes, in which insulin levels are high, and non–insulin-resistant diabetes, in which insulin levels are low

➤ Support for diagnosing pheochromocytoma as indicated by decreased levels

Nursing Care Before the Procedure

Client preparation is the same as that for the related blood glucose test (e.g., fasting blood glucose, glucose tolerance test) with which the serum insulin determination is performed (see pp. 148 to 150).

The Procedure

The general procedure is the same as that for the related blood glucose test. Blood samples for serum insulin determinations are obtained in red-topped tubes and then packed in ice. The samples should be handled gently to avoid hemolysis and sent immediately to the laboratory.

Nursing Care After the Procedure

Care and assessment after the procedure are the same as for the related blood glucose test.

➤ Assess the client for signs of hypoglycemia, which may occur in response to fasting or excessive blood glucose load.

➤ Resume foods and any medications withheld before the test.

➤ *Abnormal values:* Note and report decreased or increased levels and relation to type I or II diabetes mellitus, respectively, and response to glucose intake.

➤ *Critical values:* Notify the physician at once if fasting level is greater than 30 U/mL. Prepare client for glucose administration.

C-PEPTIDE

Measurement of C-peptide, which is accomplished through radioimmunoassay techniques, provides an index of beta-cell activity that is unaffected by the administration of exogenous insulin. As the beta cells release insulin, they also release equimolar amounts of metabolically inactive C-peptide. Injectable insulin preparations are purified to remove C-peptide. Furthermore, injected insulin elevates immunoreactive serum insulin levels and suppresses pancreatic secretion of endogenous insulin and C-peptide. That is, although exogenous insulin elevates serum insulin levels, C-peptide levels are either unaffected or decreased. C-peptide determinations may be carried out to augment or confirm results of serum insulin measurements.[53]

Reference Values

Conventional Units	SI Units
0.9–4.2 ng/mL	0.30–1.39 nmol/L

Indications for C-Peptide Test

➤ Suspected excessive insulin administration in either diabetic or nondiabetic individuals, as indicated by low C-peptide and elevated serum insulin levels
➤ Determination of beta-cell function when insulin antibodies preclude accurate measurement of serum insulin production (Insulin antibodies are most common in diabetic clients receiving exogenous insulin prepared from animal extracts.)
➤ Support for diagnosing insulinoma, especially when the tumor secretes more proinsulin than active hormone, because the normal correlation between insulin and C-peptide will be altered

Nursing Care Before the Procedure

Client preparation is the same as that for any test involving the collection of a peripheral blood sample (see Appendix I).
➤ Some laboratories may require that the client fast from food for 8 hours before the test.

The Procedure

A venipuncture is performed and the sample collected in a red-topped tube. The sample should be handled gently to avoid hemolysis and sent promptly to the laboratory. The sample also can be tested for insulin measurement.

Nursing Care After the Procedure

Care and assessment after the procedure are the same as for any study involving the collection of a peripheral blood sample.
➤ Resume usual diet.

GLUCAGON

Glucagon is secreted by the alpha cells of the islets of Langerhans in response to decreased blood glucose levels. Its actions are opposed by insulin. Elevated glucagon levels are associated with conditions that produce actual hypoglycemia or a physiological need for greater blood glucose (e.g., trauma, infection, starvation, excessive exercise) and with insulin lack. Thus, elevated glucagon levels may be found in severe or uncontrolled diabetes mellitus, despite hyperglycemia.

Reference Values

Conventional Units	SI Units
50–200 pg/mL	50–200 ng/L

Interfering Factors

➤ Trauma, infection, starvation, and excessive exercise may lead to elevated levels, as will acute pancreatitis, pheochromocytoma, uncontrolled diabetes mellitus, and uremia.
➤ Failure to follow dietary restrictions before the test may lead to falsely decreased levels.

Indications for Glucagon Determination

➤ Suspected glucagonoma as indicated by elevated levels (as high as 1000 pg/mL) in the absence of diabetic ketoacidosis, uremia, pheochromocytoma, or acute pancreatitis

➤ Confirmation of glucagon deficiency related to loss of pancreatic tissue as a result of chronic pancreatitis, pancreatic neoplasm, or surgical resection (Arginine infusion, which normally leads to elevated glucagon levels, may be used for further confirmation of the deficiency state.)

➤ Suspected renal transplant rejection, as indicated by rising plasma glucagon levels (Glucagon levels may rise markedly several days before serum creatinine begins to rise.)

Nursing Care Before the Procedure

General client preparation is the same as that for any test involving collection of a peripheral blood sample (see Appendix I).

➤ For this test, the client should fast from foods for 8 hours before the study. Water is permitted.

The Procedure

A venipuncture is performed and the sample is collected in either a green- or a lavender-topped tube, depending on the laboratory performing the test. The sample should be handled gently to avoid hemolysis and sent to the laboratory immediately.

Nursing Care After the Procedure

Care and assessment after the procedure are the same as for any test involving the collection of a peripheral blood sample.

➤ Resume usual diet as soon as possible after the sample has been obtained.

➤ *Complications and precautions:* Assess the test results in relation to insulin and glucose levels.

Gastric and Intestinal Hormones

The stomach and intestine secrete various enzymes and hormones that aid in the digestive process. The hormones secreted include gastrin, cholecystokinin, secretin, and gastric inhibitory peptide (GIP). Of these, only gastrin is currently of diagnostic significance.

Gastrin is secreted by the gastrin cells (G cells) of the gastric antrum, the pylorus, and the proximal duodenum in response to vagal stimulation and the presence of food (especially protein) in the stomach. Gastrin stimulates the secretion of acidic gastric juice and pepsin and the release of pancreatic enzymes. It also stimulates motor activities of the stomach and intestine, increases pyloric relaxation, constricts the gastroesophageal sphincter, and promotes the release of insulin.

Cholecystokinin is secreted by the duodenal mucosa in response to the presence of fats. It opposes the actions of gastrin, stimulates contraction of the gallbladder, relaxes the sphincter of Oddi, and with secretin, controls pancreatic secretions. Secretin is secreted by the duodenal mucosa in response to the presence of peptides and acids in the duodenum. It also opposes the actions of gastrin, and with cholecystokinin, controls pancreatic secretions. GIP inhibits gastric motility and secretion and stimulates secretion of insulin.

GASTRIN

Measurement of serum gastrin levels, which is accomplished through radioimmunoassay techniques, is indicated when disorders producing elevated levels are suspected. Excessive gastrin secretion occurs because of normal feedback mechanisms in disorders associated with decreased gastric acid production as a result of cellular destruction or atrophy (e.g., gastric carcinoma and age-related changes in gastric acid secretion). Elevated levels also may be seen in gastric and duodenal ulcers, in which gastric acid secretion is actually normal or low; pernicious anemia; uremia; and chronic gastritis. Decreased gastrin levels are associated with true gastric hyperacidity as may occur with stress ulcers.

Both protein ingestion and calcium infusions elevate serum gastrin levels in certain situations. Thus, these substances may be used to provoke gastrin secretion when a single serum determination is inconclusive. In the secretagogue provocation test, a fasting serum gastrin sample is drawn and the client is then given a high-protein test meal. A postprandial blood sample is then obtained. In individuals with duodenal or gastric ulcers, gastrin levels will be markedly higher than in normal persons after protein-stimulated gastrin secretion. Likewise, an infusion of calcium gluconate produces elevated serum gastrin levels in a person with gastrinoma caused by gastrin production by tumor cells. This effect is not seen in individuals with peptic ulcer disease.

Reference Values

	Conventional Units	SI Units
Fasting	50–150 pg/mL	50–150 ng/L
Postprandial	80–170 pg/mL	80–170 ng/L

Postprandial values may vary according to the test method used.

Interfering Factors

➤ Protein ingestion and calcium infusions will elevate serum gastrin levels in some situations; these substances may be used for "challenge tests" of gastrin secretion.

Indications for Serum Gastrin Test

➤ Suspected gastrinoma (Zollinger-Ellison syndrome) as indicated by markedly elevated levels (e.g., greater than 1000 pg/mL) and by marked response to calcium challenge
➤ Support for diagnosing gastric carcinoma, pernicious anemia, or G-cell hyperplasia as indicated by elevated levels
➤ Differential diagnosis of peptic ulcer disease from other disorders, because gastrin levels may be normal but will rise in response to protein challenge

Nursing Care Before the Procedure

General client preparation is the same as that for any test involving collection of a peripheral blood sample (see Appendix I).

➤ For this test, the client should fast from food for 12 hours before the study. Water is not restricted. It also is recommended that medications be withheld for 12 to 24 hours before the test, although this practice should be confirmed with the person ordering the study.

The Procedure

A venipuncture is performed and the sample collected in a red-topped tube. The sample should be packed in ice, handled gently to avoid hemolysis, and transported immediately to the laboratory.

Nursing Care After the Procedure

Care and assessment after the procedure are the same as for any test involving the collection of a peripheral blood sample.

➤ Resume usual diet and medications.

➤ *Complications and precautions:* Assess bowel sounds if levels are increased to 100 to 500 pg/mL, which indicates Zollinger-Ellison syndrome associated with peptic ulcer disease.

ELECTROLYTES

Electrolytes are substances that dissociate into electrically charged ions when dissolved. Cations carry positive charges and anions carry negative charges. Both affect the electrical and osmolal (i.e., the number of particles dissolved in a fluid) functioning of the body. Body fluids always contain equal numbers of positive and negative charges, but the nature of the ions, the number of charges present on a single molecule, and the nature and mobility of the charged molecules differ enormously among body fluid compartments (e.g., intracellular versus extracellular).

Not all charged particles are ions. Proteins, for example, carry a net negative charge. Whenever fluid contains protein, there must be accompanying cations. Similarly, not all solutes found in plasma are ions. Urea and glucose, for example, do not dissociate; they do not contribute to electrical activity of fluids and membranes, and they contribute only moderately to plasma osmolality.

Electrolyte quantities and the balance among them in the body fluid compartments are controlled by (1) oxygen and carbon dioxide exchange in the lungs; (2) absorption, secretion, and excretion of many substances by the kidneys; and (3) secretion of regulatory hormones by the endocrine glands.

Quantitatively, the most important body fluid ions are sodium, potassium, chloride, and bicarbonate. These ions are measured in routine serum electrolyte determinations. Other serum ions that may be measured include calcium, magnesium, and phosphorus.[54]

SERUM SODIUM (Na)

Sodium (Na, Na^+) is the most abundant cation in extracellular fluid and, along with its accompanying chloride and bicarbonate anions, accounts for 92 percent of serum osmolality. Sodium plays a major role in maintaining homeostasis

Table 5–22 ➤ DISORDERS AND DRUGS ASSOCIATED WITH ALTERED SERUM SODIUM AND EXTRACELLULAR FLUID (ECF) LEVELS

Increased Serum Sodium (Hypernatremia)	Decreased Serum Sodium (Hyponatremia)
Total Body Sodium Normal, ECF Volume Low Hypovolemia Dehydration Fever Thyrotoxicosis Hyperglycemic hyperosmolar nonketotic syndrome Diabetes insipidus Hyperventilation Mechanical ventilation without humidification	*Total Body Sodium and ECF Volume Low, but Total Body Sodium Proportionately Lower* Addison's disease Salt-losing renal disorders Gastrointestinal fluid loss (nasogastric suction, vomiting, diarrhea, fistula, paralytic ileus) Diaphoresis Diuresis Burns Ascites Massive pleural effusion Diabetes ketoacidosis
Total Body Sodium Increased Proportionately More Than ECF Volume Excessive salt ingestion Inappropriate or incorrect intravenous therapy with fluids containing sodium Cushing's syndrome Hyperaldosteronism	*Total Body Sodium Normal and ECF Volume Normal to High* Acute water intoxication Syndrome of inappropriate antidiuretic hormone secretion (SIADH) Glucocorticoid deficiency Severe total body potassium depletion
Total Body Sodium Low with ECF Volume Proportionately Lower Gastroenteritis Osmotic diuresis Diaphoresis	*Total Body Sodium and ECF Volume Increased, but ECF Proportionately Greater* Acute renal failure with water overload Congestive heart failure (CHF) Cirrhosis Nephrotic syndrome
Drugs Adrenocorticosteroids Methyldopa (Aldomet) Hydralazine (Apresoline) Reserpine (Serpasil) Cough medicines	*Drugs* Lithium carbonate Vasopressin Diuretics (thiazides, mannitol, ethacrynic acid, furosemide)

Note: Adapted from Sacher, RA, and McPherson, RA: Widmann's Clinical Interpretation of Laboratory Tests, ed 10. FA Davis, Philadelphia, 1991, p 389.

through a variety of functions, which include (1) maintenance of osmotic pressure of extracellular fluid, (2) regulation of renal retention and excretion of water, (3) maintenance of acid-base balance, (4) regulation of potassium and chloride levels, (5) stimulation of neuromuscular reactions, and (6) maintenance of systemic blood pressure. Serum sodium levels may be affected by a variety of disorders and drugs (Table 5–22) and are evaluated in relation to other serum electrolyte and blood chemistry results. Tests of urinary sodium and osmolality also may be necessary for complete interpretation. It should be noted that falsely decreased serum sodium levels may occur with elevated serum triglyceride levels and myeloma proteins.

Reference Values

	Conventional Units	**SI Units**
Infants	134–150 mEq/L	134–150 mmol/L
Children	135–145 mEq/L	135–145 mmol/L
Adults	135–145 mEq/L	135–145 mmol/L
Critical Values	**<120 mEq/L or >160 mEq/L**	**<120 mmol/L or >160 mmol/L**

Interfering Factors

➤ Elevated serum triglyceride levels and myeloma proteins may lead to falsely decreased levels.
➤ Adrenocorticosteroids, methyldopa, hydralazine, reserpine, and cough medicines may lead to increased levels.
➤ Lithium, vasopressin, and diuretics may lead to decreased levels.

Indications for Serum Sodium (Na) Test

➤ Routine electrolyte screening in acute and critical illness
➤ Determination of whole body stores of sodium, because the ion is predominantly extracellular
➤ Known or suspected disorder associated with altered fluid and electrolyte balance (see Table 5–22, p. 269)
➤ Estimation of serum osmolality, which is normally 285 to 310 mOsm/kg, by using the following formula:

$$\text{Serum osmolality} = 2(\text{Na}^+) + \frac{\text{glucose}}{20} + \frac{\text{BUN*}}{3}$$

• *Note:* If the value for serum osmolality is greater than 2.0 to 2.3 times the value for serum sodium, then hyperglycemia, uremia, or metabolic acidosis should be suspected.
➤ Evaluation of the effects of drug therapy on serum sodium levels (e.g., diuretic therapy)

Nursing Care Before the Procedure

Client preparation is the same as that for any study involving the collection of a peripheral blood sample (see Appendix I).
➤ Because many drugs may alter serum sodium levels, a medication history should be obtained. It is recommended that any drugs that may alter test results be withheld for 12 to 24 hours before the test, although this practice should be confirmed with the person ordering the study.

The Procedure

A venipuncture is performed and the sample collected in a red-topped tube. The sample should be handled gently to avoid hemolysis and transported promptly to the laboratory.

*Blood urea nitrogen

Nursing Care After the Procedure

Care and assessment after the procedure are the same as for any study involving the collection of a peripheral blood sample.

➤ Resume any medications withheld before the test.

➤ *Increased levels:* Note and report increased levels. Assess for symptoms associated with hypernatremia, such as fluid deficit with thirst; dry mucous membranes and skin; poor skin turgor; or fluid excess with edema, weight gain, or elevated blood pressure. Administer fluid replacement at an ordered rate and time if the client is dehydrated or if diuretics are administered for fluid excess. Instruct client in a low-sodium diet.

➤ *Decreased levels:* Note and report decreased levels. Assess for symptoms associated with hyponatremia, such as oliguria, rapid pulse, abdominal cramping, fluid retention, weight gain, edema, or elevated blood pressure. Administer ordered sodium replacement via IV or dietary intake. Instruct client in sodium intake (food, salt tablets) to replace and maintain sodium, especially if this electrolyte is lost because of vomiting, diarrhea, perspiration, or use of diuretics.

➤ *Critical values:* Notify the physician at once of levels less than 120 mEq/L or greater than 160 mEq/L.

Serum Potassium (K)

Potassium (K, K^+) is the most abundant intracellular cation; much smaller amounts are found in the blood. Potassium is essential for the transmission of electrical impulses in cardiac and skeletal muscle. In addition, it helps to maintain the osmolality and electroneutrality of cells, functions in enzyme reactions that transform glucose into energy and amino acids into proteins, and participates in the maintenance of acid-base balance.

Numerous disorders and drugs may affect serum potassium levels. As shown in Table 5–23, the clinical problems associated with altered serum potassium levels may be categorized as (1) inappropriate cellular metabolism, (2) altered renal excretion, and (3) altered potassium intake. False elevations in serum potassium may occur with vigorous pumping of the hand after tourniquet application for venipuncture, in hemolyzed samples, or with high platelet counts during clotting. Falsely decreased levels are seen in anticoagulated samples left at room temperature.

Altered serum potassium levels are of particular concern because of their effects on cardiac impulse conduction, especially when the client also is taking medications that affect cardiac conduction. The combination of low serum potassium (hypokalemia) and therapy with digitalis preparations, for example, can produce serious consequences because of increased ventricular irritability.

It should also be noted that potassium is a very changeable ion, moving easily between intracellular and extracellular fluids. An example is seen in states of acidosis and alkalosis. In acidosis (decreased serum pH), potassium moves from the cells into the blood; in alkalosis (increased serum pH), the reverse occurs.

Table 5–23 ➤ DISORDERS AND DRUGS ASSOCIATED WITH ALTERED SERUM POTASSIUM LEVELS

Increased Serum Potassium (Hyperkalemia)	Decreased Serum Potassium (Hypokalemia)
Inappropriate Cellular Metabolism Acidosis Insulin deficiency Hypoaldosteronism Cell necrosis (trauma, burns, hemolysis, antineoplastic therapy) Addison's disease	**Inappropriate Cellular Metabolism** Alkalosis Insulin excess Familial peroidic paralysis Rapid cell generation (leukemia, treated megaloblastic anemia) Chronic excessive licorice ingestion
Decreased Renal Excretion Acute renal failure Chronic interstitial nephritis Tubular unresponsiveness to aldosterone Hypoaldosteronism	**Increased Excretion** Gastrointestinal loss (vomiting, diarrhea, nasogastric suction, fistula) Excessive diuresis Hyperaldosteronism Laxative abuse Hypomagnesemia Renal tubular acidosis Diaphoresis Thyrotoxicosis Cushing's syndrome
Increased Potassium Intake Salt substitutes Potassium supplements (oral or IV) Potassium salts of antibiotics Transfusion of old banked blood	**Decreased Potassium Intake** Anorexia nervosa Diet deficient in meat and vegetables Clay eating (binds potassium and prevents absorption) IV therapy with inadequate potassium supplementation
Drugs Aldosterone antagonists Potassium preparations of antibiotics Amphotericin B Tetracycline Heparin Epinephrine Marijuana Isoniazid	**Drugs** Furosemide Ethacrynic acid Thiazide diuretics Insulin Aspirin Prednisone Cortisone Gentamicin Polymyxin B Lithium carbonate Sodium polystyrene sulfonate (Kayexalate) Ammonium chloride Aldosterone Laxatives

Note: Adapted from Sacher, RA, and McPherson, RA: Widmann's Clinical Interpretation of Laboratory Tests, ed 10. FA Davis, Philadelphia, 1991, p 390.

Reference Values

	Conventional Units	**SI Units**
Infants	4.1–5.3 mEq/L	4.1–5.3 mmol/L
Children	3.4–4.7 mEq/L	3.4–4.7 mmol/L
Adults	3.5–5.0 mEq/L	3.5–5.0 mmol/L
Critical Values	**<2.5 mEq/L or >6.5 mEq/L**	**<2.5 mmol/L or >6.5 mmol/L**

Interfering Factors

➤ False elevations may occur with vigorous pumping of the hand after tourniquet application for venipuncture, in hemolyzed samples, or with high platelet counts during clotting.

➤ Falsely decreased levels are seen in anticoagulated samples left at room temperature.

➤ Numerous drugs may produce elevated and decreased levels (see Table 5–23).

Indications for Serum Potassium (K) Test

➤ Routine electrolyte screening in acute and critical illness

➤ Known or suspected disorder associated with altered fluid and electrolyte balance, especially renal disease, disorders of glucose metabolism, trauma, and burns (see Table 5–23)

➤ Known or suspected acidosis of any etiology, because potassium moves from the cells into the blood in acidotic states

➤ Evaluation of cardiac dysrhythmias to determine whether altered serum potassium level is contributing to the problem (e.g., the combination of low serum potassium and therapy with digitalis preparations may lead to ventricular irritability)

➤ Evaluation of the effects of drug therapy (e.g., diuretics) on serum potassium levels

➤ Evaluation of response to treatment for abnormal serum potassium levels

---

➤➤ Nursing Alert

• Because of the effects of serum potassium levels on cardiac impulse conduction, abnormal values should be reported to the physician immediately so that treatment may be instituted.

Nursing Care Before the Procedure

Client preparation is the same as that for any study involving the collection of a peripheral blood sample (see Appendix I).

➤ Because many drugs may alter serum potassium levels, a medication history should be obtained. It is recommended that drugs that may alter test results be withheld for 12 to 24 hours before the test, although this practice should be confirmed with the person ordering the study.

The Procedure

A venipuncture is performed and the sample collected in a red-topped tube. Vigorous pumping of the hand after tourniquet application should be avoided, as it may lead to falsely elevated results. The sample should be handled gently to avoid hemolysis, which may also falsely elevate results, and transported immediately to the laboratory.

Nursing Care After the Procedure

Care and assessment after the procedure are the same as for any study involving the collection of a peripheral blood sample.

➤ Resume any medications withheld before the test.

➤ *Increased levels:* Note and report increased levels. Assess for symptoms associated with hyperkalemia such as oliguria, irritability, diarrhea, and ECG tracings for peaked T waves. Assess results of arterial blood gases (ABGs). Prepare client for IV administration of medications (sodium bicarbonate for acidosis, calcium gluconate if calcium level is low) or oral or enema administration of sodium polystyrene sulfonate. Instruct client in low potassium dietary intake and food restrictions (citrus juices, bananas, dried fruits, potatoes, and tomatoes).

➤ *Decreased levels:* Note and report decreased levels. Assess for symptoms of hypokalemia such as thirst, vomiting, anorexia, weak pulse, decreased blood pressure, ECG tracings for depressed T waves, or prominent U waves. Administer oral or IV potassium replacement. Instruct client in foods high in potassium, as already listed.

➤ **Critical values:** Notify the physician at once of levels less than 2.5 mEq/L or greater than 6.5 mEq/L (greater than 8.1 mEq/L in infants).

SERUM CHLORIDE (Cl)

Chloride (Cl, Cl^-) is the most abundant anion in extracellular fluid. It participates with sodium in the maintenance of water balance and aids in the regulation of osmotic pressure. It also contributes to gastric acid (HCl) for digestion and for activation of enzymes. Its most important function is in the maintenance of acid-base balance. In certain forms of metabolic acidosis, for example, serum chloride levels may rise in response to decreased serum bicarbonate levels; this condition is known as hyperchloremic acidosis. If bicarbonate levels fall and serum chloride concentration remains relatively normal, however, a gap between measured cations (i.e., sodium and potassium) and measured anions (i.e., chloride and bicarbonate) occurs. This condition often is called anion gap acidosis (see also section entitled "Anion Gap," which follows).

Chloride also helps to maintain acid-base balance through the chloride-bicarbonate shift mechanism, in which chloride ions enter red blood cells in exchange for bicarbonate. Bicarbonate leaves the red blood cells in response to carbon dioxide, which is released from the tissues into venous blood and absorbed into the red blood cells. The carbon dioxide is subsequently converted into carbonic acid, which dissociates into bicarbonate and hydrogen ions. When the bicarbonate concentration in the red blood cells exceeds that of the plasma, bicarbonate diffuses into the blood, and chloride enters the red blood cells to supply the anions necessary for electroneutrality. For this reason, the chloride content of red blood cells in venous blood is slightly higher than that of arterial red blood cells.

Numerous disorders and drugs may alter serum chloride levels (Table 5–24).

Reference Values

	Conventional Units	**SI Units**
Newborns	94–112 mEq/L	94–112 mmol/L
Infants	95–110 mEq/L	95–110 mmol/L
Children	98–105 mEq/L	98–105 mmol/L
Adults	95–105 mEq/L	95–105 mmol/L
Critical Values	**<80 mEq/L or >115 mEq/L**	**<80 mmol/L or >115 mmol/L**

Interfering Factors

➤ Drugs such as potassium chloride, ammonium chloride, acetazolamide (Diamox), methyldopa (Aldomet), diazoxide (Hyperstat), and guanethidine (Ismelin) may lead to elevated levels.

➤ Drugs such as ethacrynic acid (Edecrin), furosemide (Lasix), thiazide diuretics, and bicarbonate may lead to decreased levels.

Indications for Serum Chloride (Cl) Test

➤ Routine electrolyte screening in acute and critical illness

➤ Known or suspected disorder associated with altered acid-base or fluid and electrolyte balance, or both conditions

➤ Support for diagnosing disorders associated with altered serum chloride levels (see Table 5–24)

➤ Differentiation of the type of acidosis (hyperchloremic versus anion gap acidosis), with serum chloride levels remaining relatively normal in anion gap acidosis

➤ Evaluation of the effects of drug therapy on serum chloride levels (see Table 5–24)

Table 5–24 ➤ DISORDERS AND DRUGS ASSOCIATED WITH ALTERED SERUM CHLORIDE LEVELS

Increased Serum Chloride (Hyperchloremia)	Decreased Serum Chloride (Hypochloremia)
DISORDERS	
Acidosis	Alkalosis
Hyperkalemia	Hypokalemia
Hypernatremia	Hyponatremia
Dehydration	Gastrointestinal loss (vomiting, diarrhea, nasogastric suction, fistula)
Eclampsia	
Renal failure (severe)	Diuresis
Congestive heart failure (CHF)	Hypoventilation (especially due to chronic obstructive pulmonary disease [COPD])
Hyperventilation (especially due to neurogenic hyperventilation related to head injury)	Acute infections
Cushing's syndrome	Burns
Hyperaldosteronism	Heat stroke
Anemia	Fever
Hypoproteinemia	Diabetic ketoacidosis
Serum sickness	Pyelonephritis
Hyperparathyroidism	Addisonian crisis
Excessive dietary salt	Starvation
Jejunoileal bypass	Inadequate chloride intake
Gastric carcinoma	
DRUGS	
Potassium chloride	Ethacrynic acid (Edecrin)
Ammonium chloride	Furosemide (Lasix)
Acetazolamide (Diamox)	Thiazide diuretics
Methyldopa (Aldomet)	Bicarbonate
Diazoxide (Hyperstat)	
Guanethidine (Ismelin)	

Nursing Care Before the Procedure

Client preparation is the same as that for any study involving collection of a peripheral blood sample (see Appendix I).

➤ Because many drugs may alter serum chloride levels, a medication history should be obtained. It is recommended that those drugs that may alter test results be withheld for 12 to 24 hours before the test, although this practice should be confirmed with the person ordering the study.

The Procedure

A venipuncture is performed and the sample collected in a red-topped tube. The sample should be handled gently to avoid hemolysis and transported promptly to the laboratory.

Nursing Care After the Procedure

Care and assessment after the procedure are the same as for any study involving the collection of a peripheral blood sample.

➤ Resume any medications withheld before the test.

➤ *Increased levels:* Note and report increased levels (hyperchloremia) in relation to increased sodium and decreased bicarbonate, and assess for changes in chloride caused by or resulting in metabolic acidosis.

➤ *Decreased levels:* Note and report decreased levels (hypochloremia). Assess for possible cause (vomiting, gastric suction, diarrhea, diuretic medication regimen, chronic lung disease, increased bicarbonate and decreased potassium resulting in metabolic alkalosis).

➤ *Critical values:* Notify the physician at once of levels less than 80 mEq/L or greater than 115 mEq/L.

SERUM BICARBONATE (HCO_3, HCO_3^-)

Bicarbonate (HCO_3, HCO_3^-) is the major extracellular buffer in the blood; it functions with carbonic acid (H_2CO_3) in maintaining acid-base balance. Normally, the ratio of bicarbonate to dissolved carbon dioxide (CO_2), which derives from H_2CO_3, is $20:1$. If this ratio is altered, acid-base imbalance occurs. Additional CO_2, for example, causes increased acidity (falling pH), whereas loss of CO_2 produces alkalinity (rising pH). Similarly, additional bicarbonate leads to alkalosis, whereas loss of bicarbonate produces acidosis.

The lungs control regulation of CO_2 levels. Bicarbonate levels are under renal control; the kidneys regulate both the generation of bicarbonate ions and their rate of urinary excretion. Bicarbonate also participates with chloride in the bicarbonate-chloride shift mechanism involving red blood cells (see also p. 274).

Measurement of serum bicarbonate ion concentration may be made directly or indirectly by means of total CO_2 content, because more than 90 percent of blood CO_2 exists in the ionized bicarbonate form. Bicarbonate also is measured as part of blood gas determinations (see p. 288). Numerous disorders, especially those involving acid-base imbalance, and drugs are associated with altered serum bicarbonate levels (Table 5–25).

Table 5-25 ➤ DISORDERS AND DRUGS ASSOCIATED WITH ALTERED SERUM BICARBONATE LEVELS	
Increased Serum Bicarbonate	**Decreased Serum Bicarbonate**
DISORDERS	
Metabolic alkalosis	Metabolic acidosis
Compensated metabolic alkalosis	Compensated metabolic acidosis
Respiratory acidosis (slightly elevated or normal)	Respiratory alkalosis (slightly low or normal)
Compensated respiratory acidosis	Compensated respiratory alkalosis
Hypoventilation	Hyperventilation
Chronic obstructive pulmonary disease (COPD)	Diarrhea
Vomiting	Dehydration
Nasogastric suction	Severe malnutrition
Diuresis	Burns
Aldosteronism	Myocardial infarction
Congestive heart failure (CHF)	Acute ethanol intoxication
Hypokalemia	Shock
Cushing's syndrome	Renal disease
Pulmonary edema	Hyperthyroidism
Milk-alkali syndrome	
DRUGS	
Aldosterone	Triamterene (Dyrenium)
Adrenocorticotropic hormone (ACTH)	Acetazolamide (Diamox)
Sodium bicarbonate abuse	Calcium chloride
Adrenocorticosteroids	Ammonium chloride
Viomycin	Salicylate toxicity
Thiazide diuretics	Paraldehyde
	Sodium citrate

ANION GAP

The results of serum levels of sodium, potassium, chloride, and bicarbonate may be used to calculate the "anion gap." The anion gap refers to the normal discrepancy between unmeasured (i.e., those not routinely measured) cations and anions in the blood. Unmeasured anions include the negative charges contributed by serum proteins and those of phosphates, sulfates, and other metabolites. Unmeasured anions normally total about 24 mEq/L. Cations not routinely measured include calcium and magnesium, and together they account for about 7 mEq/L. Because there are normally more unmeasured anions than cations, the difference between the two is called the anion gap. This is normally 12 to 18 mEq/L.

The anion gap may be determined by subtracting the sum of routinely measured anions, chloride and bicarbonate, from the sum of routinely measured cations, sodium and potassium (i.e., $[Na + K] - [Cl + HCO_3]$). The concept of anion gap allows consideration of metabolic derangements without measuring specific metabolites. An increase in the anion gap is seen in acidotic states in which there is no compensatory rise in chloride levels. Examples of anion gap acidosis include diabetic ketoacidosis, lactic adicosis caused by either tissue hypoxia (type A) or renal or hepatic metabolic defect (type B), and excessive alcohol ingestion.[55]

Reference Values

	Conventional Units	**SI Units**
Peripheral vein	19–25 mEq/L	19–25 mmol/L
Arterial sample	22–26 mEq/L	22–26 mmol/L
Critical Values	**<15 mEq/L or >35 mEq/L**	**<15 mmol/L or >35 mmol/L**

Interfering Factors

➤ Numerous drugs may alter serum bicarbonate levels (see Table 5–25, p. 277).

Indications for Serum Bicarbonate (HCO_3, HCO_3^-) Test

➤ Routine electrolyte screening in acute and critical illness
➤ Known or suspected disorder associated with altered acid-base or fluid and electrolyte balance, or both
➤ Support for diagnosing disorders associated with altered serum bicarbonate levels (see Table 5–25, p. 277)
➤ Determination of the degree of compensation in acidotic and alkalotic states (Table 5–26)
➤ Evaluation of the effects of drug therapy on serum bicarbonate levels

Nursing Care Before the Procedure

Client preparation is the same as that for any study involving collection of a peripheral blood sample (see Appendix I).

➤ Because many drugs may alter serum bicarbonate levels, a medication history should be obtained. It is recommended that drugs that may alter test re-

Table 5–26 ➤ BLOOD GASES IN ACID-BASE IMBALANCES

	pH	pCO_2	HCO_3^-	Base Excess (BE)
Respiratory acidosis	↓	↑	Normal	Normal
with compensation	Sl ↓ or normal	↑	↑	↑
Respiratory alkalosis	↑		Normal	Normal
with compensation	Sl ↑ or normal	↓ ↓	↓	↓
Metabolic acidosis	↓	Normal	↓	↓
with compensation	Sl ↓ or normal	↓	↓	↓
Metabolic alkalosis	↑	Normal	↑	↑
with compensation	Sl ↑ or normal	↑	↑	↑
Mixed respiratory and metabolic acidosis	↓	↑	↓	↓

Sl = slightly.

sults be withheld for 12 to 24 hours before the test, although this practice should be confirmed with the person ordering the study.

The Procedure

A venipuncture is performed and the sample collected in a red-topped tube. The sample should be handled gently to avoid hemolysis and transported promptly to the laboratory.

Nursing Care After the Procedure

Care and assessment after the procedure are the same as for any study involving the collection of a peripheral blood sample.

➤ Resume any medications withheld before the test.

➤ *Increased levels:* Note and report increased levels or base excess in relation to hypokalemia and hypochloremia. Assess for vomiting, presence of gastric suctioning, diuretic therapy, or excessive intake of oral bicarbonate (baking soda, antacids). Assess for respiratory changes, tingling in fingers, or more severe muscular irritability symptoms. Assess for cardiac dysrhythmias if hypokalemia is present. Administer ordered oral or IV electrolyte replacement (potassium, chloride). Administer fluids (juices, broth) to replace electrolytes if decreases are not extreme.

➤ *Decreased levels:* Note and report decreased levels or base deficit in relation to other electrolytes. Assess gastrointestinal losses such as vomiting leading to acidosis and diarrhea leading to alkalosis, I&O, metabolic acidosis with change in respirations (Kussmaul's breathing), confusion, or lethargy. Prepare for IV sodium bicarbonate. Monitor I&O closely to prevent fluid and electrolyte imbalance.

➤ *Critical values:* Notify the physician at once of levels less than 15 mEq/L or greater than 35 mEq/L.

SERUM CALCIUM (Ca, Ca^{++})

Calcium (Ca, Ca^{++}) is the most abundant cation in the body and participates in virtually all vital processes. About half the total amount of calcium circulates as free ions that participate in blood coagulation, neuromuscular conduction, intracellular regulation, glandular secretion, and control of skeletal and cardiac muscle contractility. The remaining calcium is bound to circulating proteins and plays no physiological role. Serum calcium measurement includes both ionized and protein-bound calcium.

Calcium ions undergo continuous turnover, with bone serving as the major reservoir. Serum contains only a small amount at any one time, but the serum level reflects overall calcium metabolism. Calcium levels are largely regulated by the parathyroid glands and vitamin D. Other substances affecting calcium levels include estrogens and androgens, calcitonin, and ingested carbohydrates. Increased or decreased serum proteins also may affect levels of protein-bound calcium.[56]

Table 5–27 shows the various disorders and drugs associated with altered calcium levels. Abnormal serum calcium may produce cardiac dysrhythmias. Furthermore, serum calcium levels have a reciprocal relationship with serum phosphate levels; if one rises, the other tends to fall.

Table 5–27 ➤ DISORDERS AND DRUGS ASSOCIATED WITH ALTERED SERUM CALCIUM LEVELS	
Increased Levels (Hypercalcemia)	**Decreased Levels (Hypocalcemia)**
DISORDERS	
Acidosis	Alkalosis
Hyperparathyroidism	Hypoparathyroidism
Cancers involving bone	Pseudohypoparathyroidism
Paget's disease of bone	Inadequate dietary intake of calcium and/or vitamin D
Prolonged immobility	Vitamin D–resistant rickets
Leukemia	Malabsorption syndromes
Multiple myeloma	Hypoproteinemia
Lymphomas	Laxative abuse
Hyperproteinemia	Acute pancreatitis
Polycythemia vera	Burns
Bone growth or active bone formation	Osteomalacia
Vitamin D intoxication	Peritonitis
Hyperthyroidism (severe)	Pregnancy
Milk-alkali syndrome	Overwhelming infections
	Hypomagnesemia
	Renal failure
	Phosphate excess
DRUGS	
Thiazide diuretics	Barbiturates
Hormones (androgens, progestins, estrogens)	Anticonvulsants
Vitamin D	Acetazolamide (Diamox)
Calcium supplements	Adrenocorticosteroids
	Cytotoxic drugs

Reference Values

	Conventional Units	**SI Units**
Newborns	7.0–11.5 mg/dL	1.75–2.90 mmol/L
	3.7–7.0 mEq/L	
Infants	8.6–11.2 mg/dL	2.15–2.80 mmol/L
	5.0–6.0 mEq/L	
Children	<12.0 mg/dL	<3 mmol/L
	<6.0 mEq/L	
Adults	9–11 mg/dL	2.25–2.75 mmol/L
	4.5–5.5 mEq/L	
Critical Values	**<6 mg/dL or >13 mg/dL**	**<1.5 mmol/L or >3.25 mmol/L**

Interfering Factors

➤ Values are higher in children because of growth and active bone formation.
➤ Numerous drugs may alter serum calcium levels (see Table 5–27).
➤ Increased or decreased serum protein levels may alter results.

Indications for Serum Calcium (Ca, Ca^{++}) Test

➤ Evaluation of the effects of various disorders on overall calcium metabolism, especially diseases involving bone (see Table 5–27)

➤ Detection of parathyroid gland loss after thyroid or other neck surgery, as indicated by decreased levels

➤ Monitoring of the effects of renal failure on calcium levels, which are usually decreased in the disorder

➤ Evaluation of cardiac dysrhythmias to determine whether altered serum calcium level is contributing to the problem

➤ Evaluation of coagulation disorders to determine whether altered serum calcium level is contributing to the problem

➤ Monitoring for the effects of various drugs on serum calcium levels (see Table 5–27)

➤ Evaluation of the effectiveness of treatment for abnormal calcium levels, especially in deficiency states

> ## ➤➤ Nursing Alert

- Because altered serum calcium levels may produce cardiac dysrhythmias, abnormal values should be reported to the physician immediately so that treatment may be instituted.

Nursing Care Before the Procedure

Client preparation is the same as that for any study involving the collection of a peripheral blood sample (see Appendix I).

➤ Because many drugs may alter serum calcium levels, a medication history should be obtained. It is recommended that drugs that may alter test results be withheld for 12 to 24 hours before the test, although this practice should be confirmed with the person ordering the study.

The Procedure

A venipuncture is performed and the sample collected in a red-topped tube. The sample should be handled gently to avoid hemolysis and transported promptly to the laboratory.

Nursing Care After the Procedure

Care and assessment after the procedure are the same as for any study involving the collection of a peripheral blood sample.

➤ Resume any medications withheld before the test.

➤ *Increased levels:* Note and report increased levels. Assess for symptoms associated with hypercalcemia such as muscle relaxation, bone pain, nausea and vomiting, or increased intake of dietary calcium. Encourage fluid intake. Instruct client to restrict foods and medications high in calcium (milk and other dairy foods, eggs, some antacids).

➤ *Decreased levels:* Note and report decreased levels. Assess for symptoms associated with hypocalcemia such as muscular irritability (tingling in fingers and around mouth, muscle cramping or twitching, facial spasm or Chvostek's sign, carpopedal spasm or Trousseau's sign, and tetany). Instruct client to eat foods and fluids high in calcium. Administer oral calcium supplement or replacement; prepare for IV calcium replacement in more severe cases.

➤ **Critical values:** Notify the physician at once of levels less than 6 mg/dL or greater than 13 mg/dL.

SERUM PHOSPHORUS/PHOSPHATE (P)

Phosphorus (P), the dominant intracellular anion, is measured in serum as phosphate (HPO_4^{--}, $H_2PO_4^{-}$). Results are reported as inorganic phosphorus (Pi). Phosphates are vital constituents of nucleic acids, intracellular energy storage compounds, intermediary compounds in carbohydrate metabolism, and various regulatory compounds, including that which modulates dissociation of oxygen from hemoglobin. Phosphorus also aids in regulation of calcium levels and functions as a buffer in the maintenance of acid-base balance. It contributes to the mineralization of bones and teeth, promotes renal tubular reabsorption of glucose, and, as a component of phospholipids, aids in fat transport.

As with calcium, phosphorus ions undergo continuous turnover, with bone serving as the major reservoir. Serum contains a relatively small amount of phosphorus at any given time. Phosphorus levels are largely regulated by the parathyroid glands and vitamin D, and they are normally reciprocal to those of serum calcium. The equilibrium between serum phosphate levels and intracellular stores is affected by carbohydrate metabolism and blood pH. When persons with diabetic ketoacidosis are treated with insulin, for example, phosphate enters the cells along with glucose and potassium. Phosphate excretion is controlled by the kidneys. Disorders and drugs associated with altered phosphorus levels are listed in Table 5–28. Note that several disorders associated with decreased phosphorus levels are the same as those causing elevated serum calcium levels (e.g., hyperparathyroidism).

Reference Values

	Conventional Units	**SI Units**
Infants	4.5–6.7 mg/dL	1.45–2.16 mmol/L
Children	4.5–5.5 mg/dL	1.45–1.78 mmol/L
Adults	2.4–4.7 mg/dL	0.78–1.50 mmol/L
Critical Values	**<1 mg/dL**	**<0.32 mmol/L**

Phosphorus is measured in terms of phosphate; the results cannot be expressed in milliequivalents because different phosphate groups have different valences.

Interfering Factors

➤ Phosphate levels are higher in children because of bone growth and active bone formation.

➤ Values vary diurnally, being higher at night than in the morning.

➤ A number of drugs may alter serum phosphate levels (see Table 5–28, p. 283).

Table 5–28 ➤ DISORDERS AND DRUGS ASSOCIATED WITH ALTERED SERUM PHOSPHORUS/PHOSPHATE LEVELS

Increased Levels (Hyperphosphatemia)	Decreased Levels (Hypophosphatemia)
DISORDERS	
Diabetic ketoacidosis	Recovery phase of diabetic ketoacidosis
Renal failure	Renal tubular acidosis
Vitamin D intoxication	Hypocalcemia
Hypercalcemia	Vitamin D deficiency
Prolonged immobilization	Hyperparathyroidism
Hypoparathyroidism	Carbohydrate ingestion
Pseudohypoparathyroidism	Malnutrition
Bone growth or active bone formation	Malabsorption syndromes
Hyperthyroidism	Hypothyroidism
Acromegaly	Hypopituitarism
Sarcoidosis	Alcoholism
Pyloric obstruction	Prolonged vomiting and diarrhea
Milk-alkali syndrome	
DRUGS	
Sodium phosphate	Acetazolamide (Diamox)
Heparin	Aluminum hydroxide
Phenytoin (Dilantin)	Insulin
Posterior pituitary injection (Pituitrin)	Epinephrine
Androgens	

➤ Hemolysis of the sample may cause falsely elevated values resulting from release of phosphate from red blood cells.

Indications for Serum Phosphorus/ Phosphate (P) Test

➤ Support for diagnosing disorders associated with altered phosphorus/phosphate levels, especially bone disorders, parathyroid disorders, renal disease, and alcoholism (see Table 5–28)
➤ Monitoring of the effects of renal failure on phosphorus levels, which are usually increased in the disorder
➤ Support for identification of the cause of growth abnormalities in children
➤ Monitoring for the effects of various drugs on serum phosphate levels (see Table 5–28)

Nursing Care Before the Procedure

Client preparation is the same as that for any study involving the collection of a peripheral blood sample (see Appendix I).

➤ Because many drugs may alter serum phosphorus/phosphate levels, a medication history should be obtained. It is recommended that any drugs that may alter test results be withheld for 12 to 24 hours before the test, although this practice should be confirmed with the person ordering the study.

The Procedure

A venipuncture is performed and the sample collected in a red-topped tube. The sample should be handled gently to avoid hemolysis, which may falsely elevate levels, and transported promptly to the laboratory.

Nursing Care After the Procedure

Care and assessment after the procedure are the same as for any study involving the collection of a peripheral blood sample.

➤ Resume any medications withheld before the test.

➤ *Increased levels:* Note and report increased levels (hyperphosphatemia) and associated calcium levels. Instruct client to avoid foods high in phosphorus (milk and dairy products, poultry, fish, grain cereals).

➤ *Decreased levels:* Note and report decreased levels (hypophosphatemia) in relation to calcium levels. Instruct client to include foods and fluids high in phosphorus, as already listed.

➤ **Critical values:** Notify the physician at once of levels less than 1 mg/dL.

SERUM MAGNESIUM (Mg, Mg^{++})

Magnesium (Mg, Mg^{++}) is an essential nutrient found in bone and muscle. In the blood, magnesium is most abundant in the red blood cells, with relatively little found in the serum. Magnesium functions in (1) control of sodium, potassium, calcium, and phosphorus; (2) utilization of carbohydrates, lipids, and proteins; and (3) activation of enzyme systems that enable B vitamins to function. Magnesium also increases intestinal absorption of calcium and is required for bone and cartilage formation. It is essential for oxidative phosphorylation, nucleic acid synthesis, and blood clotting.

Magnesium is so abundant in foods that dietary deficiency is rare. Decreased serum magnesium levels are seen, however, in chronic alcoholism. Elevated levels most commonly occur in renal failure. A variety of other disorders and drugs also are associated with altered magnesium levels (Table 5–29). Altered magnesium levels are associated with cardiac dysrhythmias, especially decreased levels, which may lead to excessive ventricular irritability.

Reference Values

	Conventional Units	**SI Units**
Newborns	1.4–2.9 mEq/L	0.58–1.19 mmol/L
Children	1.6–2.6 mEq/L	0.65–1.07 mmol/L
Adults	1.5–2.5 mEq/L	0.61–1.03 mmol/L
	1.8–3.0 mg/dL	0.74–1.23 mmol/L
Critical Values	**<1 mg/dL or >4.9 mg/dL**	**<0.41 or >2.02 mmol/L**

Interfering Factors

➤ A number of drugs may alter serum magnesium levels (see Table 5–29, p. 285).

Table 5–29 ➤ DISORDERS AND DRUGS ASSOCIATED WITH ALTERED SERUM MAGNESIUM LEVELS	
Increased Levels (Hypermagesemia)	**Decreased Levels (Hypomagnesemia)**
DISORDERS	
Addison's disease	Hyperaldosteronism
Adrenalectomy	Hypokalemia
Renal failure	Hypocalcemia
Diabetic ketoacidosis	Diabetic ketoacidosis (resolving)
Dehydration	Alcoholism, cirrhosis
Hypothyroidism	Hyperthyroidism
Hyperparathyroidism	Hypoparathyroidism
	Acute pancreatitis
	Gastrointestinal loss (vomiting, diarrhea, nasogastric suction, fistula)
	Malabsorption syndromes
	Malnutrition
	Nephrotic syndrome
	Toxemia of pregnancy
	High-phosphate diet
DRUGS	
Antacids and laxatives containing magnesium	Thiazide diuretics
Salicylates	Ethacrynic acid (Edecrin)
Lithium carbonate	Calcium gluconate
	Amphotericin B
	Neomycin
	Insulin
	Aldosterone
	Ethanol

➤ Because magnesium is found in red blood cells, hemolysis of the sample may lead to falsely elevated values.

Indications for Serum Magnesium (Mg, Mg^{++}) Test

Determination of magnesium balance in renal failure and chronic alcoholism
➤ Evaluation of known or suspected disorders associated with altered magnesium levels (see Table 5–29)
➤ Evaluation of cardiac dysrhythmias to determine whether altered serum magnesium level is contributing to the problem (i.e., decreased magnesium levels may lead to excessive ventricular irritability)
➤ Monitoring of the effects of various drugs on serum magnesium levels (see Table 5–29)

Nursing Care Before the Procedure

Client preparation is the same as that for any study involving the collection of a peripheral blood sample (see Appendix I).
➤ Because many drugs may alter serum magnesium levels, a medication history should be obtained. It is recommended that those drugs that may alter

test results be withheld for 12 to 24 hours before the test, although this practice should be confirmed with the person ordering the study.

The Procedure

A venipuncture is performed and the sample collected in a red-topped tube. The sample should be handled gently to avoid hemolysis, which may falsely elevate levels, and transported promptly to the laboratory.

Nursing Care After the Procedure

Care and assessment after the procedure are the same as for any study involving the collection of a peripheral blood sample.

➤ Resume any medications withheld before the test.

➤ *Increased levels:* Note and report increased levels. Assess for symptoms associated with hypermagnesemia, such as a decrease in muscle activity, which can affect respiration and lead to respiratory arrest and coma. Instruct client to avoid foods high in magnesium (meats, fish, whole grains, green vegetables) and medications containing magnesium (antacids or laxatives).

➤ *Decreased levels:* Note and report decreased levels. Assess for symptoms of hypomagnesemia, such as weakness, tremors, paresthesia, and tetany, which can lead to convulsions. Assess for decreases in potassium, sodium, and calcium. Administer ordered magnesium replacement. Instruct client to eat foods high in magnesium, as already listed.

➤ *Critical values:* Notify the physician at once of levels less than 1.0 mg/dL or greater than 4.9 mg/dL.

SERUM OSMOLALITY

Osmolality refers to the concentration of solutes in plasma or serum (particle number) or in urine (number of particles). Osmolality affects the movement of fluids across body membranes and the kidney's ability to concentrate or dilute the urine. Dehydration causes an increase in osmolality, and overhydration causes a decrease. Increased osmolality causes an increase in antidiuretic hormone (ADH) secretion, which results in increased reabsorption of water by the kidneys, increased concentration in urine, and decreased concentration in serum. This lower concentration in serum osmolality normally reduces ADH secretion, which then decreases water reabsorption by the kidneys and excretion of diluted urine. Urine is normally more concentrated than plasma; the ratio of urine to serum osmolality ranges from 1 : 1 to 3 : 1 in normal states. A decrease in the 1 : 1 ratio is seen in fluid overload or in diabetes insipidus, and a ratio that does not rise above 1.2 : 1.0 indicates a loss of renal concentration function.[57]

Serum osmolality is mostly used to monitor fluid and electrolyte balance; urine osmolality is used to monitor the concentrating ability of the kidneys and fluid and electrolyte balance. Decreased levels in serum osmolality are seen in fluid excess or overhydration, hyponatremia, and syndrome of inappropriate ADH (SIADH) secretion. Decreased levels in urine osmolality are seen in diabetes insipidus, excess fluid intake or overhydration, hypokalemia, hypercalcemia, and severe renal disease. Increased levels in serum osmolality are seen in dehydration, hypercalcemia, hypernatremia, hyperglycemia, diabetes insipidus, ketosis, severe renal disease, alcohol ingestion, and mannitol therapy. Increased levels in urine osmolality are seen in Addison's disease, SIADH, hypernatremia, shock or acidotic states, and CHF.

Reference Values

	Conventional Units	**SI Units**
Children	270–290 mOsm/kg	270–290 mmol/kg
Adults	280–300 mOsm/kg	280–300 mmol/kg
Critical Values	**<240 mOsm or >360 mOsm**	**<240 or >360 mmol/kg**

Interfering Factors

➤ A delay of longer than 10 hours in testing the specimen can affect test results.
➤ Osmotic diuretics and mineralocorticoids can affect test results.
➤ Improper technique such as tourniquet in place for an extended time can cause hemostasis.

Indications for Serum Osmolality Test

➤ Screening for alcohol ingestion revealed by increase in osmolality level as the alcohol level in the blood is increased
➤ Monitoring fluid and electrolyte balance (especially sodium) and determining a state of dehydration or overhydration
➤ Evaluating ADH secretion or suppression
➤ Monitoring IV fluid replacement therapy to prevent fluid excess or overload
➤ Evaluating the effect of renal dialysis therapy and course of renal failure

Nursing Care Before the Procedure

Client preparation is the same as that for any study involving the collection of a peripheral blood sample (see Appendix I).
➤ Obtain a history of conditions affecting renal function, a medication regimen, and the results of an electrolyte panel. Any medications that may affect test results should be withheld, although this practice should be confirmed with the person ordering the study.
➤ Inform the client that a urine specimen can be collected, tested, and compared with the results of the blood test.

The Procedure

A venipuncture is performed and the sample collected in a red-topped tube. The sample should be handled gently to avoid hemolysis or hemostasis and transported promptly to the laboratory.

Nursing Care After the Procedure

Care and assessment after the procedure are the same as for any study involving the collection of a peripheral blood sample.
➤ Resume any medications withheld before the test.
➤ *Increased levels:* Note and report increased levels. Assess for symptoms associated with dehydration, such as thirst, dry skin and mucous membranes,

and poor skin turgor. Assess relationship to urine osmolality and electrolyte panel. Prepare to increase fluid intake orally or IV.

➤ *Decreased levels:* Note and report decreased levels. Assess for symptoms associated with overhydration such as edema, weight gain, dyspnea, cough, and venous distention. Assess relationship to urine osmolality and electrolyte panel. Administer ordered medications such as diuretic therapy.

➤ **Critical values:** Notify physician at once of levels less than 240 mOsm or greater than 360 mOsm.

ARTERIAL BLOOD GASES (ABGs)

Arterial blood gas (ABG) determinations are made not only to determine levels of actual blood gases (i.e., oxygen and carbon dioxide) but also to assess the client's overall acid-base balance. Thus, ABG levels may indicate hypoxia, hypercapnia or hypocapnia, acidosis, alkalosis, and physiological compensation for acid-base imbalance. The components of an ABG determination are as follows:

1. pH reflects the number of hydrogen ions in the body and is influenced primarily by the ratio of bicarbonate ions (HCO_3^-) to carbonic acid (H_2CO_3), which is essentially carbon dioxide (CO_2), in the blood. The normal HCO_3^- to CO_2 ratio is 20:1. When the hydrogen ion concentration increases (acidosis), the pH falls; when the hydrogen ion concentration decreases (alkalosis), the pH rises. Bicarbonate levels are regulated by the kidneys, whereas carbon dioxide levels are controlled by the lungs. Both the lungs and the kidneys respond to alterations in pH levels by either retaining or excreting carbon dioxide and bicarbonate, respectively.

2. pO_2 indicates the partial pressure of oxygen in the blood. When oxygen levels are lower than normal, the client is hypoxic. Hypoxemia may be caused by either low cardiac output or impaired lung function.

3. pCO_2 indicates the partial pressure of carbon dioxide in the blood, which is regulated by the lungs. Except in cases of compensation for metabolic acid-base imbalances, elevated levels (hypercapnia, hypercarbia) indicate impaired gas exchange in the lungs so that excess CO_2 is not eliminated. Decreased levels (hypocapnia, hypocarbia) indicate increased loss of CO_2 through the lungs (hyperventilation).

4. HCO_3^- indicates the bicarbonate ion concentration in the blood, which is regulated by the kidneys. Altered levels are associated with metabolic acid-base imbalances or reflect response to respiratory alterations in CO_2 levels.

5. O_2 saturation (O_2 Sat, SaO_2) indicates the oxygen content of the blood expressed as percent of oxygen capacity (the amount of oxygen the blood could carry if all of the hemoglobin were fully saturated with oxygen). If the blood is 50 percent saturated, for example, the oxygen content is one-half of the oxygen capacity.

6. Base excess (BE) usually indicates the difference between the normal serum bicarbonate (HCO_3^-) level and the client's bicarbonate level. Positive values indicate excess bicarbonate relative to normal values, whereas negative values indicate decreased HCO_3^- levels.

Reference Values

	Conventional Units	**SI Units**
pH		
Newborns	7.32–7.49	
Adults	7.35–7.45	
pO_2		
Newborns	60–70 mm Hg	
Adults	75–100 mm Hg	
pCO_2	35–45 mm Hg	
HCO_3^-		
Newborns	20–26 mEq/L	20–26 mmol/L
Adults	22–26 mEq/L	22–26 mmol/L
O_2 saturation	96–100%	
Base excess	+1 to −2	
Critical Values		
pH	**<7.2 or >7.6**	
pO_2		
Infants	**<37 mm Hg or >92 mm Hg**	
Adults	**<40 mm Hg**	
pCO_2	**<20 mm Hg or >70 mm Hg**	
HCO_3^-	**<10 mEq/L or >40 mEq/L**	**<10 mmol or >40 mmol/L**
O_2 saturation	**<60%**	

Interfering Factors

➤ Fever may falsely elevate pO_2 and pCO_2; hypothermia may lower them.
➤ Suctioning of respiratory passages within 20 to 30 minutes of the test may alter results. Excessive heparin in the sample will lower pH and pCO_2.
➤ Exposure of the sample to atmospheric air (e.g., air bubbles in the sample) may alter results. Exposure of the sample to room temperature for more than 2 minutes may alter test results.

Indications for Arterial Blood Gases (ABGs) Test

➤ Evaluation of the effectiveness of pulmonary ventilation in maintaining adequate oxygenation and in removing carbon dioxide, especially in disorders such as chronic pulmonary disease, neurologic insults, and drug intoxication
➤ Evaluation of the effectiveness of cardiac output in maintaining adequate oxygenation, especially in shock and acute myocardial infarction
➤ Determination of the need for oxygen therapy (Oxygen is generally indicated if the pO_2 is 70 mm Hg or less, except in pulmonary disorders characterized by chronic hypoxemia in which lower oxygen levels may be tolerated by the client without supplemental oxygen.)
➤ Determination of respiratory failure, which is defined as a pO_2 of 50 mm Hg or less with a pCO_2 of 50 mm Hg or more
➤ Determination of acid-base balance, type of imbalance, and degree of compensation (see Table 5–26, p. 278)

➤ Determination of need for mechanical ventilation (For example, elevated or rising pCO_2 levels may indicate the need for mechanical ventilation, especially when pO_2 is decreased.)

➤ Evaluation of effectiveness of mechanical ventilation and indication for modification of ventilator settings

➤ Evaluation of response to weaning from mechanical ventilation

Nursing Care Before the Procedure

Explain to the client:

➤ That repeat determinations may be necessary until cardiopulmonary function or acid-base balance, or both, are stabilized

➤ The method and site for obtaining the sample (e.g., arterial puncture or arterial line sample)

➤ Any anticipated discomforts (Arterial punctures cause a brief, sharp pain unless a local anesthetic is used.)

➤ That if an arterial puncture is performed, it will be necessary to maintain digital pressure on the puncture site for 5 minutes or more, after which a pressure dressing will be applied

Prepare the client for the procedure.

➤ Take the client's temperature. Fever may falsely elevate pO_2 and pCO_2; hypothermia may lower them.

➤ The client should not have had a respiratory therapy treatment, been suctioned, or had ventilator settings changed less than 20 to 30 minutes before the sample is obtained.

➤ If the test is being conducted to determine the need for oxygen therapy or response to weaning from mechanical ventilation, the client should be off oxygen, off mechanical ventilation, or on a weaning mode for a preset time, which is specified by the person ordering the test.

➤ If the sample is to be obtained by radial artery puncture, the Allen test should be performed to assess patency of the ulnar artery; in the event that thrombosis involving the radial artery occurs after the puncture:

• Extend the client's wrist over a rolled towel or similar support.

• Ask the client to clench the fist; if the client cannot clench the fist, elevate the hand above heart level.

• Apply digital pressure over both radial and ulnar arteries.

• Ask the client to unclench the fist while pressure is maintained on the arteries.

• Observe the palm for blanching, which is the expected response.

• Release pressure on the ulnar artery while continuing to maintain pressure on the radial artery.

• Observe the palm for returning pinkness, which is a positive result.

• If the palm remains blanched or if return of pinkness takes longer than approximately 5 seconds (a negative result), do not use the wrist for arterial punctures.

• Inform the client's physician of a negative response to the Allen test.

The Procedure

The procedure varies slightly with the method for obtaining the sample.

Arterial puncture. A blood gas collection kit is obtained. If prepackaged kits are not available, obtain a 3-mL syringe, heparin (usually in the concentration of 100 U/mL), 20-gauge or 21-gauge needles, povidone-iodine or alcohol swabs or sponges, gauze pads, and tape. Fill a plastic or paper cup or a small plastic bag about halfway with ice.

If the syringe is not preheparinized, draw approximately 1 mL of heparin into the syringe, pull the plunger back to about the 3-mL line, and rotate the barrel. Then expel all except approximately 0.1 mL of heparin and change the needle. Excess heparin in the syringe will lower the pH and pCO_2 of the sample.

Palpate the artery to be used. The radial artery is usually the most accessible, but the brachial or the femoral artery also may be used. If the radial artery is to be used, extend the client's wrist over a rolled towel or similar support.

Cleanse the site with povidone-iodine and allow to dry. It is recommended by some that the iodine solution be removed with an alcohol swab before arterial puncture. If the client is allergic to iodine, use only alcohol to prepare the site. Some authorities also advocate anesthetizing the puncture site with a small amount of 1 percent lidocaine (Xylocaine).

Using the heparinized syringe with needle attached, puncture the artery. A 45-degree angle is used for radial artery punctures; a 60- to 90-degree angle is used for brachial arteries. A 90-degree angle is generally used for femoral artery punctures. Advance the needle until blood begins to enter the syringe; it should not be necessary to pull back on the plunger. After 2 to 3 mL of blood have been obtained, withdraw the needle and immediately apply firm pressure to the puncture site with a sterile gauze pad. Inform the client that the discomfort felt after the puncture will disappear in a few minutes.

Meanwhile, expel any air or air bubbles from the syringe, because mixing with atmospheric air may alter test results. The needle may be plugged by inserting it into a rubber cap, or it may be removed and the rubber cap supplied in the blood gas collection kit placed on the hub of the syringe. The sample is then placed in ice to inhibit metabolic blood activity; failure to do this within 2 minutes of collecting the sample will alter test results.

The sample is sent immediately for analysis. On the ABG request form or sample label, note the time the sample was collected, the client's temperature, and whether the client was breathing room air, receiving oxygen, or using mechanical ventilation.

Arterial line sample. See Appendix III, "Indwelling Devices and Atrial/Venous Catheters."

Nursing Care After the Procedure

➤ For arterial punctures, maintain digital pressure on the site for 5 minutes and then apply a sterile pressure dressing. If the client is receiving anticoagulants or has bleeding tendencies, apply digital pressure for 10 to 15 minutes.

➤ Observe the arterial puncture site for bleeding or hematoma formation every 5 to 10 minutes for ½ hour after the pressure dressing is applied.

➤ Check for presence of pulses distal to the site when performing site observations, if the brachial or the femoral artery was used.

➤ Check for signs of nerve impairment distal to the site.

➤ Provide support when test findings are revealed and if repeated or serial testing is necessary in acute conditions.

➤ Evaluate the results of pH with electrolytes (particularly hypokalemia or hyperkalemia) and oxygen, carbon dioxide, and bicarbonate associated with respiratory or metabolic acidosis or alkalosis.

➤ Assess respiratory pattern, level of consciousness, neuromuscular irritability, fluid and electolyte imbalances, and symptoms of impaired tissue perfusion as a result of hypoxia, any of which can be associated with abnormal ABGs.

➤ Notify the physician at once of critical value levels.

VITAMINS AND TRACE MINERALS

Vitamins are essential organic substances that perform various metabolic functions. Vitamins cannot be synthesized in adequate amounts by the body and, therefore, inadequate dietary intake causes deficiency diseases. Vitamins are classified as fat-soluble and water-soluble. The fat-soluble vitamins are vitamins A, D, E, and K. Because they are stored in the body, excessive ingestion of exogenous fat-soluble vitamins may cause abnormally elevated levels. Vitamin C and the B-complex vitamins are water soluble and are not stored in the body. The B-complex vitamins include B_1 (thiamine), which is involved in carbohydrate metabolism; B_2 (riboflavin), which is involved in the transport of oxidative metabolism and fatty acids; B_3 (niacin), which is involved in the transport of cellular respiration; and B_6 (pyridoxine), which is involved as a cofactor of enzymes and in the conversion of tryptophan to nicotinic acid. A vitamin B_6 deficiency causes beriberi, and a vitamin B_3 deficiency causes pellagra.

For diagnostic purposes, blood levels of vitamins A and C and a metabolite of vitamin D are measured. Vitamin B_{12} and folic acid also are measured in studies pertaining to hematologic function (see Chap. 1).

VITAMIN A

Vitamin A is obtained from foods of animal origin, such as eggs, milk, butter, and liver. Its precursor, carotene, a yellowish pigment, is obtained from yellow or orange vegetables and fruits and from leafy green vegetables.

Vitamin A promotes normal vision by permitting visual adaptation to light and dark, and it prevents night blindness (xerophthalmia). It also contributes to the growth of bone, teeth, and soft tissues; supports the formation of thyroxine; maintains epithelial cellular membranes; aids in spermatogenesis; and maintains the integrity of skin and mucous membranes as barriers to infection.

Reference Values

	Conventional Units	**SI Units**
Vitamin A	65–275 IU/dL	—
	0.15–0.60 mg/mL	0.52–2.09 μmol/L
Carotene		
Infants	0–40 μg/dL	0–0.7 μmol/L
Children	40–130 μg/dL	0.7–2.4 μmol/L
Adults	50–300 μg/dL	0.9–5.5 μmol/L

Interfering Factors

➤ Pregnancy and oral contraceptive use may lead to falsely elevated levels, as may hyperlipidemia, hypercholesterolemia of diabetes, myxedema, and nephritis.

➤ Excessive ingestion of mineral oil, low-fat diets, and liver disease may lead to decreased levels.

➤ Failure to follow dietary and drug restrictions before the test may alter results.

➤ Excessive exposure of the sample to light may alter results.

Indications for Vitamin A and Carotene Test

➤ Evaluation of skin disorders, with vitamin A deficiency a possible cause

➤ Support for diagnosing xerophthalmia (night blindness) as indicated by decreased levels

➤ Suspected vitamin A deficiency caused by fat malabsorption or biliary tract disease

➤ Support for diagnosing excessive vitamin A or carotene ingestion, or both, as indicated by elevated blood levels

Nursing Care Before the Procedure

General client preparation is the same as that for any study involving collection of a peripheral blood sample (see Appendix I).

➤ For this test, the client should fast for 8 hours before the study. Water is not restricted.

➤ Vitamin supplements containing vitamin A should be withheld for at least 24 hours before the test.

The Procedure

A venipuncture is performed and the sample collected in a red-topped tube. The sample should be covered to protect it from light, which may alter test results; handled gently to avoid hemolysis; and sent promptly to the laboratory.

Nursing Care After the Procedure

Care and assessment after the procedure are the same as for any test involving the collection of a peripheral blood sample.

➤ Resume usual diet.

➤ Vitamin supplements may be resumed pending test results.

➤ *Decreased level:* Note and report symptoms of deficiency or decreased level. Administer ordered vitamin A supplement orally, and instruct client to eat foods high in vitamin A to correct deficiency.

➤ *Increased level:* Note and report symptoms of excesses or increased level. Discontinue the oral or topical medication administered for acne or other skin conditions.

VITAMIN C

Vitamin C (ascorbic acid) functions in many metabolic processes, especially in those related to collagen formation and the stress response. In addition, vitamin

C helps to maintain capillary strength, facilitates the release of iron from ferritin for hemoglobin formation and red blood cell maturation, and may maintain the integrity of the amniotic sac.

Elevated vitamin C levels are associated with excessive intake of the vitamin within 24 hours of the test. Decreased intake produces scurvy with low vitamin C levels.

Reference Values

	Conventional Units	**SI Units**
Children	0.6–1.6 mg/dL	34–91 μmol/L
Adults	0.2–2.0 mg/dL	11–113 μmol/L

Interfering Factors

➤ Excessive intake of vitamin C within 24 hours of the test will produce elevated levels.

➤ Failure to follow dietary restrictions before the test may alter results.

Indications for Vitamin C Test

➤ Evaluation of the effects of major stressors (e.g., pregnancy, major surgery, burns, infections, malignancies) on vitamin C levels

➤ Evaluation of the effects of malabsorption syndromes on vitamin C levels

➤ Evaluation of the effectiveness of therapy with vitamin C in treating deficiency states

Nursing Care Before the Procedure

General client preparation is the same as that for any study involving collection of a peripheral blood sample (see Appendix I).

➤ For this test, the client should fast from food for 8 hours beforehand.

➤ Vitamin C preparations also should be withheld for 24 hours before the study.

The Procedure

A venipuncture is performed and the sample collected in a black-topped tube. The sample is handled gently to avoid hemolysis and transported promptly to the laboratory.

Nursing Care After the Procedure

Care and assessment after the procedure are the same as for any test involving the collection of a peripheral blood sample.

➤ Resume usual diet.

➤ Vitamin C preparations may be resumed pending test results.

➤ *Decreased level:* Note and report symptoms of deficiency or decreased level such as bleeding and poor wound healing. Instruct client to eat foods high in vitamin C to correct deficiency. Administer oral vitamin C supplement in ordered dosage.

➤ *Increased level:* Note and report symptoms of excesses or increased level. Discontinue the oral intake to prevent overdose; high doses taken as a preventive treatment can cause renal calculi.

VITAMIN D

The form of vitamin D most easily and accurately measured is 25-hydroxy-cholecalciferol [vitamin D_3, $25(OH)D_3$, cholecalciferol], a monohydroxylated form that leaves the liver for subsequent dihydroxylation by the kidney. Indirect measurement of vitamin D by serum alkaline phosphatase, calcium, and phosphorus determinations preceded $25(OH)D_3$ assays and may still be used in the diagnosis of disorders of calcium metabolism.

Vitamin D aids in the maintenance of calcium-phosphorus balance and in the deposition of calcium and phosphorus in the bone. It also facilitates absorption of calcium and phosphorus from the small intestine and aids in the renal excretion of phosphorus.

Reference Values

	Conventional Units	**SI Units**
$25(OH)D_3$	0.7–3.3 IU/mL	
	10–55 ng/mL	25–100 pmol/L

Interfering Factors

➤ Excessive ingestion of vitamin D leads to elevated levels.
➤ Therapy with anticonvulsants and glucocorticoids may produce decreased levels.

Indications for Vitamin D Test

➤ Differential diagnosis of hypercalcemia caused by parathyroid adenoma or vitamin D toxicity
➤ Confirmation of vitamin D deficiency as the cause of bone disease
➤ Confirmation of vitamin D deficiency caused by malabsorption syndromes, hepatobiliary disease, and chronic renal failure
➤ Evidence of interference with vitamin D levels as a result of anticonvulsant or steroid therapy

Nursing Care Before the Procedure

Client preparation is the same as that for any study involving the collection of a peripheral blood sample.
➤ It is recommended that anticonvulsant and steroid medications be withheld for 24 hours before the test, although this practice should be confirmed by the person ordering the study.

The Procedure

A venipuncture is performed and the sample collected in a red-topped tube. The sample should be handled gently to avoid hemolysis and transported promptly to the laboratory.

Nursing Care After the Procedure

Care and assessment after the procedure are the same as for any study involving the collection of a peripheral blood sample.
➤ Resume medications withheld before the test.

➤ *Decreased level:* Note and report symptoms of deficiency or decreased level such as bone deformities. Instruct client to eat foods that are enriched with vitamin D. Administer ordered oral supplement.

➤ *Increased level:* Note and report symptoms of excesses or increased levels taken in medications or vitamin supplements, or both (intoxication, renal calculi, gastrointestinal intolerance). Discontinue the oral intake of vitamin D, and instruct client to avoid foods high in vitamin D.

TRACE MINERALS

Seven trace minerals are known to be essential to human function even though they are present in minute quantities in the body. These essential minerals are cobalt, copper, iodine, iron, manganese, molybdenum, and zinc.

Cobalt is a constituent of vitamin B_{12} and is essential to the formation of red blood cells. Copper participates in cytochrome oxidation of tissue cells for energy production, promotes absorption of iron from the intestines and transfer from tissues to plasma, and is essential to hemoglobin formation. It also promotes bone and brain tissue formation and supports the maintenance of myelin. Iodine is an essential component for the synthesis of thyroid hormones. Iron, which is discussed in Chapter 1, is an essential component of hemoglobin.

Manganese functions as a coenzyme in urea formation and in the metabolism of proteins, fats, and carbohydrates. Molybdenum facilitates the enzymatic action of xanthine oxidase and liver aldehyde oxidase in purine catabolism and functions in the formation of carboxylic acid. Zinc is an essential component of cellular enzymes such as alkaline phosphatase, carbonic anhydrase, lactic dehydrogenase, and carboxypeptidase, which function in protein and carbohydrate metabolism. It also aids in the storage of insulin, functions in deoxyribonucleic acid (DNA) replication, assists in carbon dioxide exchange, promotes body growth and sexual maturation, and may affect lymphocyte formation and cellular immunity.

Other trace minerals are found in the body, but their functions remain unclear. These minerals include chromium, fluorine, lithium, arsenic, cadmium, nickel, silicon, tin, and vanadium.

Deficiencies of trace minerals are likely only in individuals dependent on parenteral nutrition, because the normal diet provides adequate intake. Elevated blood levels are usually caused by environmental contamination, either in industrial settings or through water pollution.

Reference Values

	Conventional Units	**SI Units**
Cobalt	1 μg/dL	1.7 nmol/L
Copper	130–230 μg/dL	20.41–36.11 μmol/L
Iodine (protein-bound)	4–8 mg/dL	
Manganese	4–20 mg/dL	
Zinc	50–150 μg/dL	7.6–23.0 μmol/L
Chromium	0.3–0.85 μg/L	5.7–16.3 nmol/L

Indications for Trace Minerals Test

➤ Monitoring of response to parenteral nutrition, which may lead to deficiencies of trace minerals

➤ Suspected exposure to environmental toxins, which may be indicated by elevated levels of trace minerals

Nursing Care Before the Procedure

Client preparation is the same as that for any test involving the collection of a peripheral blood sample (see Appendix I).

The Procedure

A venipuncture is performed and the sample collected in a metal-free tube. The sample is handled gently to avoid hemolysis and transported immediately to the laboratory.

Nursing Care After the Procedure

Care and assessment after the procedure are the same as for any test involving the collection of a peripheral blood sample.

➤ *Abnormal values:* Note and report deficiency or decreased levels associated with anemia, poor wound healing, reduced sexual maturation, growth retardation, and the administration of total parenteral nutrition that can eliminate some trace minerals. Instruct client to eat foods high in trace minerals. Administer oral supplements as ordered.

DRUGS AND TOXIC SUBSTANCES

Blood levels of drugs are used to monitor attainment of therapeutic drug levels, compliance with therapeutic regimens, and potential excess dosing. They are also used in situations when accidental or deliberate drug overdose is suspected. In therapeutic situations, serial samples may be drawn to determine peak (highest) and trough (lowest) blood levels of drugs. Samples for peak drug levels are generally drawn within 30 to 60 minutes of drug administration. Trough levels are drawn immediately before the next dose of the drug is to be given. It is necessary to know as exactly as possible the time the drug was administered or ingested for accurate interpretation of test results.

Many potential toxins are present in the household and in industrial settings. Data regarding circulating levels of toxic substances may be used to diagnose either acute or chronic poisoning with metals or common commercial substances.

Reference Values

Therapeutic and toxic levels of various drugs are shown in Table 5–30. Toxic doses and effects of industrial and household toxins are listed in Table 5–31. For child values, refer to agency laboratory information.

Indications for Blood Levels of Drugs and Toxic Substances Test

➤ Determination of therapeutic levels of prescribed drugs, especially those with narrow therapeutic ranges or serious toxic effects, or both

Table 5–30 ➤ **BLOOD LEVELS OF DRUGS**

Drug	Peak Time	Duration of Action	Therapeutic Level	Toxic Level
Antibiotics				
Amikacin	IM: ½ hr			
	IV: 15 min	2 days	20–25 μg/mL	35 μg/mL
SI units			34–43 μmol/L	60 μmol/L
Gentamicin	IM: ½ hr	2 days	4–8 μg/mL	12 μg/mL
	IV: 15 min			
SI units			8.4–16.8 μmol/L	25.1 μmol/L
Kanamycin	½ hr	2 days	20–25 μg/mL	35 μg/mL
SI units			42–52 μmol/L	73 μmol/L
Streptomycin	½–1½ hr	5 days	25–30 μg/mL	>30 μg/mL
SI units				
Tobramycin	IV: 15 min	2 days	2–8 μg/mL	12 μg/mL
SI units			4–17 μmol/L	25 μmol/L
Anticonvulsants				
Barbiturates and barbiturate-related				
Amobarbital	IV: 30 sec	10–20 hr	7 μg/mL	30 μg/mL
SI units			30 μmol/L	132 μmol/L
Pentobarbital	IV: 30 sec	15 hr	4 μg/mL	15 μg/mL
SI units			18 μmol/L	66 μmol/L
Phenobarbital	15 min	80 hr	10 μg/mL	>55 μg/mL
SI units			43 μmol/L	>230 μmol/L
Primidone	PO: 3 hr	7–14 hr	1 μg/mL	>10 μg/mL
SI units			4 μmol/L	>45 μmol/L
Benzodiazepines				
Clonazepam (Klonopin)	1–4 hr	60 hr	5–70 ng/ml	>70 ng/mL
SI units			55–222 μmol/L	>222 μmol/L
Diazepam (Valium)	1–4 hr	1–2 days	5–70 ng/mL	>70 ng/mL
SI units			0.01–0.25 μmol/L	>0.25 μmol/L
Hydantoins				
Phenytoin (Dilantin)	3–12 hr	7–42 hr	10–20 μg/mL	>20 μg/mL
SI units			40–80 μmol/L	>80 μmol/L
Succinimides				
Ethosuximide (Zarontin)	1 hr	8 days	40–80 μg/mL	100 μg/mL
SI units			283–566 μmol/L	708 μmol/L
Miscellaneous				
Carbamazepine (Tegretol)	4 hr	2 days	2–10 μg/mL	12 μg/mL
SI units			8–42 μmol/L	50 μmol/L
Valproic acid (Depakene)	1–4 hr	24 hr	50–100 μg/mL	>100 μg/mL
SI units			350–700 μmol/L	>700 μmol/L
Bronchodilators				
Aminophylline/theophylline	PO: 2 hr	8–9 hr	10–18 μg/mL	>20 μg/mL
	IV: 15 min			

continued on page 299

Table 5–30 ➤ **BLOOD LEVELS OF DRUGS** *Continued*

Drug	Peak Time	Duration of Action	Therapeutic Level	Toxic Level
Cardiac drugs				
Disopyramide (Norpace)	PO: 2 hr	25–30 hr	2–4.5 µg/mL	>9 µg/mL
SI units			5.9–13 µmol/L	26 µmol/L
Quinidine	PO: 1 hr	20–30 hr	2.4–5 µg/mL	>6 µg/mL
	IV: immediate			
SI units			7–15 µmol/L	>18 µmol/L
Procainamide (Pronestyl)	PO: 1 hr	10–20 hr	4–8 µg/mL	>12 µg/mL
	IV: ½ hr			
SI units			17–35 µmol/L	>50 µmol/L
NAPA (*N*-acetyl procainamide, a procainamide metabolite)	—	—	2–8 µg/mL	>30 µg/mL
SI units			7–29 µmol/L	108 µmol/L
Lidocaine	IV: immediate	5–10 hr	2–6 µg/mL	>9 µg/mL
SI units			8–25 µmol/L	>38 µmol/L
Bretylium	15–30 min	6–8 hr	5–10 mg/kg	30 mg/kg
Verapamil	PO: 5 hr	8–10 hr	5–10 mg/kg	>15 mg/kg
	IV: 3–5 min	IV: ½–1 hr		
Diltiazem	PO: 2–3 hr	3–4 hr	50–200 ng/mL	>200 ng/mL
Nifedipine	1–3 hr	3–4 hr	5–10 mg	90 mg
Digitoxin	4 hr	30 days	10–25 ng/mL	30 ng/mL
SI units			13–33 nmol/L	39 nmol/L
Digoxin	2 hr	7 days	0.5–2 ng/mL	>2.5 ng/mL
SI units			0.6–2.5 nmol/L	>3.0 nmol/L
Phenytoin (Dilantin)	PO: 2 hr	96 hr	10–18 µg/mL	>20 µg/mL
SI units			40–71 µmol/L	>80 µmol/L
Quinidine	IV: 1 hr			
	—	—	2.3–5 µg/mL	>5 µg/mL
SI units			7–15 µmol/L	>15 µmol/L
Salicylates				
Aspirin	15 min	12–30 hr	2–20 mg/dL	>30 mg/dL
SI units			0.1–1.4 mmol/L	>2.1 mmol/L
			2–30 mg/dL	40 mg/dL
SI units			0.1–2.1 mmol/L	2.8 mmol/L
Narcotics				
Codeine	—	—	—	>0.005 mg/dL
SI units				>17 nmol/L
Hydromorphone (Dilaudid)	—	—	—	>0.1 mg/dL
SI units				>350 nmol/L
Methadone	—	—	—	>0.2 mg/dL
SI units				>6.46 µmol/L
Meperidine (Demerol)	—	—	—	>0.5 mg/dL
SI units				>20 µmol/L
Morphine	—	—	—	>0.005 mg/dL
Barbiturates				
Phenobarbital	—	—	10 µg/mL	55 µg/mL
SI units			43 µmol/L	230 µmol/L

continued on page 300

Table 5–30 ➤ **BLOOD LEVELS OF DRUGS** *Continued*

Drug	Peak Time	Duration of Action	Therapeutic Level	Toxic Level
Amobarbital	—	—	7 μg/mL	30 μg/mL
SI units			30 μmol/L	130 μmol/L
Pentobarbital	—	—	4 μg/mL	15 μg/mL
SI units			17 μmol/L	66 μmol/L
Secobarbital	—	—	3 μg/mL	10 μg/mL
SI units			12 μmol/L	42 μmol/L
Alcohols				
Ethanol	—	—	0.1 g/dL (legal level for intoxication)	100 mg/dL
Methanol	—	—	—	20 mg/dL
Psychiatric drugs				
Amitriptyline (Elavil)	—	—	100–250 ng/mL	>300 ng/mL
SI units			361–902 nmol/L	>1083 nmol/L
Imipramine (Tofranil)	—	—	100–250 ng/mL	>300 ng/mL
SI units			357–898 nmol/L	>1071 nmol/L
Lithium (Lithonate)	1–4 hr	—	0.8–1.4 mEq/L	1.5 mEq/L
SI units			0.8–1.4 μmol/L	1.5 μmol/L
Miscellaneous				
Acetaminophen	—	—	0–25 μg/mL	>150 μg/mL
SI units			0–170 μmol/L	>1000 μmol/L 4 hr after ingestion
Prochlorperazine	—	—	0.5 μg/mL	1.0 μg/mL
Bromides	—	—	75–150 mg/dL	>150 mg/dL
SI units			7–15 mmol/L	>15 mmol/L

➤ Evaluation of the degree of compliance with the therapeutic regimen
➤ Known or suspected drug overdose
➤ Known or suspected exposure to environmental toxins
➤ Evaluation of chronic exposure to industrial products known to be toxic

Nursing Care Before the Procedure

Client preparation is the same as that for any test involving the collection of a peripheral blood sample (see Appendix I).

The Procedure

A venipuncture is performed and the sample collected in a red-topped tube. The sample should be handled gently to avoid hemolysis and transported to the laboratory immediately. For drug levels, the name of the drug, dosage, and time administered or ingested should be noted on the laboratory request form.

Nursing Care After the Procedure

Care and assessment after the procedure are the same as for any test involving the collection of a peripheral blood sample.

Table 5–31 ➤ TOXIC DOSES AND EFFECTS OF INDUSTRIAL AND HOUSEHOLD TOXINS

Substance	Toxic Dose	Toxic Effects
Aniline	50 mg/kg	Methemoglobinemia, hepatotoxicity, nephrotoxicity
Arsenic/antimony	5 mg/kg	Gastric hemorrhage, shock
Barium salts	—	Bloody diarrhea, cardiac depression, muscle spasms, respiratory failure, renal failure
Benzene products	50 mg/kg	CNS depression, respiratory failure, cardiac arrest, bone marrow depression, liver damage
Bismuth	0.1–3.5 µg/L	Weakness, fever, anorexia, black gum line, renal damage
Cadmium	>41 ng/mL	Severe gastroenteritis, liver damage, acute renal failure; if inhaled as dust or fumes, pulmonary edema
Carbon tetrachloride	5–10 mL (total)	CNS depression, liver and kidney failure
Chlorate or bromate salts	50 mg/kg	Methemoglobinemia, intravascular hemolysis, acute renal failure
Cobalt	0.11–0.45 µg/L	Nerve damage, thyroid dysfunction
Copper salts	50 mg/kg	Generalized capillary damage, kidney and liver damage
Cyanide	>5 mg total (>0.5 mg/100 mL of blood)	Confusion, dyspnea, convulsions, death from respiratory failure
DDT	50 mg/kg	Fatigue, confusion, ataxia, convulsions, death from respiratory failure
2.4-D	—	Lethargy, diarrhea, cardiac arrest, hyperpyrexia, convulsions, coma
Ergot	5 mg/kg	Gastrointestinal inflammation, renal damage, gangrene of fingers and toes caused by persistent peripheral vasoconstriction
Ethylene glycol	>5 mg/kg	CNS depression, death from renal failure or respiratory paralysis
Iron salts	500 mg/kg	Bloody diarrhea, shock, liver damage
Fluoride	50 mg/kg (0.2–0.3 mg/dL of blood)	Hemorrhagic gastroenteritis, tremors, hypocalcemia, shock
Formaldehyde	500 mg/kg	Hemorrhagic gastroenteritis, renal failure, circulatory collapse
Hydrogen sulfide	0.1–0.2% in air	Death from respiratory paralysis

continued on page 302

Table 5–31 ➤ **TOXIC DOSES AND EFFECTS OF INDUSTRIAL AND HOUSEHOLD TOXINS** *Continued*

Substance	Toxic Dose	Toxic Effects
Sodium hypochlorite	Several ounces of household bleach	Edema of pharynx, glottis, larynx; perforation of esophagus or stomach, pulmonary edema from fumes
Iodine	5 mg/kg	Bloody diarrhea, renal damage; death from asphyxia or circulatory collapse
Ipecac, syrup or fluid extract	1–2 oz fluid extract (14 times more concentrated than syrup)	Shock caused by intractable vomiting and diarrhea, death from cardiac depression
Isopropyl alcohol	500 mg/kg	Severe CNS depression, death from respiratory failure or circulatory collapse
Kerosene	500 mg/kg if swallowed; few mL lethal if aspirated	Severe chemical pneumonitis, coma
Lead	30 g/kg (>120 μg/L blood level)	Gastrointestinal inflammation, liver and kidney damage, encephalopathy in children, paralysis of extremities, death from encephalopathy or peripheral vascular collapse
Lye, sodium and potassium hydroxide	10 g total dose may be fatal	Laryngeal or glottic edema, perforation of esophagus or stomach, severe diarrhea, shock, death
Mercury salts	5 mg/kg	*Acute:* Death from acute renal failure or peripheral vascular collapse *Chronic:* Progressive peripheral neuritis, death from renal failure
Naphthalene (mothballs)	5 g/kg	CNS excitement or depression, acute hemolytic anemia, convulsions
Nicotine	>5 mg/kg	CNS stimulation followed by depression; vomiting, diarrhea, dyspnea, death from respiratory paralysis
Oxalic acid	50 mg/kg	Shock caused by severe gastroenteritis, hypocalcemia, convulsions, renal damage, coma, death
Parathion/organophosphorus insecticides	>5 mg/kg	Vomiting, diarrhea, generalized muscle weakness, convulsions, coma, death, all caused by inhibition of acetylcholinesterase and accumulation of cholinesterase at myoneural junctions
Phosphorus	>5 mg/kg	Penetrating burns; liver, kidney, and cardiac damage

continued on page 303

Table 5–31 ➤ **TOXIC DOSES AND EFFECTS OF INDUSTRIAL AND HOUSEHOLD TOXINS** *Continued*

Substance	Toxic Dose	Toxic Effects
Quarternary ammonium germicides	5 mg/kg	CNS depression, dyspnea, death from asphyxia
Rotenone	50 mg/kg	Severe hypoglycemia, tremors, convulsions, respiratory stimulation followed by depression, death from respiratory arrest
Selenium	58–234 μg/L	Metallic taste, nausea, vomiting, headache, pulmonary disorders
Silver salts	3.5–35 g total dose	Bloody diarrhea, severe corrosion of the gastrointestinal tract, coma, convulsions, death
Strychnine	>5 mg/kg	Stimulation of spinal cord, tetanic convulsions, death in 1–3 hr (with the face fixed in a grin and the body arched in hyperextension) from anoxia
Thallium salts	5 mg/kg (>50 μg/L blood level)	Hemorrhagic gastroenteritis, encephalopathy (delirium, convulsions, coma), death
Turpentine	500 mg/kg	Aspiration pneumonitis, vomiting, diarrhea, CNS excitement (delirium), stupor, convulsions, coma, death from respiratory failure
Zinc	70–50 μg/L	Hypertension, tachycardia, nausea, vomiting, diarrhea, cough, metallic taste

➤ It may be necessary to withhold subsequent doses of drugs administered for therapeutic reasons until test results are available, but this practice should be confirmed with the person prescribing the medication.

➤ *Abnormal values:* Note and report both therapeutic and toxic values for the drug test performed. Notify the physician at once if any value is at a critical level. Prepare for immediate interventions to prevent cardiac arrest or other manifestations of toxicity, such as ECG monitoring, oxygen, or intubation and ventilation. Administer ordered antidote or other medications.

➤ *Long-term drug therapy:* Support client and instruct in long-term medication regimen, which symptoms to note and report, and when to discontinue the medication.

➤ *Medicolegal aspects:* Collection, delivery, possession, and transportation of the specimen should be witnessed by a legally responsible person, and the possession of it must remain unbroken from the time of collection to the completion of any legal court action (chain of evidence). Seal specimen to prevent tampering and label "Medicolegal Case." In some cases a number is used instead of a name for identification. Toxicology tests to determine abuse, suicide, intentional overdose, or suspected murder or attempted murder require these considerations.

Student Name _____ Class _____

Instructor _____ Date _____

CASE STUDY AND CRITICAL THINKING EXERCISE

1. Ms. Brown, age 44, is admitted to the ER. VS: T 102.8°F (39.2°C), P 134, R 28, BP 215/110. She is oriented but agitated and restless. History reveals that she had a subtotal thyroidectomy 10 days ago.

   a. What is this client's probable diagnosis?

   b. What specific lab tests do you anticipate to be ordered? What values do you expect in this client?

2. Ms. Brown is admitted to your unit for stabilization. On rounds she complains of tingling around her mouth. VS: T 100.5°F (38°C), P 92, R 18, BP 140/76.

   a. What complication may Ms. Brown be experiencing?

   b. What specific tests can you do to assess the situation?

3. Scott, a 17-year-old man, is admitted unconscious to the ER. VS: T 100°F (37.8°C), P 110, R 24, BP 100/60. ABG values are pH 7.18, HCO_3^- 12 mEq/L, pCO_2 30 mm Hg. Serum values are Na^+ 140, K^+ 5.5, Glu 760, BUN 18.

   a. What is this client's probable diagnosis?

   b. Calculate his serum osmolality.

   c. How are polydipsia, polyphagia, and polyuria (the 3 p's) associated with this problem?

   d. The nurse observes Scott's breathing and notes not only that the rate is rapid but also that it is unusually deep in inspiration and expiration. What do you interpret from these findings? Is this helpful in Scott's situation?

4. Ms. White is an elderly woman who was too ill to get out of bed for 2 days. She has a severe cough and has been unable to eat or drink during this time. On admission her laboratory values show Na^+ 156, K^+ 4.

   a. What is Ms. White's fluid problem?

   b. What clinical manifestations would you expect to find?

   c. What fluid therapies might you expect to be ordered?

5. Mr. Gray, a 45-year-old accountant, is brought to the ER. He is unconscious and a coworker reports that he has been very depressed lately. An empty pill bottle was found near his desk. Serum values are Na^+ 140, K^+ 4.4, Cl^- 100, pH 7.28, HCO_3^- 18 mEq/L, pCO_2 40 mm Hg.

   a. What is the primary acid-base disturbance?

   b. What is the probable cause?

References

1. Sacher, RA, and McPherson, RA: Widmann's Clinical Interpretation of Laboratory Tests, ed 10. FA Davis, Philadelphia, 1991, p 321.
2. Ibid, pp 322–323.
3. Ibid, p 323.
4. Ibid, p 324.
5. Ibid, p 323.
6. Ibid, p 325.
7. Ibid, p 605.
8. Ibid, p 611.
9. Ibid, p 326.
10. Ibid, pp 610–611.
11. Ibid, p 606.
12. Ibid, p 326.
13. Springhouse Corporation: Nurse's Reference Library, Diagnostics, ed 2. Springhouse, Springhouse, PA, 1986, p 242.
14. Fischbach, FT: A Manual of Laboratory Diagnostic Tests, ed 4. JB Lippincott, Philadelphia, 1992, p 303.
15. Sacher and McPherson, op cit, p 606.
16. Ibid, p 607.
17. Ibid, p 433.
18. Hillman, RS, and Finch, CA: Red Cell Manual, ed 6. FA Davis, Philadelphia, 1992, p 23.
19. Sacher and McPherson, op cit, p 328.
20. Ibid, p 329.
21. Ibid, pp 433–434.
22. Ibid, p 338.
23. Guyton, AC: Textbook of Medical Physiology, ed 6. WB Saunders, Philadelphia, 1981, pp 849–850.
24. Ibid, pp 856–857.
25. Sacher and McPherson, op cit, pp 332, 425.
26. Ibid, pp 397–398.
27. Ibid, pp 402–403.
28. Ibid, pp 400–401, 427–428.
29. Ibid, pp 406–409.
30. Ibid, pp 411–412.
31. Berkow, R (ed): The Merck Manual, ed 16. Merck Research Laboratories, Rahway, NJ, 1992, p 1839.
32. Sacher and McPherson, op cit, pp 405–406.
33. Ibid, pp 555–556.
34. Ibid, p 557.
35. Ibid, pp 557, 634.
36. Ibid, pp 583, 587, 590–591.

37. Ibid, pp 621–623.
38. Ibid, pp 617–627.
39. Ibid, pp 559–562.
40. Ibid, pp 582–583.
41. Guyton, op cit, pp 931–937, 984.
42. Sacher and McPherson, op cit, pp 585–586, 588.
43. Ibid, pp 586–587.
44. Ibid, pp 582–583, 590–592.
45. Ibid, pp 594, 598–601.
46. Ibid, pp 562, 577.

47. Ibid, pp 565–568.
48. Ibid, pp 572–573.
49. Ibid, pp 577–579.
50. Ibid, pp 631–632.
51. Ibid, pp 633–634.
52. Ibid, pp 603–604.
53. Ibid, p 604, 611.
54. Ibid, pp 367–368.
55. Ibid, pp 379, 383.
56. Ibid, pp 357, 596.
57. Ibid, pp 380–381.

Bibliography

Anderson, SC, and Cockayne, S: Clinical Chemistry: Concepts and Applications. WB Saunders, Philadelphia, 1992.

Byrne, CJ, et al: Laboratory Tests: Implications for Nursing Care, ed 2. Addison-Wesley, Menlo Park, CA, 1986.

Chernecky, CC, and Berger, BJ; Cullen, BN (ed): Laboratory Tests and Diagnostic Procedures, ed 2. WB Saunders, Philadelphia, 1996.

Corbett, JV: Laboratory Tests and Diagnostic Procedures with Nursing Diagnoses, ed 4. Appleton & Lange, Norwalk, CT, 1995.

Deglin, JH, and Vallerand, AH: Davis's Drug Guide for Nurses, ed 6. FA Davis, Philadelphia, 1999.

Henry, JB: Clinical Diagnosis and Management by Laboratory Methods, ed 19. WB Saunders, Philadelphia, 1996.

Kaplan, LA, and Pesce, AJ: Clinical Chemistry: Theory, Analysis, Correlation, ed 2. Mosby–Year Book, St Louis, 1989.

Kee, JL: Handbook of Laboratory and Diagnostic Tests with Nursing Implications, ed 3. Appleton & Lange, Norwalk, CT, 1997.

Lewis, SM, et al (eds): Medical-Surgical Nursing: Assessment and Management of Clinical Problems, ed 4. Mosby–Year Book, St Louis, 1995.

Mayne, P: Clinical Chemistry in Diagnosis & Treatment, ed 6. Edward Arnold Publication, London, 1994.

Pagana, KD, and Pagana, TJ: Diagnostic and Laboratory Test Reference, ed 3. Mosby–Year Book, St Louis, 1996.

Porth, CM: Pathophysiology: Concepts of Altered Health States, ed 4, JB Lippincott, Philadelphia, 1993.

Ravel, RR: Clinical Laboratory Medicine: Clinical Applications of Laboratory Data, ed 6. Mosby–Year Book, St Louis, 1994.

Ray, OS, and Ksir, C: Drugs, Society and Human Behavior, ed 6. Mosby–Year Book, St Louis, 1992.

Springhouse Corporation: Clinical Laboratory Tests: Values and Implications, ed 2. Springhouse, Springhouse, PA, 1995.

Tietz, NW (ed): Clinical Guide to Laboratory Tests, ed 3. WB Saunders, Philadelphia, 1995.

Tietz, NW (ed): Fundamentals of Clinical Chemistry. WB Saunders, Philadelphia, 1987.

Tilkian, SM: Clinical and Nursing Implications of Laboratory Tests, ed 5. Mosby–Year Book, St Louis, 1995.

Whaley, LF: Nursing Care of Infants and Children, ed 4. Mosby–Year Book, St Louis, 1991.

6

Studies of Urine

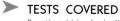 **TESTS COVERED**

Routine Urinalysis (UA), *310*

Clearance Tests and Creatinine
  Clearance, *332*

Tubular Function Tests and
  Phenolsulfonphthalein (PSP)
  Test, *334*

Concentration Tests and Dilution
  Tests, *336*

Electrolytes, *341*

Pigments, *345*

Enzymes, *349*

Hormones and Their
  Metabolites, *352*

Proteins, *364*

Vitamins and Minerals, *368*

Microbiologic Examination
  of Urine, *369*

Cytologic Examination of Urine, *370*

Drug Screening Tests of Urine, *371*

OVERVIEW OF URINE FORMATION AND ANALYSIS

Because urine results from filtration of blood, many of the substances carried in the blood are also found in the urine. The nature and amount of the substances present in urine reflect ongoing physiological processes in health and disease states. The comparative ease of obtaining urine samples ensures the continued use of urine studies as an aid to diagnosis.[1]

Urine is an ultrafiltrate of plasma from which substances essential to the body are reabsorbed and through which substances that are not needed are excreted. Normally, 25 percent of the cardiac output perfuses the kidneys each minute. This perfusion results in the production of 180 L of glomerular filtrate per day, 90 percent of which is reabsorbed. In addition to water, substances reabsorbed include glucose, amino acids, and electrolytes. Substances excreted from the body include urea, uric acid, creatinine, and ammonia. The major electrolytes lost are chloride, sodium, and potassium. Other substances found in urine include pigments, enzymes, hormones and their metabolites, vitamins, minerals, and drugs. Red blood cells, white blood cells, epithelial cells, crystals, mucus, and bacteria may also be found in urine.[2,3]

In general, the concentration of most substances normally found in the urine reflects the plasma levels of the substances. If the plasma concentration of a substance is high, more of it is lost in the urine in the presence of normal renal function. Conversely, if the plasma concentration is abnormally low, the substance is reabsorbed. The concentration of substances found in the urine is affected also by factors such as dietary intake, body metabolism, endocrine function, physical activity, body position, and time of day.[4] For these reasons, results of urine tests must be evaluated in relation to the client's history and current health status. For some studies, urine specimens are collected at certain

309

times of day or over 24-hour periods. Dietary intake may also be modified for certain studies.

Commercially prepared reagent dipsticks are available to perform simple and quick testing in hospitals, clinics, physicians' offices, and homes. They are used for routine screening of single or multiple urinary evaluations of protein, glucose, ketones, hemoglobin, urobilinogen, and nitrites as well as pH. The strips contain reagents that react with specific substances by changing color. Color change is observed and compared to a color chart for the presence of abnormal levels of substances. Special care in their use is required to prevent inaccurate results, and confirmation of quantitative tests is appropriate if results from the dipstick testing reveal abnormalities.

Urine samples for more exhaustive laboratory testing may be obtained through a variety of methods. These are described in Appendix II. Urine studies include routine urinalysis, clearance tests, tubular function tests, concentration tests, and analyses for specific substances such as electrolytes, pigments, enzymes, hormones and their metabolites, protein, and vitamins and minerals. Microbiologic and cytologic examination of urine may also be performed.

ROUTINE URINALYSIS (UA)

A routine urinalysis (UA) has two major components: (1) macroscopic analysis and (2) microscopic analysis. Macroscopic analysis includes examining the urine for overall physical and chemical characteristics. The microscopic component of a UA involves examining the sample for formed elements, also termed "urinary sediment."

Urine samples for routine analysis are best collected first thing in the morning. Urine that has accumulated in the bladder overnight is more concentrated, thus allowing detection of substances that may not be present in more dilute random samples.[5] The sample should be examined within 1 hour of collection. If this is not possible, the sample may be refrigerated until it can be examined. Failure to observe these precautions may lead to invalid results. If, for example, the sample is allowed to stand for long periods without refrigeration, the glucose level may drop and the ketones may dissipate. The color of the urine may also deepen. Similarly, urinary sediment begins deteriorating within 2 hours of sample collection. If bacteria are present, they may multiply if the sample is neither examined promptly nor refrigerated. Also, the pH of the sample may be altered, rendering it more alkaline. If the sample is exposed to light for long periods of time, bilirubin and urobilinogen may be oxidized.[6]

MACROSCOPIC ANALYSIS

Color

The color of urine is mainly a result of the presence of the pigment urochrome, which is produced through endogenous metabolic processes. Because urochrome is normally produced at a fairly constant rate, the intensity of the yellow color may indirectly indicate urine concentration and the client's state of hydration.[7,8] Pale urine with a low specific gravity may occur, for example, in a normal person after high fluid intake. It should be noted, however, that an individual with uncontrolled or untreated diabetes may also produce pale urine. The pale urine in this case is caused by osmotic diuresis resulting from the excessive glucose load. The client actually may be dehydrated. Further, the specific gravity of the urine from such an individual could be high because of the presence of excessive glucose.[9] Similarly, deeper-colored urine may not always indicate concentrated urine. The presence of bilirubin may produce darker urine in normally hydrated individuals.

Urine color may be described as pale yellow, straw, light yellow, yellow, dark yellow, and amber. For the most accurate appraisal of urine color, the sample should be examined in good light against a white background. If the sample is allowed to stand at room temperature for any length of time, the urochrome will increase and the color of the sample may deepen.[10]

Numerous factors that affect the color of urine are listed in Table 6–1.

Appearance (Clarity)

The term *appearance* generally refers to the clarity of the urine sample. Urine is normally clear or slightly cloudy. In alkaline urine, cloudiness may be caused by precipitation of phosphates and carbonates. In acidic urine, cloudiness may be caused by precipitation of urates, uric acid, or calcium oxalate. The accumulation of uroerythrin, a pink pigment normally present in urine, may produce a pinkish or reddish haze in acidic urine.

The most common substances that may cause cloudy urine are white blood cells, red blood cells, bacteria, and epithelial cells. Presence of these substances may indicate inflammation or infection of the urinary and genital tracts and must be confirmed through microscopic examination (see p. 322). Other substances that may produce cloudy urine are mucus, yeasts, sperm, prostatic fluid, menstrual and vaginal discharges, fecal material, and external substances such as talcum powder and antiseptics.[11] Proper client instruction and specimen collection may aid in reducing the presence of such substances in the urine.

Lymph and fat globules in urine may also yield cloudy specimens. The presence of lymph in the urine is most often associated with obstruction to abdominal lymph flow and rupture of lymphatic vessels into portions of the urinary tract. Fat globules in the urine are most commonly associated with nephrotic syndrome but may also be seen in clients with fractures of the long bones or pelvis.[12]

Odor

Normally, a fresh urine specimen has a faintly aromatic odor. As the specimen stands, the odor of ammonia predominates because of the breakdown of urea. Ingestion of certain foods and drugs impart characteristic odors to urine; this is especially true of asparagus.

Some unusual odors are indicative of certain disease states. Urine with a fruity odor, for example, may indicate ketonuria resulting from uncontrolled diabetes mellitus or starvation. Other abnormal odors are associated with amino acid disorders. Urine with a "mousy" smell is associated with phenylketonuria (PKU), whereas urine that smells like maple syrup is associated with maple syrup urine disease. Urine with a "fishy" or fetid odor is generally associated with bacterial infection. This odor is especially noticeable when urine is allowed to stand for some time. Occasionally, urine may lack an odor. This characteristic is seen in acute renal failure because of acute tubular necrosis and failure of normal mechanisms of ammonium secretion.[13,14]

Table 6–1 ➤ FACTORS AFFECTING THE COLOR OF URINE	
Urine Color	**Cause**
Very pale yellow	Excessive fluid intake
	Diabetes mellitus
	Diabetes insipidus
	Nephrotic syndrome
	Alcohol
	Diuretics
	Anxiety
Dark yellow, amber	Underhydration
	Bilirubin
	Urobilin
	Carrots
	Phenacetin
	Cascara
	Nitrofurantoin
	Chlorpromazine
	Quinacrine
	Riboflavin
	Sulfasalazine
Orange	Bilirubin
	Phenazopyridine (Pyridium)
	Azo-drugs
	Phenothiazine
	Oral anticoagulants
Red	Red blood cells
	Hemoglobin
	Myoglobin
	Porphyrins
	Porphobilinogen
	Many drugs and dyes
	Rifampin
	Phenolsulfonphthalein
	Fuscin
	Beets
	Rhubarb
	Senna
Green	Biliverdin
	Pseudomonas
	Vitamins
	Psychoactive drugs
	Proprietary diuretics
Blue	Nitrofurans
	Proprietary diuretics
	Methylene blue
Brown	Acid hematin
	Myoglobin
	Bile pigments
	Levodopa
	Nitrofurans
	Some sulfa drugs
	Rhubarb

continued on page 313

Table 6–1 ➤ **FACTORS AFFECTING THE COLOR OF URINE** *Continued*

Urine Color	Cause
Black, brownish black	Melanin
	Homogentistic acid
	Indicans
	Urobilin
	Red blood cells oxidized to methemoglobin
	Levodopa
	Cascara
	Iron complexes
	Phenols

Specific Gravity

The specific gravity of urine is an indication of the kidney's ability to reabsorb water and chemicals from the glomerular filtrate. It also aids in evaluating hydration status and in detecting problems related to secretion of antidiuretic hormone. By definition, specific gravity is the density of a liquid compared with that of a similar volume of distilled water when both solutions are at the same or similar temperatures. The normal specific gravity of distilled water is 1.000. The specific gravity of urine is greater than 1.000 and reflects the density of the substances dissolved in the urine. Both the number of particles present and their size influence the specific gravity of urine. Large urea molecules, for example, influence the specific gravity more than do small sodium and chloride molecules. Similarly, if large amounts of glucose or protein are present in the sample, the specific gravity will be higher.[15]

The specific gravity of the glomerular filtrate is normally 1.010 as it enters Bowman's capsule. A consistent urinary specific gravity of 1.010 usually indicates damage to the renal tubules such that concentrating ability is lost. Urine with a low specific gravity may be seen in clients with overhydration and diabetes insipidus. Urine with a high specific gravity is associated with dehydration, uncontrolled diabetes mellitus, and nephrosis. High specific gravities may also be seen in clients who are receiving intravenous (IV) solutions of dextran or other high-molecular-weight fluids and in those who have received radiologic contrast media.

The specific gravity of urine provides preliminary information. For a more thorough evaluation of renal concentrating ability, urine osmolality may be determined, and concentration tests may be performed (see p. 336).[16]

pH

The pH of urine reflects the kidney's ability to regulate the acid-base balance of the body. In general, when too much acid is present in the body (i.e., respiratory or metabolic acidosis), acidic urine (low pH) is excreted. Conversely, alkaline urine (high pH) is excreted in states of respiratory or metabolic alkalosis. Various foods and drugs also affect urinary pH.

The kidney controls the acid-base balance of the body through regulation of hydrogen ion excretion. Various acids are excreted via the glomerulus along with sodium ions. In the renal tubules, bicarbonate ions are reabsorbed and hydrogen ions are secreted in exchange for sodium ions. Additional hydrogen ions are excreted as ammonium.

Disorders involving the renal tubules affect regulation of pH. In renal tubular acidosis, for example, the ability of the distal tubules to secrete hydrogen ions and form ammonia is impaired. Metabolic acidosis results. Similarly, in proximal tubular acidosis, bicarbonate is wasted.

As noted previously, the acidity or alkalinity of the urine generally reflects that of the body. A paradoxic situation may occur, however, in clients with hypokalemic alkalosis, which may occur with prolonged vomiting or excessive use of diuretics. In this situation, an acidic urine may be produced when hydrogen ions are secreted instead of potassium ions (which are deficient) to maintain electrochemical neutrality in the renal tubules.[17]

The pH or urine samples must be evaluated in relation to the client's dietary and drug intake. A diet high in meat and certain fruits such as cranberries produces acidic urine. A diet high in vegetables and citrus fruits produces an alkaline urine. Drugs such as ammonium chloride and methamine mandelate produce an acid urine, whereas sodium bicarbonate, potassium citrate, and acetazolamide result in alkaline urine.

The changes in urinary pH that occur in relation to ingestion of certain foods and drugs are applied to the treatment of certain urinary tract disorders. Maintenance of an acidic urine may be used in the treatment of urinary tract infections (UTIs) because urea-splitting organisms do not multiply as rapidly in an acidic environment. These same organisms cause the pH of a urine specimen to rise if it is allowed to stand for a period of time.[18] Acidic urine also helps to prevent the formation of ammonium magnesium kidney stones, which are more likely to form in alkaline urine. Other types of kidney stones are more likely to be prevented if the urine is alkaline. The induction of alkaline urine may also be used in the treatment of UTIs with drugs such as kanamycin, in sulfonamide therapy, and in the treatment of salicylate poisoning.[19]

Urine is generally less acidic after a meal (the "alkaline tide") because of secretion of acids into the stomach. Urine tends to be more acidic in the morning as a result of the mild respiratory acidosis that normally occurs during sleep.[20] Thus, the time of day that the sample is collected may influence evaluation of urinary pH.

Protein

Urine normally contains only a scant amount of protein, which derives from both the blood and the urinary tract itself. The proteins normally filtered through the glomerulus include small amounts of low-molecular-weight serum proteins such as albumin. Most of these filtered proteins are reabsorbed by the proximal renal tubules. The distal renal tubules secrete a protein (Tamm-Horsfall mucoprotein) into the urine. Other normal proteins in urine include microglobulin, immunoglobulin light chains, enzymes and proteins from tubular epithelial cells, leukocytes, and other cells shed by the urinary tract. More than 200 urinary proteins have been identified.[21]

Normal protein excretion must be differentiated from that which is caused by disease states. Persons who do not have renal disease may have proteinuria after strenuous exercise or during dehydration. Functional (nonrenal) proteinuria may also be seen in congestive heart failure (CHF), cold exposure, and fever.[22]

Postural (orthostatic) proteinuria may also occur in a small percentage of normal individuals. In this situation, the client spills protein while in an upright posture but not when recumbent. Postural proteinuria is evaluated by having the client collect a urine sample on first arising and then approximately 2 hours later after having been up and about. The second sample should be positive for protein; the first should be negative. Orthostatic proteinuria is generally a benign condition, although the client should be reevaluated periodically for persistent, nonpostural proteinuria.

Persistent proteinuria is generally indicative of renal disease or of systemic disorders leading to increased serum levels of low-molecular-weight proteins. Renal disease resulting in proteinuria may be a result of damage to the glomerulus or to the renal tubules. When the glomerular membrane is damaged, greater amounts of albumin pass into the glomerular filtrate. If damage is more extensive, large globulin molecules are also excreted. Nephrotic syndrome is an example of renal disease primarily associated with a glomerular damage. In this disorder there is heavy proteinuria accompanied by decreased serum albumin. In contrast, renal disease resulting from tubular damage is characterized by loss of proteins that are normally reabsorbed by the tubules (i.e., low-molecular-weight proteins). An example of renal disease primarily associated with tubular damage is pyelonephritis. The proteinuria that occurs in disorders involving the renal tubules is generally not as profound as that associated with glomerular damage.[23,24]

Systemic disorders that result in excessive production or release of hemoglobin, myoglobin, or immunoglobulins may lead to proteinuria and may, in addition, lead to actual renal disease. Myoglobinemia, for example, which may occur with extensive destruction of muscle fibers, leads to excretion of myoglobin in the urine and may lead to acute renal tubular necrosis.[25] Multiple myeloma, a neoplastic disorder of plasma cells, is another example of a systemic disorder that may cause proteinuria. In this disorder, the blood contains excessive levels of monoclonal immunoglobulin light chains (Bence Jones protein).[26] This protein overflows through the glomerulus in quantities greater than the renal tubules can absorb. Thus, large amounts of Bence Jones protein appear in the urine. As with myoglobinuria, the excessive amounts of protein may ultimately damage the kidney itself.

Because proteinuria may indicate serious renal or systemic disease, its detection on UA must always be further evaluated for possible cause. Proteinuria occurring in the latter months of pregnancy also must be carefully evaluated because it may indicate serious complications of pregnancy.

Glucose

Normally, glucose is virtually absent from the urine. Although nearly all glucose passes into the glomerular filtrate, most of it is reabsorbed by the proximal renal tubules through active transport mechanisms. In active transport, carrier molecules attach to molecules of other substances (e.g., glucose) and transport them across cell membranes. Usually there are enough carrier molecules to transport all of the glucose from the renal tubules back to the blood. If plasma glucose levels are very high, however, so that carrier mechanisms are overwhelmed, glucose will appear in the urine. The point at which a substance appears in the urine is called its renal threshold.[27] The renal threshold for glucose ranges from 160 to 200 mg/dL, depending on the individual. That is, the blood sugar must rise to its renal threshold level before glucose appears in the urine.

The most common cause of glycosuria is uncontrolled diabetes mellitus. Because even a normal person may have elevated blood glucose levels immediately after a meal, urine samples for glucose are best collected immediately before meals, when the blood sugar should be at its lowest point. Similarly, urine that has been accumulating in the bladder overnight may contain excessive amounts of glucose resulting from increased concentration of urine and perhaps also from something eaten the previous evening. Because a negative test result for urinary sugar may not necessarily indicate a normal blood sugar level and because there is a great deal of variation in individual renal thresholds for glucose, recent trends for diabetes control have moved away from urinary glucose monitoring to blood glucose monitoring. Evaluation of glucose in routine urine specimens, however, remains a useful screening technique.

In addition to diabetes mellitus, many other disorders may result in glycosuria. In general, these disorders fall into two general categories: (1) those in which the blood sugar is elevated and (2) those in which the blood sugar is not elevated but in which renal tubular absorption of glucose is impaired. Disorders that may lead to elevated blood glucose levels and, thus, to glycosuria are listed in Table 6–2. In addition, several drugs are known to elevate the blood sugar enough to produce glycosuria. These also are listed in Table 6–2.

When renal tubular reabsorption of glucose is impaired, glucose may appear in the urine without actual hyperglycemia. In disorders involving the renal tubules, glycosuria is one of many abnormal findings. Reabsorption of amino acids, bicarbonate, phosphate, sodium, and water may also be impaired. Disorders associated with altered renal tubular function and glycosuria are listed in Table 6–2. Pregnancy represents a special case in which glycosuria may be present without hyperglycemia. During pregnancy, the glomerular filtration rate (GFR) is increased so that it may not be possible for the renal tubules to reabsorb all of the glucose presented. Glucose may appear in the urine even though blood glucose levels are within normal limits. This situation must be distinguished from actual diabetes with elevated blood sugar levels, a serious complication of pregnancy.[28]

Certain drugs are known to produce false-positive results when testing for glucose in urine, especially when copper sulfate reduction testing methods (e.g., Clinitest tablets, Benedict's solution) are used. These drugs are listed in Table 6–3. Allowing urine specimens to remain at room temperature for long periods may produce false-positive results.

The presence of nonglucose sugars in the urine may also produce false-positive results in tests for glycosuria. These sugars include lactose, fructose, galactose, pentose, and sucrose. Lactose may appear in the urine during normal pregnancy and lactation, in lactase deficiency states, and in certain disorders affecting the intestines (e.g., celiac disease, tropical sprue, and kwashiorkor). Fructose may appear in the urine after parenteral feedings with fructose and in clients with inherited enzyme deficiencies, which are generally benign in nature. Galactose in the urine also is associated with certain inherited enzyme deficiencies. Pentose may appear in the urine after ingestion of excessive amounts

Table 6-2 ➤ DISORDERS AND DRUGS THAT MAY RESULT IN GLYCOSURIA	
Glycosuria with High Blood Sugar	**Glucosuria Without High Blood Sugar**
Diabetes mellitus	Renal tubular dysfunction
Gestational diabetes	Fanconi's syndrome
Acromegaly	Galactosemia
Cushing's syndrome	Cystinosis
Hyperthyroidism	Lead poisoning
Pheochromocytoma	Multiple myeloma
Advanced cystic fibrosis	Pregnancy (must be distinguished from
Hemochromatosis	gestational diabetes)
Severe chronic pancreatitis	
Carcinoma of the pancreas	
Hypothalamic dysfunction	
Brain tumor or hemorrhage	
Massive metabolic derangement	
Severe burns	
Uremia	
Advanced liver disease	
Sepsis	
Cardiogenic shock	
Glycogen storage disease	
Obesity	
Medication-induced hyperglycemia	
Adrenal corticosteroids	
Adrenocorticotropic hormone (ACTH)	
Thiazides	
Oral contraceptives	
Excessive IV glucose	
Dextrothyroxine	

of fruits. Similarly, sucrose may be found if large amounts of sucrose are ingested, but it may also be found in clients with intestinal disorders associated with sucrase deficiency (e.g., sprue).[29]

Glycosuria may, therefore, indicate a number of pathological states or may result from drug and food ingestion. A thorough history and further evaluation through additional laboratory tests are indicated whenever glycosuria occurs.

Ketones

The term *ketones* refers to three intermediate products of fat metabolism: acetone, acetoacetic acid, and β-hydroxybutyric acid. Measurable amounts of ke-

Table 6-3 ➤ DRUGS THAT MAY PRODUCE FALSE-POSITIVE GLYCOSURIA RESULTS	
Ascorbic acid	Paraldehyde
Cephalosporins	Penicillins
Chloral hydrate	Salicylates
Metaxalone (Skelaxin)	Streptomycin
Nalidixic acid (NegGram)	Morphine
Oxytetracycline (Terramycin)	Levodopa
Para-aminobenzoic acid (PABA)	Radiographic contrast media

tones are not normally present in urine. With excessive fat metabolism, however, ketones may be found. Excessive fat metabolism may occur in several situations: (1) impaired ability to metabolize carbohydrates, (2) inadequate carbohydrate intake, (3) excessive carbohydrate loss, and (4) increased metabolic demand.[30] The disorder most commonly associated with impaired ability to metabolize carbohydrates is diabetes mellitus. As carbohydrates cannot be used to meet the body's energy needs, fats are burned, leading to the presence of ketones in the urine. A similar situation occurs when carbohydrate intake is inadequate to the body's needs. This is seen in weight-reduction diets and starvation. Excessive loss of carbohydrates (e.g., caused by vomiting and diarrhea) and increased metabolic demand (e.g., acute febrile conditions and toxic states, especially in infants and children) may also produce ketonuria. Other disorders in which ketones may be found in the urine include lactic acidosis and salicylate toxicity. Ketonuria also has been found after anesthesia and is believed to be a result of both decreased food intake before surgery and increased metabolic demand in relation to physiological stressors.

As with glucose, ketones in the urine are associated with elevated blood ketone levels. Because ketone bodies are acids, ketonuria may indicate systemic acidosis. Ketones in urine are measured most frequently in clients with diabetes mellitus and in those on weight-reduction diets. The finding of ketones on UA requires further follow-up through history and laboratory tests to determine the source. Individuals receiving levodopa, paraldehyde, phenazopyridine (Pyridium), and phthalein compounds may produce false-positive results when tested for ketonuria.

Blood

Blood may be present in the urine as either red blood cells or hemoglobin. If enough blood is present, the color of the sample may range from pink-tinged to red to brownish-black (see p. 322). Very small amounts of blood, although clinically significant, may not be detected unless the sample is tested with reagent strips ("dipsticks") or by microscopic examination (see p. 322). The dipstick approach for macroscopic UA provides a useful screening approach. Positive results require further evaluation to determine the nature and source of the blood.[31,32]

The presence of red blood cells in urine (hematuria) is relatively common, whereas the presence of hemoglobin in urine (hemoglobinuria) is seen much less frequently. Hematuria is usually associated with disease of or damage to the genitourinary tract. When hematuria is accompanied by significant proteinuria, kidney disease is generally indicated (e.g., acute glomerulonephritis). In contrast, hematuria with only small amounts of protein is associated with inflammation and bleeding of the lower urinary tract (e.g., cystitis).[33] Other disorders commonly associated with hematuria include pyelonephritis, tumors of the genitourinary tract, kidney stones, lupus nephritis, and trauma to the genitourinary tract. Nonrenal causes of hematuria include bleeding disorders and anticoagulant therapy. Hematuria may also occur in healthy individuals after excessive strenuous exercise because of damage to the mucosa of the urinary bladder.[34]

Free hemoglobin is not normally found in the urine. Instead, any hemoglobin that could be presented to the glomerulus combines with haptoglobin. The resultant hemoglobin-haptoglobin complex is too large to pass through the glomerular membrane. If the amount of free hemoglobin exceeds the amount of haptoglobin, however, the hemoglobin will pass through the glomerulus and ultimately be excreted into the urine.[35] Any disorder associated with hemolysis of red blood cells and resultant release of hemoglobin may lead to the appearance of hemoglobin in the urine. Common causes of hemoglobinuria include hemolytic anemias, transfusion reactions, trauma to red blood cells by prosthetic cardiac valves, extensive burns, trauma to muscles and blood vessels, and severe infections. Hemoglobinuria may also occur in healthy individuals and is thought to be caused by trauma to small blood vessels.[36]

It should be noted that hemoglobin is broken down in the renal tubular cells into ferritin and hemosiderin. Hemosiderin may, therefore, be found in urine a few days after an episode of acute red cell hemolysis. Hemosiderin also is found in the urine of individuals with hemochromatosis, a disorder of iron metabolism.[37]

Bilirubin and Urobilinogen

If the urine sample for UA appears dark or if the client is experiencing jaundice, the specimen may be tested for the presence of bilirubin and excessive urobilinogen. Both of these substances are bile pigments that result from the breakdown of hemoglobin (Fig. 6–1).

The average life span of red blood cells is 120 days. Old and damaged cells are broken down primarily in the spleen and to some extent in the liver. The breakdown products are iron, protein, and protoporphyrin. The body reuses the iron and protein; the protoporphyrin is converted into bilirubin and is released into the circulation, where it combines with albumin. This form of bilirubin is called unconjugated or prehepatic bilirubin. It does not pass into the urine because the complex is insoluble in water and is too large to pass through the glomerular membrane. When circulating unconjugated bilirubin reaches the liver, it is conjugated with glucuronic acid. The conjugated (posthepatic) bilirubin is normally absorbed into the bile ducts, stored in the gallbladder, and ultimately excreted via the intestine.[38] In the intestine, bilirubin is converted into urobilinogen by bacteria. Approximately half of the urobilinogen is excreted in the stools, where it is converted into urobilin; the remaining half is reabsorbed

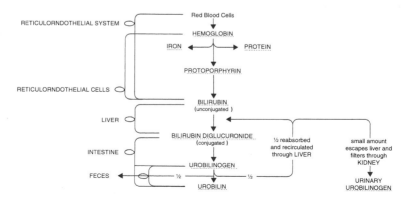

Figure 6–1 Hemoglobin degradation. (From Strasinger, SK: Urinalysis and Body Fluids, ed 3. FA Davis, Philadelphia, 1994, p 66, with permission.)

Table 6-4 ➤ URINE BILIRUBIN AND UROBILINOGEN IN JAUNDICE		
	Urine Bilirubin	**Urine Urobilinogen**
Bile duct obstruction	+++	Normal
Liver damage	+ or −	++
Hemolytic disease	Negative	+++

Note: From Strasinger, SK: Urinalysis and Body Fluids, ed 3. FA Davis, Philadelphia, 1994, p 67, with permission.

from the intestine back into the bloodstream. From the bloodstream, urobilinogen is either recirculated to the liver and excreted with bile or excreted via the kidneys. Normally, only a small amount of urobilinogen is found in the urine.[39]

Bilirubin may be found in the urine in liver disease and is usually found in clients who have biliary tract obstructions. Excessive urobilinogen may also be found in the urine of those with liver disease or hemolytic disorders. Urobilinogen is absent from the urine in disorders that cause complete obstruction of the bile ducts (Table 6-4).

Bilirubinuria may occur in clients with liver disease when the integrity of liver cells is disrupted and conjugated bilirubin leaks into the circulation; this leakage may be seen in hepatitis and cirrhosis. In fact, in these disorders, bilirubin may appear in the urine before the client actually becomes jaundiced. If liver function is impaired such that the liver cannot conjugate bilirubin, excessive bilirubin will not be found in the urine. Similarly, excessive bilirubin is not seen in the urine of clients with hemolytic disorders. These disorders have marked destruction of red blood cells with resultant high levels of unconjugated bilirubin. The normally functioning liver is unable to conjugate the excessive load, and although serum levels of unconjugated bilirubin rise, urinary bilirubin excretion remains relatively unchanged. This condition, again, is a result of the kidney's inability to excrete unconjugated bilirubin.

If there is bile duct obstruction, the conjugated bilirubin cannot pass from the biliary tract into the intestine. Instead, excess amounts are absorbed into the bloodstream and excreted via the kidneys. Also, because little or no bilirubin passes into the intestine, where urobilinogen is formed, the urine will be negative for urobilinogen. Absence of urobilinogen in urine is associated with complete obstruction of the common bile duct. When absence of urobilinogen is combined with the presence of blood in the stool, carcinoma involving the head of the pancreas may be indicated.[40]

As noted previously, approximately half of the urobilinogen formed in the intestines is reabsorbed into the bloodstream. Normally, most of this urobilinogen is circulated to the liver, where it is processed and excreted via bile. A smaller amount is excreted in the urine. When liver cells are damaged, excretion of urobilinogen in bile is decreased, whereas its urinary excretion is increased. This condition may be seen in clients with cirrhosis, hepatitis, and CHF with congestion of the liver.

Excessive urobilinogen also appears in the urine in persons with hemolytic disorders. As noted, in such disorders the amount of unconjugated bilirubin produced is more than the liver can handle, but the liver attempts to compensate, and increased amounts of urobilinogen are ultimately formed. When this urobilinogen is recirculated back to the liver, however, the liver is unable to process it further and additional amounts are excreted in the urine.

A number of factors may cause spurious results when urine is tested for bilirubin and urobilinogen. Because excessive exposure of a urine sample to light and room air may lead to false-negative results for bilirubin, only fresh urine specimens should be used. Large amounts of ascorbic acid and nitrates in the urine also cause false-negative results. It should be noted that bilirubin excretion is enhanced in alkalotic states. This also is true of urobilinogen and is a result of decreased tubular reabsorption from alkaline urine. Similarly, acidic urine results in decreased urinary levels of urobilinogen. As noted, urobilinogen is formed by bacterial action in the intestine. Broad-spectrum antibiotics impair this process and result in decreased urobilinogen production. As with bilirubin, high levels of nitrates in the urine may also cause false-negative results in tests for urobilinogen.[41,42]

Nitrite

Testing urine samples for nitrite is a rapid screening method for determining the presence of bacteria in the specimen. This test is based on the fact that nitrate, which is normally present in urine, is converted to nitrite in the presence of bacteria. The test is performed by the dipstick method and, if positive, indicates that clinically significant bacteriuria is present. Positive test results should always be followed by a regular urine culture.

Several factors may interfere with the accuracy of tests for nitrite. First, not all bacteria reduce nitrate to nitrite. Those that do so include the gram-negative bacteria, the organisms most frequently involved in UTIs. Because yeasts and gram-positive bacteria may not convert nitrate to nitrite, the presence of these organisms can cause a false-negative test result.

For bacteria to convert nitrate to nitrite, the organisms must be in contact with urinary nitrate for some period of time. Thus, freshly voided random samples or urine that is withdrawn from a Foley catheter may produce false-negative results. The best urine samples for nitrite testing are first morning samples from urine that has been in the bladder overnight. Other causes of false-negative results include inadequate amounts of nitrate in the urine for conversion (may occur in individuals who do not eat enough green vegetables), large amounts of ascorbic acid in the urine, antibiotic therapy, and excessive bacteria in the urine so that nitrite is further reduced to nitrogen, which is not detected by the test. False-positive reactions will occur if the container in which the sample is collected is contaminated with gram-negative bacteria.[43,44]

Leukocyte Esterase

Testing urine samples for the presence of leukocyte esterase is a rapid screening method for determining the presence of certain white blood cells (i.e., neutrophils) in the sample and, thus, the possibility of a UTI. This test is performed by the dipstick method and is based on the fact that the esterases present in neutrophils will convert the indoxyl carboxylic acid ester on the dipstick to indoxyl, which is converted to indigo blue by room air. Approximately 15 minutes are needed for this reaction to take place if neutrophils are present. If positive, the test should be followed by a regular urine culture.[45]

Some factors may interfere with the accuracy of tests for leukocyte esterases. False-positive results may occur if the sample is contaminated with vaginal secretions.[46] False-negative results may occur if high levels of protein and ascorbic acid are present in the urine. If the urine contains excessive amounts of yellow pigment, a positive reaction will be indicated by a change to green instead of blue.[47]

MICROSCOPIC ANALYSIS

The microscopic component of a UA involves examining the sample for formed elements, or urinary sediment, such as red and white blood cells, epithelial cells, casts, crystals, bacteria, and mucus. Microscopic analysis is performed by centrifuging approximately 10 to 15 mL of urine for about 5 minutes. The resulting sediment is then examined under the microscope. Microscopic analysis is the most time-consuming component of the UA. It involves both identifying and quantifying the formed elements present.[48]

It should be noted that the Addis count is a variation of the microscopic urinalysis. For an Addis count, all urine is collected for 12 hours and then the nature and quantity of formed elements are determined. This test, which was once used to follow the progress of acute renal disease, is seldom used today, as microscopic analysis of a single random sample usually is sufficient.[49]

Red Blood Cells

Red blood cells are too large to pass through the glomerulus; thus, the finding of red blood cells in the urine (hematuria) is considered abnormal. If red blood cells are present, damage to the glomerular membrane or to the genitourinary tract is indicated. For this test, the number of red blood cells is counted. The result may indicate the nature and severity of the disorder causing the hematuria.

Renal and genitourinary disorders associated with the presence of red blood cells in the urine include glomerulonephritis, lupus nephritis, nephritis associated with drug reactions, tumors of the kidney, kidney stones, infections, trauma to the kidney, renal vein thrombosis, hydronephrosis, polycystic kidney disease, acute tubular necrosis (occasionally), and malignant nephrosclerosis (occasionally).[50]

Red blood cells may also be seen with some nonrenal disorders: acute appendicitis; salpingitis; diverticulitis; tumors involving the colon, rectum, and pelvis; acute systemic febrile and infectious diseases; polyarteritis nodosa; malignant hypertension; and blood dyscrasias. Drugs that may lead to hematuria include salicylates, anticoagulants, sulfonamides, and cyclophosphamide. Strenuous exercise may also cause red blood cells to appear in the urine because of damage to the mucosa of the bladder.[51] Contamination of the sample with menstrual blood may lead to false-positive results.

White Blood Cells

Normally, only a few white blood cells are found in urine. Increased numbers of leukocytes in the urine generally indicate either renal or genitourinary tract disease. As with red blood cells, white blood cells may enter the urine either through the glomerulus or through damaged genitourinary tissues. In addition, white blood cells may migrate through undamaged tissues to sites of infection or inflammation. Excessive white blood cells in the urine is *pyuria*.[52]

The most frequent cause of pyuria is bacterial infection anywhere in the renal or genitourinary system (e.g., pyelonephritis, cystitis). Noninfectious inflammatory disorders, however, may also lead to pyuria. Such disorders include glomerulonephritis and lupus nephritis. In addition, tumors and renal calculi may cause pyuria because of the resultant inflammatory response.

A higher than normal number of leukocytes may be seen if the sample is contaminated with genital secretions. This finding is especially true in women. White blood cells disintegrate in dilute, alkaline urine and in samples that are allowed to stand at room temperature for more than 1 to 2 hours.[53]

Epithelial Cells

Epithelial cells found in urine samples are derived from three major sources: (1) the linings of the male and female lower urethras and the vagina (squamous epithelial cells); (2) the linings of the renal pelvis, bladder, and upper urethra (transitional epithelial cells); and (3) the renal tubules themselves. Because it is normal for old epithelial cells to slough from their respective areas, finding a few epithelial cells in a urine sample is not necessarily abnormal. Large numbers of cells, especially those of renal tubular origin, are considered pathological. When large numbers of renal tubular cells are shed, tubular necrosis is indicated. In addition to acute tubular necrosis (ATN), excessive numbers of tubular epithelial cells may be seen in renal transplant rejection, any ischemic injury to the kidney, glomerulonephritis, pyelonephritis, and damage to the kidney by drugs and toxins.[54]

Renal tubular epithelial cells may contain certain lipids and pigments. Cells that contain lipoproteins, triglycerides, and cholesterol are called *oval fat bodies*. Presence of oval fat bodies occurs in lipid nephrosis and results from lipids leaked through nephrotic glomeruli. Histiocytes are fat-containing cells that are larger than oval fat bodies and that usually can be distinguished from the latter on microscopic examination. Histiocytes may be seen in nephrotic syndrome and in lipid-storage diseases.[55]

Pigments that may be absorbed into renal tubular epithelial cells include hemoglobin that is converted to hemosiderin, melanin, and bilirubin. Hemoglobin and bilirubin have previously been discussed (see pp. 319 to 321). Melanin may be found in tubular epithelial cells in the presence of malignant melanoma that has metastasized to the genitourinary tract.

Finding increased epithelial cells from the lower genitourinary tract is generally not of major clinical significance, with one exception. If excessive numbers of transitional epithelial cells are found in large clumps, or sheets, carcinoma involving any portion of the area from the renal pelvis to the bladder may be indicated.[56]

Casts

Casts are gel-like substances that form in the renal tubules and collecting ducts. They are termed casts because they take the shape of the area of the tubule or collecting duct in which they form. Tamm-Horsfall protein, a mucoprotein secreted by the distal renal tubular cells (see p. 324), is the major constituent of

Table 6–5 ➤ SUMMARY OF URINE CASTS

Type	Origin	Clinical Significance
Hyaline	Tubular secretion of Tamm-Horsfall protein	Glomerulonephritis Pyelonephritis Chronic renal disease Congestive heart failure Stress and exercise
Red blood cell	Attachment of red blood cells to Tamm-Horsfall protein matrix	Glomerulonephritis Strenuous exercise Lupus nephritis Subacute bacterial endocarditis Renal infarction Malignant hypertension
White blood cell	Attachment of white blood cells to Tamm-Horsfall protein matrix	Inflammation or infection involving the glomerulus Pyelonephritis Lupus nephritis
Epithelial cell	Tubular cells remaining attached to Tamm-Horsfall protein fibrils	Renal tubular damage
Granular	Disintegration of white cell casts Bacteria Urates Tubular cell lysosomes Protein aggregates	Stasis of urine flow Urinary tract infection Stress and exercise Acute glomerulonephritis Renal transplant rejection Pyelonephritis Lead poisoning
Waxy	Hyaline casts in an advanced stage of development	Stasis of urine flow Renal transplant rejection Renal tubular inflammation and degeneration Chronic renal failure End-stage renal disease Nephrotic syndrome
Fatty	Renal tubular cells Oval fat bodies	Nephrotic syndrome
Broad casts	Formation in collecting ducts (i.e., casts are larger than those formed in the tubules)	Extreme stasis of urine flow Renal failure (severe) Chronic glomerulonephritis

Note: Adapted from Strasinger, SK: Urinalysis and Body Fluids, ed 3. FA Davis, Philadelphia, 1994, p 88.

casts. This protein forms a framework in which other elements may be trapped (e.g., red and white blood cells, bacteria, fats, urates). Healthy individuals may normally excrete a few casts, especially if there is a low urinary pH, increased protein in the urine, increased excretion of solutes, and decreased rate of urine flow.[57] As noted previously (p. 314), proteinuria may occur after strenuous exercise. This may lead to the formation and excretion of an increased number of casts in healthy individuals. Red blood cells may also be found in casts excreted in response to such exercise. Otherwise, excretion of an excessive number of casts is usually associated with widespread kidney disease that involves the renal tubules.[58]

Casts are classified according to the nature of the substances present in them (Table 6–5). As can be seen in the table, the finding of excessive numbers of casts requires further diagnostic follow-up, as it may indicate serious renal disease.

Crystals

Crystals form in urine because of the presence of the salts from which they are precipitated. There are numerous types of crystals (Table 6–6), many of which are not of major clinical significance. Also, several factors affect the formation of urinary crystals: (1) pH of the urine, (2) temperature of the urine, and (3) concentration of the substances from which the crystals are formed. Table 6–6 shows the pH of the urine at which the several types of crystals are most likely to be formed. In terms of the temperature of the sample, crystals are most likely to be seen in samples that have stood at room temperature for several hours or have been refrigerated, depending on the type of crystal. The concentration of various substances that lead to the formation of crystals is important in that the greater the concentration, the greater the likelihood of precipitation of the substance into the urine in crystal formation.

In analyzing crystals on microscopic examination, it is important to determine the type of crystal present. The presence of certain crystals may indicate disease states (e.g., liver disease, cystinuria). In addition, drug therapy or use of radiographic dyes may cause precipitation of crystals that may portend renal damage by blocking the tubules.[59]

Other Substances

A number of other substances may be found on microscopic urinalysis: bacteria, yeast, mucus, spermatozoa, and parasites. Bacteria are not normally present but may be seen if UTI is present or if the sample was contaminated externally. The number of bacteria will increase if the specimen is allowed to stand at room temperature for several hours. Bacteria in the urine are generally not of major significance unless accompanied by excessive numbers of white blood cells, which may indicate an infectious or inflammatory process. Yeast in the urine usually indicates contamination of the sample with vaginal secretions in women with yeast infections such as *Candida albicans.* Yeasts may also be seen in the urine of clients with diabetes. Mucus in urine generally reflects secretions from the genitourinary tract and is usually associated with contamination of the sample with vaginal secretions. Spermatozoa may be found in urine after sexual intercourse or nocturnal emissions. Parasites are frequently of vaginal origin and may indicate vaginitis caused by *Trichomonas vaginalis.* A true urinary parasite is *Schistosoma haematobium,* seen in the urine of individuals with schistosomiasis, an uncommon disorder in the United States. If pinworms and other intestinal parasites are found, contamination of the sample with fecal material is indicated.[60]

Summary

The UA, which consists of macroscopic and microscopic components, yields a great deal of information about the client. All the tests may be performed separately, especially those associated with macroscopic analysis. The most complete picture, however, is obtained by synthesizing the data obtained from the various tests.

Although a variety of disorders may be indicated by abnormal results on UA, the most common disorders indicated are the several types of renal disease. Table 6–7 shows ways in which the results of macroscopic and microscopic

Table 6–6 ▶ MAJOR CHARACTERISTICS AND CLINICAL SIGNIFICANCE OF URINARY CRYSTALS

Crystal	pH	Color	Clinical Significance	Appearance
			NORMAL	
Uric acid	Acid	Yellow-brown	Gout Leukemias and lymphomas, especially if client is receiving chemotherapy	
Amorphous urates	Acid	Brick dust or yellow-brown	Not of major clinical significance	
Calcium oxalate	Acid/neutral (alkaline)	Colorless (envelopes)	High doses of ascorbic acid Severe chronic renal disease Ethylene glycol toxicity Crohn's disease, hypercalcemia	
Amorphous phosphates	Alkaline, neutral	White, colorless	May be found in urine that has stood at room temperature for several hours	
Calcium phosphate	Alkaline, neutral	Colorless	Not of major clinical significance	
Triple phosphate	Alkaline	Colorless (coffin lids)	Not of major clinical significance	
Ammonium biurate	Alkaline	Yellow-brown (thorny apples)	Not of major clinical significance	
Calcium carbonate	Alkaline	Colorless (dumb-bells)	Not of major clinical significance	

Cystine	Acid	Colorless	Cystinuria (inherited metabolic defect that prevents reabsorption of cystine by the proximal tubules)
Cholesterol	Acid	Colorless (notched plates)	High serum cholesterol More likely to be seen in refrigerated specimens
Leucine	Acid/neutral	Yellow	Severe liver disease
Tyrosine	Acid/neutral	Colorless, yellow	Severe liver disease
Bilirubin	Acid	Yellow	Possible liver dysfunction
Sulfonamides	Acid/neutral	Green	Therapy with sulfonamides
Radiographic dye	Acid	Colorless	Dye excretion
Ampicillin	Acid/neutral	Colorless	Therapy with ampicillin

Note: Adapted from Strasinger, SK: Urinalysis and Body Fluids, ed 3. FA Davis, Philadelphia, 1994, pp 92–93.

Table 6-7 ► LABORATORY CORRELATIONS IN RENAL DISEASES

Disease	Macroscopic Examination	Microscopic Examination	Other Laboratory Findings	Remarks
Acute glomerulonephritis	Macroscopic hematuria Specific gravity ↑ Protein <5 g/day "Smoky" turbidity	RBCs RBC casts Granular casts WBCs	ASO titer ↑ GFR ↓ Sed rate ↑	Microscopic hematuria remains longer than proteinuria
Rapidly progressive (crescentic) glomerulonephritis	Macroscopic hematuria Protein	RBCs WBCs Granular casts	BUN ↑ Creatinine ↑ FDP ↑ GFR ↓	Oliguria
Chronic glomerulonephritis	Macroscopic hematuria Specific gravity 1.010 Protein	RBCs WBCs All types of casts Broad casts	Cryoglobulins ↑ BUN ↑ Creatinine ↑ Serum phosphorus ↑ Serum calcium ↓	Oliguria or anuria Nocturia Anemia
Membranous glomerulonephritis	Blood Protein	RBCs Hyaline casts	Positive ANA Positive HB_s Ag	Microscopic hematuria
Membranoproliferative (mesangioproliferative) glomerulonephritis	Macroscopic hematuria Protein	RBCs RBC casts	BUN ↑ Creatinine ↑ ASO titer ↑ Complement ↓	Hematuria may be microscopic
Focal glomerulonephritis	Blood Protein	RBCs Fat droplets	IgA deposits on membrane	Macroscopic or microscopic hematuria
Minimal change disease	Blood	RBCs Oval fat bodies Fat droplets Hyaline casts Fatty casts	Serum protein ↓ Serum albumin ↓	Hematuria may be absent
Nephrotic syndrome	Protein	RBCs Oval fat bodies Fat droplets Generalized casts Waxy casts Fatty casts	Serum lipids ↑ Serum protein ↓ Serum albumin ↓	Heavy proteinuria >5 g/day
Pyelonephritis	Cloudy Protein Nitrite Leukocytes	WBCs WBC casts Bacteria RBCs		Concentrating ability decreased in chronic cases

Note: Adapted from Strasinger, SK: Urinalysis and Body Fluids, ed 3. FA Davis, Philadelphia, 1994, pp 33–34.
ANA = antinuclear antibody, ASO = antistreptolysin O, BUN = blood urea nitrogen, FDP = fibrin degradation products, GFR = glomerular filtration rate, HB_s Ag = hepatitis B surface antigen, IgA = immunoglobulin A.

analyses are combined to indicate certain types of renal disease. Other types of disorders associated with abnormal urinalysis results are listed in the indications for UA test.

Reference Values

Macroscopic Analysis	
Color	Pale yellow to amber
Appearance	Clear to slightly cloudy
Odor	Mildly aromatic
Specific gravity	1.001–1.035 (usual range 1.010–1.025)
pH	4.5–8.0
Protein	Negative
Glucose	Negative
Other sugars	Negative
Ketones	Negative
Blood	Negative
Bilirubin	Negative
Urobilinogen	0.1–1.0 Ehrlich units/dL (1–4 mg/24 hr)
Nitrate	Negative
Leukocyte esterase	Negative
Microscopic Analysis	
Red blood cells (RBCs)	0–3 per high-power field (HPF)
White blood cells (WBCs)	0–4 per HPF
Epithelial cells	Few
Casts	Occasional (hyaline or granular)
Crystals	Occasional (uric acid, urate, phosphate, or calcium oxalate)
Critical Values:	**RBC >50, WBC, or pathological crystals, as well as grossly bloody urine, and 3+ to 4+ glucose or ketones, or both**

Interfering Factors

➤ Improper specimen collection so that the sample is contaminated with vaginal secretions or feces
➤ Use of collection containers contaminated with bacteria
➤ Therapy with medications or ingestion of foods that may alter the color, odor, or pH of the sample
➤ Delay in sending unrefrigerated samples to the laboratory within 1 hour of collection, which may lead to:
 • Deepening of the color of the sample
 • Increased alkalinity of the sample
 • Increased concentration of glucose, if already present
 • Oxidation of bilirubin, if present, and urobilinogen
 • Deterioration of urinary sediment
 • Multiplication of bacteria, if present
➤ Failure to time properly those tests done by dipstick method (e.g., glucose and ketones)

Indications for Routine Urinalysis (UA)

The routine urinalysis (UA) is a screening technique that is an essential component of a complete physical examination, especially when performed on admission to a health-care facility or before surgery. It may also be performed when renal or systemic disease is suspected. It should be noted that the components of a UA may be performed separately, if necessary. This may be done to monitor previously identified conditions. Other indications or purposes for a UA include:

➤ Detection of infection involving the urinary tract as indicated by urine with a "fishy" or fetid odor and presence of nitrite, leukocyte esterase, white blood cells, red blood cells (possibly), and bacteria

➤ Detection of uncontrolled diabetes mellitus as indicated by the presence of glucose and ketones (seen primarily in insulin-dependent diabetes mellitus) and by urine with low specific gravity

➤ Detection of gestational diabetes during pregnancy

➤ Detection of possible complications of pregnancy as indicated by proteinuria

➤ Detection of bleeding within the urinary system, as indicated by positive dipstick test for blood and detection of red blood cells on microscopic examination

➤ Detection of various types of renal disease (see Table 6–7, p. 328)

➤ Detection of liver disease as indicated by the presence of bilirubin (possibly), excessive urobilinogen, and leucine or tyrosine crystals, or both

➤ Detection of obstruction within the biliary tree as indicated by presence of bilirubin and absence of urobilinogen

➤ Detection of multiple myeloma as indicated by the presence of Bence Jones protein

➤ Monitoring of the effectiveness of weight-reduction diets as indicated by the presence of ketones in the urine

➤ Detection of excessive red blood cell hemolysis within the systemic circulation as indicated by the presence of free hemoglobin and elevated urobilinogen levels

➤ Detection of extensive injury to muscles as indicated by the presence of myoglobin in the urine

---

➤➤ Nursing Alert

- Improper collection and disposition of sample for UA may lead to spurious results (see "Interfering Factors"). The best samples, in general, are those that are collected first thing in the morning after urine has collected in the bladder overnight. The sample should be received in the laboratory within 1 hour of collection. If this is not possible, the sample may be refrigerated.
- The time of collection and the source of the sample must be noted, because this information is important in evaluating the results and in distinguishing normal from abnormal results.
- Because many drugs and foods may alter results, a thorough medication and diet history is necessary for evaluating the data obtained.

Nursing Care Before the Procedure

Explain to the client:

➤ That results are most reliable if the specimen is obtained upon arising in the morning, after urine has accumulated overnight in the bladder (*Exception:* Serial urine samples for glucose should consist of fresh urine.)

➤ The proper way to collect the sample, if the client is to do this independently (see Appendix II)

➤ The importance of the sample's being received in the laboratory within 1 hour of collection

Prepare for the procedure:

➤ The client should be provided with the proper specimen container.

➤ For women, a clean-catch midstream kit should be provided.

➤ Techniques for collecting samples from children are described in Appendix II.

➤ For catheterized specimens, a catheterization tray is needed if an indwelling catheter is not already present.

The Procedure

A voided or catheterized sample of approximately 15 mL is collected (see Appendix II).

Nursing Care After the Procedure

Care and assessment after the test include observing the color, clarity, and odor of the sample when it is obtained. Perform dipstick tests for glucose, ketones, protein, and blood on separate portions of the sample, if desired.

➤ *Hydration state:* Note and report intake and output (I&O) ratio and adequacy, changes in urinary pattern and diuresis, and dehydration and fluid shifts. Monitor I&O and effect on specimen collection and testing, urinary sample characteristics and amount, and urinary pattern changes.

➤ *Incorrect techniques:* Store dipsticks in a dry, cool, dark place. Immerse dipstick in the urine for an appropriate time and examine in a well-lit place after an appropriate time interval. Confirm all abnormal test results.

➤ *Specific gravity:* Note and report increases over 1.020. Monitor I&O. Assess for dehydration. Administer additional fluids, if allowed. Note decreases below 1.009. Monitor I&O and weight for fluid overload. Assess for renal dysfunction. Inform and instruct client in fluid intake necessary to maintain adequate hydration.

➤ *pH:* Note and report increases over 6 (alkaline urine). Assess for risk of or presence of UTI or renal calculi. Increase fluid intake and restrict foods that leave an alkaline ash (milk, citrus fruits). Administer ordered vitamin C. Note decreases below 6 (acid urine). Administer medications to promote an alkaline urine. Assess for possible metabolic or respiratory acidotic states.

➤ *Protein:* Note and report any trace or range of protein from 0 to 4+ or 10 to 1000 mg/dL. Collect another specimen and test or prepare the client for an ordered 24-hour urine analysis.

➤ *Glucose:* Note and report any trace or range of glucose from 0 to 4+. Assess blood glucose level. Also assess for drugs that cause elevations, increased urinary output and thirst, or possible dehydration state. Prepare for further testing for glucose levels in the blood and urine.

➤ *Ketones:* Note and report moderate acetone level and blood level over 50 mg/dL. Assess weight, dietary regimen, diarrhea, presence of diabetes mellitus, or possible ketoacidotic state. Administer ordered insulin or other medications.

➤ *Blood:* Note and report microscopic or macroscopic amounts of blood. Assess for anticoagulant therapy, urinary tract or renal disorders, or toxic response to drug therapy.

➤ *Bilirubin:* Note and report presence of bilirubin. Assess for jaundice of mucous membranes and sclera and for clay color of stool. Also assess for liver or biliary tract disorders and drug regimens that cause liver damage.

➤ *Nitrite:* Note and report positive result. Obtain a clean-catch urine specimen for culture tests.

➤ *Leukocyte esterase:* Note and report positive results with a positive nitrite test. Obtain a clean-catch urine specimen for culture tests.

➤ **Critical values:** Physician should be notified immediately of a positive microscopic result of high levels of red blood cells, greater than 50 white blood cells, or pathological crystals, as well as grossly bloody urine, and 3 to 4+ or 1 to 2 percent of glucose or ketones, or both, by dipstick testing.

TESTS OF RENAL FUNCTION

Renal function tests are used to evaluate the excretory, secretory, and osmolar regulation dynamics of the kidney. Broad categories of such tests include (1) clearance tests, (2) tubular function tests, and (3) concentration tests.

CLEARANCE TESTS AND CREATININE CLEARANCE

The term *clearance* refers to the relationship between the renal excretory mechanisms and the circulating blood levels of the materials to be excreted. Clearance reflects the overall efficiency of glomerular functioning.

Substances filtered through the glomerulus are (1) excreted into the urine unaltered by the renal tubules, (2) reabsorbed partially or entirely by the renal tubules, or (3) added to by the renal tubules. For the purpose of clearance tests, substances that pass through the glomerulus and are not altered by the renal tubules are analyzed. The assumption is that all of the substance is cleared from the plasma via the glomerulus and is excreted unchanged into the urine. Substances that may be measured in clearance tests include inulin, urea, para-aminohippuric acid (PAH), and creatinine.[61]

Inulin is an inert sugar that is not metabolized, absorbed, or secreted by the body. To determine renal clearance, inulin must be infused IV at a constant rate throughout the testing period. Renal clearance is then calculated by measuring the urinary excretion of inulin in relation to plasma concentration. Because this test involves administration of an exogenous substance, it is not used frequently.[62] *PAH* is similar to inulin in that it also must be administered IV for clearance tests.

Urea, an end product of protein metabolism, is formed in the liver and excreted relatively unchanged by the kidneys. Blood urea levels are affected by a variety of factors, and, therefore, it is not the ideal substance for renal clearance tests. Blood urea levels may be elevated if shock, trauma, sepsis, or tumors cause increased protein metabolism. A high-protein diet or state of dehydration will also cause elevated blood urea levels. High blood urea levels could result in normal clearance test values even though renal function is depressed.

Creatinine is the ideal substance for determining renal clearance because a fairly constant quantity is produced within the body. As discussed in Chapter 5, creatinine is the end product of creatine metabolism. Creatine resides almost exclusively in skeletal muscle, where it participates in energy-requiring metabolic reactions. In these processes, a small amount of creatine is irreversibly converted to creatinine, which then circulates to the kidneys and is excreted. The amount of creatinine generated in an individual is proportional to the mass of skeletal muscle present and remains fairly constant unless there is massive muscle damage caused by crushing injury or degenerative muscle disease.[63] As muscle mass is usually greater in men than in women, the quantity of creatinine excreted is usually greater in men.

Creatinine clearance is a sensitive indicator of glomerular function because those factors affecting creatinine clearance are primarily caused by alterations in renal function. These factors include the number of functioning nephrons, the efficiency with which they function (i.e., if there is decreased functioning of some nephrons, others may function more efficiently to compensate), and the amount of blood entering the nephrons. In general, a 50 percent reduction in functioning nephrons causes creatinine clearance to be slightly decreased. Loss of two thirds of the nephrons, however, produces a sharp decrease. It should be noted that creatinine clearance tends to decline with normal aging. Thus, it is important to know the client's age when interpreting test results.[64]

Renal disease is the major cause of reduced creatinine clearance. Other disorders that may result in decreased creatinine clearance include shock, hypovolemia, and exposure to nephrotoxic drugs and chemicals.

The creatinine clearance test is performed by collecting all urine for 24 hours, measuring the creatinine present, and calculating clearance according to the basic formula shown here. As indicated by the formula, it is necessary to determine the plasma level of creatinine at some point during the test.

$$C = \frac{UV}{P}$$

where
C = creatinine clearance
U = amount of creatinine in urine
V = volume of urine excreted per 24 hours
P = plasma creatinine level

Reference Values

Creatinine Clearance	Conventional Units	SI Units
Men	85–125 mL/min	1.41–2.08 mL/s/1.73m^2
Women	75–115 mL/min	1.21–1.91 mL/s/1.73m^2

Interfering Factors

➤ Incomplete urine collection may yield a falsely lowered value.

➤ Excessive ketones in urine and presence of substances such as barbiturates, phenolsulfonphthalein (PSP), and sulfobromophthalein (Bromsulphalein [BSP]) may cause falsely lowered values.

Indications for Clearance Tests and Creatinine Clearance

➤ Determination of the extent of nephron damage in known renal disease (i.e., at least 50 percent of functioning nephrons must be lost before values will be decreased)
➤ Monitoring for the effectiveness of treatment in renal disease
➤ Determination of renal function before administering nephrotoxic drugs or drugs that may build up if glomerular filtration is reduced

Nursing Care Before the Procedure

Explain to the client:
➤ The necessity of collecting all urine for 24 hours
➤ How to maintain the sample (e.g., on ice, refrigerated) if being collected at home
➤ That a blood sample also will be collected once during the test
Prepare for the procedure:
➤ Provide the proper collection container.
➤ Provide for proper preservation of the sample.
➤ Use the techniques for collecting a 24-hour sample as described in Appendix II.

The Procedure

Creatinine Clearance. A 24-hour urine sample is collected (see Appendix II). A preservative may be added to the collection container by the laboratory to prevent degradation of the creatinine. If a preservative is not available, the urine should be kept on ice or refrigerated throughout the collection period. A blood sample is obtained at some point during the urine collection to determine plasma creatinine level.

Nursing Care After the Procedure

Special aftercare interventions are not required for this test.
➤ *Compromised renal function:* Note and report creatinine clearance that has decreased in comparison to an increased serum creatinine and estimated GFR. Monitor I&O and fluid and protein restrictions. Instruct client in dietary, fluid, and medication inclusions and exclusions.

TUBULAR FUNCTION TESTS AND PHENOLSULFONPHTHALEIN (PSP) TEST

Tubular function tests assess the ability of the renal tubules to remove waste products and other substances (e.g., drugs) from the blood and secrete them into the urine. Normal tubular function is dependent on two main factors: (1) adequate renal blood flow and (2) effective tubular function. According to Sacher and McPherson,[65] although tests of tubular function may provide valuable physiological insight, they provide little diagnostic information in individual clinical situations. More appropriate information may be obtained by measuring blood and urine levels of substances such as glucose and electrolytes and comparing the results. Elevated serum potassium levels, for example, combined with decreased potassium in the urine indicate impaired tubular secretion of potassium. Failure to excrete an appropriate acidic or alkaline urine in relation to blood pH levels (see p. 314) also indicates disruption of normal tubular secreting mechanisms.

If tubular function tests are to be performed, they are usually carried out by injecting phenolsulfonphthalein (PSP) IV and then measuring its excretion in serial urine samples. PSP is a dye that binds to albumin in the bloodstream and, therefore, cannot be excreted through the glomerulus. To be excreted, the dye must be secreted by renal tubular cells. In the proximal renal tubules, the dye has greater affinity for the cells lining the tubules than it does for the protein. When it dissociates from the protein, it can be secreted by the tubules.[66] Because it is a dye, PSP imparts a pinkish color to alkaline urine upon excretion. Within 2 hours of injection, 75 percent of the dose is excreted if renal blood flow and tubular function are normal.

Measurement of the dye that is present is accomplished with a spectrophotometer. Thus, any substances that alter the color of urine (see Table 6–1, p. 312) may also alter test results. The client must be well hydrated so that renal perfusion is adequate and urine flow is brisk. If the urine lacks sufficient alkalinity, substances such as sodium hydroxide may be added to the sample in the laboratory to produce the necessary pH for testing.

Reference Values

Adults	After 15 min, 25% of the dose is excreted
	After 30 min, 50–60% of the dose is excreted
	After 60 min, 60–70% of the dose is excreted
	After 2 hr, 70–80% of the dose is excreted
Children	Amounts excreted are 5–10% higher at the preceding time intervals

Interfering Factors

➤ Failure to collect the urine samples at the required times (Reference values are based on these times.)

➤ Failure to completely empty the bladder each time a specimen is collected

➤ Presence in the urine of any substance that alters the color of urine (see Table 6–1, p. 312), as results are based on dye excretion

➤ Inadequately hydrated client such that the kidneys are inadequately perfused or urine flow is decreased

➤ Presence in the blood of radiographic dye, salicylates, sulfonamides, and penicillin that may lead to decreased excretion of the dye

➤ High serum protein levels, which may lead to decreased excretion of the dye

➤ Severe hypoalbuminemia, excessive albuminuria, or severe liver disease, which may lead to increased excretion of the dye

Indications for Tubular Function Tests and Phenolsulfonphthalein (PSP) Test

➤ Assessment of renal blood flow and tubular secreting ability (The PSP test is of limited clinical usefulness.)

> ➤➤ **Nursing Alert**

- The PSP excretion test should not be performed on clients who have demonstrated previous allergy to the dye.

Nursing Care Before the Procedure

Explain to the client:

➤ The importance of increased fluid intake before the test

➤ That foods and drugs that impart color to the urine (e.g., carrots, beets, rhubarb, azo- drugs) should be avoided for 24 hours before the test

➤ That a dye that circulates through the blood and then is excreted by the kidneys will be injected IV

➤ That four urine specimens will be obtained at timed intervals (i.e., 15 minutes, 30 minutes, 1 hour, and 2 hours) after injection of the dye

➤ The importance of completely emptying the bladder each time a urine sample is obtained

Obtain a signed permission consent form. Then:

➤ Ensure to the extent possible that dietary and medication restrictions are followed.

➤ Provide sufficient fluids to promote adequate hydration.

➤ Obtain four containers for the urine samples.

The Procedure

PSP Excretion Test. PSP dye is injected IV, after which a pressure dressing is applied to the injection site. Urine samples are then collected at 15-minute, 30-minute, 1-hour, and 2-hour intervals. Each specimen should consist of at least 50 mL. If the client cannot void at the required time, a Foley catheter may be inserted and the specimen obtained. The catheter is then clamped until the next specimen is due.

Nursing Care After the Procedure

Care and assessment after the test include resuming the client's foods and medications previously withheld.

➤ Monitor the dye injection site for inflammation and hematoma formation.

➤ Remove a catheter if one has been inserted for the test, and assess voiding pattern.

➤ *Allergic response:* Note and report skin rash, urticaria, and change in pulse and respirations. Administer ordered antihistamine and steroid therapy. Have resuscitation equipment and oxygen on hand.

➤ *Urinary infection:* Note and report urinary pattern changes and characteristics (cloudy, foul-smelling). Obtain urine specimen for culture. Monitor I&O. Administer antimicrobial therapy as ordered.

CONCENTRATION TESTS AND DILUTION TESTS

Concentration tests assess the ability of the renal tubules to appropriately absorb water and essential salts such that the urine is properly concentrated. The glomerular filtrate entering the renal tubules normally has a specific gravity of 1.010. If the renal tubules are damaged such that they cannot effectively reabsorb water and salt, the specific gravity of the excreted urine will remain at 1.010 (see p. 313). Loss of tubular concentrating ability is one of the earliest indicators of renal disease and may occur before blood levels of urea and creatinine rise. In addition to the various forms of renal disease, other situations in which renal concentrating ability may be impaired include failure to secrete antidiuretic hormone (central diabetes insipidus), lack of renal response to antidiuretic hormone (nephrogenic diabetes insipidus), prolonged overhydration, osmotic diuresis (especially that caused by uncontrolled diabetes mellitus), hypokalemia, hypocalcemia, lithium and ethanol use, severe hypoproteinemia, multiple myeloma, amyloidosis, sickle cell disease or trait, and psychogenic polydipsia.

The concentration of urine may be determined by measuring either the specific gravity or the osmolality of the sample. In some cases, a single early-morning specimen will suffice. In other situations, timed tests conducted over 12 to 24 hours may be necessary. Another approach is to measure both the serum and the urine osmolality and to compare the results.

Measuring the osmolality of urine is considered more accurate than determining the specific gravity. As noted previously, both the number and the size of particles present influence the specific gravity of urine (see p. 313). In contrast, osmolality is affected only by the number of particles present. Thus, smaller molecules such as sodium and chloride, which are of interest in renal concentration tests, contribute more to urine osmolality measures than they do to specific gravity determinations. In the laboratory, osmolality is reported as milliosmols (mOsm).

Normally, the kidneys can concentrate urine to an osmolality of about three to four times that of plasma (normal plasma osmolality is 275 to 300 mOsm). If the client is overhydrated, the kidneys will excrete the excess water and produce urine with an osmolality as low as one fourth or less that of plasma.[67] Because factors such as fluid intake, diet (especially protein and salt intake), and exercise influence urine osmolality, it has been difficult to establish exact reference values. It is considered more reliable to measure serum and urine osmolalities and compare the two in terms of a ratio relationship (see Chap. 5).

Timed concentration tests are performed if early-morning samples indicate inadequate overnight urine concentrating ability. In the Fishberg test, an attempt is made to maximally concentrate urine through fluid restriction. In the standard version of this test, the client consumes no fluid for 24 hours (from breakfast one day to breakfast the next). In the simplified version, fluids are restricted from the evening meal until breakfast the next morning (see "The Procedure," p. 340).[68] The 24-hour fluid restriction should produce the maximum concentration possible. The 12-hour overnight restriction will increase the concentration to about 75 percent of maximum, partly because of the normal increase in urine concentration that occurs at night.[69]

The Mosenthal test also derives from the principle of increased urine concentration at night. In this test, two consecutive 12-hour urine specimens are collected, one from approximately 8 AM to 8 PM and one from 8 PM to 8 AM. If kidney function is normal, the specific gravity of the nighttime collection should be greater than that of the daytime collection.[70]

It should be noted that tests of the kidney's ability to produce dilute urine are rarely performed. These tests involve overhydrating the client and then observing for the appearance of dilute urine with low specific gravity and osmolality. The danger is that not all clients can tolerate the fluid load needed to produce the desired results.

Reference Values

Concentration Tests	
Specific gravity	1.001–1.035 (usual range 1.010–1.025)
Osmolality	50–1400 mOsm (usual range 300–900 mOsm; average 850 mOsm)
Ratio of urine to serum osmolality	1.2:1 to 3:1
Fishberg test (standard)	Specific gravity 1.026 or higher on at least one sample
Fishberg test (simplified)	Specific gravity 1.022 or higher on at least one sample
Mosenthal test	Specific gravity 1.020 or higher with at least a 7-point difference between the specific gravities of the daytime and nighttime samples
	Dilution Tests
	Specific gravity <1.003
	or
	Osmolality <100 mOsm

Interfering Factors

Concentration Tests
➤ Failure of the client to follow the fluid restrictions necessary for the Fishberg test
➤ Ingestion of a diet with an excessive or inadequate amount of protein, sodium, or both
➤ Presence of disorders that alter serum protein or sodium levels

Dilution Tests
➤ Inability of the client to ingest the required fluids for the test
➤ Inability of the client to tolerate the fluid load required for the test

Indications for Concentration Tests and Dilution Tests

Concentration Tests
➤ Early detection of renal tubular damage (i.e., before serum levels of urea and creatinine are elevated) as indicated by loss of tubular concentrating ability
➤ Detection of disorders that impair renal concentrating ability (e.g., diabetes insipidus)
➤ Differentiation of psychogenic polydipsia from organic disease as indicated by a normal response to timed concentration tests (e.g., Fishberg test)
➤ Detection of excessive or prolonged overhydration
➤ Determination of decreased osmolality (overhydration) and increased osmolality (dehydration)

Dilution Tests
➤ Evaluation of renal tubular response to high fluid volume as indicated by production of urine with low specific gravity and osmolality

---

➤➤ Nursing Alert

- Dilution tests should not be performed on clients who may have difficulty tolerating an increased fluid load (e.g., clients with CHF).

Nursing Care Before the Procedure

Urine Osmolality
There is no specific preparation other than reviewing with the client when the specimen is to be obtained (e.g., first-voided morning urine) and providing a collection container.

Fishberg Test (Standard Version)
Explain to the client:
➤ That no fluids are to be taken after breakfast the initial morning of the test until the test is completed the next morning
➤ That solid (dry) foods are not restricted
➤ That client should completely empty the bladder at approximately 10 PM before retiring
➤ That client should remain in bed during the night (i.e., during the usual hours of sleep)
➤ That a urine specimen will be obtained at 8 PM after 24 hours without fluids
➤ That client should return to bed for 1 hour after the first specimen is collected
➤ That a second specimen will be collected at 9 PM
➤ That client should resume normal activity for 1 hour after the second specimen is collected
➤ That a third specimen will be collected at 10 PM
Prepare for the procedure:
➤ Ensure to the extent possible that fluid restrictions are followed.
➤ Provide the proper specimen containers.

Fishberg Test (Simplified Version)
Explain to the client:
➤ That no fluids should be taken from the time of the evening meal until the test is completed
➤ That client should completely empty the bladder at approximately 10 PM before retiring
➤ That urine samples will be collected at 7 AM, 8 AM, and 9 AM, after approximately 12 hours without fluids
Note: Some laboratories require that the evening meal consist of a high-protein, low-salt diet with no more than 200 mL fluid. If this is the case, the client should be so informed. Then:
➤ Ensure to the extent possible that fluid restrictions are followed.
➤ Provide the proper specimen containers.

Mosenthal Test

Explain to the client:
➤ That two consecutive 12-hour urine collections will be obtained: one from 8 AM to 8 PM in one container and one from 8 PM to 8 AM in another container
➤ The importance of collecting all urine voided during the time period
➤ That there are no diet or fluid restrictions

Prepare for the procedure:
➤ Provide the proper specimen containers.

Dilution Tests

Explain to the client:
➤ That it will be necessary to drink approximately 3 pt (1500 mL) of water in a ½-hour period
➤ That hourly urine specimens will be obtained for 4 hours after ingestion of the water
➤ That any symptoms of fluid excess (e.g., palpitations, shortness of breath) should be reported immediately

Ensure to the extent possible that the client consumes or receives the required fluids. Then:
➤ Provide the proper specimen containers.

The Procedure

Specific Gravity and Urine Osmolality. A random urine specimen of at least 15 mL is collected, preferably first thing in the morning.

Fishberg Test (Standard Version). The client eats his or her usual breakfast, after which no further fluids are ingested until the test is completed the next morning. Solid (dry) foods are allowed. The client voids at approximately 10 PM or before retiring. Urine specimens are collected the next morning at 8 AM, 9 AM, and 10 AM. The client is to remain in bed between the 8 AM and 9 AM specimens and to resume normal activities between the 9 AM and 10 AM specimens.

Fishberg Test (Simplified Version). The client eats his or her evening meal, after which no fluids are ingested until the test is completed the next morning. Some laboratories require that the evening meal consist of a high-protein, low-salt diet with no more than 200 mL of fluid. The client voids at approximately 10 PM or before retiring. Urine samples are collected the next morning at 7 AM, 8 AM, and 9 AM.

Mosenthal Test. Two separate but consecutive 12-hour urine collections are obtained, one from 8 AM to 8 PM and one from 8 PM to 8 AM the next day.

Dilution Tests. These tests, although rarely conducted, may be performed upon completion of the Fishberg tests. The client ingests 1500 mL of water over a ½-hour period. An alternative approach is to administer IV fluids, with the type and amount determined by the physician ordering the test. Urine samples are collected every hour for 4 hours after ingestion or administration of the fluid.

Nursing Care After the Procedure

Specific Gravity and Urine Osmolality. There are no special aftercare interventions.

Fishberg Tests. Resume normal fluid intake and diet.

Mosenthal Test. There are no special aftercare interventions.

Dilution Tests. Monitor response to the fluid load. Note especially increased pulse rate or difficulty breathing.
➤ *Hydration state:* Note and report I&O ratio and adequacy, changes in urinary pattern, and diuresis. Assess for dehydration signs and symptoms. Monitor I&O and effect on specimen collection and testing. Also monitor urinary amounts and characteristics.
➤ **Critical values:** Notify physician immediately if the osmolality result is less than 100 mOsm (overhydration) or greater than 800 mOsm (dehydration).

MEASUREMENT OF OTHER SUBSTANCES

A variety of substances may be measured in urine to detect alterations in physiological function. Among these are electrolytes, pigments, enzymes, hormones and their metabolites, proteins and their metabolites, vitamins, and minerals.

ELECTROLYTES

One of the major functions of the kidney is the regulation of electrolyte balance. Electrolytes are filtered through the glomerulus and reabsorbed in the renal tubules. Those electrolytes most commonly measured in urine are sodium, chloride, potassium, calcium, phosphorus, and magnesium. Tests for electrolytes in urine usually involve 24-hour urine collections. Serum determinations of electrolyte levels are, therefore, preferred to the more cumbersome urinary determinations (see Chap. 5). An exception is magnesium, which indicates deficiency earlier than does serum assay.

Sodium

Most of the sodium filtered through the glomerulus is reabsorbed in the proximal renal tubule. Additional amounts may be reabsorbed in the distal tubule under the influence of aldosterone, a hormone (mineralocorticoid) released by the adrenal cortex. Aldosterone is released in response to decreased serum sodium, decreased blood volume, and increased serum potassium. Enhanced sodium reabsorption is reflected in decreased amounts being excreted in the urine. This may be seen in situations such as hyperaldosteronism, hemorrhage, shock, CHF with inadequate renal perfusion, and therapy with adrenal corticosteroids. Increased loss of sodium into the urine is associated with excessive salt intake, diuretic therapy, diabetic ketoacidosis, adrenocortical hypofunction, toxemia of pregnancy, hypokalemia, and excessive licorice ingestion. Renal failure may cause either retention or loss of sodium. In acute renal disease involving the renal tubules (e.g., ATN), there may be excessive loss of sodium into the urine, as the tubules are too impaired to reabsorb sodium normally.

Chlorides

Chlorides are generally reabsorbed passively along with sodium. The kidney may also secrete either chloride or bicarbonate, depending on the acid-base balance of the body. Chloride excretion is directly influenced by chloride intake. It is also influenced by factors that affect sodium excretion. Chloride excretion may be impaired in certain types of renal disease.[71]

Potassium

Like sodium, potassium is filtered through the glomerulus and reabsorbed through the tubules. Adequate excretion of potassium from the body also requires that the distal tubules and collecting ducts secrete potassium into the urine. Aldosterone also influences potassium excretion in that potassium is excreted in exchange for the sodium that is reabsorbed. Urinary excretion also varies in relation to dietary intake. Causes of excessive potassium loss in the urine include diabetic ketoacidosis, therapy with diuretics, and consumption of large amounts of licorice. The most common cause of decreased potassium in the urine is chronic renal failure, in which tubular secretory activity is impaired.

Calcium

Calcium is the most abundant cation in the body, with bone its major reservoir. Only a small amount of calcium circulates in the blood, and most calcium excretion takes place via the stools. Serum calcium levels are largely regulated by the parathyroid glands and vitamin D. Urinary calcium excretion varies directly with the serum calcium level. If blood levels are high, more calcium is excreted. Blood levels of calcium vary with dietary intake, although they are more influenced by increased intake than by decreased intake. Calcium excretion is highest just after a meal and lowest at night.[72] Although many disorders may alter calcium excretion, determination of urinary calcium is made primarily to evaluate individuals with kidney stones or with suspected parathyroid disorders.

Seventy-five percent of all kidney stones contain calcium compounds. Contrary to popular belief, the most common cause of calcium-containing kidney stones is not excessive calcium intake. The hypercalcemia and increased calcium excretion associated with calcium kidney stones are the result of lack of appropriate renal tubular reabsorption of calcium, increased calcium reabsorption in the intestines, loss of calcium from bone, or low serum phosphorus levels. A variety of disorders can cause these basic defects,[73] among them hyperparathyroidism; sarcoidosis; renal tubular acidosis; cancers of the lung, breast, and bone; multiple myeloma; and metastatic cancer. Drugs that may lead to excessive calcium excretion include toxic doses of vitamin D, adrenocorticosteroids, and calcitonin.

Decreased calcium in the urine is related to hypoparathyroidism, nephrosis, acute nephritis, chronic renal failure, osteomalacia, steatorrhea, and vitamin D deficiency. Drugs associated with decreased calcium in the urine are thiazides and viomycin.

As noted, a 24-hour urine collection is made to determine the quantity of calcium lost in the urine. Sulkowitch's test, a qualitative measure, may be used to determine the presence of calcium in random urine specimens. If necessary, clients may be taught to perform this test at home.

Phosphorus

As with calcium, serum contains relatively small amounts of phosphorus, with bone serving as the major reservoir. Phosphorus levels also are regulated by the parathyroid glands and vitamin D, with excretion controlled primarily by the kidneys. Causes of increased loss of phosphorus in the urine include hyperparathyroidism and renal tubular acidosis. Causes of decreased loss in the urine are hypoparathyroidism, nephrosis, nephritis, and chronic renal failure. Toxic doses of vitamin D may also result in decreased urinary excretion of phosphorus. Dietary intake of phosphates also influences urinary excretion.

Magnesium

Magnesium is an essential nutrient found in bone, muscle, and red blood cells. Relatively little is found in serum. Magnesium participates in the control of serum electrolyte levels and increases intestinal absorption of calcium. Signs and symptoms of magnesium imbalance are manifested primarily in the central nervous and neuromuscular systems. Urinary measures of magnesium may be used instead of serum measures because changes in magnesium levels are reflected more quickly in the urine than in the blood and may facilitate prompt diagnosis of the client's problem. Causes of increased magnesium excretion include alcoholism, adrenocortical insufficiency, renal insufficiency, hypothyroidism, hyperparathyroidism, and excessive ingestion of magnesium-containing antacids. Thiazide diuretics and ethacrynic acid may also produce excessive urinary excretion of magnesium. Decreased urinary excretion is associated with malabsorption syndromes, dehydration, hyperaldosteronism, diabetic acidosis, pancreatitis, and advanced chronic renal disease. Increased calcium intake also results in decreased urinary excretion of magnesium.

Reference Values

	Conventional Units	SI Units
Sodium	30–280 mEq/24 hr	30–280 mmol/d
Chloride	110–250 mEq/24 hr	110–250 mmol/d
Potassium	40–80 mEq/24 hr	40–80 mmol/d
Calcium		
Quantitative		
Men	<275 mg/24 hr	<6.8 mmol/d
Women	<250 mg/24 hr	<6.2 mmol/d
Qualitative		
Sulkowitch's test	0 to +2 turbidity	
Phosphorus	0.9–1.3 g/24 hr	29–42.0 mmol/d
Magnesium	<150 mg/24 hr	
	6.0–8.5 mEq/24 hr	
	3.0–4.3 mmol/d	

Interfering Factors

➤ Dietary deficiency or excess of the electrolyte to be measured may lead to spurious results.
➤ Increased calcium intake may result in decreased magnesium excretion.
➤ Increased sodium and magnesium intake may cause increased calcium excretion.

➤ Diuretic therapy with excessive loss of electrolytes into the urine may falsely elevate results.

➤ Therapy with adrenocorticosteroids may lead to decreased sodium loss and increased calcium loss.

➤ Excessive ingestion of magnesium-containing antacids may lead to increased excretion of magnesium.

Indications for Measurement of Urinary Electrolytes

With the exception of magnesium, electrolytes are more likely to be measured by serum determinations than by urinary measures of the substances. General reasons for analyzing electrolytes in urine are:

➤ Suspected renal disease

➤ Suspected endocrine disorder

➤ History of kidney stones

➤ Suspected malabsorption problem

➤ Central nervous system (CNS) signs and symptoms of unknown etiology, especially if thought to be a result of magnesium imbalance, which is detected earlier in urine than in blood

Nursing Care Before the Procedure

For quantitative studies (i.e., studies to determine the amount of the electrolyte present), client preparation is the same as that for any test involving the collection of a 24-hour urine sample (see Appendix II).

➤ For calcium studies, some laboratories require that the client be on a diet with a set amount of calcium for at least 3 days before beginning the urine collection. If this is the case, the client should be instructed about the diet.

➤ Medications are not usually withheld, but the laboratory should be informed about those taken.

➤ If the Sulkowitch test, a qualitative study, is used for home monitoring of urinary calcium, the client should be instructed in the procedure.

The Procedure

Quantitative Tests. A 24-hour urine collection is obtained (see Appendix II). Check with the laboratory or individual ordering the test to see whether the diet is to be modified for calcium studies. The laboratory should be informed of any medications taken by the client that may alter test results (see "Interfering Factors" section).

Qualitative Tests (Sulkowitch's Test). A random urine specimen is obtained, 5 mL of which is poured into a test tube. Acetic acid (5 mL of a 10 percent solution) is added to the sample and the mixture is boiled to remove protein. Distilled water is then added to the sample until the original volume is restored. Sulkowitch's reagent (5 mL), which contains oxalic acid and ammonium oxalate, is then added. This reagent reacts with the calcium in the sample and produces turbidity (cloudiness) in the sample. Turbidity is graded on a scale of 0 to +4.[74,75]

Nursing Care After the Procedure

Care and assessment after the test include resuming the client's diet after the specimen collection is completed.

PIGMENTS

Pigments that may be found in urine consist primarily of those substances involved in the synthesis and breakdown of hemoglobin. These substances consist of hemoglobin, hemosiderin, bilirubin, urobilinogen, and porphyrins. Myoglobin, which is related to hemoglobin but found primarily in skeletal muscle, is another type of pigment, as is melanin, which is found in hair and skin. With the exceptions of urobilinogen and porphyrins, these substances are not normally found in urine.

Hemoglobin, hemosiderin, bilirubin, and urobilinogen were previously discussed (see pp. 319 to 321). Myoglobin is discussed on page 315. Its presence is associated with extensive damage to skeletal muscles. Melanin, which may be incorporated into tubular epithelial cells, is seen in malignant melanoma (see p. 315). The focus of this section, therefore, is on the porphyrins.

Porphyrins

Porphyrins are produced during the synthesis of heme (Fig. 6–2). If heme synthesis is deranged, these precursors accumulate and are excreted in the urine in excessive amounts. Conditions producing increased levels of heme precursors are called porphyrias. The two main categories of genetically determined porphyrias are erythropoietic porphyrias, in which major diagnostic abnormalities occur in red cell chemistry, and hepatic porphyrias, in which heme precursors are found in urine and feces. Erythropoietic and hepatic porphyrias are very rare. Acquired porphyrias are characterized by greater accumulation of precursors in urine and feces than in red blood cells. Lead poisoning is the most common cause of acquired porphyria.

Those prophyrins for which urine may be tested include aminolevulinic acid (ALA), porphobilinogen (PBG), uroporphyrin, and coproporphyrin. Knowing the type of porphyrin excreted in excess aids in diagnosing specific disorders. Tests for porphyrins usually involve collection of 24-hour urine samples to determine the quantity of the specific substance present. Screening tests on random specimens to determine the presence of excessive amounts of porphyrins (i.e., qualitative studies) also are available.

The presence of ALA in the urine is associated with lead poisoning. It is also found in liver disease (e.g., hepatic carcinoma and hepatitis) and in acute intermittent and variegate porphyria. PBG is found in the same disorders and may also be seen in clients taking griseofulvin. Rifampin, elevated urobilinogen, and light exposure may falsely elevate values. Uroporphyrin and coproporphyrin also are seen in clients with lead poisoning and liver disease as well as in those with uroporphyria and porphyria cutanea tarda. Uroporphyrin may be found in hemochromatosis, a disorder of iron metabolism that affects the liver and certain other body organs. Coproporphyrin is associated with obstructive jaundice and exposure to toxic chemicals.

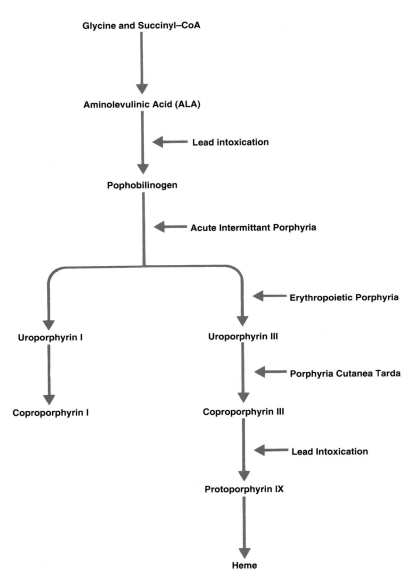

Figure 6–2   Pathway of heme formation, including stages affected by the major disorders of porphyrin metabolism. (From Strasinger, SK: Urinalysis and Body Fluids, ed 3. FA Davis, Philadelphia, 1994, p 125, with permission.)

Porphyrins are reddish fluorescent compounds. Depending on the type of porphyrin present, therefore, the urine may be reddish or the color of port wine (see Table 6–1, p. 312). The presence of congenital porphyria may be suspected when an infant's wet diapers show a red discoloration. PBG is excreted as a colorless compound. If a sample containing PBG is acidic and is exposed to air for several hours, however, a color change may occur.[76]

Reference Values

	Conventional Units	SI Units
Hemoglobin	Negative	Negative
Hemosiderin	Negative	Negative
Bilirubin	Negative	Negative
Urobilinogen		
Random specimen	0.1–1.0 Ehrlich U/dL	Negative
24-hr urine	1–4 mg/24 hr	
Myoglobin	Negative	Negative
Melanin	Negative	Negative
Porphyrins		
Aminolevulinic acid (ALA)		
Random specimen		38.1 μmol/L
Children	<0.5 mg/dL	7.6–45.8 μmol/L
Adults	0.1–0.6 mg/dL	
24-hr urine	1.5–7.5 mg/dL/24 hr	11.15–57.2 μmol/d
Porphobilinogen (PBG)		
Random specimen	Negative	Negative
24-hr urine	0–1.5 mg/24 hr	0–66 μmol/d
Uroporphyrin		
Random specimen	Negative	Negative
24-hr urine	10–30 μg/24 hr	12–37 nmol/d
	(Values may be slightly higher in men than in women.)	
Coproporphyrin		
Random specimen		
Adults	0.045–0.30 μmol/L	
24-hr urine		
Children	0–80 μg/24 hr	0–0.12 μmol/d
Adults	50–160 μg/24 hr	0.075–0.24 μmol/d
	(Values may be slightly higher in men than in women.)	

Interfering Factors

➤ For random samples, delay in sending the specimen to the laboratory within 1 hour of collection may lead to oxidation of bilirubin, if present, and of urobilinogen; random samples for porphyrin tests must be fresh and, thus, must be sent to the laboratory immediately upon collection.

➤ For 24-hour samples, failure to collect the specimen in a dark container or in a container covered with aluminum foil or dark plastic bag may result in invalid results. The specimen must also be refrigerated or kept on ice throughout the collection period unless a preservative has been added to the container by the laboratory. (If the client has a Foley catheter, the drainage bag must be covered with a dark plastic bag and placed in a basin of ice.)

➤ Therapy with griseofulvin, rifampin, and barbiturates may falsely elevate values in tests for porphyrins.

Indications for Analysis of Urinary Pigments

➤ Detection of liver disease as indicated by the presence of bilirubin (possible), excessive urobilinogen, and elevated porphyrins

➤ Diagnosis of the source of obstructive jaundice (i.e., obstruction in the biliary tree) as indicated by presence of bilirubin, absence of urobilinogen, and elevated coproporphyrins

➤ Detection of suspected lead poisoning as indicated by elevated porphyrins, especially ALA and PBG

➤ Detection of excessive red blood cell hemolysis within the systemic circulation as indicated by the presence of free hemoglobin, elevated urobilinogen levels, and presence of hemosiderin a few days after the acute hemolytic episode

➤ Detection of extensive injury to muscles as indicated by the presence of myoglobin in the urine

➤ Detection of malignant melanoma as indicated by the presence of melanin in the urine

Nursing Care Before the Procedure

For quantitative studies, client preparation is the same as that for any test involving collection of a 24-hour urine sample (see Appendix II).

➤ The client should receive the proper container and instructions for maintaining the collection (e.g., refrigerated, protected from light).

➤ For studies involving the porphyrins, medications such as griseofulvin, rifampin, and barbiturates may be withheld. This practice should be confirmed with the person ordering the test.

➤ For random samples, there is no specific preparation other than informing the client that the sample must be protected from light and sent to the laboratory within 1 hour of collection. The proper container should be provided to the client.

The Procedure

Quantitative Tests. A 24-hour urine collection is obtained in a dark container or in one covered with aluminum foil or dark plastic bag. The sample must be kept refrigerated or on ice throughout the collection period unless a preservative has been added to the container by the laboratory. If the client has a Foley catheter, the drainage bag must be covered with a dark plastic bag and placed in a basin of ice.

Random Specimens (Qualitative Tests). A random sample is collected and sent promptly (within 1 hour) to the laboratory. The specimen must be protected from excessive exposure to light.

Nursing Care After the Procedure

Care and assessment after the tests include resuming the client's withheld medications after the specimen collection has been completed.

ENZYMES

As noted in Chapter 5, enzymes are catalysts that enhance reactions without directly participating in them. Enzymes are normally intracellular molecules. When the cells and tissues in which these molecules are found are damaged, enzymes are released. Increased levels will be found in the blood and the urine. Because some enzymes are specific to only certain tissues, elevated levels may aid in pinpointing the source of pathophysiological problems.

Although many enzymes may be measured in blood, only a few are analyzed in urine, including amylase, arylsulfatase A (ARS A), lysozyme (muramidase), and leucine aminopeptidase (LAP). All studies of urinary enzymes involve the collection of 24-hour urine samples, with the exception of amylase, which may be evaluated in timed specimens over shorter periods of time (e.g., 1 or 2 hours).

Amylase

Amylase is a digestive enzyme that splits starch into disaccharides such as maltose. Although many cells have amylase activity, amylase circulating in serum (and ultimately excreted in urine) derives from the parotid glands and the pancreas. Unlike many other enzymes, amylase activity is primarily extracellular; it is secreted into saliva and the duodenum, where it splits large carbohydrate molecules into smaller units for further digestive action by intestinal enzymes.

Urinary amylase levels generally parallel the levels found in blood. There is, however, a lag time between the rise of blood levels and urinary levels. Elevated urine levels also return to normal more slowly than blood levels. This difference between blood and urinary levels of amylase aids in diagnosing and monitoring disorders associated with elevated amylase levels.

Arylsulfatase A (ARS A)

Arylsulfatase A (ARS A) is a lysosomal enzyme found in all body cells except mature red blood cells. Its main sites of activity are in the liver, pancreas, and kidney.

Lysozyme (Muramidase)

Lysozyme is a bactericidal enzyme present in tears, saliva, mucus, and phagocytic cells. Lysozyme is produced in granulocytes and monocytes.

Leucine Aminopeptidase (LAP)

Leucine aminopeptidase (LAP) is an isoenzyme of alkaline phosphatase, an enzyme that cleaves phosphate from compounds and is optimally active at a pH of 9. Although widely distributed in body tissues, LAP is most abundant in hepatobiliary tissues, pancreas, and small intestine.

Reference Values

	Conventional Units	**SI Units**
Amylase	10–80 amylase U/hr (Mayo Clinic)	265–680 U/d*
	35–260 Somogyi U/hr	SI U/hr
		6.5–48.1*
Arylsulfatase A (ARS A)		
Children	>1 U/L	
Men	1.4–19.3 U/L	
Women	1.4–11 U/L	
Lysozyme (Muramidase)	1.3–3.6 mg/24 hr	
Leucine aminopeptidase (LAP)	2–28 U/24 hr	

*These values reflect routine testing methods used in many laboratories, not those under Conventional Units.

Interfering Factors

➤ Incomplete specimen collection and improper specimen maintenance may lead to spurious results.

Amylase

➤ Ingestion of drugs that may falsely elevate values (morphine, codeine, meperidine, pentazocine, chlorothiazides, aspirin, corticosteroids, oral contraceptives, alcohol, indomethacin, bethanechol (Urecholine), secretin, and pancreozymin)
  • Inadvertent addition of salivary amylase to the sample because of coughing or talking over it may falsely elevate values.

Arylsulfatase A (ARS A)

➤ Contamination of the sample with blood, mucus, and feces may falsely elevate levels.
➤ Abdominal surgery within 1 week of the collection may falsely elevate levels.

Lysozyme (Muramidase)

➤ Presence of bacteria in the sample, which will falsely decrease levels
➤ Presence of blood and saliva in the sample, which will falsely elevate levels

Leucine Aminopeptidase (LAP)

➤ Advanced pregnancy and therapy with drugs containing estrogen and progesterone may falsely elevate levels.

Indications for Urinary Enzyme Tests

Amylase

➤ Retrospective diagnosis of acute pancreatitis when serum amylase levels have returned to normal but urine levels remain elevated for 7 to 10 days[77]
➤ Diagnosis of chronic pancreatitis revealed by persistently elevated urinary amylase levels
➤ Monitoring for response to treatment for pancreatitis
➤ Assistance in identifying the cause of "acute abdomen"

➤ Differentiation between acute pancreatitis and perforated peptic ulcer (Urinary amylase levels are higher in pancreatitis.)

➤ Diagnosis of macroamylasemia, a disorder seen in alcoholism and malabsorption syndromes, as revealed by elevated serum amylase and normal urinary amylase

➤ Confirmation of the diagnosis of salivary gland inflammation

Arylsulfatase A (ARS A)

➤ Suspected malignancy involving the bladder, colon, or rectum as indicated by elevated levels

➤ Suspected granulocytic leukemia as indicated by elevated levels

➤ Family history of lipid storage diseases (e.g., mucolipidoses II and III), with support for the diagnosis indicated by elevated levels

➤ Suspected metachromatic leukodystrophy as indicated by decreased levels

Lysozyme (Muramidase)

➤ Suspected acute granulocytic or monocytic leukemia as indicated by elevated levels

➤ Monitoring for the extent of destruction of monocytes and granulocytes in known leukemias

➤ Suspected renal tubular damage as indicated by elevated levels

➤ Monitoring of response to renal transplant with rejection indicated by elevated levels[78]

Leucine Aminopeptidase (LAP)

➤ Elevated serum alkaline phosphatase or LAP levels of unknown etiology

➤ Suspected liver (cirrhosis, hepatitis, cancer), pancreatic (pancreatitis, cancer), and biliary diseases (obstruction caused by gallstones, strictures, atresia), especially when serum LAP levels are normal (Urinary elevations lag behind serum elevations.)

Nursing Care Before the Procedure

Amylase. Client preparation is the same as that for any study involving a 24-hour or timed urine collection. The proper container and instructions for maintaining the collection (e.g., refrigerated, protected from exposure to salivary secretions) should be provided.

➤ Drugs that may alter test results (see "Interfering Factors") may be withheld during the test, although this practice should be confirmed with the person ordering the study.

Arylsulfatase A (ARS A). Client preparation is the same as that for any study involving a 24-hour urine collection (see Appendix II). The proper container and instructions for maintaining the collection (e.g., refrigerated, placed on ice) should be provided.

Lysozyme (Muramidase). Client preparation is the same as that for any study involving a 24-hour urine collection. The proper container and instructions for maintaining the collection (e.g., refrigerated, placed on ice) should be provided. The client should be cautioned to avoid touching the inside of the collection container to avoid bacterial contamination of the sample. The client also should be cautioned to avoid contaminating the sample with saliva (e.g., coughing over the specimen) or blood.

Leucine Aminopeptidase (LAP). Client preparation is the same as that for any study involving a 24-hour urine collection. The proper container and instructions for maintaining the collection (e.g., refrigerated, placed on ice) should be provided. Because drugs containing estrogens and progesterone may falsely elevate levels, a medication history regarding these types of drugs should be obtained.

The Procedure

Amylase. A timed urine collection is obtained. The collection may be made over 1-, 2-, 6-, 8-, and 24-hour periods. The sample must be kept refrigerated or on ice throughout the collection period unless the laboratory has added a preservative to the container. If the client has a Foley catheter, the drainage bag must be placed in a basin of ice. Care must be taken to avoid adding salivary secretions to the sample by coughing or talking over the specimen. The sample should be sent promptly to the laboratory when the collection is completed.

Arylsulfatase A (ARS A). A 24-hour urine collection is obtained. The sample must be kept refrigerated or on ice throughout the collection period unless a preservative has been added to the container by the laboratory. If the client has a Foley catheter, the drainage bag must be placed in a basin of ice. Care must be taken not to contaminate the sample with blood, mucus, or feces. The sample should be sent promptly to the laboratory when the collection is completed.

Lysozyme (Muramidase). A 24-hour urine collection is obtained. The sample must be kept refrigerated or on ice throughout the collection period unless a preservative has been added to the container by the laboratory. If the client has a Foley catheter, the drainage bag must be placed on ice. Care must be taken not to contaminate the sample with bacteria, blood, or saliva. The sample should be sent promptly to the laboratory when the collection is completed.

Leucine Aminopeptidase (LAP). A 24-hour urine collection is obtained. The sample must be kept refrigerated or on ice throughout the collection period unless a preservative has been added to the container by the laboratory. If the client has a Foley catheter, the drainage bag must be placed on ice. The sample should be sent promptly to the laboratory when the collection is completed.

Nursing Care After the Procedure

Care and assessment after the test include resuming any withheld medications after the specimen collection has been completed.

HORMONES AND THEIR METABOLITES

Hormones are chemicals that control the activities of responsive tissues. Some hormones exert their effects in the vicinity of their release; others are released into the extracellular fluids of the body and affect distant tissues. Numerous hormones may be measured in blood (see Chap. 5). Most urinary measures focus on the hormones secreted by the adrenal cortex, the adrenal medulla, the gonads, and the placenta. Either the hormone itself or the metabolites thereof may be measured.

Urinary measures of hormones and their metabolites usually involve collection of 24-hour urine specimens. The advantage of such quantitative measures over single blood level determinations is that overall levels of hormone secretion are reflected. This is important because blood levels of hormones tend to vary, depending on time of day.

Cortisol

The adrenal cortex secretes three types of steroids: (1) glucocorticoids, which affect carbohydrate metabolism; (2) mineralocorticoids, which promote potassium excretion and sodium retention by the kidneys; and (3) adrenal androgens, which the liver converts primarily to testosterone. Cortisol is the predominant glucocorticoid. It is produced and secreted in response to adrenocorticotropic hormone (ACTH), which is secreted by the adenohypophysis. Ninety percent of cortisol is bound to cortisol-binding globulin (CBG) and albumin. The "free" (unbound) portion is responsible for its physiological activity and also is the portion excreted into the urine. Cortisol stimulates gluconeogenesis, mobilizes fats and proteins, antagonizes insulin, and suppresses inflammation.

The purpose of urinary measures of cortisol is to detect elevated levels of free cortisol, which may not be apparent in random blood samples. Elevated cortisol levels occur in Cushing's syndrome, in which there is excessive production of adrenocorticosteroids. Cushing's syndrome may be caused by pituitary adenoma, adrenal hyperplasia, benign or malignant adrenal tumors, and nonendocrine malignant tumors that secrete ectopic ACTH. Therapy with adrenal corticosteroids may also produce cushingoid signs and symptoms. Elevated cortisol levels are additionally associated with stress, hyperthyroidism, obesity, diabetic ketoacidosis, pregnancy, and excessive exercise. Other drugs that may elevate cortisol levels include estrogens, oral contraceptives, lithium carbonate, methadone, alcohol, phenothiazines, amphetamines, morphine, and reserpine.

Aldosterone

Aldosterone, the predominant mineralocorticoid, is secreted by the zona glomerulosa of the adrenal cortex in response to decreased serum sodium, decreased blood volume, and increased serum potassium. Aldosterone is released in response to direct stimulation by altered serum sodium and potassium levels. In addition, decreased blood volume and altered sodium and potassium levels stimulate the juxtaglomerular apparatus of the kidney to secrete renin. Renin is subsequently converted to angiotensin II, which then stimulates the adrenal cortex to secrete aldosterone. In normal states, ACTH does not play a major role in aldosterone secretion. In disease states, however, ACTH may also enhance aldosterone secretion.

Aldosterone increases sodium reabsorption in the renal tubules, gastrointestinal tract, salivary glands, and sweat glands. This subsequently results in increased water retention, blood volume, and blood pressure. Aldosterone also increases potassium excretion by the kidneys in exchange for the sodium ions that are retained.

Excessive aldosterone levels are categorized as primary and secondary hyperaldosteronism. Primary hyperaldosteronism represents inappropriate aldosterone secretion, which is usually caused by benign adenomas or bilateral hyperplasia of the aldosterone-secreting zona glomerulosa cells. In primary aldosteronism, aldosterone is secreted independently of the renin-angiotensin system. A hallmark of primary aldosteronism is low plasma renin levels.

Secondary hyperaldosteronism indicates an appropriate response to pathological changes in blood volume and electrolytes. Common causes of secondary hyperaldosteronism include CHF, cirrhosis, nephrotic syndrome, chronic obstructive pulmonary disease (COPD), and renal artery stenosis. Other causes of elevated aldosterone levels are stress, excessive exercise, pregnancy, and several drugs (diuretics, apresoline, diazoxide, and nitroprusside). In secondary hyperaldosteronism, plasma renin levels are elevated.

Decreased aldosterone levels are associated with Addison's disease, hypernatremia, hypokalemia, diabetes mellitus, toxemia of pregnancy, excessive licorice ingestion, and certain drugs (propranolol and fludrocortisone).

17-Hydroxycorticosteroids (17-OHCS)

All glucocorticoids are degraded by the liver to metabolites, which as a group are called 17-hydroxycorticosteroids (17-OHCS). These steroid metabolites also are called Porter-Silber chromogens because of the method used to measure them in urine. Because 80 percent of urinary 17-OHCS are metabolites of cortisol, those disorders that are associated with elevated cortisol levels also are associated with elevated 17-OHCS (e.g., Cushing's syndrome). Decreased levels of 17-OHCS are associated with Addison's disease, hypopituitarism, and myxedema. As with cortisol, numerous drugs may alter urinary excretion of 17-OHCS. Thus, a thorough medication history is necessary. Some medications may be withheld before and during the test.

When adrenocortical hypofunctioning or hyperfunctioning is suspected, 17-OHCS may be measured in urine as part of the diagnostic process. It should be noted, however, that measurement of urinary cortisol levels provides more accurate quantification than does measurement of 17-OHCS levels in individuals receiving drugs that alter hepatic metabolism of steroids.

17-Ketosteroids (17-KS)

17-Ketosteroids (17-KS) are metabolized from androgenic hormones. In men, two thirds of 17-KS originate in the adrenal cortex and one third derive from the testes. In women, virtually all 17-KS originate in the adrenal cortex. 17-KS do not include testosterone. Components of 17-KS, which may be measured individually, include androsterone, dehydroepiandrosterone, etiocholanolone, 11-hydroxyandrosterone, 11-hydroxyetiocholanolone, 11-ketoandrosterone, 11-ketoetiocholanolone, pregnanediol, pregnanetriol (see following section), 5-pregnanetriol, and 11-ketopregnanetriol.

Levels of 17-KS are elevated in clients having adrenogenital syndrome (congenital adrenal hyperplasia), Cushing's syndrome, hormone-secreting tumors of the adrenal glands or gonads, adrenocortical carcinoma, hyperpituitarism, and stressful conditions. Decreased levels of 17-KS are associated with Addison's disease, liver disease, hypopituitarism, hypothyroidism, gout, nephrotic syndrome, and starvation. As with other urinary hormones, drugs may alter the excretion of 17-KS. Thus, a thorough medication history is necessary.

17-Ketogenic Steroids (17-KGS)

Cortisol and its many metabolites can be manipulated in the laboratory to form 17-ketosteroids. The substances thus formed are called 17-ketogenic steroids (17-KGS) and may be studied as an index of overall glucocorticoid metabolism. Before urinary 17-KGS can be evaluated, the 17-KS of androgenic origin must be either removed or measured separately.[79] Because such a large array of steroid metabolites is reflected in 17-KGS measures, this test provides for a good overall assessment of adrenal function.

Pregnanetriol

Pregnanetriol is a metabolite of the cortisone precursor 17-hydroxyprogesterone. It should not be confused with pregnanediol, which is a metabolite of the hormone progesterone, secreted by the corpus luteum and the placenta (see p. 354). Elevated pregnanetriol levels are associated with adrenogenital syndrome. In this disorder, cortisol synthesis is impaired at the point of 17-hydroxyprogesterone conversion. The substance accumulates and its metabolite, pregnanetriol, is excreted in the urine in increased amounts. Excessive amounts of 17-hydroxyprogesterone, and the resultant pregnanetriol, are produced in response to feedback mechanisms. Because cortisol synthesis is impaired, serum cortisol levels are low. This, in turn, stimulates the adenohypophysis to secrete ACTH, which normally causes cortisol levels to rise. Because cortisol synthesis is impaired, however, pregnanetriol accumulates instead. Furthermore, the feedback mechanism continues to stimulate ACTH production. It should be noted that excessive 17-hydroxyprogesterone may be converted to androgens. This conversion plus excessive androgen secretion in response to ACTH may result in virilization in women and in sexual precocity in boys.

Catecholamines

The adrenal medulla, a component of the sympathetic nervous system, secretes epinephrine and norepinephrine, which are collectively known as the catecholamines. A third catecholamine, dopamine, is secreted in the brain, where it functions as a neurotransmitter. Dopamine is a precursor of epinephrine and norepinephrine. Serotonin, an amine related to the catecholamines, is found in the platelets and in the argentaffin cells of the intestines.

Epinephrine (adrenalin) and norepinephrine are normally secreted in response to generalized sympathetic nervous system stimulation. Epinephrine increases the metabolic rate of all cells, heart rate, arterial blood pressure, blood glucose, and free fatty acids. Norepinephrine, the predominant catecholamine, decreases heart rate while increasing peripheral vascular resistance and arterial blood pressure.

The most clinically significant disorder involving the adrenal medulla is the catecholamine-secreting tumor, pheochromocytoma. Pheochromocytomas may release catecholamines—primarily epinephrine—continuously or intermittently. For this reason, urinary measurements are helpful in quantifying overall excretory levels. Because the most common sign of pheochromocytoma is arterial hypertension, measurement of either plasma (see Chap. 5) or urinary catecholamines and their metabolites is indicated in new-onset hypertension of unknown etiology.

Total catecholamines may be measured in either random or 24-hour urine specimens. The individual catecholamines, epinephrine and norepinephrine, may be measured in 24-hour urine collections, as may metanephrine, a metabolite of epinephrine. Numerous drugs may alter blood and urine levels of catecholamines, and stress, smoking, and strenuous exercise may produce elevated levels. Thus, a thorough health history is required before testing.

Vanillylmandelic Acid (VMA)

Vanillylmandelic acid (VMA) is the predominant catecholamine metabolite found in urine. VMA is easier to detect by laboratory methods than are the catecholamines themselves. Therefore, this test is more frequently used when pheochromocytoma is suspected.

A disadvantage of the test is the need for a special diet for 2 days before the study as well as on the day the 24-hour urine specimen is collected. The following foods are restricted on a "VMA diet": bananas, nuts, cereals, grains, tea, coffee, gelatin foods, citrus fruits, chocolate, vanilla, cheese, salad dressing, jelly, candy, chewing gum, cough drops, most carbonated beverages, licorice, and foods with artificial flavoring or coloring. Ingestion of such foods will falsely elevate VMA levels. It should be noted, however, that, as laboratory methods become more precise, it may be possible to dispense with the VMA diet in urinary measures of VMA.[80]

Homovanillic Acid (HVA)

Homovanillic acid (HVA) is a metabolite of dopamine, a major catecholamine itself, as well as a precursor to the catecholamines epinephrine and norepinephrine. HVA is synthesized in the brain and is associated with disorders involving the nervous system. As with other metabolites, numerous drugs, stress, and excessive exercise may alter HVA levels.

5-Hydroxyindoleacetic Acid (5-HIAA)

5-Hydroxyindoleacetic acid (5-HIAA) is a metabolite of serotonin, which is normally present only in the platelets and in the argentaffin cells of the intestines.

Estrogens and Estrogen Fractions

Estrogens are secreted in large amounts by the ovaries and, during pregnancy, by the placenta. Minute amounts are secreted by the adrenal glands and, possibly, by the testes. Estrogens induce and maintain the female secondary sex characteristics, promote growth and maturation of the female reproductive organs, influence the pattern of fat deposition that characterizes the female form, and cause early epiphyseal closure. They also promote retention of sodium and water by the kidneys and sensitize the myometrium to oxytocin.

Total estrogens as well as the estrogen fractions (estrone, estradiol, and estriol) may be measured in urine. In blood tests, only the fractions are routinely measured (see Chap. 5). Estrone (E_1) is the immediate precursor of estradiol (E_2), which is the most biologically potent fraction. Estriol (E_3), in addition to ovarian sources, is secreted in large amounts by the placenta during pregnancy. It is also secreted by maternal and fetal adrenal glands. Normally, estriol levels should rise steadily during pregnancy.

In addition to advancing and multiple pregnancy, elevated estrogen levels are associated with ovarian and adrenal tumors as well as estrogen-producing tumors of the testes. Drugs that elevate estrogen levels include estrogen-containing drugs, adrenocorticosteroids, tetracyclines, ampicillin, and phenothiazines.

Decreased estrogen levels are seen with primary and secondary ovarian failure, Turner's syndrome, hypopituitarism, adrenogenital syndrome, Stein-Leventhal syndrome, anorexia nervosa, and menopause. Low or steadily decreasing levels of estriol during pregnancy may indicate placental insufficiency, impending fetal distress, fetal anomalies (e.g., anencephaly), and Rh isoimmunization. Decreased estriol levels are associated also with diabetes, hypertensive disorders, and other maternal complications of pregnancy.

It should be noted that, in ovulating women, estrogen levels vary in relation to the menstrual cycle. Thus, the date of the last menstrual period should be noted when analysis of urinary estrogens is performed.

Pregnanediol

Pregnanediol is the chief metabolite of progesterone, which is secreted by the corpus luteum and by the placenta during pregnancy. Progesterone also is secreted in minute amounts by the adrenal cortex in both men and women. Progesterone prepares the endometrium for implantation of the fertilized ovum, decreases myometrial excitability, stimulates proliferation of the vaginal epithelium, and stimulates growth of the breasts during pregnancy. During pregnancy, after implantation of the embryo, progesterone production increases, thus sustaining the pregnancy. This increased production continues until about the 36th week of pregnancy, after which levels begin to diminish.

Although serum determination of progesterone may be made (see Chap. 5), the study of its metabolite, pregnanediol, in urine reflects overall progesterone levels, which may not be apparent in single blood measures. In addition to pregnancy, elevated pregnanediol levels may be associated with ovarian tumors and cysts, adrenocortical hyperplasia and tumors, precocious puberty, and therapy with adrenocorticosteroids. Biliary tract obstruction may also produce elevated levels.

Decreased levels of pregnanediol are associated with placental insufficiency, fetal abnormalities or demise, threatened abortion, and toxemia of pregnancy. Other causes of decreased levels include panhypopituitarism, ovarian failure, Turner's syndrome, adrenogenital syndrome, and Stein-Leventhal syndrome. Therapy with drugs containing progesterone may also lead to decreased pregnanediol levels.

In ovulating women, pregnanediol levels vary in relation to the menstrual cycle. Thus, the date of the last menstrual period should be noted when analysis of pregnanediol is performed.

Human Chorionic Gonadotropin (hCG)

Human chorionic gonadotropin (hCG) is produced only by the developing placenta, and its presence in blood (see Chap. 5) and urine has been used for decades to detect pregnancy. Human chorionic gonadotropin is secreted at increasingly higher levels during the first 2 months of pregnancy, declining during the third and fourth months, and then remaining relatively stable until term.

Qualitative screening test kits for hCG are available for home use to determine pregnancy as early as 8 to 10 days after conception. These screening kits have almost eliminated quantitative testing for hCG to confirm pregnancy. A positive result indicates that a visit to a physician is necessary to obtain confirmation tests and prenatal care, and a negative result in the presence of symptoms of pregnancy indicates that a visit to a physician is necessary for further evaluation.

Elevated levels may be seen in nonendocrine tumors that produce hCG ectopically (e.g., carcinomas of the stomach, liver, pancreas, and breast; multiple myeloma; and malignant melanoma). Decreased levels of hCG are associated with ectopic pregnancy, fetal demise, threatened abortion, and incomplete abortion. Drugs that may alter test results include phenothiazines and anticonvulsants.

Reference Values

	Conventional Units	SI Units
Cortisol	20–90 μg/24 hr	55–230 μmol/d
Aldosterone	2–26 μg/24 hr	5.6–72 nmol/d
17-Hydroxycorticosteroids (17-OHCS)		
Children	1.5–4.0 mg/24 hr (age-related: the younger the child, the less hormone secreted)	4.1–11.0 μmol/d
Men	5.5–14.4 mg/24 hr	15.2–39.7 μmol/d
Women	4.9–12.9 mg/24 hr	13.5–35.6 μmol/d
17-Ketosteroids (17-KS)		
Children	<1–3 mg/24 hr (age-related: the younger the child, the less hormone secreted)	3–10 μmol/d
Men	8–25 mg/24 hr	27–85 μmol/d
Women	5–15 mg/24 hr	17–52 μmol/d
Elderly persons	4–8 mg/24 hr	13.5–28 μmol/d
17-Ketogenic steroids (17-KGS)		
Children	<2–6 mg/24 hr (age-related: the younger the child, the less hormone secreted)	6–17 μmol/d
Men	5–23 mg/24 hr	17–80 μmol/d
Women	3–15 mg/24 hr	10–52 μmol/d
Elderly persons	3–12 mg/24 hr	10–42 μmol/d
Pregnanetriol		
Children, <6 yr	Up to 0.2 mg/24 hr	0.6 μmol/d
Children, 7–16 yr	0.3–1.1 mg/24 hr	0.9–3.3 μmol/d
Adults	<3.5 mg/24 hr	<10.4 μmol/d

Catecholamines
  Total
      Random urine   0–14 μg/dl   0.73 nmol/d
      24-hour urine   <100 g/24 hr   160 nmol/d
    Epinephrine   <10 ng/24 hr   55 nmol/d
    Norepinephrine   <100 ng/24 hr   591 nmol/d
    Metanephrines   0.1–1.6 mg/24 hr   0.5–8.7 μmol/d
Vanillylmandelic acid (VMA)   0.7–6.8 mg/24 hr   3–34 μmol/d
Homovanillic acid (HVA)
  Children
      1–2 yr   0–25 mg/24 hr   1–126 μmol/d
      2–10 yr   0.5–10 mg/24 hr   3–55 μmol/d
      10–15 yr   0.5–12 mg/24 hr   3–66 μmol/d
    Adult   <8 mg/24 hr   1–14 μmol/d
5-Hydroxyindoleacetic acid (5-HIAA)   2–9 mg/24 hr   10.4–46.8 μmol/d
Estrogens
  Total
    Adult men   4–24 μg/24 hr   4–24 μg/d
    Nonpregnant women
      Preovulatory phase   5–25 μg/24 hr   5–25 μg/d
      Ovulatory phase   24–100 μg/24 hr   24–100 μg/d
      Luteal phase   12–80 μg/24 hr   12–80 μg/d
    Postmenopausal women   <10 μg/24 hr   <10 μg/d
  Estrone (E₁)
    Children   0.2–1 g/24 hr   0.7–4 nmol/d
    Men   3.4–8.2 g/24 hr   12–37 nmol/d
    Nonpregnant women
      Early in cycle   4–7 g/24 hr   1.6–3.5 mmol/mol
      Luteal phase   11–31 g/24 hr   4.6–15.7 mmol/mol
    Postmenopausal women   0.8–7.1 g/24 hr
  Estradiol (E₂)
    Children   0–0.2 μg/24 hr   0–0.69 nmol/d
    Men   0–0.4 μg/24 hr   0–1.39 nmol/d
    Nonpregnant women
      Early in cycle   0–3 μg/24 hr   0–10.4 nmol/d
      Luteal phase   4–14 μg/24 hr   13.9–49.6 nmol/d
    Postmenopausal women   0–2.3 μg/24 hr   0–8.0 nmol/d
  Estriol (E₃)
    Children   0.3–2.4 μg/24 hr   1.04–8.33 nmol/d
    Men   0.8–7.5 μg/24 hr   2.8–26.0 nmol/d
    Nonpregnant women
      Early in cycle   0–15 μg/24 hr   0–52.0 nmol/d
      Luteal phase   13–54 μg/24 hr   6.1–187.4 nmol/d
    Postmenopausal women   0.6–6.8 μg/24 hr   2.08–23.6 nmol/d
    Pregnant women   Up to 28 mg/24 hr   Up to 97 μmol/d
                              (When plotted on a
                              graph, levels should
                              steadily rise during
                              pregnancy.)

Pregnanediol		
Men	<1.5 mg/24 hr	<4.7 μmol/d
Nonpregnant women		
Proliferative phase	0.5–1.5 mg/24 hr	1.6–4.7 μmol/d
Luteal phase	2–7 mg/24 hr	6.2–22 μmol/d
Postmenopausal women	0.2–1 mg/24 hr	0.6–3.1 μmol/d
Pregnant women		
16 wk	5–21 mg/24 hr	15–65 μmol/d
20 wk	6–26 mg/24 hr	18–81 μmol/d
24 wk	12–32 mg/24 hr	37–100 μmol/d
28 wk	19–51 mg/24 hr	59–160 μmol/d
32 wk	22–66 mg/24 hr	68–206 μmol/d
36 wk	22–77 mg/24 hr	40–240 μmol/d
40 wk	23–83 mg/24 hr	72–197 μmol/d
Human chorionic gonadotropin (hCG)		
Random urine	Negative if not	Negative if not
24-hr urine	pregnant	pregnant
Men	Not measurable	Not measurable
Nonpregnant women	Not measurable	Not measurable
Pregnant women		
1st trimester	Up to 500,000 IU/24 hr	Up to 500,000 IU/L[6]
2nd trimester	10,000–25,000 IU/24 hr	10,000–25,000 IU/L[6]
3rd trimester	5,000–15,000 IU/24 hr	5,000–15,000 IU/L[6]

Interfering Factors

➤ Improper specimen collection and improper specimen maintenance may lead to spurious results.

➤ Numerous drugs may alter test results. A thorough medication history should be obtained before testing. Some medications may be withheld.

Cortisol

➤ Excessive exercise and stressful situations during the testing period may lead to falsely elevated levels.

Aldosterone

➤ Ingestion of certain foods may lower levels (e.g., licorice and excessive sodium intake).

➤ Excessive exercise and stressful situations during the testing period may falsely elevate levels.

➤ Radioactive scans within 1 week of the study may alter results because urinary aldosterone determinations are made by radioimmunoassay method.

17-Hydroxycorticosteroids (17-OHCS)

➤ Excessive exercise and stressful situations during the testing period may falsely elevate levels.

17-Ketosteroids (17-KS)
➤ Blood in the specimen may alter test results; the test should be postponed if the female client is menstruating.
➤ Excessive exercise and stressful situations during the testing period may falsely elevate levels.

17-Ketogenic Steroids (17-KGS)
➤ Excessive exercise and stressful situations during the testing period may falsely elevate levels.

Pregnanetriol
➤ None, except drugs and improper specimen collection and maintenance

Catecholamines
➤ Excessive exercise and stressful situations during the testing period may falsely elevate levels.

Vanillylmandelic Acid (VMA)
➤ Numerous foods may falsely elevate levels (see p. 356); the client must follow a special diet for this test.
➤ Excessive exercise and stressful situations during the testing period may falsely elevate levels.

Homovanillic Acid (HVA)
➤ Excessive exercise and stressful situations during the testing period may falsely elevate levels.

5-Hydroxyindoleacetic Acid (5-HIAA)
➤ Certain foods (bananas, plums, pineapples, avocados, eggplants, tomatoes, and walnuts) will falsely elevate levels and must be withheld for 4 days before the test.[81]
➤ Severe gastrointestinal disturbance or diarrhea may alter test results.

Estrogens and Estrogen Fractions
➤ Maternal disorders (e.g., hypertension, diabetes, anemia, malnutrition, hemoglobinopathy, liver disease, intestinal disease) may result in decreased estriol levels during pregnancy.
➤ Threatened abortion, ectopic pregnancy, and early pregnancy may result in falsely decreased estriol levels.

Pregnanediol
➤ None, except drugs and improper specimen collection.

Human Chorionic Gonadotropin (hCG)
➤ Proteinuria and hematuria may lead to falsely elevated levels.

Indications for Measurement of Urinary Hormones and Their Metabolites

Cortisol
➤ Diagnostic evaluation of signs of Cushing's syndrome without definitive elevation of plasma cortisol levels (Adrenal hyperplasia raises the urinary cortisol level more significantly than it does the plasma cortisol level.)

➤ Diagnostic evaluation of obesity of undetermined etiology (Obesity may raise plasma cortisol levels but does not significantly elevate free cortisol levels in urine.)

➤ Quantification of cortisol excess, regardless of its source

➤ More accurate quantification than 17-hydroxycorticosteroids (17-OHCS) in individuals receiving drugs that alter hepatic metabolism of steroids

Aldosterone

➤ Suspected hyperaldosteronism, especially when serum aldosterone levels are not definitive for the diagnosis

17-Hydroxycorticosteroids (17-OHCS)

➤ Signs and symptoms of adrenocortical hypofunctioning or hyperfunctioning

➤ Suspected Cushing's syndrome as indicated by elevated levels

➤ Suspected Addison's disease as indicated by decreased levels

17-Ketosteroids (17-KS)

➤ Suspected adrenocortical dysfunction, especially if urinary levels of 17-OHCS are normal

➤ Suspected Cushing's syndrome as indicated by elevated levels

➤ Suspected adrenogenital syndrome as indicated by elevated levels

➤ Monitoring of response to therapy for adrenogenital syndrome

17-Ketogenic Steroids (17-KGS)

➤ Suspected adrenal hypofunctioning or hyperfunctioning (The test provides a good overall assessment of adrenal function.)

➤ Suspected Cushing's syndrome as indicated by elevated levels

➤ Suspected Addison's disease as indicated by decreased levels

➤ Monitoring for response to therapy with corticosteroid drugs or other drugs that alter adrenal function

Pregnanetriol

➤ Suspected adrenogenital syndrome (virilization in women, precocious sexual development in boys) as indicated by elevated levels

➤ Family history of adrenogenital syndrome

➤ Monitoring of response to cortisol therapy for adrenogenital syndrome[82]

➤ Suspected testicular tumors as indicated by elevated levels

➤ Suspected Stein-Leventhal syndrome as indicated by elevated levels

Catecholamines

➤ Hypertension of unknown etiology

➤ Suspected pheochromocytoma as indicated by elevated levels

➤ Acute hypertensive episode (A random sample is collected in such cases.)

➤ Suspected neuroblastoma or ganglioneuroma as indicated by elevated levels

Vanillylmandelic Acid (VMA)

➤ Hypertension of unknown etiology

➤ Suspected pheochromocytoma as indicated by elevated levels

➤ Suspected neuroblastoma or ganglioneuroma as indicated by elevated levels

Homovanillic Acid (HVA)

➤ Suspected neuroblastoma or ganglioneuroma as indicated by elevated levels

➤ Diagnosis of benign pheochromocytoma as indicated by normal HVA levels with elevated VMA levels

➤ Diagnosis of malignant pheochromocytoma as indicated by elevated HVA and VMA levels

5-Hydroxyindoleacetic Acid (5-HIAA)

➤ Detection of early carcinoid tumors (argentaffinomas) of the intestine as indicated by elevated levels

Estrogens and Estrogen Fractions

➤ Suspected tumor of the ovary, testicle, or adrenal gland as indicated by elevated total estrogens and fractions

➤ Suspected ovarian failure as indicated by decreased total estrogens and fractions

➤ Detection of placental and fetal problems as indicated by estriol levels that fail to show a steady increase over several days or weeks (A sharp decline over several days indicates impending fetal demise; consistently low levels may indicate fetal anomalies.)

➤ Detection of maternal disorders of pregnancy as indicated by estriol levels that fail to show a steady increase over several days or weeks

Pregnanediol

➤ Verification of ovulation in planning a pregnancy or in determining the cause of infertility as indicated by normal values in relation to the menstrual cycle

➤ Diagnosis of placental dysfunction, as indicated by either low levels or failure of levels to progressively increase, and identification of the need for progesterone therapy to sustain the pregnancy

➤ Detection of fetal demise as indicated by decreased levels, although levels may remain within normal limits if placental circulation is adequate

Human Chorionic Gonadotropin (hCG)

➤ Confirmation of pregnancy within 8 to 10 days after conception, especially in women with a history of infertility or habitual abortion or in women who may desire a therapeutic abortion

➤ Suspected hydatidiform mole as indicated by elevated levels

➤ Suspected choriocarcinoma or testicular tumor as indicated by elevated levels

➤ Suspected nonendocrine tumor that produces hCG ectopically as indicated by elevated levels

➤ Threatened abortion as indicated by decreased levels

Nursing Care Before the Procedure

All urine studies for hormones and their metabolites involve collecting 24-hour urine samples (see Appendix II); exceptions are catecholamines and hCG, which may also be analyzed in random samples. The client should, therefore, be instructed on how to collect the sample. The proper container and instructions for maintaining the collection (e.g., refrigerated or on ice) should be provided.

➤ Drugs that may alter test results may be withheld during the test, although this practice should be confirmed with the person ordering the study.

➤ The client should be cautioned to avoid excessive exercise and stress during the following studies: cortisol, aldosterone, 17-OHCS, 17-KS, 17-KGS, catecholamines, VMA, and HVA.

➤ The client also should be instructed on the following dietary restrictions in relation to specific tests: (1) aldosterone—maintain a normal salt intake; (2) VMA—maintain a "VMA diet" (see p. 356) for 2 days before the test and for the day of the test; and (3) 5-HIAA—maintain a diet low in serotonin (see p. 356) for 4 days before the test.

➤ For gonadal and placental hormone studies, the date of the last menstrual period should be noted.

The Procedure

All urine studies for hormones and their metabolites involve collecting 24-hour urine specimens; exceptions are catecholamines and hCG, which may also be analyzed in random samples. For 24-hour collections, an acidifying preservative is added to the container by the laboratory. In addition, some laboratories require that the sample be refrigerated or placed on ice throughout the collection period. Special diets may be required before collection of 24-hour urines for VMA and 5-HIAA (see the previous "Nursing Care Before the Procedure" section).

Random samples for catecholamines may be collected at any time but frequently are obtained after a hypertensive episode. Random samples for hCG are more reliable if collected first thing in the morning because dilute urine may lead to false-negative results.

All specimens should be sent promptly to the laboratory when the collection is completed.

Nursing Care After the Procedure

Care and assessment after the test include resuming the client's usual diet, medications, or activities at completion of specimen collection.

PROTEINS

Normally, the urine contains only a scant amount of protein. Excessive amounts of protein in the urine are generally associated with renal disease. Thus, part of the screening process in a UA is to test the sample for protein (see p. 314). If increased amounts are found, a quantitative 24-hour urine collection is performed. The presence of certain types of proteins in urine also is diagnostic of specific disease states. The presence of Bence Jones protein in the urine, for example, is associated with multiple myeloma (see p. 315).

Protein metabolites such as creatinine and uric acid may also be measured in urine. Creatinine, which is produced at a fairly constant rate within the body, is a sensitive indicator of glomerular function because factors affecting creatinine clearance are primarily the result of alteration in renal function (see p. 333). Creatinine levels may also be measured along with 24-hour measures of other substances in urine (e.g., protein) as an indicator of the accuracy of the collection because the amount excreted in 24 hours should be fairly constant. Measurement of urinary levels of uric acid are discussed later. Amino acids are also products of protein metabolism. As is discussed later, abnormal metabolism and congenital disorders (e.g., phenylketonuria) are associated with excessive levels of certain amino acids.

Uric Acid

Uric acid is an end product of purine metabolism. Purines are constituents of nucleic acids in the body and appear in the urine in the absence of dietary sources of purines. Dietary sources of purines include organ meats, legumes, and yeasts. Uric acid is filtered, absorbed, and secreted by the kidneys and is a common constituent of urine (see p. 309).

The amount of uric acid produced in the body and the efficiency of renal excretion affect the amount of uric acid found in urine. Excessive amounts of uric acid may be found in excessive dietary intake of purines, in massive cell turnover with degradation of nucleic acids, and in disorders of purine metabolism. The body's ability to filter, reabsorb, and secrete uric acid affects the amount of uric acid ultimately found in urine.[83]

Elevated urinary uric acid is commonly associated with neoplastic disorders such as leukemia and lymphosarcoma. It may be found also in individuals with pernicious anemia, sickle cell anemia, and polycythemia. Disorders associated with impaired renal tubular absorption (e.g., Fanconi's syndrome and Wilson's disease) also lead to elevated uric acid levels in urine.[84]

Drugs used to treat elevated serum uric acid levels frequently work by increasing urinary excretion of the substance. Such drugs include probenecid and sulfinpyrazone. Allopurinol also decreases serum uric acid levels but without necessarily leading to excessive urinary levels.[85] It should be noted that colchicine, a drug frequently used to treat gout, does not alter urinary levels of uric acid. Other drugs associated with elevated urinary uric acid include aspirin (large doses), adrenocorticosteroids, coumarin anticoagulants, and estrogens.

Although gout is associated with elevated serum uric acid levels (see Chap. 5), decreased amounts of uric acid are often found in urine because of impaired tubular excretion. Decreased amounts of urinary uric acid also are associated with various renal diseases for the same reason. Decreased urinary uric acid levels are associated with lactic acidosis and ketoacidosis because of impaired renal excretion and also with ingestion of alcohol, aspirin (small doses), and thiazide diuretics.

Amino Acids

Elevated amino acid levels in urine are associated with congenital defects and disorders of amino acid metabolism. The major inherited disorders include phenylketonuria (PKU), tyrosyluria, and alkaptonuria. PKU occurs when the normal conversion of phenylalanine to tyrosine is impaired, leading to the excretion of increased keto acids such as phenylpyruvate in the urine, which can be detected on screening tests. If undetected and untreated, PKU results in severe mental retardation. Blood tests for PKU may also be performed.

Tyrosyluria occurs because of either inherited disorders or metabolic defects. It is most frequently seen in premature infants with underdeveloped liver function, but it seldom results in permanent damage. Acquired severe liver disease also leads to tyrosyluria, as well as to the appearance of tyrosine crystals in the urine (see p. 327).

Alkaptonuria represents another defect in the phenylalanine-tyrosine conversion pathway. In this disorder, homogentisic acid accumulates in the urine. Alkaptonuria generally manifests in adulthood and leads to deposition of brown pigment in the body, arthritis, liver disease, and cardiac disorders.[86]

Urine Hydroxyproline

A special urinary test for a specific amino acid is measurement of urine hydroxyproline, a component of collagen in skin and bone. Foods such as meat, poultry, fish, and foods containing gelatin falsely elevate levels and must, therefore, be restricted for at least 24 hours before the test. Drugs such as ascorbic acid, vitamin D, glucocorticoids, aspirin, mithramycin, and calcitonin will also elevate levels, as will skin disorders such as burns and psoriasis.[87]

Reference Values

	Conventional Units	**SI Units**
Protein	0–150 mg/24 hr	0–150 mg/d
Creatinine		
Men	1–1.9 g/24 hr	8.8–17.6 mmol/d
Women	0.8–1.7 g/24 hr	7–15.8 mmol/d
Bence Jones protein	Negative	Negative
Uric acid	250–750 mg/24 hr	1.5–4.5 mmol/d
Amino acids		
Screening tests (e.g., for PKU, tyrosyluria, alkaptonuria, cystinuria, maple syrup urine disease)	Negative	Negative
Urine hydroxyproline		
2-hour sample		
Men	0.4–5mg/2 hr	3.1–38 μmol/2h
Women	0.4–2.9 mg/2 hr	3.1–22 μmol/2h
24-hour sample		
Adults	14–45 mg/24 hr	0.11–0.36 mmol/d
Critical Values	**Notify physician of protein levels >4 g/24 hr.**	**Notify physician of protein levels >50 nmol/d**

Note: Values are higher in children and during the third trimester of pregnancy

Interfering Factors

➤ Improper specimen collection and improper specimen maintenance.
➤ Ingestion of foods and drugs that may alter test results (see p. 366) or failure to ingest certain foods (e.g., a low-purine diet leads to decreased levels of urinary uric acid; lack of protein intake may lead to false-negative PKU test results in infants).
➤ Skin disorders such as psoriasis and burns may falsely elevate urine hydroxyproline levels.

Indications for Measurement of Urinary Proteins

Protein
➤ Detection of various types of renal disease as indicated by elevated levels
➤ Detection of possible complications of pregnancy as indicated by elevated levels

Bence Jones Protein
➤ Detection of multiple myeloma

Creatinine
➤ Assessment of glomerular function with decreased levels indicating impairment (see also "Reference Values" section, p. 366)
➤ Assessment of the accuracy of 24-hour urine collections for other substances

Uric Acid
➤ Monitoring for urinary effects of disorders that cause hyperuricemia (see p. 365)
➤ Monitoring for response to therapy with uricosuric drugs
➤ Comparison of urine levels with serum uric acid levels to provide for an index of renal function

Amino Acid Screening Tests
➤ Detection of inherited and metabolic disorders such as PKU, tyrosyluria, alkaptonuria, cystinuria, and maple syrup urine disease

Urine Hydroxyproline
➤ Detection of disorders associated with increased bone reabsorption (e.g., Paget's disease, metastatic bone tumors, and certain endocrine disorders)
➤ Monitoring of treatment for Paget's disease

Nursing Care Before the Procedure

The client should be instructed in the method to be used for obtaining the sample (e.g., 24-hour urine, 2-hour urine, clean-catch midstream sample).
➤ A medication history should be obtained.
➤ Drugs that may alter test results may be withheld during the test, although this practice should be confirmed with the person ordering the study.
➤ The client also must be instructed in any dietary modifications needed for the test. Such dietary modifications may be necessary in uric acid and urine hydroxyproline tests.

The Procedure

Protein, Creatinine, and Uric Acid. A 24-hour urine specimen is collected. For creatinine measures, a preservative is usually added to the collection container by the laboratory. It may be necessary also to refrigerate the sample.

Bence Jones Protein. An early morning sample of at least 60 mL is collected. The sample should be sent promptly to the laboratory. It is recommended that the sample be collected using the clean-catch midstream technique (see Appendix II) to avoid contaminating the sample with other proteins from bodily secretions.

Amino Acid Screening Tests. A random urine specimen of at least 20 mL is collected. In infants, collection involves application of a urine-collecting device. The specimen should be sent immediately to the laboratory. The PKU (phenylpyruvic acid) test is performed in no fewer than 3 days after birth. It is performed by pressing a Phenistix reagent strip on a wet diaper or by dipping the strip into a sample obtained with a urine-collecting device, waiting 30 seconds, and comparing it to a color chart. The chart is scaled at milligram concentrations of the substance, ranging from 0 to 100.

Urine Hydroxyproline. A 2- or 24-hour urine specimen is collected in a container to which preservative has been added. It may also be necessary to refrigerate the sample.

Nursing Care After the Procedure

Care and assessment after the test include resuming the client's diet and medications if previously withheld or modified.

➤ *Compromised renal function:* Note and report presence of or increases in proteins. Monitor I&O and fluid and protein restrictions. Instruct in dietary and fluid inclusions and exclusions.

➤ **Critical values:** Notify physician immediately of a protein level of greater than 4 g/24 hr.

VITAMINS AND MINERALS

The functions and serum assays of vitamins and minerals are discussed in Chapter 5. In general, serum assays are preferred to the more cumbersome urine level determinations, which require 24-hour urine collections.

Vitamins

Fat-soluble vitamins are not readily excreted in the urine, and therefore urinary determinations focus on water-soluble vitamins B and C. Urinary determinations for vitamins B_1 (thiamine), B_2 (riboflavin), and C may be made in suspected deficiency states. The Schilling test for vitamin B_{12} absorption is discussed in Chapter 20, as it is used to diagnose an abnormality of hematopoiesis.

Minerals

Minerals are essential to normal body metabolism. In urine, three commonly measured minerals include iron (found in hemosiderin, see p. 319), copper, and oxalate. Copper aids in the formation of hemoglobin and is a component of certain enzymes necessary for energy production.[88] Elevated urinary copper levels are associated with Wilson's disease, an inherited disorder of copper metabolism. Oxalate is found in combination with calcium in certain kidney stones. Elevated urinary oxalate levels are seen in hyperoxaluria, a disorder in which oxalate accumulates in soft tissues, especially those of the kidney and bladder.[89] Oxalate levels may also be elevated by excessive ingestion of strawberries, tomatoes, rhubarb, or spinach.

Reference Values

	Conventional Units	**SI Units**
Vitamins		
B₁ (thiamine)	100–200 μg/24 hr	
B₂ (riboflavin)		
Men	0.51 mg/24 hr	1356 nmol/d
Women	0.39 mg/24 hr	1037 nmol/d
C (absorbic acid)	30 mg/ 24 hr	
Minerals		
Copper	15–60 μg/24 hr	0.24–0.94 μmol/d
Oxalate	<40 mg/24 hr	456 μmol/d

Interfering Factors

➤ Improper specimen collection and maintenance may affect test results.
➤ Ingestion of strawberries, tomatoes, rhubarb, or spinach may falsely elevate oxalate levels.

Indications for Measurement of Vitamins and Minerals in Urine

➤ Detection of vitamin deficiency states
➤ Screening for and detection of Wilson's disease as indicated by elevated urinary copper levels
➤ Detection of hyperoxaluria as indicated by elevated oxalate levels

Nursing Care Before the Procedure

The client should be instructed in the method of obtaining the sample (i.e., usually a 24-hour urine collection).

The Procedure

A 24-hour urine specimen is collected. Samples for oxalate should be collected in containers that have been protected from light and to which hydrochloric acid has been added.

Nursing Care After the Procedure

Care and assessment after the test include resuming the client's usual diet, medications, or activities at completion of specimen collection.

MICROBIOLOGIC EXAMINATION OF URINE

Urine tests for culture and sensitivity (C&S) indicate the type and number of organisms present in the specimen (culture) and the antibiotics to which the organisms are susceptible (sensitivity). In urine, it is common to culture out only one organism, although polymicrobial infections may be seen in individuals with Foley catheters. Most organisms infecting the urinary tract are derived from fecal flora that have ascended the urethra. Organisms commonly found in urine include *Escherichia coli, Enterococcus, Klebsiella, Proteus,* and *Pseudomonas.*[90]

After treatment with the appropriate antibiotic, as indicated by sensitivity tests, follow-up urine cultures may be undertaken to determine the effectiveness of treatment.

Reference Values

Negative for pathologic organisms
➤ *Critical value:* Notify physician if the culture result is greater than 100,000 organisms/mL (S1 = 1,000,000 CFU/L).

Interfering Factors

➤ Improper specimen collection so that the sample is contaminated with nonurinary organisms
➤ Delay in sending the specimen to the laboratory (Bacteria may multiply in nonrefrigerated samples.)

Indications for Microbiologic Examination of Urine

➤ Suspected UTI
➤ Identification of antibiotics to which the cultured organism is sensitive
➤ Monitoring for response to treatment for UTIs

Nursing Care Before the Procedure

Client preparation is the same as that for any test involving the collection of either a clean-catch midstream urine specimen, a catheterized specimen, or a suprapubic aspiration (see Appendix II).

The Procedure

A sample of at least 5 to 10 mL is obtained either by clean-catch technique, catheterization, or suprapubic aspiration. The sample is placed in a sterile container and is transported to the laboratory immediately.

Nursing Care After the Procedure

Care and assessment after the test include assessing the suprapubic site for inflammation if the specimen was obtained by aspiration. Cover the area with a sterile dressing.
➤ **Critical value:** Notify physician immediately if the culture result is greater than 100,000 organisms/mL (S1 = 1,000,000 CFU/L).

CYTOLOGIC EXAMINATION OF URINE

Cytology is the study of the origin, structure, function, and pathology of cells. In clinical practice, cytologic examinations are generally performed to detect cell changes caused by malignancies or inflammatory conditions.

Cytologic examination of urine is performed when cancer or inflammatory disorders of the urinary tract are suspected. It is especially indicated to detect cancer of the bladder and cytomegalic inclusion disease.[91] In these disorders, abnormal cells are shed into the urine and can be detected upon examination of the sample.

Reference Values

Negative for abnormal cells and inclusions

Interfering Factors

➤ Improper specimen collection such that the sample is contaminated with extraneous cells

➤ Delay in sending the sample to the laboratory (Cells may begin to disintegrate.)

Indications for Cytologic Examination of Urine

➤ Suspected cancer of the bladder or other urinary tract structure, especially in individuals exposed to environmental carcinogens

➤ Suspected infection with cytomegalovirus

Nursing Care Before the Procedure

Client preparation is the same as that for any test involving the collection of a clean-catch midstream urine specimen, a catheterized specimen, or a suprapubic aspiration (see Appendix II).

The Procedure

A sample of at least 180 mL in adults and 10 mL in children is obtained either by clean-catch technique, catheterization, or suprapubic aspiration. Depending on the laboratory, a special container or preservative, or both, may be needed. The sample must be transported to the laboratory immediately.

Nursing Care After the Procedure

Care and assessment after the test include assessing the suprapubic site for inflammation if the specimen was obtained by aspiration.

➤ Cover the area with a sterile dressing.

DRUG SCREENING TESTS OF URINE

Toxicological analysis of urine is performed to identify drugs that have been used and abused. Urine is preferred for drug screening because most drugs are detectable in urine but not in blood. The exception is testing for alcohol concentration. The screening tests are performed in groups according to the pharmacological classification of the drugs. Commonly used substances that involve a risk for psychological, physical, or both psychological and physical dependence and are tested are the following:

Sedatives: benzodiazapines, methaqualone

Depressants: alcohol, barbiturates, opiates (codeine, morphine, methadone)

Stimulants: amphetamines, cocaine, "crack," methylphenidate

Hallucinogens: cannabinoids (marijuana, hashish), phencyclidine (PCP), lysergic acid diethylamide (LSD), mescaline[92]

Drug abuse includes the recreational use of drugs (illicit use); unwarranted use of drugs to relieve problems or symptoms, leading to dependence and later continued use; and therapeutic use to prevent the consequences of withdrawal. These substances act on the CNS to reduce anxiety and tension, produce euphoria and other pleasurable mood changes, increase mental and physical ability, and alter sensory perceptions and change behaviors.[93] Detection of levels varies with the time of the last dose of a specific drug and can range from hours to days to weeks.

Anabolic steroids (synthetic derivatives of testosterone) are used to enhance athletic performance primarily in power-related sports and, in some instances, to improve appearance. Its use (known as "sports doping") results in a change in body bulk, strength, and energy. Psychological effects include mood swings, aggressiveness, and irrational behavior. Physical effects include liver dysfunction and cardiovascular dysfunction that result from hypertension and increased low-density lipoproteins (LDL). Anabolic steroid metabolites can be detected in the urine for up to 6 months after drug use.[94]

Reference Values

- Negative for drugs in group tested

Interfering Factors

➤ High or low pH of urine (alkaline or acid levels)
➤ Blood or other abnormal constituents in the urine
➤ Urine that has a low specific gravity, causing dilution

Indications for Drug Screening Tests of Urine

➤ Determination of abuse of drugs before or during employment in which public welfare is at stake
➤ Identification of use of drugs to enhance athletic ability and success
➤ Detection and identification of specific drugs when use and abuse is suspected so as to differentiate it from other causes of a set of signs and symptoms
➤ Confirmation of a diagnosis of drug overdose after death
➤ Detection of drug use before prescribing a medication or treatment regimen

Nursing Care Before the Procedure

Client preparation is the same as for any test involving the collection of a random urine specimen (see Appendix II).
➤ If drug abuse is suspected, the collection and delivery of the urine sample should be witnessed by a legally responsible person and labeled with a code instead of a name and other personal information.
➤ The client should be informed of the procedure to collect and test the specimen, the reporting protocol, and possible implications of the results.

The Procedure

A random sample of 50 to 100 mL of urine is collected in a clean container and covered with a lid and labeled with a code while a trained witness observes to ensure that the specimen has been obtained from the correct client. The specimen container is placed in a plastic bag and sealed to ensure that any tampering with the package will be revealed. A signature of the individual who collects the specimen and anyone who handles it in any way is required on a document. The specimen is examined by enzyme immunoassay or fluorescence polarization immunoassay procedures. Confirmation tests are performed to ensure that false-positive results are resolved. Because of the legal implications, documented testing procedures for a positive, negative, or unconfirmed result with evidence to support the result should accompany the test report. After the complete testing of the specimen, the sample is resealed in the labeled bag and stored for 30 days or as long as needed.[95]

Nursing Care After the Procedure

No specific care is needed after these tests. Inform the client of the possible economic, psychological, and legal implications of a confirmed positive test.

➤ *Abnormal test results:* Note and report effect of results on client's psychological and physical health, economic status (work, sports), and legal status (illicit drug use). Ensure that correct testing and confirmation were performed and reported. Advise client to consider drug abuse counseling or educational programs, or both, provided by school officials, coaches, physicians, and other health-care professionals.

(Case Study follows on page 375)

Student Name _____ Class _____

Instructor _____ Date _____

CASE STUDY AND CRITICAL THINKING EXERCISE

Eddie, age 9, had a severe sore throat 10 days ago. Because he was on a camping trip, he sought no attention at that time. He has come to the ER because his "urine was a dark color, not yellow as usual." He also had had some back pain for a week. VS: T 101.2°F (38.5°C), P 108, R 20, BP 140/102. Urine labs reveal color dark amber, SG 1.038, RBCs 10 per HPF, protein 2.8 g/day.

a. Interpret all lab values.

b. What is the probable diagnosis?

c. How did you differentiate from other renal pathology?

References

1. Strasinger, SK: Urinalysis and Body Fluids, ed 3. FA Davis, Philadelphia, 1994, pp 1–2.
2. Ibid, pp 2–3.
3. Bullock, BL, and Rosendahl, PP: Pathophysiology: Adaptations and Alterations in Function. Little, Brown & Co, Boston, 1984, p 10.
4. Strasinger, op cit, p 2.
5. Ibid, p 7.
6. Sacher, RA, and McPherson, RA: Widmann's Clinical Interpretation of Laboratory Tests, ed 10. FA Davis, Philadelphia, 1991, p 699.
7. Ibid, p 699.
8. Strasinger, op cit, p 43.
9. Schweitzer, GB, and Schumann, GB: Examination of urine. In Henry, JB: Clinical Diagnosis and Management by Laboratory Methods, ed 18. WB Saunders, Philadelphia, 1991, p 393.
10. Strasinger, op cit, p 43.
11. Ibid, pp 45–46.
12. Schweitzer and Schumann, op cit, p 394.
13. Ibid, p 395.
14. Strasinger, op cit, p 50.
15. Ibid, pp 46–47.
16. Ibid, p 50.
17. Schweitzer and Schumann, op cit, p 400.
18. Strasinger, op cit, p 61.
19. Schweitzer and Schumann, op cit, p 399.
20. Ibid, p 399.
21. Ibid, p 400.
22. Ibid, p 402.
23. Ibid, p 401.
24. Strasinger, op cit, p 62.
25. Schweitzer and Schumann, op cit, p 401.
26. Strasinger, op cit, p 62.
27. Hole, JW: Human Anatomy and Physiology, ed 4. William C Brown, Dubuque, Iowa, 1987, p 760.
28. Schweitzer and Schumann, op cit, p 405.
29. Ibid, pp 407-408.
30. Strasinger, op cit, p 67.
31. Ibid, p 70.
32. Schweitzer and Schumann, op cit, p 409.
33. Ibid, p 410.
34. Ibid, p 410.
35. Strasinger, op cit, p 69.
36. Schweitzer and Schumann, op cit, p 410.
37. Ibid, p 410.
38. Strasinger, op cit, p 71.
39. Ibid, p 74.
40. Schweitzer and Schumann, op cit, p 415.
41. Ibid, p 415.
42. Strasinger, op cit, pp 74–76.
43. Ibid, p 76.
44. Schweitzer and Schumann, op cit, p 416.
45. Strasinger, op cit, p 77.
46. Schweitzer and Schumann, op cit, p 417.
47. Strasinger, op cit, p 77.
48. Ibid, pp 88–89.
49. Schweitzer and Schumann, op cit, p 421.
50. Strasinger, op cit, p 93.
51. Schweitzer and Schumann, op cit, p 421.
52. Strasinger, op cit, p 93.
53. Schweitzer and Schumann, op cit, p 423.
54. Ibid, p 424.
55. Ibid, p 424.
56. Ibid, p 424.
57. Strasinger, op cit, p 95.
58. Schweitzer and Schumann, op cit, p 425.
59. Strasinger, op cit, p 98.
60. Ibid, p 98.
61. Sacher and McPherson, op cit, pp 711–712.
62. Strasinger, op cit, p 23.
63. Sacher and McPherson, op cit, p 711.
64. Ibid, p 712.
65. Ibid, p 713.
66. Strasinger, op cit, p 30–31.
67. Sacher and McPherson, op cit, p 714.
68. Strasinger, op cit, p 27.
69. Sacher and McPherson, op cit, p 715.
70. Strasinger, op cit, p 27.
71. Corbett, JV: Laboratory Tests and Diagnostic Procedures with Nursing Diagnoses, ed 3. Appleton & Lange, Norwalk, Conn, 1992, p. 127.
72. Sacher and McPherson, op cit, p 721.
73. Schweitzer and Schumann, op cit, p 433.
74. Ibid, p 459.
75. Strasinger, op cit, p 129.
76. Strasinger, op cit, p 125.
77. Springhouse Corporation: Nurse's Reference Library: Diagnostics, ed 2. Springhouse, Springhouse, Pa, 1986, p 374.
78. Ibid, pp 376–377.
79. Sacher and McPherson, op cit, p 564.
80. Ibid, p 581.
81. Ibid, pp 403–404.
82. Ibid, pp 394–396.
83. Ibid, p 330.
84. Nurse's Reference Library, op cit, p 423.
85. Sacher and McPherson, op cit, p 331.
86. Strasinger, op cit, p 122.
87. Nurse's Reference Library, op cit, pp 418–419.
88. Ibid, p 451.
89. Ibid, pp 464–465.
90. Sacher and McPherson, op cit, p 499.
91. Fischbach, FT: A Manual of Laboratory Diagnostics Tests, ed 4. JB Lippincott, Philadelphia, 1992, pp 709–710.
92. Sacher and McPherson, op cit, pp 686–688.
93. Berkow, R (ed): The Merck Manual, ed 16. Merck Sharp and Dohme Research Laboratory, Rahway, NJ, 1992, p 1549.
94. Ibid, p 2277.
95. Fischbach, op cit, p 186.

Bibliography

Brenner, H, et al: Clinical Nephrology. WB Saunders, Philadelphia, 1987.

Byrne, CJ, et al: Laboratory Tests: Implications for Nursing Care, ed 2. Addison-Wesley, Menlo Park, Calif, 1986.

Chernecky, CC, and Berger, BJ; Cullen, BN (ed): Laboratory Tests and Diagnostic Procedures, ed 2. WB Saunders, Philadelphia, 1996.

Coe, FL: Hypercalciuric States. WB Saunders, Philadelphia, 1984.

Deglin, JH, and Vallerand, AH: Davis's Drug Guide for Nurses, ed 6. FA Davis, Philadelphia, 1999.

Fowler, JE: Urinary Tract Infections and Inflammation. Mosby – Year Book, St Louis, 1988.

Kee, JL: Handbook of Laboratory and Diagnostic Tests with Nursing Implications, ed 3. Appleton and Lange, Norwalk, Conn, 1997.

Lewis, SM, et al (eds): Medical-Surgical Nursing: Assessment and Management of Clinical Problems, ed 4. Mosby – Year Book, St Louis, 1995.

Muther, RS, et al: Manual of Nephrology. Mosby – Year Book, St Louis, 1990.

Pagana, KD, and Pagana, TJ: Diagnostic and Laboratory Test Reference, ed 3. Mosby – Year Book, St Louis, 1996.

Porth, CM: Pathophysiology: Concepts of Altered Health States, ed 4. JB Lippincott, Philadelphia, 1993.

Springhouse Corporation: Clinical Laboratory Tests: Values and Implications, ed 2. Springhouse, Springhouse, Pa, 1995.

Stamey, TA, and Kindrachuck, RW: Urinary Sediment and Urinalysis: A Practical Guide for the Health Science Professional. WB Saunders, Philadelphia, 1985.

Tietz, NW (ed): Clinical Guide to Laboratory Tests, ed 3. WB Saunders, Philadelphia, 1997.

Tilkian, SM: Clinical and Nursing Applications of Laboratory Tests, ed 5. Mosby – Year Book, St Louis, 1995.

Whaley, LF: Nursing Care of Infants and Children, ed 4. Mosby – Year Book, St Louis, 1991.

7

Sputum Analysis

➤ TESTS COVERED

Gram Stain and Other Stains, *380*
Culture and Sensitivity (C&S), *383*

Acid-Fast Bacillus (AFB) Smear and
    Culture, *385*
Cytologic Examination, *386*

OVERVIEW OF SPUTUM PRODUCTION AND ANALYSIS

Sputum is the material secreted by the tracheobronchial tree and, by definition, brought up by coughing. The submucosal glands and secretory cells of the tracheobronchial mucosa normally secrete up to 100 mL of mucus per day as part of bronchopulmonary cleansing. The secretions form a thin layer over the ciliated epithelial cells and travel upward toward the oropharynx, carrying inhaled particles away from the bronchioles. From the oropharynx the secretions are swallowed; therefore, the healthy person does not produce sputum.

In addition to its mechanical cleansing action, mucus attacks inhaled bacteria directly. This antibacterial effect is primarily the result of antibodies, which are predominantly IgA, but also of lysozymes and slightly acid pH. Normally, the contents of the lower respiratory tract are sterile.

Environmental factors, drugs, and respiratory tract disease alter tracheobronchial secretions and may lead to sputum production. Tobacco smoke, cold air, alcohol, and sedatives depress ciliary action and may cause stasis of secretions. Respiratory infections cause an increase in secretions and may lead to a more acidic pH and changes in the chemical composition. A pH below 6.5 inhibits ciliary action, as does increased sputum viscosity. Leukocytes present in respiratory secretions also rise during infection, and membrane permeability increases because of the normal inflammatory response. Thus, antibiotics and other elements normally found in the blood may be present in the sputum. The quantity of sputum produced in pathological states is roughly parallel to the severity of the problem. Specific characteristics and constituents of sputum help to determine the nature of the disorder.[1]

The most common laboratory tests performed on sputum are (1) Gram stain and other staining tests, (2) culture and sensitivity (C&S), (3) examination for acid-fast bacilli (AFB), and (4) cytologic examination. The gross appearance of the specimen should, however, be observed and documented before sending the sample to the laboratory. Respiratory secretions are normally clear, colorless, odorless, and slightly watery.

Abnormal sputum may be described as mucoid (consisting of mucus), mucopurulent (consisting of mucus and pus), and purulent (consisting of pus). Expectoration of mucoid sputum is seen in chronic bronchitis and asthma. A

379

change from mucoid to mucopurulent sputum indicates infection superimposed on the chronic inflammatory condition.[2] Purulent sputum may indicate acute bacterial pneumonia, bronchiectasis, or rupture of a pulmonary abscess. Foul-smelling sputum is associated also with bronchiectasis and lung abscess, as well as with cystic fibrosis. Viscous (tenacious) secretions are seen in clients with cystic fibrosis, *Klebsiella* pneumonia, and dehydration.

Purulent sputum is yellow to green. Gray sputum may indicate inhaled dust; grayish-black sputum is seen after smoke inhalation. Frothy pink or rusty-colored sputum is associated with congestive heart failure (CHF). It is abnormal to expectorate blood (hemoptysis), whether the quantity involves only a few scant streaks or a life-threatening hemorrhage. In addition to being associated with CHF, rusty-colored sputum may be seen also in pneumococcal pneumonia, whereas bright streaks of blood are associated with *Klebsiella* pneumonia. Dark blood in small amounts is associated with tuberculosis, tumors, and trauma caused by instrumentation. Bright blood in moderate to large amounts is associated with cavitary tuberculosis, broncholithiasis, and pulmonary thrombosis.

SPUTUM TESTS

GRAM STAIN AND OTHER STAINS

Gram staining is one of the oldest and most useful microbiologic staining techniques. It involves smearing a small amount of sputum on a slide and then exposing it to gentian or crystal violet, iodine, alcohol, and safranine, a red dye. This technique allows for morphologic examination of the cells contained in the specimen and differentiates any bacteria present into either gram-positive organisms, which retain the iodine stain, or gram-negative organisms, which do not retain the iodine stain but can be counterstained with safranine.

Gram staining may be used to differentiate true sputum from saliva and upper respiratory tract secretions. True sputum contains polymorphonuclear leukocytes and alveolar macrophages. It should also contain a few squamous epithelial cells. Excessive squamous cells or absence of polymorphonuclear leukocytes usually indicates that the specimen is not true sputum.

Another stain used in sputum examinations is polychromase chain reaction, used when pulmonary alveolar proteinosis or *Pneumocystis carinii* pneumonia is suspected. A characteristic of pulmonary alveolar proteinosis is compacted protein, which may be found either inside mononuclear cells, free in round or laminated clumps, or in aggregates with cleftlike spaces. The round and laminated clumps may resemble the cysts of *P. carinii*.

Reference Values

Normal sputum contains polymorphonuclear leukocytes, alveolar macrophages, and a few squamous epithelial cells.

Interfering Factors

➤ Improper specimen collection
➤ Delay in sending specimen to the laboratory

Indications for Gram Stain and Other Stains Tests

Gram Stain

➤ Differentiation of sputum from upper respiratory tract secretions, the latter being indicated by excessive squamous cells or absence of polymorphonuclear leukocytes

➤ Determination of types of leukocytes present in sputum (e.g., neutrophils indicating infection and eosinphils seen in asthma)

➤ Differentiation of gram-positive from gram-negative bacteria in respiratory infections

➤ Identification of Curschmann's spirals, which are associated with asthma, acute bronchitis, bronchopneumonia, and lung cancer[4]

Wright's Stain

➤ Confirmation of the types of leukocytes present in sputum

Polychromase Chain Reaction

➤ Identification of compacted proteins associated with pulmonary alveolar proteinosis

➤ Identification of cysts associated with *P. carinii* infections

➤ Confirmation of the presence of cysts associated with *P. carinii* infections

Nursing Care Before the Procedure

Explain to the client:

➤ That results are most reliable if the specimen is obtained in the morning upon arising, after secretions have accumulated overnight

➤ That a sample of secretions from deep in the respiratory tract, not saliva or postnasal drainage, is needed

➤ The methods by which the specimen will be obtained (i.e., by coughing or by tracheal suctioning)

➤ That increasing fluid intake before retiring for the night aids in liquefying secretions and may make them easier to expectorate

➤ That humidifying inspired air also helps to liquefy secretions

➤ That, if feasible, the client should brush the teeth or rinse the mouth before obtaining the specimen to avoid excessive contamination of the specimen with organisms normally found in the mouth

➤ Proper handling of the container and specimen, if the client is to obtain the specimen independently

➤ The number of samples to be obtained, as it may be necessary to analyze more than one sample for accurate diagnosis

Prepare for the procedure:

➤ Assist in providing extra fluids, unless contraindicated, and proper humidification.

➤ Assist with mouth care as needed.

➤ Provide sputum collection container(s).

➤ If the specimen is to be obtained by tracheal suctioning, it is recommended that oxygen be administered for 20 to 30 minutes before the procedure.

➤ Hyperventilation with 100% O_2 should be performed before and after suctioning.

The Procedure

The procedure varies with the method for obtaining the sputum specimen. The nurse should wear gloves, face mask, and possibly glasses or goggles when obtaining the sputum sample.

Expectorated Specimen. The client should sit upright, with assistance and support (e.g., with an overbed table) as needed. The client should then take two or three deep breaths and cough deeply. Any sputum raised should be expectorated directly into a sterile container. The client should not touch the lip or the inside of the container with the hands or mouth. A 10- to 15-mL specimen is adequate.

If the client is unable to produce the desired amount of sputum, several strategies may be attempted. One approach is to have the client drink two glasses of water and then assume the positions for postural drainage of the upper and middle lung segments. Support for effective coughing may be provided by placing the hands or a pillow over the diaphragmatic area and applying slight pressure. Another approach is to place a vaporizer or other humidifying device at the bedside. After sufficient exposure to adequate humidification, postural drainage of the upper and middle lung segments may be repeated before attempting to obtain the specimen.

It may also be helpful to obtain an order for an expectorant and administer it along with additional water approximately 2 hours before attempting to obtain the specimen. In addition, chest percussion and postural drainage of all lung segments may be used. If the client still is unable to raise sputum, the use of an ultrasonic nebulizer ("induced sputum") may be necessary. This is usually undertaken by a respiratory therapist.

Tracheal Suctioning. Suction equipment, a suction kit, and a Lukens tube or in-line trap are obtained. The client is positioned with head elevated as high as tolerated. Sterile gloves are applied, with the dominant hand maintained as "sterile" and the nondominant hand as "clean." The suction catheter is attached with the "sterile hand" to the rubber tubing of the Lukens tube or in-line trap. The suction tubing is then attached to the male adapter of the trap with the "clean" hand. The suction catheter is lubricated with sterile saline.

Nonintubated clients should be instructed, if feasible, to protrude the tongue and take a deep breath as the suction catheter is passed through the nostril. When the catheter enters the trachea, a reflex cough is stimulated; the catheter is immediately advanced into the trachea, and suction is applied.

Suction should be maintained for approximately 10 seconds and never for more than 15 seconds. The catheter is then withdrawn without applying suction. The suction catheter and suction tubing are separated from the trap, and the rubber tubing is placed over the male adapter to seal the unit. The specimen is labeled and sent to the laboratory immediately.

For clients who are intubated or have a tracheostomy, the aforementioned procedure is followed, except that the suction catheter is passed through the existing endotracheal or tracheostomy tube rather than through the nostril. The client should be hyperoxygenated before and after the procedure in accordance with usual protocols for suctioning such clients.

Nursing Care After the Procedure

For specimens obtained by expectoration or nasotracheal suctioning, care and assessment after the procedure include mouth care offered or provided after the specimen has been obtained.

➤ Provide a cool beverage to aid in relieving throat irritation caused by coughing and suctioning.

➤ Assess the client's color and respiratory rate, and administer supplemental oxygen as necessary.

➤ For specimens obtained by endotracheal tube or tracheostomy, hyperoxygenate the client after the procedure according to usual protocols. Additional suctioning may be necessary to clear secretions raised during suctioning to obtain the specimen.

➤ The characteristics (e.g., color, consistency, volume) of the sample should be noted and documented.

➤ *Infection or hypoxemia:* Note and report tachypnea, dyspnea, diminished breath sounds, change in skin color (cyanosis), and elevated temperature. Administer oxygen and have emergency intubation equipment on hand.

➤ *Transmission of respiratory pathogens:* Place on respiratory precautions. Use mask when in contact with client. Dispose of used articles according to standard precautions and transmission-based isolation procedures.

➤ **Critical values:** Notify physician immediately if test result is positive.

CULTURE AND SENSITIVITY (C&S)

Sputum tests for culture and sensitivity (C&S) indicate the type and number of organisms in the specimen (culture) and the antibiotics to which the organisms are susceptible (sensitivity). Although examination of the organisms found in sputum by microscopy or stain may lend support in the diagnosis of suspected infectious disorders, growth of a pathogen in culture is more definitively diagnostic.

The pathogenic organisms most often cultured from the sputum of individuals with bacterial pneumonia are *Streptococcus pneumoniae, Haemophilus influenzae, Staphylococcus,* and gram-negative bacilli. Other pathogens that may be identified in sputum cultures include *Klebsiella pneumoniae, Mycobacterium tuberculosis,* fungi such as *Candida* and *Aspergillus, Corynebacterium diphtheriae,* and *Bordetella pertussis.* In contrast, other organisms that may cause pneumonia, such as mycoplasmas, respiratory viruses, and rickettsiae, are not detected on routine culture.[5] Sputum collected by expectoration or suctioning with catheters and by bronchoscopy cannot be cultured for anaerobic organisms. Instead, transtracheal aspiration or lung biopsy must be used.[6]

Interpretation of the results of sputum cultures requires knowledge of the client's symptomatology and the nature of the pathogen cultured. Pathogens may be identified in the sputum of individuals who do not have pneumonia or whose pneumonia is actually caused by an organism not identified on culture. Similarly, a person may be diagnosed as having pneumonia on the basis of sputum cultures, when the infection is caused by an obstruction by tumors or foreign bodies, pulmonary infarction, or pulmonary hemorrhage. If *Candida* or *Aspergillus* is found on culture, the client must be further evaluated, as these environmental contaminants may be the cause of serious pulmonary disease.[7] In legionnaires' disease, sputum cultures and Gram staining are negative, despite clinical signs of severe pneumonia. When this disease is suspected, confirmation must be obtained through immunologic blood tests (see Chap. 3).[8]

Rapidity of results from sputum cultures varies according to the rate of growth of the organisms. Routine cultures of *M. tuberculosis,* for example, may take weeks to become positive. To provide more rapid and reliable diagnostic information, some laboratories use immunologic methods such as counterimmunoelectrophoresis (CIEP) to identify microbial pathogens. In CIEP, antibodies specific to the suspected organisms are used, and rapid confirmation of significant tissue involvement is possible.[9]

Reference Values

Normal respiratory flora include *Moraxella catarrhalis, Candida albicans,* diphtheroids, α-hemolytic streptococci, and some staphylococci.

Interfering Factors

➤ Improper specimen collection
➤ Delay in sending specimen to the laboratory
➤ C&S should be performed before antimicrobial therapy to evaluate effectiveness of therapy.

Indications for Culture and Sensitivity (C&S) Test

➤ Support for diagnosing the cause of respiratory infection as indicated by presence or absence (e.g., viral infections, legionnaires' disease) of organisms in culture
➤ Confirmatory diagnosis of tuberculosis (see also AFB smear and culture)
➤ Monitoring for response to treatment for respiratory infections, especially tuberculosis
➤ Identification of antibiotics to which the cultured organism is sensitive

Nursing Care Before the Procedure

Client preparation is the same as that for any test involving the collection of sputum or lower respiratory secretions (see p. 382).

The Procedure

The procedures for obtaining the specimen are the same as those described on page 382.

Nursing Care After the Procedure

Care and assessment after the procedure are the same as for any test involving collection of sputum or lower respiratory secretions.
➤ Depending on the nature of the suspected or confirmed infection, respiratory isolation or drainage and secretion precautions may be used, although these infection-control protocols may have been already implemented before obtaining sputum cultures.
➤ *Abnormal test results, complications, and precautions:* Respond the same as for stains (see p. 383). The client should be informed that culture results for the more common pathogenic microorganisms can be obtained in 24 to

48 hours and that sensitivity results can cause a change in antimicrobial therapy.

ACID-FAST BACILLUS (AFB) SMEAR AND CULTURE

The acid-fast staining method is used primarily to identify tubercle bacilli (*M. tuberculosis*). Acid-fast bacilli have a cell wall that resists decolorization by acid treatment[10]; that is, they retain the stain applied to the specimen, a small portion of which is smeared on a slide, even after treatment with an acid-alcohol solution.

Because the tubercle bacillus is slow growing and culture results may take weeks, an acid-fast bacillus (AFB) smear aids in early detection of the organism and timely initiation of antituberculosis therapy. In addition to organisms of the *Mycobacterium* genus, *Nocardia* spp. and *Actinomyces* spp. may also be identified by acid-fast techniques.

AFB cultures are used to confirm both positive and negative results of AFB smears. By specifying that AFB is the organism to be detected on culture, the laboratory is alerted to the fact that several weeks may be needed for conclusive results. As noted, immunologic methods may also be used in diagnosing tuberculosis by sputum analysis.

Reference Values

Negative for AFB

Interfering Factors

➤ Improper specimen collection
➤ Delay in sending specimen to the laboratory

Indications for Acid-Fast Bacillus (AFB) Smear and Culture

➤ Suspected pulmonary tuberculosis
➤ Monitoring for response to treatment for pulmonary tuberculosis

Nursing Care Before the Procedure

Client preparation is the same as that for any test involving the collection of sputum or lower respiratory secretions (see p. 382).
➤ The client should be informed that it may be several weeks before culture results are available.

The Procedure

The procedures for obtaining the specimen are the same as those described on page 382.

Nursing Care After the Procedure

Care and assessment after the procedure are the same as for any test involving the collection of sputum or lower respiratory secretions.
➤ If tuberculosis is suspected, the client may be placed on AFB or respiratory isolation, pending AFB smear results.

CYTOLOGIC EXAMINATION

Cytology is the study of the origin, structure, function, and pathology of cells. In clinical practice, cytologic examinations are generally performed to detect cell changes resulting from malignancies or inflammatory conditions. Lipid droplets contained in macrophages may be found on cytologic examination and may indicate lipoid or aspiration pneumonia.[11]

Sputum specimens for cytologic examination may be collected by expectoration alone, during bronchoscopy, or by expectoration after bronchoscopy. The method of reporting results of cytologic examinations varies according to the laboratory performing the test. Terms used to report results include negative (no abnormal cells), inflammatory, benign atypical, suspect for malignancy, and positive for malignancy.

Reference Values

Negative for abnormal cells, Curschmann's spirals, fungi, ova, and parasites.

Interfering Factors

➤ Improper specimen collection
➤ Delay in sending specimen to the laboratory

Indications for Cytologic Examination

➤ Suspected lung cancer
➤ History of cigarette smoking, which may lead to metaplastic (nonmalignant) cellular changes
➤ History of acute or chronic inflammatory or infectious lung disorders, which may lead to benign atypical or metaplastic cellular changes
➤ Known or suspected viral disease involving the lung
➤ Known or suspected fungal or parasitic infection involving the lung

Nursing Care Before the Procedure

Client preparation is the same as that for any test involving the collection of sputum or lower respiratory secretions (see p. 381).

The Procedure

The procedures for obtaining the specimen are the same as those described on page 382. It is common practice to collect three sputum specimens for cytologic examination, usually on three separate mornings. After bronchoscopy, however, serial specimens may be obtained from sputum expectorated within 12 to 24 hours of the procedure. Specimens are collected in either sterile containers or sterile containers to which 50 percent alcohol has been added, depending on specific laboratory procedures.

Nursing Care After the Procedure

Care and assessment after the procedure are the same as for any test involving the collection of sputum or lower respiratory secretions.

➤ *Abnormal test results, complications, and precautions:* The client should be offered additional support if the diagnostic findings indicate a premalignant or malignant condition and if further diagnostic procedures or chemotherapy/radiation therapy is advised.

Student Name _____ Class _____

Instructor _____ Date _____

CASE STUDY AND CRITICAL THINKING EXERCISE

Mr. Jones, age 68, is admitted to the hospital complaining of fever, chills, and a productive cough. VS: T 101.5°F (38.8°C), P 102, R 22, and BP 160/92. WBC is 17,500 and sputum is rust colored.

a. What diagnostic test should be ordered?

b. What is the probable diagnosis?

References

1. Sacher, RA, and McPherson, RA: Widmann's Clinical Interpretation of Laboratory Tests, ed 10. FA Davis, Philadelphia, 1991, p 747.
2. Ibid, p 748.
3. Ibid, p 749.
4. Ibid, p 749.
5. Ibid, p 749.
6. Ibid, p 453.
7. Ibid, p 749.
8. Ibid, p 456.
9. Ibid, pp 460–461.
10. Ibid, pp 460-461.
11. Ibid, p 749.

Bibliography

Baron, EJ, et al: Bailey and Scott's Diagnostic Microbiology, ed 9. Mosby–Year Book, St Louis, 1994.

Byrne, CJ, et al: Laboratory Tests: Implications for Nursing Care, ed 2. Addison-Wesley, Menlo Park, Calif, 1986.

Chernecky, CC, and Berger, BJ; Cullen, BN (ed): Laboratory Tests and Diagnostic Procedures, ed 2. WB Saunders, Philadelphia, 1996.

Corbett, JV: Laboratory Tests and Diagnostic Procedures with Nursing Diagnoses, ed 4. Appleton & Lange, Norwalk, Conn, 1995.

Fischbach, FT: A Manual of Laboratory Diagnostic Tests, ed 5. Lippincott-Raven, Philadelphia, 1995.

Kee, JL: Handbook of Laboratory and Diagnostic Tests with Nursing Implications, ed 3. Appleton & Lange, Norwalk, Conn, 1997.

Lewis, SM, et al (eds): Medical-Surgical Nursing: Assessment and Management of Clinical Problems, ed 4. Mosby–Year Book, St Louis, 1995.

Pagana, KD, and Pagana, TJ: Diagnostic Testing and Nursing Implications: A Case Study Approach, ed 4. Mosby–Year Book, St Louis, 1993.

Porth, CM: Pathophysiology: Concepts of Altered Health States, ed 4. JB Lippincott, Philadelphia, 1993.

Springhouse Corporation: Nurse's Reference Library: Diagnostics, ed 2. Springhouse, Springhouse, Pa, 1986.

Tietz, NW (ed): Clinical Guide to Laboratory Tests, ed 3. WB Saunders, Philadelphia, 1997.

8

Cerebrospinal Fluid Analysis

➤ TESTS COVERED

Routine Cerebrospinal Fluid (CSF)
   Analysis, *391*
Microbiologic Examination of
   Cerebrospinal Fluid (CSF), *396*

Cytologic Examination of
   Cerebrospinal Fluid (CSF), *398*
Serologic Tests for
   Neurosyphilis, *399*

OVERVIEW OF CEREBROSPINAL FLUID FORMATION AND ANALYSIS

Cerebrospinal fluid (CSF) is secreted into the ventricles of the brain by specialized capillaries called choroid plexuses. Most of the CSF arises in the lateral ventricles, although additional amounts are secreted in the third and fourth ventricles. CSF formed in the ventricles circulates into the central canal of the spinal cord and also enters the subarachnoid space through an opening in the wall of the fourth ventricle near the cerebellum, after which it circulates around the brain and spinal cord. Although 500 to 800 mL of CSF are formed daily, only 125 to 140 mL are normally present. Thus, almost all of the CSF formed is reabsorbed via arachnoid granulations, which project from the subarachnoid space into the venous sinuses, and is subsequently returned to the venous circulation. The functions of CSF include cushioning the brain against shocks and blows, maintaining a stable concentration of ions in the central nervous system (CNS), and providing for removal of wastes.[1,2]

CSF is produced by the processes of filtration, diffusion, osmosis, and active transport. Initially, sodium is actively transported into the CSF; then water follows passively by osmosis. Facilitated diffusion allows glucose to move between the blood and CSF. Although similar in composition to plasma, CSF generally contains more sodium and chloride and less potassium, calcium, and glucose. Most constituents of CSF, however, parallel those found in plasma and are found in amounts equal to or slightly less than those in the blood.[3,4]

In addition to entering CSF via the choroid plexuses, substances may pass into CSF from the blood through capillaries in the parenchyma and meninges of the brain and spinal cord. "Barriers" exist between the blood and the CSF and between the brain and the CSF; that is, substances do not pass as readily into the CSF as they would pass into extracellular fluid through other capillary beds. Water, carbon dioxide, oxygen, glucose, small molecules, lipid-soluble substances, nonionized substances, and some drugs (e.g., erythromycin and sulfadiazine) pass rapidly into CSF, whereas large molecules, ionized substances, various toxins, and certain other drugs (e.g., chlortetracyclines and penicillins) do not pass readily into CSF.[5]

Under pathological conditions, elements normally held back by the blood-brain barrier may enter CSF. Red cells and white cells can enter the CSF either from rupture of vessels or from meningeal reaction to irritation. Unconjugated (prehepatic) bilirubin may be found after intracranial hemorrhage, whereas conjugated bilirubin may be found if the circulating plasma contains large amounts. Fibrinogen, which is normally absent from CSF, may be found along with albumin and globulins when inflammatory disorders cause increased permeability of the blood-brain barrier. Urea, lactic acid, and glutamine levels in CSF will rise if plasma levels of these or related substances are elevated. Bacteria and fungi found in CSF indicate infection with these organisms.[6]

As a general rule, routine CSF analysis includes a cell count and differential as well as determinations of protein and glucose levels. In addition, CSF may be analyzed for electrolytes, lactic acid, urea, glutamine, and enzymes. Microbiologic studies of CSF include culture and sensitivity (C&S), Gram stain and other stains, acid-fast bacillus (AFB) smear and culture, and the Limulus assay for gram-negative bacteria. Cytologic examination for malignant cells, as well as serologic tests for syphilis, may be performed on CSF.

The gross appearance, opening pressure, and closing pressure should be noted during the procedure and documented. The pH of the sample may also be noted. CSF is normally clear, colorless, and of the consistency of water. Turbidity indicates the presence of a significant number of leukocytes (i.e., greater than 200 to 500 white cells per cubic millimeter). Yellowish discoloration of CSF (xanthochromia) usually indicates previous bleeding but may also be seen when CSF protein levels are greatly elevated. Fresh blood in the specimen may be due to traumatic spinal tap, although clearing should be noted as the second and third tubes are withdrawn in such a case. Bleeding from a traumatic tap adds approximately one to two white cells and 1 mg/dL of protein for every 1000 red cells per cubic millimeter contained in the sample. If blood does not clear as subsequent samples are obtained, bleeding due to subarachnoid hemorrhage is usually indicated. Brown CSF generally indicates a chronic subdural hematoma with CSF stained from methemalbumin.[7]

As fibrinogen is normally absent from CSF, the sample should not clot. Clotting may occur, however, when the protein content of the sample is elevated. In conditions involving spinal subarachnoid block, CSF may be yellow and have a tendency toward rapid spontaneous clotting. The pH of CSF is normally slightly lower than that of blood, with a range of 7.32 to 7.35 when arterial blood pH is within normal limits.[8]

CSF specimens must be transported to the laboratory immediately. Within 1 hour of collection, any red cells contained in the sample begin to lyse and may cause spurious coloration of the specimen. Neutrophils and malignant cells may also disintegrate in a short time. Bacteria and other cells will continue to metabolize glucose, such that delays in analysis may alter chemical values.[9]

The opening CSF pressure (OP) is measured after the spinal needle is determined to be in the subarachnoid space. CSF pressure may be elevated if clients are anxious and hold their breath or tense their muscles. It may also be elevated if there is venous compression such as may occur if the client's knees are flexed too firmly against the abdomen. Significant elevations in CSF pressure may occur with intracranial tumors and with purulent or tuberculous meningitis. Less marked increases (i.e., 250 to 500 mm of water) are associated with low-grade inflammatory processes, encephalitis, or neurosyphilis. Decreases in CSF pressure are rare but may occur with dehydration, high obstruction to CSF flow, or previous aspiration of spinal fluid.[10]

The closing pressure (CP) is recorded before removal of the spinal needle from the subarachnoid space. Normally, CSF pressure decreases 5 to 10 mm of water for every milliliter of CSF withdrawn. The expected decrease in CSF pressure does not occur in disorders in which the total quantity of CSF is increased (e.g., hydrocephalus). In contrast, a large drop in pressure indicates a small CSF pool and is seen in tumors or spinal block.[11]

CEREBROSPINAL FLUID TESTS

ROUTINE CEREBROSPINAL FLUID (CSF) ANALYSIS

Routine CSF analysis includes a cell count and differential, as well as determinations of protein and glucose levels. CSF may also be analyzed for electrolytes, lactic acid, urea, glutamine, and enzymes.

Cell Count and Differential

Normal spinal fluid is free of cells. It should be noted that cryptococcal organisms in the sample may be mistaken for small lymphocytes.

Proteins

CSF normally contains very little protein because most proteins cannot cross the blood-brain barrier. In addition to determining the amount of protein present in CSF, levels of certain types of protein may also be measured. Albumin, for example, is a relatively small molecule and may pass more easily into CSF. For this reason, the albumin-globulin (A-G) ratio is normally higher in CSF than in serum. Protein electrophoresis may also be performed on CSF samples.

The protein concentration in CSF may rise as a result of increased permeability of the blood-brain barrier because of inflammation and infection. CSF protein levels may also be elevated in clients with diabetes mellitus and cardiovascular disease because of increased permeability of the blood-brain barrier.[12]

Glucose

The glucose concentration of CSF is altered by the presence of microorganisms. Because all types of organisms consume glucose, levels will be decreased if the CSF contains bacteria, fungi, protozoa, or tubercle bacilli. However, this decrease is not as pronounced or may not be seen at all in viral meningitis.

Bacterial and other cells present in CSF continue to metabolize glucose even after the sample has been collected. Thus, spuriously low glucose levels may be found in CSF if analysis is delayed.

Other Substances

Other substances for which CSF may be analyzed include electrolytes, lactic acid, urea, glutamine, and enzymes. The electrolyte levels found in CSF are similar to those of plasma, with the exceptions of sodium and chloride, which are higher, and potassium and calcium, which are lower. The significance of electrolyte levels in CSF is questionable. Some writers, for example, indicate that chlorides are decreased in tuberculosis and bacterial meningitis.[13,14] Others state that chloride levels provide no specific diagnostic information.[15] The calcium found in CSF is that fraction not bound by protein and is about half that of serum levels. Calcium levels rise with CSF protein levels; it is more important to determine the protein level in such cases, however, than to measure calcium.[16]

Lactic acid in CSF reflects local glycolytic activity and adds to diagnostic information when results of other analyses are inconclusive. Severe systemic lactic acidosis causes CSF lactate to rise accordingly. Elevated CSF lactate without a parallel elevation in serum level indicates increased CSF glucose metabolism, which is usually due to bacterial or fungal meningitis. In early or partially treated bacterial or fungal meningitis, CSF cell count and glucose levels may be similar to those found in viral meningitis or noninfectious conditions. Lactate levels above 35 mg/dL rarely occur, however, unless the client has bacterial or fungal meningitis. Lactate levels remain elevated until the individual has received effective antibiotic therapy for several days. Persistent elevation of CSF lactate levels indicates inadequate treatment of meningitis.[17]

Urea levels in CSF and blood are approximately equal; thus, CSF urea levels rise when blood levels are elevated, as in uremia. Urea is sometimes administered intravenously (IV) to lower intracranial pressure. In such cases, the subsequent elevation in CSF urea levels causes fluid to shift from the brain to the CSF. CSF urea levels may remain elevated for 24 to 48 hours after IV administration of urea. Glutamine is synthesized in the CNS from ammonia and glutamic acid. CSF glutamine levels rise when blood ammonia levels are high, a situation seen in cirrhosis with altered hepatic blood flow and encephalopathy. It has been found that glutamine levels in CSF correlate as well or better than blood ammonia levels with the degree of hepatic encephalopathy. Enzymes that have been measured in CSF include lactic dehydrogenase (LDH), alanine aminotransferase (ALT, SGPT), and aspartate aminotransferase (AST, SGOT). Levels of these enzymes are normally lower than those found in the blood. CSF enzymes may rise in inflammatory, hemorrhagic, or degenerative diseases of the CNS. CSF enzyme levels are not measured under routine conditions, however, and may not add to the diagnostic information obtained from more routinely available tests.[18]

Reference Values

	Conventional Units	**SI Units**
Color	Clear	
Pressure		
Children	50–100 mm H_2O	
Adults	75–200 mm H_2O (120 mm H_2O, average)	
Cell count and differential		
Children	Up to 20 small lymphocytes per mm^3	
Adults	Up to 5 small lymphocytes per mm^3	
	No RBC or granulocytes	

Protein		
Total proteins		
Infants	30–100 mg/dL	0.30–1.0 g/L
Children	14–45 mg/dL	0.14–0.45 g/L
Adults	15–45 mg/dL (lumbar area) or less than 1% of serum levels	0.15–0.45 g/L
Albumin-globulin (A-G) ratio	8:1	
IgG	3–12% of total protein	
Glucose		
Infants	20–40 mg/dL	1.11–2.22 mmol/L
Children	35–75 mg/dL	1.94–4.16 mmol/L
Adults	40–80 mg/dL or less than 50–80% of blood glucose level 30–60 min earlier	2.22–4.44 mmol/L
Electrolytes		
Chloride	118–132 mEq/L	118–132 mmol/L
Calcium	2.1–2.7 mEq/L	1.05–1.35 mmol/L
Sodium	144–154 mEq/L	144–154 mmol/L
Potassium	2.4–3.1 mEq/L	2.4–3.1 mmol/L
Lactic acid (lactate)	10–20 mg/dL	1.1–2.2 mmol/L
Urea	10–15 mg/dL	3.6–5.3 mmol/L
Glutamine	Less than 20 mg/dL	<1370.0 μmol/L
Lactic dehydrogenase (LDH)	1/10 that of serum level	

Interfering Factors

➤ Delay in transporting sample to the laboratory (may cause spurious discoloration as a result of lysis of any red cells present, disintegration of any neutrophils present, and false decrease in glucose as a result of continued utilization by cells in the sample)

➤ Blood in the sample caused by traumatic tap (adds one to two white cells and 1 mg/dL of protein for every 1000 red cells per cubic millimeter contained in the sample)

Indications for Routine Cerebrospinal Fluid (CSF) Analysis

➤ Suspected viral meningitis, cerebral thrombosis, or brain tumor as indicated by a cell count of 10 to 200 per cubic millimeter, consisting mostly of lymphocytes, a mild elevation (to 300 mg/dL) in total proteins, and normal or slightly decreased glucose level

➤ Suspected multiple sclerosis or neurosyphilis as indicated by a normal or slightly elevated cell count, consisting mostly of lymphocytes, slightly elevated protein (less than 100 mg/dL), slightly elevated globulins, elevated IgG on protein electrophoresis, and a normal or slightly decreased glucose level

➤ Suspected acute bacterial or syphilitic meningitis, herpes infection of CNS as indicated by a cell count of greater than 500 per cubic millimeter, consisting largely of granulocytes, moderately or pronounced elevation in protein (greater than 300 mg/dL), pronounced decrease in glucose, and decreased chloride[19]

➤ Suspected tuberculous meningitis as indicated by a cell count of 200 to 500 per cubic millimeter, consisting of lymphocytes or mixed lymphocytes and granulocytes, moderate or pronounced elevation in proteins, pronounced reduction in glucose, and decreased chloride

➤ Suspected early bacterial or fungal meningitis as indicated by CSF lactate level above 35 mg/dL, even when cell count and glucose level are only slightly altered

➤ Evaluation of effectiveness of treatment for bacterial or fungal meningitis, with effective treatment indicated by decreasing lactate levels after several days of antimicrobial therapy

➤ Suspected CNS leukemia as indicated by a cell count of 200 to 500 per cubic millimeter, consisting mainly of blast cells and a moderate reduction in glucose

➤ Suspected spinal cord tumor as indicated by a cell count of 10 to 200 per cubic millimeter, moderate or pronounced elevation in protein, and normal or slightly decreased glucose

➤ Support for diagnosing subarachnoid hemorrhage as indicated by the presence of red blood cells, elevated proteins, and a moderate reduction in glucose

➤ Support for diagnosing hepatic encephalopathy as indicated by elevated glutamine levels

➤ Support for diagnosing Guillain-Barré syndrome (ascending polyneuritis) as indicated by pronounced elevation in proteins

Nursing Care Before the Procedure

Explain to the client:

➤ That the procedure will be performed by a physician and requires 20 to 30 minutes

➤ The positioning used for the procedure and the necessity of remaining still while the procedure is being performed

➤ That a local anesthetic will be injected at the needle insertion site

➤ That the needle is inserted below the end of the spinal cord (for lumbar punctures)

➤ That a sensation of pressure may be felt when the needle is inserted

➤ The necessity of remaining flat in bed for 6 to 8 hours after the procedure (for lumbar punctures) and that turning from side to side is permitted as long as the head is not raised

➤ That taking fluids after the procedure will aid in returning the CSF volume to normal (provided that this is not contraindicated for the particular client)

Prepare the client for the procedure:

➤ Have the client void.

➤ Provide a hospital gown.

➤ Take and record vital signs, assess legs for neurological status (strength, movement, and sensation) for comparision with postprocedure assessment.

Obtain a signed informed consent if required by the agency.

The Procedure

The necessary equipment is assembled (e.g., lumbar puncture tray). The client is assisted to a side-lying position, with the head flexed as far as comfortable and the knees drawn up toward, but not pressing on, the abdomen. Support in maintaining this position may be provided by placing one hand on the back of the client's neck and the other behind the knees. Lumbar punctures may also be performed with the client seated while leaning forward with arms resting on an overbed table or other support.

The lumbar area is cleansed with an antiseptic and protected with sterile drapes. The skin is infiltrated with a local anesthetic and the spinal needle with stylet is inserted into a vertebral interspace between L2 to S1, usually L3-4 or L4-5. The stylet is then removed and, if the needle is properly positioned in the subarachnoid space, spinal fluid will drip from the needle. A sterile stopcock and manometer are then attached to the needle. The opening pressure is read (see p. 390) and, if indicated, Queckenstedt's test is performed. When the needle and manometer are properly positioned, the CSF level should fluctuate several millimeters with respiration.[20]

Queckenstedt's test is based on the principle that a change in pressure in one area of the closed system—composed of the ventricular spaces, intracranial subarachnoid space, and vertebral subarachnoid space—will be reflected in other areas of the system as well. The test is indicated when total or partial spinal block (e.g., due to tumor) is suspected, and it is performed by compressing both jugular veins while monitoring lumbar CSF pressure. Temporary occlusion of the jugular veins impairs the absorption of intracranial fluid and produces an acute rise in CSF pressure. If CSF flow is unimpeded, the pressure elevation will be transmitted to the lumbar area, and the fluid level in the manometer will rise. Total or partial spinal block is diagnosed if the CSF pressure fails to rise or if more than 20 seconds is required for the pressure to return to the pretest level after pressure on the jugular veins is released. Queckenstedt's test is risky in clients with increased intracranial pressure of highly reactive carotid body receptors. Radiologic examinations such as myelograms and computed axial tomography (CAT) scans may give more information and carry less risk.[21]

The manometer is then removed and CSF is allowed to drip into three sterile test tubes, 3 to 10 mL per tube. The tubes are numbered in order of filling, labeled with the client's name, and sent to the laboratory immediately. The manometer may then be reattached and the closing pressure recorded. The spinal needle is removed, and pressure is applied to the site. If no excessive bleeding or CSF leakage is noted, an adhesive bandage is applied to the site and the client is assisted to a recumbent position.

Alternatives to the lumbar puncture include cisternal and ventricular punctures. These procedures may be used when lumbar puncture is not feasible because of bony abnormalities or infection at the lumbar area. For a cisternal puncture, the client is assisted to a side-lying position with the neck flexed and the head resting on the chest. The back of the neck may require shaving before the procedure. After the skin is infiltrated with local anesthetic, the needle is inserted at the base of the occiput, between the first cervical vertebra and the foramen magnum. CSF samples are then obtained in the same manner as for lumbar punctures. Cisternal punctures are considered somewhat hazardous, as the needle is inserted close to the brainstem; however, clients are said to be less likely to experience postprocedure headaches and may resume usual activities within a few hours of the procedure.[22]

Ventricular punctures are surgical procedures (i.e., usually performed in an operating room) in which CSF samples are obtained directly from one of the lateral ventricles in the brain. For this procedure, a scalp incision is made and a burr hole is drilled in the occipital area of the skull. The needle is then inserted through the hole and into the lateral ventricle, and CSF samples are obtained. This procedure is rarely performed.[23]

The cell count and protein content of CSF samples obtained by cisternal or ventricular punctures are normally lower than those found in lumbar samples. The higher levels of cells and protein found in CSF from lumbar punctures are thought to be caused by stagnation of CSF, which occurs in the lumbar sac.[24]

Nursing Care During the Procedure

Note any distress, especially dyspnea, that may be caused by positioning.
➤ Observe for signs of brainstem herniation such as decreased level of consciousness, irregular respirations, and a unilaterally dilating pupil (uncal herniation).

Nursing Care After the Procedure

Care and assessment after the procedure include assisting the client to a recumbent position and having the client maintain a flat position for 6 to 8 hours to prevent the occurrence of headache.
➤ Remind the client that turning from side to side is permitted, as long as the head is not raised.
➤ Assist the client in taking liberal amounts of fluids to replace the CSF loss, unless otherwise contraindicated.
➤ A dressing can be applied after pressure to the puncture site.
➤ Care after cisternal and ventricular punctures is essentially the same as that for lumbar punctures. For cisternal punctures, provide bed rest for only 2 to 4 hours, after which usual activities may be resumed. For ventricular punctures, maintain bed rest for 24 hours.
➤ Take and record vital signs every hour for the first 4 hours and then every 4 hours for 24 hours (for hospitalized clients).
➤ Perform a neurological check each time vital signs are taken to determine nerve damage affecting the legs.
➤ Assess the puncture site for bleeding, CSF drainage, and inflammation each time vital signs are taken during the first 24 hours and daily thereafter for several days. (Family members or support persons should be instructed to do this for nonhospitalized clients.)
➤ Observe for signs of meningeal irritation such as fever, nuchal rigidity, and irritability indicating infection.
➤ Assess the client's comfort level, noting presence or absence of headache. Administer an ice bag to the head and a mild analgesic if ordered.

MICROBIOLOGIC EXAMINATION OF CEREBROSPINAL FLUID (CSF)

Microbiologic studies of CSF include C&S, Gram stain and other stains, AFB smear and culture, and the Limulus assay for gram-negative bacteria.

Numerous microorganisms may cause meningitis, encephalitis, and brain abscess. Thus, whenever CNS infection is suspected, CSF should be tested for the presence of bacteria, fungi, protozoa, and tubercle bacilli, as it is possible that more than one organism is present.[25] The CSF is also tested for bacterial antigens in addition to culturing for bacteria. CSF rarely contains abundant organisms, so specimens for microbiologic examination must be collected and handled with strict aseptic technique. The usual laboratory procedure is to centrifuge a few milliliters of CSF to concentrate any organisms present. After culture plates with several different media are inoculated, the remaining CSF sediment is examined with Gram staining and AFB staining techniques (see Chap. 7).[26]

Failure to isolate organisms on stained smear does not necessarily mean that organisms are absent from the CSF sample. Reliably positive results are obtained only when at least 10^5 bacteria per milliliter are present. Gram stains, for example, are positive in only 80 to 90 percent of individuals with untreated meningitis. CSF is almost routinely examined and cultured for AFB when the cause of the CNS disorder is unknown, because tuberculous meningitis can develop insidiously and presents with few clear diagnostic indicators.[27]

When infection with the fungus *Cryptococcus* is suspected, the specimen may be examined by testing for cryptococcal antigen.[28] The cryptococcal antigen test, in which a strong anticryptococcal antibody is used, may elicit antigenic elements even when cryptococcal organisms are undetected by other methods.[29]

Amebae may also cause meningitis, especially in individuals who swim in lakes or indoor swimming pools. A wet-mount preparation of CSF is examined for motile cells when such an infection is suspected.[30]

Spinal fluid is normally cultured on several different media to test for different organisms. The meningococcal organism (*Neisseria meningitidis*), for example, prefers to grow in a medium with a high carbon dioxide atmosphere. Counterimmunoelectrophoresis (CIEP) may also be used to detect bacterial antigens when usual techniques fail to demonstrate bacteria in CSF.[31]

The presence of gram-negative organisms in CSF may be demonstrated rapidly with the Limulus assay. This test uses the bloodlike fluid of the horseshoe crab of the genus *Limulus,* which is coagulated by gram-negative endotoxins. This test, therefore, provides a quick means of diagnosing gram-negative infections of the CNS and gram-negative endotoxemia. The test is more reliable when performed on CSF than when performed on blood.[32]

Acute bacterial meningitis occurs most commonly in children younger than age 5 years and in adults who have experienced head trauma. Gram-negative bacilli (*Escherichia coli, Klebsiella, Enterobacter, Proteus*) are the usual etiologic agents of meningitis in premature infants and newborns. In infants, the causative agents include *Streptococcus agalactiae* (group B) and *Listeria monocytogenes.* In young children, meningitis is most frequently caused by gram-negative bacilli (*Haemophilus influenzae*). In adolescents, the agent is most likely to be *N. meningitidis.* In adults, meningitis may also be caused by *Streptococcus pneumoniae.* In elderly persons, the agent is a gram-negative bacillus. Viral infections, tuberculous meningitis, and fungal and protozoal infections may occur at any age and often present as insidious or misleading syndromes.[33]

Reference Values

Organisms are not normally present in CSF.

Interfering Factors

➤ Delay in transporting the sample to the laboratory (organisms may disintegrate if the sample is held at room temperature for more than 1 hour)
➤ Contamination of the sample with normal skin flora or other organisms because of improper collection or handling of the sample

Indications for Microbiologic Examination of Cerebrospinal Fluid (CSF)

➤ Suspected meningitis, encephalitis, or brain abscess
➤ CNS disorder of unknown etiology without clear diagnostic indicators
➤ Head trauma with possible resultant CNS infection

Nursing Care Before the Procedure

Client preparation is the same as that for any test involving the collection of CSF samples (see p. 394).

The Procedure

The procedures for obtaining the specimen are the same as those described on pages 394 to 395. Extreme care must be used in obtaining and collecting the sample, so as not to contaminate the sample or introduce organisms into the CNS.

Nursing Care After the Procedure

Care and assessment after the procedure are the same as for any test involving the collection of a CSF sample (see p. 396).
➤ Depending on the nature of the suspected or confirmed infection, use infectious disease precautions.
➤ *Complications and precautions:* Note and report signs and symptoms of brain disorder such as fever, irritability, or headache. Perform neurological checks and take and record vital signs. Notify physician immediately of a positive stain result.

CYTOLOGIC EXAMINATION OF CEREBROSPINAL FLUID (CSF)

Cytologic examination of CSF is performed primarily to detect malignancies involving the CNS. Cellular changes caused by malignancies whose primary site is the CNS (e.g., brain tumors) or malignancies that have metastasized to the CNS from other sites (e.g., breast and lung) may be detected. Abnormal cells resulting from acute leukemia involving the CNS may also be seen.

Reference Values

No abnormal cells

Interfering Factors

➤ Delay in transporting the sample to the laboratory (Cells may disintegrate if the sample is held at room temperature for more than 1 hour.)
➤ Contamination of the sample with skin cells

Indications for Cytologic Examination of Cerebrospinal Fluid (CSF)

➤ Suspected malignancy with primary site in the CNS
➤ Suspected metastasis of malignancies to the CNS
➤ Suspected CNS involvement in acute leukemia

Nursing Care Before the Procedure

Client preparation is the same as that for any test involving the collection of CSF samples (see p. 394).

The Procedure

The procedures for obtaining the specimen are the same as those described on pages 394 to 395. Care must be taken not to contaminate the sample with skin cells.

Nursing Care After the Procedure

Care and assessment after the procedure are the same as for any test involving the collection of a CSF sample (see p. 396).

SEROLOGIC TESTS FOR NEUROSYPHILIS

When syphilis involving the CNS (neurosyphilis) is suspected, serologic tests are performed on samples of CSF. Blood tests for syphilis (see Chap. 3) consist of two main types: (1) nonspecific tests that demonstrate syphilitic reagin and (2) specific tests that demonstrate antitreponemal antibodies. Reagin tests include the Wassermann and Reiter complement fixation tests and the Venereal Disease Research Laboratory (VDRL) and rapid plasma reagin (RPR) flocculation tests. The best specific test is the fluorescent treponemal antibody (FTA) test.

Nonspecific reagin tests are usually used for routine testing of CSF because they are cheaper and more readily available than the FTA test. The false-positive results that may occur when blood is tested with reagin tests occur fairly rarely in CSF specimens. Nonspecific tests are, however, less sensitive than the FTA test. Thus, if neurosyphilis is a serious diagnostic consideration, the FTA is the test of choice.[34]

Reference Values

Negative

Interfering Factors

➤ Delay in transporting the sample to the laboratory (organisms may disintegrate if the sample is held at room temperature for more than 1 hour.)

Indications for Serologic Tests for Neurosyphilis

➤ Suspected neurosyphilis

Nursing Care Before the Procedure

Client preparation is the same as that for any test involving the collection of CSF samples (see p. 394).

The Procedure

The procedures for obtaining the specimen are the same as those described on pages 394 to 395.

Nursing Care After the Procedure

Care and assessment after the procedure are the same as for any test involving the collection of a CSF sample (see p. 396).

Student Name _____ Class _____

Instructor _____ Date _____

CASE STUDY AND CRITICAL THINKING EXERCISE

Sara, age 14, is admitted to the ER complaining of a severe headache. She states that she had a "bad cold" 2 weeks ago. On examination she demonstrates nuchal rigidity. A lumbar puncture is ordered along with routine blood work.

a. What is the probable diagnosis?

b. What do you expect the CSF analysis to reveal?

References

1. Hole, JW: Human Anatomy and Physiology, ed 4. Wm C Brown, Dubuque, Iowa, 1987, p 366.
2. Bullock, BL, and Rosendahl, PP: Pathophysiology: Adaptations and Alterations in Function. Little, Brown & Co, Boston, 1984, pp 647–650.
3. Ibid, p 647.
4. Sacher, RA, and McPherson, RA: Widmann's Clinical Interpretation of Laboratory Tests, ed 10. FA Davis, Philadelphia, 1991, p 537.
5. Bullock and Rosendahl, op cit, pp 651–652.
6. Sacher and McPherson, op cit, pp 731, 735.
7. Ibid, p 729.
8. Ibid, p 732.
9. Ibid, p 733.
10. Ibid, p 730.
11. Ibid, p 731.
12. Ibid, pp 732–733.
13. Fischbach, FT: A Manual of Laboratory Diagnostic Tests, ed 4. JB Lippincott, Philadelphia, 1992, p 255.
14. Springhouse Corporation: Nurse's Reference Library: Diagnostics, ed 2. Springhouse, Springhouse, Pa, 1986, p 776.
15. Sacher and McPherson, op cit, p 735.
16. Ibid, p 735.
17. Ibid, p 733. 18.
18. Ibid, pp 733, 735. 19.
19. Ibid, pp 731–732. 30.
20. Ibid, p 730. 31.
21. Ibid, pp 730–731. 32.
22. Nurse's Reference Library, op cit, p 779. 33.
23. Ibid, p 779. 34.
24. Sacher and McPherson, op cit, p 732.
25. Ibid, p 735. 20.
26. Ibid, p 495. 21.
27. Ibid, p 735. 22.
28. Ibid, p 735. 23.
29. Ibid, p 735. 24.
30. Ibid, p 735. 25.
31. Ibid, p 735. 26.
32. Ibid, p 734. 27.
33. Ibid, p 734. 28.
34. Ibid, p 736. 29.

Bibliography

Baron, EJ, and Finegold, SM: Bailey and Scott's Diagnostic Microbiology, ed 9. Mosby–Year Book, St Louis, 1994.

Byrne, CJ, et al: Laboratory Tests: Implications for Nursing Care, ed 2. Addison-Wesley, Menlo Park, Calif, 1986.

Chernecky, CC, and Berger, BJ; Cullen, BN (ed): Laboratory Tests and Diagnostic Procedures, ed 2. WB Saunders, Philadelphia, 1996.

Corbett, JV: Laboratory Tests and Diagnostic Procedures with Nursing Diagnoses, ed 4. Appleton & Lange, Norwalk, Conn, 1995.

Fishman, RA: Cerebrospinal Fluid in Diseases of the Nervous System, ed 2. WB Saunders, Philadelphia, 1992.

Kee, JL: Handbook of Laboratory and Diagnostic Tests with Nursing Implications, ed 3. Appleton & Lange, Norwalk, Conn, 1997.

Lambert, HP: Infections of the Central Nervous System. Mosby–Year Book, St Louis, 1992.

Lewis, SM, and Collier, IC: Medical-Surgical Nursing: Assessment and Management of Clinical Problems, ed 3. Mosby–Year Book, St Louis, 1992.

Liu, PI: Blue Book of Diagnostic Tests. WB Saunders, Philadelphia, 1986.

Pagana, KD, and Pagana, TJ: Diagnostic and Laboratory Test Reference, ed 3. Mosby–Year Book, St Louis, 1996.

Pagana, KD, and Pagana, TJ: Diagnostic Testing and Nursing Implications: A Case Study Approach, ed 4. Mosby–Year Book, St Louis, 1993.

Porth, CM: Pathophysiology: Concepts of Altered Health States, ed 4. JB Lippincott, Philadelphia, 1993.

Tietz, NW (ed): Clinical Guide to Laboratory Tests, ed 3. WB Saunders, Philadelphia, 1997.

Whaley, LF: Nursing Care of Infants and Children, ed 4. Mosby–Year Book, St Louis, 1991.

Wood, M, and Anderson, M: Neurological Infections. WB Saunders, Philadelphia, 1989.

9

Analysis of Effusions

> **TESTS COVERED**
> Pericardial Fluid Analysis, *405*
> Pleural Fluid Analysis, *408*

Peritoneal Fluid Analysis, *412*
Synovial Fluid Analysis, *415*

OVERVIEW OF EFFUSIONS

Effusions are excessive accumulations of fluid in body cavities lined with serous or synovial membranes. Such cavities normally contain only small amounts of fluid (i.e., less than 50 mL). Serous membranes line the closed cavities of the thorax and abdomen and cover the organs within them. Membranes lining cavities are termed parietal membranes; membranes covering organs are called visceral membranes. Serous membranes consist of a layer of simple squamous epithelium (mesothelium) that covers a thin layer of connective tissue.[1] Serous membranes secrete a small amount of watery fluid into the potential space between the parietal and visceral membranes. Serous fluid serves as a lubricant, allowing the internal organs to move without excessive friction. Although there is no actual space between visceral and parietal serous membranes, the potential space between them is called a cavity. In certain disease states, these cavities may contain large amounts of fluid (i.e., effusions). Three such serous cavities are the pericardial cavity, the pleural cavity, and the peritoneal cavity.

Synovial membranes line the cavities of most joints, the bursae, and the synovial tendon sheaths. These membranes consist of fibrous connective tissue, which overlies loose connective tissue and adipose tissue.[2] Synovial cells are found in layers one to three cells thick; wide gaps are often found between adjacent synovial cells. Synovial membranes secrete a thick, colorless fluid with a high mucin content. As with serous fluid, synovial fluid acts as a lubricant in joint cavities. It also provides nourishment to articular cartilage.[3]

Serous fluid is formed by diffusion from adjacent capillaries via interstitial fluid and may be described as an ultrafiltrate of plasma. Thus, substances that normally diffuse from capillaries (e.g., water, electrolytes, glucose) diffuse into serous fluid. Similarly, substances can diffuse from serous fluid back into the capillaries. Protein may also collect in serous cavities because of capillary leakage. Protein and excess fluids are normally removed from these cavities by the surrounding lymphatics.

Synovial fluid is formed in a manner similar to that of serous fluid but additionally contains a hyaluronate-protein complex (i.e., a mucopolysaccharide containing hyaluronic acid and a small amount of protein) that is secreted by the connective tissue cells of the synovial membrane.[4] As with serous cavities,

403

excess proteins and fluids are normally drained from synovial cavities by the lymphatics.

Changes in fluid production and drainage may lead to the development of effusions in serous and synovial cavities. Mechanical factors that may cause effusions include increased capillary permeability, increased capillary hydrostatic pressure, decreased capillary colloidal osmotic pressure, increased venous pressure, and blockage of lymphatic vessels. Damage to the serous and synovial membranes (e.g., caused by inflammation or infection) may also cause excessive fluid buildup.

Effusions involving serous cavities may be differentiated as transudates or exudates. Transudates occur because of abnormal mechanical factors and are generally characterized by low-protein, cell-free fluids. Exudates are caused by infection or inflammation and contain cells and excessive amounts of protein. Pleural and peritoneal effusions may be either transudates or exudates; pericardial effusions, however, are almost always exudates.[5] Chylous effusions caused by the escape of chyle from the thoracic lymphatic duct may form in the pleural and peritoneal cavities. Accumulation of large amounts of fluid in the peritoneal cavity is termed *ascites.*

Samples of effusions for laboratory analysis are obtained by needle aspiration. *Centesis* is a suffix denoting "puncture and aspiration of."[6] Thus, aspiration of pericardial fluid is called *pericardiocentesis,* aspiration of pleural fluid is called *thoracentesis,* aspiration of peritoneal fluid is called *paracentesis,* and aspiration of synovial fluid is called *arthrocentesis.*

Serous fluids are normally clear and pale yellow, occurring in amounts of 50 mL or less in the pericardial and peritoneal cavities and 20 mL or less in the pleural cavity. Cloudy (turbid) fluid suggests an inflammatory process that may be caused by infection. Milky fluid is associated with chylous effusions or chronic serous effusions (pseudochylous effusions). Bloody fluid may indicate a hemorrhagic process or a traumatic tap. Bloody pericardial fluid is associated with a number of disorders, including hemorrhagic and bacterial pericarditis, postmyocardial infarction and postpericardiectomy syndromes, metastatic cancer, aneurysms, tuberculosis, systemic lupus erythematosus (SLE), and rheumatoid arthritis. Bloody pleural effusions are most often the result of malignancies involving the lung but may also be seen in pneumonia, pulmonary infarction, chest trauma, pancreatitis, and postmyocardial infarction syndrome. Bloody pleural transudates also have been noted in congestive heart failure (CHF) and cirrhosis of the liver. Bloody peritoneal fluid is associated primarily with malignant processes and abdominal trauma. Greenish peritoneal fluid is seen in perforated duodenal ulcers, intestines, and gallbladders, as well as with cholecystitis and acute pancreatitis.[7]

As with serous fluid, synovial fluid is normally clear and pale yellow, occurring in amounts of approximately 3 mL or less per joint cavity. Synovial fluid is more viscous than is serous fluid because of the presence of the hyaluronate-protein complex secreted by the synovial cells. Arthritis and other inflammatory conditions involving the joints may affect the production of hyaluronate and lead to decreased viscosity of synovial fluid. The mucin clot test (Ropes test), in which synovial fluid is added to a 2 to 5 percent acetic acid solution, may be used to assess the viscosity of synovial fluid in relation to the type of clot formed (e.g., solid, soft, friable, or none).[8] This test is not as accurate as specific synovial fluid cell counts and other analyses, however.[9]

Cloudy synovial fluid suggests an inflammatory process. Substances such as crystals, fibrin, amyloid, and cartilage fragments may also result in cloudy synovial fluid. Milky synovial fluid is associated with various types of arthritis as well as with SLE. Purulent fluid may be seen in acute septic arthritis, whereas greenish fluid may occur in *Haemophilus influenzae* septic arthritis, chronic rheumatoid arthritis, and acute synovitis caused by gout. Bloody synovial fluid may be the result of a traumatic tap but is most commonly associated with fractures or tumors involving the joint and traumatic or hemophilic arthritis.[10]

Tests of serous and synovial effusions include cell count and differential, measurement of substances normally found in the fluid (e.g., glucose), culture and sensitivity (C&S) testing, and cytologic examination. These tests are discussed subsequently in relation to the cavity from which the fluid is obtained.

TESTS OF EFFUSIONS

PERICARDIAL FLUID ANALYSIS

Pericardial effusions are most commonly caused by pericarditis, malignancy, or metabolic damage. As noted previously, most pericardial effusions are exudates. Tests commonly performed on pericardial fluid include red cell count, white cell count and differential, determination of glucose level, and cytologic examination. Gram stains and cultures of pericardial fluid are not routinely performed unless bacterial endocarditis is suspected.[11]

Cytologic examination of pericardial fluid is undertaken to detect malignant cells. Gram stain and culture reveal the causative agent when infection is suspected.

Reference Values

Red blood cells	None normally present
White blood cells	$<1000/mm^3$
Glucose	80–100 mg/dL or essentially the same as the blood glucose level drawn 2 to 4 hr earlier
Cytologic examination	No abnormal cells
Gram stain and culture	No organisms present
Critical Values	**Positive Gram stain or culture**

Interfering Factors

➤ Blood in the sample because of traumatic pericardiocentesis
➤ Undetected hypoglycemia or hyperglycemia
➤ Contamination of the sample with skin cells and pathogens

Indications for Pericardial Fluid Analysis

➤ Pericardial effusion of unknown etiology
➤ Suspected hemorrhagic pericarditis as indicated by the presence of red cells and an elevated white cell count
➤ Suspected bacterial pericarditis as indicated by the presence of red cells, elevated white cell count with a predominance of neutrophils, and decreased glucose

➤ Suspected postmyocardial infarction syndrome (Dressler's syndrome) as indicated by the presence of red cells and elevated white cell count with a predominance of neutrophils

➤ Suspected tuberculous or fungal pericarditis as indicated by the presence of red cells and an elevated white cell count with a predominance of lymphocytes

➤ Suspected viral pericarditis as indicated by the presence of red cells and an elevated white cell count with neutrophils predominating

➤ Suspected rheumatoid disease or SLE as indicated by the presence of red cells, elevated white cell count, and decreased glucose levels

➤ Suspected malignancy as indicated by the presence of red cells, decreased glucose, and presence of abnormal cells on cytologic examination

Nursing Care Before the Procedure

Explain to the client:

➤ That the procedure will be performed by a physician and will require approximately 20 minutes

➤ Where the test will be performed (i.e., it is sometimes performed in the cardiac laboratory)

➤ Any dietary restrictions (fasting for 6 to 8 hours before the test may be required)

➤ That an intravenous (IV) infusion will be started before the procedure and discontinued afterward

➤ That a sedative may be administered before the procedure

➤ That the skin will be injected with a local anesthetic at the chest needle insertion site and that this may cause a stinging sensation

➤ That, after the skin has been anesthetized, a needle will be inserted through the chest wall below and slightly to the left of the breast bone into the fluid-filled sac around the heart

➤ That a sensation of pressure may be felt when the needle is inserted to obtain the pericardial fluid

➤ That heart rate and rhythm will be monitored during the procedure

➤ The importance of remaining still during the procedure

➤ Any activity restrictions after the test (usually a few hours of bed rest)

Prepare for the procedure:

➤ Withhold anticoagulant medications and aspirin as ordered.

➤ Have the client void.

➤ Provide a hospital gown.

➤ Take and record vital signs.

➤ Administer premedication as ordered.

The Procedure (Pericardiocentesis)

The necessary equipment is assembled, including a pericardiocentesis tray with solution for skin preparation, local anesthetic, 50-mL syringe, needles of various sizes including a cardiac needle, sterile drapes, and sterile gloves. Sterile test tubes (same as those used for collecting blood samples) also are needed; at least one red-topped, one green-topped, and one lavender-topped tube should be available. Containers for culture and cytologic analysis of pericardial fluid samples may also be needed. Cardiac monitoring equipment should be obtained, along with an alligator clip for attaching a precordial (V) lead to the cardiac needle.

The client is assisted to a supine position with the head elevated 45 to 60 degrees. The limb leads for the cardiac monitor are attached to the client, and the IV infusion is started. The skin is cleansed with an antiseptic solution and protected with sterile drapes. The skin at the needle insertion site is then infiltrated with local anesthetic. Strict aseptic technique is used during the entire procedure.

The precordial (V) cardiac lead wire is attached to the hub of the cardiac needle with the alligator clip. The needle is then inserted just below and slightly to the left of the xiphoid process. Gentle traction is sustained on the plunger of the 50-mL syringe until fluid appears, indicating that the needle has entered the pericardial sac. Fluid can be aspirated with ultrasound guidance. Fluid samples are then withdrawn and placed in appropriate tubes. The samples are labeled and sent promptly to the laboratory.

When the desired samples have been obtained, the cardiac needle is withdrawn. Pressure is applied to the site for 5 minutes. If there is no evidence of bleeding or other drainage, a sterile bandage is applied. If the client's cardiac rhythm is stable, cardiac monitoring is discontinued.

Nursing Care During the Procedure

Observe the client for respiratory or cardiac distress. Possible complications of a pericardiocentesis include cardiac dysrhythmias (atrial or ventricular), laceration of the pleura, laceration of the cardiac atrium or coronary vessels, injection of air into a cardiac chamber, and contamination of pleural spaces with infected pericardial fluid.

➤ Monitor the electrocardiograph (ECG) for position of the needle tip to note any puncture of the right atrium.

Nursing Care After the Procedure

Care and assessment after the procedure include assisting the client to a position of comfort and reminding the client of any activity restrictions.

➤ Resume any foods or fluids withheld before the test and any medications withheld upon the physician's order.

➤ Continue IV fluids until vital signs are stable and the client is able to resume normal fluid intake.

➤ Take and record vital signs as for a postoperative client (i.e., every 15 minutes for the first hour, every 30 minutes for the second hour, every hour for the next 4 hours, and then every 4 hours for 24 hours). Assess for abnormalities in ECG patterns.

➤ Assess the puncture site for bleeding, hematoma formation, and inflammation each time vital signs are taken and daily thereafter for several days.

➤ Observe the client for any cardiac or respiratory distress.

➤ Provide support when diagnostic findings are revealed.

➤ Note relief of symptoms of cardiac tamponade or pericarditis: absence of distended neck veins; normal cardiac output, heart rate, and heart sounds; absence of chest pain and pulsus paradoxus.

➤ Administer antibiotics specific to the causative agent and anti-inflammatory drugs to reduce the inflammatory response.

➤ Notify physician immediately if the Gram stain and culture are positive.

PLEURAL FLUID ANALYSIS

Pleural effusions are most commonly caused by CHF, hypoalbuminemia (e.g., resultng from cirrhosis of the liver), hypoproteinemia (e.g., resulting from nephrotic syndrome), neoplasms, and pulmonary infections (e.g., pneumonia, tuberculosis). Other causes include trauma and pulmonary infarctions, both of which are associated with hemorrhagic effusions, rheumatoid disease, SLE, pancreatitis, and ruptured esophagus. Chylous pleural effusions occur when there is damage or obstruction to the thoracic lymphatic duct. Pleural effusions may be either transudates or exudates.

Tests commonly performed on pleural fluid include red cell count, white cell count and differential, Gram stain, culture and sensitivity (C&S), and cytologic examination. The pH of the sample is usually determined, and the fluid is tested for levels of glucose, protein, lactic dehydrogenase (LDH), and amylase. Triglycerides and cholesterol may also be measured when chylous effusion is suspected.

Gram stain and C&S tests are generally performed to identify the causative organism when infection is suspected. Cytologic examination is undertaken to detect malignant cells.

Pleural effusions may also be tested for levels of immunoglobulins, complement components, and carcinoembryonic antigen (CEA) (see Chap. 3) when disorders of immunologic and malignant origin are suspected. Elevated immunoglobulins and CEA or decreased complement levels, or both, are seen in inflammatory or neoplastic reactions involving the pleural membranes.[12]

Reference Values

Red blood cells	0–<1000/mm^3
White blood cells	0–<1000/mm^3, consisting mainly of lymphocytes
Gram stain and culture	No organisms present
Cytologic examination	No abnormal cells
pH	7.37–7.43 (usually >7.40)
Glucose	Parallels serum levels
Protein	3.0 g/dL
Pleural fluid : serum protein ratio	0.5 or less
Lactic dehydrogenase (LDH)	71–207 IU/L
Pleural fluid : serum LDH ratio	0.6 or less
Amylase	<180 Somogyi U/dL or <200 dye U/dL
Triglycerides	
Cholesterol	
Immunoglobulins	Parallel serum levels
Carcinoembryonic antigen (CEA)	
Complement	
Critical Values	**Positive Gram stain or culture**

Interfering Factors

➤ Blood in the sample because of traumatic thoracentesis
➤ Undetected hypoglycemia or hyperglycemia
➤ Contamination of the sample with skin cells and pathogens

Indications for Pleural Fluid Analysis

➤ Pleural effusion of unknown etiology
➤ Differentiation of pleural transudates from exudates (Table 9–1)
➤ Suspected traumatic hemothorax as indicated by bloody pleural fluid, elevated red cell count, and hematocrit similar to that found in whole blood
➤ Suspected pleural effusion caused by pulmonary tuberculosis as indicated by presence of red blood cells (less than 10,000 per cubic millimeter); white cell count of 5,000 to 10,000 per cubic millimeter, consisting mostly of lymphocytes; presence of acid-fast bacilli (AFB) on smear and culture; pH of less than 7.30, decreased glucose (sometimes); and elevated protein, pleural fluid : serum protein ratio, LDH, and pleural fluid:serum LDH ratio
➤ Suspected pleural effusion caused by pneumonia (parapneumonic effusion) as indicated by presence of red blood cells (<5000 per cubic millimeter); white cell count of 5,000 to 25,000 per cubic millimeter, consisting mainly of neutrophils and sometimes including eosinophils; pH less than 7.40; and elevated protein, pleural fluid : serum protein ratio, LDH, and pleural fluid : serum LDH ratio. (If the pneumonia is of bacterial origin, the organism may be demonstrated on culture and the pleural fluid glucose level may be decreased.)
➤ Suspected bacterial or tuberculous empyema as indicated by red cell count of less than 5,000 per cubic millimeter; white cell count of 25,000 to 100,000 per cubic millimeter, consisting mostly of neutrophils; pH less than 7.30; decreased glucose; and increased protein, LDH, and related ratios[13]
➤ Suspected pleural effusion caused by carcinoma as indicated by presence of red blood cells (1,000 to more than 100,000 per cubic millimeter); white cell count of 5,000 to 10,000 per cubic millimeter, consisting mostly of

Table 9–1 ➤ **DIFFERENTIATION OF PLEURAL TRANSUDATES FROM EXUDATES**

	Transudates	**Exudates**
Appearance	Clear	Cloudy; may be bloody
Red blood cells	<1000/mm³	>1000/mm³ (usually)
White blood cells	<1000/mm³	>1000/mm³
pH	7.40 or higher	<7.40
Glucose	Parallels serum level	May be less than serum level
Protein	<3.0 g/dL	>3.0 g/dL
Pleural fluid : serum protein ratio	<0.5	>0.5
Lactic dehydrogenase (LDH)	<200 IU/L	>200 IU/L
Pleural fluid : serum LDH ratio	<0.6	>0.6
Common causes	Congestive heart failure (CHF) Cirrhosis Nephrotic syndrome	Pneumonia Tuberculosis Empyema Pulmonary infarction Rheumatoid disease Systemic lupus erythematosus (SLE) Carcinoma Pancreatitis

lymphocytes and sometimes including eosinophils; detection of malignant cells on cytologic examination; pH less than 7.30; decreased glucose (sometimes); increased protein, LDH, and related ratios; elevated CEA and immunoglobulins; and decreased complement[14]

➤ Suspected pleural effusion caused by pulmonary infarction as indicated by red cell count of 1,000 to 100,000 per cubic millimeter; white cell count of 5,000 to 15,000 per cubic millimeter, consisting mainly of neutrophils and sometimes including eosinophils; pH greater than 7.30; normal glucose; and elevated protein, LDH, and related ratios[15]

➤ Suspected pleural effusion caused by rheumatoid disease as indicated by a normal red cell count; a white cell count of 1,000 to 20,000 per cubic millimeter with either lymphocytes or neutrophils predominating; pH less than 7.30; decreased glucose; elevated protein, LDH, and related ratios; and elevated immunoglobulins[16]

➤ Suspected pleural effusion caused by SLE as indicated by findings similar to those in rheumatoid disease, except that glucose is not usually decreased

➤ Suspected pleural effusion caused by pancreatitis as indicated by red cell count of 1,000 to 10,000 per cubic millimeter; white cell count of 5,000 to 20,000 per cubic millimeter, consisting mostly of neutrophils; pH greater than 7.30; normal glucose; elevated protein, LDH, and related ratios; and elevated amylase

➤ Suspected pleural effusion caused by esophageal rupture as indicated primarily by a pH as low as 6.0 and elevated amylase[17]

➤ Differentation of chylous pleural effusions caused by thoracic lymphatic duct blockage from pseudochylous (chronic serous) effusions, with chylous effusions indicated primarily by a triglyceride level two to three times that of serum; decreased cholesterol; and markedly elevated chylomicrons

Nursing Care Before the Procedure

Explain to the client:

➤ That the procedure will be performed by a physician and requires approximately 20 minutes

➤ That there are no food or fluid restrictions before the test

➤ That a sedative is not usually given before the procedure, although a cough suppressant may be given to prevent coughing

➤ The positioning used for the procedure (supported sitting or side-lying)

➤ That the skin will be injected with a local anesthetic at the chest needle insertion site and that the injection may cause a stinging sensation

➤ That, after the skin has been anesthetized, a needle will be inserted through the posterior chest into the space near the lungs where excessive fluid has accumulated

➤ That a sensation of pressure may be felt when the needle is inserted

➤ The importance of remaining still during the procedure and the need to control breathing, coughing, and movement

➤ Any activity restrictions after the test (usually 1 hour of bed rest)

Prepare for the procedure:

➤ Withhold anticoagulant medications and aspirin as ordered.

➤ Have the client void.

➤ Provide a hospital gown.

➤ Take and record vital signs.
➤ Administer cough suppressant, if ordered.

The Procedure (Thoracentesis)

The necessary equipment is assembled, including a thoracentesis tray with solution for skin preparation, local anesthetic, 50-mL syringe, needles of various sizes including a thoracentesis needle, sterile drapes, and sterile gloves. Sterile collection bottles and containers for culture and cytologic examination also are needed.

The client is assisted to the position that will be used for the test. The usual position is sitting on the side of a bed or treatment table, leaning slightly forward to spread the intercostal spaces, with arms supported on an overbed table with several pillows. Alternatively, the client may sit on the bed or table with legs extended on it and arms supported as described earlier. If the client cannot assume either sitting position, the side-lying position is used. In such situations, the client lies on the unaffected side.

The skin is cleansed with an antiseptic solution and protected with sterile drapes. The skin at the needle insertion site is then infiltrated with local anesthetic. The thoracentesis needle is inserted. When fluid appears, a stopcock and 50-mL syringe are attached to the needle and the fluid is aspirated. The pleural fluid samples are placed in appropriate containers, labeled, and sent promptly to the laboratory.

If the thoracentesis is being performed for therapeutic as well as diagnostic reasons, additional pleural fluid may be withdrawn. When the desired amount of fluid has been removed, the needle is withdrawn, and slight pressure is applied to the site for a few minutes. If there is no evidence of bleeding or other drainage, a sterile bandage is applied to the site.

Nursing Care During the Procedure

Observe the client for signs of respiratory distress or pneumothorax (e.g., anxiety, restlessness, dyspnea, cyanosis, tachycardia, and chest pain). Possible complications of a thoracentesis include pneumothorax, mediastinal shift, and excessive reaccumulation of pleural fluid.

Nursing Care After the Procedure

Care and assessment after the procedure include assisting the client in lying on the unaffected side and reminding the client that this position should be maintained for approximately 1 hour.

➤ Elevate the head for client comfort.
➤ Prepare for a post-thoracentesis chest x-ray examination ordered to ensure that a pneumothorax as a result of the tap has not occurred and to evaluate the amount of fluid removed.
➤ Take and record vital signs as ordered (e.g., every 15 minutes for the first half hour, every 30 minutes for the next hour, and then every 4 hours for 24 hours or until stable).
➤ Observe the client for respiratory distress or hemoptysis, diaphoresis, or skin color changes.
➤ Auscultate breath sounds. Absent or diminished breath sounds on the side used for the thoracentesis may indicate pneumothorax.
➤ Assess the puncture site for bleeding, hematoma formation, and inflammation each time vital signs are taken and daily thereafter for several days.

➤ Provide support when diagnostic findings are revealed and information is given about subsequent therapy based on the findings.

➤ Note relief of chest pain, dyspnea, or diminished breath sounds.

➤ Note response to antibiotic or cytotoxic drugs if injected into the cavity after fluid removal.

➤ Notify physician immediately if the Gram stain or culture is positive.

PERITONEAL FLUID ANALYSIS

Peritoneal transudates are most commonly caused by CHF, cirrhosis of the liver, and nephrotic syndrome. Peritoneal exudates occur with neoplasms including metastatic carcinoma, infections (e.g., tuberculosis, bacterial peritonitis), trauma, pancreatitis, and bile peritonitis. Chylous peritoneal effusions occur when there is damage or obstruction to the thoracic lymphatic duct. Accumulation of large amounts of fluid in the peritoneal cavity is termed *ascites,* and the peritoneal fluid is referred to as *ascitic fluid.*

Peritoneal fluid is removed by paracentesis or by paracentesis and lavage with normal saline or Ringer's lactate. Lavage involves instilling the desired solution over 15 to 20 minutes, then removing it and analyzing it for cells and other constituents.

Tests commonly performed on peritoneal or ascitic fluid include red cell count, white cell count and differential, Gram stain, C&S, AFB smear and culture, and cytologic examination. The fluid may also be tested for glucose, amylase, ammonia, alkaline phosphatase, and carcinoembryonic antigen (CEA). Urea and creatinine may be measured if there is suspicion of ruptured or punctured urinary bladder.

Gram stain C&S tests are generally performed to identify the causative organism when infection is suspected. If tuberculous effusion is suspected, an AFB smear and culture may be performed, although positive results are seen in only 25 to 50 percent of cases.[18] Cytologic examination is used to detect malignant cells.

Reference Values

Red blood cells	<100,000/mm³
White blood cells	<300/mm³ (undiluted peritoneal fluid)
	<500/mm³ (lavage fluid)
Neutrophils	<25%
Absolute granulocyte count	<250/mm³
Gram stain and culture	No organisms present
AFB smear and culture	No AFB present
Cytologic examination	No abnormal cells present
Glucose	
Amylase	
Ammonia	
Alkaline phosphatase	Parallel serum levels
Creatinine	
Urea	
Carcinoembryonic antigen (CEA)	
Critical Values	**Positive Gram stain or culture**

Interfering Factors

➤ Blood in the sample as a result of traumatic paracentesis
➤ Undetected hypoglycemia or hyperglycemia
➤ Contamination of the sample with skin cells and pathogens

Indications for Peritoneal Fluid Analysis

➤ Ascites of unknown cause
➤ Suspected peritoneal effusion caused by abdominal malignancy as indicated by elevated red cell count, decreased glucose, elevated CEA, and detection of malignant cells on cytologic examination
➤ Suspected abdominal trauma as indicated by elevated red cell count of greater than 100,000 per cubic millimeter[19]
➤ Suspected ascites caused by cirrhosis of the liver as indicated by elevated white cell count, neutrophil count of greater than 25 percent but less than 50 percent, and an absolute granulocyte count of less than 250 per cubic millimeter
➤ Suspected bacterial peritonitis as indicated by elevated white cell count, neutrophil count greater than 50 percent, and an absolute granulocyte count of greater than 250 per cubic millimeter[20]
➤ Suspected tuberculous peritoneal effusion as indicated by elevated lymphocyte count, positive AFB smear and culture in about 25 to 50 percent of cases, and decreased glucose
➤ Suspected peritoneal effusion caused by pancreatitis, pancreatic trauma, or pancreatic pseudocyst as indicated by elevated amylase levels
➤ Suspected peritoneal effusion caused by gastrointestinal perforation, strangulation, or necrosis as indicated by elevated amylase, ammonia, and alkaline phosphatase levels[21]
➤ Suspected rupture or perforation of the urinary bladder as indicated by elevated ammonia, creatinine, and urea levels

Nursing Care Before the Procedure

Explain to the client:
➤ That the test will be performed by a physician and takes approximately 30 minutes
➤ That there are no food or fluid restrictions before the test
➤ The positioning used for the procedure (seated or in high-Fowler's position)
➤ That the skin will be injected with a local anesthetic at the abdominal needle insertion site and that this injection may cause a stinging sensation
➤ That, after the skin has been anesthetized, a large needle will be inserted through the abdominal wall
➤ That a "popping" sensation may be experienced as the needle penetrates the peritoneum
➤ The importance of remaining still during the procedure
➤ Any activity restrictions after the test (usually an hour or more of bed rest)
Prepare for the procedure:
➤ Withhold anticoagulant medications and aspirin as ordered.
➤ Have the client void, or catheterize if the client is unable to void to ensure an empty bladder that is not as likely to be punctured by the needle.

➤ Provide a hospital gown and have the client put it on with the opening in the front.

➤ Take and record vital signs.

➤ If the client has ascites, obtain weight and measure abdominal girth.

➤ If the abdomen is hirsute, it may be necessary to shave the area of the puncture site.

The Procedure (Paracentesis)

The necessary equipment is assembled, including a paracentesis tray with solution for skin preparation, local anesthetic, 50-mL syringe, needles of various sizes including large-bore paracentesis needle or trocar and cannula, sterile drapes, and sterile gloves. Specimen collection tubes and bottles for the tests to be performed also are needed.

The client is assisted to the position that will be used for the test. The usual position is sitting on the side of a bed or treatment table, with the feet and back supported. An alternative approach is to place the client in bed in a high-Fowler's position.

The skin is cleansed with an antiseptic solution and protected with sterile drapes. The skin at the needle or trocar insertion site is then infiltrated with local anesthetic. The paracentesis needle is inserted approximately 1 to 2 inches below the umbilicus. If a trocar with cannula is to be used, a small skin incision may be made to facilitate insertion. The 50-mL syringe with stopcock is attached to the needle or cannula after the trocar has been removed. Gentle suction may be applied with the syringe to remove fluid. For peritoneal lavage, sterile normal saline or Ringer's lactate may be infused via the needle or cannula over 15 to 20 minutes. The client is then turned from side to side before the lavage fluid is removed.

Samples of peritoneal or ascitic fluid are obtained, placed in appropriate containers, labeled, and sent promptly to the laboratory. If the paracentesis is being performed for therapeutic as well as diagnostic reasons, additional fluid is removed. No more than 1000 to 1500 mL of fluid should be removed at any one time to avoid complications such as hypovolemia and shock resulting from abdominal pressure changes and massive fluid shifts into the space that has been drained by paracentesis.

When the desired amount of fluid has been removed, the needle or cannula is withdrawn and slight pressure is applied to the site for a few minutes. If there is no evidence of bleeding or other drainage, a sterile dressing is applied to the site.

Nursing Care During the Procedure

If feasible, check the client's vital signs every 15 minutes during the procedure.

➤ Observe the client for pallor, diaphoresis, vertigo, hypotension, tachycardia, pain, or anxiety. Rapid removal of fluid may precipitate hypovolemia and shock.

Nursing Care After the Procedure

Care and assessment after the procedure include assisting the client to a position of comfort and reminding the client of any activity restrictions.

➤ Redress the puncture site using sterile technique if excessive drainage is present.

➤ Take and record vital signs as for a postoperative client (i.e., every 15 minutes for the first hour, every 30 minutes for the next 2 hours, every hour for the next 4 hours, and then every 4 hours for 24 hours). Take temperature every 4 hours for 24 hours. Monitor intake and output (I&O) for at least 24 hours.

➤ Assess the puncture site for bleeding, excessive drainage, and signs of inflammation each time the vital signs are taken and daily thereafter for several days.

➤ Continue to observe the client for pallor, vertigo, hypotension, tachycardia, pain, or anxiety for at least 24 hours after the procedure.

➤ If a large amount of fluid was removed, measure abdominal girth and weigh the client.

➤ Provide support when diagnostic findings are revealed and information is given about subsequent therapy (antibiotics) based on findings.

➤ Have IV fluids and albumin on hand if hypotension results from the fluid shift from the vascular space.

➤ Note severe abdominal pain. Rigid abdominal muscles indicate that peritonitis is developing from the paracentesis.

➤ Notify physician immediately of a positive Gram stain or culture.

SYNOVIAL FLUID ANALYSIS

Synovial fluid is a clear, pale yellow, and viscous liquid formed by plasma ultrafiltration and by secretion of a hyaluronate-protein complex by synovial cells (see pp. 403 and 404). It is secreted in small amounts (i.e., 3 mL or less) into the cavities of most joints. Synovial effusions are associated with disorders or injuries involving the joints. Samples for analysis are obtained by aspirating joint cavities. The most commonly aspirated joint is the knee, although samples may also be obtained from the shoulder, hip, elbow, wrist, and ankle if clinically indicated.

Synovial fluid analysis is used primarily to determine the type or cause of joint disorders. Joint disorders may be classified according to five categories based on synovial fluid findings: (1) noninflammatory (e.g., degenerative joint disease), (2) inflammatory (e.g., rheumatoid arthritis, SLE), (3) septic (e.g., acute bacterial or tuberculous arthritis), (4) crystal-induced (e.g., gout or pseudogout), and (5) hemorrhagic (e.g., traumatic or hemophilic arthritis).[22]

Tests commonly performed on synovial fluid include red cell count, white cell count and differential, white cell morphology, microscopic examination for crystals, Gram stain, and C&S. Determination of protein, glucose, and uric acid levels also aids in diagnosis. Various immunologic tests such as determination of complement, rheumatoid factor, and antinuclear antibodies also have been used in synovial fluid analysis. In the recent past, the mucin clot test (see p. 404) has been used in analyzing synovial fluid, but this test is not considered as reliable as specific cell counts and other measurements of synovial fluid constituents. Lactate and pH measurements may be used as nonspecific indicators of inflammation and to differentiate between infection and inflammation.[23]

Table 9–2 lists the types of white blood cells and inclusions seen in synovial fluid, along with the disorders with which the presence of such cells is associated.

Examination of synovial fluid for crystals is used in diagnosing crystal-induced arthritis. The several types of crystals that may be identified are listed in Table 9–3. Monosodium urate (MSU) crystals are associated with arthritis caused by gout, whereas calcium pyrophosphate (CPP) crystals are seen in

Table 9–2 ➤ WHITE BLOOD CELLS AND INCLUSIONS SEEN IN SYNOVIAL FLUID

Cell/Inclusion	Description	Significance
Neutrophil	Polymorphonuclear leukocyte	Bacterial sepsis Crystal-induced inflammation
Lymphocyte	Mononuclear leukocyte	Nonseptic inflammation
Macrophage (monocyte)	Large mononuclear leukocyte; may be vacuolated	Normal Viral infections
Synovial lining cell	Similar to macrophage but may be multinucleated, resembling a mesothelial cell	Normal
LE cell	Neutrophil containing characteristic ingested "round body"	Lupus erythematosus
Reiter cell	Vacuolated macrophage with ingested neutrophils	Reiter's syndrome Nonspecific inflammation
RA cell (ragocyte)	Neutrophil with dark cytoplasmic granules containing immune complexes	Rheumatiod arthritis Immunologic inflammation
Cartilage cells	Large, multinucleated cells	Osteoarthritis
Rice bodies	Macroscopically resemble polished rice Microscopically show collagen and fibrin	Tuberculosis, septic and rheumatoid arthritis
Fat droplets	Refractile intracellular and extracellular globules Stain with Sudan dyes	Traumatic injury
Hemosiderin	Inclusions within synovial cells	Pigmented villonodular synovitis

Note: From Strasinger, SK: Urinalysis and Body Fluids, ed 3. FA Davis, 1994, p 168, with permission.

pseudogout. Cholesterol crystals are associated with chronic joint effusions, which may be caused by tuberculous or rheumatoid arthritis. Arthritis associated with the presence of apatite crystals is commonly recognized as a cause of synovitis. Corticosteroid crystals may be seen for a month or more after intra-articular injections of steroids and may induce acute synovitis. Although usually of a rhomboid shape, corticosteroid crystals are sometimes needle-shaped and may be confused with MSU or CPP crystals. Not shown in Table 9–3 are talcum crystals. These crystals, which are shaped like Maltese crosses, are most commonly seen after joint surgery and reflect contamination of the joint with talcum powder from surgical gloves.[24]

Gram stain and C&S tests are used to identify the causative organisms when infection is suspected. AFB smear and culture may be performed when tuberculous arthritis is suspected, but results are frequently negative. When the results of microbiologic tests of synovial fluid are inconclusive, synovial biopsy may be necessary to establish the diagnosis.[25]

The need to perform immunologic tests of synovial fluid is indicative of the association of the immune system with inflammatory joint disorders. Substances measured include rheumatoid factor (RF), antinuclear antibodies (ANA), and complement, all of which may also be measured in serum (see Chap. 3).

Determination of complement levels in synovial fluid aids in differentiating arthritis of immunologic origin from that with nonimmunologic causes. Decreased synovial fluid complement levels are seen in approximately 60 to

Table 9–3 ➤ SYNOVIAL FLUID CRYSTALS	
Crystal	**Shape**
Monosodium urate	Needles
Calcium pyrophosphate	Rods Needles Rhombics
Cholesterol	Notched rhombic plates
Apatite	Small needles
Corticosteroid	Flat, variable-shaped plates

Note: Adapted from Strasinger, SK: Urinalysis and Body Fluids, ed 3. FA Davis, 1994, p 169.

80 percent of individuals with rheumatoid arthritis and SLE. Decreased complement levels are occasionally seen in rheumatic fever, gout, pseudogout, and bacterial arthritis; however, synovial complement levels may be high in these disorders if serum levels also are elevated. Complement levels in synovial fluid may be measured as total complement (CH_{50}) or as individual components (C1q, C4, C2, and C3). Because synovial fluid complement levels parallel synovial fluid protein levels, complement levels may be expressed as ratios in relation to protein levels to ensure that abnormal findings are not caused by changes in synovial fluid membrane filtration.[26,27]

Reference Values

Red blood cells	$<2000/mm^3$
White blood cells	$<200/mm^3$
Neutrophils	$<25\%$
White cell morphology	No abnormal cells or inclusions (see Table 9–2)
Crystals	None present (see Table 9–3)
Gram stain and culture	No organisms present
Acid-fast bacillus (AFB) smear and culture	No AFB present
Protein	<3 g/dL
Glucose	Not <10 mg/dL of blood level or not <40 mg/dL
Uric acid	Parallels serum level
Lactate	0.6–2.0 mmol/L or 5–20 mg/dL
Antinuclear antibodies (ANA) Rheumatoid factor (RF) Complement	Parallel serum levels
Critical Values	**Positive Gram stain or culture**

Interfering Factors

➤ Blood in the sample caused by traumatic arthrocentesis
➤ Undetected hypoglycemia or hyperglycemia or failure to comply with dietary restrictions before the test, or both
➤ Contamination of the sample with pathogens
➤ Improper handling of the specimen (Refrigeration of the sample may result in an increase in MSU crystals because of decreased solubility of uric acid. Exposure of the sample to room air with a resultant loss of carbon dioxide and rise in pH encourages the formation of calcium CPP crystals.)[28]

Indications for Synovial Fluid Analysis

➤ Joint effusion of unknown etiology
➤ Suspected trauma, tumors involving the joint, or hemophilic arthritis as indicated by an elevated red cell count, elevated protein level, and possibly fat droplets if trauma is involved (see Table 9–2, p. 416)
➤ Suspected joint effusion caused by noninflammatory disorders (e.g., osteoarthritis, degenerative joint disease) as indicated by a white cell count of less than 5000 per cubic millimeter with a normal differential and the presence of cartilage cells (see Table 9–2)
➤ Suspected rheumatoid arthritis as indicated by a white cell count of 2,000 to 100,000 per cubic millimeter with an elevated neutrophil count (i.e., 30 to 50 percent), presence of rheumatoid arthritis cells and possibly rice bodies (see Table 9–2), cholesterol crystals if effusion is chronic, elevated protein level, decreased glucose level, moderately elevated lactate level (i.e., 2 to 7.5 mmol/L), decreased pH, presence of RF (60 percent of cases), and decreased complement
➤ Suspected SLE involving the joints as indicated by a white cell count of 2,000 to 100,000 per cubic millimeter with an elevated neutrophil count (i.e., 30 to 40 percent), presence of LE cells (see Table 9–2), elevated protein level, decreased glucose level (i.e., 2 to 7.5 mmol/L), decreased pH, presence of ANA (20 percent of cases), and decreased complement
➤ Suspected acute bacterial arthritis as indicated by a white cell count of 10,000 to 200,000 per cubic millimeter with a markedly elevated neutrophil count (i.e., as high as 90 percent), positive Gram stain (50 percent of cases), positive cultures (30 to 80 percent of cases), possible presence of rice bodies (see Table 9–2), decreased glucose, lactate level greater than 7.5 mmol/L, pH less than 7.3, and complement levels paralleling those found in serum (i.e., may be elevated or decreased)[29]
➤ Suspected tuberculous arthritis as indicated by a white cell count of 2,000 to 100,000 per cubic millimeter with an elevated neutrophil count (i.e., 30 to 60 percent), possible presence of rice bodies (see Table 9–2), cholesterol crystals if effusion is chronic, positive AFB smear and culture in some cases (results are frequently negative), decreased glucose, elevated lactate levels, and decreased pH
➤ Suspected joint effusion caused by gout as indicated by a white cell count of 500 to 200,000 per cubic millimeter with an elevated neutrophil count (i.e., approximately 70 percent), presence of MSU crystals (see Table 9–3, p. 417), decreased glucose, elevated uric acid levels, and complement levels paralleling those of serum (may be elevated or decreased)[30,31]

➤ Differentiation of gout from pseudogout as indicated primarily by finding CPP crystals (see Table 9–3), which are associated with pseudogout (Other findings in pseudogout are similar to those of gout except that the white cell count may not be as high.)

Nursing Care Before the Procedure

Explain to the client:
➤ The purpose of the test
➤ That it will be performed by a physician and requires approximately 20 minutes
➤ Any dietary restrictions (fasting for 6 to 12 hours before the test is recommended if the synovial fluid is to be tested for glucose)
➤ The positioning to be used (seated or supine for knee, shoulder, elbow, wrist, or ankle aspiration; supine for hip joint aspiration)
➤ That the skin at the site will be injected with a local anesthetic and that it may cause a stinging sensation
➤ That, after the skin has been anesthetized, a large needle will be inserted into the joint capsule
➤ That discomfort may be experienced as the joint capsule is penetrated
➤ The importance of remaining still during the procedure
➤ Any activity restrictions after the test (The client usually is advised to avoid excessive use of the joint for several days after the procedure to prevent pain and swelling.)
➤ That ice packs or analgesics or both may be prescribed after the procedure to prevent swelling and alleviate discomfort

Prepare for the procedure:
➤ Withhold anticoagulant medications and aspirin as ordered.
➤ Ensure to the extent possible that any dietary restrictions are followed.
➤ Have the client void.
➤ Provide a hospital gown if necessary to allow access to the site without unduly exposing the client.
➤ Take and record vital signs.
➤ If the client is extremely hirsute, it may be necessary to shave the area of the puncture site.

The Procedure (Arthrocentesis)

The necessary equipment is assembled, including an arthrocentesis tray with solution for skin preparation, local anesthetic, a 20-mL syringe, needles of various sizes, sterile drapes, and sterile gloves. Specimen collection tubes and containers for the tests to be performed also are obtained. For cell counts and differential, lavender-topped tubes containing ethylenediaminetetra-acetic acid (EDTA) are used. Green-topped tubes containing heparin are used for certain immunologic and chemistry tests, whereas samples for glucose are collected in either plain red-topped tubes or gray-topped tubes containing potassium oxalate. Plain sterile tubes (e.g., red-topped tubes) are recommended for microbiologic testing and crystal examination.[32]

The client is assisted to the position that will be used for the test (sitting or supine). The skin is cleansed with antiseptic solution, protected with sterile drapes, and infiltrated with local anesthetic. The aspirating needle is inserted into the joint space and as much fluid as possible is withdrawn. The specimen should contain at least 10 mL of synovial fluid, but more may be removed to reduce swelling. Manual pressure may be applied to facilitate fluid removal.

If medication is to be injected into the joint, the syringe containing the sample is detached from the needle and replaced with the one containing the drug. The medication is injected with gentle pressure. The needle is then withdrawn and digital pressure is applied to the site for a few minutes. If there is no evidence of bleeding, a sterile dressing is applied to the site. An elastic bandage may also be applied to the joint.

The samples of synovial fluid are placed in the appropriate containers, labeled, and sent to the laboratory immediately.

Nursing Care After the Procedure

Care and assessment after the procedure include assisting the client to a position of comfort.

➤ Apply an ice pack to the site and administer analgesics as needed.

➤ Resume any foods, fluids, or medications withheld before the test upon the physician's order.

➤ Remind the client of any activity restrictions and, if indicated, site care requirements.

➤ Apply an elastic bandage to the joint to provide support and to minimize edema formation.

➤ Take and record vital signs.

➤ Assess comfort level and response to measures such as ice packs and analgesics.

➤ Assess the puncture site for bleeding, bruising, inflammation, and excessive drainage of synovial fluid approximately every 4 hours for 24 hours and then daily thereafter for several days.

➤ Provide support when diagnostic findings are revealed and information is provided about subsequent treatment based on findings (anti-inflammatory drugs, immobilization of the joint, analgesics).

➤ Notify physician immediately of a positive Gram stain or culture.

Student Name _____ Class _____

Instructor _____ Date _____

Case Study and Critical Thinking Exercise

Ms. Brown, age 45, is admitted to the ER complaining of shortness of breath. She also states that "it hurts to take a breath." VS: T 101°F (38.5°C), P 112, R 32, and BP 164/88. Lung auscultation reveals diminished breath sounds of the left lower lobe. A chest x-ray is ordered.

a. What is the probable diagnosis?

b. How does a mediastinal shift occur with this problem?

References

1. Hole, JW: Human Anatomy and Physiology, ed 4. Wm C Brown, Dubuque, Iowa, 1987, p 158.
2. Ibid, p 158.
3. Kjeldsberg, CR, and Krieg, AF: Cerebrospinal fluid and other body fluids. In Henry, JB: Clinical Diagnosis and Management by Laboratory Methods, ed 18. WB Saunders, Philadelphia, 1991, p 457.
4. Strasinger, SK: Urinalysis and Body Fluids, ed 3. FA Davis, Philadelphia, 1994, p 166.
5. Kjeldsberg and Krieg, op cit, p 463.
6. Miller, BF, and Keane, CB: Encyclopedia and Dictionary of Medicine, Nursing and Allied Health, ed 4. WB Saunders, Philadelphia, 1987, p 226.
7. Kjeldsberg and Krieg, op cit, p 468.
8. Strasinger, op cit, p 168.
9. Kjeldsberg and Krieg, op cit, p 461.
10. Ibid, p 458.
11. Strasinger, op cit, p 177.
12. Ibid, p 177.
13. Ibid, p 176.
14. Ibid, p 177.
15. Kjeldsberg and Krieg, op cit, p 464.
16. Strasinger, op cit, p 178.
17. Kjeldsberg and Krieg, op cit, p 465.
18. Ibid, p 469.
19. Ibid, p 468.
20. Strasinger, op cit, p 179.
21. Kjeldsberg and Krieg, op cit, p 469.
22. Strasinger, op cit, pp 167–168.
23. Kjeldsberg and Krieg, op cit, pp 461–462.
24. Ibid, pp 459–460.
25. Ibid, pp 462–463.
26. Ibid, p 462.
27. Strasinger, op cit, p 173.
28. Ibid, p 169.
29. Ibid, p 172.
30. Ibid, p 169.
31. Kjeldsberg and Krieg, op cit, p 462.
32. Strasinger, op cit, p 167.

Bibliography

Byrne, CJ, et al: Laboratory Tests: Implications for Nursing Care, ed 2. Addison-Wesley, Menlo Park, Calif, 1986.

Chernecky, CC, and Berger, BJ; Cullen, BN (ed): Laboratory Tests and Diagnostic Procedures, ed 2. WB Saunders, Philadelphia, 1996.

Corbett, JV: Laboratory Tests and Diagnostic Procedures with Nursing Diagnoses, ed 4. Appleton & Lange, Norwalk, Conn, 1995.

Fischbach, FT: A Manual of Laboratory Diagnostic Tests, ed 5. Lippincott-Raven, Philadelphia, 1995.

Henry, JB: Clinical Diagnosis and Management by Laboratory Methods, ed 19. WB Saunders, Philadelphia, 1996.

Kee, JL: Handbook of Laboratory and Diagnostic Tests with Nursing Implications, ed 3. Appleton & Lange, Norwalk, Conn, 1997.

Lewis, SM, et al (eds): Medical-Surgical Nursing: Assessment and Management of Clinical Problems, ed 4. Mosby–Year Book, St Louis, 1995.

Pagana, KD, and Pagana, TJ: Diagnostic and Laboratory Test Reference, ed 3. Mosby–Year Book, St Louis, 1996.

Porth, C: Pathophysiology: Concepts of Altered Health States, ed 4. JB Lippincott, Philadelphia, 1993.

Sokoloff, L (ed): The Joints and Synovial Fluid, Vol 1. Academic Press, New York, 1978.

Springhouse Corporation: Clinical Laboratory Tests: Values and Implications, ed 2. Springhouse, Springhouse, Pa, 1995.

Springhouse Corporation: Nurse's Reference Library: Diagnostics, ed 2. Springhouse, Springhouse, Pa, 1986.

Tietz, NW (ed): Clinical Guide to Laboratory Tests, ed 3. WB Saunders, Philadelphia, 1997.

Tilkian, SM: Clinical and Nursing Implications of Laboratory Tests, ed 5. Mosby–Year Book, St Louis, 1995.

Wallach, J: Interpretation of Diagnostic Tests: A Synopsis of Laboratory Medicine, ed 6. Little, Brown & Co, Boston, 1996.

10

Amniotic Fluid Analysis

➤ **TESTS COVERED**
Tests for Genetic and Neural Tube
  Defects, *424*

Tests for Hemolytic Disease of the
  Newborn, *426*
Tests for Fetal Maturity, *427*

OVERVIEW OF AMNIOTIC FLUID FORMATION AND ANALYSIS

Amniotic fluid is produced in the membranous sac that surrounds the developing fetus. This sac appears during the second week of gestation and arises from a membrane called the *amnion*. Amniotic fluid is derived from the exchange of water from maternal blood across fetal membranes, from fetal cellular metabolism, and later in pregnancy from fetal urine. Amniotic fluid serves several purposes. It prevents the amniotic membranes from adhering to the embryo and protects the fetus from shocks and blows. It also aids in controlling the embryo's body temperature and permits the fetus to move freely, thus aiding in normal growth and development.[1] Amniotic fluid may be thought of as an extension of the extracellular fluid space of the fetus.[2] Testing samples of amniotic fluid for various constituents and substances may, therefore, be used to assess fetal well-being and maturation. Specifically, amniotic fluid analysis is used to test for various inherited disorders, anatomic abnormalities such as neural tube defects, hemolytic disease of the newborn, and fetal maturity.

Amniotic fluid is normally clear and colorless in early pregnancy. Later in pregnancy, it may appear slightly opalescent because of the presence of particles of vernix caseosa and may be pale yellow because of fetal urine. The presence of meconium in amniotic fluid is normal in breech presentations but abnormal in vertex presentations and indicates relaxation of the anal sphincter from hypoxia. Amniotic fluid stained the color of port wine generally indicates abruptio placentae.

As the fetus begins to produce urine, it also swallows amniotic fluid in amounts that nearly equal urinary output (i.e., 400 to 500 mL per day).[3] Failure to swallow sufficient amounts of amniotic fluid results in excessive accumulation of fluid in the amniotic sac (polyhydramnios). This occurrence is commonly associated with anencephaly and esophageal atresia but may also occur in the presence of maternal diabetes and hypertensive disorders of pregnancy. Excessive amounts of amniotic fluid also are seen with fetal edema, which is associated with fetal heart failure, hydrops fetalis, and multiple births. Excessive swallowing of amniotic fluid results in decreased volume (oligohydramnios) and is associated with chronic illness of the fetus, placental insufficiency, fetal urinary tract malformations, and multiple births.[4] By the 14th to

423

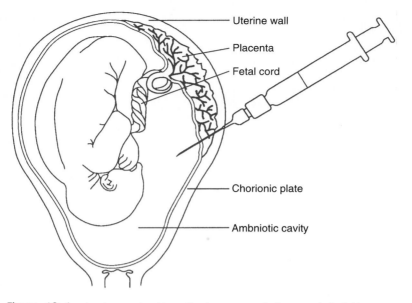

Uterine wall

Placenta

Fetal cord

Chorionic plate

Ambniotic cavity

Figure 10–1 Amniocentesis with needle placement to obtain an amniotic fluid sample.

16th weeks of pregnancy, the amniotic sac normally contains at least 50 mL of fluid; at term, the sac contains 500 to 2500 mL of amniotic fluid, with an average volume of 1000 mL.

Samples of amniotic fluid are obtained by needle aspiration (Fig. 10–1). As noted in Chapter 9, *centesis* is a suffix denoting "puncture and aspiration of"; thus, aspiration of fluid from the amniotic sac is called *amniocentesis*. For suspected genetic and neural tube defects, amniocentesis is generally performed early in the second trimester of pregnancy (i.e., 14th to 16th weeks), when there is sufficient amniotic fluid for sampling yet enough time for safe abortion, if desired. For hemolytic disease of the newborn, a series of amniocenteses may be performed beginning with the 26th week. Tests for fetal maturity usually are not performed until at least the 35th week of gestation.

TESTS OF AMNIOTIC FLUID

Tests of amniotic fluid are discussed hereafter in relation to the three general purposes for which they are performed: (1) to detect genetic and neural tube defects, (2) to test for hemolytic disease of the newborn, and (3) to assess fetal maturity.

TESTS FOR GENETIC AND NEURAL TUBE DEFECTS

Tests for genetic and neural tube defects include gender determination, chromosome analysis, and measurement of α-fetoprotein (AFP) and acetylcholinesterase levels. Determination of the gender of the fetus is indicated when sex-linked inherited disorders are suspected (e.g., hemophilia, Duchenne's muscular dystrophy). In such disorders, the abnormal gene is carried by women, although the disorder itself is inherited only by male offspring. Although no specific tests for these disorders are currently available, knowing the gender of the fetus may aid in deciding whether to continue the pregnancy. Some couples carrying these disorders, for example, choose to abort all male fetuses, even though some would have been normal.[5]

Determining the chromosomal makeup (karyotype) of the fetus may also assist in the prenatal diagnosis of disorders such as Down syndrome (trisomy 21) and Tay-Sachs disease. Karyotyping, especially when augmented by staining techniques, includes determination of the number of chromosomes as well as specific morphologic changes in the chromosomes that may indicate various genetic disorders. Karyotyping is performed by culturing fetal cells and then photographing individual chromosomes during the metaphase of mitosis.[6] Among the disorders that may be detected are alterations in carbohydrate, lipid, and amino acid metabolism. Karyotyping may take from 2 to 4 weeks before results are available to the client. Specimens for chromosome analysis must be delivered promptly to the laboratory performing the test. If immediate culturing is not possible, the sample must be incubated at normal body temperature for no longer than 2 days.[7]

Neural tube and other anatomic defects in the fetus may be determined by measuring levels of AFP and acetylcholinesterase in amniotic fluid. In the embryo, the central nervous system develops from the neural tube, which begins to form at about 22 days of gestation. Failure of the neural tube to close properly may result in disorders such as anencephaly, spina bifida, and myelomeningocele. During gestation, the major fetal serum protein is AFP. Similar to albumin, this protein is manufactured in large quantities by the fetal liver until the 32nd week of gestation, with peak production occurring at 13 weeks (see Chap. 3). With a severe neural tube defect, higher than normal amounts of AFP escape into the amniotic fluid as well as into the maternal circulation. Routine prenatal screening includes determination of the mother's serum AFP level at 13 to 16 weeks of pregnancy. Causes of elevated maternal AFP levels are listed in Table 10–1. If maternal levels are elevated on two samples obtained 1 week

Table 10–1 ➤ CONDITIONS ASSOCIATED WITH INCREASES IN MATERNAL SERUM α-FETOPROTEIN (AFP)

Gestational age underestimated	Hydrocephaly
Open neural tube defects	Hydrops fetalis
Fetomaternal hemorrhage	Twin pregnancy
Omphalocele	Turner's syndrome
Congenital proteinuric nephropathies	Cystic hygroma
Sacrococcygeal teratoma	Cyclopia
Duodenal atresia	Microcephaly
Intrauterine death	Gastroschisis
Esophageal atresia	Maternal malignancy producing α-fetoprotein (AFP)
Tetralogy of Fallot	Cancer

Note: Adapted from Wenk, RE, and Rosenbaum, JM: Analyses of amniotic fluid. In Henry, JB: Clinical Diagnosis and Management of Laboratory Methods, ed 18. WB Saunders, Philadelphia, 1991, p 484, with permission.

apart, an ultrasound is performed to determine gestational age and to check for twins or gross fetal anomalies. If the ultrasound is normal, amniotic fluid samples are obtained and analyzed for AFP levels.[8,9] If AFP levels are elevated in amniotic fluid, the presence of acetylcholinesterase in the fluid may be determined to confirm the presence of a neural tube defect. Using electrophoretic methods, the isoenzyme of acetylcholinesterase, which originates in fetal spinal fluid, may also be demonstrated and is more specific to the diagnosis of neural tube defect.[10]

AFP and acetylcholinesterase may be falsely elevated if the sample is contaminated with fetal blood. The level of the fetal spinal fluid isoenzyme of acetylcholinesterase is not, however, so affected.

TESTS FOR HEMOLYTIC DISEASE OF THE NEWBORN

One of the oldest uses of amniotic fluid analysis is in evaluating suspected hemolytic disease of the newborn, in which the mother builds antibodies against fetal red blood cell antigens (isoimmunization). The result is hemolysis of fetal erythrocytes with release of bilirubin into the amniotic fluid. The most common causes are ABO and Rh incompatibilities (e.g., an Rh-negative mother carrying an Rh-positive fetus), although other red cell antibodies may also be involved. Maternal IgG antibodies may cross the placenta to react with fetal red blood cells as early as the 16th week of pregnancy. As fetal red blood cells are broken down, bilirubin is released and can be detected in the amniotic fluid.[11]

Normally, the bilirubin level in amniotic fluid is highest between the 16th and 30th weeks of gestation. Much of this bilirubin is in the unconjugated form and can be excreted by the placenta. As the fetal liver matures, it begins to conjugate the bilirubin; this may occur as early as 28 weeks of gestation. The conjugated bilirubin is not, however, cleared by the placenta; instead, it is excreted by the fetal biliary tract and absorbed by the intestine. After the 30th week of gestation, the bilirubin level in amniotic fluid normally decreases as pregnancy progresses. This is partly because of dilution of any bilirubin present by the normal increase in amniotic fluid volume. At term, bilirubin is nearly absent from amniotic fluid.[12]

In hemolytic disease of the newborn, fetal red cell destruction leads to excessive bilirubin levels, which overwhelm both placental and fetal liver mechanisms for its clearance. Bilirubin levels in amniotic fluid continue to rise throughout the pregnancy and consist primarily of unconjugated bilirubin.[13] The amount of bilirubin present in the amniotic fluid indicates the degree of fetal red hemolysis and, indirectly, the degree of fetal anemia.

When hemolytic disease of the newborn is suspected or if maternal IgG levels are elevated, or both, serial amniocenteses for bilirubin determinations are performed beginning at approximately the 26th week of pregnancy. Bilirubin measurement in amniotic fluid is performed by spectrophotometric analysis, with the optical density (OD) of the fluid measured at wavelength intervals between 365 μm and 550 μm. When excessive bilirubin is present, a rise in OD at 450 μm, the wavelength of maximum bilirubin absorption, is seen.[14] The results of spectrophotometric analysis may be compared with the

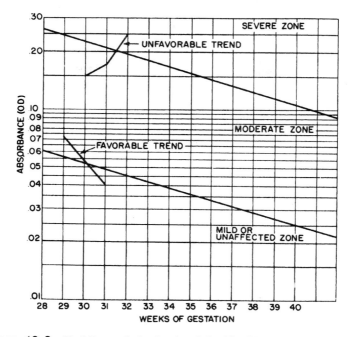

Figure 10–2   The Liley graph showing the relationship of duration of pregnancy and net optical density of amniotic fluid at 450 μm. (From Wenk, RE, Rosenbaum, JM, and Statland, BE: Assessment of fetal condition and amniotic fluid analysis. In Henry, JB [ed]: Clinical Diagnosis and Management by Laboratory Methods, ed 17. WB Saunders, Philadelphia, 1984, p 502, with permission.)

Liley graph (Fig. 10–2) to predict fetal outcome or to plan medical management of the problem.

Substances other than bilirubin may cause abnormal spectrophotometric results. Maternal hemoglobin from a traumatic amniocentesis, methemalbumin, and meconium in amniotic fluid may cause false elevations, as will fetal acidosis. Fetal hemoglobin may be differentiated from maternal hemoglobin by staining and cytologic techniques. The presence of methemalbumin indicates marked hemolysis and impending fetal demise.[15] Falsely decreased bilirubin levels may occur if the amniotic fluid sample is exposed to light or if excessive amniotic fluid volume causes dilution. Other disorders that may cause elevated amniotic fluid bilirubin levels include anencephaly and intestinal obstruction.[16]

TESTS FOR FETAL MATURITY

Tests for fetal maturity are generally performed after the 35th week of pregnancy, when preterm delivery is being considered because of fetal or maternal problems. The lungs are the last of the fetal organs to mature; therefore, the most common complication of early delivery is newborn respiratory distress syndrome (RDS). Tests of amniotic fluid for fetal maturity focus on determining fetal lung maturity and include the lecithin : sphingomyelin (L : S) ratio, as well as measures of other lung surface lipids such as phosphatidylglycerol and phosphatidylinositol. If the lungs are found to be mature by these tests, the other body organs also are assumed to be mature.[17,18] Tests of amniotic fluid, which may be used to indicate maturity of other fetal organ systems, include creatinine and bilirubin determinations, as well as examination of fetal cells for type and lipid content.

During the last trimester of pregnancy, fetal lung enzyme systems initiate the production of surfactant by type II pneumocytes, which line the alveoli. Surfactant, a phospholipid mixture, lowers the surface tension in the alveoli and prevents them from collapsing during exhalation. The phospholipid components of surfactant are (1) lecithin (phosphatidylcholine), (2) sphingomyelin, (3) phosphatidyl glycerol (PG), (4) phosphatidylethanolamine (PE), (5) phosphatidylinositol (PI), and (6) phosphatidylserine (PS). Surfactant appears in amniotic fluid as a result of fetal respiratory movements that cause it to diffuse from fetal airways.[19]

L : S RATIO

Lecithin constitutes about 75 percent of surfactant in mature lungs and is responsible for most of the surface activity of surfactant. The saturated form of lecithin, α-palmitic β-myristic lecithin, is seen early in the third trimester; the desaturated form, dipalmitic lecithin (L), begins to appear at approximately 35 weeks' gestation and continues to increase throughout the remainder of the pregnancy. Sphingomyelin, a surfactant component without major surface activity properties, remains fairly constant during pregnancy. The L : S ratio measures the relationship between lecithin and sphingomyelin; if the increasing amount of lecithin over the relatively constant amount of sphingomyelin produces a ratio of 2 : 1 or more, fetal lung maturity is generally indicated, as long as the pregnancy is uncomplicated and the amniotic fluid sample is not contaminated with blood or meconium.[20]

PHOSPHATIDYL GLYCEROL

A more reliable measure of fetal lung maturity is the "lung profile," in which the concentrations of the several lung surface lipids (i.e., PG, PI, PS, and PE) are measured in addition to lecithin and sphingomyelin. Next to lecithin, PG is the second major constituent of surfactant and is believed to aid in maintaining alveolar stability. PG appears in amniotic fluid at about 36 weeks' gestation and indicates secretion of mature surfactant. It has been found that, if PG is present in amniotic fluid, RDS in the newborn will not occur. PI is found in amniotic fluid before the appearance of PG and indicates immature fetal lungs. PI has a peak concentration at approximately 5 weeks before term and decreases thereafter. Measurement of PG and PI are most useful because they are unaffected by the presence of blood and meconium, although PG is affected by dilution of the specimen with water and by variations in test performance techniques. In addition to their usefulness in evaluating bloody or meconium-stained samples of amniotic fluid, lung profiles aid in determining lung maturity in fetuses of diabetic mothers. In maternal diabetes, the L : S ratio may indicate fetal lung maturity even though PG is not present. If the infant were delivered, RDS would be likely to occur. Measurement of PG in such situations aids in determining whether delivery should be attempted.[21,22] The significance of measures of PS and PE in lung profiles has not yet been determined.

SHAKE TEST

A bedside test to estimate fetal lung maturity may be performed when immediate results are needed. The shake test is based on the ability of surfactant to form stable foam, even in the presence of alcohol, which impairs foaming of most other biologic compounds. In this test, equal amounts of 95 percent ethanol and amniotic fluid are shaken together vigorously for 15 seconds and then allowed to stand undisturbed for 15 minutes. If a complete ring of bubbles is present at the meniscus, the test result is reported as positive, which indicates that sufficient lecithin is available for fetal lung maturity.[23] The sample of amniotic fluid for the shake test may also be diluted with saline to various concentrations to estimate fetal lung maturity more accurately. There should be a positive test result even when amniotic fluid has been diluted with two parts of saline.[24]

CREATININE BILIRUBIN

Other tests of amniotic fluid for fetal maturity include creatinine and bilirubin determinations and examination of fetal cells for type and lipid content. Creatinine appears in increased amounts in amniotic fluid at about the 36th week of gestation because of urinary excretion by the fetal kidneys and increased fetal muscle mass. A creatinine concentration of greater than 2.0 mg/dL indicates a fetal age of at least 36 to 37 weeks.[25,26] As noted previously, bilirubin levels decline throughout the last several weeks of pregnancy. Thus, a bilirubin level of less than 0.025 mg/dL at term is considered an indication of fetal maturity. It should be noted, however, that bilirubin levels may not be used to assess fetal maturity in isoimmunized mothers, because levels will be elevated as a result of hemolytic disease involving the fetus.

During the second and third trimesters, fetal epithelial cells are shed into the amniotic fluid. As the fetus matures, the percentage of cells containing lipids increases. The test is performed by staining the cells with Nile blue stain. Cells containing lipid appear orange.[27] Although only 1 percent of the cells contain lipid at 34 weeks' gestation, 10 to 50 percent contain lipid at 38 to 40 weeks.[28] Fetal maturity may also be evaluated by examining the types of cells present. Whereas basal cells are present until about 32 weeks' gestation, cornified cells appear at 36 weeks and are the predominant cell type after 38 weeks.[29]

Reference Values

	Conventional Units	**SI Units**
Color	Light straw or colorless	
Chromosome analysis	Normal karyotype	
α-Fetoprotein (AFP)	13–41 μg/mL at 13–14 wk	1–4 g/L
	0.2–3.0 μg/mL at term	0.02–0.03 g/L at term
Acetylcholinesterase	Absent	
Bilirubin	<0.075 mg/dL early in pregnancy	1.28 μmol/L
	<0.025 mg/dL at term	<0.43 μmol/L
L:S ratio	<1.6:1 before 35 wk	
	>2.0:1 at term	
Phosphatidylglycerol (PG)	Present at approximately 36 wk	
Phosphatidylinositol (PI)	Peak amounts present 5 wk before term, followed by a decline	
Shake test	Positive	
Creatinine	1.8–4.0 mg/dL at term	159–354 μmol/L

Interfering Factors

➤ Failure to promptly deliver samples for chromosomal analysis to the laboratory performing the test or improper incubation of the sample, or both, such that cells do not remain alive, make karyotyping impossible to perform. Sample should also be protected from light.

➤ AFP and acetylcholinesterase may be falsely elevated if the sample is contaminated with fetal blood.

➤ Bilirubin may be falsely elevated if maternal hemoglobin, methemalbumin, or meconium are present in the sample. Fetal acidosis may also lead to falsely elevated bilirubin levels.

➤ Bilirubin may be falsely decreased if the sample is exposed to light or if amniotic fluid volume is excessive.

➤ Contamination of the sample with blood or meconium may yield inaccurate L:S ratios.

Indications for Amniotic Fluid Tests

➤ Familial or parental history of genetic disorders such as Tay-Sachs disease, mental retardation, chromosome or enzyme anomalies, or inherited hemoglobinopathies

➤ Advanced maternal age (Chromosomal analysis is routine in mothers aged 35 or older.)

➤ Prenatal gender determination when the mother is a known carrier of a sex-linked abnormal gene that could be transmitted to male offspring

➤ In utero diagnosis of metabolic disorders such as cystic fibrosis, diabetes mellitus, or other errors of lipid, carbohydrate, or amino acid metabolism

➤ Suspected neural tube defect as indicated by elevated AFP and acetylcholinesterase levels

➤ Known or suspected hemolytic disease involving the fetus as indicated by rising bilirubin levels, especially after the 30th week of gestation

➤ Determination of fetal maturity when preterm delivery is being considered, with fetal maturity indicated by L:S ratio of 2:1 or greater, presence of PG, positive shake test, creatinine greater than 2.0 mg/dL, and bilirubin less than 0.025 mg/dL (nonisoimmunized mother)

Contraindications

➤ History of premature labor or incompetent cervix
➤ Presence of placenta previa or abruptio placentae

Nursing Care Before the Procedure

Explain to the client:
➤ That the procedure will be performed by a physician and requires 20 to 30 minutes
➤ The precautions taken to avoid injury to the fetus (i.e., careful palpation, localization of the fetus and placenta by ultrasound, and use of strict aseptic technique)
➤ The positioning used for the procedure and the necessity of remaining still while it is taking place
➤ That the skin will be injected with a local anesthetic at the needle insertion site and that this injection may cause a stinging sensation
➤ That a sensation of pressure may be felt when the needle is inserted for the amniotic fluid sample
➤ How to use focusing and controlled breathing for relaxation during the procedure
➤ That slight cramping may occur after the procedure
➤ That, if the test is being conducted for chromosomal studies, it may be 2 to 4 weeks before results are available

Prepare for the procedure:
➤ If an ultrasound is to be performed immediately before the amniocentesis to localize the fetus and placenta, hydrate the client to ensure a full bladder.
➤ After the ultrasound, have the client empty the bladder to prevent perforation during the amniocentesis. (The most common nonamniotic fluid obtained during the procedure is maternal urine.[30])
➤ Provide a hospital gown.
➤ Record maternal vital signs and fetal heart rate.

The Procedure (Amniocentesis)

The necessary equipment is assembled, including an amniocentesis tray with solution for skin preparation, local anesthetic, 10- or 20-mL syringe, needles of various sizes (including a 22-gauge, 5-inch spinal needle), sterile drapes, and sterile gloves. Special specimen collection tubes (either brown or foil-covered) also are needed.

The client is assisted to a supine position. The head or legs may be raised slightly to promote client comfort and to relax abdominal muscles. If the uterus is large, a pillow or rolled blanket is placed under the client's right side to prevent hypotension resulting from great vessel compression.

The skin of the lower abdomen is prepared with an antiseptic solution and protected with sterile drapes. The local anesthetic is injected. A 5-inch, 22-gauge spinal needle is inserted, usually at the midline, through the abdominal and uterine walls. The stylet is withdrawn and a plastic syringe of sufficient volume for the sample to be obtained is attached. A sample of at least 10 mL of amniotic fluid is withdrawn and placed in appropriate containers.

When the desired amount of fluid has been removed, the needle is withdrawn and slight pressure applied to the site. If there is no evidence of bleeding or other drainage, a sterile adhesive bandage is applied to the site. The specimens should be sent to the laboratory immediately.

Nursing Care After the Procedure

Care and assessment after the procedure include assisting the client to a position of comfort.

➤ If the client is Rh-negative, administer Rh_o (D) immune globulin (RhoGAM) intramuscularly (IM) to prevent potential sensitization to fetal blood.

➤ Remind the client to report fever, leaking amniotic fluid, vaginal bleeding, or uterine contractions to her physician.

➤ Changes in fetal activity — either an increase or a decrease — should also be reported.

➤ Take and record maternal vital signs and fetal heart sounds every 15 minutes for ½ to 1 hour.

➤ Assess the client for contractions, pain, and vaginal bleeding each time vital signs are checked.

➤ Observe the puncture site for bleeding or other drainage.

➤ Notify the physician if client experiences abdominal pain, fever, chills, vaginal bleeding, or change in fetal activity.

➤ Provide support when diagnostic findings are revealed, especially if fetal abnormality is determined.

➤ If appropriate and timely, offer information about genetic counseling or pregnancy termination counseling, or both.

Student Name _____ Class _____

Instructor _____ Date _____

CASE STUDY AND CRITICAL THINKING EXERCISE

Ms. Brown is para 2 gravida 1 and is Rh-negative. Her first child was Rh-positive. She is at 30 weeks of gestation. At her clinic appointment, a routine amniocentesis was performed, which revealed the following: Color amber, Chromosome analysis normal, Bilirubin 0.950 mg/dL.

a. What is the probable diagnosis?

b. If Ms. Brown was given RhoGAM at her first delivery, how could this problem have developed?

c. What are some possible treatment options?

References

1. Moore, ML: Realities in Childbearing, ed 2. WB Saunders, Philadelphia, 1983, p 762.
2. Wenk, RE, and Rosenbaum, JM: Analyses of amniotic fluid. In Henry, JB: Clinical Diagnosis and Management by Laboratory Methods, ed 18. WB Saunders, Philadelphia, 1991, p 482.
3. Strasinger, SK: Urinalysis and Body Fluids, ed 3. FA Davis, Philadelphia, 1994, p 175.
4. Wenk and Rosenbaum, op cit, p 482.
5. Sacher, RA, and McPherson, RA: Widmann's Clinical Interpretation of Laboratory Tests, ed 10. FA Davis, Philadelphia, 1991, p 644.
6. Ibid, p 643.
7. Strasinger, op cit, p 176.
8. Wenk and Rosenbaum, op cit, pp 483–484.
9. Sacher and McPherson, op cit, p 650.
10. Wenk and Rosenbaum, op cit, p 484.
11. Ibid, p 485.
12. Ibid, p 485.
13. Ibid, p 485.
14. Strasinger, op cit, p 177.
15. Wenk and Rosenbaum, op cit, pp 488–489.
16. Fischbach, FT: A Manual of Laboratory Diagnostic Tests, ed. 4. JB Lippincott, Philadelphia, 1992, p 946.
17. Wenk and Rosenbaum, op cit, p 490.
18. Strasinger, op cit, p 177.
19. Wenk and Rosenbaum, op cit, p 490.
20. Ibid, pp 490–492.
21. Ibid, p 492.
22. Strasinger, op cit, pp 177–178.
23. Wenk and Rosenbaum, op cit, p 491.
24. Moore, op cit, p 430.
25. Strasinger, op cit, p 178.
26. Moore, op cit, p 430.
27. Pagana, KD, and Pagana, TJ: Diagnostic Testing and Nursing Implications: A Case Study Approach, ed 2. CV Mosby, St Louis, 1986, p 175.
28. Moore, op cit, p 430.
29. Ibid, p 430.
30. Wenk and Rosenbaum, op cit, p 489.

Bibliography

Byrne, CJ, et al: Laboratory Tests: Implications for Nursing Care, ed 2. Addison-Wesley, Menlo Park, Calif, 1986.

Callen, PW (ed): Ultrasonography in Obstetrics and Gynecology, ed 3. WB Saunders, Philadelphia, 1993.

Chernecky, CC, and Berger, BJ; Cullen, BN (ed): Laboratory Tests and Diagnostic Procedures, ed 2. WB Saunders, Philadelphia, 1996.

Corbett, JV: Laboratory Tests and Diagnostic Procedures with Nursing Diagnoses, ed 4. Appleton & Lange, Norwalk, Conn, 1995.

Kee, JL: Handbook of Laboratory and Diagnostic Tests with Nursing Implications, ed 3. Appleton & Lange, Norwalk, Conn, 1997.

Krieg, AF, and Wenk, RE: Pregnancy tests and evaluation of placental function. In Henry, JB: Clinical Diagnosis and Management by Laboratory Methods, ed 17. WB Saunders, Philadelphia, 1984.

Ladewig, PA, et al: Essentials of Maternal-Newborn Nursing, ed 3. Benjamin-Cummings, Menlo Park, Calif, 1994.

Pagana, KD, and Pagana, TJ: Diagnostic and Laboratory Test Reference, ed 3. Mosby–Year Book, St Louis, 1996.

Springhouse Corporation: Clinical Laboratory Tests: Values and Implications, ed 2. Springhouse, Springhouse, Pa, 1995.

Springhouse Corporation: Nurse's Reference Library: Diagnostics, ed 2. Springhouse Corporation, Springhouse, Pa, 1986.

Tietz, NW (ed): Clinical Guide to Laboratory Tests, ed 3. WB Saunders, Philadelphia, 1997.

Whaley, LF: Nursing Care of Infants and Children, ed 4. Mosby–Year Book, St Louis, 1991.

11

Semen Analysis

➤ **TESTS COVERED**
Tests for Fertility, *437*
Tests for the Presence of Semen, *439*

OVERVIEW OF SEMEN FORMATION AND ANALYSIS

Semen is a fluid that consists of sperm suspended in seminal plasma. It is composed of four main fractions that are contributed by (1) the testis and epididymis, (2) the seminal vesicle, (3) the prostate gland, and (4) the bulbourethral and urethral glands (Fig. 11-1). Sperm, which are less than 5 percent of the volume of semen, are produced in the testis and mature in the epididymis. It is thought that the epididymis secretes a number of proteins that are essential to the fertilizing capability of sperm. Most mature sperm are stored in the vas deferens until released by emission and ejaculation. While in the vas deferens, sperm are relatively inactive because of the diminished oxygen supply and acid environments; they can, however, survive for up to 1 month in this location.[1,2]

The seminal vesicles, which contribute approximately 60 percent to the volume of semen, are attached to the vas deferens near the base of the urinary bladder. They secrete a viscous, slightly alkaline fluid with high levels of fructose, flavin, potassium, and citric acid. Fructose provides the major nutrient for sperm after emission. (Sperm may survive in the vagina for more than 72 hours after sexual intercourse.[3]) Flavin is responsible for the fluorescence of semen in ultraviolet light, thus allowing detection of semen on clothing or other fabrics in rape cases. The significance of the high potassium and citric acid levels in seminal fluid has not yet been established. The fluid secreted by the seminal vesicles also contains prostaglandins, which are thought to stimulate muscular contractions in female reproductive organs, and a fibrinogen-like substance that causes semen to coagulate after ejaculation.[4,5]

The prostate gland, which contributes about 20 percent to the volume of semen, secretes a milky fluid with a pH of 6.5, due largely to its high citric acid content. Prostatic fluid also is high in proteolytic enzymes and acid phosphatase. The proteolytic enzymes are believed to act upon seminal fluid, causing coagulation and, subsequently, liquefaction of the ejaculate.[6,7] The bulbourethral and urethral glands secrete a clear, mucus-like fluid that cleanses the urethra and lubricates the end of the penis in preparation for intercourse. This fluid contributes less than 10 to 15 percent to the volume of semen.[8,9]

When ejaculation occurs, the components of semen enter the urethra individually but in rapid succession. Secretion from the bulbourethral and urethral

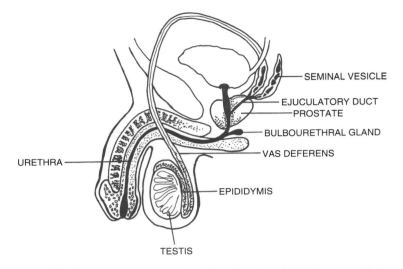

Figure 11–1 Diagram of male genitalia. (From Strasinger, SK: Urinalysis and Body Fluids, ed 3. FA Davis, Philadelphia, 1994, p. 160, with permission.)

glands occurs first, followed by prostatic secretion and most of the sperm. Note that the first two components contribute only about 40 percent of the total ejaculate. Finally, the seminal vesicles empty, contributing the bulk of the fluid. The sequence in which these fluids appear is an important consideration in the method of specimen collection for semen analysis. If, for example, coitus interruptus is practiced, it is possible that the sperm-rich portion will be missed and that the sample will consist primarily of fluid from the seminal vesicles.[10]

Freshly ejaculated semen is viscous, opaque, and white or grayish white. It coagulates almost immediately but within 10 to 30 minutes liquefies to become a translucent fluid that pours in droplets and does not appear clumped or stringy. The pH of semen is slightly alkaline (average 7.7). A pH of less than 7.0 is indicative of a sample consisting mainly of prostatic secretions and may indicate congenital aplasia of the seminal vesicles. Increased turbidity after liquefaction may indicate the presence of leukocytes and inflammation. Blood in the sample is abnormal. The usual volume of the ejaculate is 2 to 5 mL, although the amount may range from 0.7 to 6.5 mL and still be considered normal. Extending the time between ejaculations does not lead to an increase in volume. Increased volumes of sperm-poor semen are associated with male infertility, whereas greatly decreased volumes may impair penetration of the cervical mucus by those sperm present.[11,12]

Semen is examined in the laboratory for four main reasons: (1) to investigate infertility, (2) to evaluate the effectiveness of vasectomy, (3) to support or disprove sterility in a paternity suit, and (4) to investigate alleged or suspected rape. For fertility studies, the optimal method of obtaining a specimen is masturbation, with collection of the ejaculate in a clean glass or plastic container. Other approaches include obtaining the specimen by coitus interruptus and collection of the sample by using a condom. The problems associated with collecting the specimen by coitus interruptus have been noted previously. The use of condoms presents problems because many of them contain spermicides. If used, the condom should be thoroughly washed and dried first.

When rape is alleged or suspected, the specimen may be swabbed from the vagina with a Papanicolaou stick or cotton-tipped applicator or may be obtained by aspiration with a bulb syringe to which a rubber catheter is attached, or with saline lavage. Samples of dried semen on the skin may be obtained by sponging the site with saline-moistened gauze. Sections of clothing and other fabric samples containing semen may be soaked in saline for 1 hour. The resulting solution is then subjected to semen analysis.[13,14]

TESTS OF SEMEN

Tests of semen are discussed in relation to those used to determine fertility and those used when rape is suspected.

TESTS FOR FERTILITY

In addition to examining the sample for appearance, viscosity, and pH (see p. 436), fertility tests include assessment of sperm count, sperm motility, and sperm morphology. Other tests include determination of the viability of sperm, presence of fructose in the sample, presence of antibodies to sperm, and ability of sperm to penetrate the cervical mucus after coitus.

The sperm count is performed in a manner similar to that used for blood counts. With the liquefied specimen diluted to immobilize the sperm, the number of sperm in a given microscopic area is counted and the result multiplied by a factor of either 100,000 or 1 million to obtain the sperm count. The normal sperm count ranges from 40 to 160 million per mL, with counts of 20 to 40 million per mL considered borderline normal. For postvasectomy tests, only the sperm count is necessary. It should eventually be negative for sperm on two consecutive monthly examinations.

Because sperm must migrate through the cervical mucus and the fallopian tubes, sperm motility is a key indicator of fertility. For this test, the motility of at least 200 sperm is examined microscopically. The percentage of sperm showing progressive forward motion is recorded and should normally be greater than 60 percent within 3 hours of collecting the sample. Those sperm showing progressive motility may also be graded according to the quality of the movement observed (Table 11–1).[15]

Table 11–1 ➤ GRADES OF SPERM MOTILIITY	
Grade I	Minimal forward progression
Grade II	Poor to fair activity
Grade III	Good activity with tail movements
Grade IV	Full activity with tail movements difficult to visualize

Note: From Cannon, DC: Seminal fluid. In Henry, JB: Clinical Diagnosis and Management by Laboratory Methods, ed 18. WB Saunders, Philadelphia, 1990, p 518, with permission.

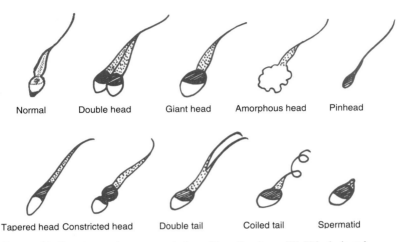

Normal   Double head   Giant head   Amorphous head   Pinhead

Tapered head Constricted head   Double tail   Coiled tail   Spermatid

Figure 11–2   Abnormal sperm morphology. (From Strasinger, SK: Urinalysis and Body Fluids, ed 3. FA Davis, Philadelphia, 1994, p. 164, with permission.)

Sperm morphology involves microscopic examination of sperm to detect abnormal forms and shapes that may render the sperm incapable of fertilization. The appearance of both the head and the tail of a minimum of 200 sperm is evaluated. Normally, the sperm has an oval head, which measures about 3×5 μm, and a long, tapering tail.[16] Abnormal head structures (Fig. 11–2) are associated with failure to penetrate the ovum. Abnormal tail structures are associated with poor sperm motility. The finding of numerous immature sperm (spermatids) is also considered abnormal because sperm usually mature in the epididymis. In a normal specimen, fewer than 30 percent abnormal sperm will be found.[17]

If abnormalities in sperm count, motility, or morphology are detected, additional tests may be performed. Tests for sperm viability are indicated when the sperm count is normal but motility markedly decreased. Sperm viability is tested by staining the sample such that dead and living sperm appear different on microscopic examination.[18] If the sperm count is low, the sample may be examined for the presence of fructose. As noted previously (p. 435), the fluid secreted by the seminal vesicles is high in fructose, a major nutrient for sperm. Thus, presence of fructose in the sample indicates that adequate support medium is available for the sperm and also that the ejaculatory ducts are patent.[19,20]

Both men and women may produce antibodies to sperm. Male antibodies are suspected when semen analysis shows decreased sperm motility with clumping. Female antibodies are suspected when semen analysis is normal and assessment of the woman reveals no cause for continuing infertility. The test is performed by mixing sperm with serum from either the man or the woman and then observing for agglutination or immobilization of the sperm. The quantity of antibodies present may be determined through radioimmunoassay techniques.[21]

Postcoital tests of semen are performed to determine both the quality of cervical mucus and the ability of sperm to penetrate the cervical mucus and still remain active. The test, known as Sims-Huhner, is performed during the ovulatory phase of the menstrual cycle, within 6 to 8 hours of coitus. Normally, at least 10 motile sperm should be present per high-power microscopic field. During the ovulatory phase, cervical mucus should be clear and somewhat watery with a spinnbarkeit of 10 cm. A spinnbarkeit is a measure of tenacity of the cervical mucus and is determined by grasping a portion of the cervical mucus with a forceps and seeing how far it can be drawn before breaking.[22,23]

The sperm penetration assay (SPA) assesses the qualitative aspects of sperm function. Oocytes from an animal such as a hamster are used to determine the ability of the sperm to penetrate the egg for possible in vitro fertilization of a human egg.[24]

TESTS FOR THE PRESENCE OF SEMEN

Tests for the presence of semen are performed when rape is alleged or suspected. These tests include examination for sperm, determination of acid phosphatase, and detection of blood group substances.

As noted previously (p. 435), the flavin content of semen is responsible for the fluorescence of semen in ultraviolet light. Thus, a preliminary scan of the victim's clothing may help in identifying specific areas that may yield samples for analysis. The presence of sperm in samples obtained from clothing as well as in vaginal secretions may be detected with various staining techniques and microscopic examination. It should be noted, however, that sperm will not be detected if the man has had a vasectomy or is sterile for some other reason.

A more sensitive test to ascertain the presence of semen is the acid phosphatase test, because semen is the only body fluid high in this substance. The acid phosphatase test specifically indicates the presence of prostatic fluid and does not depend on the presence of sperm for a positive result. Vaginal samples as well as clothing stains may be examined. It has been found that acid phosphatase can be detected in semen stains that are several months old.[25]

If the presence of semen is positively determined, testing for the presence of A, B, or H blood group substances may be used to ascertain whether the semen sample is of the same of a different blood group as that of the suspect. Inheritance of the H gene is necessary for the normal expression of the ABO genes and the subsequent development of A, B, and H antigens and related blood groups. The H gene is found in more than 99 percent of the population. Inheritance of the A gene leads to conversion of nearly all the H antigen on the red blood cell surface to A antigen sites. Similarly, inheritance of the B gene leads to conversion of H antigen to B antigen sites. When both the A and B genes are inherited, somewhat more H antigen sites are changed to B than to A. Inheritance of the O gene does not produce such changes in the H structure. Thus, blood group O has the highest level of H antigen. In addition to their presence on red blood cells, A, B, and H antigens may be found on white blood cells and platelets, and in all body secretions—including semen—in 80 percent of the population.[26,27]

Reference Values

pH	>7.0 (average 7.7)
Volume	0.7–6.5 mL/ejaculate (usually 1.5–5 mL)
Sperm count	40–160 million/mL (20–40 million/mL = borderline normal)
Sperm motility	>60% within 3 hr of specimen collection
	Quality greater than grade II (see Table 11–1, p. 437)
Sperm morphology	<30% abnormal sperm
Fructose	Present and/or >150 mg/dL
Sperm antibodies	Negative for male and female antibodies
Postcoital test	At least 10 motile sperm per high-power microscopic field within 6 to 8 hr of coitus
Acid phosphatase	2500 King-Armstrong U/mL (average)
	SI units: 42μkat/L
	Prostatic-enzymatic (SI units): 0.0–1.0 U/L
	Prostatic-immunologic (SI units): 0.0–3.0 μg/L

Interfering Factors

➤ Improper specimen collection (e.g., use of condoms containing spermicide, loss of sperm-rich portion of the sample through use of coitus interruptus)
➤ Failure to deliver the ejaculated sample to the laboratory within 1 hour
➤ Failure to maintain the ejaculated specimen at body temperature until liquefaction occurs (20 to 60 minutes)

Indications for Semen Analysis

➤ Investigate infertility
➤ Evaluate the effectiveness of vasectomy as indicated by two sperm-free samples collected 1 month apart
➤ Support or disprove sterility in a paternity suit
➤ Investigate alleged or suspected rape

Nursing Care Before the Procedure

Male Clients

Explain to the client:
➤ The various procedures that may be used to obtain the sample
➤ The desirability of abstaining from sexual activity for approximately 3 days before sample collection, to promote the highest sperm count
➤ The importance of transporting the sample promptly to the laboratory, while maintaining it at body temperature, if the sample is collected at home

Prepare for the procedure:
➤ Provide appropriate specimen collection containers.

Female Clients

Explain to the client:
➤ That samples will be collected through vaginal examination
➤ That the use of lubricant during intercourse and of douching after intercourse should be avoided
➤ The positioning on the pelvic examination table

➤ That, if saline lavage is used to collect the sample, the client may experience a sensation of coldness

Prepare for the procedure:

➤ The rape victim may need additional support to cope with undergoing a vaginal examination.

➤ Assist the client in donning an examination gown. If rape is suspected, handle the client's clothes carefully because additional specimens may be obtained from them.

➤ Advise the client to void before the procedure. Rape victims should not wipe after voiding, so as not to remove possible semen.

The Procedure

Ejaculated Sample. The ideal sample is obtained in the laboratory by masturbation and is collected in a glass or plastic specimen container. If the sample is collected at home by masturbation, it must be transported to the laboratory within 1 hour of collection and must be maintained at body temperature.

If the client is unable to produce the specimen by masturbation for either religious or psychological reasons, the specimen may be obtained during the sexual act through the use of condoms or coitus interruptus. If a condom is used, it must be washed and dried thoroughly before use to rid it of possible spermicides. If coitus interruptus is used, the client must be informed of the potential for loss of the sperm-rich portion of the sample (see p. 440).

If none of the aforementioned approaches is acceptable to the client, a final alternative is to obtain postcoital samples from the cervical canal and vagina of his partner.

Cervical/Vaginal Samples. The necessary equipment is assembled, including vaginal speculums, Papanicolaou sticks, cotton-tipped applicators, gloves, saline and syringes for lavage (if necessary), slides, and small jars containing 95 percent ethanol.

The client is assisted to the lithotomy position on the pelvic examination table. A vaginal speculum is inserted and the specimen obtained by direct smear, aspiration, or saline lavage. The specimens are labeled and sent immediately to the laboratory.

Samples from Skin and Clothing. Samples of dried semen on the skin may be obtained by sponging the site with saline-moistened gauze. Sections of clothing and other fabric samples containing semen may be soaked in saline for 1 hour. The resulting solution is then subjected to semen analysis.

Nursing Care After the Procedure

There is no specific aftercare unless postejaculatory or postcoital cleansing is desired.

➤ Administer a spermicidal douche in addition to the prescribed medication for prevention of pregnancy.

➤ A supportive, nonjudgmental attitude can assist a client through the experience of evaluation of infertility or sexual function.

➤ *Grieving, loss of desired child:* Offer counseling for dealing with infertility. Assist client in developing coping strategies for feelings of inadequacy. Anticipate client's need to resolve grief and express feelings. Offer information about support groups and alternatives that can be explored.

(Case Study follows on page 443)

Student Name _____ Class _____

Instructor _____ Date _____

CASE STUDY AND CRITICAL THINKING EXERCISES

Jim, age 27, and Mary, age 26, have been married for 2 years and have been trying to conceive a child. The couple is being evaluated for infertility. The following are results of Jim's semen analysis: pH 7.5, Volume 0.4 ml, Sperm count 40 million/mL, Sperm motility 30% within 2 hours of specimen collection, Quality grade 2, Morphology 20% abnormal, Negative for antibodies, Fructose 160 mg/dL.

a. What is likely to be Jim's problem?

b. Jim has also complained of headaches the past 6 months that are progressively worsening. An MRI reveals a pituitary tumor. How is a pituitary tumor related to Jim's problem with infertility?

c. What is the probable prognosis for Jim?

References

1. Cannon, DC: Seminal fluid. In Henry, JB: Clinical Diagnosis and Management by Laboratory Methods, ed 18. WB Sanders, Philadelphia, 1991, pp 497–498.
2. Strasinger, SK: Urinalysis and Body Fluids, ed 3. FA Davis, Philadelphia, 1994, p 161.
3. Springhouse Corporation: Nurse's Reference Library: Diagnostics, ed 2. Springhouse, Springhouse, Pa, 1986, p 701.
4. Cannon, op cit, pp 497–498.
5. Hole, JW: Human Anatomy and Physiology, ed 4. Wm C Brown, Dubuque, Iowa, 1987, p 815.
6. Strasinger, op cit, p 161.
7. Cannon, op cit, p 498.
8. Hole, op cit, p 815.
9. Cannon, op cit, p 498.
10. Ibid, p 498.
11. Ibid, pp 498–499.
12. Strasinger, op cit, p 162.
13. Nurse's Reference Library, op cit, p 701.
14. Cannon, op cit, p 502.
15. Ibid, pp 499–500.
16. Strasinger, op cit, p 164.
17. Ibid, pp 164–165.
18. Ibid, p 165.
19. Ibid, p 165.
20. Sacher, RA, and McPherson, RA: Widmann's Clinical Interpretation of Laboratory Tests, ed 10. FA Davis, Philadelphia, 1991, p 629.
21. Strasinger, op cit, p 165.
22. Cannon, op cit, p 501.
23. Nurse's Reference Laboratory, op cit, pp 700, 703.
24. Sacher and McPherson, op cit, p 630.
25. Cannon, op cit, p 502.
26. Ibid, p 502.
27. Pittiglio, DH: Modern Blood Banking and Transfusion Practices. FA Davis, Philadelphia, 1983, pp 94–96.

Bibliography

Byrne, CJ, et al: Laboratory Tests: Implications for Nursing Care, ed 2. Addison-Wesley, Menlo Park, Calif, 1986.

Chernecky, CC, and Berger, BJ; Cullen, BN (ed): Laboratory Tests and Diagnostic Procedures, ed 2. WB Saunders, Philadelphia, 1996.

Corbett, JV: Laboratory Tests and Diagnostic Procedures with Nursing Diagnoses, ed 4. Appleton & Lange, Norwalk, Conn, 1995.

Fischbach, FT: A Manual of Laboratory and Diagnostic Tests, ed 5. Lippincott-Raven, Philadelphia, 1995.

Kee, JL: Handbook of Laboratory and Diagnostic Tests with Nursing Implications, ed 3. Appleton & Lange, Norwalk, Conn, 1997.

Lewis, SM, et al (eds): Medical-Surgical Nursing: Assessment and Management of Clinical Problems, ed 4. Mosby–Year Book, St Louis, 1995.

Overstreet, J: Male infertility. In Infertility and Reproductive Medicine Clinics of North America, April 1992.

Pagana, KD, and Pagana, TJ: Diagnostic and Laboratory Test Reference, ed 3. Mosby–Year Book, St Louis, 1996.

Porth, C: Pathophysiology: Concepts of Altered Health States, ed 4. JB Lippincott, Philadelphia, 1993.

Tietz, NW (ed): Clinical Guide to Laboratory Tests, ed 3. WB Saunders, Philadelphia, 1997.

Wallach, J: Interpretation of Diagnostic Tests: A Handbook Synopsis of Laboratory Medicine, ed 6. Little, Brown & Co, Boston, 1996.

12

Analysis of Gastric and Duodenal Secretions

➤ TESTS COVERED
Analysis of Gastric Contents, *447*
Tests of Gastric Acidity, *450*

Analysis of Duodenal Contents, *454*
Duodenal Stimulation Tests, *457*

OVERVIEW OF GASTRIC AND DUODENAL SECRETIONS

The stomach secretes 1500 to 3000 mL of gastric juice each day in response to ingestion of food; the sight, smell, or thought of food; and excessive stress, alcohol, and caffeine. Normally, stomach secretions aid in preparing ingested food for absorption in the small intestine, initiate the digestion of proteins, and promote absorption of vitamin B_{12}.

The chief cells of the stomach secrete digestive enzymes. The major enzyme secreted is pepsinogen, which is converted to pepsin in the presence of hydrochloric acid. Hydrochloric acid is secreted by the parietal cells of the stomach in a highly concentrated form with a pH of approximately 0.8. Pepsin, which functions in the initial digestion of proteins, is most active in an acidic environment. It functions optimally at a pH of 2.0 and a pH of not greater than 5.0.[1] In addition to hydrochloric acid, the parietal cells secrete intrinsic factor, which aids in the absorption of vitamin B_{12}. The goblet cells and mucous glands of the stomach secrete a viscous alkaline material that protects the stomach lining from damage by the acidic gastric juices.[2] Gastric juices also contain other substances such as electrolytes (sodium, potassium, chloride, and bicarbonate) and other enzymes such as gastric lipase, urease, lysozyme, and carbonic anhydrase.[3]

Gastric juices are produced continuously, although amounts vary in relation to food intake and other factors that stimulate or inhibit gastric secretion. The production of gastric juices is normally lowest early in the morning. Gastric secretion is mediated by the autonomic nervous system via the vagus nerve. When an individual ingests food—or thinks of, sees, or smells food—parasympathetic impulses travel via the vagus nerve to the stomach and stimulate the G cells of the stomach to secrete the hormone gastrin. Gastrin then stimulates the various cells in the stomach to increase their secretions.[4] In addition to distention of the stomach with food, exposure of the gastric mucosa to substances called secretagogues also stimulates the secretion of gastrin. Examples of such substances are alcohol, caffeine, meat extracts, and spices.

Because parasympathetic impulses increase gastric secretions, sympathetic nervous system activity inhibits them. Gastric secretion, for example, is inhibited when food enters the small intestine. This inhibition is thought to be caused by sympathetic impulses that are triggered when acidic gastric contents come into contact with the upper part of the small intestine. These sympathetic impulses ultimately inhibit those of the vagus nerve. Hormones secreted by the small intestine also inhibit gastric secretion. These include enterogastrone, secretin, and cholecystokinin-pancreozymin (CCK-PZ).

In addition to the normal neural and humoral mechanisms involved in gastric secretion, numerous other substances, including many drugs, may stimulate or inhibit gastric secretion. Substances that stimulate gastric secretion include histamine, nicotine, adrenocorticotropic steroids, insulin, and parasympathetic agents such as acetylcholine, reserpine, and pilocarpine. Substances that inhibit gastric secretion include belladonna alkaloids (e.g., atropine), anticholinergic drugs (e.g., propantheline bromide [Probanthine]), and histamine receptor antagonists (e.g., cimetidine, ranitidine). Aspirin causes changes in the gastric mucosa and decreases the secretion of mucus by the stomach, resulting in insufficient protection of the stomach lining from gastric juices.[5]

In the small intestine, digestion and absorption of nutrients are completed. This process is accomplished by a combination of intestinal juices, pancreatic juices, and bile. As with the stomach, intestinal secretions consist of enzymes, hormones, and mucus. Intestinal enzymes include peptidases, sucrase, maltase, lactase, intestinal lipase, intestinal amylase, and nucleases that break down ingested proteins, carbohydrates, and fats so that they may be absorbed from the small intestine into the blood. In addition, enterokinase is secreted. This enzyme activates trypsin, a peptidase secreted by the pancreas. Other pancreatic enzymes include chymotrypsin, carboxypeptidase, pancreatic amylase, pancreatic lipase, and nuclease.

Normally, 1200 to 1500 mL of duodenal juices are secreted each day. Digestive juices are clear, have a high bicarbonate content, and range in pH from 8.0 to 8.5. As noted previously, hormones secreted by the small intestine include secretin and CCK-PZ. When acidic gastric contents enter the duodenum, the resultant decrease in pH stimulates the mucosal cells of the small intestine to produce secretin. Secretin stimulates secretion of pancreatic juices that have a high bicarbonate content. CCK-PZ also stimulates the pancreas to release its juices, especially enzymes, although the source of the stimulation in this case is thought to be from the presence of polypeptides or fatty acids in the small intestine.[6]

Tests of gastric and intestinal secretions include analysis of contents and tests of normal function (e.g., tests that stimulate gastric and duodenal secretions). Most of these tests involve insertion of a nasogastric (NG) or intestinal tube and may be quite uncomfortable for the client. Newer nonlaboratory procedures are beginning to replace tests of gastric and intestinal secretions, as they are more accurate, less time-consuming, and less uncomfortable for the client because they do not require long-term tube insertion. These newer procedures include endoscopy; various radiologic techniques; measurement of hydrogen ion concentration (pH) via electrodes in the endoscopy tube; radioimmunoassay of serum gastrin levels; cytologic examination of gastric contents for malignant cells; and serum analysis of intrinsic factor, anti-intrinsic factor antibodies, and antiparietal cell antibodies.[7,8] Many of these tests are not widely used at this time; only those tests in more common use are discussed in this chapter.

TESTS OF GASTRIC SECRETIONS

ANALYSIS OF GASTRIC CONTENTS

Gastric fluid analysis has two major components: (1) macroscopic analysis and (2) microscopic analysis. Macroscopic analysis includes examination of the specimen for overall physical and chemical characteristics such as color, presence of mucus and blood, and pH determination. Microscopic analysis involves examination of the specimen for organisms such as bacteria and parasites. Cytologic examination for abnormal (i.e., malignant) exfoliated cells may also be undertaken, although special techniques must be used so that the cells are not destroyed before analysis.

Specimens for gastric analysis are normally collected in the morning after the client has been fasting for 12 hours. Approximately 20 to 100 mL of gastric fluid should be present in the stomach at that time. If digestion is normal and the client has observed fasting instructions, no food particles should be present.[9]

Macroscopic Analysis

Color. Gastric juice is normally a translucent, pale gray, slightly viscous fluid. If the gastric aspirate is yellow to green, the presence of bile is indicated. This finding may be a result of reflux of bile from excessive gagging when the NG tube was inserted for the test or it may indicate an obstruction in the small intestine distal to the ampulla of Vater, the site of bile secretion into the small intestine.[10] Pink, red, or brownish gastric secretions indicate the presence of blood (see further on).

Mucus. Mucus is normally present in gastric secretions and derives mainly from the mucus secreted by the gastric glands. The mucus content is responsible for the viscosity of gastric secretions. Saliva may also contribute to the mucus content, but it is frothy and tends to float on top of the sample. In tests of gastric secretions, clients are instructed to expectorate saliva during the test so as not to contaminate the sample. If mucus from the respiratory tract is present, it tends to be more tenacious than are gastric secretions and sometimes contains dust particles. Small amounts of mucus from duodenal reflux may also be present in the sample.[11]

Blood. Blood is not normally present in gastric secretions. Small particles or streaks of fresh blood may be present because of trauma during NG intubation. Larger amounts of blood or "coffee-ground" material indicates bleeding of a greater magnitude and is usually a result of some type of gastric lesion (e.g., ulcer, gastritis, carcinoma). Blood swallowed from the mouth, nasopharynx, or lungs may also be present in the sample. Regardless of whether overt blood appears in the sample, the specimen should always be tested for blood.[12]

pH. The pH of gastric secretions is usually less than 2.0 and is not normally greater than 6.0 if gastric secretion is normal. Lack of normal gastric acidity is seen in pernicious anemia; gastric carcinoma; aplastic or hypochromic anemia;

and immune-related disorders of the thyroid, stomach, and connective tissue. Elevated pH in gastric juice also supports ruling out peptic ulcer disease as a diagnosis.[13] In addition to peptic ulcer disease, low pH levels are seen in Zollinger-Ellison syndrome (non–beta-cell adenomas of the pancreas that produce excessive gastrin).

Microscopic Analysis

Red Blood Cells. As noted earlier, the presence of a few red blood cells may be a result of the trauma of gastric intubation. Larger numbers, however, may indicate serious disorders and require additional diagnostic follow-up.

White Blood Cells. Normally, a few white blood cells are present in gastric juices. Elevated numbers may indicate inflammation of the gastric mucosa, mouth, paranasal sinuses, or respiratory tract. White blood cells found in gastric aspirates may also be present because of inflammation of the duodenum, pancreas, or biliary tract, although it is a less common finding.[14]

Epithelial Cells. A few epithelial cells are normally present because of sloughing from mucosal surfaces. The presence of clumps of cells may be caused by dislodgment during intubation. Gastritis may also lead to the finding of increased epithelial cells in gastric fluid.

Bacteria and Yeasts. Because of the highly acidic environment of the stomach, bacteria are not normally found in gastric contents. In most cases, those bacteria (and yeasts) that are cultured from gastric fluid are normal flora of the mouth or respiratory tract. Increased numbers of bacteria may be found in gastric contents that have an abnormally high pH. Excessive numbers of yeasts are associated with retention of gastric contents because of some type of blockage (e.g., pyloric obstruction).[15] Cultures for *Mycobacterium tuberculosis* are made in individuals who are suspected of having pulmonary tuberculosis but who are unable to expectorate sputum effectively for analysis. Gastric samples for cytology are best collected through procedures designed to cause cells to exfoliate (i.e., exfoliative cytology). In addition to gastric aspiration, samples may be obtained by gastroscopy and use of balloons and brushes. The best method is said to be gastric lavage with a solution containing chymotrypsin.[16]

Parasites. Parasites may be found in gastric fluid, mainly resulting from reflux of duodenal contents. Such parasites include *Giardia lamblia,* trophozoites or cysts, *Strongyloides* larvae, and hookworm ova.

Reference Values

Macroscopic Analysis	
Volume (fasting)	20–100 mL
Color	Pale gray, translucent
Mucus	Present such that the sample is slightly viscous
Blood	Negative
pH	<2.0 **(never >6.0)**
Microscopic Analysis	
Red blood cells	Negative to a few
White blood cells	Negative to a few

Epithelial cells	Few
Bacteria	Absent to few
Yeasts	Absent to few
Parasites	Absent
Abnormal cells	Absent

Interfering Factors

➤ Failure to follow dietary restrictions so that food particles are present
➤ Exposure to the sight, smell, or thought of food immediately before the test
➤ Ingestion of drugs that may alter gastric secretions (e.g., alcohol, histamine, nicotine, adrenocorticotropic steroids, insulin, parasympathetic agents, belladonna alkaloids, anticholinergic drugs, histamine receptor antagonists, aspirin)
➤ Contamination of the sample with saliva and respiratory secretions, which should be expectorated rather than swallowed during the procedure
➤ Failure to send the samples to the laboratory promptly for analysis of cells, which may disintegrate in gastric juices

Indications for Analysis of Gastric Contents

➤ Suspected peptic ulcer disease, as indicated by low to normal pH and (possibly) the presence of blood
➤ Suspected Zollinger-Ellison syndrome, as indicated by low to normal pH
➤ Suspected gastric carcinoma, as indicated by lack of normal gastric acidity, blood (possibly), and abnormal cells on cytologic examination
➤ Suspected pernicious anemia as indicated by lack of normal gastric acidity
➤ Suspected pulmonary tuberculosis, as indicated by positive cultures for *M. tuberculosis*
➤ Suspected parasitic infestation of the gastrointestinal tract

Nursing Care Before the Procedure

Explain to the client:
➤ The purpose of the test (*Note:* Gastric analysis is often performed as a component of specific tests for gastric acidity.)
➤ That fasting for 12 hours before the test is necessary, although water may be permitted up to 8 hours before the test
➤ That smoking is not permitted for 8 hours before the test
➤ That certain medications may be withheld, upon the physician's order, for up to 24 hours before the test
➤ That a stomach tube will be passed through the nose or mouth into the stomach
➤ That the client will be asked to swallow periodically when the tube is passed, as swallowing facilitates tube passage
➤ That the tube may cause a sensation of burning or irritation as it is passed and that gagging may occur when the tubing touches the back of the throat
➤ That saliva and respiratory secretions should be expectorated rather than swallowed during the test
➤ That a sample of stomach juices will be removed via the tube
➤ That the tube will be removed on completion of the test

Prepare for the procedure:
> Ensure to the extent possible that dietary, smoking, and medication restrictions are followed.
> Provide the client with a hospital gown.
> Ensure that an informed consent has been obtained and signed, if required.

The Procedure

The equipment needed is assembled, including an NG tube, lubricant, gloves, 50-mL syringe adapted for use with NG tube, saline, and specimen containers with appropriate labels. Tissues and an emesis basin also should be available for expectoration of secretions by the client.

With the client seated comfortably, the NG tube is passed into the stomach and the syringe is attached. All gastric contents are aspirated, placed in a container, and labeled. If a specimen for tubercle bacilli is to be obtained, gastric washings with saline may be performed to obtain the sample. This procedure is accomplished by irrigating the NG tube with saline and withdrawing the contents.

When all needed samples are obtained, the NG tube is removed. The samples should be sent to the laboratory immediately.

Nursing Care After the Procedure

Care and assessment after the test include assisting the client to a position of comfort. Provide mouth and nose care. Resume any foods and medications withheld for the test.
> Administer lozenges to alleviate sore throat caused by irritation by the tube.
> Assess the client's comfort level.
> Assess the client's ability to resume normal food and fluid intake.
> Assess for sore throat, abdominal pain, and nausea; administer gargle, lozenge, or ordered medication to control nausea or pain.

TESTS OF GASTRIC ACIDITY

Tests of gastric acidity are used to determine the presence and amount of hydrochloric acid in the stomach and to diagnose disorders associated with altered secretion of gastric acids. Three main types of tests are used to evaluate gastric acidity: (1) basal gastric acidity test, (2) gastric acid stimulation tests, and (3) tubeless gastric analysis test. The basal gastric acidity test usually is performed with tests of gastric acid stimulation.

Basal Gastric Acidity Test

This test is used to determine elevated gastric acidity, which is seen in Zollinger-Ellison syndrome and peptic ulcer disease. The sample is examined for volume, pH, and total acid secretion in each specimen as well as in the total sample. Total acid secretion is expressed as basal acid output (BAO) in milliequivalents per hour. The BAO is somewhat lower in elderly people and in women and varies directly with body weight.[17]

Gastric Acid Stimulation Tests

Gastric acid stimulation tests are performed to determine the response to substances that are administered to induce increased gastric acid secretion. Elevated acid output is associated with peptic ulcer disease and Zollinger-

Ellison syndrome. Decreased acid output is usually associated with pernicious anemia and gastric carcinoma; however, it may also be seen in a variety of other disorders, including hypochromic anemia, nutritional megaloblastic anemia, steatorrhea, rheumatoid arthritis, and myxedema.

Substances used to induce gastric secretion in these tests include histamine, betazole, and pentagastrin, with the latter being the drug of choice. Histamine is a substance that occurs naturally in the body and is implicated in various allergic and inflammatory responses. It also has the effect of stimulating gastric acid secretion. Unfortunately, when used for gastric acid stimulation tests, histamine produces numerous unpleasant side effects such as flushing, bradycardia, headache, nasal stuffiness, lacrimation, and alterations in blood pressure.[18] Betazole is an analogue of histamine that also produces increased gastric acid secretion but more slowly. It has minimal side effects but requires a longer testing period when used for gastric acid stimulation tests. Pentagastrin is a synthetic compound that induces gastric secretion as rapidly as histamine but without major side effects. For these reasons, it is the current drug of choice for gastric acid stimulation tests.

As with basal gastric acidity tests, samples obtained from gastric acid stimulation tests are examined for volume, pH, and amount of acid secreted. First, basal acid output (BAO) is determined. Maximum acid output (MAO) is also determined by adding the total milliequivalents of acid secreted in all samples after injection of the gastric acid stimulant.[19] Peak acid output (PAO) may also be determined by adding the greatest acid output in two consecutive 15-minute samples. Finally, BAO and MAO are compared as a ratio, which normally ranges from 0.3 to 0.6. That is, the maximum output should be 1½ to 3 times the basal output.[20]

Hollander Insulin Test. This test is used to evaluate the effectiveness of vagotomy (i.e., severing vagal nerve connections to the stomach) as a treatment for persistent peptic ulcer disease and involves stimulation of the vagus nerve through insulin-induced hypoglycemia. Hypoglycemia is normally a potent stimulator of gastric secretions and causes impulses to be transmitted via the vagus nerve. If the vagus nerve has been severed, however, the normal physiological response does not occur.

This test is not used very frequently, as it may be dangerous for the client (i.e., a blood sugar of less than 45 to 50 mg/dL is needed to provoke gastric secretion). In addition, data from the test do not always provide a clear distinction between normal and abnormal results; false-positive and false-negative results are common, and the results do not correlate strongly with recurrent ulcer disease.

Reference Values

Volume	20–100 mL (usually 30–60 mL)
Basal acid output (BAO)	2–6 mEq/hr (Values may be slightly lower in women and elderly persons; values vary directly with body weight.)
Maximum acid output (MAO) (after stimulation tests)	16–26 mEq/hr or at least 1½–3 times the BAO
BAO:MAO ratio	0.3–0.6 (usually <0.4)

Interfering Factors

➤ Failure to follow dietary restrictions, resulting in stimulation of gastric secretions

➤ Exposure to the sight, smell, or thought of food immediately before and during the test

➤ Ingestion of drugs that may alter gastric secretions (e.g., alcohol, histamine, nicotine, adrenocorticotropic steroids, insulin, parasympathetic agents, belladonna alkaloids, anticholinergic drugs, and histamine receptor antagonists) unless administered as part of the testing procedure

➤ Dilution of the samples with saliva and respiratory secretions, which should be expectorated during the test

Indications for Tests of Gastric Acidity

➤ Suspected duodenal ulcer as indicated by elevated BAO (5 to 7 mEq/hr) and MAO (greater than 40 mEq/hr) (Individuals with stomach ulcers may have low to normal BAO and MAO.)

➤ Suspected Zollinger-Ellison syndrome as indicated by elevated BAO, normal or elevated MAO (elevated MAO after gastric stimulation is frequently not seen in these individuals because gastric acid output is already at maximum levels), and high BAO:MAO ratio

➤ Suspected pernicious anemia as indicated by decreased or absent gastric acid output with BAO, MAO, and BAO:MAO ratio frequently at 0

➤ Suspected gastric carcinoma as indicated by decreased BAO (e.g., 1.0 mEq/hr), decreased MAO (e.g., 4.0 mEq/hr), and decreased BAO:MAO ratio (e.g., 0.25)

➤ Evaluation of effectiveness of vagotomy in the treatment of peptic ulcer disease as indicated by absence of response to gastric stimulation with insulin (Hollander insulin test)

Nursing Care Before the Procedure

Client preparation is essentially the same as that for analysis of gastric contents (see pp. 449 to 450).

➤ For gastric stimulation tests using pentagastrin, betazole, and histamine, the client should be informed that a medication will be injected to increase stomach secretions and that the test requires 2 to 3 hours for completion.

➤ The client should be advised to report unusual symptoms such as flushing, headache, nasal stuffiness, dizziness, faintness, and nausea.

➤ For the insulin test, the client should be informed that insulin will be injected intravenously (IV) to lower the blood sugar and should be reassured that glucose will be available for administration if necessary.

➤ The client should also be advised that it may be necessary to insert an intermittent venous access device (e.g., heparin lock).

➤ The client should be informed that it takes approximately 4 hours to complete this test.

➤ Vital signs should be monitored.

➤ Depending on the institution, signed consents may be required for gastric acid stimulation tests because they involve injection of drugs.

The Procedure

Equipment needed for the tests subsequently discussed is essentially the same as for analysis of gastric secretions (see p. 450). In some institutions, the serial gastric aspirates are obtained by connecting the NG tube to a suction device. Manual aspiration of gastric contents is, however, the preferred approach. For the Hollander insulin test, equipment to insert an intermittent venous access device (i.e., heparin lock) will be needed, as well as a syringe of 50 percent glucose.

Basal Gastric Acidity Test. An NG tube is inserted and the stomach contents aspirated. The tube is clamped. After 15 minutes, the tube is opened and the gastric contents aspirated. This procedure is continued until a total of four samples have been obtained. Each sample is labeled with the time and sequence of collection. The samples should be transported promptly to the laboratory.

Gastric Acid Stimulation Tests. A basal gastric acidity test is performed; then the gastric stimulant (pentagastrin, betazole, or histamine) is injected subcutaneously (SC). For pentagastrin and histamine tests, gastric samples are obtained at 15-minute intervals for 1 hour after injection of the drug; for betazole, the samples are obtained at 15-minute intervals for 2 hours after drug injection. If side effects of the drugs become severe, epinephrine or ephedrine may be administered. These drugs antagonize the effects of histamine, except for effects on gastric secretions.[21]

Hollander Insulin Test. A 2-hour basal gastric acidity test is performed. A baseline blood sugar level is then measured. An intermittent venous access device (i.e., heparin or saline lock) may also be inserted for administration of insulin and for glucose, if extreme hypoglycemia should occur. This device may also be used to obtain blood sugar samples during the test. Regular insulin is then administered in a dosage of 15 to 20 units or 0.2 units per kilogram of body weight. Gastric aspirates are then obtained every 15 minutes for 2 hours. Blood glucose determinations also are made at 30, 60, and 90 minutes after injection of the insulin.

A syringe of 50 percent glucose should be available for administration if extreme hypoglycemia occurs. Sweetened orange juice or milk may also be administered orally, if necessary. Note that a blood sugar level of 45 to 50 mg/dL is needed to provoke gastric secretions.

All specimens are labeled with the time and sequence of collection. The NG tube and venous access device are removed upon completion of the test.

Nursing Care After the Procedure

Care and assessment after the test are the same as for analysis of gastric contents (see p. 450).

➤ *Gastric stimulation tests:* Monitor vital signs after the test and assess the client for side effects of drugs administered to induce gastric secretions.
➤ *Hollander insulin test:* Monitor for hypoglycemia and resume dietary intake immediately at the conclusion of the test.

TESTS OF DUODENAL SECRETIONS

ANALYSIS OF DUODENAL CONTENTS

Duodenal fluid analysis is used mainly to evaluate clients with chronic pancreatitis or suspected carcinoma of the pancreas. It may also be used in evaluating infants with suspected cystic fibrosis or with diarrhea or steatorrhea of unknown etiology.[22]

Duodenal fluid samples are more difficult and time-consuming to obtain than are gastric samples. Duodenal samples are obtained by inserting a double-lumen tube. One lumen opens into the stomach and drains gastric secretions so that they do not interfere with duodenal fluid analysis. The end of the tube is positioned near the ampulla of Vater so that the second lumen actually drains duodenal and pancreatic fluids. Correct tube placement must be confirmed by fluoroscopic radiologic procedures. Duodenal samples may be obtained during endoscopic procedures.

Specimens for duodenal analysis are usually collected in the morning, after the client has been fasting for 12 hours. Approximately 20 mL of duodenal fluid should be obtained at that time. If digestion is normal and if the client has observed fasting instructions, no food particles should be present.

Macroscopic Analysis

Color. Duodenal secretions are normally pearly gray, translucent, and moderately viscous. Yellow or green coloration indicates that bile is present, but this finding is generally of no major clinical significance. Pink, red, or brownish secretions may indicate the presence of blood (see further on). If food particles are present, it may indicate failure to follow dietary restrictions, intestinal obstruction, or duodenal diverticula.[23]

Blood. Blood is not normally present in duodenal secretions. Small particles or streaks of fresh blood may be present because of the trauma of intubation. Larger amounts of blood suggest pancreatic carcinoma.

pH. The pH of duodenal fluid normally ranges from 8.0 to 8.5. Increased pH is associated with chronic pancreatitis.

Bicarbonate. Bicarbonate may be measured as part of a routine analysis but is more likely to be determined as part of stimulation tests. Decreased bicarbonate levels are seen in chronic pancreatitis.

Microscopic Analysis

Red Blood Cells. As previously noted, the finding of red blood cells may indicate intubation trauma or carcinoma of the pancreas.

White Blood Cells and Epithelial Cells. Normally, a few white blood cells and epithelial cells are present in duodenal aspirates. Larger amounts are associated with inflammation of the duodenum, bile ducts, or pancreas.

Bacteria. Bacteria are not normally present in duodenal secretions because of the effects of gastric acid. Samples for routine analysis are rarely cultured for bacteria.

Parasites. Parasites are rarely seen in duodenal secretions. When present, they usually consist of the following: (1) larvae of *Strongyloides stercoralis,* (2) cysts or trophozoites of *Giardia lamblia* or *Entamoeba histolytica,* and (3) ova of *Necator, Ancylostoma,* or *Ascaris.*[24]

Reference Values

	Conventional Units	SI Units
Macroscopic Analysis		
Volume (fasting)	20 mL	
Color	Pearl gray, translucent	
Blood	Negative	
pH	8.0–8.5	
Bicarbonate	145 mEq/L	145 mmol/L
Microscopic Analysis		
Red blood cells	Negative	
White blood cells	Few	
Epithelial cells	Few	
Bacteria	Negative	
Parasites	Negative	

Interfering Factors

➤ Failure to follow dietary restrictions, resulting in the presence of food particles in the aspirate
➤ Improper tube placement, resulting in aspiration of gastric secretions

Indications for Analysis of Duodenal Contents

➤ Suspected carcinoma of the pancreas as indicated by decreased volume, presence of blood (possibly), and normal bicarbonate
➤ Known or suspected chronic pancreatitis as indicated by decreased volume, pH, and bicarbonate
➤ Suspected cystic fibrosis as indicated by decreased volume, pH, and bicarbonate
➤ Suspected infestation with parasites, especially *Giardia lamblia*

Nursing Care Before the Procedure

Explain to the client:
➤ The purpose of the test (*Note:* Analysis of duodenal contents is often performed as a component of duodenal stimulation tests.)
➤ That fasting from foods and fluids for 12 hours before the test is necessary
➤ That smoking is not permitted for 8 to 12 hours before the test
➤ That a tube will be passed through the mouth or nose into the small intestine
➤ That various positions may be required (e.g., sitting, lying on side or back) while the tube is passed (see "The Procedure" section next)
➤ That the client may be asked to swallow or deep-breathe periodically as the tube is passed
➤ That a mild sedative may be administered before insertion of the tube
➤ That the tube may cause a sensation of burning as it is passed and that gagging may occur when the tube touches the back of the throat
➤ That tube placement will be checked by an x-ray examination
➤ That a sample of juices from the small intestine will be removed from the tube by using a suction apparatus
➤ That the tube is removed upon completion of the test

Prepare for the procedure:

➤ Assess the client's degree of mobility, as the client must assume various positions (sitting, side-lying, back-lying) while the tube is passed. If the client's mobility is impaired, the individual performing the test should be so informed so that sufficient assistance is available for client positioning.

➤ A signed consent may be required for this test, depending on the institution.

➤ Ensure to the extent possible that dietary and smoking restrictions are followed.

➤ Provide the client with a hospital gown.

The Procedure

The needed equipment is assembled, including a double-lumen intestinal tube to aspirate duodenal contents, lubricant, gloves, 20- or 50-mL syringe adapted for use with the intestinal tube, and specimen containers. Tissues and an emesis basin also should be available for client use. A mechanical suction device for removing gastric secretions continuously during the test will be needed, as will a suction device for removing duodenal secretions.

With the client seated comfortably, the double-lumen tube is passed into the upper part of the stomach. The client is then positioned on the left side and the tube is passed into the lower part of the stomach. The client is then assisted to a sitting position and asked to lean forward from the waist as far as possible. He or she also is instructed to take several deep breaths at this time, which should move the tip of the tube into the portion of the stomach near the pyloric sphincter. The client is then assisted to lie on the right side; this position, along with normal peristalsis, should move the tube into the duodenum. The client is then assisted to a back-lying position and the tube advanced another 10 to 15 cm. Approximately 15 minutes are required to pass the tube in this manner. Under fluoroscopic visualization, the tube is positioned so that the tip is in the middle of the third portion of the duodenum, distal to the ampulla of Vater.[25] When proper location of the tube is ascertained, the tube is secured to the client's face with tape.

The gastric lumen of the tube is connected to a suction device throughout the procedure. Duodenal secretions are collected by mechanical suction for 20 minutes and then sent to the laboratory for analysis. The gastric aspirate is discarded. If tests of duodenal stimulation are to be made, they will be performed before removal of the intestinal tube.

Nursing Care After the Procedure

Care and assessment after the test are the same as that for analysis of gastric contents (see p. 450).

➤ If a sedative has been administered, delay resumption of diet, fluid intake, and activity until the medication has worn off.

➤ Assess the client's comfort level.

➤ Assess the client's degree of sedation and take appropriate safety measures.

➤ Assess the client's ability to resume normal food and fluid intake.

➤ Provide support when diagnostic findings are revealed, and assist the client in coping with possible acute or chronic disorder and therapy.

DUODENAL STIMULATION TESTS

Duodenal stimulation tests involve administering substances that stimulate pancreatic secretion and then measuring the pancreatic substances as they appear in duodenal aspirates. Two such tests are performed: (1) secretin test and (2) cholecystokinin-pancreozymin (CCK-PZ) test.

Secretin Test

Secretin is a hormone normally secreted by the small intestine (see p. 446). It acts to stimulate the pancreas to secrete increased volumes of pancreatic juices with high bicarbonate content. In this test, secretin is administered IV (1 clinical unit per kilogram of body weight) and three duodenal samples are aspirated at 20-minute intervals. A decreased response to secretin is seen in any disorder characterized by chronic inflammation and scarring of the pancreas (e.g., chronic pancreatitis). This test may also aid in diagnosing carcinoma of the pancreas, as bicarbonate values in this disorder are higher than in chronic pancreatitis after stimulation with secretin. Deficiency in pancreatic secretion is associated also with cystic fibrosis. The main use of this test, however, is to monitor declining pancreatic function in individuals with chronic pancreatitis.[26]

Cholecystokinin-Pancreozymin (CCK-PZ) Test

Cholecystokinin-pancreozymin (CCK-PZ) is a hormone normally secreted by the small intestine. It acts to stimulate the pancreas to secrete increased amounts of pancreatic enzymes. This test, which is sometimes performed after the secretin test, involves administration of CCK-PZ and then aspiration of duodenal secretions. The aspirated samples are then assayed for the pancreatic enzymes amylase, lipase, or trypsin, with amylase the enzyme most commonly measured. The results of this test generally parallel those of the secretin test; that is, if overall pancreatic function is decreased, enzyme production is also decreased.

Reference Values

	Conventional Units	**SI Units**
Volume	2–4 mL/kg body weight	
Bicarbonate	90–130 mEq/L	90–130 mmol/L
Pancreatic amylase	6.6–35.2 U/kg body weight	

Interfering Factors

➤ Failure to follow dietary restrictions, resulting in stimulation of pancreatic secretion by food particles
➤ Improper tube placement, resulting in aspiration of gastric secretions

Indications for Duodenal Stimulation Tests

➤ Monitoring of the progression of chronic pancreatitis, with worsening disease indicated by decreased volume, decreased bicarbonate, and decreased enzyme secretion

➤ Suspected cancer of the pancreas as indicated by decreased volume, normal bicarbonate, and decreased enzyme secretion

Nursing Care Before the Procedure

Client preparation is the same as that for routine analysis of duodenal contents (see p. 455).

➤ The client should be informed that a medication will be administered to stimulate pancreatic secretion.

➤ Intradermal skin tests to determine sensitivity to secretin or CCK-PZ, or both, may be performed before the test.

➤ Because secretin is administered IV, an intermittent venous access device (i.e., heparin lock) may be inserted for the test.

The Procedure

The procedure begins with aspiration of baseline (fasting) duodenal secretions (see p. 456). For the secretin test, secretin is administered IV in the amount of 1 clinical unit per kilogram of body weight. Three samples of duodenal aspirate are then obtained at 20-minute intervals. For the CCK-PZ test, the hormone is administered and samples for pancreatic enzymes (usually amylase) are withdrawn.

Nursing Care After the Procedure

Care and assessment after the procedure are the same as for analysis of duodenal contents (see p. 456).

➤ Monitor for allergic reactions to the hormones even though skin tests have been negative.

Student Name _____ Class _____

Instructor _____ Date _____

CASE STUDY AND CRITICAL THINKING EXERCISE

Mr. Green, age 68, is seen at the clinic complaining of stomach fullness and loss of appetite. He reports a 10-lb weight loss. An analysis of gastric contents is ordered and reveals Volume 20 mL, Color translucent, Mucus present, Blood positive, pH 6.4.

a. What is the probable diagnosis?

b. What additional tests will be conducted to confirm the diagnosis?

References

1. Bullock, BL, and Rosendahl, PP: Pathophysiology: Adaptations and Alterations in Function. Little, Brown & Co, Boston, 1984, p 489.
2. Hole, JW: Human Anatomy and Physiology, ed 4. Wm C Brown, Dubuque, Iowa, 1987, p 506.
3. Bullock and Rosendahl, op cit, p 488.
4. Hole, op cit, p 507.
5. Bullock and Rosendahl, op cit, p 490.
6. Sacher, RA, and McPherson, RA: Widmann's Clinical Interpretation of Laboratory Tests, ed 10. FA Davis, Philadelphia, 1991, p 754.
7. Strasinger, SK: Urinalysis and Body Fluids, ed 3. FA Davis, Philadelphia, 1994, p 192.
8. Kao, YS, and Liu, FJ: Laboratory diagnosis of gastrointestinal tract. In Henry, JB: Clinical Diagnosis and Management by Laboratory Methods, ed 18. WB Saunders, Philadelphia, 1991, p 519.

9. Ibid, p 521.
10. Ibid, p 521.
11. Ibid, p 521.
12. Ibid, p 521.
13. Sacher and McPherson, op cit, p 752.
14. Kao and Liu, op cit, p 522.
15. Ibid, p 522.
16. Ibid, p 524.
17. Sacher and McPherson, op cit, pp 751–752.
18. Kao and Liu, op cit, p 522.
19. Ibid, p 520.
20. Sacher and McPherson, op cit, pp 751–752.
21. Bergensen, BS: Pharmacology in Nursing, ed 14. CV Mosby–Year Book, 1979, p 700.
22. Kao and Liu, op cit, p 526.
23. Ibid, p 525.
24. Ibid, pp 525–526.
25. Kao and Liu, op cit, p 525.
26. Sacher and McPherson, op cit, p 754.

Bibliography

Byrne, CJ, et al: Laboratory Tests: Implications for Nursing Care, ed 2. Addison-Wesley, Menlo Park, Calif, 1986.
Chernecky, CC, and Berger, BJ; Cullen, BN (ed): Laboratory Tests and Diagnostic Procedures, ed 2. WB Saunders, Philadelphia, 1996.
Corbett, JV: Laboratory Tests and Diagnostic Procedures with Nursing Diagnoses, ed 4. Appleton & Lange, Norwalk, Conn, 1995.
Fischbach, FT: A Manual of Laboratory Diagnostic Tests, ed 5. Lippincott-Raven, Philadelphia, 1996.
Kee, JL: Handbook of Laboratory and Diagnostic Tests with Nursing Implications, ed 3. Appleton & Lange, Norwalk, Conn, 1997.
Kuhn, M: Pharmacotherapeutics: A Nursing Process Approach, ed 4. FA Davis, Philadelphia, 1997.
Lewis, SM, et al (eds): Medical-Surgical Nursing: Assessment and Management of Clinical Problems, ed 4. Mosby–Year Book, St Louis, 1995.
Pagana, KD, and Pagana, TJ: Diagnostic and Laboratory Test Reference, ed 3. Mosby–Year Book, St Louis, 1996.
Porth, C: Pathophysiology: Concepts of Altered Health States, ed 4. JB Lippincott, Philadelphia, 1993.
Sleisenger, MH, and Fordtran, JS (eds): Gastrointestinal Diseases, ed 4. WB Saunders, Philadelphia, 1989.
Springhouse Corporation: Clinical Laboratory Tests: Values and Implications. Springhouse, Springhouse, Pa, 1991.
Springhouse Corporation: Nurse's Reference Library: Diagnostics, ed 2. Springhouse, Springhouse, Pa, 1986.
Tietz, NW (ed): Clinical Guide to Laboratory Tests, ed 3. WB Saunders, Philadelphia, 1997.

13

Fecal Analysis

➤ TESTS COVERED
Microscopic Analysis of Feces, *463*
Tests for Specific Substances in
    Feces, *466*

Microbiologic Tests of Feces, *472*

COMPOSITION AND CHARACTERISTICS OF FECES

Feces consist mainly of cellulose and other undigested foodstuffs, bacteria, and water (as much as 70 percent). Other substances normally found in stools include epithelial cells shed from the gastrointestinal tract, small amounts of fats, bile pigments in the form of urobilin (see Fig. 6–1, p. 312), gastrointestinal and pancreatic secretions (see Chap. 12), and electrolytes.[1,2] The average adult excretes 100 to 300 g of fecal material per day, the residue of approximately 10 L of liquid material that enters the intestinal tract each day.[3]

Feces are normally brown because of bacterial degradation of bile pigments to stercobilin. The characteristic odor of feces is caused by bacterial action on proteins and other residues that produce substances such as indole, skatole, phenol, hydrogen, sulfide, and ammonia.[4] The normal consistency of feces is described as "plastic"; that is, stools should not normally be liquid, mushy, or hard.[5] The shape and caliber of normal stools is the same as that of the distal colon.

Alterations in color, odor, consistency, or shape may indicate the presence of disease. Although these characteristics are not always specifically studied in the laboratory, the nurse may observe them when providing care. Feces that are abnormal in terms of gross characteristics require additional diagnostic follow-up. Table 13–1 depicts normal and abnormal characteristics that may be observed and possible causes of alterations.

Laboratory analysis of feces includes microscopic examinations, chemical tests for specific substances, and microbiologic tests. Laboratory analysis of feces is performed much less frequently than are studies of blood, urine, and other body fluids. One reason for this is that clients and health-care providers dislike collecting stool specimens. Furthermore, fecal samples cannot usually be collected on demand the way blood samples can, with the possible exception of small samples obtained during rectal examination, which may be sufficient for screening tests (e.g., occult blood). Despite these disadvantages, analysis of fecal material aids in diagnosing gastrointestinal and other disorders.[6]

Table 13–1 ➤ NORMAL AND ABNORMAL GROSS CHARACTERISTICS OF FECES

Characteristic	Normal	Alterations	Possible Causes of Alterations
Volume	100–300 g	Large volume, malodorous, floating	Malabsorption of fats or proteins
Odor	Pungent		Cystic fibrosis, pancreatitis, postgastrectomy syndrome, bile duct obstruction, primary small bowel disease
Shape/caliber	Shape and caliber of the distal colon	Large caliber	Dilatation of the colon
		Small, ribbonlike	Decreased elasticity of the colon
			Partial bowel obstruction
Color	Brown	Red	Lower gastrointestinal (GI) tract bleeding
			Red beet ingestion
			Bromsulphalein (BSP) dye, phenazopyridine (Pyridium) compounds
		Black	Upper GI tract bleeding
			Charcoal, licorice, iron, or bismuth ingestion
		Dark brown	Hemolytic anemia
			Diet high in meat
			Prolonged exposure of the sample to air
		Gray	Chocolate and cocoa ingestion
		Gray, silvery	Steatorrhea
		Pasty, gray-white	Barium ingestion
			Bile duct obstruction
		Very pale gray	Diet high in milk products
		Green, yellow-green	Ingestion of spinach, other greens, laxatives of vegetable origin, indomethacin
			Rapid transit time through the intestine, preventing oxidation of bile pigments
		Green-black	Meconium, infant
		Green-yellow (watery)	Transitional stool, infant
		Yellow, pasty	Breast-fed infant
		Yellow-brown	Cow's milk–fed infant
Consistency	Plastic	Small, round, hard masses	Habitual constipation
		Mucoid, watery but without blood	Irritable bowel syndrome, diffuse superficial bowel inflammation, villous adenoma
		Mucoid, bloody	Inflammatory bowel syndrome, carcinoma, typhoid, *Shigella*, amebae
		Sticky, tarry, black	Upper GI tract bleeding

(continued on page 463)

Table 13–1 ➤ NORMAL AND ABNORMAL GROSS CHARACTERISTICS OF FECES *(Continued)*			
Characteristic	**Normal**	**Alterations**	**Possible Causes of Alterations**
		Voluminous, watery, little-formed material	Osmotic catharsis
			Noninvasive infections (cholera toxigenic, *Escherichia coli,* staphylococcal food poisoning)
		Loose, purulent, or with necrotic tissue	Diverticulitis, abscess, necrotic tumor, parasites
Mucus	Absent	Present	Colitis, bacillary dysentery, diverticulitis, carcinoma

Note: Adapted from Sacher, RA, and McPherson, RA: Clinical Interpretation of Laboratory Tests, ed 10. FA Davis, Philadelphia, 1991, pp 739–740.

TESTS OF FECES

MICROSCOPIC ANALYSIS OF FECES

Microscopic analysis of stool specimens includes examining the sample for leukocytes, epithelial cells, qualitative fat, meat fibers, and parasites. These tests may be performed singly, in combination with other tests, or as routine screening tests.

Leukocytes

Examination of feces for leukocytes, especially neutrophils and monocytes, is usually performed in the initial evaluation of diarrhea of unknown etiology. Testing for the presence or absence of leukocytes can provide important diagnostic clues, and these tests yield results faster than do stool cultures.

Epithelial Cells

Normally small to moderate numbers of epithelial cells are present in feces. Large numbers of epithelial cells (or large amounts of mucus), however, indicate that the intestinal mucosa is irritated.[7]

Qualitative Fats

Fats are found in the feces primarily in the forms of triglycerides (neutral fats), fatty acids, and fatty acid salts. Their presence is determined through various staining techniques before microscopic examination. Through these methods, the number of fat droplets and their size can be determined, and the type of fat can be identified. The finding of more than 60 fat droplets per high-power field (HPF) usually indicates steatorrhea, which simply means excess fat in the stool. The size of the droplet also must be considered in arriving at a diagnosis. The fat droplets in steatorrhea are usually larger than normal.

Excess fat in the stool is usually caused by either malabsorption syndromes or deficiency in pancreatic enzymes. Microscopic examination for fecal fat may aid in differentiating between these two disorders. An increase in triglycerides generally indicates a deficiency of pancreatic enzymes that normally break down triglycerides to fatty acids. In contrast, individuals with malabsorption syndromes usually have normal amounts of triglycerides in their stools but excessive fatty acids because these clients are unable to absorb the fats once they are broken down.[8] Other causes of excessive fecal fat include surgical resection or fistulas of the intestines and recent intake of excessive amounts of dietary fats. False-negative results may occur in individuals with malabsorption problems who restrict their fat intake because of anorexia.

Microscopic tests for fecal fats are essentially qualitative in nature. The test simply indicates whether excessive fat is present and, if so, the nature of that fat. The definitive test for evaluating steatorrhea is quantitative analysis for fecal fat. This evaluation is accomplished through a 72-hour stool collection while the client is on a diet containing 100 g of fat per day (see p. 469).[9]

Meat Fibers

Microscopic examination of stool specimens for meat fibers aids in evaluating the efficiency of digestion. If protein digestion is adequate, meat fibers will not be found. If they are present, inadequate proteolysis is indicated. The finding of meat fibers in feces usually correlates positively with the finding of steatorrhea.[10] Individuals who have difficulty in digesting proteins also have difficulty in digesting fats.

Parasites

Microscopic tests for parasites and their ova augment observation of gross characteristics of stools; that is, certain types of parasites (e.g., tapeworm segments) may be apparent in stool samples without the aid of a microscope.[11] Microscopic analysis for parasites is usually indicated in individuals with intestinal disorders of unknown etiology, history of possible exposure to parasites, or eosinophilia of unknown cause that could be a result of parasitic infestation.

Parasites commonly found in stools include roundworms (e.g., *Ascaris lumbricoides*), tapeworms (e.g., *Diphyllobothrium latum, Taenia saginata*), hookworms (e.g., *Necator americanus*), ameba (e.g., *Entamoeba histolytica*), and protozoa (e.g., *Giardia lamblia*).[12] In collecting specimens for parasites, it is important that the sample be transported immediately to the laboratory. The best samples are considered to be those that contain blood and mucus because they are also most likely to contain parasites.

Reference Values

Leukocytes	Negative
Epithelial cells	Few to moderate
Fat (qualitative)	<60 normal-sized droplets per HPF
Triglycerides (neutral fats)	1–5%
Fatty acids	5–15%
Meat fibers	Negative
Parasites	Negative

Interfering Factors

➤ A diet too high or too low in fat may alter results of qualitative tests for fats.
➤ Failure to send fresh stool specimens immediately to the laboratory, thereby avoiding excessive exposure to room temperature and air, may damage any parasites so that they cannot be identified microscopically.
➤ Contamination of the sample with urine or toilet bowl water.
➤ Use of laxatives for several days before the tests.
➤ Presence of barium in the stool after x-ray procedures.
➤ Antibiotic therapy.

Indications for Microscopic Analysis of Feces

➤ Abnormal appearance of stools (see Table 13–1, pp. 462 to 463)
➤ Diarrhea of unknown etiology
  • Diarrhea resulting from disorders involving the intestinal wall (e.g., ulcerative colitis and bacterial infection with *Salmonella, Shigella, Yersinia,* and invasive *Escherichia coli*) is associated with the presence of leukocytes in the sample.
  • Diarrhea resulting from organisms that cause diarrhea by toxin rather than by intestinal wall damage (e.g., viruses, *Staphylococcus,* noninvasive *E. coli, Clostridium perfringens, Vibrio cholerae, Giardia, Entamoeba*) is associated with absence of leukocytes in the sample.[13,14]
➤ Suspected inflammatory bowel disorder as indicated by large numbers of epithelial cells
➤ Suspected pancreatitis as indicated by excessive fecal fat (steatorrhea) with elevated triglycerides (neutral fats)
➤ Suspected malabsorption syndromes as indicated by steatorrhea, normal triglycerides, and elevated fecal fatty acids
➤ Suspected alteration in protein digestion as indicated by the presence of meat fibers
➤ Suspected infestation with intestinal parasites, ova, and viruses
➤ Eosinophilia of unknown etiology, with suspicion of parasitic infestation

Nursing Care Before the Procedure

Explain to the client:
➤ The importance of following a normal diet for several days before the collection or notifying the physician if this requirement cannot be met
➤ The importance of not taking laxatives for several days before the collection or notifying the physician if this avoidance is not possible
➤ The method for collecting a sample of a bowel movement (see under "The Procedure")
➤ The method for transferring the sample from the specimen pan to the sample container (e.g., using tongue blades; obtaining the sample from the midportion of the stool, including any portion of the stool with visible blood, mucus, pus, or parasites such as tapeworms)
➤ The importance of not contaminating the specimen with urine or water
➤ The importance of delivering the sample to the laboratory within 30 to 60 minutes of collection or refrigerating the sample if it must be stored longer than 60 minutes (*Exception:* Samples for parasites may not be refrigerated and must be received in the laboratory while still warm.)

> The importance of placing the sample in a tightly covered container

Prepare for the procedure:

> Ensure to the extent possible that the client has followed a relatively normal diet and has not used laxatives for several days before testing.
> Provide a specimen collection container (e.g., a plastic "hat" device, which is placed under the toilet seat), gloves, and tongue blades.
> Provide the specimen container in which the sample is to be sent to the laboratory.

The Procedure

The sample is collected in either a plastic hat-type receptacle, which is placed under the toilet seat, or in a bedpan. It is important that the hat or bedpan be clean and dry and that the sample not be contaminated with urine or water. Gloves are worn, and two clean tongue blades are used to transfer the midportion of the sample to a clean, dry plastic container with a tightly fitting lid. Any visible blood, mucus, pus, or parasites should be included in the sample. The container should be covered tightly as soon as the sample is obtained.

The tongue blades should be double-wrapped in paper towels, and they may be inserted into one of the gloves when they are removed. The collection container (e.g., plastic hat or bedpan) should be thoroughly cleansed or disposed of, preferably in a large plastic bag. Hands should be washed thoroughly.

In infants and young children, samples may be obtained from diapers, provided that contact with urine is avoided. To avoid contact, apply a urine collection bag to catch the urine. Check the bag frequently because the urine may spill and contaminate the feces.

The sample should be sent, properly labeled, to the laboratory within 30 to 60 minutes. If this is not possible, the sample may be refrigerated unless it is to be tested for parasites, in which case it must be sent to the laboratory while still warm.

Nursing Care After the Procedure

Care and assessment after collection of a feces specimen include hand washing to prevent transmission of pathogens to others and disposal of the articles used according to standard precautions and transmission-based isolation procedures.

> *Diarrhea:* Note and report frequency and gross characteristics of bowel eliminations. Examine perianal area for irritation. Administer ordered antidiarrheal or antibiotic therapy, or both. Monitor for fluid deficit and replace fluid losses. Cleanse perianal area after each episode of diarrhea and apply a soothing ointment. Inform client that follow-up testing is conducted to evaluate therapy, and instruct the client in the collection, frequency, and transportation of specimens to the laboratory. Report a positive result for parasites to the physician immediately.

TESTS FOR SPECIFIC SUBSTANCES IN FECES

Fecal samples can be chemically analyzed for a variety of substances including occult (hidden) blood, qualitative fats, trypsin, urobilinogen, and bile. In addition, estimates of carbohydrate utilization can be made.

Occult Blood

The most frequently performed test of feces is chemical screening for occult blood. The purpose of the test is to detect pathological lesions (e.g., carcinoma) before they produce symptoms and while the condition is still amenable to treatment. Indeed, such testing is widely used in mass screening programs for colorectal cancer, with 75 percent of such cancers detected while still localized.[15]

A number of easy-to-use test kits for detection of occult blood are available. Before the existence of such kits, the traditional method was to expose the sample to a sequence of solutions that included glacial acetic acid, gum guaiac solution, and hydrogen peroxide. A blue color indicated a positive test result. The test kits use these same principles, with some using paper impregnated with guaiac. For these reasons, analysis of feces for occult blood is sometimes still referred to as a "stool for guaiac."

One of the main problems of testing stools for occult blood is the number of false-positive results that occur. A diet high in meat, for example, may cause stools to test positive for blood, as do diets high in certain vegetables (e.g., horseradish and turnips) and bananas. In addition, bleeding from the gums or nasal passages may produce positive results for occult blood in stools. Therapy with many drugs may lead to positive results because of direct or indirect drug effects on the gastrointestinal tract. These drugs include aspirin (as little as one 300-mg tablet per day), iron preparations, anticoagulants, adrenocorticosteroids, colchicine, and phenylbutazone. In contrast, ascorbic acid may lead to false-negative results.

Numerous pathological conditions may cause bleeding into the intestinal tract. Table 13–2 details these disorders, including severity of bleeding and other clinical features.

Sometimes bleeding appears so obvious that one may be tempted not to confirm visual observations with appropriate testing. Stools that are grossly red or black are usually assumed to contain blood. Such assumptions, however, must always be confirmed because certain foods and medications may also impart these colors to stools (see Table 13–1, pp. 462 to 463). If blood is present in sufficient quantity, the color of the stool reflects the source of the bleeding or the length of time the blood was in the gastrointestinal tract, or both. Black stools, for example, are associated with upper GI bleeding when the hemoglobin has come in contact with gastric acid and has been converted to acid hematin. In such cases, stools may remain black for as long as 5 days after the initial bleeding occurred. If, however, upper GI bleeding is massive and the volume increases GI motility (e.g., as occurs in bleeding from esophageal varices), stools may be red or maroon and somewhat liquid in consistency. Generally, though, bright red stools are associated with lower GI bleeding from hemorrhoids, ulcerative colitis, and carcinomas.[16]

For occult blood studies, samples are obtained from rectal examination or portions of bowel movements. It is recommended that the client follow a meat-free, high-bulk diet for 3 days before testing and that drugs that may alter test results be withheld. In practice, however, these restrictions frequently are not applied.

Quantitative Fats

As noted previously (p. 464), the definitive test for excessive fecal fat is the 72-hour quantitative measure, with the amount of fat present expressed as a per-

Table 13-2 ➤ CONDITIONS ASSOCIATED WITH GASTROINTESTINAL BLEEDING

Condition	Usual Age of Occurrence	Severity	Other Features
UPPER GI TRACT			
Peptic ulcer (gastric or duodenal)	Any, including young children	Variable, from occult to life-threatening	Pain, typical history often absent
Erosive gastritis	Usually adults over age 25	Usually mild; may be very severe	Aspirin, alcohol use often predispose Severe uremia, chronic liver disease predispose
Atrophic gastritis	Adults over age 25	Usually mild	Associated with pernicious anemia, autoantibodies, decreased gastric acidity
Esophageal varices	Adults; children with portal hypertension	Massive, sudden	Common in alcoholic liver disease Cirrhosis or portal hypertension always present
Mallory-Weiss tears at gastroesophageal junction	Any, but usually older adults	Variable, depending on depth, location of tear	Common in alcohol abusers
Hiatal hernia, esophagitis	Progressively increasing incidence over age 40	Usually mild	Persistent, painless bleeding a common cause of iron-deficiency anemia in elderly people
SMALL AND LARGE BOWEL			
Meckel's diverticulum	Most common in children and young adults	Moderate; stools red or maroon	Caused by peptic ulceration of ectopic gastric mucosa
Polyps	Any age	Usually mild; often intermittent	Diarrhea, mucus in stools sometimes accompany
Infections diarrheas	Any age	Usually mild or moderate	Ameba, *Shigella, Clostridium difficile*
Inflammatory bowel disease (Crohn's disease, ulcerative colitis)	Adolescents, adults under age 60	Usually mild but may be massive	Diarrhea, pain, weight loss more common in Crohn's disease than in ulcerative colitis Bleeding more prominent in ulcerative colitis
Diverticular disease	Progressively increasing incidence over age 40	Usually mild, frequently occult	Often asymptomatic, unless inflammation or abscess develops
Vascular malformations	Older adults	Usually mild; may be life-threatening in ~15%	Bleeding often recurrent Often misdiagnosed as peptic ulcer or diverticular disease
Carcinoma	Older adults	Variable, from occult to moderate	Common cause of iron-deficiency anemia in older adults Red blood more common with distally located tumors

(continued on page 469)

Table 13–2 ➤ CONDITIONS ASSOCIATED WITH GASTROINTESTINAL
BLEEDING *(Continued)*

Condition	Usual Age of Occurrence	Severity	Other Features
		RECTUM AND ANUS	
Hemorrhoids	Older adults	Usually mild; blood is bright red	May be painless or symptomatic Often associated with constipation
Anorectal fissure	Any age	Usually mild; blood is bright red	Nearly always painful Crohn's disease, anal intercourse may predispose

Note: Adapted from Sacher, RA, and McPherson, RA: Widmann's Clinical Interpretation of Laboratory Tests, ed 10. FA Davis, Philadelphia, 1991, pp 744–745, with permission.

centage of solid material. Because fat output may vary on a day-to-day basis, the 3-day collection is believed to be the most reliable approach. In adults, a controlled fat diet of 100 g per day also is followed during the collection. In infants and children, for whom such a diet could not be used, results of the collection are based on the estimated intake of dietary fat. Thus, it is important to know which foods were ingested during the test period.[17]

Trypsin

Trypsin is an enzyme secreted by the pancreas. It is normally not present in stools, except in children under the age of 2 years. If it is absent from the stools of children under age 2, pancreatic deficiency is indicated. It should be noted that trypsin may not be detected if the child is constipated, because of the prolonged action of normal intestinal bacteria on the enzyme.[18]

Carbohydrate Utilization

Individuals with various disorders related to malabsorption (e.g., celiac disease, tropical sprue, disorders involving the small intestine) may have difficulty with carbohydrate absorption as well as fat absorption. Thus, a thorough investigation of the finding of steatorrhea (excess fat in the stool) includes evaluation of carbohydrate metabolism. Such an evaluation includes performing oral and intravenous (IV) glucose tolerance tests (see Chap. 5) and comparing the results. Persons with carbohydrate malabsorption have normal results on IV glucose tolerance tests but not on oral glucose tolerance tests.[19]

If carbohydrates cannot be absorbed normally, excessive amounts appear in the stool. This condition can be tested by placing a Clinitest tablet (Ames Company, Elkhart, Ind.) in a portion of stool that has been emulsified with water. It should be noted that Clinitest tablets are one of the methods used to detect excess sugar in urine. When performed on fecal samples, a positive Clinitest result indicates carbohydrate malabsorption. This test is easily performed and may be used as a screening test to detect metabolic and intestinal disorders.

Urobilinogen

Urobilinogen is produced from bilirubin, a breakdown product of red blood cells, and normally appears in urine (see Chap. 6) and feces. Because blood and urine samples for products of bilirubin metabolism are more easily obtained than stool samples, this test is rarely used. Factors that may lead to falsely decreased values include antibiotic therapy and exposure of the sample to light.[20]

Bile

Bile should not be present in feces of adults because it is broken down in the intestines during normal digestion; however, tests for bile may normally be positive in children. Bile may appear in the stools of adults if there is rapid transit through the gastrointestinal tract (e.g., diarrhea). It may also be found in clients with hemolytic anemias that produce jaundice.[21]

Reference Values

Occult blood	Negative (0.5–2 mL/day)
	5–7% of dietary intake
Quantitative fat (72-hr collection)	<5 g/24 hr
	10–25% of dry fecal matter
Neutral fat	1–5% of dry fecal matter
Fatty acids	5–15% of dry fecal matter
Trypsin	Positive (2+ to 4+)
Carbohydrates (Clinitest)	Negative
Urobilinogen	
Random sample	Negative
24-hr collection	40–200 mg/24 hr
	80–280 Ehrlich units/24 hr
Bile	
Children	Positive
Adults	Negative

Interfering Factors

➤ Ingestion of a diet high in meat, certain vegetables (e.g., horseradish and turnips), and bananas may cause false-positive results in tests for occult blood.
➤ Therapy with numerous medications may lead to positive results in tests for occult blood because of direct or indirect drug effects; examples of such drugs are aspirin, anticoagulants, adrenocorticosteroids, iron preparations, colchicine, and phenylbutazone.
➤ Ingestion of ascorbic acid may lead to false-negative results in tests for occult blood.
➤ A diet too high or too low in fats or failure to follow the prescribed diet (100 g of fat per day) may alter results of quantitative fat tests.
➤ Constipation may lead to false-negative results in tests for fecal trypsin in children.
➤ Ingestion of antibiotics and exposure of the fecal sample to light may produce false-negative results in tests for fecal urobilinogen.

Indications for Tests for Specific Substances in Feces

Occult Blood

➤ Known or suspected disorder associated with gastrointestinal bleeding (see Table 13–2, pp. 468 to 469)

➤ Therapy with drugs that may lead to gastrointestinal bleeding (e.g., aspirin, anticoagulants)

Quantitative Fats
➤ Suspected intestinal malabsorption or pancreatic insufficiency as indicated by elevated fat levels (see p. 467)
➤ Monitoring of effectiveness of therapy for intestinal malabsorption or pancreatic insufficiency

Trypsin
➤ Suspected pancreatic insufficiency in very young children as indicated by negative or decreased results

Carbohydrate Utilization (Clinitest)
➤ Suspected malabsorption syndromes as indicated by positive results

Urobilinogen
➤ Suspected anemias characterized by decreased red blood cell production as indicated by decreased levels
➤ Suspected liver and biliary tract disorders as indicated by decreased levels
➤ Suspected hemolytic anemias as indicated by increased levels

Bile
➤ Suspected hemolytic anemias, which lead to excessive levels

Nursing Care Before the Procedure

Client preparation is essentially the same as that for microscopic analysis of feces (see p. 465).
➤ For tests for occult blood, the client should eat a high-bulk, meat-free diet for 3 days before testing.
➤ Medications that may alter test results (e.g., aspirin) may also be withheld for 3 or more days before the test, although this practice should be confirmed with the person ordering the study.
➤ For qualitative fat studies, the client should follow a diet containing 100 g of fat for 3 days before testing as well as during the test.
➤ Alcohol, antacids, laxatives, and antibiotics may also be withheld.
➤ The client should be provided with a large container (usually a gallon paint can) and should be instructed to refrigerate the sample.
➤ If the test is for urobilinogen, the client should not be taking antibiotics and should be supplied with a light-protected container.

The Procedure

The procedure is essentially the same as that described on page 466. Fecal specimens for analysis of specific substances are usually obtained on random samples, although the test for quantitative fats requires a 72-hour collection. Such a study is usually begun early in the morning of a given day and continued for 3 consecutive days. The sample is maintained in a large, refrigerated container (usually a gallon paint can). Fecal studies for urobilinogen may be carried out on a 24-hour basis.

When random samples are used, the tests are often repeated on a serial basis, especially in studies for occult blood. When this approach is used, it is desirable to obtain the samples on 3 different days.

Nursing Care After the Procedure

Care and assessment are the same as for any fecal specimen collection and analysis (see p. 466).

➤ Instruct the client in sample collection procedures according to the client's ability to perform the procedure.

➤ Resume dietary and medication regimens after the specimen is collected if they were modified to prepare for the test.

➤ *Hemorrhage or anemia:* Note and report blood loss and characteristics; occult blood; pallor, weakness, and other symptoms of anemia; and possible site of blood loss. Administer ordered whole blood or packed red blood cell transfusion. Monitor vital signs and assist with care activities to conserve energy.

➤ *Malabsorption syndromes:* Note and report presence of steatorrhea in feces and dietary intake of fats and carbohydrates. Administer ordered medications to treat pancreatic, liver, or biliary disorders.

MICROBIOLOGIC TESTS OF FECES

Stool Cultures

Certain bacteria are normally found in feces (i.e., the "normal flora" of the bowel). The presence of pathological types of bacteria may, however, produce diarrhea and other signs of systemic infection. Thus, most stool cultures are undertaken to evaluate diarrhea of unknown etiology to identify possible causative bacteria. Bacteria produce diarrhea in three main ways: (1) The organisms invade the intestinal wall, damaging tissue; (2) the organisms produce toxins within the intestine that alter gastrointestinal motility; and (3) toxins produced by bacteria are ingested (e.g., via foods) and produce diarrhea, although the organisms themselves are not detected in feces.[22] Table 13–3 lists the types of diarrhea associated with specific conditions. The primary purpose of stool cultures is to identify organisms that cause damage to intestinal tissue.

Samples for stool cultures may be obtained either by rectal swab or by collection of a bowel movement sample. It is important that such samples not be exposed to air or to room temperature more than necessary, as these conditions may damage bacteria so that they cannot be grown in culture. Thus, samples obtained by rectal swab must be placed in preservative, whereas those obtained from bowel movements must be placed in tightly sealed containers.

Reference Values

Stool culture	Normal flora

Interfering Factors

➤ Therapy with antibiotics may decrease the type and amount of bacteria present.

➤ Excessive exposure of the sample to air or to room temperature may damage bacteria so that they will not grow in culture.

➤ Failure to transport the sample to the laboratory within 1 hour of collection may affect results.

Table 13-3 ➤ TYPES OF DIARRHEA

Category	Specific Condition	Other Features
Osmotic	Disaccharidase deficiency (lactose intolerance)	Symptoms follow ingestion of dairy products.
	Indigestible oligosaccharides in beans, other legumes	Abdominal distention, "gas" very common.
	Saline laxatives	Patient may alternate constipation with laxative abuse
		History of peptic ulcer symptoms.
Secretory	Nondigestible sugars in artificial sweeteners	Dietary history is crucial.
	Bacterial toxins (cholera, *Escherichia coli,* staphylococcal food poisoning)	Epidemiology is more revealing than stool culture.
	Enteroactive hormones (gastrin in Zollinger-Ellison syndrome; serotonin, others in carcinoid syndrome)	Other systemic symptoms are common.
	Malabsorption syndromes: fat, protein	
	Irritation by bile acids	
Altered structure or function	Intestinal resection	Follows ileal resection.
		Bacterial overgrowth in small intestine.
		Apparent from history.
	Enterocolonic fistula	Complication of diverticular disease or inflammatory bowel disease.
	Irritable bowel syndrome	Pathophysiology remains unclear.
Mucosal damage	Inflammatory bowel disease (Crohn's disease, ulcerative colitis)	Bleeding, pain, weight loss may accompany.
	Invasive organisms (some shigella, some salmonella, amebae, campylobacter)	Stool cultures useful early in disease.
	Pseudomembranous colitis	Often follows use of broad-spectrum antibiotics
		May complicate uremia, antibiotic use, congestive heart failure; intestinal ischemia.

Note: Adapted from Sacher, RA, and McPherson, RA: Widmann's Clinical Interpretation of Laboratory Tests, ed 10. FA Davis, Philadelphia, 1991, pp 741, with permission.

Indications for Stool Cultures

➤ Diarrhea of unknown etiology that may be caused by bacteria that damage intestinal tissue (see Table 13-3)

Nursing Care Before the Procedure

Client preparation is essentially the same as that for other tests of feces (p. 465).

➤ If the sample is to be obtained by rectal swab, explain to the client how this will be accomplished.

The Procedure

If the sample is to be obtained by rectal swab, a clean or sterile swab and preservative are needed. Prepackaged sterile swabs with cylinders containing preservative are commercially available for obtaining various types of samples for culture (e.g., wound drainage, throat secretions). The swab is inserted into the rectum (*without* the use of a lubricant) past the anal sphincter. It is rotated gently and then withdrawn.[23]

For samples of portions of bowel movements, the procedure is the same as that described on page 466. The sample should be placed in a clean, dry container. As certain nonpathological bacteria are normally present in feces, it is not necessary for the container to be sterile.

All samples should be protected from air and sent to the laboratory within 1 hour of collection. Samples should not be refrigerated.

Nursing Care After the Procedure

Care and assessment are the same as that for any fecal specimen collection and analysis (see p. 466).

➤ Assist or instruct client, or both, in collecting the specimen, according to his or her ability to perform the procedure.

➤ Notify physician immediately of a positive culture for pathogenic microorganisms.

Student Name _____ Class _____

Instructor _____ Date _____

CASE STUDY AND CRITICAL THINKING EXERCISE

Dr. White is a 55-year-old professor whose department chair is an unrelenting harasser. Dr. White's family investments have failed and his plan for early retirement is no longer possible. He has had persistent upper abdominal pain for the past 2 months. History reveals smoking 1 pack of cigarettes per day for 25 years, irregular eating habits, four to six aspirin tablets for mild arthritis, and a 10-lb weight loss the last 2 months. He reports a pain-antacid-relief pattern because the pain is more intense after eating.

a. What is his probable diagnosis?

b. What are the contributing factors in this diagnosis?

c. What is the significance of "tarry" stools?

References

1. Hole, JW: Human Anatomy and Physiology, ed 4. Wm C Brown, Dubuque, Iowa, 1987, pp 527–528.
2. Strasinger, SK: Urinalysis and Body Fluids, ed 3. FA Davis, Philadelphia, 1994, p 200.
3. Sacher, RA, and McPherson, RA: Widmann's Clinical Interpretation of Laboratory Tests, ed 10. FA Davis, Philadelphia, 1991, p 737.
4. Hole, op cit, p 528.
5. Sacher and McPherson, op cit, p 738.
6. Ibid, p 737.
7. Ibid, p 743.
8. Strasinger, op cit, p 202.
9. Kao, YS, and Liu, FJ: Malabsorption, diarrhea, and examination of feces. In Henry, JB: Clinical Diagnosis and Management by Laboratory Methods, ed 18. WB Saunders, Philadelphia, 1991, p 544.
10. Ibid, p 540.
11. Sacher and McPherson, op cit, p 742.
12. Springhouse Corporation: Nurse's Reference Library: Diagnostics, ed 2. Springhouse, Springhouse, Pa, 1986, p 526.
13. Strasinger, op cit, p 201.
14. Kao and Liu, op cit, p 536.
15. Strasinger, op cit, p 202.
16. Sacher and McPherson, op cit, pp 744–745.
17. Kao and Liu, op cit, p 544.
18. Fischbach, FT: A Manual of Laboratory and Diagnostic Tests, ed 4. JB Lippincott, Philadelphia, 1992, p 240.
19. Sacher and McPherson, op cit, p 746.
20. Nurse's Reference Library, op cit, p 808.
21. Fischbach, op cit, p 240.
22. Sacher and McPherson, op cit, pp 739–740.
23. Nurse's Reference Library, op cit, p 509.

Bibliography

Berk, JE, and Haubrich, WS: Gastrointestinal Symptoms: Clinical Interpretation. Mosby–Year Book, St Louis, 1991.

Byrne, CJ, et al: Laboratory Tests: Implications For Nursing Care, ed 2. Addison-Wesley, Menlo Park, Calif, 1986.

Chernecky, CC, and Berger, BJ; Cullen, BN (ed): Laboratory Tests and Diagnostic Procedures, ed 2. WB Saunders, Philadelphia, 1996.

Corbett, JV: Laboratory Tests and Diagnostic Procedures with Nursing Diagnoses, ed 4. Appleton & Lange, Norwalk, Conn, 1995.

Johnson, LR: Gastrointestinal Physiology, ed 4. Mosby–Year Book, St Louis, 1991.

Kee, JL: Handbook of Laboratory and Diagnostic Tests with Nursing Implications, ed 3. Appleton & Lange, Norwalk, Conn, 1997.

Lewis, SM, et al (eds): Medical-Surgical Nursing: Assessment and Management of Clinical Problems, ed 4. Mosby–Year Book, St Louis, 1995.

Ming, SC, and Goldman, H: Pathology of the Gastrointestinal Tract. WB Saunders, Philadelphia, 1991.

Pagana, KD, and Pagana, TJ: Diagnostic and Laboratory Test Reference, ed 3. Mosby–Year Book, St Louis, 1996.

Porth, C: Pathophysiology: Concepts of Altered Health States, ed 4. JB Lippincott, Philadelphia, 1993.

Sleisenger, MH, and Fordtran, JS (eds): Gastrointestinal Diseases, ed 4. WB Saunders, Philadelphia, 1989.

Tietz, NW (ed): Clinical Guide to Laboratory Tests, ed 3. WB Saunders, Philadelphia, 1997.

Treseler, KM: Clinical Laboratory and Diagnostic Tests, ed 3. Appleton & Lange, Norwalk, Conn, 1994.

Wallach, J: Interpretation of Diagnostic Tests: A Synopsis of Laboratory Medicine, ed 6. Little, Brown & Co, Boston, 1996.

14

Analysis of Cells and Tissues

➤ **TESTS COVERED**

Papanicolaou Smear (Pap Smear), *478*
Skin Biopsy, *481*
Bone Biopsy, *482*
Breast Biopsy, *484*
Cervical Punch Biopsy, *485*
Biopsy of Bladder/Ureter, *487*
Renal Biopsy (Kidney Biopsy), *489*
Chorionic Villus Biopsy (CVB), *492*

Liver Biopsy, *494*
Muscle Biopsy, *496*
Lymph Node Biopsy, *497*
Intestinal Biopsy (Small Intestine), *498*
Lung Biopsy, *501*
Pleural Biopsy, *503*
Prostate Gland Biopsy, *505*
Thyroid Gland Biopsy, *507*

OVERVIEW OF CYTOLOGIC AND HISTOLOGICAL METHODS

The cells and tissues of the body may be analyzed through cytologic and histological methods. *Cytology* refers to the study of the structure, function, and pathology of cells. *Histology* deals with the study of the structure, function, and pathology of tissues. Both methods are used primarily to detect cancer.

Cytologic methods are used mainly as screening procedures to detect precancerous or malignant cells. Laboratory techniques were developed by George Papanicolaou, who identified characteristics that allowed for differentiation of normal from neoplastic cells. This differentiation is based on changes that occur in the relationships between the cytoplasm and the nucleus of cells.[1] In performing cytologic examinations, slides with cells are stained with various substances and are then examined microscopically. Malignant cells may show large, darkly stained irregular nuclei.[2]

The most common site examined through cytologic methods is the uterine cervix and endometrium (site of the "Pap smear"). Cells from the respiratory tract are also frequently examined. Samples of such cells may be obtained through sputum specimens (see Chap. 7), bronchial brushings or washings obtained during bronchoscopic examinations, or from postbronchoscopy sputum specimens. Various body fluids may also be examined for abnormal cells. Such fluids include urine (see Chap. 6); cerebrospinal fluid (see Chap. 8); and pleural, peritoneal, pericardial, and synovial effusions (see Chap. 9).

The method of reporting results of cytologic examinations varies somewhat with the laboratory. Papanicolaou developed a numerical classification system for the various types of cells found on cytologic examination. Because of problems with overlapping classes and variation in laboratory interpretation, narrative descriptions of the cells are now more likely to be used.[3]

It should be noted that cellular changes that mimic neoplastic changes may occur in response to inflammatory processes. Thus, the cytologist should be provided with information about the client so that accurate interpretation of the cell types present may be made.[4]

In addition to its use in cancer detection, cytologic study may provide other types of diagnostic information. By examining cells obtained from the oral cavity, female sexual chromosomes (Barr bodies) may be identified. Various Papanicolaou stains may elicit cell types associated with viral or fungal infections. Analysis of cells from effusions may also demonstrate cell types associated with collagen vascular diseases such as systemic lupus erythematosus (SLE) and rheumatoid arthritis. The nature of the cells present in vaginal smears may indicate the client's estrogen levels.[5]

Histological methods are used primarily to confirm the diagnosis of cancer when screening tests are positive for abnormal cells. Histological techniques involve obtaining samples of tissue by biopsy and examining them microscopically. Such an evaluation involves examining the structure of the tissues and may also include cytologic study of the cells through the use of various staining techniques. Electron microscopy methods also have been used.[6]

If the tissue sample is that of a tumor, it is examined in relation to anatomic size, position, and extent of the tumor. Whether malignant cells have invaded blood or lymphatic channels also is assessed.[7] Sections of tissue obtained at surgery may be frozen (i.e., "frozen sections") and analyzed during the surgical procedure to determine whether more extensive surgery is needed, thus avoiding the client's being subjected to a second procedure.

In addition to samples obtained during surgery, biopsies of tissues may be performed by local excision, needle aspiration, or biopsy (Fig. 14–1) or with special instruments such as tissue punches and curettes. Tissue samples may also be obtained during various endoscopic procedures (see Chap. 16). Common sites for biopsies are the skin, mucous membranes, serous membranes (e.g., pleurae), synovial membranes lining joints, various organs (e.g., liver, kidney, lung), glands (e.g., thyroid, prostate), lymph nodes, bone, muscle, and female reproductive tissues. Bone marrow biopsies also are performed (see Chap. 1).

TESTS OF CELLS AND TISSUES

PAPANICOLAOU SMEAR (PAP SMEAR)

The Papanicolaou (Pap) smear is used primarily in the early detection of cervical cancer. Results of Pap smears are reported in various ways, depending on the laboratory's preference. The traditional method for reporting results is shown here:

Class I	Normal cells only
Class II	Atypical cells but not malignant/inflammatory
Class III	Atypical cells, suspicious of malignancy/mild cervical dysplasia
Class IV	Atypical cells, suggestive of malignancy/severe cervical dysplasia
Class V	Cancer cells present, conclusive for malignancy/cancer

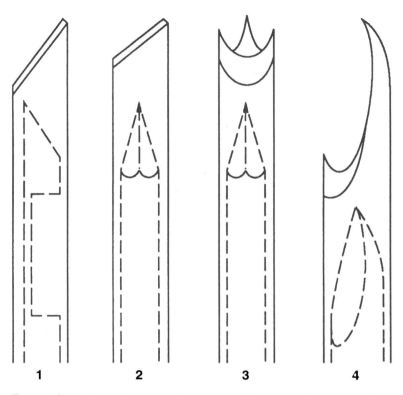

Figure 14–1 Types of biopsy needles: 1. Tru-cut; 2. Turner; 3. Franseen; 4. Shark Jaw.

Abnormal results of Pap smears should be followed by either repeat Pap smears or cervical biopsies. It is recommended that women between the ages of 20 and 40 have a Pap smear at least every 3 years. Women over 40 should have a Pap smear every year. More frequent examinations may be performed in women who are at high risk for developing cervical cancer (e.g., positive family history).

Reference Values

No abnormal cells (class I Pap smear)

Interfering Factors

➤ Douching within 24 hours of the test, which may wash away cells that would have been obtained on sampling
➤ Use of lubricating jelly on the vaginal speculum, which may alter the sample
➤ Improper specimen collection (Samples for cancer screening are obtained from the posterior vaginal fornix and from the cervix; samples for hormonal evaluation are obtained from the vagina.)

➤ Improper preservation of the specimen upon collection
➤ Collection of the sample during menstruation; blood in the sample may impair identification of abnormal cells

Indications for Papanicolaou Smear (Pap Smear)

➤ Routine screening for cervical cancer
➤ Evaluation of estrogen levels and response to therapy with estrogen
➤ Identification of inflammatory tissue changes
➤ Detection of viral and fungal vaginal infections

Nursing Care Before the Procedure

Explain to the client:
➤ That the test should not be performed when the client is menstruating
➤ That the client should not douche or have sexual intercourse for at least 24 hours before the test
➤ That, if she has been using antibiotic vaginal medication, she should discontinue it and the test should be delayed for 1 month
➤ That all clothing below the waist must be removed, except for the shoes, which may be kept on (If the Pap smear is to be performed along with a breast examination, it may be necessary to remove all clothing and don an examination gown.)
➤ That the examination will be performed with the client positioned on a gynecologic examination table
➤ That a metal or plastic vaginal speculum will be inserted to visualize the cervix
➤ That slight discomfort may be experienced when the speculum is inserted
➤ That relaxation and controlled breathing aid in reducing discomfort during the examination
➤ That samples of vaginal and cervical cells will be obtained with a small wooden spatula or with a cotton-topped applicator
➤ That the examiner may perform a bimanual examination involving the vagina, rectum, and pelvic cavity as part of the examination
➤ That a breast examination may also be performed as part of the gynecologic evaluation
➤ That the entire procedure should take approximately 15 minutes
Prepare for the procedure:
➤ Ensure that the client voids immediately before the examination.
➤ Obtain a brief gynecologic history that includes the date of the last menstrual period, frequency of periods, duration of periods, type of menstrual flow, date of last Pap smear, and use of birth control pills or other medications containing hormones.

The Procedure

The equipment needed is assembled, including vaginal speculum, gloves, wooden spatulas or cotton-tipped applicators, slides, preservative or spray fixative, marking pens for labeling the samples, and lubricant if a bimanual examination is to be performed after the Pap smear has been obtained.

The client is positioned on the examination table. The feet should not be placed in the stirrups until immediately before the Pap smear is to be obtained.

When the feet have been positioned, the client should be instructed to allow her legs to "drop" to each side and to attempt to relax as much as possible. The client's legs should be draped to avoid excessive and unnecessary exposure and chilling and to reduce embarrassment.

The speculum may be dipped or rinsed in water to aid in insertion but should not be lubricated. With the speculum positioned, vaginal and cervical samples are obtained and placed on slides. The slides should be fixed with spray or placed in preservative immediately.

The speculum is removed. If a bimanual pelvic examination is to be performed, it takes place at this time. However, a breast examination is usually performed before obtaining the Pap smear.

Nursing Care After the Procedure

Care and assessment after the procedure include assisting the client in removing the legs from the stirrups and allowing the client to rest in a supine position for a period of time.

➤ Cleanse or allow client to cleanse excess lubricant or secretions from the perineal area.

➤ Provide a perineal pad if cervical bleeding occurs.

➤ *Follow-up examination:* Note and report results of the Pap smear, and advise client of the timing and importance of the next examination. Explain treatment of dysplasia if it is present.

SKIN BIOPSY

Skin biopsies are performed to detect malignancies and are indicated when skin lesions have suspicious appearance or when they change in size, color, or texture. Skin biopsies may be performed with a biopsy punch or by scraping or excising the lesion using a scalpel.

Reference Values

No abnormal cells or tissue present

Indications for Skin Biopsy

➤ Evaluation of skin lesions that are suspected of malignancy

➤ Diagnosis of keratoses, warts, moles, keloids, fibromas, cysts, or inflammatory lesions

Nursing Care Before the Procedure

Explain to the client:

➤ That the test involves removing a small skin sample or portion of a skin lesion

➤ That the test will be performed by a physician

➤ That it may be necessary to shave the site before the biopsy

➤ That a local anesthetic will be either sprayed onto or injected at the biopsy site to prevent pain

➤ That one or two sutures may be necessary to close the biopsy site, depending on its extent

➤ That a dressing or Band-Aid will be applied to the site after the procedure

The Procedure

The equipment needed is assembled, including sterile drapes (depending on the site and the extent of the lesion), materials for cleansing the skin, equipment for obtaining the sample, local anesthetic, jar with formalin to preserve the specimen, suture or other material to close the biopsy site, sterile gloves, and dressings or Band-Aids.

The client is assisted to a position of comfort and the area to be biopsied is adequately supported and exposed. The area is then cleansed with antiseptic solution. A local anesthetic is applied by either topical spray or needle infiltration. Depending on the size of the lesion to be biopsied, the area may be draped with sterile drapes.

If the sample is to be obtained by curettage, the surface of the lesion is scraped with a curette until adequate tissue samples are obtained. The scrapings are placed on a microscope slide and preserved with an appropriate fixative. The sample is sent to the laboratory immediately. If bleeding occurs, a Band-Aid is applied to the site.

If the sample is to be obtained by shave or excision, a scalpel is used to remove the portion of the lesion that protrudes above the epidermis. Bleeding is controlled with digital pressure. A sterile dressing or Band-Aid is applied to the site. The sample is placed in an appropriate fixative (usually in formalin) and sent to the laboratory immediately.

If the sample is to be obtained by punch biopsy, a small round "cookie-cutter" punch, 4 to 6 mm in diameter, is rotated into the skin to the desired depth. The cylinder of skin is pulled upward with a forceps and separated at its base with a pointed scalpel or scissors. The site may then be closed using sutures or other material, and a sterile dressing is applied. The specimen is placed in an appropriate fixative and sent to the laboratory immediately.

Nursing Care After the Procedure

Care and assessment after the procedure include allowing the client to rest for a period of time, if needed.
➤ Assess dressing or Band-Aid for excessive bleeding.
➤ Instruct client in care and assessment of the site.
➤ Inform client of follow-up appointment to remove sutures, if any are present.
➤ *Pain or infection, or both, at site:* Note and report excessive bleeding, redness, edema, or pain at the biopsy site. Instruct the client to maintain a dry and clean site until it is healed. Change dressing as needed. Administer ordered mild analgesic and antibiotic therapy.

BONE BIOPSY

A bone biopsy consists of removing a plug of bone with a special serrated needle or surgically excising a sample of bone for examination before further surgery for bone disease. If performed by surgical excision (i.e., "open" biopsy), the preparation and procedure are the same as for any orthopedic surgical procedure requiring general anesthesia. Bone biopsies are generally indicated when x-ray examination shows evidence of a lesion involving bone.

Reference Values

No abnormal cells or tissue present

Indications for Bone Biopsy

➤ Radiographic evidence of a bone lesion
➤ Differentiation of benign from malignant bone lesions
➤ Identification of the source of a metastatic lesion involving bone

Nursing Care Before the Procedure

Explain to the client:

➤ The method that will be used to obtain the sample (needle biopsy or surgical excision)
➤ That the procedure will be performed by a physician
➤ That foods and fluids are usually not restricted before a needle biopsy but are restricted before an open biopsy
➤ That special skin preparation may be required (e.g., shave, orthopedic skin prep), especially for an open biopsy
➤ The type of anesthetic to be administered (local infiltration for needle biopsies, general anesthesia for open biopsies)
➤ That, if a needle biopsy is to be performed, momentary discomfort may be experienced when the periosteum is penetrated
➤ That a dressing will be applied to the site
➤ That analgesics may be administered after the procedure to alleviate any discomfort

Prepare for the procedure:

➤ For an open biopsy, the physical preparation is the same as for any surgical procedure requiring general anesthesia. A shave or orthopedic skin prep, or both, may be required before the procedure.
➤ For a needle biopsy, a shave and orthopedic skin prep may be required. The client should be assisted to disrobe as necessary and should be provided with a hospital gown.

The Procedure

For an open biopsy, the samples are obtained through surgical excision during the operative procedure.

For a needle biopsy, the client is assisted to a position of comfort, and the biopsy site is supported and exposed. The skin is cleansed with an antiseptic solution, injected with local anesthetic, and draped with sterile drapes. A small incision is made, and the biopsy needle is inserted to obtain a plug of bone. The sample is placed in formalin and sent to the laboratory immediately. The incision may be closed with sutures or other material and a sterile dressing applied.

Nursing Care After the Procedure

Care and assessment after the procedure are the same as for skin biopsy (see p. 482).

➤ After open biopsy, perform care in the same manner as for anyone who has had surgery with general anesthesia.

BREAST BIOPSY

Breast lesions can be localized by palpation, mammography, or ultrasound, but the nature of the lesion can be confirmed only by biopsy. The tissue sample may be obtained by needle aspiration or by open incision. Many physicians perform only open biopsies, excising the entire lesion rather than aspirating only a small sample.

A mammotest is a more recently developed type of breast biopsy performed for early detection and diagnosis of breast malignancy. It is performed in the x-ray department using a special instrument to assist in obtaining a core biopsy (small amount of tissue) of the breast. The site is anesthetized with a local injection and a small incision is made to introduce the needle to obtain the biopsy. Several areas can be biopsied if indicated. The method is considered to be as accurate as an open biopsy if the proper protocol is followed.

Reference Values

No abnormal cells or tissue present

Indications for Breast Biopsy

➤ Evidence of a breast lesion by palpation, mammography, or ultrasound
➤ Observable breast changes such as "peau d'orange" skin, scaly skin of nipple or areola, drainage from nipple, or ulceration of skin
➤ Differentiation of benign from malignant breast lesions

Nursing Care Before the Procedure

Explain to the client:
➤ That the procedure will be performed by a physician
➤ The method that will be used to obtain the sample (needle biopsy or surgical excision)
➤ That foods and fluids are not usually restricted before a needle biopsy but are restricted before an open biopsy
➤ The type of anesthetic to be administered (local infiltration for a needle biopsy, general anesthesia for an open biopsy)
➤ That a dressing will be applied to the site
➤ That analgesics may be administered after the procedure to alleviate any discomfort
Prepare for the procedure:
➤ For an open biopsy, the physical preparation is the same as for any surgical procedure requiring general anesthesia.
➤ For a needle biopsy, the client should disrobe from the waist up and should be provided with a hospital gown with the opening in the front.

The Procedure

For an open biopsy, the sample is obtained through surgical excision during the operative procedure.

For a needle biopsy, the client is assisted to a supine position and the area to be biopsied is exposed. The skin is cleansed with antiseptic, injected with local anesthetic, and draped with sterile drapes. A needle (either a Vim-Silverman biopsy needle or an 18-gauge needle) is inserted into the mass. A plug of tissue or bolus of fluid is aspirated via a syringe connected to the needle. The tissue is placed in a specimen container with normal saline; fluid is gently expelled into a green-topped (heparinized) blood collection tube. The samples should be sent to the laboratory immediately. A sterile dressing is applied to the biopsy site.

Nursing Care After the Procedure

Care and assessment after the procedure are the same as for skin biopsy (see p. 482).

➤ After an open biopsy, perform care in the same manner as for anyone who has had surgery with general anesthesia.

➤ *Pain or infection:* Note and report degree of pain after the procedure. Apply an ice bag to the site. Inform client to assess for and report redness, edema, or drainage at the biopsy site. Advise client to wear a bra with good support 24 hr/day after the procedure until healing is complete. Administer ordered analgesic and antibiotic therapy.

➤ *Breast self-examination:* Instruct client to perform monthly breast self-examination (BSE) and to have mammography annually to ensure early detection of breast malignancy. Offer literature from the American Cancer Society about the prevention and treatment of breast pathology.

CERVICAL PUNCH BIOPSY

Punch biopsy of the uterine cervix may be performed during a routine pelvic examination if abnormal areas are noted, or it may be indicated by abnormal results of a Pap smear (see p. 479) or a positive Schiller test. The Schiller test involves applying iodine solution to the cervix. Normal tissues stain dark brown, but abnormal tissues fail to pick up the color. Both the Schiller test and punch biopsy of the cervix are performed using a colposcope, a specialized binocular microscope that allows direct visualization of the cervix. Punch biopsy results may indicate the need for the more extensive cone biopsy of the cervix. This operative procedure involves excision of cervical tissue and requires general anesthesia.

Reference Values

No abnormal cells or tissue present

Indications for Cervical Punch Biopsy

➤ Abnormal Pap smear
➤ Schiller test positive for abnormal cells or tissue (see p. 479)
➤ Appearance of abnormal cells or tissue (e.g., ulceration, leukoplakia, polyps) on colposcopic examination
➤ Differentiation of benign from malignant cells or tissue

Contraindications

➤ Acute pelvic inflammatory disease
➤ Cervicitis
➤ Bleeding disorder

Nursing Care Before the Procedure

Explain to the client:
- ➤ That the test should not be performed when the client is menstruating and is best performed approximately 1 week after her period has ended
- ➤ That all clothing below the waist needs to be removed, except for the shoes, which may be kept on
- ➤ That the procedure will be performed with the client positioned on a gynecologic examination table
- ➤ That a metal or plastic vaginal speculum will be inserted to visualize the cervix
- ➤ That slight discomfort may be experienced when the speculum is inserted
- ➤ That relaxation and controlled breathing aid in reducing discomfort during the examination
- ➤ That the cervix may be swabbed with iodine to aid in identification of abnormal cells (If the client is allergic to iodine, it should be noted before the test.)
- ➤ That a microscope-like device will be used to more clearly visualize the cervix but that it is not inserted into the vagina
- ➤ That a small sample of cervical tissue will be obtained with forceps
- ➤ That mild discomfort may be experienced when the sample is removed as well as after the test
- ➤ That the entire procedure should take approximately 15 minutes
- ➤ That a small amount of cervical bleeding may occur after the procedure
- ➤ That a gray-green vaginal discharge may persist for a few days to a few weeks after the procedure
- ➤ That strenuous exercise should be avoided for 8 to 24 hours after the procedure
- ➤ That douching and intercourse should be avoided for approximately 2 weeks after the procedure or as directed by the physician

Prepare for the procedure:
- ➤ Ensure that the client voids immediately before the procedure.

The Procedure

The client is positioned on the examination table. The legs are draped and the external genitalia cleansed with an antiseptic solution. The vaginal speculum is inserted using water as a lubricant if a Pap smear is to be performed before the biopsy (see p. 481).

For the biopsy, the cervix is swabbed with 3 percent acetic acid to remove mucus and improve the contrast between tissue types. If the Schiller test is to be performed, the cervix is swabbed with iodine solution to aid in identification of abnormal cells. The colposcope is inserted through the speculum and is focused on the cervix. If an area is identified as abnormal, the biopsy forceps are inserted through the speculum or colposcope, and tissue samples are obtained. The samples are placed in specimen containers with formalin solution. The containers should be labeled with the source of the samples.

Bleeding, which is not uncommon after a cervical punch biopsy, may be controlled by cautery or suturing or by applying silver nitrate or ferric subsulfate to the site. If bleeding persists, a tampon may be inserted by the physician after removal of the speculum.

Nursing Care After the Procedure

Care and assessment after the procedure include assisting the client to remove the legs from the stirrups and allowing the client to rest for a period of time.

➤ Assist client in cleansing excess lubricant, solutions, or secretions from the perineal area and in dressing, if needed.

➤ Inform the client that she should remove the vaginal tampon in 8 to 24 hours and wear a pad if bleeding or drainage is present.

➤ Remind the client that a gray-green vaginal discharge can persist for a few days to a few weeks and that strenuous activity should be avoided for 8 to 24 hours and douching and intercourse for 2 weeks or as otherwise directed by the physician.[8]

➤ *Hemorrhage:* Note and report excessive and prolonged vaginal bleeding after the removal of the tampon. Instruct the client to assess for and report excessive bleeding.

BIOPSY OF BLADDER/URETER

Biopsies of the bladder and ureter are usually performed during cystoscopic examinations of the bladder. Such biopsies are indicated if a bladder tumor is visualized radiologically, if the symptoms persist after excision of bladder polyps or tumors, and if a hydroureter without kidney stones is evident.

Reference Values

No abnormal cells or tissue present

Indications for Biopsy of Bladder/Ureter

➤ Differentiation between benign and malignant lesions involving the bladder or ureter, or both, especially if bladder tumor is evident on radiologic examination or if hydroureter is present without stones

➤ Monitoring of recurrent lesions of the bladder or ureter for malignant changes

Contraindications

➤ Acute cystitis
➤ Bleeding disorders

Nursing Care Before the Procedure

Explain to the client:

➤ That the procedure will be performed by a urologist during a cystoscopic examination of the bladder

➤ That a sedative may be administered before the procedure to promote relaxation

➤ The type of anesthetic to be administered (local or general anesthesia may be used)

➤ That, if general anesthesia is to be used, foods and fluids are withheld for 8 hours before the procedure

➤ That, if local anesthesia is to be used, only clear liquids may be taken for 8 hours before the test

➤ That the test will be performed with the client positioned on a special urologic table and that the legs will be elevated in stirrups

➤ That after he or she is positioned on the table, the legs will be draped and the external genitalia will be cleansed with antiseptic solution

➤ That a special microscope-like instrument will be inserted into the urethra to visualize the bladder

➤ That, if local anesthesia is used, a sensation of pressure or of having to void, or both sensations, may be experienced

➤ That a small amount of tissue will be removed from the bladder or ureter, or from both, with a special brush or forceps inserted through the cystoscope

➤ That, after tissue removal and inspection of the bladder and urethra, the cystoscope will be removed

➤ That vital signs and urinary output will be monitored closely after the test

➤ That burning or discomfort on urination may be experienced for the first few voidings after the test

➤ That urine may be blood tinged for the first and second voidings after the test

Prepare for the procedure:

➤ Assist the client to disrobe from at least the waist down and provide a hospital gown, if necessary.

➤ Ensure to the extent possible that dietary or fluid restrictions, or both, are followed before the test.

➤ If general anesthesia is to be used, the physical preparation is the same as for any surgical procedure requiring general anesthesia.

➤ If local anesthesia is to be used, the client's vital signs are checked and premedication is administered as ordered.

The Procedure

The client is positioned on the examination table, and the legs are placed in the stirrups and draped. If general anesthesia is to be used, it is administered before positioning the client on the table. The external genitalia are cleansed with antiseptic solution. If a local anesthetic is to be used, it is instilled into the urethra and retained for 5 to 10 minutes. A penile clamp may be used for male clients to aid in retention of the anesthetic.

The cystoscope alone may be used for the examination or a urethroscope may be used to examine the urethra before cystoscopy. The urethroscope has a sheath that may be left in place and the cystoscope may be inserted through it, thus avoiding multiple instrumentations. After the cystoscope is inserted, the bladder is irrigated and then inspected. Urine samples may be obtained before bladder irrigation.

The area of the bladder to be biopsied is identified and tissues are removed by cytology brush or biopsy forceps. If a tumor is found and if it is small and localized, it may be excised. Bleeding may be controlled using electrocautery. If ureteral samples are needed, small catheters may be inserted into the ureters via the cystoscope. Specimens obtained for biopsy are placed in appropriate containers and sent to the laboratory immediately.

On completion of cystoscopy and collection of tissue samples, the cystoscope is withdrawn. The client's legs are removed from the stirrups, and the supine position is assumed.

Nursing Care After the Procedure

Care and assessment after the procedure are the same as for skin biopsy (see p. 482).

➤ If local anesthesia was used, monitor vital signs and compare with baseline values.

➤ If a general anesthesia was used, perform care in the same manner as for anyone who has had this type of anesthesia. Resume food and fluid withheld before the procedure. Encourage a fluid intake of 3000 mL per 24 hours unless contraindicated.

➤ *Hemorrhage:* Note and report change in vital signs or hematuria, or both, after the second voiding. Collect and send urine specimen to the laboratory. Test urine for occult blood with dipstick. Monitor intake and output (I&O) for 24 hours.

➤ *Urinary pattern changes:* Note and report resumption of normal voiding pattern, time and amount of voidings as well as urine characteristics, bladder distention, incomplete emptying of the bladder, suprapubic or flank pain, chills, fever, or bladder spasms. Administer ordered analgesic and warm sitz or hip baths to alleviate discomfort. Administer prophylactic antibiotic therapy, if ordered. Instruct client in monitoring urinary output and instruct to report pain, chills, bleeding, and fever to physician if client is an outpatient.

RENAL BIOPSY (KIDNEY BIOPSY)

Renal biopsy involves obtaining a sample of kidney tissue for histological and cytologic evaluation. The test may be performed by percutaneous needle biopsy (closed biopsy) or through surgical incision (open biopsy). Lesions of the kidney may be localized by renal computed axial tomography (CAT) scan or ultrasound.

Renal biopsy, especially when performed by the percutaneous method, is not without its attendant risks. Bleeding within the kidney, damage to renal tissue, and infection may occur. Therefore, this procedure is performed only when absolutely necessary to obtain data not otherwise available through blood, urine, and noninvasive radiologic tests.

Reference Values

No abnormal cells or tissue present

Indications for Renal Biopsy (Kidney Biopsy)

➤ Determination of the nature of lesions of the kidney identified by renal CAT scan or ultrasound (e.g., benign versus malignant lesions)

➤ Hematuria, proteinuria, or urinary casts, or a combination of these conditions, of unknown etiology, to determine the nature of the renal disorder

➤ Monitoring of the progression of nephrotic syndrome

➤ Acute or rapidly progressing renal failure of unknown etiology

➤ Systemic lupus erythematosus (SLE) with urinary abnormalities, to determine the extent of renal involvement

➤ Suspected renal cysts to confirm the diagnosis

➤ Monitoring of the function of a transplanted kidney

Contraindications

> Bleeding disorders
> Advanced renal disease with uremia
> Severe, uncontrolled hypertension
> Solitary kidney (except transplanted kidney)
> Gross obesity and severe spinal deformity (contraindicates percutaneous needle biopsy)
> Inability of the client to cooperate during the procedure (contraindicates percutaneous needle biopsy)

➤➤ Nursing Alert

- Renal biopsy, especially when performed by the percutaneous method, may result in bleeding within the kidney, damage to renal tissue, and infection.
- Before the procedure the client's hematologic status and blood clotting ability must be assessed; therefore, a complete blood count (CBC), platelet level, prothrombin time (PT), partial thromboplastin time (PTT), clotting time, and bleeding time should be performed before the test. (In addition, a type and cross-match for 2 units of blood may be ordered.)
- After the procedure, the client's vital signs, amount of urine output, characteristics of urine output, and comfort level must be monitored closely for early detection of possible complications.

Nursing Care Before the Procedure

Explain to the client:
> That the procedure will be performed by a physician
> The method that will be used to obtain the sample (percutaneous [closed] biopsy or surgical [open] biopsy)
> The type of anesthesia to be administered (local infiltration for needle biopsies, general anesthesia for open biopsies)
> That foods and fluids are withheld for 6 to 8 hours before the procedure
> That a sedative may be administered before the procedure
> That, if a needle biopsy is performed, it will be necessary to remain motionless and breathe as instructed during certain portions of the procedure
> That, if a needle biopsy is performed, a pressure dressing will be applied to the site
> That, after a needle biopsy, the client will be required to lie on the biopsied side for at least 30 minutes, with a pillow or a sandbag under the site to prevent bleeding
> That bed rest is required for 24 hours after the procedure
> That vital signs and urinary output will be monitored closely for at least 24 hours after the test
> That, unless medically contraindicated, the client should have a fluid intake of approximately 3 qt (3000 mL) for at least the first 24 hours after the test

➤ That strenuous activity, sports, and heavy lifting should be avoided for at least 2 weeks after the test

➤ That any discomfort, especially in the area of the kidneys, shoulders, or abdomen, should be reported immediately

Prepare for the procedure:

➤ Ensure that a signed consent for the procedure has been obtained.

➤ If the skin at the biopsy site is unusually hirsute, it may be necessary to shave the site before the procedure.

➤ Ensure to the extent possible that dietary and fluid restrictions are followed before the test.

➤ If an open biopsy is to be performed, the physical preparation is the same as for any surgical procedure requiring general anesthesia.

➤ For a percutaneous needle biopsy, the client's vital signs are taken and compared with baseline levels. The client should void immediately before the procedure and be provided with a hospital gown. (The premedication, if ordered, is administered 30 to 60 minutes before the procedure).

The Procedure

For an open biopsy, the samples are collected during the operative procedure.

For a percutaneous needle biopsy, the client is assisted to the prone position. A sandbag may be placed beneath the abdomen to aid in moving the kidneys to the posterior and in maintaining the desired position. The biopsy site is exposed, cleansed with antiseptic, and draped with sterile drapes. The skin and subcutaneous tissues are then infiltrated with a local anesthetic.

To facilitate downward movement and subsequent immobilization of the kidneys, the client is instructed to take a deep breath and hold it as the biopsy needle (usually a Vim-Silverman needle) is inserted. As the needle enters the kidney, the client is instructed to exhale. The needle is rotated to obtain a plug of tissue and then withdrawn. Manual pressure is applied to the site for 5 to 20 minutes. If there is no evidence of bleeding, a pressure dressing is applied. The tissue sample is placed in a container with buffered saline and sent immediately to the laboratory.

Nursing Care After the Procedure

Care and assessment after an open biopsy are the same as for anyone who has had surgery requiring general anesthesia.

➤ For a percutaneous biopsy, place the client on the biopsied side and maintain the position with a small pillow or sandbag under the biopsy site for at least 30 minutes.

➤ Maintain complete bed rest for 24 hours after the test.

➤ Resume foods and fluids withheld before the test.

➤ Unless medically contraindicated, encourage the client to take in 3000 mL of fluid during the first 24 hours after the procedure.

➤ Collect a urine specimen for culture and sensitivity (C&S) 24 hours after the test.

➤ Remind client that heavy lifting or any strenous activities should be avoided for 1 week after the procedure.

➤ Take and record vital signs as for a postoperative client whether the biopsy was performed by open or closed technique (i.e., every 15 minutes for the

first hour, every 30 minutes for the next 2 hours, every hour for the next 4 hours, and then every 4 hours for 24 hours).
➤ Assess the biopsy site for bleeding, hematoma formation, and inflammation each time vital signs are taken.
➤ Assess the client's comfort level, and report immediately any complaints of perirenal, shoulder, or abdominal pain.
➤ Monitor time and amount of each voiding.
➤ Assess each voiding for the presence of blood. This assessment may involve using dipsticks to detect microscopic blood. Report immediately any grossly bloody urine.
➤ Monitor temperature for several days and instruct client to report burning and frequency of urination or any other change in urinary pattern.

CHORIONIC VILLUS BIOPSY (CVB)

Chorionic villus biopsy (CVB) is used to detect fetal abnormalities caused by various genetic disorders. The advantage of CVB over amniocentesis (see Chap. 10) is that CVB can be performed as early as the 8th week of pregnancy, thus permitting earlier decisions to retain or terminate the pregnancy.

Chorionic villi are fingerlike projections that cover the embryo and anchor it to the uterine lining before development of the placenta. Because chorionic villi are of embryonic origin, samples provide information about the developing baby. Chorionic villi samples are best obtained between the 8th and 10th weeks of pregnancy. After 10 weeks of pregnancy, the villi are overgrown with maternal cells.

CVB can be used to detect hundreds, and potentially even thousands, of genetic defects. It cannot, however, be used to detect neural tube defects such as spina bifida. For the latter condition, amniocentesis is still the test of choice.

CVB is performed in a manner similar to an amniocentesis, although entry into the amniotic sac is not necessary. The test carries with it the risks of damage to the chorionic membrane, bleeding, and possible spontaneous abortion even as late as 18 to 20 weeks of pregnancy. The number of spontaneous abortions attributed to CVB is estimated to be as low as 2 percent.[9]

In addition to the CVB's advantage of being performed earlier than amniocentesis, results are also available more quickly — many times within 48 hours of the study.

The developing embryo and chorion may be localized before or during the procedure by ultrasound or endoscopic tests.

Reference Values

No chromosomal abnormalities detected

Indications for Chorionic Villus Biopsy (CVB)

➤ Family history of genetic disorders (e.g., chromosomal abnormalities, enzyme deficiencies, sickle cell anemia or other hemoglobinopathies, Tay-Sachs disease)
➤ Maternal age over 35 years to screen for disorders such as Down syndrome
➤ Prenatal gender determination when the woman is a known carrier of a sex-linked disorder such as hemophilia

➤ Need for early decision to terminate or maintain pregnancy when fetal abnormality is suspected

Contraindications

➤ History of incompetent cervix

Nursing Care Before the Procedure

Explain to the client:
➤ That the procedure will be performed by a physician and requires approximately 15 minutes
➤ The precautions taken to avoid injury to the fetus (e.g., localization of the embryo by ultrasound)
➤ That all clothing below the waist must be removed, except for the shoes, which may be kept on
➤ That the procedure will be performed with the client positioned on a gynecologic examination table
➤ That a metal or plastic vaginal speculum will be inserted to visualize the cervix
➤ That slight discomfort may be experienced when the speculum is inserted
➤ That relaxation and controlled breathing aid in reducing discomfort during the examination
➤ That a small catheter will be inserted through the cervix to a site between the wall of the uterus and the developing embryo
➤ That a small amount of tissue will be removed by gentle suction
➤ That the suction catheter and speculum will then be removed
Prepare for the procedure:
➤ Ensure that the client voids immediately before the procedure.
➤ Take and record vital signs and compare with baseline readings.
➤ Obtain history of genetic disorders and counseling received.

The Procedure

The client is positioned on the examination table. The legs are draped, and the external genitalia may be cleansed with an antiseptic solution. The vaginal speculum is then inserted. For the biopsy, a suction catheter is inserted via the speculum through the cervical os to the biopsy site. The catheter is then connected to a 20-mL syringe, and approximately 10 mL of suction is applied. The suction is maintained as the catheter is withdrawn to avoid introducing cervical secretions into the uterus. The outside of the catheter is wiped to remove maternal secretions, and the tissue sample is flushed onto Petri dishes with an appropriate culture medium. The samples are labeled and sent to the laboratory immediately to be examined for chromosomal abnormalities.

Nursing Care After the Procedure

Care and assessment after the procedure are the same as for cervical biopsy (see p. 487).
➤ *Abnormal results:* If appropriate and timely, offer information about genetic counseling or pregnancy termination counseling, or both.
➤ *Hemorrhage or infection, or both:* Note and report vital sign and fetal heart rate changes, abdominal pain, temperature and chills, or excessive vaginal

bleeding. Inform the client to monitor and report these changes to the physician.

LIVER BIOPSY

Liver biopsy involves obtaining a sample of hepatic tissue for histological and cytologic evaluation. The test may be performed by percutaneous needle biopsy (closed biopsy) or through surgical incision (open biopsy). This test is indicated when liver disease is suspected but is not evidenced by less invasive procedures such as ultrasounds and CAT scans.

Liver biopsy, especially when performed by the percutaneous method, is not without its attendant risks: Bleeding within the liver, damage to hepatic tissue, and infection may occur. Therefore, this procedure is performed only when absolutely necessary.

Reference Values

No abnormal cells or tissue present

Indications for Liver Biopsy

➤ Suspected disease of the liver parenchyma (e.g., cirrhosis, malignancy, hemochromatosis, sarcoidosis, hepatitis, amyloidosis) to determine nature of the pathological problem
➤ Hepatomegaly (enlarged liver) or jaundice of unknown etiology
➤ Persistently elevated liver enzymes of unknown etiology

Contraindications

➤ Bleeding disorders
➤ Suspected vascular tumor of the liver
➤ Ascites, which may obscure location of the liver for percutaneous biopsy
➤ Subdiaphragmatic or right hemothoracic infection
➤ Infection involving the biliary tract
➤ Inability of the client to cooperate during the procedure (contraindicates percutaneous needle biopsy)

➤➤ Nursing Alert

- Liver biopsy, especially when performed by the percutaneous route, may result in bleeding within the liver, damage to hepatic tissue, and infection.
- Clients with liver disease frequently have impaired blood coagulation and are especially at risk for bleeding during or after this procedure.
- Before the procedure the client's hematologic status and blood clotting ability must be assessed; therefore, a CBC, platelet level, PT, PTT, clotting time, and bleeding time should be performed before the study.
- After the procedure the client's vital signs must be monitored closely; in addition, the client's comfort level must be assessed: Complaints of right shoulder or pleuritic chest pain should be reported immediately. (Respiratory distress caused by bleeding within the liver or inadvertent pneumothorax may also occur.)

Nursing Care Before the Procedure

Explain to the client:

➤ That the procedure will be performed by a physician
➤ The method that will be used to obtain the sample (percutaneous [closed] biopsy or surgical [open] biopsy)
➤ The type of anesthesia to be administered (local infiltration for needle biopsies, general anesthesia for open biopsies)
➤ That foods and fluids are withheld for 6 to 8 hours before the procedure
➤ That, if a needle biopsy is performed, it will be necessary to remain motionless and breathe as instructed during certain portions of the procedure (Allow client to practice holding the breath after an expiration.)
➤ That, if a needle biopsy is performed, the client may experience slight discomfort in the area of the right shoulder when the biopsy needle is introduced
➤ That, if a needle biopsy is performed, a pressure dressing will be applied to the site
➤ That, after a needle biopsy, the client must lie on the right side with a rolled towel or small pillow under the site to create pressure and prevent bleeding and that this position must be maintained for at least 2 hours
➤ That bed rest is required for 24 hours after the procedure
➤ That vital signs will be monitored closely for at least 24 hours after the test
➤ That any unusual or persistent discomfort or any difficulty breathing should be reported immediately

Prepare for the procedure:

➤ Ensure that a signed consent for the procedure has been obtained.
➤ If the skin at the biopsy site is unusually hirsute, it may be necessary to shave the site before the procedure.
➤ If an open biopsy is to be performed, the physical preparation is the same as for any surgical procedure requiring general anesthesia.
➤ For a percutaneous needle biopsy, the client's vital signs are taken and compared with baseline readings. The client should void immediately before the procedure and be provided with a hospital gown.
➤ Administer a sedative, if necessary, as ordered.

The Procedure

For an open biopsy, the samples are collected during the operative procedure.

For a percutaneous needle biopsy, the client is assisted to the supine or the left lateral position with the right hand under the head. The biopsy site is exposed, cleansed with antiseptic, and draped with sterile drapes. The skin and subcutaneous tissues are then infiltrated with a local anesthetic. The syringe is attached to the biopsy needle. The client is then instructed to take a deep breath, exhale forcefully, and hold his or her breath. The biopsy needle is then inserted, rotated to obtain a core of liver tissue, and quickly removed. It is important that the client remain motionless during biopsy needle insertion. After the needle is removed, the client may resume normal breathing. A pressure dressing is applied to the site. The sample is expelled from the needle into a container with formalin solution and sent to the laboratory immediately.

Nursing Care After the Procedure

Care and assessment after an open biopsy include care in the same manner as for anyone who has had surgery requiring general anesthesia.

➤ For a percutaneous biopsy, position client on the right side with a rolled towel or small pillow under the biopsy site to create pressure and prevent bleeding.

➤ Maintain this position for at least 2 hours.

➤ Maintain complete bed rest for 24 hours after the test.

➤ Resume foods and fluids withheld for the test.

➤ If ordered, administer analgesics for postbiopsy discomfort.

➤ Advise the client not to cough or strain after the procedure because it can increase intra-abdominal pressure.

➤ Take and record vital signs as for a postoperative client, whether the biopsy was performed by open or closed technique (i.e., every 15 minutes for the first hour, every 30 minutes for the next 2 hours, every hour for the next 4 hours, and then every 4 hours for 24 hours).

➤ Assess the biopsy site for bleeding, hematoma formation, bile leakage, and inflammation each time vital signs are taken.

➤ Assess the client's comfort level and immediately report pleuritic pain, persistent right shoulder pain, or abdominal pain.

➤ Assess the client's respiratory status and immediately report any signs or symptoms of respiratory distress.

MUSCLE BIOPSY

A muscle biopsy consists of obtaining a sample of tissue, usually from the deltoid or gastrocnemius muscle, for histological study. Muscle biopsies are indicated for suspected neuropathy or myopathy.

Reference Values

No abnormal cells or tissue present

Indications for Muscle Biopsy

➤ Family history of Duchenne's muscular dystrophy

➤ Diagnosis of suspected fungal or parasitic infestation of muscle

➤ Neuromuscular disorders of unknown etiology to differentiate between neuropathy and myopathy

Interfering Factors

➤ Electromyography (EMG), if performed before muscle biopsy, may produce residual inflammation leading to false-positive biopsy findings.

Nursing Care Before the Procedure

Explain to the client:

➤ That the procedure will be performed by a physician and takes approximately 15 minutes

➤ The site from which the sample will be obtained (usually the deltoid or gastrocnemius muscle)

➤ That it may be necessary to shave the biopsy site before the study
➤ That the procedure involves making a small incision over the muscle and removing a small bit of muscle tissue with a biopsy forceps
➤ That a local anesthetic will be injected at the biopsy site to alleviate discomfort
➤ That suture or other material may be necessary to close the biopsy site
➤ That a dressing will be applied to the biopsy site
➤ That the muscle will be tender to touch and movement for several days after the procedure
➤ That, if the area to be biopsied is hirsute, it may be necessary to shave it before the biopsy

The Procedure

The client is assisted to the necessary position (supine for deltoid biopsy, prone for gastrocnemius biopsy). The biopsy site is exposed, cleansed with antiseptic, and draped with sterile drapes. The skin and subcutaneous tissues are then infiltrated with a local anesthetic. A small incision is made over the muscle with a scalpel, and a bit of muscle tissue is then grasped with a forceps and excised. The sample is placed in normal saline and sent to the laboratory immediately. The incision is closed with sutures or other material, and a sterile dressing is applied.

Nursing Care After the Procedure

Care and assessment after the procedure are the same as for skin biopsy (see p. 482).

LYMPH NODE BIOPSY

Lymph node biopsies are performed when there is persistent enlargement of lymph nodes or signs and symptoms of systemic disease that may indicate malignant or infectious processes. The lymph nodes most commonly biopsied are the cervical, axillary, and inguinal nodes. Cervical lymph nodes drain the scalp and face; axillary lymph nodes drain the arms, breasts, and upper chest; and inguinal nodes drain the legs, external genitalia, and lower abdominal wall.

Lymph node biopsies may be performed by needle aspiration or by surgical excision. The latter approach is preferred when the node is deeper and when a larger or more complete sample of the node is required.

Reference Values

No abnormal cells or tissue present

Indications for Lymph Node Biopsy

➤ Persistent enlargement of one or more lymph nodes of unknown etiology, especially if accompanied by signs of systemic illness such as weight loss, fever, night sweats, cough, edema, and pain
➤ Differentiation between benign (e.g., sarcoidosis) and malignant (e.g., lymphomas, leukemias) disorders that may lead to enlarged lymph nodes
➤ Suspected fungal or parasitic infections involving the lymph nodes

➤ Staging of metastatic carcinomas, with the stage indicated by the extent of lymph node involvement

Nursing Care Before the Procedure

Explain to the client:

➤ The method that will be used to obtain the sample (needle biopsy or surgical excision)

➤ That foods and fluids are usually not restricted before a needle biopsy but are restricted before an excisional biopsy

➤ That the procedure will be performed by a physician

➤ The type of anesthesia to be administered (local infiltration for needle biopsies, general anesthesia for excisional biopsies if deeper nodes are to be removed)

➤ That, if an excisional biopsy is performed, sutures or other material may be used to close the biopsy site

➤ That a dressing will be applied to the biopsy site

➤ That analgesics may be administered after the procedure to alleviate any discomfort

➤ That, if the skin at the biopsy site is unusually hirsute, it may be necessary to shave the site before the procedure

Prepare for the procedure:

➤ Take and record vital signs and compare with baseline readings.

➤ Provide a hospital gown.

The Procedure

The site to be biopsied is exposed, cleansed with antiseptic, and draped with sterile drapes. If the biopsy is to be performed under local anesthesia, the skin and subcutaneous tissues are so infiltrated.

For surgical excision of the node, a small incision is made over the node. The lymph node is then grasped with forceps and placed in normal saline solution. The biopsy site is closed with sutures or other materials and a sterile dressing is applied.

For a needle biopsy, the lymph node is grasped with the fingers and a needle with syringe attached is inserted directly into the node. A specimen is then aspirated and placed in a container with normal saline solution. Pressure is applied to the site. If there is no bleeding, a sterile dressing is applied.

All specimens are sent to the laboratory immediately.

Nursing Care After the Procedure

Care and assessment after the procedure are the same as for skin biopsy (see p. 482).

➤ If general anesthesia was used, care is the same as for anyone who has had this type of anesthetic.

➤ Administer ordered analgesic therapy, if needed.

INTESTINAL BIOPSY (SMALL INTESTINE)

Biopsies of the small intestine are generally performed during endoscopic procedures. During these tests, samples of intestinal tissue may be obtained via the endoscope if abnormal lesions are visualized.

Reference Values

No abnormal cells or tissue present

Indications for Intestinal Biopsy (Small Intestine)

➤ Suspected malignant or premalignant tissue change on endoscopic visualization
➤ Differentiation between benign and malignant disorders involving the small intestine
➤ Diagnosis of various intestinal disorders such as lactose intolerance, enzyme deficiencies, sprue, and parasitic infestations

Interfering Factors

➤ Barium swallow within the preceding 48 hours

Contraindications

➤ Aneurysm of the aortic arch
➤ Inability of the client to cooperate during the procedure
➤ Bleeding disorders

Nursing Care Before the Procedure

Explain to the client:
➤ That the procedure will be performed during an endoscopic examination of the stomach and small intestine
➤ That foods and fluids are withheld for 6 to 8 hours before the procedure
➤ That a sedative may be administered before the procedure to promote relaxation
➤ That full or partial dentures should be removed before the procedure
➤ That the test may be performed with the client in a sitting or semireclining position
➤ That a flexible, microscope-like instrument will be inserted through the mouth and passed into the stomach and small intestine
➤ That the throat will be sprayed with a local anesthetic to make passage of the tube less uncomfortable
➤ That this anesthetic will have a bitter taste, may create a sensation of warmth, and may impair swallowing
➤ That a device may be inserted into the mouth to protect the teeth and prevent biting the endoscope
➤ That saliva will be removed by suctioning during the procedure (similar to dental suctioning)
➤ That, after the tube is inserted, the client may be assisted to a side-lying position
➤ That air may be injected into the stomach during the test to aid in visualization and that it may cause a sensation of fullness or bloating
➤ That the procedure may take from 45 minutes to an hour
➤ That, after the stomach and intestine have been visualized and tissue samples obtained, the endoscope and mouth device will be removed
➤ That vital signs will be monitored closely after the procedure
➤ That the client will not be permitted to eat or drink until the local anesthetic has worn off

➤ That activity may be restricted until the premedication has worn off
➤ That the client should report immediately any chest pain or upper abdominal pain, pain on swallowing, difficulty in breathing, and expectoration of blood

Prepare for the procedure:

➤ Remove full or partial dentures. If the client has any permanent crowns on the teeth (i.e., "caps"), the physician performing the test should be so informed.
➤ Provide a hospital gown.
➤ Have the client void.
➤ Take and record vital signs, and compare with baseline values.
➤ Administer premedication as ordered. (It may consist of an analgesic or a tranquilizer to reduce discomfort and promote relaxation, as well as atropine to reduce secretions.)

The Procedure

With the client seated in a semireclining position, a local anesthetic is sprayed into the throat and may also be swabbed in the mouth. A protective guard is inserted to cover the teeth. A bite block may also be inserted to maintain adequate opening of the mouth without client effort.

The endoscope is passed through the mouth, and the client is assisted to the left lateral position. The dental suction device is inserted to drain saliva. The esophagus may be examined and then the scope is advanced into the stomach. Gastric lavage may be performed to clear the stomach of residual. After the stomach is examined, the scope is advanced into the duodenum. Air may be injected through the endoscope to aid in visualizing structures. A cytology brush or biopsy forceps is introduced through the endoscope to obtain tissue samples. Specimens are placed in appropriate containers and are sent to the laboratory immediately. The dental suction device is removed, the endoscope is withdrawn, and the tooth guard and bite block are removed.

Nursing Care After the Procedure

Care and assessment after the procedure include assisting the client to a position of comfort and allowing the client to rest for a few minutes.

➤ Maintain side-lying position for 1 to 2 hours to prevent aspiration of secretions.
➤ Remind the client not to eat or drink until the local anesthetic has worn off and normal swallowing ability has returned.
➤ Remind the client to report immediately any chest or upper abdominal pain, pain on swallowing, difficulty in breathing, and expectoration of blood.
➤ Take and record vital signs. Additional readings may be required until vital signs are stable.
➤ Assess and record breath sounds and characteristics of respirations.
➤ Assess the client's ability to swallow.
➤ Assess the client's recovery from the premedication.
➤ Assess the client's comfort level and report immediately any complaints of chest pain, epigastric pain, periumbilical pain, and pain on swallowing.
➤ Assess the client's ability to resume usual food and fluid intake.

LUNG BIOPSY

Lung biopsy is the removal of a sample of lung tissue for cytologic and histological study. The sample may be obtained through "closed" methods, such as insertion of a needle through the chest wall and fiberoptic bronchoscopy, or by "open" biopsy, which entails a thoracotomy and general anesthesia.

This test should be performed with caution and only when necessary to obtain diagnostic information not otherwise available through less invasive procedures.

Reference Values

No abnormal cells or tissue present

Indications for Lung Biopsy

➤ Determination of the cause of diffuse pulmonary disease of unknown etiology
➤ Diagnosis of suspected malignancy, infection, or parasitic infestation
➤ Inconclusive results of less invasive tests such as chest x-ray examinations, computed tomography (CT) scans, and sputum analyses

Contraindications

➤ Bleeding disorders
➤ Hyperinflation of the lung
➤ Cor pulmonale
➤ Inability of the client to cooperate for the procedure (contraindicates needle biopsies and bronchoscopies performed under local anesthesia)

➤➤ Nursing Alert

- Lung biopsies may result in bleeding into lung tissue, pneumothorax, hemothorax, and infection.
- Before the procedure, the client's hematologic status and blood clotting ability must be assessed; therefore, a CBC, platelet level, PT, PTT, clotting time, and bleeding time should be performed.
- After the procedure, the client's vital signs, lung sounds, and comfort level are monitored closely for early detection of possible complications.

Nursing Care Before the Procedure

Explain to the client:
➤ That the procedure will be performed by a physician
➤ The method that will be used to obtain the sample (needle biopsy, bronchoscopy, or thoracotomy)
➤ The type of anesthesia to be administered (local anesthesia for needle biopsies, topical or general anesthesia for bronchoscopy, general anesthesia for thoracotomy)

➤ That foods and fluids are withheld for 6 to 8 hours before the procedure, especially if bronchoscopy is to be performed or general anesthesia is to be used
➤ That a sedative may be administered before the procedure
➤ That, if the specimen is to be obtained by bronchoscopy or thoracotomy, full or partial dentures should be removed before the procedure
➤ That, if a needle biopsy is to be performed, the client should remain as still as possible and refrain from coughing after the biopsy needle is inserted
➤ That, if a bronchoscopy is to be performed, a microscope-like instrument will be inserted through the mouth and passed into the trachea ("windpipe")
➤ That, if a thoracotomy is to be performed, a chest incision will be made and a chest tube will be inserted before the incision is closed
➤ That, after the procedure, vital signs and respiratory status will be monitored closely
➤ That, after the procedure, the client should report immediately any difficulty in breathing or other discomforts
➤ That sputum samples may be collected after bronchoscopy
➤ The type of activity restrictions that may be necessary after the procedure
Prepare for the procedure:
➤ For bronchoscopy or thoracotomy, remove full or partial dentures. If the client has any permanent crowns on the teeth (i.e., "caps"), the physician performing the procedure should be so informed.
➤ Provide a hospital gown.
➤ Have the client void.
➤ Take and record vital signs and compare with baseline readings.
➤ Administer premedication as ordered.

The Procedure

For a needle biopsy, the client is assisted to a sitting position with arms supported on a pillow on an overbed table. The needle insertion site is cleansed with an antiseptic solution, infiltrated with a local anesthetic, and draped with sterile drapes. The client is reminded to remain as still as possible and to avoid coughing during the procedure. The needle is inserted through the posterior chest wall into the selected intercostal space. A small incision may be made before needle insertion. After insertion, the needle is rotated to obtain the sample and is then withdrawn. Pressure is applied to the biopsy site. If there is no bleeding, a pressure dressing is applied. The sample is placed in formalin solution and sent to the laboratory immediately. If cultures are desired, the sample may be divided into two portions, with the portion for culture placed in a sterile container.

For a bronchoscopy, the client is initially positioned in relation to the type of anesthesia to be used. If general anesthesia is to be administered, the client is placed in the supine position and anesthetized. The neck is hyperextended and the bronchoscope introduced through the mouth. If local anesthesia is used, the client is seated and the tongue and oropharynx are sprayed and swabbed with anesthetic. The client is then assisted to a supine or a side-lying position and the bronchoscope is introduced through the mouth. Additional anesthetic is applied through the scope as it approaches the vocal cords and the carina, eliminating reflexes in these sensitive areas. After inspection through the bronchoscope, the samples are collected by bronchial brush or biopsy forceps. Specimens are placed in appropriate containers and sent to the laboratory immediately.

Open biopsies are performed in the operating room under general anesthesia. A thoracotomy is performed to obtain the sample, and a chest tube is inserted after the procedure.

Nursing Care After the Procedure

Care and assessment after a needle biopsy or bronchoscopy using local or topical anesthesia include positioning the client in a semi-Fowler's position to permit maximum ventilation and allowing the client to rest for a few minutes.

➤ Monitor vital signs and compare with baseline levels. Repeat at 15- to 30-minute intervals for 1 to 2 hours or until stable.

➤ If a needle biopsy was performed, assess the biopsy site for bleeding each time vital signs are taken.

➤ Assess breath sounds and observe for any signs of respiratory distress. Evaluate the client's comfort level.

➤ Resume foods and fluids withheld for the procedure if assessment data indicate that the client is stable.

➤ If a bronchoscopy was performed using local anesthesia, monitor vital signs and observe for signs of laryngospasm, bronchospasm, and laryngeal edema as indicated by wheezing, stridor, absence of air movement at the mouth or nares, anxiety, and cyanosis.

➤ Provide gargles or lozenges for throat discomfort.

➤ For an open biopsy, perform care and observation in the same manner as for anyone who has had a thoracotomy under general anesthesia.

➤ *Pneumothorax or hemothorax:* Note and report rapid and shallow respirations, dyspnea, air hunger, chest pain, cough, hemoptysis, or absence of breath sounds over the area. Prepare for needle aspiration of air or fluid or for insertion of a chest tube.

➤ *Infection:* Note and report change in respiratory status, chest pain, sputum that is yellow or other color, or elevated temperature. Monitor vital signs, administer ordered antibiotic therapy, and obtain sputum cultures for laboratory analysis.

PLEURAL BIOPSY

Pleural biopsy is the removal of a sample of pleural tissue for cytologic and histological study. It is usually performed by needle biopsy and may be undertaken as part of a thoracentesis (see Chap. 9). Open biopsy, requiring a thoracotomy using general anesthesia, may also be performed.

This test should be performed with caution and only when necessary to obtain diagnostic information not otherwise available through less invasive procedures.

Reference Values

No abnormal cells or tissue present

Indications for Pleural Biopsy

➤ Evidence of pleural effusion of unknown etiology

➤ Suspected tumor involving the pleura

➤ Differentiation between benign and malignant disorders involving the pleurae
➤ Determination of the cause of infection involving the pleurae (i.e., viral, fungal, bacterial, and parasitic infections)
➤ Diagnosis of fibrosis or collagen vascular disease involving the pleurae

Contraindications

➤ Bleeding disorders
➤ Inability of the client to cooperate in the procedure (contraindicates needle biopsies)

➤➤ Nursing Alert

- Pleural biopsies may result in bleeding into lung tissue, pneumothorax, hemothorax, and infection.
- Before the procedure, the client's hematologic status and blood clotting ability must be assessed. Therefore, a CBC, platelet level, PT, PTT, clotting time, and bleeding time should be performed.
- After the procedure, the client's vital signs, lung sounds, and comfort level are monitored closely for early detection of possible complications.

Nursing Care Before the Procedure

Explain to the client:
➤ That the procedure will be performed by a physician
➤ The method that will be used to obtain the sample (needle biopsy or open biopsy via thoracotomy)
➤ The type of anesthesia to be administered (local anesthesia for needle biopsy, general anesthesia for open biopsy)
➤ That foods and fluids are generally not withheld before a needle biopsy but are restricted for 6 to 8 hours before an open biopsy
➤ That a sedative may be administered before the procedure
➤ That, if a thoracotomy is to be performed, full or partial dentures should be removed before the procedure
➤ That, if a needle biopsy is to be performed, the client should remain as still as possible and refrain from coughing after the biopsy needle is inserted
➤ That, if a thoracotomy is performed, a chest incision will be made and a chest tube will be inserted before the incision is closed
➤ That, after the procedure, vital signs and respiratory status will be monitored closely
➤ That, after the procedure, the client should immediately report any difficulty in breathing or other discomfort
➤ The type of activity restrictions that may be necessary after the procedure
Prepare for the procedure:
➤ For thoracotomy, remove full or partial dentures.
➤ Assist the client to disrobe, and provide a hospital gown.
➤ Have the client void.
➤ Take and record vital signs and compare with baseline readings.
➤ Administer premedication as ordered.

The Procedure

For a needle biopsy, the client is assisted to a sitting position with arms supported on a pillow on an overbed table. The needle insertion site is cleansed with an antiseptic solution, infiltrated with a local anesthetic, and draped with sterile drapes. The client is reminded to remain as still as possible and to avoid coughing during the procedure. The needle is inserted through the posterior chest wall into the selected intercostal space, rotated to obtain the sample, and then withdrawn. Pressure is applied to the biopsy site. If there is no bleeding, a pressure dressing is applied. The sample is placed in formalin solution and sent to the laboratory immediately.

Open biopsies are performed in the operating room under general anesthesia. A thoracotomy is performed to obtain the sample, and a chest tube is inserted after the procedure.

Nursing Care After the Procedure

Care and assessment after a needle biopsy include positioning the client in a semi-Fowler's position to permit maximum ventilation.

➤ Monitor vital signs and compare with baseline levels. Repeat at 15- to
➤ 30-minute intervals for 1 to 2 hours or until stable.
➤ Assess the biopsy site for bleeding each time vital signs are taken.
➤ Evaluate breath sounds and observe for any signs of respiratory distress.
➤ Evaluate the client's comfort level.
➤ Resume foods and fluids withheld before the procedure if assessment data indicate that the client is stable.
➤ For an open biopsy, provide care and observation as for anyone who has had a thoracotomy under general anesthesia.

PROSTATE GLAND BIOPSY

Prostate gland biopsy involves the removal of a sample of prostatic tissue for histological and cytologic examination. Several approaches to obtaining the sample are possible: transurethral, transrectal, and perineal. Possible complications include bleeding and infection at the biopsy site, although they are not frequent problems.

Reference Values

No abnormal cells or tissue present

Indications for Prostate Gland Biopsy

➤ Prostatic hypertrophy of unknown etiology
➤ Suspected cancer of the prostate gland

Contraindications

➤ Bleeding disorders

Nursing Care Before the Procedure

Explain to the client:
➤ That the procedure will be performed by a physician
➤ That foods and fluids are usually not restricted before the test

➤ That a sedative may be administered to promote relaxation

➤ The method that will be used to obtain the sample

➤ The type of positioning that may be used for the test (see "The Procedure")

➤ That a local anesthetic will be administered to prevent pain but that the client may feel a "pinching" or "pulling" sensation during the procedure

➤ The importance of remaining still during the procedure

➤ That an antibiotic may be administered to prevent infection

➤ That vital signs and urinary output will be monitored closely after the procedure

➤ That, after the procedure, any rectal pain or bleeding, blood in the urine, or fever should be reported immediately

➤ Any special site care necessary (e.g., a dressing is applied when the perineal approach is used)

Prepare for the procedure:

➤ Administer enemas, if ordered—if the perineal or transurethral approach is to be used, one enema is usually ordered; if the transrectal approach is to be used, saline enemas until clear may be ordered.

➤ Provide a hospital gown.

➤ Have the client void.

➤ Take and record vital signs and compare with baseline readings.

➤ Administer premedication as ordered.

The Procedure

For the transurethral approach, the client is positioned on a urologic examination table as for a cystoscopy (see p. 561). The external genitalia are cleansed with antiseptic solution and a local anesthetic is instilled into the urethra. The endoscope is then inserted. The prostate gland is visualized, and the tissue for biopsy is removed with a cutting loop. The sample is placed in formalin solution and sent to the laboratory immediately. The disadvantage of this approach is that malignant nodules or tissue may not be included in the sample, even though the endoscope is under direct visual guidance.

For the transrectal approach, the client is assisted to the Sims' position, and a rectal examination is performed to locate potentially malignant nodules. A biopsy needle guide is then passed along the examining finger and the stylet removed. The biopsy needle is inserted through the needle guide and rotated to obtain a core of tissue. The needle is then withdrawn and the sample placed in formalin solution. The disadvantage of this approach is the perforation of the rectum and the creation of a tract through which cells from the nodule may be seeded. Possible complications include infection, hemorrhage, and perforation of the bladder.

For the perineal approach, the client is assisted to the position desired by the physician, usually the jack-knife or the lithotomy position, both achieved by using a special examination or operative-type table. The client is draped appropriately with the perineum exposed. The perineum is cleansed with an antiseptic solution and infiltrated with a local anesthetic. A small incision is made and either a biopsy needle or a biopsy punch inserted. Samples are taken from several locations and placed in formalin solution. Digital pressure is applied to the site. If there is no bleeding, a sterile dressing is applied.

Nursing Care After the Procedure

Care and assessment after the procedure include assisting the client to a comfortable position and allowing the client to rest for a few minutes.

➤ Monitor vital signs and compare with baseline readings; repeat every 4 hours for 24 hours.
➤ If the perineal approach was used, observe the biopsy site for bleeding or other drainage.
➤ If the transurethral approach was used, monitor for resumption of usual voiding patterns.
➤ Observe the appearance of the urine.
➤ Remind the client to report immediately any rectal pain or bleeding, blood in the urine, or fever.

THYROID GLAND BIOPSY

Thyroid gland biopsy involves the removal of a sample of thyroid tissue for histological and cytologic examination. Thyroid tissue samples may be obtained by needle aspiration (closed biopsy) or surgical incision (open biopsy). Needle biopsies require local anesthesia, whereas open biopsies are performed in a manner similar to that used for a thyroidectomy.

Reference Values

No abnormal cells or tissue present

Indications for Thyroid Gland Biopsy

➤ Abnormal thyroid scan
➤ Thyroid gland enlargement of unknown etiology
➤ Signs and symptoms of thyroiditis or hyperthyroidism
➤ Presence of thyroid nodules of unknown etiology to differentiate between benign and malignant nodules
➤ Differentiation between thyroid cysts and solid tumors
➤ Differentiation between inflammatory thyroid diseases (Hashimoto's thyroiditis versus granulomatous thyroiditis)
➤ Confirmation of the diagnoses of hyperthyroidism and nontoxic nodular goiter

Contraindications

➤ Bleeding disorders

Nursing Care Before the Procedure

Explain to the client:

➤ That the procedure will be performed by a physician
➤ The method that will be used to obtain the sample (needle biopsy or open biopsy)
➤ The type of anesthesia to be administered (local anesthesia for needle biopsy, general anesthesia for open biopsy)
➤ That foods and fluids are generally not withheld before a needle biopsy but are restricted for 6 to 8 hours before an open biopsy

➤ That a sedative may be administered before the procedure

➤ That, if a needle biopsy is to be performed, the client will be positioned on an examining table with a pillow, sandbag, or folded blanket under the shoulders to make the thyroid gland more accessible

➤ That, if a needle biopsy is to be performed, the client should remain as still as possible and should refrain from swallowing as the local anesthetic is injected

➤ That, if an open biopsy is to be performed, an incision will be made at the front of the neck

➤ That, after the procedure, vital signs and respiratory status will be monitored carefully

➤ That the client may have a sore throat after the procedure

Prepare for the procedure:

➤ For a needle biopsy, the client is assisted to the supine position and a small pillow, sandbag, or folded blanket is placed under the shoulders; the skin is cleansed with an antiseptic solution, injected with a local anesthetic, and draped with sterile drapes. The client is reminded not to swallow as the local anesthetic is injected. The biopsy needle is inserted, the specimen obtained, and the needle withdrawn. Pressure is applied to the biopsy site. If there is no bleeding, a pressure dressing is applied to the site. The sample is placed in formalin solution and sent to the laboratory immediately.

➤ For an open biopsy, the sample is obtained through surgical excision during the operative procedure.

Nursing Care After the Procedure

Care and assessment after a needle biopsy include allowing the client to rest for a few minutes after the procedure.

➤ Monitor vital signs and compare with baseline readings; repeat every 15 minutes for 1 hour, every hour for 4 hours, and then every 4 hours for 24 hours.

➤ Assess the biopsy site for bleeding each time the vital signs are taken.

➤ Evaluate the client for dyspnea, hoarseness, and difficulty swallowing.

➤ Monitor comfort level and administer analgesics for throat discomfort.

➤ For an open biopsy, provide care and observation as for a client who has had a thyroidectomy.

Student Name _____ Class _____

Instructor _____ Date _____

CASE STUDY AND CRITICAL THINKING EXERCISE

Ms. Smith, age 53, comes to the clinic and reports vaginal bleeding. She is 2 years postmenopausal and has been on estrogen therapy since menopause. A Pap smear is ordered and the results are class IV.

a. What is the probable diagnosis?

b. What other diagnostic tests will be ordered in this case?

References

1. Halsted, JA, and Halsted, CH (eds): The Laboratory in Clinical Medicine: Interpretation and Application, ed 2. WB Saunders, Philadelphia, 1981, p 138.
2. Ibid, p 139.
3. Ibid, p 138.
4. Ibid, p 138.
5. Ibid, pp 138–139.
6. Ibid, pp 140–141.
7. Ibid, p 141.
8. Springhouse Corporation: Nurse's Reference Library: Diagnostics, ed 2. Springhouse, Springhouse, Pa, 1986, p 493.
9. Packer, B: Early prenatal testing—a chorionic villus update. Mothers Today, May/June 1987, p 12.

Bibliography

Atkinson, BF: Atlas of Diagnostic Cytopathology. WB Saunders, Philadelphia, 1992.

Bibbo, M; Day, L (ed): Comprehensive Cytopathology, ed 2. WB Saunders, Philadelphia, 1996.

Byrne, CJ, et al: Laboratory Tests: Implications for Nursing Care, ed 2. Addison-Wesley, Menlo Park, Calif, 1986.

Chernecky, CC, and Berger, BJ; Cullen, BN (ed): Laboratory Tests and Diagnostic Procedures, ed 2. WB Saunders, Philadelphia, 1996.

Corbett, JV: Laboratory Tests and Diagnostic Procedures with Nursing Diagnoses, ed 4. Appleton & Lange, Norwalk, Conn, 1995.

Craigmyle, MBL: Color Atlas of Histology, ed 2. Mosby–Year Book, St Louis, 1986.

Donegan, WL, and Spratt, JS: Cancer of the Breast, ed 4. WB Saunders, Philadelphia, 1995.

Dubowitz, V: Muscle Biopsy, ed 2. WB Saunders, Philadelphia, 1985.

Frable, WJ: Thin needle aspiration biopsy. Major Problems in Pathology Series, Vol 14. WB Saunders, Philadelphia, 1983.

Henry, JB (ed): Clinical Diagnosis and Management by Laboratory Methods, ed 19. WB Saunders, Philadelphia, 1996.

Kee, JL: Handbook of Laboratory and Diagnostic Tests with Nursing Implications, ed 3. Appleton & Lange, Norwalk, Conn, 1997.

Lewis, SM, et al (eds): Medical-Surgical Nursing: Assessment and Management of Clinical Problems, ed 4. Mosby–Year Book, St Louis, 1995.

McDowell, EM, and Beals, TF: Biopsy Pathology of the Bronchi. WB Saunders, Philadelphia, 1987.

Pagana, KD, and Pagana, TJ: Diagnostic and Laboratory Test Reference, ed 3. Mosby–Year Book, St Louis, 1996.

Porth, CM: Pathophysiology: Concepts of Altered Health States, ed 4. JB Lippincott, Philadelphia, 1993.

Striker, LJ, et al: The renal biopsy. Major Problems in Pathology, Vol 8. WB Saunders, Philadelphia, 1986.

Weinstein, RS: Advances in Pathology and Laboratory Medicine. Mosby–Year Book, St Louis, 1996.

Whitehead, R: Mucosal Biopsy of the Gastrointestinal Tract, ed 5. WB Saunders, Philadelphia, 1996.

15

Culture and Sensitivity Tests

➤ **TESTS COVERED**

Blood Culture, *513*
Eye and Ear Cultures, *515*
Nose and Throat Cultures, *516*

Wound Culture, *518*
Skin Culture, *519*
Genital and Anal Cultures, *521*

INTRODUCTION

Cultures are the laboratory cultivation of substances collected from a body site, using appropriate techniques and methods specific to the type of material to be examined. For most infections, culture is considered the most effective method of laboratory testing in obtaining a definitive diagnosis. Other methods used to detect and identify infectious microorganisms include microscopic examination (Gram, acid-fast, and other stains) and immunologic techniques (microbial antigen detection).

CULTURES

A culture involves the introduction of material to an artificial growth culture medium such as liquid (broth), solid (agar), or cell culture lines, which are classified as selective, nonselective, or differential, depending on the growth support needed by the suspected microorganisms. Liquid and solid media are used to cultivate bacteria and fungi, whereas cell lines are used to culture viruses and chlamydiae.[1] Material to be cultured can be streaked along the culture medium or injected into it. Culture media are contained in Petri dishes, test tubes, and dilution containers. After the material is introduced into the proper medium, the culture is incubated for a specific length of time (usually 48 to 72 hours for agar and 3 to 7 days for broth media), at a specific temperature (usually 95.0°F [35°C]), and under other conditions suitable for the suspected microorganism (e.g., CO_2 for anaerobic culture).[2] Another 24 hours is needed to identify the pathogen that is causing a particular infectious disease.

Any excreted or secreted body fluid, drainage, or tissue sample can be cultured for microorganism identification. The types of materials collected and the procedures followed for culture of sputum, bronchial washings, feces, urine, tissue biopsy, cerebrospinal fluid, bone marrow, amniotic fluid, semen, gastrointestinal materials, and body fluids such as pleural, synovial, peritoneal, and pericardial effusions are discussed in their respective chapters. This chapter is confined to the materials collected for culture tests of blood and from the fol-

511

lowing sites: eye and ear; nose and throat; wounds; skin, nails, and hair; and genital and anal areas.

ANTIMICROBIAL SUSCEPTIBILITY

In conjunction with the culture, microorganisms are tested for sensitivity to specific antibiotics. This is known as culture and sensitivity (C&S) testing. Bacteria are classified according to their reaction to a number of antibiotics as (1) resistant (growth not inhibited), (2) sensitive (growth inhibited), or (3) intermediately sensitive (some inhibition).

The most common sensitivity test is the agar diffusion test. A special agar plate is inoculated with bacteria, filter disks prepared with antibiotics are applied to the agar surface, and the plates are incubated. As the numbers of bacteria increase and the antimicrobial agent concentration changes during incubation, a zone of inhibition develops around each disk. The diameters of the inhibition zones are measured and compared to a sensitivity reference chart.[3]

Some sensitivity tests are made using a blood sample containing the infectious agent cultured in a liquid medium to determine the concentration of an added antibiotic to inhibit bacterial growth (minimal inhibitory concentration). Penicillins and cephalosporins are tested for effectiveness using the β-lactamase assay. Some bacteria produce an enzyme (penicillinase) that renders these antimicrobials ineffective.[4]

SPECIMEN COLLECTION REQUIREMENTS

In most instances, the nurse is responsible for collecting specimens for C&S testing. To obtain the most accurate diagnostic information, the nurse should observe these requirements:

1. Use gloves and observe standard precautions and transmission-based isolation procedures (see Appendix III). Avoid contaminating the sample with the flora indigenous to skin and mucosa.
2. Collect the specimen from the site with the most viable and active microorganisms.
3. Collect the specimen at a time when the microorganisms are present in large numbers, preferably early in the disease, before antibiotic therapy is begun.
4. Collect a sufficient quantity for a complete analysis.
5. Collect the correct number of specimens at the same time or at the correct time intervals.
6. Collect the specimen in sterile, disposable containers or introduce into a container without contaminating either the specimen or the outer surfaces of the container.
7. Take into consideration the microorganism's special needs for survival, such as an anaerobic environment or particular media requirements. Use special kits for collection of such specimens.
8. Label all specimens correctly with all pertinent information regarding the client's history and status, site, time, suspected infectious agent, and tests ordered.

9. Transport the specimen to the laboratory immediately to avoid overgrowth or death of the microorganisms.

BLOOD CULTURE

Blood cultures are microbiologic tests undertaken to assist in the diagnosis of bacteremia, septicemia, or infectious diseases such as typhoid fever, plague, and malaria. When bacteria or fungi enter the bloodstream, an infection of greater or lesser severity may result. Pathogens entering the bloodstream from soft tissue infection sites, contaminated intravenous (IV) lines, or invasive procedures such as minor surgery, tooth extraction, or cystoscopy usually do not result in infections severe enough to cause sepsis. But if the infection is persistent or recurrent, it can lead to septicemia, a more life-threatening condition that is manifested by severe signs and symptoms of infection. In adults, the most common microorganisms causing septicemia are *Staphylococcus aureus,* the gram-negative rods such as *Escherichia coli, Aerobacter* spp., and *Klebsiella* spp.; in infants, the microorganisms are *E. coli* and β-hemolytic streptococcus.[5] In clients who have received antimicrobial therapy before the test, an antimicrobial removal device containing a resin is used to remove the inhibitory effects of antibiotics from the blood sample before culturing. This practice allows for more rapid growth and identification of the organism. Test results are recorded as negative with no growth or as positive if growth occurs.

Reference Values

Negative, no growth of pathogens in a specific time span

Interfering Factors

➤ Pretest antimicrobial therapy, which delays growth of pathogens
➤ Contamination of the specimen by the skin's resident flora
➤ Inadequate amount of blood or number of blood specimens drawn for examination
➤ Specimens that are tested more than 1 hour after collection

Indications for Blood Culture

➤ Determination of the cause of sudden change in pulse and temperature with or without chills and diaphoresis
➤ History of persistent, intermittent fever associated with a heart murmur
➤ Intermittent or continuous temperature elevation of unknown origin
➤ Suspected bacteremia after invasive procedures
➤ Identification of the cause of shock in the postoperative period
➤ Immunosuppression, which predisposes to invasion by microorganisms that rarely invade a healthy host
➤ Fever and chills in debilitated or elderly persons receiving hyperalimentation or antibiotic therapy
➤ Determination of sepsis in the newborn as a result of prolonged labor, early rupture of the membranes, maternal infection, or neonatal aspiration[6]

Contraindications

➤ None

>> **Nursing Alert**

- Absolute sterile technique must be used in performing the venipuncture and obtaining the blood samples to prevent possible contamination. Measures must be taken during the procedure to prevent transmission of infectious agents to the client or personnel.

Nursing Care Before the Procedure

Client preparation is the same as for any study involving the collection of a peripheral blood sample (see Appendix I).

➤ The client should be informed that a sample is being obtained from the site and that the test results can take 1 to 3 weeks, depending on the suspected or underlying conditions.

➤ A history should be obtained regarding the presence of fever of unknown origin, suspected bacterial or fungal infections, and antibiotic therapy.

The Procedure

The venipuncture site is cleansed with povidone-iodine and allowed to dry. The venipuncture is performed using strict sterile technique and gloves. Blood in the amount of 20 mL (30 mL if an infection is suspected, or 1 to 3 mL in an infant or young child) is withdrawn without allowing air to be aspirated into the syringe. The needle is replaced by a new sterile needle on the syringe. The caps of the two culture bottles are removed and the tops cleansed with povidone-iodine, allowed to dry, and then cleansed with alcohol. Half of the blood is injected into each bottle of aerobic media and anaerobic media and gently mixed with the culture media. The bottles should contain a 1 : 10 dilution of blood and media. The bottles can also contain an adsorbent resin to remove previously administered antibiotics that can inhibit growth of the microorganisms. If the blood is not inoculated after withdrawal, it can be transported in a sterile tube containing a preservative and placed in the bottles of media in the laboratory. The procedure is repeated at a different site immediately and in 3 hours or during a septic episode. Within 24 hours as many as four cultures can be obtained to isolate the etiologic agent.[7] Cultures to isolate parasites in blood require blood collected in a lavender-topped tube or blood smears for microscopic examination.

Use standard precautions and transmission-based isolation procedures for blood-borne pathogens in handling and disposing of all articles used in blood culture collection (see Appendix III).

Nursing Care After the Procedure

Care and assessment after the procedures are the same as for any study involving the collection of a peripheral blood sample (see Appendix I).

➤ *Abnormal values:* Note and report to the physician immediately any positive culture result and microorganisms indicating bacteremia or septicemia. Assess for fever, chills, hypotension, and other signs and symptoms associated with acute infection. Assess blood glucose and bilirubin in an infant with suspected sepsis. Administer ordered antimicrobial and antipyretic therapy orally or intravenously (IV). Monitor vital signs and

temperature, and provide care and comfort measures for elevated
temperature, fatigue, and other complaints.

➤ *Disease transmission:* Note and report type of infection, infectious agent,
and client status (age, immunosuppression). Observe preventive standards
for blood-borne pathogens for hand protection, personal protection, and
needles and sharps (see Appendix III).

EYE AND EAR CULTURES

Eye cultures are performed on pus, corneal scrapings, or aspirate of intraocular
fluid to establish the bacterial or viral infectious agent involved in orbital cellulitis, conjunctivitis, keratitis, and blepharitis.[8] The specimen is obtained with
a swab and Culturette. Among the pathogens causing eye infectious disease are
Haemophilus aegyptius, Neisseria gonorrhoeae, Chlamydia, adenovirus, and
herpesvirus.

Ear cultures are made on material from the outer, middle, or inner ear to
identify a microorganism involved in a chronic infectious disease, local lesion
infections, and abscess formation. The specimen is obtained with a swab and
Culturette. The outer ear and external ear canal are usually associated with skin
conditions, whereas the middle and inner ear are usually associated with either
the spread of infections from the nasopharynx or a systemic infection.[9] Among
the pathogens causing ear infections are *E. coli, Chlamydia* spp., *Proteus* spp.,
β-hemolytic streptococci, *S. aureus, P. aeruginosa, C. albicans,* and *Aspergillus*
spp. Test results for eye and ear cultures are recorded as negative with no
growth or as positive with the infectious agent identified.

Reference Values

Negative, no growth of pathogens

Interfering Factors

➤ Pretest antimicrobial therapy, which will delay growth of pathogens
➤ Contamination of the specimen by the surrounding skin or mucous
membrane
➤ Failure to collect an adequate amount of material for culture

Indications for Eye and Ear Cultures

➤ Ear pain, drainage, changes in hearing
➤ Suspected infection in the outer, middle, or inner ear
➤ Eye redness, drainage, changes in vision
➤ Determination of the causative agent of infection of parts of the eye
➤ Determination of effective local or systemic antimicrobial therapy specific
to identified microorganism and sensitivity

Contraindications

➤ None

Nursing Care Before the Procedure

Client preparation includes informing the client of the reason for the procedure
and the method of obtaining the specimen (swab and Culturette).

➤ A history should include information regarding the presence of pain, redness, drainage from the area, and antimicrobial therapy administered before the test.

The Procedure

The client is placed in a sitting position with the head tilted slightly backward for an eye culture or turned to the side, exposing the ear to be cultured.

To obtain an ear culture, cleanse the area surrounding the site with a swab containing a cleansing solution to remove contaminating material or flora that has collected in the external ear. Cerumen in the ear canal can be removed before obtaining a specimen. A Culturette swab is inserted into the external canal of the ear ¼ inch and rotated in the exudate. The swab is removed without touching the sides of the canal and is placed in the tube; the end of the tube is squeezed to allow for dispersion of the medium.

To obtain an eye culture, the client is requested to look upward, and a sterile swab is placed in the inner canthus of the eye or on the affected surface of the eye; the swab is then rotated to collect the drainage material. The swab is placed in a Culturette tube and the end of the tube is squeezed to allow for dispersion of the medium, or the swab is placed in a special bottle of medium depending on the suspected microorganism to be isolated.

Nursing Care After the Procedure

Care and assessment after the procedure include resuming eye or ear care and treatments.

➤ *Abnormal values:* Note and immediately report to the physician any positive culture results and the microorganisms identified. Administer ordered antimicrobial therapy. Provide eye or ear care and treatments. Instruct client to wear dark glasses, if they are needed. Instruct client in the procedure for using eyedrops or eardrops and inform of the need to avoid rubbing the eyes and the importance of hand washing to prevent transmission of the microorganism to the other eye or other body sites.

NOSE AND THROAT CULTURES

Culture sites of the upper respiratory tract include the nares and the nasopharynx or throat. The culture material is obtained by swab and Culturette. The cultures are made to identify suspected infections or carrier states caused by *S. aureus,* group A streptococci, *N. gonorrhoeae, Corynebacterium diphtheriae, Bordetella pertussis, C. albicans,* and *Haemophilus influenzae.* The tests are commonly performed on health personnel to screen for carriers.[10] Test results are recorded as negative with normal flora or as positive with the infectious agent identified.

Reference Values

Negative, no growth of pathogens

Interfering Factors

➤ Pretest antimicrobial therapy, which delays the growth of pathogens
➤ Contamination of the specimen by the surrounding skin or mucosa
➤ Improper technique or inadequate amount of material to be tested

Indications for Nose and Throat Cultures

➤ Screen for carriers of *S. aureus* or *H. influenzae* and differentiate between these states and actual infection.

➤ Diagnose upper respiratory viral infections causing bronchitis, pharyngitis, croup, and influenza.

➤ Diagnose bacterial infections such as tonsillitis, diphtheria, thrush, gonorrhea, pertussis, or streptococcal throat infection.

➤ Determine the cause of scarlet fever, rheumatic fever, and acute glomerulonephritis.

➤ Obtain sputum specimens from children, as necessary.

➤ Determine effective antimicrobial therapy specific to identified microorganism and sensitivity.

Contraindications

➤ None

Nursing Care Before the Procedure

Client preparation includes informing the client or caregiver, or both, of the reason for the procedure and the method of obtaining the specimen (swab and Culturette).

➤ A history should include information regarding the presenting signs and symptoms, past immunizations, and antimicrobial therapy administered before the test.

The Procedure

The client is placed in a sitting position or, if a child, on the caregiver's lap with the head and body held to immobilize while the procedure takes place.

To obtain a nasal culture, gently raise the tip of the nose, insert a flexible swab into the nares and rotate it in place against the sides. Then remove the swab and place it in the appropriate medium to be transported to the laboratory for immediate examination.

To obtain a nasopharyngeal culture, gently raise the tip of the nose, insert a flexible swab along the bottom of the nares, and guide it along until it reaches the posterior pharynx. Rotate the swab in place to obtain the secretions and then remove. Then place the swab in the culture tube with the appropriate medium and transport it to the laboratory.

To obtain a throat culture, tilt the head slightly backward, depress the tongue with a tongue blade, and insert the swab through the mouth to the pharyngeal and tonsillar area without touching any part of the oral cavity. Rub the areas, including any lesions, inflammation, or exudate, with the swab. Remove the swab and squeeze the Culturette tube before the swab is introduced into the medium. Transport the specimen to the laboratory for immediate testing.

Nursing Care After the Procedure

Care and assessment after the procedure include resumption of the treatment regimen for signs and symptoms of upper respiratory infections.

➤ *Abnormal values:* Note and report positive culture results to the physician. Administer ordered antimicrobial therapy. Provide comfort measures and treatment such as antiseptic gargles; warm, moist applications; and inhalants.

➤ *Disease transmission:* Practice standard precautions and transmission-based isolation procedures in collection and transportation of specimens and disposal of used articles (see Appendix III). Instruct client in covering mouth and nose when coughing or sneezing; advise regarding tissue disposal and frequent hand washing. Manage identified carriers among personnel according to agency policy to prevent transmission to ill clients.

WOUND CULTURE

Wound culture is used to isolate and identify pathogens that cause infection so that the physician can prescribe the appropriate therapy. Wound exudates and drainage as well as tissue samples can be obtained from the actual site of infection. Specimens are collected from a superficial wound with a cotton-tipped sterile swab and Culturette tube containing the medium. From a deep wound, specimens are obtained by aspirating drainage with a syringe and needle and injecting the material into a tube of culture medium. Wound debridement or excised tissue specimens can also be collected and cultured.

Wound infections are most likely to occur after trauma, surgical incision, or any other condition that results in abscess or skin breaks, for example, decubitus ulcer. Both aerobic and anaerobic microorganisms can be identified in wound culture specimens. Some bacterial infectious agents found in wounds are *S. aureus,* group A streptococci; *Clostridium perfringens, Klebsiella* spp., *Proteus* spp., *Pseudomonas* spp., *Mycobacterium* spp., and the fungal infectious agents *Candida albicans* and *Aspergillus* spp.[11] Test results are recorded as either normal flora and negative for growth or positive with the infectious agent identified.

Reference Values

Negative or no growth of pathogens

Interfering Factors

➤ Pretest antimicrobial therapy, which will delay growth of pathogens
➤ Specimens that are tested more than 1 hour after collection
➤ A dried specimen, which cannot be effectively cultured for microorganism isolation

Indications for Wound Culture

➤ Determination of an infectious agent as the cause of redness, warmth, or edema with drainage at a site
➤ Presence of pus or other exudate in an open wound
➤ Suspected abscess or deep wound infectious process
➤ Suspected wound infection after trauma that causes break in the first line of defense (skin)
➤ Stage III and IV decubitus ulcers to determine presence of infectious agents
➤ Determination of effective antimicrobial therapy specific to identified microorganism and sensitivity

Contraindications

➤ None

Nursing Care Before the Procedure

Client preparation includes informing the client of the reason for the procedure and the method of obtaining the culture specimen (swab or aspiration).

➤ A history should include the presence of pain, edema, redness, warmth, and drainage of an area; trauma or invasive procedures; and antimicrobial therapy administered before the suspected infection.

The Procedure

The client is placed in a comfortable position and draped; the site to be cultured should be exposed. The area around the wound is cleansed to remove flora indigenous to the skin. A Culturette swab is placed in the most excessive exudate in a superficial wound without touching the wound edges. The swab soaked with the exudate is placed in the tube and the tube is squeezed to allow for dispersion of the medium. More than one swab and Culturette tube can be used to obtain specimens from other areas in the wound. A deep wound specimen is obtained by aspiration with a sterile syringe and needle inserted directly into the wound. After the aspiration, the air is expelled from the syringe and the needle covered with a rubber stopper or the material injected into a tube containing an anaerobic culture medium.

Nursing Care After the Procedure

Care and assessment after the procedure include dressing the wound as appropriate and leaving the client in a comfortable position.

➤ *Abnormal values:* Note and immediately report to the physician any positive culture results and the microorganisms identified. Assess for signs and symptoms associated with an infectious process. Administer ordered antimicrobial therapy. Provide wound care and treatments and nutritional requirements to promote wound healing.

➤ *Disease transmission:* Note and report type of infection, infectious agent, and need for wound precaution measures. Observe standard precautions and transmission-based isolation procedures in the care of the wound and articles used to collect and test specimens (see Appendix III).

SKIN CULTURE

Skin culture is performed on skin scrapings or exudate, nail scrapings, or hair stubs. Skin culture is used to identify bacterial and fungal infections as well as to perform antimicrobial sensitivity testing. Cultural identification is made from the growth of a microorganism on a specialized agar or broth medium incubated at a specific temperature. Direct slide preparations are made from scrapings spread on a slide and stained or unstained for microscopic viewing. Normally, the hair, skin, and nails contain nonpathogenic surface contaminants in low numbers. The same resident microorganisms can be pathogenic when present in large numbers. Positive culture results are reported with the name of the pathogen and the number of colonies. Stains are reported for the presence and type of inflammatory cells and their staining characteristics. Pathogens found on the hair include *Blastomyces, Coccidioides, Candida, Trichophyton,* and *Microsporum.* Pathogens found on the nails include *Candida, Cephalosporium, Epidermophyton,* and *Trichophyton.* Pathogens found on the skin include *Bacteroides, Clostridium,*

Corynebacterium, Candida, Trichophyton, Epidermophyton, Trichophyton, Aspergillus, Pseudomonas, the common *Staphylococcus,* and group A streptococcal organisms.

Reference Values

Normally low numbers of microorganisms on the skin, hair, and nails

No evidence of large quantities of pathogens identified

Interfering Factors

➤ Failure to obtain a specimen from the proper location or a sufficient quantity of scrapings, fluid, or other material to be cultured
➤ Failure to transport the specimen as soon as it is collected
➤ Drying of specimens or use of an improper container for the specimen

Indications for Skin Culture

➤ Diagnosis of superficial or cutaneous infections of the integument
➤ Skin eruptions such as pustules, vesicles, or lesions; scalp or nail abnormality
➤ Determination of sensitivity to specific antimicrobials for use in treatment of the infection

Contraindications

➤ None

Nursing Care Before the Procedure

Inform the client of the reason for the procedure and the method of obtaining the culture specimen.
➤ Advise the client that the culture is collected by the physician or nurse in 5 to 10 minutes and that results should be available in 48 to 72 hours.
➤ Inform the client that little or no pain is associated with the procedure.
➤ The history should include information about acute and chronic skin conditions, signs and symptoms indicating a need for a culture, other skin tests, and the results.

The Procedure

The client is placed in a comfortable position with the culture site exposed. The area is gently cleansed with sterile saline and alcohol and allowed to air-dry. Hair stubs, including the shaft and root, or scrapings from the area affected are clipped or plucked with a sterile forceps and sent to the laboratory in a Petri dish for incubation and identification of the organism. Nail scrapings are obtained with a sterile scalpel or clippings with a sterile scissors and placed in a Petri dish or clean envelope. The specimen is transported to the laboratory for incubation and examination. Skin scrapings from several lesion edges are obtained with a sterile scalpel and placed in a Petri dish or spread on a slide for smear examination. Fluid from a vesicle or pus from a pustule is obtained by aspiration with a sterile needle and tuberculin syringe and the exudate flushed on the culture medium in a Petri dish. If fluid is not present, the lesion is opened with a sterile applicator and swabbed for collection of the material; then the applicator is placed in a sterile culture tube to be transported to the laboratory for examination. Dark, warm, and moist areas in the folds of the skin (axillary, groin, submammary) or nares can also be cultured to identify causes of rashes with well-defined borders (usually fungal). The result of skin cultures reveals the specific bacterial, fungal, or viral infectious agent in sufficient quantities to indicate pathology.

Nursing Care After the Procedure

Care and assessment after the procedure include telling the client that test results can be expected in 48 to 72 hours and that treatment (topical or systemic medications) can be prescribed by the physician at that time.

GENITAL AND ANAL CULTURES

Most genital and anal specimens are cultured to identify possible sexually transmitted diseases (STDs). The specimen is obtained with a swab and Culturette or cultured on various media, depending on the suspected organism. Immunoassay methods are also used to detect and identify specific infectious agents. Specimens can be obtained from the mouth-throat, anal-rectal, urethral, cervical, and vaginal sites. Tests help to identify infectious processes associated with herpes simplex virus, *Chlamydia, Candida, Mycoplasma,* and *Gardnerella vaginalis,* as well as other infections caused by *N. gonorrhoeae, Treponema pallidum,* and *Trichomonas vaginalis.* Tests are also performed to detect toxin-producing strains of *S. aureus* in vaginal infections associated with toxic shock syndrome.[12] Test results are recorded as negative with normal flora or as positive with the infectious agent identified.

Reference Values

Negative or no growth of pathogens

Interfering Factors

➤ Pretest antimicrobial therapy, which delays growth of pathogens
➤ Contamination of the specimen by the surrounding skin, mucosa, or feces
➤ Improper collection technique or inadequate amount of material to be tested

Indications for Genital and Anal Cultures

➤ Genital itching and purulent drainage
➤ Diagnosis of STDs in those with the signs and symptoms associated with the mouth and throat (caused by oral sexual practices), anus (caused by anal sexual practices), and vagina or penis (caused by traditional sexual practices)

Contraindications

➤ None

Nursing Care Before the Procedure

Client preparation includes informing the client of the reason for the procedure and the method of obtaining the specimen (swab).
➤ A history should include information regarding sexual practices, itching and drainage of the affected site, and antimicrobial therapy administered before the test.

The Procedure

Place the client in a lithotomy position and drape for privacy. Observe standard precautions and transmission-based isolation procedures including the use of gloves in specimen collection, handling, transporting, and testing of body drainage materials.

To obtain an anal culture, insert the swab 1 inch into the anal canal; rotate and move the swab from side to side to allow it to come in contact with the microorganisms. Then remove the swab, place it in the appropriate transport medium, and send it to the laboratory for immediate testing.

To obtain a urethral culture in men, insert the loop swab into the penile meatus to obtain a sample of the discharge by gently scraping the anterior mucosa. Then place the swab in the appropriate transport medium and send it to the laboratory for immediate testing.

To obtain a vaginal and endocervical culture in women, insert a vaginal speculum and gently cleanse mucus from the cervix with cotton. Then insert the swab into the endocervical canal. Rotate the swab to collect the secretions containing the microorganisms, remove, and place in the appropriate culture medium, depending on the suspected pathogen. Vaginal material can also be collected by moving the swab along the sides of the mucosa and then placing it in a tube of saline medium and transporting it to the laboratory for immediate testing.

Nursing Care After the Procedure

Care and assessment after the procedure include resumption of treatment regimen for STDs or other inflammatory or infectious states of the genitoreproductive tract.

➤ *Abnormal values:* Note and report positive culture results to the physician and to the health department, if appropriate. Administer ordered antimicrobial therapy. Provide a comfortable, sensitive, nonjudgmental environment for the client, who may experience embarrassment with the diagnosis.

➤ *Disease transmission:* Practice standard precautions and transmission-based isolation procedures in collection and transportation of specimens (see Appendix III). Inform client of safe sex practices for client and partner. Instruct in vaginal suppository and douche procedures and topical medication administration to treat specific conditions.

Student Name _____ Class _____

Instructor _____ Date _____

Case Study and Critical Thinking Exercise

Mr. Black, age 45, has been hospitalized for 5 days and has a central line for administration of TPN and medications. VS: T 102.2°F (39°C), P 96, R 28, and BP 108/64. WBC is 25,000.

a. What complication has Mr. Black developed?

b. If this situation is not corrected, what serious problem can he develop?

References

1. Sacher, RA, and McPherson, RA: Widmann's Clinical Interpretation of Laboratory Tests, ed 10. FA Davis, Philadelphia, 1991, p 467.
2. Ibid, pp 471–472.
3. Ibid, pp 479-480.
4. Corbett, JV: Laboratory Tests and Diagnostic Procedures with Nursing Diagnoses, ed 3. Appleton & Lange, Norwalk, Conn, 1992, p 415.
5. Ibid, p 423.
6. Ibid, p 423.
7. Washington, JA: Medical bacteriology. In Henry, JB: Clinical Diagnosis and Management by Laboratory Methods, ed 18. WB Saunders, Philadelphia, 1991, pp 1027–1028.
8. Sacher and McPherson, op cit, p 515.
9. Ibid, p 515.
10. Ibid, p 429.
11. Fischbach, FT: A Manual of Laboratory and Diagnostic Tests, ed 4. JB Lippincott, Philadelphia, 1992, p 434.
12. Corbett, op cit, p 434.

Bibliography

Ackerman, V, and Dunk-Richards, G: Microbiology: An Introduction for the Health Sciences. WB Saunders, Philadelphia, 1990.

Anhalt, JP: Pocket Manual of Antimicrobial Agents, ed 11. Mosby–Year Book, St Louis, 1989.

Baron, EJ, et al: Bailey and Scott's Diagnostic Microbiology, ed 9. Mosby–Year Book, St Louis, 1994.

Byrne, CJ, et al: Laboratory Tests: Implications for Nursing Care, ed 2. Addison-Wesley, Menlo Park, Calif, 1986.

Chernecky, CC, and Berger, BJ; Cullen, BN (ed): Laboratory Tests and Diagnostic Procedures, ed 2. WB Saunders, Philadelphia, 1996.

Deglin, JH, and Vallerand, AH: Davis's Drug Guide for Nurses, ed 6. FA Davis, Philadelphia, 1999.

Ellner, PD, and Neu, HC: Understanding Infectious Disease. Mosby–Year Book, St Louis, 1992.

Henry, JB: Clinical Diagnosis and Management by Laboratory Methods, ed 19. WB Saunders, Philadelphia, 1996.

Howard, BJ: Clinical and Pathogenic Microbiology, ed 2. Mosby–Year Book, St Louis, 1993.

Kee, JL: Handbook of Laboratory and Diagnostic Tests with Nursing Implications, ed 3. Appleton & Lange, Norwalk, Conn, 1997.

Krugman, PR, et al: Infectious Diseases of Children, ed 9. Mosby–Year Book, St Louis, 1992.

Lewis, SM, et al (eds): Medical-Surgical Nursing: Assessment and Management of Clinical Problems, ed 4. Mosby–Year Book, St Louis, 1995.

Markell, EK, and John, DT: Medical Parasitology, ed 7. WB Saunders, Philadelphia, 1992.

Murray, PR: Medical Microbiology, ed. 3. Mosby-Year Book, St Louis, 1997.

Pagana, KD, and Pagana, TJ: Diagnostic and Laboratory Test Reference, ed 3. Mosby–Year Book, St Louis, 1996.

Schulman, ST: The Biologic and Clinical Basis of Infectious Diseases, ed 4. WB Saunders, Philadelphia, 1992.

Tietz, NW (ed): Clinical Guide to Laboratory Tests, ed 3. WB Saunders, Philadelphia, 1997.

Whaley, LF: Nursing Care of Infants and Children, ed 4. Mosby–Year Book, St Louis, 1991.

Diagnostic Tests and Procedures

16

Endoscopic Studies

➤ **PROCEDURES COVERED**

Laryngoscopy, *529*
Bronchoscopy, *533*
Mediastinoscopy, *540*
Thoracoscopy, *542*
Esophagogastroduodenoscopy
  (EGD), *544*
Endoscopic Retrograde
  Cholangiopancreatography
  (ERCP), *548*

Proctosigmoidoscopy, *552*
Colonoscopy, *555*
Cystoscopy, *559*
Colposcopy, *563*
Culdoscopy, *565*
Amnioscopy, *567*
Laparoscopy, *569*
Arthroscopy, *576*

INTRODUCTION

Internal body structures can be visualized directly using an endoscope, a tubular instrument with a light source and a system of lenses through which body organs and hollow cavities can be observed. The endoscope can be inserted through a natural body orifice or through a small incision.[1]

Endoscopes are of two basic types: rigid metal tubes (Fig. 16–1) and flexible fiberoptic scopes (Fig. 16–2). Rigid metal tubes are the earliest type of endoscope available and are still used in certain situations, usually when a larger tube diameter is needed, depending on the body structures to be visualized and the purpose of the procedure. Flexible fiberoptic scopes involve the transmission of images over flexible, light-carrying bundles of glass fibers. Because flexible fiberoptic scopes are capable of transmitting light around curves, they can provide views of body areas that are inaccessible with rigid scopes. The scopes contain a part for the insertion of medications, instruments for suctioning, and other instruments that can be used in the procedure. Specialized instrument accessories give these scopes additional capabilities, such as obtaining biopsy specimens, coagulating bleeding vessels, removing foreign objects, and obtaining photographs for future reference and comparisons. A cross-section of the bending portion of a fiberoptic scope is shown in Figure 16–3. Because they cause less discomfort, the fiberoptic scopes have better client acceptance and can be used with local rather than general anesthesia in adults.

Specialized endoscopes of varying diameters and lengths are available, depending on the type of procedure to be performed and whether the client is an adult or child. Emerging technical applications include the use of lasers, video systems, and computers with endoscopic devices.

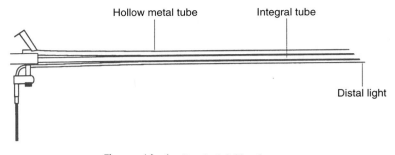

Figure 16-1 Standard rigid endoscope.

Endoscopic procedures are generally considered invasive, and a signed informed consent is required unless specified otherwise in some of the procedures. Client preparation for an adult is similar to that of a minor surgical procedure with local anesthesia and for a child it is the same as a surgical procedure requiring general anesthesia. Endoscopic examinations or surgical procedures are performed in specially equipped endoscopy rooms, operating room, or outpatient department, or at the bedside, depending on the study. Physicians with special training and expertise in procedures related to their specialties perform the procedures; that is, a bronchoscopy is performed by a pulmonologist and a colonoscopy, by a gastroenterologist. Procedures and treatments by endoscopy are performed using sterile technique and standard precautions and transmission-based isolation procedures.

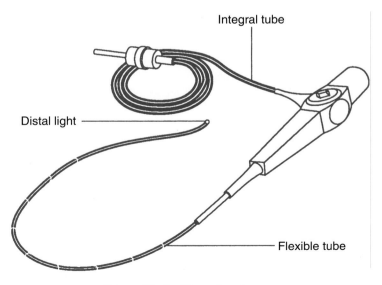

Figure 16-2 Fiberoptic endoscope.

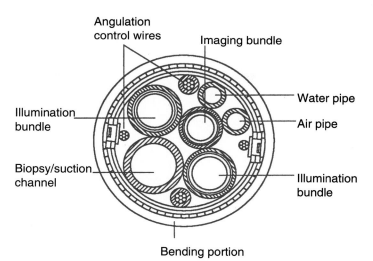

Figure 16–3 Cross-section view of the fiberoptic endoscope.

ENDOSCOPIC PROCEDURES

Endoscopic procedures are named for the organ or body area to be examined or treated, including the larynx, trachea, bronchi, pleurae, mediastinum, pericardium, esophagus, stomach, duodenum, pancreas, bile ducts, liver, colon, rectum/sigmoid colon, bladder, urethra, ureters, prostate, vagina, cervix, uterus, fetus, fallopian tubes, ovaries, and joints.

LARYNGOSCOPY

Laryngoscopy is the visualization of the larynx. It can be performed by indirect or direct technique. The larynx is an organ that connects the pharnyx with the trachea. It is associated with speech and protects the lungs as the epiglottis covers the larynx during swallowing, preventing foods and fluids from entering the trachea and lungs.

Indirect Laryngoscopy

Indirect laryngoscopy is the visualization of the reflected image of the larynx using a laryngeal mirror, a head mirror, and a light source[2] (Fig. 16–4). This procedure can be performed by a nurse, physician, or other health-care professional in almost any setting. A signed informed consent is required only if tissue is to be removed.

Direct Laryngoscopy

Direct laryngoscopy is performed with a rigid laryngoscope or a flexible fiberoptic endoscope and permits a more prolonged and thorough visualization of the larynx than does an indirect laryngoscopy. It is usually performed by a physician, but it can be carried out by a nurse anesthetist in an emergency if a

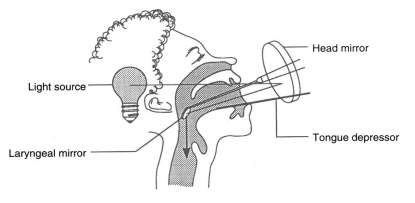

Figure 16–4 Indirect laryngoscopy.

laryngoscope is used. In an emergency, the procedure can be performed in almost any setting provided that the necessary equipment is available.

Reference Values

Normal larynx with no inflammation, abnormal growths, or foreign objects

Interfering Factors

Indirect Laryngoscopy

➤ Inability to cooperate in the procedure
➤ Excessive gagging
➤ Large oropharyngeal mass or severe hypertrophy of tonsillar tissue

Indications for Laryngoscopy

Indirect Laryngoscopy

➤ History of ingestion or inhalation of a foreign body, with removal if visualized and accessible
➤ Determination of the source of laryngeal stridor of unknown etiology in presence of actual or risk for airway obstruction
➤ Persistent cough, hemoptysis, throat pain, hoarseness or irritation, to identify possible cause such as lesions or inflammation of the larynx
➤ Simple excision of laryngeal polyps

Direct Laryngoscopy

➤ History or symptoms, or both, of laryngeal obstruction or disease (see previous section)
➤ Determination of the presence of strictures, edema, or other abnormalities
➤ Suspected tumor to aid in the diagnosis of a malignancy
➤ Removal of a benign lesion or foreign body in the larynx[3]
➤ Removal of tissues or secretions, or both, for laboratory examination
➤ Examination of areas that cannot be visualized as clearly by the indirect laryngoscopy method

➤ Examination of the larynx in children and adults who require general anesthesia or who are otherwise unable to cooperate in an indirect laryngoscopy
➤ Examination of the larynx in clients who have a strong gag reflex
➤ Suspected congenital laryngeal stridor, subglottic stenosis, laryngeal webs, or Pierre Robin syndrome in infants[4]

Contraindications

Indirect Laryngoscopy

➤ Presence of epiglottitis in children with its potential for edema and airway obstruction after the procedure (*Note:* If absolutely necessary, this examination can be performed by a physician if supplies and equipment for intubation or tracheostomy are available.)

➤➤ Nursing Alert

* Attempts to visualize the larynx or epiglottis using a tongue depressor or any other article in children with epiglottitis can precipitate laryngospasm, complete obstruction, and death.

Nursing Care Before the Procedure

Explain to the client:
➤ The location for the procedure and the person performing it
➤ The method by which the examination will be performed (direct or indirect)
➤ That, after the procedure, the client should immediately report any difficulty in breathing
➤ That discomfort will be minimized by local or general anesthesia (age and mentation dependent)

If indirect laryngoscopy is to be performed:
➤ That there are no fluid and food restrictions before the procedure
➤ That the procedure requires 5 minutes or less
➤ That the client will be requested to maintain a sitting position and protrude the tongue as far as possible
➤ That the tongue can be held in the protruded position by the client or an assistant to maintain the tongue's position throughout the procedure
➤ That the client will be observed after the procedure and offered comfort measures, if needed

If direct laryngoscopy is to be performed:
➤ That the procedure requires about 15 to 30 minutes
➤ That food and fluids are restricted for 6 to 8 hours before the procedure
➤ That anesthesia can be achieved by spraying or swabbing the throat while in a sitting position or that a general anesthetic can be administered, if warranted, depending on the client's age and condition
➤ That the local anesthetic has a bitter taste and can cause sensations such as a thickened tongue and difficulty in swallowing

➤ That a sedative or antianxiety agent can be administered before the procedure to promote relaxation and that, possibly, a medication can be administered to reduce secretions

➤ That the client will be observed and activities restricted after the procedure until the medication or anesthesia has worn off

➤ That foods and fluids will be withheld until the ability to swallow has returned (usually about 2 hours after the procedure)

➤ That comfort measures and medications will be administered to alleviate throat discomfort after the procedure

Prepare for the procedure:

➤ Obtain a history of allergies to medications or anesthetics and known or suspected upper respiratory disorders.

➤ Ensure that dietary and fluid restrictions have been followed before the procedure.

➤ Remove full or partial dentures and inform the person performing the test whether the client has any permanent crowns on the teeth (caps).

If direct laryngoscopy is performed:

➤ Have the client disrobe from the waist up and provide a hospital gown.

➤ Have the client void.

➤ Obtain and record baseline vitals signs for later comparison readings.

➤ Administer premedications, if ordered, subcutaneously (SC) or orally with a small amount of water 30 to 60 minutes before the procedure. (Premedications can include an analgesic such as meperidine [Demerol] to reduce discomfort, a sedative or an antianxiety agent such as diazepam [Valium] to promote relaxation, or an anticholinergic such as atropine sulfate to reduce secretions.)

The Procedure

The procedure varies with the type of endoscopic study to be performed and the type of anesthesia used.

Indirect Laryngoscopy. The client is seated in a chair and the light source is positioned to reflect the light from the operator's head mirror into the mouth (see Fig. 16–4, p. 530). The throat is sprayed or swabbed with a local anesthetic. The client is instructed to concentrate on controlled breathing to prevent gagging. A laryngeal mirror is placed in the mouth as far posteriorly as possible and rotated to reflect light into the larynx. If the examination requires more than 2 to 3 minutes, the client is permitted to swallow, and the examination is resumed. Tissue can be excised for examination and foreign bodies can be removed during the procedure. Specimens that are collected are placed in appropriate containers, properly labeled, and promptly sent to the laboratory.

Direct Laryngoscopy. The initial portion of the procedure can vary, depending on the type of anesthesia used. If general anesthesia is used, the client is placed in the supine position and the anesthesia administered. If local anesthesia is used, the client is placed in a sitting position and the mouth and throat swabbed or sprayed, or both, with the anesthetic. When loss of sensation is adequate after the local administration, the client is placed in the supine position with the neck extended and supported by an assistant. A laryngoscope or flexible endoscope is introduced into the mouth and advanced through the pharynx into the larynx for visualization. Tissue can be excised and foreign objects removed. Specimens are placed in appropriate containers, properly labeled, and promptly sent to the laboratory. The scope is removed and the client, if conscious, is placed in a semi-Fowler's position. The client who has received a general anesthetic is placed in a side-lying position with the head slightly elevated.

Nursing Care After the Procedure

Indirect Laryngoscopy. Provide the client with a cool drink or mouthwash to alleviate dryness of the tongue and lozenges for any postprocedure discomfort when the gag reflex returns.

➤ If a local anesthetic is used, monitor the ability to swallow until sensation returns.

Direct Laryngoscopy. Maintain the client for about 2 hours in the position appropriate to the type of anesthesia used. Monitor vital signs, compare with baselines, and assess swallowing ability continuously.

➤ Advise the client to refrain from smoking for several hours after the procedure and to withhold food and fluids until swallowing ability returns.

➤ Apply cool compresses to the throat to reduce any laryngeal edema resulting from trauma of the scope or removal of tissue.

➤ Provide warm saline gargles, lozenges, or viscous lidocaine (Xylocaine) to alleviate throat discomfort.

➤ Remind the client to report any excessive bleeding or breathing difficulty immediately.

➤ Assist with client's transportation home if the test is performed in an ambulatory care setting.

➤ *Reaction to anesthetic agent:* Note and report tachycardia, palpitations, hyperpnea, or hypertension. Administer ordered antihistamine. Initiate intravenous (IV) line and resuscitation procedure if needed.

➤ *Persistent bleeding:* Note and report amount of excessive hemoptysis or changes in vital signs for potential hypovolemia. Provide tissues and an emesis basin, and caution client against coughing and throat clearing, which can dislodge a clot at the tissue excision site and precipitate bleeding. Initiate IV line and prepare to replace fluid loss. Prepare client for laryngeal examination to control bleeding at the site.

➤ *Tracheal perforation during the procedure:* Note and report difficulty in breathing or subcutaneous crepitus on the face or neck indicating subcutaneous emphysema. Assist to initiate resuscitation or tracheostomy procedures to maintain ventilation.

BRONCHOSCOPY

Bronchoscopy is the direct visualization of the larynx, trachea, and bronchial tree by means of either a rigid or a flexible bronchoscope. Its purposes are both diagnostic and therapeutic (Fig. 16–5). The trachea divides into the left and right primary bronchi, with the right shorter and wider and the left longer and narrower. The primary bronchi divide into the secondary bronchi, which divide to form the segmental bronchi. Branching continues until the terminal bronchioles are formed.[5] Bronchial smooth muscle tone is controlled by the autonomic

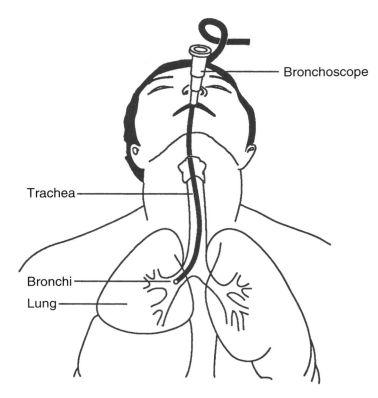

Figure 16−5 Bronchoscopy with fiberoptic endoscope.

nervous system. The narrowing of bronchioles caused by bronchospasm of these muscles results in impaired airflow and ineffective breathing pattern and airway clearance.

The rigid bronchoscope is designed to allow visualization of the larger airways, including the lobar, segment, and subsegment bronchi, while maintaining effective gas exchange. The lumen of the bronchoscope is large enough to allow for the insertion of instruments such as biopsy forceps and electrocautery devices. A rigid bronchoscope is used with laser therapy to remove lesions. A specialized attachment allows for mechanical ventilation during the procedure. Although it can require general anesthesia, rigid bronchoscopy is preferred for aspirating large volumes of blood or secretions, or both; for removing foreign bodies; for obtaining larger-sized biopsy specimens than possible with fiberoptic bronchoscope; and for performing most bronchoscopies in children.[6]

The flexible fiberoptic bronchoscope has a smaller lumen than that of the rigid bronchoscope and is designed to allow for visualization of all segments of the bronchial tree, entry into all third-order bronchi and half of the sixth-order bronchi, and visualization of the openings of most sixth-order bronchi. Some now allow for visualization of tenth-order bronchi. It is in the smaller airways that bronchogenic carcinomas arise; therefore, this type of bronchoscope allows for the detection and biopsy of tissues that could not be visualized with a rigid bronchoscope via an accessory lumen. In general, they are less traumatic to the surrounding tissues than are the larger rigid scopes. Most fiberoptic bronchoscopies are performed under local anesthesia, and client tolerance is better than for rigid bronchoscopy.[7]

Bronchoscopies can be performed in almost any setting. In an emergency, a bedside bronchoscopy can be performed, provided that equipment is available for oxygen delivery, cardiac monitoring, and cardiopulmonary resuscitation.[8]

Reference Values

Normal larynx, trachea, bronchi, bronchioles, and alveoli; absence of tracheo-esophageal fistula in infant if contrast studies are performed with the bronchoscopy

Interfering Factors

➤ Inability to cooperate during the procedure if it is performed under local anesthesia
➤ Failure to follow dietary and fluid restrictions
➤ Improper handling and care of a specimen removed for examination

Indications for Bronchoscopy

➤ Determination of the cause of persistent cough, hemoptysis, or hoarseness of unknown etiology
➤ Determination of the cause of unexplained chest x-ray abnormalities such as pulmonary infiltrates or tumor
➤ Coughing, choking, or cyanosis during feeding of an infant
➤ Respiratory distress and tachypnea if secretions are aspirated in an infant to rule out tracheoesophageal fistula or other congenital anomaly
➤ Determination of the cause of unexplained abnormal cytologic findings in sputum
➤ Suspected bronchogenic carcinoma to obtain samples by bronchial washings or brushings or by biopsy for cytologic analysis
➤ Determination of the stage of known bronchogenic carcinoma to assist in determining the approach to treatment protocols
➤ Local treatment of known lung cancer through instillation of chemotherapeutic agents, implantation of radioisotopes, or laser palliative therapy
➤ Abnormal exudate secured by thoracentesis to determine the cause (cancer, infection, tuberculosis) by performing a pleuroscopy via bronchoscopy into the pleural space[9]
➤ Identification of hemorrhagic and inflammatory changes seen in endobronchial Kaposi's sarcoma associated with acquired immunodeficiency syndrome (AIDS)
➤ Diagnosis of opportunistic lung infections caused by *Pneumocystis, Nocardia,* cytomegalovirus, invasive fungi, and parasites, especially in immunosuppressed clients
➤ Diagnosis of tuberculosis, abscesses, pulmonary infections (coccidioidomycosis, histoplasmosis, blastomycosis, phycomycosis)

➤ Inhalation of a foreign body, with removal if visualized and accessible

➤ Smoke inhalation injury or other traumatic injury to the tracheobronchial tree to determine the nature and extent of tissue damage

➤ Evaluation of airway patency in clients suspected of having stenosis, strictures, tumors, or abnormal bifurcation of the bronchi

➤ Identification of bleeding sites within the tracheobronchial tree, with removal of blood and clots, and the tamponade or coagulation of bleeding sites

➤ Aspiration of deep or retained secretions or mucus plugs to improve airway patency, especially in clients with atelectasis

➤ Evaluation of possible airway obstruction in clients with a known or suspected sleep apnea condition

➤ Intubation of clients in situations using the fiberoptic bronchoscope as a guide for the endotracheal tube when technical difficulties can be encountered, as in cervical spine injuries or massive upper airway edema

➤ Evaluation of endotracheal tube placement

➤ Evaluation of possible adverse sequelae of intubation or tracheostomy

Contraindications

➤ Bleeding disorders, especially those associated with uremia and cytotoxic chemotherapy

➤ Hypoxemic or hypercapnic states that require continuous oxygen administration

➤ Pulmonary hypertension that can be associated with an increased risk of hemorrhage from the procedure

➤ Cardiac conditions or dysrhythmias that can be exacerbated as a result of the procedure

➤ Disorders that limit extension of the neck that can be contraindicated if the procedure is to be performed with the rigid bronchoscope

➤ Severe obstructive tracheal conditions such as stenosis that prevent passage of the scope or prevent air passage around the scope for ventilation during the procedure

➤ Presence of or potential for respiratory failure, because introduction of the bronchoscope alone can cause a 10 to 20 mm Hg drop in arterial pO_2.[10] (If the procedure must be performed, the client should be intubated and mechanically ventilated before the procedure, which should then be accomplished with a ventilating bronchoscope.)

➤➤ Nursing Alert

- The smaller airway lumen in children is further compromised by a bronchoscope that causes some edema and can result in hypoxia. Resuscitation equipment should be on hand for use if needed.
- The use of morphine sulfate in clients with asthma or other pulmonary disease in which bronchospasms are common can further exacerbate the spasms and respiratory impairment.

Nursing Care Before the Procedure

Explain to the client:

➤ The location for the procedure and the fact that a physician will explain and perform the procedure

➤ That the procedure requires about 30 to 45 minutes

➤ That foods and fluids are withheld for 6 to 8 hours before the procedure

➤ That an analgesic, sedative, or antianxiety agent will be administered before the procedure to promote relaxation and alleviate potential discomfort

➤ That a medication can also be given before the procedure to reduce secretions and cause the mouth to feel dry

➤ The type of anesthesia to be administered, usually general for rigid bronchoscopies and local for fiberoptic bronchoscopies

➤ That the mouth and throat can be sprayed or swabbed with the local anesthetic while the client is in a sitting position, but the procedure itself is performed in a supine position

➤ That the local anesthetic has a bitter taste and can cause sensations such as a thickened tongue and difficulty in swallowing and that additional anesthetic is applied as the scope is advanced through the airway passages

➤ That a microscope-like instrument will be inserted through the mouth or nose and passed into the trachea ("windpipe")

➤ That the client will be able to breathe through the nose during the procedure even though he or she feels uncomfortable; an opportunity will be provided for the client to practice nose breathing with the mouth open before the procedure

➤ That oxygen can be administered and secretions removed via the bronchoscope

➤ That vital signs and respiratory status will be monitored closely during and after the procedure and that an instrument will be attached to a finger to monitor oxygen saturation

➤ That, if needed, heart activity can be monitored during and after the procedure

➤ That measures will be provided to treat any discomfort resulting from the procedure

Prepare for the procedure:

➤ Obtain a history of allergies to medications or anesthetics, known or suspected respiratory disorders, and treatment regimen.

➤ Ensure that dietary and fluid restrictions have been followed before the procedure.

➤ Ensure that, before the procedure, hematologic status and blood clotting ability have been assessed to include complete blood count (CBC), platelet level, prothrombin time (PT), partial thromboplastin time (PTT), clotting time, and bleeding time as well as arterial blood gases (ABGs).

➤ Note and record results of electrocardiogram (ECG), chest x-ray, and pulmonary function studies if the client is over 40 years of age and if a heart or lung disease is present.

➤ Remove full or partial dentures, and inform the person performing the test whether the client has any permanent crowns on the teeth (caps).

➤ Remove glasses, contact lenses, or eye prosthesis if applicable, and store in a safe place.

➤ Provide mouth care to reduce bacterial flora in the oral cavity.

➤ Provide hospital gown.

➤ Obtain and record baseline vital signs for later comparison readings.

➤ Have the client void.

➤ Administer premedications SC or intramuscularly (IM) as ordered. (Premedications can include an analgesic such as meperidine [Demerol] to reduce discomfort, a sedative, an antianxiety agent such as diazepam [Valium] to promote relaxation, or an anticholinergic such as atropine sulfate to reduce secretions and prevent vagal stimulation that can cause bradycardia.[11])

The Procedure

The procedure varies with the type of bronchoscope and the type of anesthesia used. If needed, cardiac monitoring and cardiopulmonary equipment should be available during both types of bronchoscopy procedures. Specimens obtained during the procedures should be placed in appropriate containers, properly labeled, and promptly sent to the laboratory for cytologic or microbiologic study.

Rigid Bronchoscopy. The client is placed in the supine position and general anesthesia is administered. The neck is hyperextended and the lightly lubricated bronchoscope is inserted orally and advanced through the glottis. If necessary, the bronchoscope can be inserted via a laryngoscope. The segments of the tracheobronchial tree accessible with a rigid bronchoscope are visualized. The client's head can be turned or repositioned to aid visualization of various segments as in turning the head to the left to evaluate the right tracheobronchial tree.[12] After inspection, the bronchial brush, suction catheter, or biopsy forceps can be introduced to obtain tissue or sputum specimens for cytologic or microbiologic study. Specimens can also be obtained by bronchial washing, a procedure that entails the instillation of small amounts of solution into the airways and then removing it. Bronchial washing is a useful technique for the identification of occult malignancies and opportunistic infections in immunocompromised clients.[13] When the examination is completed, the bronchoscope is removed and the client placed in a side-lying position with the head slightly elevated.

Fiberoptic Bronchoscopy. This procedure is usually performed using local anesthesia. The client is placed in a sitting position and the tongue and oropharynx sprayed or swabbed with the local anesthetic. When the loss of sensation is established, the client is placed in the supine position. The fiberoptic scope is introduced into the nose, the mouth, an endotracheal tube, a tracheostomy tube, or a rigid bronchoscope. The most common insertion site is the nose. Clients who have copious secretions or massive hemoptysis or who are more likely to have airway complications can be intubated before the bronchoscopy.[14]

Additional local anesthetic is applied through the scope as it approaches the vocal cords and the carina, eliminating reflex activity in these sensitive areas. The right lung is usually examined first, followed by the left lung. In contrast to rigid bronchoscopy, the fiberoptic approach allows for visualization of airway segments without having to move the client's head through various positions. After inspection, specimens can be obtained for cytologic and microbiologic study. It should be noted that fiberoptic bronchoscopies can be performed with the aid of fluoroscopy if biopsies of small airways or lung parenchyma are to be obtained. When the examination is completed, the bronchoscope is removed. The client who receives a local anesthetic is placed in a semi-Fowler's position.

Nursing Care After the Procedure

If the bronchoscopy is performed under general anesthesia, care and assessment after the procedure are the same as for anyone who is recovering from this type of anesthesia.

➤ If local anesthesia is used, maintain the client in a semi-Fowler's position for about 2 hours and turn to the side as needed.

➤ Monitor vital signs including lung sounds and cardiac rhythm; compare with baselines, and continually assess swallowing ability.

➤ Administer oxygen and monitor for hypoxemia (oxygen saturation) by the oximeter attached to a finger.

➤ Supply tissues and an emesis basin for expectoration of secretions.

➤ If postbronchoscopy sputum samples are to be obtained, provide the client with the appropriate containers and instruct in the procedure to secure the specimens.

➤ Advise the client to refrain from smoking for several hours after the procedure and to withhold food and fluids for 4 to 6 hours until swallowing ability returns.

➤ Inform the client that activities can be resumed when the anesthesia and medications have worn off.

➤ Remind the client that some soreness and possibly hoarseness can be expected after the procedure and that these are of short duration.

➤ Provide warm saline gargles, throat lozenges, and a cool compress to the neck to alleviate throat pain or hoarseness.

➤ Provide pencil and paper for those clients who find it difficult to speak to enable them to communicate.

➤ When the gag reflex and swallowing return, provide soft foods and warm, soothing fluids.

➤ Encourage fluids to assist in easier expectoration or removal of secretions.

➤ Remind the client to report immediately any excessive bleeding, breathing difficulty, or unusual discomforts or sensations.

➤ If the procedure is performed in an ambulatory care setting, assist with arrangements for the client's transportation home.

➤ *Reaction to anesthetic agent or medications:* Note and report tachycardia, palpitations, hyperpnea, or hypertension. Administer ordered antihistamine. Initiate IV line and resuscitation procedure if needed.

➤ *Persistent bleeding:* Note and report amount of excessive hemoptysis and changes in vital signs for potential hypovolemia; caution against coughing and throat clearing that can dislodge a clot at the excision site and precipitate bleeding. Initiate IV line and prepare to replace fluid loss. Prepare the client for bronchoscopy examination to control bleeding at the site.

➤ *Infection:* Note and report elevated temperature, yellowish or other abnormal color of sputum, or changes in breathing pattern. Administer ordered antibiotic therapy.

➤ *Respiratory depression, pneumothorax:* Note and report laryngospasm or bronchospasm, chest pain, increased anxiety, dyspnea, cyanosis, audible wheezing, stridor, or other changes in respiratory pattern, abnormal or absent breath sounds, or hypoxemia. Initiate oxygen and IV line. Prepare and administer ordered medications. Arrange for ABG monitoring. Prepare the client for chest x-ray. Have resuscitation and tracheostomy equipment on hand for immediate use.

➤ *Subcutaneous emphysema:* Note and report subcutaneous crepitus on the face or neck or any changes in breathing pattern. Prepare the client for thoracentesis. Prepare to initiate resuscitation or tracheostomy to maintain ventilation.

➤ *Cardiopulmonary arrest, cardiac dysrhythmias:* Note and report ECG rhythm changes, chest pain, or alterations in vital signs. Administer ordered medications. Prepare to initiate resuscitation procedure and secure assistance.

MEDIASTINOSCOPY

Mediastinoscopy is the direct visualization of the structures that lie beneath the sternum and between the lungs. These structures include the trachea, the esophagus, the heart and its major vessels, the thymus gland, and the lymph nodes that receive drainage from the lungs. The procedure is performed primarily to palpate and biopsy the mediastinal lymph nodes through a small incision at the base of the neck (suprasternal notch).

The lymph nodes in the right side of the mediastinum are those most accessible and safest to biopsy with this procedure. The nodes on the left side are more difficult to explore and biopsy because of the proximity to the aorta.[15] Nodes in the left side of the mediastinum may require biopsy by mediastinotomy, involving a left anterior thoracotomy procedure.[16]

Reference Values

Normal appearance of mediastinal structures; no abnormal lymph node tissue

Interfering Factors

➤ None

Indications for Mediastinoscopy

➤ Lack of confirmation of a diagnosis by bronchoscopy, x-ray, scan, or sputum examination[17]

➤ Radiologic or cytologic evidence of carcinoma or sarcoidosis to confirm the disease

➤ Radiologic evidence of a thoracic infectious process of an indeterminate nature to establish the diagnosis of granulomatous infections, histoplasmosis, coccidiodomycosis, or tuberculosis[18]

➤ Support for diagnosis of Hodgkin's disease involving the lymph nodes[19]

➤ Determination of the stage of known bronchogenic carcinoma as evidenced by the extent of mediastinal lymph node involvement

➤ Support for diagnosis of metastasis of a malignancy into the anterior mediastinum or extrapleurally into the chest

➤ Signs and symptoms of obstruction of mediastinal lymph flow in clients with a history of head or neck malignancy, or both, to determine recurrence or spread of the cancer

Contraindications

➤ Previous mediastinoscopy that resulted in scarring and could make insertion of the scope and biopsy of lymph nodes difficult or impossible

---

➤➤ Nursing Alert

- Inadvertent puncture of the trachea, esophagus, or major blood vessels during mediastinoscopy requires an immediate thoracotomy.

Nursing Care Before the Procedure

Explain to the client:
➤ The location for the procedure (operating room) and the fact that a physician will explain and perform the procedure
➤ That the procedure requires about 1 hour
➤ That food and fluids are withheld for at least 8 hours before and after the procedure until recovery from anesthesia
➤ That the skin at the incisional site can be shaved before the procedure
➤ That a sedative is administered before the procedure to promote relaxation and an IV infusion is started to administer fluids and medications
➤ That general anesthesia is administered and the client is asleep during the procedure
➤ That a small incision is made at the base of the neck for insertion of a microscope-like instrument to examine the structures under the breastbone and between the lungs
➤ That the incision is sutured closed after the examination and a small dressing applied to the area
➤ That vital signs and respiratory status are monitored closely during and after the procedure, that an instrument can be attached to the finger to monitor oxygen saturation, and that cardiac activity is monitored, if needed
➤ That some chest and throat discomfort can be experienced after the procedure and that an analgesic will be administered for these discomforts
Prepare for the procedure:
➤ Obtain a history of allergies to medications or anesthetics, thoracic or hematologic disorders, and treatment regimen.
➤ Ensure that blood typing and cross-matching are obtained and recorded before the procedure in the event that an emergency thoracotomy must be performed.
➤ Shave and prepare the site of insertion, if needed and ordered.

The Procedure

The client is placed in a supine position and an IV infusion is started. General anesthesia is administered via an endotracheal tube. An incision is made at the suprasternal notch, and a path for the mediastinoscope is made using finger dissection. The lymph nodes can be palpated at this time, followed by insertion of the scope through the incision into the superior mediastinum. The area is then inspected and can be photographed for future reference and comparison. Biopsy and culture specimens are obtained, placed in their appropriate containers, properly labeled, and promptly sent to the laboratory. The scope is removed and the incision closed. If the client is stable and no further surgery is immediately indicated, the endotracheal tube is removed.

Nursing Care After the Procedure

Care and assessment after the procedure are the same as for anyone who is recovering from general anesthesia, including monitoring of vital signs, breath sounds, and comfort level.

➤ Observe the incision site for excessive bleeding or drainage. Assess for pain and administer analgesics accordingly.

➤ Administer warm gargles or lozenges for throat soreness resulting from endotracheal tube insertion for general anesthesia.

➤ Resume any foods or fluids withheld before the procedure, as well as other activities, when the client has recovered from anesthesia.

➤ Instruct the client in the observation and care of the incision site.

➤ *Infection:* Note and report elevated temperature, yellowish or other abnormal color of sputum, changes in breathing pattern, redness, pain, edema, and drainage at the incision site. Administer ordered antibiotic therapy. Perform wound care and dressing change.

➤ *Pneumothorax:* Note and report difficulty in breathing and abnormal breath sounds or chest pain. Administer ordered medications. Prepare the client for portable chest x-ray for confirmation and for chest tube insertion.

➤ *Left recurrent laryngeal nerve damage:* Note and report dysphagia, hoarseness, or changes in vocal patterns. Advise the client not to use the voice. Provide the client with pencil and paper for communication.

➤ *Tracheal perforation during the procedure:* Note and report subcutaneous crepitus on face or neck or changes in breathing pattern. Provide for and assist with resuscitation or tracheostomy.

➤ *Puncture of esophagus or major blood vessels during the procedure:* Note and report hemoptysis and amount or changes in vital signs for potential hypovolemia. Provide for post-thoracotomy care with chest tubes in place.

THORACOSCOPY

Thoracoscopy is the direct visualization of the thoracic cavity, which includes the examination of the parietal and visceral pleurae, pleural spaces, thoracic walls, mediastinum, and pericardium of the heart. It can be undertaken as a means of performing laser procedures.[20] Thoracoscopy allows more accurate diagnosis of pulmonary conditions than other diagnostic methods. It requires the insertion of a chest tube connected to negative thoracic suction and a drainage system until the lung reinflates.

Reference Values

Normal appearance of thoracic cavity; no abnormality of the parietal and visceral pleurae, pleural spaces, chest cavity wall, mediastinum, or pericardium

Interfering Factors

➤ None

Indications for Thoracoscopy

➤ Radiologic evidence of pleural effusion to establish the diagnosis of inflammatory processes

➤ Evaluation of lung involvement in sarcoidosis

➤ Obtaining of tissue for biopsy to support diagnosis of malignancy and size of tumor, extent of growth, and metastasis within the thoracic cavity

➤ Confirmation of cause or predisposing factors associated with pneumothorax

➤ Evidence of emphysema, empyema, or other chronic pulmonary disease by x-ray, scan, or sputum examination

➤ Performance of laser procedure to reduce the size of a tumor

Contraindications

➤ Severely compromised respiratory status caused by obstructive or restrictive pulmonary disease

➤ Presence of or risk for respiratory failure as indicated by ABG levels for pO_2 and CO_2

➤➤ Nursing Alert

• Respiratory distress after the procedure requires resuscitation equipment to be on hand.

Nursing Care Before the Procedure

Client teaching is the same as for mediastinoscopy (see p. 541).

➤ The client should also be informed that a local anesthetic can be used instead of a general anesthetic and that the incision is made in the chest with the scope inserted through the incision to examine the structures in the chest cavity and possibly to obtain a biopsy.

➤ The client should be informed that a chest tube is inserted and connected to a suction apparatus after the procedure and will remain in place for about 24 hours or until the lung has re-expanded.

➤ The client should be instructed and provided with an opportunity to practice coughing and breathing exercises to assist with lung re-expansion and prevent atelectasis after general anesthesia.

➤ Physical preparation is the same as that outlined for bronchoscopy and mediastinoscopy (see pp. 537 to 538).

➤ Additional diagnostic test and procedure results should be recorded before the procedure, such as ABGs, routine blood tests and urinalysis, and chest x-ray and ECG for those over 40 years of age or with cardiac or pulmonary conditions.

➤ An IV line should be initiated to administer fluids and medications if needed.

The Procedure

The client is positioned to expose the insertion site, and local anesthetic is injected or general anesthetic administered via an endotracheal tube. An incision is made to allow insertion of the scope into the thoracic cavity. The areas are inspected and specimens obtained or treatment performed by laser or other method. The tissue biopsy or culture material, or both, are placed in appropriate containers, properly labeled, and promptly sent to the laboratory. A chest tube is inserted and connected to negative pressure suction after the scope is removed. The client is extubated when the condition is determined to be stable; he or she is then taken to a hospital room.

Nursing Care After the Procedure

Care and assessment after the procedure are the same as for anyone who is recovering from general anesthesia, including monitoring of vital signs, breath sounds, and comfort level.

➤ Monitor the amount and color of drainage from the chest tube, chest tube patency, and suction functioning in removing the fluid. Assess respiratory status based on ABG determinations and breathing.

➤ Assist with a chest x-ray if performed to determine whether air or fluid is present in the pleural space.

➤ Observe the incision site for excessive bleeding or drainage, and assess for pain and administer analgesics accordingly.

➤ Encourage coughing and deep-breathing exercises, with splinting of the incision site.

➤ Resume any foods or fluids withheld before the procedure when the client has recovered from general anesthesia.

➤ Resume other activities after removal of the chest tube and healing of the incision wound.

➤ *Infection (empyema):* Note and report temperature elevation and changes in sputum color and breathing pattern indicating infection. Administer antibiotic therapy.

➤ *Hemorrhage:* Note and report hemoptysis and amount, blood loss in chest drainage bottle, or changes in vital signs indicating hypovolemia. Initiate IV fluid replacement. Prepare for invasive procedure to stop bleeding, if necessary.

➤ *Respiratory distress:* Note and report dyspnea, hypoxia based on ABG levels, or abnormal breath sounds. Administer oxygen and ordered medications. Prepare for intubation and assisted ventilation.

Esophagogastroduodenoscopy (EGD)

Esophagogastroduodenoscopy (EGD) is the direct visualization of the mucosa of the upper gastrointestinal tract, which includes the esophagus, stomach, and upper duodenum, using a flexible fiberoptic endoscope (Fig. 16–6). Any or all of the three structures can be included in the examination and can be referred to as esophagoscopy, gastroscopy, or duodenoscopy, or a combination of these, that is, esophagogastroduodenoscopy. The upper small intestinal tract procedure, referred to as enteroscopy, can also be performed with a longer scope to obtain biopsies and diagnose pathologies in this area of the tract.[21]

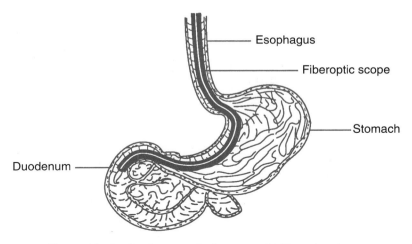

Figure 16-6 Esophagogastroduodenoscopy with fiberoptic endoscope.

Direct visualization yields greater diagnostic data than is possible through radiologic procedures such as upper gastrointestinal (UGI) x-ray studies and is gradually replacing them as the diagnostic study of choice.[22] The EGD procedure can be performed for therapeutic as well as diagnostic purposes.

The standard flexible fiberoptic endoscope used for EGD contains one to three channels that allow for passage of various instruments needed to perform therapeutic or diagnostic procedures. Smaller endoscopes are available for use in children and in adults in whom passage of a larger endoscope can be difficult; however, technical capabilities of the instrument are often correspondingly reduced.[23]

Reference Values

Normal appearance of the mucosa of the esophagus, stomach, and duodenum; no inflammation, ulceration, stricture, or other abnormality

Interfering Factors

➤ Inability to cooperate in the procedure
➤ Failure to follow dietary restrictions before the procedure, although some gastric contents can be aspirated via the endoscope
➤ Barium swallow within the preceding 48 hours, because the retained barium can hinder adequate visualization
➤ Severe UGI bleeding,; blood and clots can interfere with visualization (Gastric lavage is performed before endoscopy in this instance.)

Indications for Esophagogastroduodenoscopy (EGD)

➤ Signs and symptoms of reflux esophagitis or esophageal strictures to confirm the diagnosis
➤ Signs and symptoms of hiatal hernia to confirm the diagnosis
➤ Signs and symptoms of gastric or duodenal ulcer to confirm the diagnosis, especially when radiologic studies yield unsatisfactory or equivocal results

➤ Persistent symptoms of peptic ulcer disease, despite therapy, to determine the nature of the problem

➤ Bleeding from the UGI tract to determine the source, such as esophageal varices, Mallory-Weiss tears, peptic ulcer, stress ulcer, and stoppage of bleeding, if possible, by sclerotherapy or coagulation. (*Note:* If a perforated viscus is suspected, EGD is contraindicated, and surgery is performed.)

➤ Suspected immunologic, anatomic, and neoplastic disorders involving the UGI tract to confirm diagnosis through tissue biopsy[24]

➤ Suspected strictures involving the antrum or pylorus of the stomach to confirm diagnosis, with dilatation if indicated

➤ Diagnosis of tumors, malformation, and other pathology of the upper small intestine

➤ History of ingestion of a foreign body that cannot or has not passed through the gastrointestinal system, with removal if visualized and accessible

➤ History of ingestion of chemicals that can injure the esophagus or stomach to determine the extent of damage

➤ Suspected inflammatory or infectious process involving the esophagus, such as *Candida* esophagitis, to confirm the diagnosis through microbiologic analysis

➤ Evaluation of client status after surgery on the UGI tract

➤ Performance of endoscopic surgery with a laser beam

Contraindications

➤ Aneurysm of the aortic arch because of the risk of rupture during EGD instrumentation

➤ Unstable cardiac status, because mild hypoxemia can be induced by EGD (If it is absolutely necessary to perform the procedure, the client can be intubated and mechanically ventilated before and during the procedure.)

➤ Known or suspected perforated viscus, because the situation indicates surgery, not endoscopy, and because endoscopic instrumentation can further aggravate the situation

➤ Large Zenker's diverticulum involving the esophagus, as perforation can occur during instrumentation

➤ Suspected aortoduodenal fistula with persistent or major bleeding, because surgical intervention is indicated

➤ History of dysphagia, unless previous radiologic studies such as esophagram indicate the nature of the problem and potential hazards involved in passing the endoscope

➤ Recent gastrointestinal surgery in which anastomosis can be disrupted by the insufflation of the organ with air

Nursing Care Before the Procedure

Client teaching and physical preparation are the same as for bronchoscopy (see pp. 537 to 538).

➤ Inform the client that the procedure takes at least 1 hour, that an IV line is initiated to administer fluid and additional medications immediately before the procedure, and that the type of anesthesia is usually local but can be general if the client is unduly apprehensive.

➤ Inform the client that the instrument is inserted through the mouth and passed into the stomach and small intestine.

➤ Obtain a history that includes known and suspected gastrointestinal tract disorders, treatment regimen, and other diagnostic tests and procedures.

The Procedure

The client is seated in a semireclining position and the oropharynx is sprayed or swabbed with a topical local anesthetic. It should be noted that not all endoscopists use local anesthesia, because it is not thought to be necessary in the adequately sedated client.[25] The client is then assisted to the left lateral position, with the right hand at the side, the left hand under the pillow at the head, the neck slightly flexed, and the knees drawn up at a right angle to the body. Additional IV sedation can be given, usually diazepam (Valium), at this time. Depending on the client's condition, vital signs and cardiac rhythm can be monitored throughout the procedure. Cardiopulmonary resuscitation equipment is available for use if needed. In an emergency such as bleeding esophageal varices, EGD can be performed at the bedside provided that cardiac status is monitored continuously and equipment is on hand for resuscitation if needed.

A protective guard is inserted into the mouth to cover the teeth, and a bite block can also be inserted to maintain an open mouth without client effort or control. The client is informed that speaking is not possible but that breathing is not affected. Advise the client that breathing deeply will help to allay gagging and choking. The endoscope is then directed through the mouth and down the pharynx. A dental-type suction device is used to drain secretions from the mouth. The esophagus is examined, and the scope is advanced into the stomach. If the client retches or vomits when the scope is introduced into the esophagus, the emesis is removed by the suction apparatus attached to the endoscope. Air can be introduced through the endoscope to inflate and smooth out the folds of the stomach for more thorough visualization, and the client should be informed that it causes a feeling of fullness or bloating. Excessive introduction of air causes client discomfort and leads to uncontrollable belching.[26] The endoscope is then advanced through the pyloric sphincter, and the duodenum is visualized.

At any point in the examination of the organs, accessory equipment such as a cytology brush, biopsy forceps, and camera can be introduced to obtain specimens or photographs. Specimens are placed in appropriate containers, properly labeled, and promptly sent to the laboratory. When the examination is completed, the dental suction device is removed, the endoscope is withdrawn, and the tooth guard and bite block are removed.

Nursing Care After the Procedure

If the procedure is performed under general anesthesia, care and assessment are the same as for anyone who is recovering from this type of anesthesia, including monitoring of vital signs, breath sounds, and comfort level.

➤ After local anesthesia, assist the client to a position of comfort with the head slightly elevated, and encourage the client to expectorate any accumulated secretions.

➤ Maintain the client in a side-lying position for 1 to 2 hours to prevent aspiration of secretions.

➤ Monitor vital signs and cardiac rhythm as well as respiratory status, and compare with baselines. Assess swallowing ability, site, and degree of pain continuously.

➤ Advise the client to withhold food and fluids for 4 to 6 hours, until swallowing ability returns.

➤ Restrict activities until the sedative or anesthetic has worn off and the client is awake and alert.

➤ Provide warm saline gargles or throat lozenges to alleviate throat discomfort.

➤ When the gag reflex and swallowing return, provide soft foods and warm, soothing fluids.

➤ Remind the client that belching, bloating, or flatulence is the result of air insufflation.

➤ Instruct the client to report immediately any postprocedural discomfort or pain in the chest, neck, back, or upper abdomen; pain upon swallowing; difficulty in breathing; or blood expectoration.

➤ *Reaction to anesthetic agent or medications:* Note and report tachycardia, palpitations, hyperpnea, or hypertension. Administer ordered antihistamines. Initiate IV line and resuscitation procedure if needed.

➤ *Perforation of esophagus:* Note and report neck pain or pain on swallowing, hemoptysis and amount (bleeding at the cervical level), substernal or epigastric pain, chest pain that increases with breathing (bleeding at the thoracic level), or changes in vital signs for potential hypovolemia. Initiate IV line for fluid replacement. Prepare for intervention to repair damaged area.

➤ *Perforation of diaphragm or stomach:* Note and report pain in the shoulder, dyspnea (diaphragm), abdominal or back pain (stomach), or changes in vital signs for potential hypovolemia. Initiate IV line for fluid replacement. Prepare for intervention to repair damaged area.

➤ *Persistent bleeding:* Note and report hemoptysis; hematemesis and amounts; black, tarry stools; or changes in vital signs for potential hypovolemia if bleeding is excessive. Initiate IV line for fluid volume replacement or transfusion of whole blood or packed red blood cells as ordered.

➤ *Pulmonary aspiration:* Note and report dyspnea, cyanosis, abnormal breath sounds, hypoxemia, or signs and symptoms of aspiration pneumonia or pleural effusion. Maintain the client in a side-lying position and suction airway; provide resuscitation procedure as needed for immediate interventions. Administer antibiotic therapy if pneumonia is present.

➤ *Cardiac abnormalities:* Note and report dysrhythmias, chest pain, or alterations in blood pressure and pulse. Administer ordered cardiac medications. Monitor cardiac activity via ECG.

ENDOSCOPIC RETROGRADE CHOLANGIOPANCREATOGRAPHY (ERCP)

Endoscopic retrograde cholangiopancreatography (ERCP) is the visualization of the pancreatic and biliary ducts after they have been injected with dye (Fig. 16–7). The study involves both endoscopic and radiologic procedures. A side-

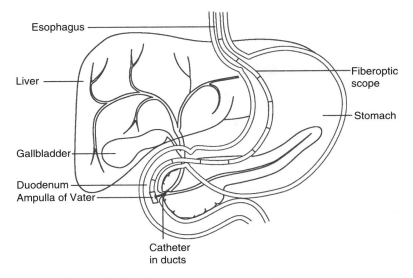

Esophagus

Liver

Gallbladder

Duodenum

Ampulla of Vater

Fiberoptic
scope

Stomach

Catheter
in ducts

Figure 16-7   Endoscopic retrograde cholangiopancreatography.

viewing flexible fiberoptic endoscope is passed into the duodenum and a small
cannula is inserted into the duodenal papilla (ampulla of Vater), through which
pancreatic juices and bile normally drain into the duodenum. Radiographic contrast medium is injected through the cannula, and the pancreatic and biliary ducts
are visualized by fluoroscopic x-ray. Manometry to measure the pressure of the
ducts can be obtained by insertion of a catheter into the channel of the scope and
placing it at the sphincter of Oddi. Another procedure that provides visualization
of the ducts is percutaneous transhepatic cholangiography (PTHC), an invasive
procedure associated with significant morbidity.[27] The ERCP procedure can be
performed for therapeutic as well as diagnostic purposes, usually in a special endoscopy suite or in the radiology department.

Reference Values

Normal appearance of the duodenal papilla upon visualization; patent common
bile and pancreatic ducts when visualized by fluoroscopic x-ray; no gallstones,
strictures, or abnormal tissue

Interfering Factors

➤ Inability to cooperate during the procedure, although it can be performed
    under general anesthesia, if necessary
➤ Failure to follow dietary restrictions before the procedure, although some
    gastric and duodenal contents can be aspirated via the endoscope
➤ Previous surgery involving the stomach or duodenum, or both, that can
    cause difficulty in locating the duodenal papilla
➤ Barium remaining in the stomach or bowel when gastrointestinal series has
    been performed before the procedure

Indications for Endoscopic Retrograde Cholangiopancreatography (ERCP)

➤ Jaundice of unknown etiology to differentiate biliary tract obstruction from liver disease
➤ Identification of obstruction caused by calculi, cysts in the ducts, strictures, stenosis, and anatomic abnormalities
➤ Retrieval of small gallstones from the distal common bile duct, release of strictures by dilatation within the biliary tree, performance of therapeutic procedures such as sphincterotomy (sphincter of Oddi), and placement of biliary drains[28]
➤ Suspicion of carcinoma involving the duodenal papilla, head of the pancreas, or biliary tract when results of other studies such as ultrasound, scans, or radiography are negative or inconclusive
➤ Signs and symptoms of chronic pancreatitis to confirm the diagnosis
➤ Signs and symptoms of sclerosing cholangitis to confirm the diagnosis
➤ Persistent abdominal pain of unknown etiology when the only alternative to ERCP is exploratory surgery
➤ Obtaining of tissue biopsy for cytologic analysis

Contraindications

➤ Unstable cardiopulmonary status because ERCP could precipitate cardiac dysrhythmias and hypoxemia
➤ Blood coagulation defects, especially if sphincterotomy is to be performed
➤ Cholangitis unless the client received antibiotic therapy before the procedure
➤ Acute pancreatitis unless there are specific indications for the procedure such as suspicion of hemorrhagic pancreatitis, recurrent acute pancreatitis of unknown etiology, or acute pancreatitis caused by gallstone blockage[29]
➤ Pancreatic pseudocyst except when ultrasound and computed tomography (CT) scans have aided in localizing the cyst and when follow-up surgery is anticipated[30]
➤ Large Zenker's diverticulum involving the esophagus because the scope can find its way into the diverticulum and perforation can occur with instrumentation

---

➤➤ Nursing Alert

• Resuscitation equipment should be available to treat respiratory depression with hypoxemia, cardiac complications, or adverse effects of drugs used before and during the procedure.

Nursing Care Before the Procedure

Client teaching is the same as for bronchoscopy and esophagogastroduodenoscopy (see pp. 537 to 538).

➤ Inform the client that an x-ray can be taken before the procedure and several x-ray films during the procedure after the endoscope has been inserted and that additional medication can be administered to relax the sphincter of the duodenal papilla.

➤ Advise the client that the position will be changed to prone after the endoscope reaches the small intestine to accommodate the visualization of the duodenal papilla and injection of a dye into the ducts. Inform the client that a flushed feeling can be experienced when the dye is injected.

➤ Physical preparation is the same as for a client being prepared for bronchoscopy or esophagogastroduodenoscopy (see pp. 537 to 538).

➤ Obtain a history that includes known or suspected gastrointestinal disorders, treatment regimen, information about sensitivity to iodine to prevent possible reaction to the dye, and the date of the last menstrual period to determine the possibility of pregnancy to prevent exposure of the developing fetus to x-ray.

➤ Administer morphine sulfate instead of meperidine (Demerol) as a preprocedural medication.

The Procedure

The client is placed on an x-ray table in the supine position and a plain film (flat plate) of the abdomen is taken to observe for any residual contrast media from previous studies, such as barium studies or scans using contrast media, which can interfere with a successful procedure. Because the client will lie on the table for approximately 1 to 2 hours, it is desirable that the table be padded and that measures be taken to ensure client comfort. The oropharynx is sprayed or swabbed with a topical local anesthetic. If an IV access such as a heparin lock or IV line has not been established, it is done at this time. The IV access device or line is placed in the right hand or arm because the client will be positioned on the left side during the procedure until the endoscope is passed into the duodenum.[31] Cardiac rhythm and pulse oximetry for oxygen saturation and vital signs should be monitored throughout the procedure, and cardiopulmonary resuscitation equipment should be available.

The client is then assisted to the left lateral position with the left arm positioned behind the back, the right hand at the side, and the neck slightly flexed. A protective guard is inserted into the mouth to cover the teeth, and a bite block can also be inserted to maintain an adequate opening of the mouth without client effort or control. Additional sedative and analgesic medications are administered through the IV line at this time. The endoscope is passed through the mouth with a dental suction device in place to drain secretions. The scope is then advanced down the esophagus and into the stomach. Air can be introduced to smooth out the folds of the stomach for better visualization of all areas. When the endoscope reaches the duodenum, medications such as simethicone (Mylicon) can be instilled via the scope to reduce the bubbling caused by bile secretions. Atropine sulfate and glucagon can be administered through the IV line at this time to relax the duodenum and reduce motility to allow for cannulation of the ampulla of Vater.

The client is then turned to the prone position, and the duodenal papilla is visualized and cannulated with a catheter. The client is requested to remain very still during this phase of the procedure. Occasionally the client can be turned slightly to the right side to aid in visualization of the papilla. Dye (contrast medium) is injected into the pancreatic and biliary ducts via the catheter, and a series of fluoroscopic x-ray films are taken. ERCP manometry can also be performed to measure the pressure in the bile duct, pancreatic duct, and sphincter of Oddi at the papilla area via the catheter as it is placed in the area before the dye is injected.[32]

Specimens and biopsies for cytologic analysis can be obtained during the procedure. These are placed in appropriate containers, properly labeled, and promptly sent to the laboratory. When the examination is completed, the dental suction device is removed, the endoscope is withdrawn, and the tooth guard and bite block are removed.

Nursing Care After the Procedure

Care and assessment after the procedure are the same as for esophagogastro-duodenoscopy (see p. 547).

➤ Assess the ability to resume usual voiding patterns because anticholinergics (atropine sulfate) can cause urinary retention.

➤ *Reaction to medications or anesthetic agent:* Note and report tachycardia, palpitations, hyperpnea, hypertension, or reactions to the dye, such as pallor, hypotension, restlessness, and diaphoresis. Administer ordered antihistamines. Initiate resuscitation procedure if needed.

➤ *Perforation of pharynx or esophagus:* Note and report neck or chest pain, pain on swallowing, hemoptysis, or changes in vital signs for potential hypovolemia. Initiate IV line for fluid volume replacement. Prepare for intervention to repair damaged area.

➤ *Respiratory depression:* Note and report breathing difficulty, apnea, cyanosis, hypoxemia, hypotension, bradycardia, or bronchospasm. Administer oxygen or narcotic antagonist (naloxone), if ordered. Perform resuscitation and mechanical ventilation if needed.

➤ *Cholangitis, septicemia:* Note and report temperature elevation, upper abdominal pain, culture results identifying *Escherichia coli* or *Pseudomonas* spp. from release of organisms in infected bile into the bloodstream.[33] Administer ordered antibiotic and analgesic therapy.

➤ *Acute pancreatitis:* Note and report severe epigastric and abdominal pain radiating to the back, abdominal distention, hypoactive bowel sounds, jaundice, or temperature elevation. Administer ordered analgesia. Obtain blood specimen for amylase and bilirubin as levels rise in pancreatitis, although they are usually elevated as a result of the procedure itself from the pressure and volume of the dye injected into the pancreatic duct.[34,35]

➤ *Cardiac abnormalities:* Note and report dysrhythmias, chest pain, or alterations in blood pressure and pulse. Administer cardiac medications. Monitor cardiac activity via ECG.

PROCTOSIGMOIDOSCOPY

Proctosigmoidoscopy is the direct visualization of the mucosa of the anal canal (anoscopy), the rectum (proctoscopy), and the distal sigmoid colon (sigmoidoscopy). The procedure can be performed using a rigid or flexible fiberoptic endoscope, although the flexible instrument is generally preferred.

Either procedure can be performed in any setting, and a signed informed consent is not required for anoscopy if performed as a single procedure, but it is required for proctosigmoidoscopy if tissue is to be removed. Some type of bowel preparation is always needed before the procedure to clear the rectum and sigmoid colon of feces to enhance visualization.

Reference Values

Normal mucosa of the anal canal, rectum, and sigmoid colon; no polyps or other abnormal tissue, bleeding, or inflammation

Interfering Factors

➤ Inability to cooperate with the procedure
➤ Severe rectal bleeding or inadequate bowel preparation

Indications for Proctosigmoidoscopy

➤ Cancer screening with identification and polyp removal in individuals over 40 to 45 years of age who are asymptomatic, as part of a complete physical examination[36,37]
➤ Examination of the distal colon before a barium enema x-ray to obtain a better view of the area[38]
➤ Determination of pathology after a barium enema x-ray with uncertain findings
➤ Excision of tissue for cytologic analysis
➤ Blood, pus, or mucus in the feces, or a combination of these conditions, to determine the cause of the problem, such as inflammatory bowel disease
➤ Determination of the cause of pain or tissue prolapse on defecation to determine the cause of the problem, such as rectal prolapse, abscess, fistula, or fissure
➤ History of rectal itching, pain, or burning to determine the cause of the problem, such as hemorrhoids
➤ Signs and symptoms of diverticular disease involving the sigmoid colon to confirm the diagnosis
➤ Signs and symptoms of Hirschsprung's disease and colitis in children to confirm the diagnosis
➤ Treatment to reduce volvulus of the sigmoid colon
➤ Removal of hemorrhoids by laser therapy

Contraindications

➤ Suspected bowel perforation, acute peritonitis, acute fulminant colitis, diverticulitis, toxic megacolon, or ischemic bowel necrosis
➤ Severe cardiopulmonary disease
➤ Large abdominal aortic or iliac aneurysm
➤ Severe bleeding or blood coagulation abnormality
➤ Advanced pregnancy

➤➤ Nursing Alert

- A preparation that includes a laxative or enemas should not be administered to pregnant women or clients with inflammatory colon diseases unless the physician is notified and special orders are obtained.

Nursing Care Before the Procedure

Explain to the client:

➤ The location for the procedure and the fact that a physician will perform the procedure

➤ That the procedure requires about 15 to 30 minutes

➤ That a light meal the evening before and liquids the morning of the procedure are allowed

➤ That a laxative and enema can be administered the night before and that two sodium phosphate-sodium biphosphate (Fleet) small-volume enemas can be given 1 hour before the procedure to remove feces for better visualization (This instruction varies with physician or hospital depending on the procedure to be performed and whether it is performed in conjunction with other studies, such as barium enema x-ray.)

➤ That the client will be placed in a knee-chest position for the rigid proctoscopic examination or a left lateral position for the flexible fiberoptic procedure; that drapes will be used to avoid exposure and prevent embarrassment; and that the lubricated scope will be inserted into the rectum after the physician performs a digital rectal examination

➤ That the urge to defecate can be experienced when the scope is inserted; that slow, deep breathing through the mouth can help to alleviate this feeling; that the client will be allowed to practice this breathing technique beforehand

➤ That specimens can be obtained and suctioning performed through the scope to remove excess materials during the examination to enhance visualization

➤ That slight rectal bleeding can be experienced after the procedure if polyps or tissue is excised but that it should not persist for longer than 2 days

Prepare for the procedure:

➤ Obtain a history of bowel disorders, pregnancy status, and blood studies that indicate a coagulation disorder.

➤ Ensure that dietary and fluid restrictions have been followed (light meal in the evening and liquids in the morning before the procedure).

➤ Ensure that bowel preparation has been implemented (laxatives or enema, or both, in the evening and one or two enemas in the morning before the study).

➤ Provide the client with a hospital gown to wear as needed.

➤ Have the client void.

➤ Obtain and record baseline vital signs for later comparison readings.

The Procedure

Depending on the type of instrument to be used, the client is assisted to either the left lateral position with the buttocks at or extending slightly beyond the edge of the examination table or bed (fiberoptic scope) or the knee-chest position on a special examining table that tilts the client into the desired position (rigid scope). The client is draped for warmth and privacy.

After visual inspection of the perianal area, a preliminary digital rectal examination is performed with a well-lubricated gloved finger. A fecal specimen can be obtained from the glove when the finger is removed from the rectum. A lubricated anoscope is then inserted and the anal canal inspected (anoscopy).

The anoscope is then removed, and a lubricated proctoscope or flexible sigmoid-oscope is inserted. The lubricant is used to ease passage of the scope and de-crease discomfort. The scope is manipulated gently to facilitate passage, and air can be injected to improve visualization. Inform the client that this portion of the procedure can cause flatus to be expelled. Suction and cotton swabs are used to remove excess blood, mucus, or liquid feces that can hinder visualiza-tion. Examination also takes place as the scope is gradually withdrawn. Speci-mens of tissue or exudate can be obtained, polyps excised, or photographs taken via accessories to the endoscope. Additional examination of the rectal and anal areas can also be performed. When the examination is completed, the scope is completely withdrawn and residual lubricant is cleansed from the anal area.

Nursing Care After the Procedure

Care and assessment after the procedure include assisting the client to the supine position and allowing him or her to rest for a few minutes or as needed.

➤ Take vital signs and compare with preprocedure readings.

➤ Gradually assist the client to a sitting position to avoid possible orthostatic hypotension. Take vital signs again, and report to the physician any changes from the baselines.

➤ Assist the client in cleansing any remaining lubricant from the anal area with commercial wipes or mild soap and warm water, if needed.

➤ Provide a sitz bath that can soothe and relieve discomfort.

➤ Remind the client that slight rectal bleeding or blood in the stool can be noted for up to 2 days.

➤ Instruct the client to report to the physician any abdominal pain or distention or pain on defecation.

➤ *Persistent bleeding:* Note and report amount of bleeding from the rectum or changes in vital signs for potential hypovolemia. Prepare for procedure to control bleeding at the biopsy or polyp removal site.

➤ *Colon perforation:* Note and report abdominal pain and distention, fever, or mucopurulent drainage or bleeding from the rectum. Initiate IV line. Prepare the client for surgical repair of the colon.

COLONOSCOPY

Colonoscopy is the direct visualization of the mucosa of the entire colon and terminal ileum by means of a flexible fiberoptic colonoscope (Fig. 16–8). Fluoroscopy can be used to assist in guiding the advancement of the scope.[39] Colonoscopes used for this procedure vary in length, depending on the extent of the colon to be examined and the size and age of the client, with more than 20 different types of scopes available commercially.[40] When the colonoscope has been inserted as far as the cecum, nearly the entire tube is contained within the colon.[41] The procedure is similar to that for a proctosigmoidoscopy, except that it takes longer to perform (as long as 2 or more hours).

Reference Values

Normal intestinal mucosa with no polyps or other abnormal tissues; no bleed-ing or inflammation.

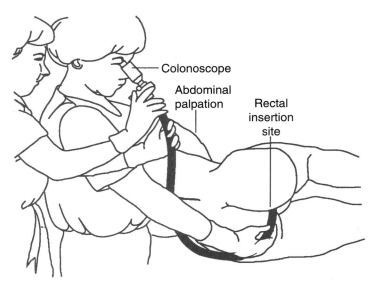

Figure 16–8 Colonoscopy with fiberoptic endoscope.

Interfering Factors

➤ Inability to cooperate in the procedure
➤ Severe gastrointestinal bleeding or inadequate bowel preparation

Indications for Colonoscopy

➤ Signs and symptoms of lower gastrointestinal disorders, especially when barium enema x-rays and proctosigmoidoscopy have failed to provide a definitive diagnosis
➤ Determination of the cause of rectal bleeding, such as in polyps, diverticular disease, cancer, vascular abnormalities, with possible hemostasis by coagulation
➤ Suspicion of cancer involving any part of the colon
➤ Follow-up of clients previously treated for cancer of the colon
➤ Follow-up of clients who have had surgery for recurrence of polyps or lesions
➤ Signs and symptoms of inflammatory bowel disease such as Crohn's disease, ulcerative colitis, infectious colitis
➤ Follow-up of clients who have previously received radiation therapy to detect radiation colitis
➤ Further evaluation and sclerosis of strictures in the colon by laser if needed
➤ Evaluation or diagnosis of Hirschsprung's disease in children
➤ Evaluation of clients with endometriosis, which can involve the colon in 30 to 35 percent of those examined
➤ Removal of polyps and foreign bodies from the colon
➤ Reduction of sigmoid volvulus and intussusceptions of the colon[42]

Contraindications

➤ Suspected bowel perforation, acute peritonitis, acute fulminant colitis or other type of colitis, ischemic bowel necrosis
➤ Recent bowel surgery
➤ Advanced pregnancy
➤ Severe cardiac or pulmonary disease
➤ Recent myocardial infarction
➤ Known or suspected pulmonary embolus
➤ Large abdominal aortic or iliac aneurysm
➤ Severe bleeding or blood coagulation abnormality

➤➤ Nursing Alert

- A preparation that includes laxatives or enema should not be administered to pregnant women or to clients with inflammatory colon disease unless the physician is notified and special orders are obtained.

Nursing Care Before the Procedure

Client teaching is the same as for proctosigmoidoscopy (see p. 554).

➤ Inform the client that the procedure requires 30 to 60 minutes to complete and that meals should consist of a clear liquid diet for 24 to 48 hours before the examination.
➤ Inform the client that bowel preparation consists of a laxative during the late afternoon of the day before the procedure and that warm tap water or saline enemas until clear are administered 2 hours before the procedure.
➤ Medications are administered to promote relaxation, alleviate potential discomfort, and reduce secretions 30 minutes before the procedure, and an IV line can be started to administer fluids and additional medications for sedation and relaxation before insertion of the scope.
➤ Obtain history of bowel, anal, or rectal disorders; blood coagulation disorder; pregnancy status; and medications such as aspirin or iron preparation taken 1 week before the procedure, as such medications affect blood clotting and cause black, sticky stool that is difficult to remove with bowel preparation.
➤ Ensure that hematologic status and blood clotting ability have been assessed to include CBC, platelet level, PT, PTT, clotting time, and bleeding time before the procedure.
➤ Ensure that clients with heart valve disorders have had prophylactic antibiotic therapy.
➤ Ensure that client follows dietary and fluid restrictions of a liquid diet for 24 to 48 hours before the study and ingests no solid foods for at least 2 hours before oral bowel preparation.
➤ Ensure that the bowel preparation has been implemented. (This includes 1 day of oral bowel preparation except in those clients with ulcers, colitis, or obstructions or in children. It also includes administering laxatives or enemas, or both, until clear and free from any solid material.)

➤ Initiate an IV line or venous access device if ordered.

➤ Provide a hospital gown.

➤ Have the client void.

➤ Obtain and record baseline vital signs for later comparison readings.

➤ Administer premedications SC or IM as ordered. (Premedications can include an analgesic such as meperidine [Demerol] to reduce discomfort, a sedative or an antianxiety agent such as diazepam [Valium] to promote relaxation, or an anticholinergic such as atropine sulfate to reduce secretions.)

The Procedure

The client is assisted to the left lateral position and draped for privacy with the buttocks exposed. Every effort should be made to prevent client embarrassment. Cardiac monitoring and cardiopulmonary resuscitation equipment are available during and after the procedures. If an IV access such as a heparin lock or an IV line has not been established, it is made at this time in the right hand or arm because the client is positioned on the left side initially. Additional sedation such as diazepam (Valium) can be administered through the IV at this time. After visual inspection of the perianal area, a preliminary digital rectal examination is performed with a well-lubricated finger. The fiberoptic colonoscope is well lubricated to ease passage of the scope and reduce discomfort and is then inserted into the anus. The client is requested to bear down as the scope is advanced into the rectum to ease passage of the tube. Gentle abdominal pressure can be applied as the scope is advanced through the sigmoid colon. As the transverse colon is entered, the client can be assisted to the supine position to facilitate passage of the scope. Small amounts of air can be insufflated throughout the procedure to aid in visualization, and sometimes air is removed to promote passage of the scope. The client should be informed that this practice can cause flatus during and after the study. Abdominal pressure can be applied again when the scope reaches the splenic flexure. As the scope reaches the hepatic flexure, the client is requested to take deep breaths to aid in the movement of the scope downward through the ascending colon to the cecum. Finally, the scope is inserted into the terminal portion of the ileum.[43]

The bowel lumen is studied as the scope is withdrawn and, if indicated, biopsy specimens, cultures, and smears are obtained and polyps or foreign bodies removed. Photographs can also be taken for future reference. Tissue samples are placed in appropriate containers, properly labeled, and promptly sent to the laboratory.

Nursing Care After the Procedure

Care and assessment after the procedure include assisting the client to a position of comfort and allowing time to rest.

➤ Take vital signs and compare them with preprocedure readings to assess for changes caused by vasovagal reflex and other complications as outlined later in this section.

➤ Monitor respiratory status and cardiac rhythm as well as comfort level, and report changes to the physician.

➤ Provide a sitz bath to relieve discomfort.

➤ Restrict foods and fluids for approximately 2 hours after the procedure as well as activities until the sedation has worn off.

➤ Discontinue the IV line or access device when the client is stable.

➤ Remind the client that slight bleeding can cause blood in the feces for about 2 days if polyps or biopsy tissues have been excised and to report immediately any abdominal pain, excessive bleeding, fever, or unusual sensations.

➤ *Reactions to medications:* Note and report changes in vital signs (hypotension and bradycardia) or respiratory depression (cyanosis, changes in breathing pattern, and breath sounds). Administer ordered antihistamines and other medications. Initiate oxygen administration or resuscitation procedure as needed.

➤ *Postcolonoscopy distention syndrome:* Note and report abdominal distention and cramping from air injected into the bowel during the procedure. Insert rectal tube, perform position changes, and encourage walking with assistance.

➤ *Hemorrhage:* Note and report excessive and persistent bleeding from the rectum if polyps were removed or biopsy was performed. Also note and report increased pulse and decreased blood pressure or grossly bloody feces. Initiate IV line for fluid volume replacement or blood transfusion as appropriate.

➤ *Colon perforation:* Note and report abdominal pain, distention, and rigidity or fever. Administer ordered medication. Prepare the client for possible surgical repair of the colon.

➤ *Cardiac dysrhythmias, myocardial infarction:* Note and report chest pain or changes in pulse rate and rhythm. Monitor cardiac activity via ECG. Initiate IV line and administer ordered medications.

CYSTOSCOPY

Cystoscopy is the direct visualization of the urethra, urinary bladder, and ureteral orifices by means of a rigid cystoscope inserted through the urethra (Fig. 16–9). It contains an obturator to assist in the insertion (which is removed after the scope is in place) and a telescope with a lens and light system. Flexible fiberoptic cystoscopes are also available and are used in different sizes and varieties depending on the reason for the procedure. The purpose of cystoscopy is primarily to diagnose pathological conditions, but it can also be therapeutic to perform or evaluate treatment protocols. The procedure allows a view of areas not usually observable with x-ray procedures, and it can be performed with or after ultrasonography or radiography.

Reference Values

Normal urethra, bladder, and ureters; no polyps or other abnormal tissues, inflammation or bleeding, or strictures or anatomic abnormalities

Interfering Factors

➤ None

Indications for Cystoscopy

➤ Inspection of the lower urinary tract when radiologic studies are abnormal or inconclusive, especially flat plate and excretory urography, to diagnose the problem

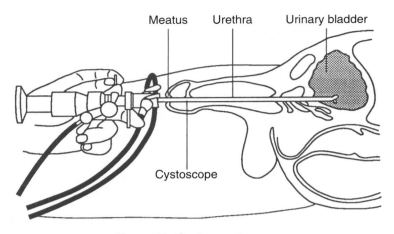

Figure 16-9 Cystourethroscopy.

➤ Differentiation of benign and malignant lesions involving the bladder through tissue biopsy and laboratory analysis
➤ Evaluation of changes in urinary elimination patterns that include frequency, nocturia, urgency, dysuria, dribbling, hesitancy, and incontinence
➤ Hematuria of unknown etiology to determine the source of the problem
➤ Persistent urinary tract infections (UTIs) that do not respond to medications to determine the source of the problem
➤ View of the urethra and neck of the bladder area to identify prostatic hyperplasia and degree of obstruction and to perform transurethral prostatectomy
➤ Identification of tumors, polyps, congenital anomalies such as duplicate ureters, ureteroceles, urethral or ureteral strictures, diverticula, and areas of inflammation or ulceration
➤ Removal of small renal calculi from the bladder or ureters
➤ Removal of polyps and small tumors (including fulguration) from the bladder
➤ Evaluation of function of each kidney by obtaining urine samples from each ureteral catheter
➤ Dilation of strictures of the urethra or ureters
➤ Placement of ureteral catheters (ureteroscopy) to drain urine from the renal pelvis or for retrograde pyelography; placement of ureteral stents before surgical procedures such as colon resection
➤ Evaluation of blood clots and fulguration of bleeding sites within the lower urinary tract
➤ Implantation of radioactive seeds into bladder tumors

Contraindications

➤ Bleeding disorders, because instrumentation can lead to excessive bleeding from the lower urinary tract
➤ Acute cystitis or urethritis, because instrumentation can allow bacteria to enter the bloodstream and cause septicemia

Nursing Care Before the Procedure

Explain to the client:
- ➤ The location for the procedure (cystoscopy suite)
- ➤ That a physician will perform the procedure
- ➤ That the study can take 30 minutes or more, depending on the purpose and type of procedures to be performed, such as retrograde pyelogram or transurethral prostatectomy
- ➤ That food and fluids are withheld for 8 hours before the procedure if general or spinal anesthesia is used and that intake is restricted to clear fluids for 8 hours before the procedure if local anesthesia is used
- ➤ That an anesthetic will be administered, such as local, general, or spinal, depending on the age of the client and the procedure to be performed
- ➤ That, to prevent infection, an antibiotic can be administered before and after the procedure
- ➤ That a special microscope-like instrument will be inserted into the urethra to visualize the bladder
- ➤ That, if a local anesthetic is administered, a sensation of pressure or need to void or both can be experienced as the procedure is performed
- ➤ That, if general anesthesia is to be used, the client will be instructed in deep-breathing technique and other postoperative activities and that time will be allowed to practice techniques
- ➤ That vital signs and urinary output will be monitored closely after the procedure
- ➤ That, if a transurethral prostatectomy is performed, a catheter will remain in place and possibly an irrigation system attached
- ➤ That a burning sensation or discomfort on urination can be experienced during the first few voidings and that the urine will be blood-tinged the first and second voidings after the procedure

Prepare for the procedure:
- ➤ Obtain history of genitourinary infections, bleeding disorders, or other disorders of the urinary tract.
- ➤ Ensure that hematologic status and blood clotting ability have been assessed to include CBC, platelet count, PT, PTT, and urinalysis results for abnormal results.
- ➤ Ensure that dietary and fluid restrictions have been followed based on the type of anesthesia to be administered.
- ➤ Administer enema if ordered.
- ➤ Provide a hospital gown.
- ➤ Have client void.
- ➤ Obtain and record baseline vital signs for later comparison readings.
- ➤ Administer ordered antibiotic therapy.
- ➤ Administer premedications SC or IM as ordered, depending on the type of anesthesia to be used. Such premedications include meperidine (Demerol) to promote relaxation and atropine sulfate to decrease secretions.

The Procedure

The client is positioned on the special cystoscopy table with the legs placed in stirrups and draped for privacy. A general or spinal anesthetic is administered before positioning. The external genitalia are cleansed with an antiseptic solution. If a local anesthetic is used, it is instilled into the urethra and retained for 5 minutes. A penile clamp can be used for male clients to aid in the retention of the anesthetic.

The cystoscope alone can be used for the examination or an urethroscope can be used to examine the urethra before the cystoscopy. The urethroscope has a sheath that can be left in place and the cystoscope inserted through it, avoiding the need for multiple instrumentation. After the insertion of the cystoscope, any urine remaining in the bladder can be drained or a sample of residual urine can be obtained for culture or other analyses. The bladder is irrigated using an irrigation system attached to the scope, usually sterile water unless an isotonic solution such as mannitol is used during the transurethral resection procedure. The isotonic solution is used because of the possibility of the solution's entering the circulation. Solution instilled into the bladder aids in visualization to ensure thorough examination.

If a tumor is found, it can be biopsied by use of a cytology brush or biopsy forceps inserted through the scope. A tumor that is small and localized can be excised and fulgurated. This procedure is termed *transurethral resection of the bladder* (*TURB*). Polyps can also be excised if identified.

Other procedures that can be performed via the cystoscope are fulguration of ulcers or bleeding sites using electrocautery, crushing and removal of small renal calculi from the ureters or bladder, dilation of ureteral or urethral strictures, and instillation of chemotherapeutic agents. Ureteral catheters can also be inserted to obtain urine samples from each kidney for comparative analysis and radiologic studies.

On completion of the examination or treatments, or both, the cystoscope is withdrawn, the legs lowered from the stirrups, and the supine position assumed. Any specimens obtained are placed in the appropriate container, properly labeled, and promptly sent to the laboratory.

Nursing Care After the Procedure

Care and assessment after the procedure are the same as for anyone who is recovering from general anesthesia and include monitoring vital signs, breath sounds, and comfort level.

➤ If a local anesthetic has been administered, allow the client to rest in the supine position for several minutes, and then assist him or her from the table.

➤ Assess for the resumption of normal voiding patterns, the time and amount of voiding, and the appearance of the urine.

➤ If bladder spasms occur, administer an anticholinergic.

➤ Administer an analgesic such as phenazopyridine (Pyridium) for dysuria caused by edema, and provide warm sitz or hip baths for adults or tub baths for children.

➤ Resume foods and fluids withheld before the procedure and, if not medically contraindicated, encourage fluid intake.

➤ Remind the client to report flank or suprapubic pain, persistent blood-tinged or bloody urine, any persistent difficulty or change in urinary pattern, or fever and chills.

➤ *UTI:* If bacteremia is suspected, note and report burning on urination; voiding frequency; cloudy or foul-smelling urine, or both; positive culture results; or chills and fever. Administer antimicrobial therapy as ordered. Increase fluid intake to 3000 mL within 24 hours of the procedure to dilute the urine. Instruct the client as to which foods and medications irritate the bladder and which fluids promote an acidic urine.

➤ *Urinary retention:* Note and report dribbling, hesitancy, frequency of small amounts of urinary output, or bladder distention. Prepare for catheterization for residual. Administer cholinergic such as bethanechol (Urecholine) to stimulate contraction of the bladder. Increase fluid intake to 3000 mL, if appropriate, and monitor intake and output (I&O) for at least 24 hours after the procedure.

➤ *Hemorrhage:* Note and report hematuria (excessive and persistent) and amount if biopsy was performed; report changes in vital signs indicating hypovolemia. If biopsy was performed, maintain bed rest for 4 hours, if possible.

➤ *Bladder perforation:* Note and report suprapubic pain or excessive hematuria. Administer ordered medications. Prepare for surgical repair.

➤ *Ureteral or urethral catheter obstruction:* Note and report drainage difficulty. Maintain patency and connection to a closed collecting system. Avoid kinking or tension on catheter. Irrigate only with order, using proper amount of solution based on type of catheter. Maintain sterile closed system, and provide catheter insertion site care as appropriate.

COLPOSCOPY

Colposcopy is the direct visualization of the vagina and cervix by means of a special binocular microscope and light system. It allows more accurate early diagnostic findings in the prevention of cancer as well as in the identification and extent of cervical lesions. Another source of detection of cervical pathology is cervicography, a photograph of the cervix that can be made during routine gynecologic examinations or with colposcopy. The photographs are made into slides that allow visualization of the entire cervix and can be used with or without other tests to detect malignancy.[44]

Colposcopy can be an alternative to cone biopsy (conization) of the cervix, a surgical procedure. If the results of the biopsy obtained from colposcopy are inconclusive, the conization is performed.

Reference Values

Normal appearance of the vagina and cervix; no abnormal cells or tissues

Interfering Factors

➤ Inability to cooperate with the procedure
➤ Failure to adequately cleanse the cervix of secretions and medications
➤ Heavy menstrual flow
➤ Scarring of the cervix

Indications for Colposcopy

➤ Abnormal Papanicolaou (Pap) smear to determine presence of malignant cells
➤ Schiller test positive for abnormal cells

➤ Identification of existing lesions and monitoring of postsurgical removal of lesions

➤ Monitoring for the development of cancer in women whose mothers took diethylstilbestrol (DES) during pregnancy

➤ Localization of the area from which cervical biopsy samples can be obtained because such areas are not always visible to the naked eye

➤ Evaluation of the male genitalia for diagnosis of sexually transmitted diseases (STDs), condylomata, and papillomavirus[45]

Contraindications

➤ Bleeding disorders, especially if cervical biopsy specimens are to be obtained

Nursing Care Before the Procedure

Explain to the client:

➤ The location for the procedure and the fact that a physician or nurse practitioner will perform the procedure

➤ That the procedure should take about 15 minutes

➤ That there are no food or fluid restrictions

➤ That a vaginal speculum will be inserted to visualize the cervix, causing only slight discomfort, followed by clearer visualization through the speculum with a microscope-like device focused on the cervix

➤ That a small sample of cervical tissue can be obtained, causing slight discomfort and a minimal amount of bleeding, for laboratory analysis

Prepare for the procedure:

➤ Ensure that the client is not menstruating at the time of the procedure.

➤ Obtain a history of the last menstrual period, because the procedure is best performed 1 week after the end of a period. Also obtain the results of blood clotting laboratory tests such as CBC, platelet count, PT, or PTT.

➤ Provide a gown or drape as appropriate.

➤ Have the client void immediately before the procedure.

The Procedure

The client is placed on the gynecologic examination table, legs flexed at the knees, or placed in stirrups and draped for privacy as for a routine pelvic examination. The external genitalia are cleansed with an antiseptic solution, and a lubricated metal or plastic speculum is inserted into the vagina. Water is used as a lubricant if a Pap smear is also to be collected.

For colposcopy, the cervix is swabbed with 3 percent acetic acid to remove mucus or cream medications and to improve the contrast between tissue types. The scope is positioned at the speculum and is focused on the cervix (the scope itself is not inserted into the vagina). The client is advised to relax and control breathing to reduce any discomfort during the procedure. The area is carefully examined using light and magnification. Photographs can be taken for future reference.

Tissues that appear abnormal, such as whitish epithelia (leukoplakia) or atypical or irregular blood vessels, are biopsied with forceps inserted through the speculum. The samples are placed in appropriate containers with a special preservative solution, properly labeled, and promptly taken to the laboratory.

Bleeding, not uncommon after cervical biopsy, can be controlled by cautery, suture, or application of silver nitrate or ferric subsulfate to the site. The vagina is rinsed with sterile saline or water to remove the acetic acid and prevent burning after the procedure. If bleeding persists, a tampon can be inserted by the physician after removal of the speculum.

Nursing Care After the Procedure

Care and assessment after the procedure include cleansing the excess lubricant, solutions, or secretions from the perineal area.

➤ Assist the client to slowly assume a sitting or standing position and to dress. If cramping occurs, administer a mild analgesic.

➤ If a biopsy was performed and a vaginal tampon inserted, inform the client as to when it can be removed (usually 8 to 24 hours) and that pads can be worn afterward if there is bleeding or drainage.

➤ Inform clients who have had a biopsy procedure that a gray-green vaginal discharge can persist for a few days to a few weeks, that strenuous exercise should be avoided for 8 to 24 hours, and that douching and intercourse should be avoided for 2 weeks or as otherwise directed by the physician.

➤ Remind the client to report excessive vaginal bleeding or abnormal vaginal discharge, abdominal pain, or fever to the physician.

➤ *Hemorrhage:* Note and report excessive or persistent vaginal bleeding if biopsy was performed. Also note and report changes in vital signs. Weigh pads to determine blood loss.

➤ *Pelvic inflammation:* Note and report abdominal pain or fever. Administer ordered antibiotic and analgesic therapy. Remind client to avoid douching or intercourse for 2 weeks.

CULDOSCOPY

Culdoscopy is the direct visualization of the cul-de-sac of Douglas by means of a culdoscope, a rigid endoscope that is introduced through a small incision in the posterior vaginal fornix (Fig. 16–10). The procedure permits visualization of the pelvic surfaces of the sigmoid colon and rectum, pelvic ligaments, fallopian tubes, ovaries, and uterus. It has been largely replaced by laparoscopy (see pp. 569 to 576), a procedure that provides a view of a wider field with less risk of infection. It can still be used, however, for very obese women.[46]

Reference Values

Normal appearance of ovaries, fallopian tubes, uterus, and pelvic ligaments; normal appearance of pelvic surfaces of sigmoid colon and rectum

Interfering Factors

➤ Inability to assume the knee-chest position
➤ Presence of pelvic adhesions

Indications for Culdoscopy

➤ Suspected ectopic pregnancy or tubal abnormalities leading to fertility problem in obese clients who are not candidates for laparoscopy
➤ Pelvic pain or masses of unknown etiology
➤ Tubal ligation procedure in obese clients

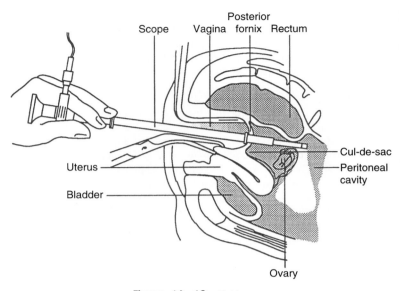

Figure 16–10 Culdoscopy.

Contraindications

➤ Acute infections involving the vulva or vagina
➤ Acute peritonitis
➤ Pelvic masses that involve the cul-de-sac of Douglas

Nursing Care Before the Procedure

Client teaching is the same as for colposcopy (see p. 564).

➤ Inform the client that foods and fluids are withheld for 6 to 8 hours before the procedure.
➤ Inform the client that a local or spinal anesthesia will be used and that medications will be administered by injection before the procedure to promote relaxation and comfort.
➤ Explain that a small incision will be made in the vaginal wall and the scope inserted through the vagina into the pelvic cavity to examine the organs but that no sutures are required to close the incision, which usually heals within 1 week.

Prepare for the procedure:

➤ Provide a hospital gown.
➤ Administer enema or vaginal irrigation, or both, as ordered.
➤ Perform partial perineal shave as ordered.
➤ To provide venous access during the procedure, initiate an IV line or access device such as a heparin lock if ordered.
➤ Obtain and record baseline vital signs for later comparison readings.
➤ Have the client void.
➤ Administer premedications SC or IV as ordered, such as an analgesic (meperidine [Demerol]) and a sedative (diazepam [Valium]).

The Procedure

The client is placed on the operating room table in a supported knee-chest position and draped for privacy. The table is tilted to shift the abdominal contents toward the diaphragm. If a spinal anesthesia is used, it is administered before the client is placed in this position. If a local anesthesia is used, it is injected into the posterior vaginal fornix either before or after the knee-chest position is assumed. A vaginal speculum or retractors are inserted into the vagina to provide visualization of the posterior fornix. A small incision is made in the posterior vaginal wall, and the culdoscope is inserted into the vagina and through the incision. The pelvic organs are examined with the microscope-like instrument and therapeutic procedures are completed. The scope is then removed. No sutures are required to close the incision.

Nursing Care After the Procedure

Care and assessment after the procedure include assisting the client to the supine position and allowing her time to rest.

➤ Take vital signs and compare them with baselines.

➤ Cleanse the perineal area of any blood and apply a clean perineal pad.

➤ Resume foods, fluids, and activities when the client has stabilized, the sedative has worn off, and no signs of complications exist.

➤ Administer a mild analgesic to alleviate any discomfort.

➤ Inform the client that a small amount of "spotting" can occur for 1 to 2 days and that a pad can be worn after the procedure.

➤ Instruct the client to refrain from douching or intercourse for 2 weeks or as directed by the physician.

➤ Remind the client to report to the physician any excessive vaginal bleeding, blood in the feces or urine, fever, or unusual discomfort.

➤ *Hemorrhage:* Note and report amount of excessive vaginal bleeding and change in vital signs, which includes increased pulse and decreased blood pressure. Weigh pads to determine blood loss. Initiate IV line to replace fluid volume loss.

➤ *Pelvic infection:* Note and report fever or abdominal pain. Administer ordered analgesic and antibiotic therapy. Remind client to refrain from douching or intercourse for 2 weeks.

➤ *Rectal, bladder, or intestinal perforation:* Note and report abdominal pain or blood in urine or feces. Administer ordered medication. Prepare client for possible surgical repair.[47]

Amnioscopy

Amnioscopy is the direct visualization of the amniotic fluid by means of an amnioscope inserted into the cervical canal after dilatation of the cervix. The procedure allows visualization of the amniotic fluid through the intact membrane to detect and evaluate meconium staining. Meconium in the amniotic fluid is an indication of fetal distress.[48] Blood samples can also be obtained through the amnioscope from the scalp of the fetus to determine pH level, oxygen, carbon dioxide, and bicarbonate levels if fetal distress is suspected.[49]

Reference Values

Normal amniotic fluid color with no meconium staining

Interfering Factors

➤ None

Indications for Amnioscopy

➤ To evaluate for possible fetal hypoxia by noting change in color of amniotic fluid caused by passage of meconium from the rectum of the fetus
➤ To secure a fetal scalp blood sample to determine fetal acid-base and blood gases status in the diagnosis of fetal hypoxia and distress

Contraindications

➤ Clients that are in active labor
➤ Clients with ruptured membranes
➤ Clients with cervical infection or STD such as gonorrhea

Nursing Care Before the Procedure

Explain to the client:
➤ The location for the procedure
➤ That a physician will explain the benefits, risks, and precautions taken during the procedure to prevent complications
➤ That the procedure requires 15 minutes
➤ That food and fluid are not restricted nor will medications be administered before the procedure
➤ That an amnioscope is inserted into the dilated cervical canal to view the amniotic sac to evaluate the color of the fluid and obtain a blood sample from the scalp of the fetus
➤ That pressure is applied to the puncture site and that no fluid will be removed
➤ That some discomfort is experienced during the procedure

Prepare for the procedure:
➤ Obtain history for presence of cervical or vaginal infections or other abnormalities to report before the procedure.
➤ Provide a gown or drape as appropriate.
➤ Have client void immediately before the procedure.

The Procedure

The client is placed in the lithotomy position with the legs supported in stirrups and draped for privacy. The external genitalia are cleansed with an antiseptic solution and the vaginal speculum is inserted. The cervix is dilated to 2 cm, and the scope is inserted into the cervical canal. The amniotic sac is viewed with the lighted amnioscope for color. Fluid is not removed from the sac for analysis.

If a fetal scalp blood sample is to be obtained, the fetal scalp is cleansed with an antiseptic through the scope and gently dried. A small amount of petrolatum is placed on the scalp, and the skin of the scalp is pierced with a small lancet. The fetal blood beads on the site with the assistance of the petrolatum, and a long capillary tube collects the blood. Firm pressure is applied to the puncture site, and the capillary tube is sealed with wax, placed on ice, and promptly labeled and sent to the laboratory.[50]

The amnioscope is removed after the examination or collection of the specimen, and a perineal pad is applied, if needed.

Nursing Care After the Procedure

Care and assessment after the procedure include cleansing the perineal area, assisting the client in removing her legs from the stirrups, and allowing her time to rest in the supine position.

➤ Assess uterine contractions, and, if a scalp specimen has been obtained, assess the fetus for condition at the site and apply an antibiotic ointment.

➤ Remind the client that some vaginal and cramping discomfort can be experienced for 24 hours after the procedure.

➤ Inform her that excessive pain or rupture of membranes should be reported immediately.

➤ *Premature membrane rupture:* Note and report amniotic fluid leakage and amount of loss. Assess contractions. Provide pads. Instruct to avoid walking and to report any changes in contractions. Provide support to allay anxiety.

➤ *Bleeding from fetal scalp puncture:* Note and report condition of the site and presence of hematoma or other abnormality.

LAPAROSCOPY

Laparoscopy is the direct visualization of the abdominal and pelvic contents by means of a rigid laparoscope that is introduced into the body cavity through a small periumbilical incision about 1 to 2 cm in length. The procedure has replaced the laparotomy as a method of diagnosis and treatment of abdominal and pelvic organ disorders. Three types of laparoscopies can be performed: (1) gastrointestinal, (2) gynecologic, and (3) those associated with surgical procedures such as vaginal hysterectomy, cholecystectomy, or splenectomy.

Gastrointestinal laparoscopy, also known as peritoneoscopy, allows for viewing the liver, gallbladder, spleen, and stomach (greater curvature) after insufflation with nitrous oxide.[51] It is performed on a special endoscopy table that can be tilted to various positions to improve visualization. Figure 16–11 depicts a typical gastrointestinal laparoscopy with the scope positioned in the pneumoperitoneum. Premedication with sedatives and analgesics as well as the local anesthetic injection are administered to minimize discomfort associated with the procedure.[52]

Gynecologic laparoscopy, also known as pelviscopy, is performed to view the ovaries, fallopian tubes, and uterus within the pelvic cavity. At this time, the procedure has generally replaced culdoscopy. Figure 16–12 depicts a typical gynecologic laparoscopy with the instruments in place to manipulate and view the pelvic organs. For this test, the abdomen is insufflated with carbon dioxide. Despite the fact that carbon dioxide can lead to more discomfort than nitrous oxide and can cause hypercarbia and cardiac dysrhythmias, it is used whenever general anesthesia and electrocoagulation are used during the procedure because it is less likely to support combustion.[53]

Another endoscopic procedure is the fetoscopy. It allows for the direct visualization of the fetus through a fiberoptic scope with a light source and telescopic lens inserted through the abdomen and into the uterus. Ultrasonography is performed to identify the area of the fetus to be viewed for insertion of the fetoscope.[54] The procedure takes place at about 18 weeks' gestation at the time the vessels of the placental surface are of adequate size and areas of the fetus

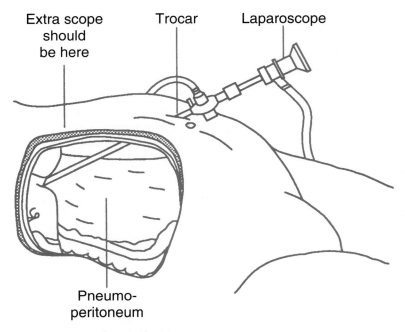

Extra scope should be here

Trocar

Laparoscope

Pneumo-peritoneum

Figure 16–11 Gastrointestinal laparoscopy.

are more easily identified.[55] A signed informed consent that specifically identifies which procedure is to be performed is required.

Reference Values

Gastrointestinal laparoscopy: Normal appearance of the liver, spleen, gallbladder, pancreas, and other abdominal contents

Gynecologic laparoscopy: Normal appearance of the ovaries, fallopian tubes, uterus, and other pelvic contents

Fetoscopy: Absence of fetal distress, congenital malformation, or blood disorders

Interfering Factors

➤ Inability to cooperate in the procedure, if it is performed with local anesthesia
➤ Obesity
➤ Abdominal or pelvic adhesions

Indications for Laparoscopy

Gastrointestinal Laparoscopy

➤ Evaluation of abdominal pain of unknown etiology when other diagnostic studies are inconclusive

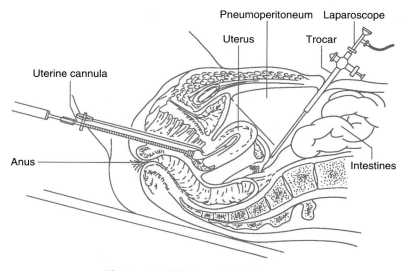

Figure 16–12   Gynecologic laparoscopy.

➤ Evaluation for possible appendicitis
➤ Evaluation of an abdominal mass of unknown etiology
➤ Suspected benign or malignant liver disease to determine the nature of the problem by obtaining a biopsy of tissue rather than by performing a "blind" percutaneous liver biopsy in which malignant cells can be missed[56]
➤ Diagnosis of cirrhosis of the liver
➤ Determination of stage of malignant disorders such as Hodgkin's disease, lymphomas, and hepatic carcinoma[57]
➤ "Second look" for possible metastases after surgery for cancer of the colon[58]
➤ Evaluation of jaundice of unknown etiology to determine the cause, such as liver disease; gallstones; malignancies involving the gallbladder, bile ducts, or liver
➤ Assistance in performing surgical cholecystectomy via the laparoscopic procedure
➤ Diagnosis of disorders involving the pancreas, such as acute and chronic pancreatitis or cancer of the pancreas
➤ Evaluation of problems involving the spleen, especially splenomegaly caused by portal hypertension
➤ Evaluation of problems involving the peritoneum, such as ascites caused by portal hypertension; tuberculosis; and metastatic cancer from primary sites such as the ovaries, colon, pancreas, lung, and breast[59]
➤ In emergency situations, evaluation of abdominal trauma such as blunt injury or stab wounds to determine the extent of intra-abdominal bleeding and the need for exploratory surgery, especially in clients who are poor surgical risks[60]

Gynecologic Laparoscopy

➤ Evaluation of amenorrhea and infertility to determine the possible cause

➤ "Second look" after therapy for fertilization

➤ Evaluation of fallopian tubes and anatomic defects to determine the cause of infertility

➤ Tubal sterilization[61]

➤ Suspected ectopic pregnancy to determine the need for surgery

➤ Determination of the cause of pelvic pain or masses or unknown etiology

➤ Evaluation of known or suspected endometriosis

➤ Treatment of endometriosis through electrocautery or laser vaporization

➤ Diagnosis of pelvic inflammatory disease

➤ Diagnosis of uterine fibroids, ovarian cysts, and uterine malformation with aspiration of ovarian cysts during the procedure

➤ Assistance in performing surgical vaginal hysterectomy via the laparoscopic procedure

➤ Diagnosis of pelvic malignancies by obtaining tissue biopsy for laboratory analysis during the procedure

➤ Evaluation for possible removal of adhesions or foreign bodies such as intrauterine devices (IUDs)[62]

Fetoscopy

➤ Diagnosis of severe fetal malformations such as neural tube defect

➤ Obtaining of fetal blood samples for examination to detect congenital blood disorders such as hemophilia or sickle cell anemia

➤ Obtaining of fetal skin biopsy for examination to determine the presence of skin disorders[63]

Contraindications

➤ Peritoneal adhesions that could prevent adequate visualization or lead to bleeding or perforation of the bowel[64]

➤ History of peritonitis, because dense adhesions could have resulted

➤ Presence of peritonitis, palpable abdominal mass, or large abdominal hernia

➤ History of multiple abdominal operations, because dense adhesions could have resulted

➤ Acute infection involving the abdominal wall, because organisms can be introduced into the normally sterile peritoneal cavity

➤ Intestinal obstructions, because dilated loops of bowel can be inadvertently perforated

➤ Severe ascites or extreme obesity, because the procedure would be technically very difficult to perform

➤ Coagulation disorders, especially those that cannot be adequately corrected, as the control of abdominal wall bleeding can be affected[65]

➤ Unstable cardiopulmonary status or chronic tuberculosis

➤ Gestation of less than 18 weeks for fetoscopy because the fetal parts cannot be identified until this time, and the blood vessels in the placental surface are not of the appropriate size to secure blood samples[66]

> ➤➤ **Nursing Alert**

- Preparation to initiate laparotomy care is required for uncontrolled bleeding or other complications of the procedure that can lead to surgical intervention.
- Premature delivery or change in the status of the fetus requires monitoring of fetal heart rate (FHR) and fetal and uterine activity during and after the procedure.

Nursing Care Before the Procedure

Explain to the client:
➤ The location for the procedure
➤ That a physician will explain the benefits, risks, and precautions taken during the procedure to prevent complications
➤ That the procedure requires 30 to 60 minutes to complete or 1 to 2 hours for fetoscopy
➤ That foods and fluids are withheld for 8 hours before the procedure regardless of the anesthesia used
➤ That a local anesthesia is usually used for gastrointestinal laparoscopy and fetoscopy; a general anesthesia is usually used for gynecologic laparoscopy
➤ That, if the laparoscopy is to be performed under general anesthesia, preparation includes the usual preoperative activities and instruction
➤ That a sedative is administered before the procedure to promote relaxation and that, if fetoscopy is to be performed, a medication is administered to quiet the fetus and facilitate the procedure
➤ That a special microscope-like instrument is inserted into the abdomen through a small incision near the umbilicus; for fetoscopy, a smaller instrument is inserted through the abdominal wall and into the uterine cavity
➤ That vital signs and fetal well-being are monitored during and after the procedure
➤ That the incision is closed with sutures, slips, or Steri-Strips and a small dressing is applied
Prepare for the procedure:
➤ Obtain a history of gestational age if fetoscopy is to be performed; medical disorders that could prevent performing gynecologic laparoscopy or fetoscopy; blood clotting ability with results of CBC, platelet count, PT, and PTT; and typing, cross-matching, and Rh factor if fetoscopy is to be performed.
➤ Provide a hospital gown.
➤ Remove full or partial dentures and glasses or contact lenses, and perform other preoperative activities if general anesthesia is to be administered.
➤ Initiate IV line or venous access device such as heparin lock, or both, as ordered.
➤ Have the client void. Insert an indwelling catheter to maintain an empty bladder if gynecologic laparoscopy is to be performed.
➤ Shave abdomen if unusually heavy hair growth is present.
➤ Take and record vital signs and FHR as applicable for later comparison readings.

➤ Administer premedications SC or IM as ordered. (Premedications can include antibiotic therapy as a preventive measure, an analgesic such as meperidine [Demerol] to reduce discomfort, a sedative such as diazepam [Valium] to promote relaxation, and an anticholinergic such as atropine sulfate to reduce secretions.)

The Procedure

Gastrointestinal Laparoscopy. The client is positioned on the laparoscopy table and shoulder braces, footrest, and safety belts are applied to prevent falling or slipping as the table is tilted into various positions. If not already initiated, an IV infusion is begun and maintained at a "keep-vein-open" (KVO) rate to avoid overdistention of the bladder. Additional sedation can be administered via the IV line at this time. The abdomen is cleansed with antiseptic solution and sterile drapes are placed in position around the incision site.

The site for insertion of the scope is identified and infiltrated with local anesthetic. After the skin is anesthetized, deeper layers of the abdominal wall are injected with anesthetic. Inform the client that this causes a stinging sensation. A small skin incision about 10 mm in length is made, and a Veress needle is inserted into the incision. The Veress (pneumoperitoneum) needle is a special needle with a blunt inner needle that protrudes beyond a pointed, sharp outer needle with a beveled edge. During the insertion, the blunt needle is pushed back, allowing the sharp needle to penetrate the layers of the abdominal wall. After insertion, the blunt needle is pushed beyond the sharp one to prevent damage to the abdominal viscera.[67] Before the insertion of the Veress needle, the client is requested to tense the abdomen and perform Valsalva's maneuver, so that the abdominal wall is elevated, allowing for maximal distance between the visceral and parietal peritoneums.[68]

Nitrous oxide or other gas is injected into the abdomen to create pneumoperitoneum. This condition separates the abdominal wall from the abdominal viscera to improve visualization and protect the organs from possible injury and damage from the laparoscope. An average of 3 L of gas is necessary to allow for the space required to insert the scope without damage to the abdominal organs. If the client has ascites, it may be necessary to remove 1 or 2 L of fluid before instilling the gas.

The Veress needle is then removed and a trocar is inserted through the incision. The trocar provides a sleeve through which the scope is inserted (see Fig. 16–11, p. 570). In addition, some physicians insert a second trocar in the upper right portion of the abdomen through which accessory instruments such as needles can be inserted to perform liver biopsies. This type of procedure requires an additional injection of local anesthetic.[69] The abdomen is then thoroughly explored via the laparoscope, with the table tilted slightly in various positions such as head up, head down, and lateral. Tissue samples for biopsy can be obtained from the liver, peritoneum, and spleen during the procedure.

When the examination is completed, the laparoscope is removed. Most of the air that was instilled into the abdomen is then expelled through a valve on the trocar. The trocar is removed and the skin incision closed with sutures, clips, or Steri-Strips. A small dressing or Band-Aid is applied to the incision site and to the accessory trocar site if used. In an emergency situation the procedure can be performed in 15 to 30 minutes, because the primary purpose is to assess for intra-abdominal bleeding.[70]

Gynecologic Laparoscopy. The client is placed on the laparoscopy table and general anesthesia is administered. The client is then placed in a modified lithotomy position with the head tilted downward. The external genitalia are cleansed with an antiseptic solution and draped. The client can be catheterized at this time if an indwelling catheter is not in place. A bimanual pelvic examination can be performed before a uterine manipulator is inserted through the vagina and cervix and then into the uterus to permit organs such as the ovaries, fallopian tubes, and uterus to be moved for better visualization[71] (see Fig. 16–12, p. 571).

The abdomen is cleansed with antiseptic solution and sterile drapes positioned around the incision site. A small incision is made and a pneumoperitoneum created, using a technique similar to the one used for the gastrointestinal procedure except that the gas used for insufflation is usually carbon dioxide. The pneumoperitoneum needle is removed, and the trocar and laparoscope are inserted through the incision. The pelvic organs are visualized and examined, tissue samples collected, and therapeutic procedures performed such as tubal sterilization. The scope is withdrawn, carbon dioxide is evacuated via the trocar, and then the trocar is removed. The skin incision is closed as outlined previously, the uterine manipulator is removed, and a perineal pad is applied after the perineum is cleansed.

Fetoscopy. The client is given meperidine (Demerol) by injection to quiet the fetus and facilitate the procedure. The client is placed in the supine position on the examining table and draped with the abdomen exposed. Ultrasound is performed to locate the fetus and placenta and to identify the incision site. It also ensures that the fetus and placenta are normal and will not be affected by the study. The site is cleansed with antiseptic solution and a local anesthetic injected. The fetoscope, a very small telescopic instrument, is then inserted through the incision and passed into the uterine cavity near the placental site. Visualization of the fetus is performed to view abnormalities present at this stage of fetal development. Accessory instruments are inserted to obtain blood samples from the vessels of the umbilical cord or skin samples from the fetus.

After the examination and collection of specimens, the scope is withdrawn. The skin incision is closed as outlined for the other laparoscopies.

Nursing Care After the Procedure

Care and assessment after laparoscopy performed under local or general anesthesia include placing the client on a stretcher and transporting to a recovery area.

➤ Cardiac monitoring and cardiopulmonary resuscitation equipment are available after, as well as during, the procedure.

➤ Monitor vital signs, cardiac rhythm, respiratory status, and comfort level, and compare them with baseline readings.

➤ If a liver biopsy was performed, place the client on bed rest for 24 hours.

➤ If fetoscopy has been performed, assess FHR, and monitor the mother and fetus for changes in blood pressure, pulse, uterine activity, fetal activity, vaginal bleeding, and loss of amniotic fluids.[72]

➤ Resume food, fluid, and activities when the client has stabilized and no immediate signs of complications are present (usually within 2 hours after the procedure).

➤ Administer a mild analgesic and cold applications for shoulder pain caused by the elevation of the diaphragm from the air injected into the abdomen.

➤ Administer $Rh_o(D)$ immune globulin (RhoGAM) to Rh-negative mothers unless fetal blood is found to be Rh-negative.

➤ Caution the client to report persistent shoulder or abdominal pain, blood in the urine or feces, vaginal bleeding, leakage of amniotic fluid, fever, painful contractions, or changes at the incision site, depending on the procedure performed.

➤ Inform the client who has had a fetoscopy to avoid strenuous activity for 1 to 2 weeks and to keep her appointment to have ultrasonography the next day to ensure that the fetus and placenta are normal and unaffected by the procedure.

➤ *Reaction to anesthetic agent or medications:* Note and report tachycardia or bradycardia, hyperpnea, hypertension, or hypotension. Administer ordered antihistamine. Initiate IV line and resuscitation procedure if needed.

➤ *Bleeding (abdominal wall, organ, or blood vessel laceration):* Note and report abdominal pain, blood in urine or feces, guarding or tenderness, decreased bowel sounds, or decreased blood pressure and increased pulse. Administer ordered medications and IV fluid to replace fluid loss. Prepare the client for surgical repair.

➤ *Perforation of the gastrointestinal tract or damage to organs:* Note and report signs and symptoms outlined for laceration or fever if peritonitis is present. Administer ordered antibiotic therapy and other medications. Prepare for surgical repair.

➤ *Cardiac or pulmonary abnormalities:* Note and report cardiac dysrhythmias, chest pain, tachycardia, signs and symptoms of air embolism, subcutaneous emphysema such as respiratory difficulty, change in breathing pattern and breath sounds, tachypnea, or hypercarbia if carbon dioxide is used to create pneumoperitoneum.[73] Initiate oxygen. Administer ordered medications. Monitor ECG and respiratory status.

➤ *Premature membrane rupture or fluid leakage:* Note and report rupture and amount of fluid loss, FHR, and fetal and uterine activity. Provide pad and maintain bed rest. Provide support to allay anxiety.

➤ *Premature birth, abortion, intrauterine death:* Note and report fetal and uterine activity and spontaneous abortion and condition of fetus. Provide support and monitor postdelivery condition of mother for hemorrhage and infection.

ARTHROSCOPY

Arthroscopy is the direct visualization of the internal structures of a joint by means of a rigid fiberoptic arthroscope. The procedure can be preceded by an arthrography that has indicated some abnormality to be investigated, but this is not always the case. The knee is the joint most commonly examined (Fig. 16–13). Other joints that can be evaluated by arthroscopy include the shoulder, elbow, hip, ankle, and wrist.[74] This procedure is becoming the study of choice in the diagnosis of injuries and disorders of the knee, especially when the problem is not readily identified by plain x-rays. Moreover, arthroscopy allows 30 percent more visibility in the knee than does an exploratory arthrotomy.[75] Arthroscopy can be performed for both diagnostic and therapeutic purposes.

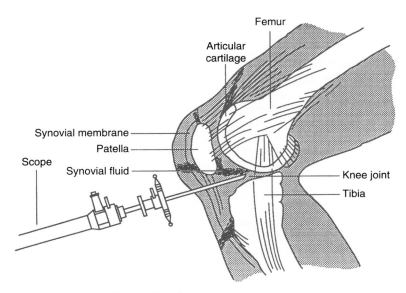

Figure 16–13 Arthroscopy of the knee.

Reference Values

Normal appearance of synovial membranes, cartilage, ligaments, and tendons; no degenerative changes, inflammation, injury, or foreign loose bodies.

Interfering Factors

➤ Inability to cooperate or maintain a position of the joint to be examined if the procedure is to be performed under local anesthetic
➤ Arthrography performed within 7 to 10 days of the procedure if contrast medium remains in the joint

Indications for Arthroscopy

➤ Suspected injury to the joint, such as torn meniscus in the knee or ruptured or torn ligaments, especially when other studies such as plain x-rays or arthrograms (radiologic visualization of a joint after dye is injected) are inconclusive[76]
➤ Suspected disorder involving the synovial membrane, such as in synovitis
➤ Diagnosis of acute and chronic joint disorders, such as arthritis
➤ Diagnosis of inflammatory disorders of the bone or cartilage, such as osteochondritis dissecans
➤ Evaluation of disorders involving the patella, such as chondromalacia
➤ Aspiration of fluid or obtaining of tissue biopsy for laboratory analysis
➤ Monitoring of the response to therapy for various joint disorders[77]
➤ Correction of disorders involving the knee, such as torn cartilage (closed meniscectomy) and removal of degenerative patellar cartilage (patellar shaving)[78]

➤ Removal of loose bodies consisting of bone and cartilage that result from inflammation, degeneration, or injury[79]

Contraindications

➤ Severe ankylosis of the joint (stiffness usually caused by adhesions), because it can impair adequate manipulation of the knee (flexion of 40 degrees) and scope for complete visualization of the area
➤ Superficial infection at or near the arthroscope insertion site, because infectious organisms can be introduced into the joint and possibly the bloodstream by instrumentation

Nursing Care Before the Procedure

Client teaching and physical preparation are the same as for laparoscopy (see pp. 573 to 574).

➤ Inform the client of the site of scope insertion and the fact that some discomfort is experienced when the local anesthetic is injected, that a tourniquet can be applied to the extremity, and that activities and weight bearing can be restricted, depending on the procedure.
➤ Teach crutch-walking, and provide the client with an opportunity to practice.
➤ Inform the client to report fever, swelling of the joint, or redness or swelling of the incision site to the physician.
➤ Obtain a history of known or suspected musculoskeletal disorders, treatment regimen, and tests and procedures associated with this system.
➤ Perform an orthopedic prep that includes scrubbing the site, applying a sterile wrap, and shaving the area 6 inches above and below the arthroscopy site as ordered.

The Procedure

The procedure varies with the physician and the joint being examined or treated. Anesthesia can be local or general, depending on the extent of the procedure to be performed, with general anesthesia administered for surgical procedures. After the client is positioned on the table with the site exposed, the skin is prepared with an antiseptic solution and draped. Sterile technique is used throughout the procedure.

For arthroscopies of the knee (the most common site examined), the entire leg can be wrapped with an elastic bandage and elevated to drain blood from the leg.[80] Other measures to control bleeding include the application of a pneumatic tourniquet and the addition of epinephrine to the local anesthetic or to the saline solution used to irrigate and distend the joint during the procedure.

After the desired anesthesia has been achieved, a small incision is made and a sharp trocar inserted. Fluid can be aspirated from the joint at this time. The trocar is removed and the proper-sized scope inserted, usually with the knee in a flexed position (see Fig. 16–13). The diameter of the scope depends on the joint to be examined and the purpose of the procedure. Saline is injected via the arthroscope to distend the joint. The arthroscope is also maneuvered within the joint and the extremity manipulated by the examiner as necessary for maximal visualization of all structures. Culture, biopsy, surgical repair, and removal of loose bodies can take place as indicated. The joint is irrigated and medication instilled before the scope is withdrawn and after the irrigating fluid has been removed by placing pressure on the knee.

For certain procedures such as closed meniscectomy and patellar shaving, the irrigating catheter can be inserted via a second puncture wound, and a third puncture site can be used to introduce surgical instruments into the area.

The wounds are closed at the conclusion of the procedure with a single suture or with Steri-Strips. A sterile dressing is applied and the area wrapped with an elastic bandage. Depending on the extent of the procedure, the joint can be immobilized with padding, plaster splints, or commercially made immobilizers.

Nursing Care After the Procedure

Care and assessment after the procedure include placing the client on a stretcher and transporting to a recovery area for additional monitoring of vital signs, peripheral pulses, and comfort level.

➤ Administer a mild analgesic for pain and apply an ice pack to the site to reduce swelling.

➤ Provide the client with assistive devices such as crutches or arm sling if needed, and remind the client of the correct use or application.

➤ Review and instruct the client in any activity and weight-bearing restrictions, as well as in exercising and positioning of the joint.

➤ Instruct the client in the care of immobilizing devices that have been applied to the joint and in the care of the incision area.

➤ Remind the client to report fever, swelling of the joint, pain at the site, changes in color or sensation in the extremity, or changes in the incision area.

➤ *Reaction to medications or anesthetic:* Note and report changes in vital signs (hypotension, bradycardia) or respiratory changes (cyanosis, changes in breathing pattern and breath sounds). Administer ordered antihistamine. Initiate oxygen or resuscitation procedure, or both, as needed.

➤ *Infection:* Note and report fever, swelling of the joint, redness or swelling of the incision site, or pain at the site or in the joint. Administer ordered antibiotic and analgesic therapy. Apply ordered heat treatments.

➤ *Thrombophlebitis:* Note and report pain or redness and warmth of the calf area. Elevate leg, refrain from massaging the area, apply ordered moist heat, and administer ordered analgesic and anticoagulant.

➤ *Hemarthrosis or joint injury:* Note and report joint pain or swelling. Immobilize limb. Administer ordered medication for pain.[81]

➤ *Neurovascular damage:* Note and report changes in color, peripheral pulse, capillary refill, sensation, and temperature of the extremity. Perform neurological and circulatory checks. Monitor dressing tightness. Instruct in precautions to take to prevent trauma to the extremity.

(Case Study follows on page 581)

Student Name _____ Class _____

Instructor _____ Date _____

CASE STUDY AND CRITICAL THINKING EXERCISE

Mr. Jones, age 72, comes to the clinic complaining of shortness of breath and a productive cough. He states a 1 pack per day smoking history for 50 years. A bronchoscopy is ordered.

a. While you are explaining the procedure to Mr. Jones, he asks you, "How will I breathe during this test?" How would you respond?

b. What might the results of the bronchoscopy reveal?

References

1. Thomas, CL (ed): Taber's Cyclopedic Medical Dictionary, ed 17. FA Davis, Philadelphia, 1993, p 644.
2. Springhouse Corporation: Nurse's Reference Library: Diagnostics, ed 2. Springhouse, Springhouse, Pa, 1986, p 641.
3. Ibid, p 641.
4. Smith, MJ, et al: Child and Family: Concepts of Nursing Practice. McGraw-Hill, NY, 1982, p 635.
5. Porth, CM: Pathophysiology: Concepts of Altered Health States, ed 4. JB Lippincott, Philadelphia, 1993, p 337.
6. Haponik, EF, et al: Bronchoscopy and related procedures. In Fishman, AP: Pulmonary Diseases and Disorders, ed 2, vol 1. McGraw-Hill, NY, 1988, pp 437–440.
7. Ibid, p 437.
8. Ibid, p 440.
9. Pagana, KD, and Pagana, TJ: Mosby's Diagnostic and Laboratory Test Reference. Mosby–Year Book, St Louis, 1992, p 570.
10. Haponik, op cit, p 461.
11. Pagana and Pagana, op cit, p 130.
12. Haponik, op cit, p 442.
13. Ibid, p 445.
14. Ibid, p 441.
15. Nurse's Reference Library, op cit, p 646.
16. Fischbach, FT: A Manual of Laboratory and Diagnostic Tests, ed 4. JB Lippincott, Philadelphia, 1992, p 728.
17. Nurse's Reference Library, op cit, p 646.
18. Fischbach, op cit, p 278.
19. Nurse's Reference Library, op cit, p 646.
20. Ibid, p 733.
21. Pagana and Pagana, op cit, p 321.
22. Carey, WD: Indications, contraindications, and complications of upper gastrointestinal endoscopy. In Sivak, MV: Gastroenterologic Endoscopy. WB Saunders, Philadelphia, 1987, p 296.
23. Sivak, MV: Technique of upper gastrointestinal endoscopy. In Sivak, MV: Gastroenterologic Endoscopy. WB Saunders, Philadelphia, 1987, pp 276–277.
24. Carey, op cit, p 297.
25. Sivak, op cit, p 274.
26. Ibid, p 288.
27. Pagana and Pagana, op cit, p 305.
28. Ferguson, DR, and Sivak, MV: Indications, contraindications, and complications of ERCP. In Sivak, MV: Gastroenterologic Endoscopy. WB Saunders, Philadelphia, 1987, p 586.
29. Ibid, p 589.
30. Ibid, pp 588–589.
31. Vennes, JA: Techniques of ERCP. In Sivak, MV: Gastroenterologic Endoscopy. WB Saunders, Philadelphia, 1987, p 565.
32. Fischbach, op cit, p 738.
33. Ferguson and Sivak, op cit, p 593.
34. Ibid, p 594.
35. Nurse's Reference Library, op cit, p 836.
36. Fischbach, op cit, p 746.
37. Manier, JW: Flexible sigmoidoscopy. In Sivak, MV: Gastroenterologic Endoscopy. WB Saunders, Philadelphia, 1987, p 983.
38. Ibid, p 983.
39. Kee, JL: Laboratory and Diagnostic Tests with Nursing Implications, ed 3. Appleton & Lange, Norwalk, Conn, 1997, p 364.
40. Sakai, Y: Technique of colonoscopy. In Sivak, MV: Gastroenterologic Endoscopy. WB Saunders, Philadelphia, 1987, p 842.
41. Ibid, p 863.
42. Rankin, GB: Indications, contraindications, and complications of colonoscopy. In Sivak, MV: Gastroenterologic Endoscopy. WB Saunders, Philadelphia, 1987, pp 868–873.
43. Sakai, op cit, pp 850–865.
44. Fischbach, op cit, p 745.
45. Ibid, p 742.
46. Pagana and Pagana, op cit, p 254.
47. Ibid, p 254.
48. Ibid, p 41.
49. Ibid, p 345.
50. Ibid, p 346.
51. Nord, JH: Technique of laparoscopy. In Sivak, MV: Gastroenterologic Endoscopy. WB Saunders, Philadelphia, 1987, p 996.
52. Ibid, p 1008.
53. Ibid, p 996.
54. Fischbach, op cit, p 929.
55. Pagana and Pagana, op cit, p 347.
56. Lightdale, CJ: Indications, contraindications, and complications of laparoscopy. In Sivak, MV: Gastroenterologic Endoscopy. WB Saunders, Philadelphia, 1987, p 1032.
57. Ibid, p 1030.
58. Ibid, p 1034.
59. Ibid, p 1038.
60. Berci, G: Emergency laparoscopy. In Sivak, MV: Gastroenterologic Endoscopy. WB Saunders, Philadelphia, 1987, p 1120.
61. Yuzpe, AA: Gynecologic laparoscopy for the gastroenterologist. In Sivak, MV: Gastroenterologic Endoscopy. WB Saunders, Philadelphia, 1987, p 1125.
62. Ibid, p 1125.
63. Pagana and Pagana, op cit, p 347.
64. Lightdale, op cit, p 1038.
65. Ibid, p 1039.
66. Pagana and Pagana, op cit, p 347.
67. Nord, op cit, pp 994–995.
68. Ibid, p 1007.
69. Ibid, pp 1016–1018.

70. Berci, op cit, p 1122.
71. Pagana and Pagana, op cit, p 456.
72. Ibid, p 348.
73. Lightdale, op cit, pp 1038–1040.
74. Fischbach, op cit, p 761.
75. Farrell, J: Illustrated Guide to Orthopedic Nursing, ed 3. JB Lippincott, Philadelphia, 1986, p 229.

76. Nurse's Reference Library, op cit, p 679.
77. Pagana and Pagana, op cit, p 75.
78. Farrell, op cit, p 230.
79. Ibid, p 233.
80. Nurse's Reference Library, op cit, p 681.
81. Pagana and Pagana, op cit, p 75.

Bibliography

Andrews, JR, and Soffer, SR: Elbow Arthroscopy. Mosby–Year Book, St Louis, 1993.

Becker, HD, et al: Atlas of Bronchoscopy. Mosby–Year Book, St Louis, 1991.

Berci, G, and Cuschieri, A: Practical Laparoscopy. WB Saunders, Philadelphia, 1986.

Black, JM, and Matassarin-Jacobs, E: Luckmann and Sorensen's Medical-Surgical Nursing: A Psychophysiologic Approach, ed 4. WB Saunders, Philadelphia, 1993.

Chernecky, CC, and Berger, BJ; Cullen, BN (ed): Laboratory Tests and Diagnostic Procedures, ed 2. WB Saunders, Philadelphia, 1996.

Corbett, JV: Laboratory Tests and Diagnostic Procedures with Nursing Diagnoses, ed 4. Appleton & Lange, Norwalk, Conn, 1995.

du Bois, RM, and Clarke, SW: Fiberoptic Bronchoscopy in Diagnosis and Management. WB Saunders, Philadelphia, 1988.

Huffman, JL, et al: Ureteroscopy. WB Saunders, Philadelphia, 1987.

Johnson, LJ: Diagnostic and Surgical Arthroscopy of the Shoulder. Mosby–Year Book, St Louis, 1992.

Kato, H, and Horai, T: In Harubumikato (ed): A Color Atlas of Endoscopic Diagnosis in Early Stage Lung Cancer. Mosby–Year Book, St Louis, 1992.

Katon, RM, et al: Flexible Sigmoidoscopy. WB Saunders, Philadelphia, 1985.

Kitamura, S: Color Atlas of Clinical Applications of Fiberoptic Bronchoscopy. Mosby–Year Book, St Louis, 1990.

Pagana, KD, and Pagana, TJ: Diagnostic Testing and Nursing Implications: A Case Study Approach, ed 4. Mosby–Year Book, St Louis, 1993.

Ponsky, JL: Atlas of Surgical Endoscopy. Mosby–Year Book, St Louis, 1992.

Saleh, JN: Laparoscopy: A Clinical Companion. WB Saunders, Philadelphia, 1988.

Schonebeck, J, and Hakansson, LJ (eds): Atlas of Cystoscopy. WB Saunders, Philadelphia, 1985.

Scott, WN: Arthroscopy of the Knee: Diagnosis and Treatment. WB Saunders, Philadelphia, 1990.

Silverstien, FE, and Tytgat, GNJ: Atlas of Gastrointestinal Endoscopy. WB Saunders, Philadelphia, 1987.

Springhouse Corporation: Nurse's Reference Library: Diagnostic Tests. Springhouse, Springhouse, Pa, 1991.

Tilkian, SM: Clinical and Nursing Implications of Laboratory Tests, ed 5. Mosby–Year Book, St Louis, 1995.

Whaley, LF: Nursing Care of Infants and Children, ed 4. Mosby–Year Book, St Louis, 1991.

White, RA, and Klein, SR: Endoscopic Surgery. Mosby–Year Book, St Louis, 1991.

Wyllie, R: Colonoscopy in the pediatric patient. In Sivak, MV: Gastroenterologic Endoscopy. WB Saunders, Philadelphia, 1987, pp 966–974.

Wyllie, R: Esophagogastroduodenoscopy in the pediatric patient. In Sivak, MV: Gastroenterologic Endoscopy. WB Saunders, Philadelphia, 1987, pp 307–320.

17

Radiologic Studies

➤ **PROCEDURES COVERED**

Skull Films, *589*
Orbital Films, *591*
Paranasal Sinus Films, *592*
Chest Films (CXR), *593*
Abdominal Films (KUB), *596*
Obstruction Series, *598*
Pelvimetry, *599*
Spinal Films, *600*
Extremity Films, *602*
Cardiac Films, *603*
Chest Tomography, *605*
Paranasal Sinus Tomography, *606*
Mammography, *607*
Barium Swallow, *609*
Upper Gastrointestinal (UGI)
   Series, *612*
Barium Enema (BE), *614*

Oral Cholecystography (OCG), *617*
Intravenous Cholangiography
   (IVC), *620*
T-Tube Cholangiography, *621*
Operative Cholangiography, *623*
Percutaneous Transhepatic
   Cholangiography (PTHC), *624*
Antegrade Pyelography, *627*
Retrograde Urethrography, *630*
Retrograde Cystography, *631*
Retrograde Ureteropyelography, *633*
Intravenous Pyelogram (IVP), *635*
Voiding Cystourethrography, *636*
Sialography, *638*
Arthrography, *638*
Bronchography, *640*
Hysterosalpingography, *642*
Myelography, *644*

INTRODUCTION

Radiographs (also called x-rays and roentgenograms) are used to evaluate the bones and soft tissues of the body. The x-rays are produced by applying an electron beam to a vacuum tube containing tungsten. The resulting rays have a shorter wavelength than that of visible light rays and are able to penetrate many substances that are opaque to visible light.

In photographic film, x-rays cause silver to precipitate. This precipitation causes the film to turn black when it is developed. Objects placed between the beam of x-rays and the photographic film absorb some of the x-rays and cause a shadow to be cast upon the film.[1] The amount of x-rays absorbed varies with the thickness and composition of the object. Metal, for example, absorbs all of the x-rays and no silver is precipitated; when the film is developed, the object appears solid white. In contrast, soft tissues absorb only part of the x-rays and cause a grayish shadow to be cast on the film.[2] The usefulness of diagnostic radiography is based on the differences in the absorption of rays by various substances or objects.

Because x-rays precipitate silver in photographic film slowly, clients may potentially be exposed to unduly long studies and excessive radiation. To avoid these problems, special film cassettes are used. These cassettes contain a fluo-

585

rescent screen that is activated by the x-rays and emits light rays that augment the effects of x-rays on the photographic film.[3]

For many body parts, such as bones and air-filled soft structures, differences in composition and density produce natural contrasts that are sufficient for "plain" films of diagnostic quality. Solid organs and hollow structures that do not normally contain air, however, require either special filming techniques such as tomography or use of radiopaque contrast media such as barium sulfate or iodinated dyes for accurate imaging.

Radiographic procedures can be either invasive or noninvasive, and client preparation varies accordingly. In the case of noninvasive procedures such as plain-film x-rays, tomography, and those using barium sulfate as a contrast medium, the client should be told what to expect, but a signed consent form is not required. The only exception to this is mammography, which uses xeroradiography to create its images. A signed consent form is required for invasive procedures that use iodinated dyes administered intravenously (IV) or directly into an organ or area to be examined. The procedures are usually performed in the radiology department or a special room with x-ray equipment, but some can be performed at the bedside, in the physician's office, or at an imaging agency. Such studies can be performed by a qualified radiologist, urologist, or x-ray technician. All invasive radiologic procedures are performed under sterile conditions using Standard Precautions and transmission-based isolation procedures.

TOMOGRAPHY

Tomography (laminography, planigraphy, stratigraphy) is an imaging technique in which a selected body plane is isolated from the tissues on either side. The x-ray source and the film are moved in opposite directions, resulting in a two-dimensional slice a few millimeters thick that is imaged with a clarity superior to plain films. Tomography is especially valuable in visualizing air-filled structures such as the lungs, paranasal sinuses, and kidneys. Used alone, tomography provides two-dimensional gray-scale images; when combined with computers in computed scans or CTs, tomography produces three-dimensional images. A disadvantage of tomography is the high level of radiation exposure to the client.

FLUOROSCOPY

Fluoroscopy is an imaging technique in which x-rays are passed through the client to a fluorescent viewing screen coated with calcium tungstate. The viewer is able to observe movement in the area being filmed while the study is in progress, making fluoroscopy particularly useful in evaluating movement of the diaphragm, heart, and digestive system (esophagus, stomach, small bowel, colon). It is also used in catheter guidance for placement during angiography, needle insertion for biopsy or removal of fluid from a body cavity, and nasogastric (NG) tube insertion for precise placement in the stomach or small bowel. Fluoroscopy can be used with single films (spot films) or with videotape if a record of movement is desired. Fluoroscopy is also often used in combination with other radiologic procedures and techniques, such as plain films or cineradiography, and is frequently augmented by the addition of a contrast medium such as barium sulfate.

The viewer faces the screen during fluoroscopy and thus can be exposed to x-rays. For this reason, the viewer must wear special lead-shielded glasses, gloves, and aprons for protection. Fluoroscopy delivers much larger doses of radiation than conventional x-rays. Newer fluoroscopy equipment, which has image intensifiers that amplify the pictures electronically, allows the studies to be performed in lighted rooms, thus exposing the client and fluoroscopist to less radiation.[4]

CINERADIOGRAPHY

Cineradiography is a rapid-sequence filming technique similar to that used to make motion pictures. When used with fluoroscopy, it creates a photographic record of the motion under study, such as swallowing. The resulting film is comparable to photographs taken with a 16- or 35-mm camera at speeds of 30 to 200 frames per second. A recording for later replay allows study in greater detail.

XERORADIOGRAPHY

Xeroradiography is an x-ray imaging technique that uses a photoelectric process rather than the photochemical process of conventional x-rays; this process reduces the amount of radiation exposure to the client. The images are printed on paper in a manner similar to that of a typical office copier.[5] Xeroradiography produces very distinct images with excellent contrast. Because it is especially useful in studying soft tissues for small-point abnormalities, it is used primarily for x-ray studies of the breasts.

CONTRAST-MEDIATED STUDIES

Soft tissues produce poor images on x-ray, and contrast media are added to enhance the viewing of structural details. A contrast medium can be administered orally, rectally, IV, intrathecally, or by insufflation. When contrast media are injected to visualize blood vessels and lymphatics, the studies are referred to as angiography.

The most commonly used contrast media are barium sulfate, organic iodides, and iodized oils. These substances are radiopaque and block the passage of x-rays. Gases such as oxygen, carbon dioxide, helium, nitrogen, and air have been used to render body spaces radiolucent as the spaces partially block the passage of x-rays. Many of the studies in which gases are used have now been replaced by safer, noninvasive computed tomography (CT) and other imaging techniques.

In addition to the radiation hazards inherent in all x-ray studies, contrast-mediated procedures pose the additional risk of severe allergic reaction to the iodinated contrast medium, including vomiting, laryngospasm, anaphylactic shock, and cardiac arrest (Table 17–1). Emergency equipment should be at hand so that resuscitative measures can be initiated immediately.

Table 17–1 ➤ ADVERSE REACTIONS TO IODINATED CONTRAST MEDIA
Manifestations of Reaction
Anxiety
Tachycardia
Diaphoresis
Sneezing, rhinorrhea
Urticaria, rash
Angioneurotic edema
Coughing
Dyspnea, wheezing
Hoarseness
Laryngeal stridor
Hypotension
Pulmonary edema
Shock state
Cardiopulmonary failure
Cardiopulmonary arrest
Medications to Counteract Reactions
Dyphenhydramine (Benadryl): PO (orally), IM for mild reactions
Epinephrine (adrenalin): IV for severe reactions
Aminophylline: IV for severe reactions
Hydrocortisone (Solu-Cortef): IV for severe reactions

Barium sulfate is a chalky emulsion that is flavored and aerated to the consistency of a milk shake. Oral ingestion of this medium can lead to nausea and vomiting as well as to prolonged retention of the barium within the intestinal tract, leading to constipation and impaction. The color of the feces will be white or much lighter than usual until the barium is eliminated from the tract.

RADIATION EXPOSURE RISKS

All radiation studies carry risks of exposure to radiation. Radiation can have adverse effects on both gonadal and somatic cells. The cells of the developing embryo are especially sensitive to radiation. Children are at higher risk than adults, so this diagnostic method should be used only when absolutely necessary. Possible adverse effects of radiation include genetic mutations, cancer, and congenital anomalies.[6]

X-ray studies should not be performed more often than necessary for diagnosis. Clients should be adequately prepared so that the need for repeat films and studies is reduced. Newer x-ray equipment and film should be used because they expose clients and personnel to less radiation than older equipment. Personnel and clients should be shielded from unnecessary exposure by lead aprons and gloves. Women who are pregnant should not be x-rayed, and women of childbearing age should be assessed for the date of the last menstrual period to reduce the possibility of having radiographic studies performed during pregnancy. If undiagnosed pregnancy is a risk or if a pregnancy is not confirmed, the study is generally not performed unless it is an extreme necessity.[7]

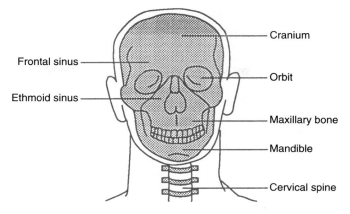

Figure 17–1   Cranial and facial bones; cervical spine.

PLAIN FILMS

Plain films are radiologic studies that use external beams and are performed without contrast media or augmentation with other techniques. They are used for "routine" examinations of areas such as the skull, chest, abdomen, pelvis, spine, extremities, and bony structures in other parts of the body. Plain x-rays are contraindicated in pregnant clients unless the benefits of performing the procedure far outweigh any risks to the fetus.

SKULL FILMS

Skull films involve radiographic examination of the cranial vault and facial bones (Fig. 17–1). A variety of abnormalities can be identified on skull films, such as fractures, tumors, and changes in bone structure or size. Several views are taken, depending on the signs and symptoms and the suspected pathology. In cases involving fractures of the cervical vertebrae, positioning to obtain varied views is limited.

Reference Values

Normal skull, facial, and jaw bones; normal brain tissue; normal suture lines and fontanels in infant

Interfering Factors

➤ Improper positioning to achieve the desired views
➤ Limitations in positioning from known or suspected fractures of the cervical vertebrae
➤ Metal objects such as dentures, hearing aids, and eyeglasses within the x-ray field

Indications for Skull Films

➤ Known or suspected trauma to the face or cranium to reveal a fracture
➤ Suspected increased intracranial pressure revealed by abnormal markings on the inside of the cranial vault
➤ Suspected pituitary tumor revealed by increased size and erosion of the sella turcica
➤ Suspected metastatic tumor involving the small bones or brain tissue revealed by a shift of intracranial contents
➤ Suspected acromegaly revealed by an enlarged mandible
➤ Suspected tumor or inflammation involving the paranasal sinuses
➤ Suspected Paget's disease revealed by a thickening of the skull bones
➤ Suspected vascular abnormalities such as chronic subdural hematoma revealed by calcifications in brain tissue
➤ Suspected perinatal injury or congenital defect involving the skull
➤ Evaluation of thinning of bones, separation of suture lines, widened fontanels, and an enlarged cranium in the diagnosis of hydrocephalus in infants
➤ Evaluation of premature closing of the cranial sutures in the diagnosis of craniostenosis in infants

Contraindications

➤ Pregnancy, unless benefits of performing the procedure greatly outweigh the risks to the fetus

Nursing Care Before the Procedure

Explain to the client:
➤ The location for the procedure and the fact that a technician or radiologist will perform it
➤ That the procedure takes about 15 minutes
➤ That foods, fluids, and medications are not restricted before the procedure
➤ That no sedation or anesthetic is administered before the procedure
➤ That views may be taken with the client in various positions on the x-ray table or in an x-ray chair
➤ That the area to be examined will be immobilized or the client will be asked to remain still during the procedure
➤ That the procedure should not cause discomfort, except possibly from lying on the hard table
Prepare for the procedure:
➤ Obtain a history of known underlying medical conditions or trauma and (for women) date of last menstrual period to determine the possibility of pregnancy.
➤ Ensure that all dental prostheses, jewelry, eyeglasses, or other metal objects such as hair clips are removed.
➤ Provide a hospital gown, if needed.
➤ Perform baseline neurological check and vital signs for later comparison readings.

The Procedure

The client is placed on the x-ray table or seated in a chair. Various views of the skull are taken with the client repositioned and the head stabilized with a headband, sandbags, or foam pads for each change of position. For lateral (left and right sides), posterior and anterior (back to front), and basilar (inferior to superior) views, the client is placed in the prone position; for anterior-posterior (front to back) and axial (crown to chin) views, the client is in the supine position. Varying degrees of neck flexion are used for the different views. The client is requested to remain very still while the x-rays are taken. The positions are maintained while the films are developed and checked in case more filming is needed.[8]

Nursing Care After the Procedure

➤ Perform neurological checks and vital signs and compare with baselines.
➤ *Complications and precautions:* Note and report suspected fracture or injury to the cervical spine or neck pain. Consider this limitation when positioning the neck during the x-ray procedure.

ORBITAL FILMS

Orbital films involve examination of the bony orbits of the eyes (see Fig. 17–1, p. 589). The procedure is indicated to diagnose fracture, tumor, or foreign body in the orbit or in the eye itself as well as craniofacial anomalies. As with skull films, several views are taken, depending on known or suspected pathology or abnormal conditions.

Reference Values

Orbits of normal size; no fractures, bony abnormalities, or foreign bodies

Interfering Factors

➤ Improper positioning of the client to obtain the desired views
➤ Metal objects such as eyeglasses, eye prosthesis, dentures, or jewelry within the x-ray field

Indications for Orbital Films

➤ Identification of fractures after known or suspected trauma to the eyes or face
➤ Suspected tumor involving the orbit, hypophysis, retina, or optic nerve revealed by alterations in the size of the orbit
➤ Suspected foreign body in the eye or in the orbit itself
➤ Suspected Paget's disease revealed by an increased density of the bone
➤ Suspected congenital microphthalmia or other craniofacial anomalies revealed by alterations in the size of the orbit

Contraindications

➤ Pregnancy, unless benefits of performing the procedure greatly outweigh the risks to the fetus

Nursing Care Before the Procedure

Client teaching and physical preparation are the same as for any plain x-ray procedure (see p. 590).

The Procedure

The client is placed on the x-ray table in a supine position or seated in an x-ray chair. Different views of the orbits are taken such as posterior-anterior, inferior-superior (basilar), and projections through the optical canal.[9] The client is repositioned for each view, and headbands, sandbags, and foam blocks are used to stabilize the head for each position during the procedure. The client is requested to remain very still during the procedure and to wait while the films are developed and checked before leaving the department.[10]

Nursing Care After the Procedure

Care and assessment after the procedure are the same as for any plain x-ray procedure (see p. 591).

PARANASAL SINUS FILMS

Paranasal sinuses are air-filled cavities lined with mucous membrane in the frontal, ethmoid, sphenoid, and maxillary bones (see Fig. 17–1, p. 589). Films are taken to diagnose and evaluate the sinuses for fracture, inflammation, cysts, tumors, and foreign bodies.

Reference Values

Normal sinus bones and soft tissues; no fractures, tumors, or inflammation

Interfering Factors

➤ Inability of client to remain still and maintain position during filming
➤ Improper positioning for the desired views
➤ Metal objects such as eyeglasses, dental or eye prostheses, or jewelry within the x-ray field

Indications for Paranasal Sinus Films

➤ Detection of fractures to the head or face after trauma
➤ Suspected acute or chronic sinusitis revealed by inflammation of the mucous membranes
➤ Suspected cyst, polyp, or tumor involving the sinuses revealed by soft tissue changes, bony abnormalities, or both

Contraindications

➤ Pregnancy, unless benefits of performing the procedure greatly outweigh the risks to the fetus

Nursing Care Before the Procedure

Client teaching and physical preparation are the same as for any plain x-ray procedure (see p. 590).

The Procedure

The client is seated in a special x-ray chair. The head is immobilized in a padded brace or vise to maintain the desired position. The client is requested to remain very still to prevent any blurring of the image while films are taken in different angles. Several views can be taken, and the client is requested to remain in the position until the films are developed and checked.[11] The brace is then removed and the client is allowed to leave the department.

Nursing Care After the Procedure

Care and assessment after the procedure are the same as for any plain x-ray procedure (see p. 591).

CHEST FILMS (CXR)

Chest x-rays (CXR) are among the most frequently performed radiologic studies and yield a great deal of information about the pulmonary and cardiac systems. The lung fields, the clavicle and ribs, the cardiac border, the mediastinum, the diaphragm, and the thoracic spine can all be studied using CXRs.

Although generally performed in the radiology department, chest x-rays using portable equipment can be taken at the client's bedside in more acute or critical situations. Although only a single view is obtained, critical problems such as pneumonia, atelectasis, pneumothorax, pulmonary edema, and pleural effusion can be identified. In addition, portable chest x-ray equipment is often used to evaluate the placement of various tubes, such as central venous catheters.[12]

Chest x-ray studies can include several views. In the posterior-anterior (PA) view (Fig. 17–2), the x-ray beam passes through the client from back to front. This is a preferred view because it results in less magnification of the heart than does the anterior-posterior (AP) view.[13] The farther away from the x-ray film an object is situated, such as the heart in the AP view, the more magnified and less distinct will be its image.[14] It should be noted, however, that portable chest x-rays are performed using the AP view. The lateral view (Fig. 17–3) is performed with the client's left side placed against the film and the

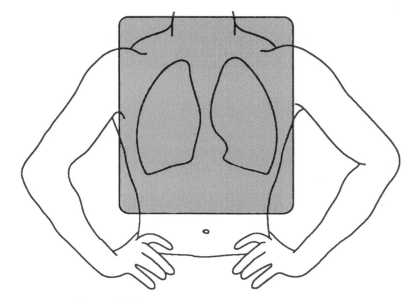

Figure 17–2   Posterior-anterior view for chest radiograph.

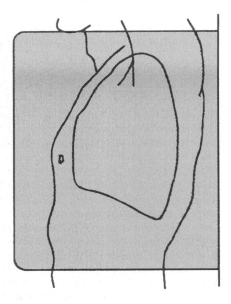

Figure 17–3 Left lateral view for chest radiograph.

arms positioned to avoid interference with the chest view. The rationale for this position is the same as for the PA view; that is, the heart lies toward the left side of the chest and is less magnified in the left lateral view.[15] Lateral views add information that cannot be obtained through PA filming. Two areas seen more clearly on lateral views are the anterior portion of the lungs closest to the mediastinum and the vertebral column.[16]

Oblique chest films are made by angling the x-ray beam between the PA and the lateral views.[17] Oblique views are helpful in evaluating pulmonary masses and infiltrates, especially those involving the mediastinum. These views can be supplemented with barium swallow studies, because barium in the esophagus aids in identifying mediastinal abnormalities.[18]

Lateral decubitus chest films are made by directing the x-ray beam parallel to the floor with the client in a side-lying, supine, or prone position.[19,20]

Lordotic chest films are taken with the client leaning backward against the x-ray film with the abdomen protruding.[21] This position allows better visualization of the apices of the lungs, the area most commonly involved in pulmonary tuberculosis.

Fluoroscopic studies of the chest can also be performed to evaluate movement of the chest and diaphragm during breathing and coughing. It provides information about bronchiolar obstruction, loss of elasticity, or paralysis of the diaphragm.[22]

Reference Values

Normal lung fields, cardiac size, mediastinal structures, and thoracic spine; no masses, infiltrates, areas of collapse, pleural effusion, fractures of clavicles or ribs, or abnormal elevation or flattening of the diaphragm

Interfering Factors

➤ Improper positioning, especially for views such as the oblique and lordotic films or for portable chest x-rays
➤ Inability of client to take and hold deep breaths during the filming
➤ Improper adjustment of the x-ray equipment to accommodate obese and thin clients, causing overexposure or underexposure and poor-quality films
➤ Metal objects such as closures on undergarments or hospital gown within x-ray field

Indications for Chest Films (CXR)

➤ Known or suspected pulmonary infectious disorders such as pneumonia, tuberculosis, or lung abscess
➤ Diagnosis of obstructive pulmonary lung diseases such as atelectasis, emphysema, or chronic bronchitis
➤ Diagnosis of interstitial lung diseases such as sarcoidosis, silicosis, or asbestosis
➤ Diagnosis of pneumothorax or fractures of the ribs or clavicles resulting from known or suspected chest trauma
➤ Known or suspected cardiovascular disorders such as congestive heart failure (CHF), pericarditis, or aortic aneurysm
➤ Monitoring of pulmonary or cardiac disease to evaluate the effectiveness of therapy
➤ Suspected diaphragmatic hernia
➤ Suspected neoplasm (benign or malignant) involving the mediastinum, lungs, or chest wall
➤ Suspected pleural effusion or other abnormalities involving the pleurae or fluid accumulation in the lungs, as in pulmonary edema
➤ Diagnosis of cystic fibrosis in children
➤ Diagnosis of bronchopulmonary dysplasia, air leak syndrome, hyaline membrane disease, and meconium aspiration syndrome in infants
➤ Evaluation of the placement and positioning of endotracheal tubes, tracheostomy tubes, central venous catheters, Swan-Ganz catheters, chest tubes, NG feeding tubes, pacemaker wires, and intra-aortic balloon pumps[23]

Contraindications

➤ Pregnancy, unless benefits of performing the procedure greatly outweigh the risks to the fetus

Nursing Care Before the Procedure

Client teaching and physical preparation are the same as for any plain x-ray procedure (see p. 590).

The Procedure

For Routine Films. The client is positioned in front of the x-ray machine and against the film holder. The client can be seated if unable to stand. For the PA view, the client stands or sits facing the film with the hands on the hips, neck extended, and shoulders forward and touching the film holder. The client is requested to inspire deeply and hold the breath while the x-ray is taken. For the lateral view, the client is positioned with the side (usually the left) against the film holder with the arms raised over the head and away from the x-ray field. The client is again requested to hold the breath while the x-ray is taken.

For Oblique, Decubitus, or Lordotic Views. The client is assisted to the proper position. If fluoroscopic examination is being performed to visualize movement of the thoracic contents, especially the diaphragm and lung expansion and contraction, the client is asked to breathe and cough as the films are taken. Tissues are supplied for client use if coughing is required during the study.

For Portable Chest X-Rays. The client is moved toward the head of the bed as far as possible. The head of the bed is raised as high as possible (preferably a 90-degree angle) or to the limit of the client's tolerance. Any metal objects on the gown or other objects (electrodes, tubing) that can interfere with the visualization of the chest are removed. The client is helped to lean forward while the film cassette is placed between the back and the mattress. If the client cannot maintain a position for filming, a staff member may assist if he or she wears a lead apron. The client is eased back onto the cassette and checked for proper positioning. The client is requested to hold the breath, if possible, while the x-ray is obtained.

Nursing Care After the Procedure

Care and assessment after the procedure are the same as for any plain x-ray procedure.

ABDOMINAL FILMS (KUB)

A plain film of the kidneys, ureters, and bladder (KUB), also called a scout film or flat plate, consists of a single AP view of the abdomen (Fig. 17–4). The abdominal film is commonly taken to assist in the diagnosis of urologic and gastrointestinal abnormalities.

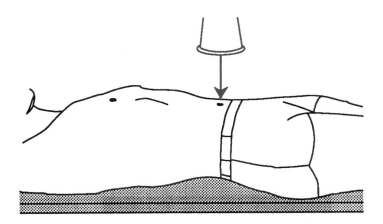

Figure 17–4   Supine position for abdominal radiograph.

Reference Values

Normal shape and size of kidneys, with the right kidney positioned slightly lower than the left; normal bladder, if visualized; no renal calculi, abdominal masses, abnormal accumulation of air or fluid, or foreign objects within the gastrointestinal tract

Interfering Factors

➤ Feces, barium or other radiopaque substances, gas, or ascites
➤ Extreme obesity, uterine and ovarian tumors or lesions[24]
➤ Metal objects such as belts or girdles within the x-ray field

Indications for Abdominal Films (KUB)

➤ Diagnosis of intestinal obstruction and acute abdominal pain of unknown etiology
➤ Evaluation of palpable abdominal mass
➤ Determination of size, shape, and position of kidneys to aid in the diagnosis of congenital anomalies and diseases such as absence of kidney or horseshoe kidney, hypoplasia, polycystic kidney disease, hydronephrosis, or atrophic kidney
➤ Determination of the size, shape, and position of liver and spleen in liver cirrhosis, splenomegaly, and tumors
➤ Suspected abnormal air, fluid, or objects in the abdomen
➤ Evaluation of size, shape, and location of renal calculi, revealed by visualization of opaque bodies
➤ Differentiation between the cause of urologic symptoms and gastrointestinal symptoms
➤ Initial component of a contrast-mediated study of the renal/urinary and gastrointestinal tract[25]

Contraindications

➤ Pregnancy, unless benefits of performing the procedure greatly outweigh the risks to the fetus

Nursing Care Before the Procedure

Client teaching and physical preparation are the same as for any plain x-ray procedure (see p. 590).

The Procedure

The client is placed on the x-ray table in the supine position with the arms extended over the head. A protective shield is placed over the testicular area of male clients. Usually a single AP film of the abdomen is taken, although a film with the client in a sitting or standing position can be performed, depending on the reason for the study.[26] During the filming, the client is requested to take a deep breath and hold it or exhale and not breathe. Visualization of the bladder depends on its density and whether it contains urine.[27]

Nursing Care After the Procedure

Care and assessment after the procedure are the same as for any plain x-ray procedure (see p. 591).
➤ Monitor bowel sounds in clients who experience abdominal pain.

OBSTRUCTION SERIES

For an obstruction series, a plain film of the abdomen is followed by abdominal films in varying positions. An obstruction series is performed to reveal bowel obstruction as well as a variety of other abdominal disorders, such as paralytic ileus. In mechanical bowel obstruction the small bowel and colon become distended with air. This distention is proximal to the obstruction, as air tends to be cleared from the portion of the bowel distal to the obstruction because of peristalsis. In paralytic ileus both the small and large bowels are distended with air as peristalsis is decreased. Free air can be detected in the abdomen if the bowel ruptures.[28]

Reference Values

Normal small and large intestines; no abnormal distention, mechanical bowel obstruction, paralytic ileus, or perforation

Interfering Factors

➤ Feces, barium or other radiopaque substances, gas, or ascites
➤ Extreme obesity
➤ Metal objects such as belts and girdles within the x-ray field

Indications for Obstruction Series

➤ Evaluation of acute abdominal pain of unknown etiology such as appendicitis or abdominal abscess
➤ Suspected bowel perforation revealed by free air under the diaphragm
➤ Suspected bowel obstruction revealed by air and fluid within the intestine that cause bowel distention proximal to the obstruction
➤ Suspected paralytic ileus revealed by small-bowel and colon distention with air as peristalsis decreases
➤ Suspected renal calculi revealed by calcification in the kidney or a ureter
➤ Monitoring of the course of renal or gastrointestinal disease
➤ Suspected abdominal aortic aneurysm revealed by calcification, especially in older clients[29]

Contraindications

➤ Pregnancy, unless benefits of performing the procedure greatly outweigh the risks to the fetus

Nursing Care Before the Procedure

Client teaching and physical preparation are the same as for any plain x-ray procedure (see p. 590).

The Procedure

The client is placed in a standing position. If the client is unable to stand, he or she is helped into a side-lying position on the x-ray table, and a left lateral decubitus film is taken. A second film can be taken with the client in the supine position with the arms extended upward over the head for an AP view of the abdomen. A third film can be taken for a cross-table lateral view of the abdomen if an aortic disorder is suspected.[30] A single chest x-ray can also be included in the series. Either a PA or an AP view can be taken, depending on the client's ability to stand for the x-ray. If the client is unable to be transported to the radiology department, the study can be performed at the bedside with a portable unit.

Nursing Care After the Procedure

Care and assessment after the procedure are the same as for any plain x-ray procedure (see p. 591).
➤ Monitor bowel sounds and assist with positioning for comfort if the client is experiencing pain.
➤ Reapply dressings as needed.

PELVIMETRY

Pelvimetry involves x-ray of the pelvis of a pregnant woman at or near term. It is performed to determine whether the pelvis is adequate in size relative to the fetal head. The study is rarely used, but it is helpful in determining whether a vaginal birth will be possible.[31] Because this study does not take place until the client is at or near term or during labor, the risk to the fetus is minimal. However, the procedure should not be performed unless absolutely necessary.

Reference Values

Normal pelvic diameters with size adequate in relation to the fetal head

Interfering Factors

➤ Excessive fetal activity
➤ Metal objects within the x-ray field

Indications for Pelvimetry

➤ Maternal history of problems involving pelvic bones or birthing process
➤ Abnormal pelvic measurements
➤ Suspected abnormal fetal presentation[32]
➤ Failure of the fetal head to engage during the labor phase
➤ Possible administration of oxytocin (Pitocin) to induce labor in the absence of labor progression
➤ Confirmation of the need for a cesarean birth

Contraindications

➤ None

Nursing Care Before the Procedure

Client teaching and physical preparation are the same as for any plain x-ray procedure (see p. 590).
➤ Obtain baseline fetal heart rate (FHR) for postprocedure comparison, if indicated.
➤ Assess trimester of pregnancy, as study is performed only at term or during labor phase.

The Procedure

The client is helped to a standing position and a lateral view is taken to assess the lowest level of the head in the birth canal. A second film can be taken with the client in the supine position, supine position with knees flexed (semirecumbent), or side-lying position.[33] When the client is in the supine position and an anterior view is to be obtained, a metal ruler (pelvimeter) can be placed at the level of the ischial tuberosities, or it can be placed between the gluteal folds when the side-lying position is assumed. While the filming is taking place, the client is requested to breathe rapidly and then hold the breath.[34]

Nursing Care After the Procedure

Care and assessment after the procedure are the same as for any plain x-ray procedure (see p. 591).

➤ Assess fetal heart sounds and signs of progression of labor, if appropriate.

SPINAL FILMS

Various segments of the spine can be examined radiologically, including the cervical, thoracic, and lumbosacral spine (Fig. 17–5). In most cases, such x-rays are taken because the client is experiencing pain. If spinal films are negative for abnormality, additional diagnostic procedures, such as CT or contrast-mediated studies, can be performed. If a fracture is suspected, appropriate measures must be taken when positioning the client for x-rays so that spinal cord injury (SCI) does not inadvertently occur. The physician who ordered the study should be consulted before removing braces or other immobilizing devices.

Reference Values

Normal vertebral bodies; no abnormal curvatures or fracture of the spine

Interfering Factors

➤ Problems with positioning when fractures are suspected or if immobilizing devices are in place
➤ Metal objects such as jewelry or clothing fasteners within the x-ray field

Indications for Spinal Films

➤ Evaluation of back or neck pain of unknown etiology for possible arthritis, spondylosis, or spondylolisthesis
➤ Diagnosis of tumor or destruction of vertebral bodies caused by malignancy or evidence of spread of cancer to the spine[35]
➤ Suspected or known vertebral fracture
➤ Abnormal curvatures of the spine, such as scoliosis and kyphosis, in children
➤ Monitoring of progression or treatment of scoliosis or lordosis
➤ Determination of congenital spinal cord defects in infants

Contraindications

➤ Pregnancy, unless benefits of performing the procedure greatly outweigh the risks to the fetus

Nursing Care Before the Procedure

Client teaching and physical preparation are the same as for any plain x-ray procedure (see p. 590).

➤ Consult the physician before removing braces or other immobilizing devices.

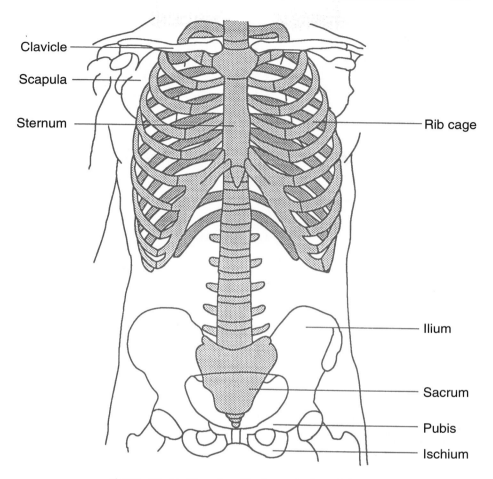

Clavicle

Scapula

Sternum

Rib cage

Ilium

Sacrum

Pubis

Ischium

Figure 17–5   Thoracic and lumbosacral spine and rib cage.

The Procedure

The client is placed on the x-ray table in a supine position. First, an AP film is taken. The client is then placed in the side-lying position and additional lateral and oblique views are filmed.[36] The oblique is performed by angling the x-ray beam between AP and lateral views. Fracture sites are immobilized during the procedure to prevent further injury to the spine. The client should be instructed to report any discomfort during the study.

Nursing Care After the Procedure

Care and assessment after the procedure are the same as for any plain x-ray procedure (see p. 591).

➤ Reapply braces or other appliances or devices, and inform the client of any activity restrictions.

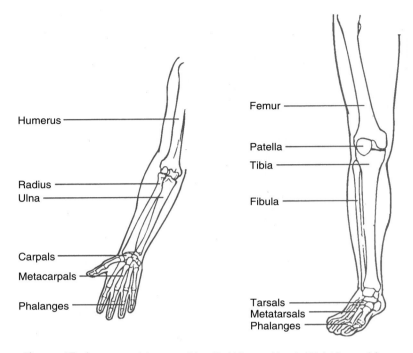

Figure 17–6 Bones of the extremities. *(Left)* Arm and hand. *(Right)* Leg and foot.

EXTREMITY FILMS

Films of all or part of the arms and legs are used to diagnose a variety of skeletal conditions, including fractures and other bone and joint disorders (Fig. 17–6). Positioning is important to obtain the desired views; in some cases, orthopedic devices, joint mobility, and client discomfort can interfere with filming and clear imaging. The physician who ordered the study should be consulted before splints or other immobilizing devices are removed.

Reference Values

Normal bone, bone ossification, and joint structure; no fractures, dislocations, or congenital anomalies involving bones or joints

Interfering Factors

➤ Problems with positioning caused by orthopedic devices, joint mobility, or client discomfort
➤ Metal objects within the x-ray field

Indications for Extremity Films

➤ Evaluation of bone and joint pain of unknown etiology for possible arthritis or other degenerative or malignant disorders of the bone

➤ Suspected fracture of a bone, joint dislocation, or fluid accumulation
➤ Monitoring of fracture reduction and healing process
➤ Detection of changes in bone caused by infectious diseases such as osteomyelitis
➤ Monitoring of response to treatment for various bone and joint disorders
➤ Evaluation of skeletal trauma in younger children
➤ Evaluation of growth pattern revealed by wrist ossification
➤ Determination of alterations in alignment and configuration of the epiphysis after skeletal injury
➤ Diagnosis and monitoring of improvement after corrective interventions for congenital hip dysplasia and talipes deformities in infants

Contraindications

➤ Pregnancy, unless benefits of performing the procedure greatly outweigh the risks to the fetus

Nursing Care Before the Procedure

Client teaching and physical preparation are the same as for any plain x-ray procedure (see p. 590).
➤ Consult the physician before removing any splits or immobilizing devices.

The Procedure

The client is placed on the x-ray table with the extremity to be studied in an appropriate position. Films can also be taken with the client is a sitting position. All injured parts are handled gently and supported when moved or repositioned. A shield is placed over the abdomen and testicular area to protect the reproductive organs from radiation. Pillows, sandbags, and other immobilizing devices are used to position or immobilize a body part. Usually several different views of an area are filmed.

Nursing Care After the Procedure

Care and assessment after the procedure are the same as for any plain x-ray procedure (see p. 591).
➤ Reapply any immobilizing devices.
➤ Administer a mild analgesic for discomfort and heat application to a painful joint if ordered.[37]
➤ Inform the client of any activity restrictions after the procedure.

CARDIAC FILMS

Cardiac films involve the evaluation of cardiac diseases and disorders by providing images of the size, position, and contour of the heart and great vessels. The cardiac series includes a barium swallow with subsequent views of the heart with the client in various positions, which provides a constant view, by fluoroscopy, of the heart in motion and of pulsations of the heart and great vessels during systole and diastole phases.[38] Filming of the heart in motion exposes the client to a higher level of radiation and has generally been replaced by echocardiography.

Reference Values

Normal size, shape, and position of the heart and great vessels; normal movement of the heart during systole and diastole

Interfering Factors

➤ Improper positioning, especially for views taken by portable x-ray equipment with the client in bed
➤ Improper adjustment of the x-ray equipment to accommodate obese and thin clients, resulting in overexposure or underexposure and poor-quality films
➤ Inability of client to take deep breaths during filming or to maintain a position without moving
➤ Metal objects such as jewelry or clothing fasteners within the x-ray field

Indications for Cardiac Films

➤ Evaluation of heart size, contour, and position for abnormalities indicating a cardiac disorder
➤ Observation of heart motion and pulsations by fluoroscopic viewing to determine the presence of aneurysm, congenital heart disorder, or valve disorder
➤ Evaluation of prosthetic valve function
➤ Determination of calcifications within the heart, especially of the valves
➤ Suspected pericardial effusion or other abnormalities involving the area surrounding the heart
➤ Evaluation of the placement and positioning of pacemaker wires and cardiac catheters[39]

Contraindications

➤ Pregnancy, unless benefits of performing the procedure greatly outweigh the risks to the fetus

Nursing Care Before the Procedure

Client teaching and physical preparation are the same as for any plain x-ray procedure (see p. 590).
➤ Inform the client that a barium contrast medium is administered orally if a cardiac series is to be performed.

The Procedure

For routine, plain cardiac films or portable cardiac films, the procedure is the same as for routine or portable chest x-rays (see p. 595). Films of infants are taken in the supine position. If fluoroscopic examination is performed to visualize movement of the heart or to verify pacemaker wires or catheter placement, the client is assisted to the best positions for viewing heart movement from four directions.[40] If a cardiac series is to be performed, a barium swallow is given and PA, lateral, right oblique, and left oblique views are taken.[41] The series allows better visualization of the aortic arch and left heart enlargement, revealed by esophageal deviations.[42]

Nursing Care After the Procedure

Care and assessment after the procedure are the same as for any plain x-ray procedure (see p. 591).

➤ Place the client in a position of comfort and replace all tubes or wires in their proper position if a portable film is taken.

➤ If the cardiac series was performed, administer a laxative to assist in the elimination of the barium.

TOMOGRAPHY

Tomography provides a two-dimensional image with clarity superior to that of plain films. It is especially valuable in visualizing air-filled structures such as the lungs and paranasal sinuses. The studies are contraindicated during pregnancy, unless the benefits of performing the procedure far outweigh the risks to the fetus.

CHEST TOMOGRAPHY

Tomograms of the chest are valuable when the nature of lesions seen on routine chest x-rays must be determined or when routine films are negative but an abnormality is suspected. Tomography provides an image of the organ at different depths and angles and reveals parts not seen on plain radiographs. Because the client is exposed to more radiation than with plain x-ray filming, tomography is used only when absolutely necessary. This procedure has been replaced by computed tomography (CT) of the chest.[43,44]

Reference Values

Normal lung fields, mediastinal structures, ribs, and thoracic spine

Interfering Factors

➤ Inability of client to maintain required positioning and remain still during the study

➤ Improper positioning of the client

➤ Metal objects such as jewelry or clothing fasteners within x-ray field

Indications for Chest Tomography

➤ Further evaluation of abnormal pulmonary vasculature seen on chest x-ray

➤ Suspected lung tumor when plain chest films are negative

➤ Further evaluation of abnormal results of plain films of the chest that can include tuberculous cavitation, lung abscess, or calcifications

➤ Suspected tumor involving mediastinal structures, ribs, and spine[45]

Contraindications

➤ Pregnancy, unless benefits of performing the procedure greatly outweigh the risks to the fetus

Nursing Care Before the Procedure

Client teaching and physical preparation are the same as for any plain x-ray procedure (see p. 590).

The Procedure

The client is placed on the x-ray table in a supine position. Side-lying or prone positions can also be used for this study. The x-ray tube overhead is moved back and forth in a circular or a figure 8 motion while the films are being taken. The client is requested to remain very still on the table but to breathe in a normal pattern.

Nursing Care After the Procedure

Care and assessment after the procedure are the same as for any plain x-ray procedure (see p. 591).

Paranasal Sinus Tomography

Tomograms of the paranasal sinuses produce images in sections, making views possible that are not obstructed by structures surrounding the sinuses.

Reference Values

Normal sinuses; no bony abnormalities, masses, or foreign bodies

Interfering Factors

➤ Inability of client to remain motionless during the study while filming is taking place
➤ Improper positioning for the desired views
➤ Metal objects such as dental or eye prostheses or eyeglasses within the x-ray field

Indications for Paranasal Sinus Tomography

➤ Further evaluation of abnormal results of plain films that reveal evidence of tumors, cysts, or fracture
➤ Suspected fracture or tumor of the nasal bones and bones surrounding the sinuses when plain films are negative[46]
➤ Detection of foreign bodies in the sinuses

Contraindications

➤ Pregnancy, unless benefits of performing the procedure greatly outweigh the risks to the fetus

Nursing Care Before the Procedure

Client teaching and physical preparation are the same as for any plain x-ray procedure (see p. 590).

The Procedure

The client is seated in a special chair with the head immobilized in a padded brace or vise to maintain a proper position. The client is requested to remain very still while an x-ray tube overhead is moved in different directions around a pivot point during filming. Several views can be taken, depending on the purpose of the study.

Nursing Care After the Procedure

Care and assessment after the procedure are the same as for any plain x-ray procedure (see p. 591).

XERORADIOGRAPHY

The technique for xeroradiography, as described in the "Introduction" section of this chapter, provides a photoelectric view of the organ tissue, especially soft tissue of the type found in the breasts.

MAMMOGRAPHY

Mammograms are performed primarily to detect malignancy of the breast. They can also be performed to aid in determining the nature of palpable lesions and to detect breast lesions in women whose breasts are large, pendulous, and difficult to examine adequately by palpation. A signed informed consent form is required for this procedure.

Mammography is usually performed using xeroradiography, which is believed to have a comparatively low radiation exposure level, although newer conventional x-ray filming now allows minimal exposure to radiation. The method selected is mostly a matter of physician preference. Mammography allows detection of breast tumors less than 0.5 cm in diameter 2 to 3 years before they are clinically evident; it carries an 85 percent accuracy rate and less than a 10 percent false-positive rate in the diagnosis of carcinoma.[47] Positive mammography results are confirmed by biopsy but can be further studied by ultrasonography or diaphanography (transillumination).[48] Transillumination is not as reliable as conventional mammography in the diagnosis of breast malignancy but is valuable in the diagnosis of benign tumors and fibrocystic disease, as well as in the evaluation of silicone-injected or -augmented breasts.[49]

The American Cancer Society recommends that all women between the ages of 35 and 40 have a baseline mammogram. From ages 40 to 49, a mammogram should be performed every 1 to 2 years, depending on the client's history. For example, women with fibrocystic breast disease, previous mastectomy, cancer of other organs, or family history of breast cancer are advised to have yearly mammograms. After the age of 50, it is recommended that all women have an annual mammogram.

Many women find mammography an embarrassing and uncomfortable procedure. Those who have cystic disease should have the procedure performed 1 week after menses, when tenderness is decreased. For some who find the procedure painful, a mild analgesic can be administered before the study. Also, many women are anxious about the procedure because of the possibility of malignancy. Effective client preparation and support are essential. The importance of performing breast self-examination (BSE) and having regular mammograms should also be stressed. If detected early enough, breast cancer has a high cure rate.

It should be noted that, if a disease involving the mammary ducts is suspected, mammography can be performed after a contrast medium is injected into the ducts. This is done to identify papillomas or ductal obstruction.

Reference Values

Normal breast tissue; no cysts, tumors, or abnormal calcifications

Interfering Factors

➤ Powder, creams, perfumes, lotions, or underarm deodorant on the skin
➤ Extremely nodular breasts or previous surgery on the breasts[50]
➤ Inability to adequately compress the breasts or to include all of the breast tissue in the films
➤ Hematoma, mastitis, or papillomatosis if a transillumination study is performed[51]
➤ Metal objects such as jewelry or clothing fasteners within the x-ray field

Indications for Mammography

➤ Early detection of malignant tumors of the breast before they are large enough to be palpated
➤ Previous surgery for breast cancer, history of cancer involving other organs, or both
➤ Family history of breast cancer, cancer involving other organs, or both
➤ Evaluation of lumps or areas of thickening tissue detected on BSE or by health-care practitioner on clinical examination
➤ Determination of cause of painful breasts
➤ Diagnosis of breast cancer revealed by irregular masses with poorly defined borders, extension into surrounding tissue, or both conditions, or abnormal calcifications in breast or ductal tissue[52,53]
➤ Diagnosis of fibrocystic disease of the breasts with benign cysts revealed by round, smooth masses with well-defined borders
➤ Diagnosis of mastitis and breast abscess when symptoms are evident
➤ Evaluation of nipple and skin changes on breast and association with malignancy
➤ Routine screening procedure for breast cancer

Contraindications

➤ Pregnancy, unless the benefits of performing the study greatly outweigh the risks to the fetus

Nursing Care Before the Procedure

Client teaching and physical preparation are the same as for any plain x-ray procedure (see p. 590).
➤ Instruct the client to avoid application of any substance to the skin of the breasts, chest, or underarms, and administer a mild analgesic if pain is experienced when breasts are manipulated or compressed.

The Procedure

The client is placed in front of the x-ray machine in a standing or a sitting position. The machine is adjusted to the level of the breasts. One at a time, the client's breasts are positioned on a flat plastic or metal holder and compressed without creases or wrinkles under the compression apparatus. If xeroradiography is used, four views can be taken, including oblique, lateral, chest wall, or vertical (craniocaudal). A minimum of two views of each breast is taken; one is usually chest wall. If conventional x-ray is used, three views can be taken, including oblique, lateral, or vertical, with a minimum of two views of each breast, of which one view is usually oblique. The arm is positioned upward and out of range of the area to be x-rayed. The actual filming takes place while the client takes a deep breath and holds it. The client is requested to wait while the films are developed and checked to be sure that all the breast tissue was included in the views.

Diaphanography or transillumination is performed in a dark room with the client in a sitting position and the torso leaning forward. The examiner directs an infrared lighting device over each breast. The light is filtered by the breast and densities are converted into images. The images produced by the light are photographed by a computerized camera that is focused on the area.[54] Films are developed and reviewed to provide diagnostic information.

Nursing Care After the Procedure

Care and assessment after the procedure are the same as for any plain x-ray procedure (see p. 591).

➤ Teach the client BSE and provide brochures outlining the procedure and the signs and symptoms to report. Stress the importance of regular mammography, depending on the client's age.

CONTRAST-MEDIATED STUDIES

Contrast-mediated studies are performed to visualize soft tissues that produce poor images on x-ray unless they are enhanced in some way. The most commonly used contrast media are barium sulfate and the organic iodides. These substances are radiopaque and block the passage of the x-rays, resulting in the images on film. Signed informed consent forms are not obtained for procedures using a barium contrast medium but are required for those using iodinated contrast medium. The risks or complications associated with the use of either medium are outlined in the "Introduction" section of the chapter.

BARIUM SWALLOW

A barium swallow (esophagography) involves the recording of radiographic images of the esophageal lumen while the client swallows barium solution. The test is performed using fluoroscopic and cineradiographic techniques and is recorded on film or videotape to evaluate both motion and anatomic structures. A barium swallow is often performed along with an upper gastrointestinal (UGI) series. It is also performed as part of a cardiac series to visualize the size and shape of the heart and great vessels (see p. 603).

Barium sulfate solutions of both thick and thin consistencies are given. A swallowed small cotton ball soaked in barium can be used to detect foreign bodies in the esophagus, because swallowing liquid barium occurs too rapidly for such objects to be visualized.[55] Food items can also be coated with barium to evaluate both chewing and swallowing. Barium is not used if perforation or obstruction of the esophagus is suspected, because deposition of the barium in soft tissues can cause a serious inflammatory response. In such cases, a water-soluble solution of an iodinated contrast medium such as diatrizoate meglumine

(Gastrografin) is used. It should be noted, however, that some of these materials are irritating to the mucosa of the tracheobronchial tree and should not be used when tracheoesophageal fistula is suspected.[56]

Reference Values

Normal peristalsis through the esophagus into the stomach with normal size and shape of the esophagus; no inflammation, strictures, ulcerations, polyps, tumors, rupture, foreign bodies, varices, or hiatal hernia

Interfering Factors

➤ Inability of client to assume or remain in the proper position during the procedure
➤ Inability of client to swallow radiopaque substance or barium-coated items
➤ Foods and fluids ingested within 8 hours of the study
➤ Metal objects within the x-ray field

Indications for Barium Swallow

➤ Chronic difficult or painful swallowing (dysphagia), heartburn, or regurgitation of food[57]
➤ Suspected esophageal motility disorders such as achalasia, spasms of the esophageal muscles
➤ Diagnosis of esophageal reflux revealed by barium returning to the esophagus from the stomach
➤ Suspected strictures, polyps, Zenker's diverticula, benign or malignant tumor of the esophagus
➤ Determination of whether sharp foreign object is caught in the esophagus after accidental swallowing
➤ Diagnosis of inflammatory or infectious process such as acute or chronic esophagitis
➤ Suspected congenital abnormality in infants such as tracheoesophageal fistula or atresia
➤ Suspected rupture of the esophagus (the study must be performed with extreme caution)
➤ Suspected esophageal varices, although they are more likely to be detected by endoscopic procedures

Contraindications

➤ Pregnancy, unless benefits of performing the procedure greatly outweigh the risks to the fetus
➤ Allergy to iodine, if an iodinated contrast medium is used
➤ Suspected presence of intestinal obstruction
➤ Suspected esophageal rupture, unless water-soluble iodinated contrast medium is used
➤ Suspected tracheoesophageal fistula, unless barium sulfate is used

Nursing Care Before the Procedure

Explain to the client:
➤ That a physician or a technician will perform the study
➤ That the procedure requires about 45 minutes to 1 hour

➤ That foods and fluids are withheld for at least 8 hours before the procedure and should continue to be restricted until the study has been completed

➤ That the client will be requested to swallow a flavored barium solution while standing in front of a fluoroscopy x-ray screen and that films will be taken while the barium moves down the esophagus

➤ That no pain is associated with the procedure, although swallowing of the contrast medium can be unpleasant

Prepare for the procedure:

➤ Obtain a history to ascertain the date of the last menstrual period and pregnancy status, possible allergy to iodine if an iodinated contrast medium is to be used, assessment of gastrointestinal system for signs and symptoms, treatment and medication regimen, and associated diagnostic tests and procedures.

➤ Ensure that dietary and fluid restrictions have been followed.

➤ Ensure that all jewelry and clothing are removed from the waist up and provide the client with a gown without metal closures.

➤ Assess baseline vital signs to compare with later readings or to determine any deviations that can warrant postponement of the study.

The Procedure

The client is helped onto the x-ray table in a supine position or into a standing position in front of the x-ray screen. An initial plain film is taken. The client stands in front of a fluoroscopic screen and is requested to swallow a barium solution with or without a straw. If the client has problems with chewing or swallowing, small food items coated with barium can be offered. A water-soluble iodinated contrast medium can be used if a rupture of the esophagus is suspected. Barium sulfate, which does not react with the surrounding mucosa, is used if tracheoesophageal fistula is suspected.[58]

The passage of the contrast material through the esophagus is evaluated using fluoroscopic and cineradiologic techniques, and spot films are taken at different angles. The upright position facilitates the diagnosis of strictures or obstructions of the esophagus.[59] The client is then strapped to the table and the table rotated or tilted into the head-down position, or the client is placed in the prone, supine, and lateral positions for additional films. The client may be requested to drink additional barium as these films are taken. Delayed films can also be taken to evaluate esophageal abnormalities caused by failure of the barium to completely pass through the esophagus into the stomach.

Nursing Care After the Procedure

➤ Resume food and fluids if no additional films are to be taken.

➤ Monitor vital signs and compare with baselines for changes that indicate complications.

➤ Administer, or advise client to take, a mild laxative and increase fluid intake to aid in the elimination of the barium.

➤ Inform the client that feces will be whitish or light in color for 2 to 3 days and to notify the physician if the normal color does not return or if the client is unable to eliminate the barium.

➤ *Reaction to iodinated contrast medium:* Note and report tachycardia, hyperpnea, palpitations, or hypertension. Administer ordered antihistamine or steroid. Initiate IV line and resuscitation procedure, if needed (see Table 17–1, p. 588).

UPPER GASTROINTESTINAL (UGI) SERIES

An upper gastrointestinal (UGI) series involves radiologic examination of the lower esophagus, stomach, duodenum, and upper jejunum after ingestion of a solution of barium sulfate. The entire small bowel can also be evaluated by this study. The procedure is then referred to as a UGI with small-bowel follow-through. A combination of x-ray and fluoroscopic techniques are used to perform the study. Fluoroscopic techniques are used to visualize passage of the barium from the esophagus into the stomach and from the stomach into the duodenum. A complete examination of the small intestine by fluoroscopy can also be made in addition to the UGI. This study involves visualization of the small bowel up to the ileocecal valve by taking films at specific time intervals (usually every 10 minutes) as the barium passes through the small intestine. A more detailed evaluation of the small bowel can be accomplished by a procedure known as the small-bowel enema. X-ray filming can also be used to obtain spot films of various areas of the UGI tract. As with barium swallow, solutions of barium should not be used if perforation of the stomach or duodenum is suspected, because deposition of barium in soft tissues can cause a serious inflammatory response. In such cases, a water-soluble solution of an iodinated contrast medium, diatrizoate meglumine, is used.

Reference Values

Normal esophageal, stomach, and small intestine motility; normal size and shape of the stomach and small intestine; no ulcerations, inflammation, tumors, strictures, ruptures, foreign bodies, or hiatal hernia

Interfering Factors

➤ Inability of client to assume or remain in the desired position for the procedure
➤ Inability of client to ingest the radiopaque substance
➤ Foods and fluids ingested within 8 hours of the study that affect peristalsis
➤ Medications such as anticholinergics and narcotics that affect motility
➤ Barium remaining in the tract from other studies using the contrast medium
➤ Metal objects within the x-ray field

Indications for Upper Gastrointestinal (UGI) Series

➤ Persistent epigastric pain or heartburn of unknown etiology
➤ Possible strictures or varices in the lower esophagus
➤ Hematemesis or presence of blood in the feces
➤ Unexplained weight loss, anorexia, nausea, or vomiting
➤ Palpable mass in the epigastric area[60]
➤ Persistent abdominal pain or diarrhea of unknown etiology
➤ Possible peptic ulcer disease
➤ Suspected tumor of the stomach or small bowel
➤ Inflammatory disorder or the stomach or small bowel
➤ Diagnosis of obstruction or malabsorption syndrome and fistula or

ulcerations of the small bowel revealed by diminished or increased motility[61]

➤ Congenital anomalies such as pyloric stenosis in children

➤ Malrotation causing bowel obstruction in infants

➤ Suspected hiatal hernia

➤ Suspected foreign body in the UGI tract

➤ Evaluation of treatment regimen for gastrointestinal diseases

Contraindications

➤ Pregnancy, unless benefits of performing the procedure greatly outweigh the risks to the fetus

➤ Allergy to iodine, if an iodinated contrast medium is used

➤ Clients who are combative or generally uncooperative

➤ Evidence of or suspected intestinal obstruction

➤ Suspected rupture involving the stomach or small intestine, unless the study is performed with caution and with a water-soluble iodinated contrast medium

Nursing Care Before the Procedure

Client teaching and physical preparation are the same as for barium swallow (see p. 610).

➤ Inform the client that medications that interfere with gastric motion are withheld for 12 to 24 hours, that filming can take as long as 5 hours, and that it may continue the next day to evaluate small-bowel function in those with decreased peristalsis.

The Procedure

The procedure varies slightly, depending on the institution. The client can be placed on the x-ray table in a supine position for an initial plain abdominal film. The client is then assisted to a sitting or standing position or is strapped to the table, tilted into a vertical position, and given 8 to 16 oz of barium solution to drink. The client is informed that the solution is flavored and chalky in consistency and not too pleasant to drink. The passage of the barium through the esophagus, stomach, and duodenum is filmed and evaluated by fluoroscopy as the client drinks the barium solution. Visualization can be improved by using both air and barium as contrast agents ("double-contrast" study). For this method, the client sips the barium through a perforated straw, which allows both barium and air to be introduced into the stomach and promotes viewing by smoothing the ridges of the gastric rugae.[62]

After the complete ingestion of the barium solution, films are taken in various positions, including supine, side-lying, and prone. PA, AP, lateral, and oblique views are taken. Pressure can be applied to the epigastric area to ensure adequate coating of the stomach with the barium or to straighten overlapping bowel loops. Filming takes place throughout the procedure, and additional barium can be given to ensure adequate coating of the small intestine if a small-bowel series is done. Small-bowel filming is performed at 15- to 30-minute intervals until the barium reaches the cecum.

If a small-bowel enema study is conducted, a barium solution is injected into an enteral tube placed into the duodenum via the mouth or endoscope and films taken as in the small-bowel series.

Nursing Care After the Procedure

Care and assessment after the procedure are the same as for barium swallow (see p. 611).

➤ Advise the client that diarrhea can occur if a water-soluble contrast medium was administered.

➤ *Barium aspiration:* Note and report choking or any change in respiratory pattern. Perform orotracheal suction. Provide ordered oxygen. Prepare for intubation, if needed.

BARIUM ENEMA (BE)

Barium enema (BE), or lower gastrointestinal (LGI) series, involves radiologic examination of the colon after the instillation of barium via a rectal tube inserted into the rectum or an existing ostomy. A combination of x-ray and fluoroscopic techniques are used to perform the study. Fluoroscopic techniques are used to visualize passage of the barium through the large intestine. X-rays are taken to obtain spot films of various areas of the colon. Visualization can be improved by using both air and barium as the contrast agents. This procedure is known as a double-contrast study and is especially useful in improving detection of small lesions and polyps. As with the barium swallow and UGI series, barium solutions should not be used if perforation of the colon is suspected, because leakage of barium can cause a serious inflammatory response. In such instances, a water-soluble solution of an iodinated contrast medium such as diatrizoate meglumine is used.

For the procedure to be successful, the bowel must be cleared of fecal matter or barium from previous studies. Various approaches are used to cleanse the bowel, as outlined in the "Nursing Care Before the Procedure" section, with modifications made for young children, elderly clients, and clients with an ostomy or a history of colitis.[63]

The proper sequencing of the gastrointestinal studies in which barium is used as the contrast medium is also important. Barium enema should be performed before the UGI series, which in turn should be performed before the barium swallow, if the UGI series and barium swallow are performed as separate studies. Privacy and comfort are preserved: Most clients find barium enemas uncomfortable and embarrassing procedures. Effective preparation and support for this study are essential to ensure that the procedure will not require repetition.

Reference Values

Normal size, shape, and motility of the colon; no inflammation, tumors, polyps, diverticulae, congenital anomalies, or foreign bodies

Interfering Factors

➤ Inability of client to assume or remain in the desired position

➤ Inability of client to tolerate introduction of or to retain barium, air, or both, in the bowel

➤ Residual barium or excessive feces in the bowel resulting from inadequate cleansing or failure to restrict food intake before the study

➤ Colon spasms that impair visualization[64]
➤ Metal objects within the x-ray field

Indications for Barium Enema (BE)

➤ Rectal bleeding of unknown etiology
➤ Unexplained blood, pus, or mucus in the feces
➤ Change in bowel patterns that leads to chronic diarrhea, constipation, or caliber of feces
➤ Unexplained weight loss or anemia
➤ Persistent abdominal pain or distention of unknown etiology
➤ Identification of benign and malignant polyps and tumors
➤ Evaluation of genitourinary malignancies to determine metastasis to the colon
➤ Identification of diverticula, megacolon, or other structural changes
➤ Suspected inflammatory process of the colon and of the terminal ileum, such as colitis, ulcerative colitis, or Crohn's disease
➤ Suspected abnormality in bowel motility and obstructions of the bowel
➤ Suspected congenital anomaly involving the bowel
➤ Reduction of intussusception in children
➤ Suspected foreign body in the colon
➤ Evaluation of colon surgery

Contraindications

➤ Pregnancy, unless benefits of performing the procedure greatly outweigh the risks to the fetus
➤ Allergy to iodine, if an iodinated contrast medium is used
➤ Evidence of intestinal obstruction
➤ Evidence of toxic megacolon, acute ulcerative colitis, acute diverticulitis, or other acute colon disorder[65]
➤ Suspected rupture involving the colon, unless performed with caution using a water-soluble iodinated contrast medium

---

➤➤ Nursing Alert

- A client scheduled for several studies using barium should have the barium enema performed first because residual barium from other studies can necessitate repeated bowel preparation if an LGI series is performed as a second study.
- Lack of adequate fluid intake before or after the study can cause dehydration if excessive fluids are removed from the colon during bowel preparation.
- Use of laxatives or cathartics in bowel preparation can cause a life-threatening complication in the presence of obstruction, acute ulcerative colitis, or diverticulitis.

Nursing Care Before the Procedure

Client teaching and preparation are the same as for barium swallow (see p. 610), except that this study requires 45 to 90 minutes.

➤ Dietary regimen and bowel preparation vary with institutions.
➤ Instruct the client to follow a low-residue diet for several days before the

procedure, to increase fluids the day before, to ingest a clear liquid diet the evening before, and to take nothing by mouth, including medications, on the day of the procedure.

➤ Instruct the client to take magnesium citrate liquid and a bisacodyl tablet the evening before; inform client that this preparation can cause cramping and diarrhea.

➤ Administer suppositories and cleansing enemas before the procedure and evaluate their effectiveness (clear return of the enemas).

➤ Be cautious in the use of enemas and laxatives on children and elderly people, who are more prone to fluid and electrolyte imbalances.

➤ Inform clients with an ostomy to follow the same dietary preparations, to take laxatives the evening before, and to administer a colostomy irrigation before the study.

➤ Advise clients with an ostomy that the barium enema is administered through a Foley catheter introduced into the ostomy; clients should bring an appliance and pouch system with them if they are outpatients.[66]

The Procedure

The procedure varies slightly, depending on the institution and approaches for children, elderly clients, and clients with ostomies. The client is placed on the x-ray table in a supine position for an initial plain abdominal film. The client is then assisted to a side-lying position and draped with the anus exposed or to a comfortable supine position and draped with the stoma exposed. A lubricated rectal tube is inserted into the anus and a balloon on the end of the tube is inflated after it is situated against the anal sphincter.[67] A Foley catheter is inserted into the stoma if an ostomy is present. For children or elderly clients, the buttocks can be taped together or a special inflatable retention device can be used.[68]

Barium is instilled into the colon. The client should be informed that this procedure can cause cramping, sensations of abdominal fullness, and the urge to defecate. Encourage controlled breathing and relaxation to aid in tolerance and retention of the barium. The tube can be left in place after the instillation is completed to assist in retention of the barium until all the films are taken. Movement of the barium through the colon into the ileocecal valve and then into the terminal ileum is observed by fluoroscopy. The client is assisted into supine, prone, side-lying, and erect positions while spot films are taken for different views.

The procedure for performing double-contrast studies to improve visualization varies with institutions. Double-contrast studies have a higher rate of accuracy in detecting small lesions and polyps of the colon. One method allows some of the barium to be expelled or aspirated and for air to be injected to distend the colon. Another method involves instilling barium into the descending colon and then forcefully injecting air without removing any of the barium.

When the films are completed, the barium is aspirated and the tube removed. The client is assisted to the bathroom or placed on a bedpan to expel the barium remaining in the colon. Another film can be taken after the elimination of the barium.

Nursing Care After the Procedure

Care and assessment after the procedure are the same as for barium swallow (see p. 611).

➤ Encourage the client to increase fluid intake and to rest if feeling fatigued.
➤ Administer a tap water colostomy irrigation to assist in the removal of the barium.
➤ *Fluid imbalance:* Note and report signs and symptoms of dehydration such as decreased urinary output; warm, dry skin; or poor skin turgor. Administer fluid orally or IV to replace losses. Monitor electrolytes.
➤ *Perforation of colon:* Note and report acute abdominal pain, nausea, vomiting, or abdominal distention. Administer ordered analgesic and antibiotic therapy. Insert NG tube and attach to suction. Prepare for possible surgery.

ORAL CHOLECYSTOGRAPHY (OCG)

For an oral cholecystogram (OCG), the dye, usually iopanoic acid (Telepaque) or ipodate sodium (Oragrafin), is administered orally in tablet form. The dye is subsequently absorbed in the small bowel, transported to the liver, excreted by the liver into bile, and concentrated in the gallbladder.[69] Approximately 12 to 14 hours are required for this process to occur.[70] The dye is administered the evening before the study. A low-fat diet is also given so that the gallbladder does not contract and empty.

Gallstones are usually not visualized on plain films unless they are calcified, which occurs in approximately 10 percent of all cases of cholelithiasis.[71] The concentration of dye in the gallbladder allows the gallstones to appear as shadows on the x-ray film.[72] In addition to the actual appearance of gallstones on x-ray, gallstones can be suspected if the gallbladder is not visualized after administration of the dye; that is, gallstones can obstruct the bile ducts and prevent the dye from reaching the gallbladder. Failure to visualize the gallbladder can also be caused by inflammation of the bile ducts, impaired liver function, impaired absorption from the small intestine, or inadequate dosage of the contrast medium. Jaundice with elevated bilirubin levels is also associated with diminished excretion of the dye and impaired visualization of the gallbladder.[73]

The study is performed after any study involving the measurement of iodinated compounds and before any gastrointestinal study involving the use of barium as the contrast medium. Ultrasound examination of the gallbladder is more sensitive than the OCG in detecting gallstones and is replacing this procedure as the diagnostic test of choice. Magnetic resonance imaging (MRI) and CT scanning are also used in selected situations.[74]

Reference Values

Normal appearance of gallbladder; no calcification of the gallbladder wall, stones, filling defects, or abnormal accumulation of gas

Interfering Factors

➤ Inability of client to maintain the required positions
➤ Barium in the gastrointestinal tract
➤ Inadequate dose of the oral contrast medium
➤ Vomiting or diarrhea after administration of the contrast medium
➤ Failure to follow dietary restrictions
➤ Impaired absorption of the dye from the gastrointestinal tract

➤ Impaired liver function, resulting in failure to excrete the dye into the bile

➤ Cystic duct obstruction, preventing dye from entering the gallbladder

➤ Inability of the gallbladder to concentrate the dye for visualization

➤ Jaundice with bilirubin levels over 2 mg/dL and with impaired excretion of the dye

➤ Metal objects within the x-ray field

Indications for Oral Cholecystography (OCG)

➤ Upper right quadrant (URQ) pain, right epigastric pain, or both, of unknown etiology

➤ Evaluation of symptoms of cholecystitis and gallbladder function revealed by the gallbladder's ability to accumulate, concentrate, and expel the dye

➤ Suspected malignant tumor revealed by calcification of the gallbladder wall[75]

➤ Suspected gallstones in the gallbladder or obstructed cystic duct with gallstones, or both conditions

➤ Determination of the presence of papillomas, adenomas, and diverticula of the gallbladder

➤ Diagnosis of fistula between the biliary system and the gastrointestinal tract revealed by gas in the gallbladder or ducts[76]

➤ Determination of congenital anomalies of the gallbladder

Contraindications

➤ Pregnancy, unless benefits of performing the procedure greatly outweigh the risks to the fetus

➤ Allergy to iodine or history of allergy to contrast material

➤ Jaundice with bilirubin of greater than 2 mg/dL

➤ Severe renal or hepatic insufficiency

➤ Severe vomiting, diarrhea, or conditions that affect absorption of the dye

---

➤➤ Nursing Alert

- A client scheduled for barium studies should have oral cholecystography first to prevent interference from possible residual barium.
- Clients who are scheduled for studies such as thyroid procedures that involve the measurement of iodinated compounds should have oral cholecystography after these tests.
- Inadequate fluid intake before the study can lead to impaired renal function and excretion of the dye.
- Assessment and observations for allergic reactions to iodinated contrast medium should be made on all clients (see Table 17–1, p. 588).

Nursing Care Before the Procedure

Explain to the client:

➤ That the procedure requires about 1 hour but that additional films can be taken 30 to 60 minutes after a high-fat meal

➤ That a low-fat diet is to be eaten the evening before the procedure and foods and fluids withheld after midnight
➤ That the contrast material is ingested 2 hours after the evening meal, with six tablets taken with a full glass of water, one at a time, every 5 minutes[77]
➤ That fluid intake should be increased during the evening before midnight
➤ That the tablets can cause vomiting, diarrhea, abdominal cramping, and epigastric pain and that any of these conditions should be reported immediately, as they can cause postponement of the study
➤ That any symptoms such as palpitations, difficult breathing, or other complaints after ingestion of the tablets should be reported immediately
➤ That no pain is associated with the procedure

Prepare for the procedure:

➤ Obtain a history to ascertain the date of the last menstrual period and possible pregnancy, allergy to iodine, known or suspected gallbladder or liver disorders, treatment regimen, associated diagnostic tests and procedures that include a serum bilirubin for levels greater than 2 mg/dL.
➤ Ensure that the dietary requirements have been followed and that fluid intake has been sufficient.
➤ Ensure that the full dose of contrast material has been ingested and retained; that is, no vomiting or diarrhea has been experienced to indicate that the dose is not adequate for the study to be performed.
➤ Administer an ordered suppository or enema to clear the gastrointestinal tract of solid material, even if a laxative was taken the evening before the study.

The Procedure

The client is placed on the x-ray table in the supine position. A sequence of films of the URQ of the abdomen is taken in prone, left side-lying, and standing positions. The client can be given a high-fat meal or a fatty substance to stimulate contraction and emptying of the gallbladder. The response of the gallbladder to the fat stimulus is evaluated by fluoroscopy. Additional plain films are also taken to evaluate emptying of the gallbladder and movement of the dye through the common bile duct.

Nursing Care After the Procedure

➤ Care and assessment after the procedure include monitoring for adequate fluid intake and urinary output and allergic response to the dye.
➤ Encourage extra fluid intake in clients with an ostomy if bowel output increases as a result of the laxative or enema effect of the dye.[78]
➤ Instruct the client to resume a normal diet if the study has been concluded.
➤ Also, inform the client that the dye is excreted through the kidneys but that the urine does not change color.
➤ *Reaction to iodinated contrast medium:* Note and report anxiety, tachycardia, hyperpnea, or palpitations. Administer ordered antihistamines and steroids. Provide oxygen and initiate resuscitation, if needed (see Table 17–1, p. 588).
➤ *Fluid-electrolyte imbalance:* Note and report excessive vomiting, diarrhea, and signs and symptoms of dehydration such as decreased urinary output; hot, dry skin; and poor skin turgor. Increase fluid intake orally or initiate IV fluid replacement as ordered. Monitor electrolytes.

Intravenous Cholangiography (IVC)

The intravenous cholangiogram (IVC) allows visualization of the biliary ducts. It is performed if the gallbladder is not visualized on an oral cholecystogram (OCG), if the client cannot tolerate or is unable to absorb the oral preparation for OCG, or if symptoms persist after cholecystectomy. For this study, the iodinated contrast medium iodipamide (Cholografin) is administered IV. A combination of plain and tomographic films are taken 15 minutes after the injection and periodically for up to 8 hours. The dye aids in the visualization of the hepatic and common bile ducts for stones, strictures, or tumors.[79]

Reference Values

Normal hepatic and common bile ducts; no stones, strictures, or tumors

Interfering Factors

➤ Inability of client to maintain positions required for the procedure
➤ Barium or feces in the gastrointestinal tract
➤ Failure to refrain from eating or drinking 8 to 12 hours before the procedure
➤ Jaundice with a bilirubin level of greater than 2 mg/dL[80]
➤ Metal objects within the x-ray field

Indications for Intravenous Cholangiography (IVC)

➤ Failure to visualize the gallbladder with oral cholecystography (OCG)
➤ Inability of client to tolerate the oral preparation or its absorption in the gastrointestinal tract with OCG
➤ Persistence of symptoms after cholecystectomy
➤ Evaluation of the hepatic and bile ducts for patency, which can be affected by the presence of stones, tumor, or stricture

Contraindications

➤ Pregnancy, unless benefits of performing the procedure greatly outweigh the risks to the fetus
➤ Allergy to iodine or history of allergy to contrast material
➤ Severe renal or hepatic insufficiency
➤ Jaundice with a bilirubin level of greater than 2 mg/dL

➤➤ Nursing Alert

• A client scheduled for gastrointestinal studies that use barium should have the IVC first to prevent interference in imaging caused by residual barium in the tract.
• A client scheduled for studies involving the measurement of iodinated compounds as in thyroid tests should have the IVC study performed after such tests.
• Inadequate fluid intake before the study can lead to impaired renal excretion of the dye and can adversely affect renal function.
• Assessment and observation for allergic reactions to iodinated contrast medium should be made on all clients (see Table 17–1, p. 588).

Nursing Care Before the Procedure

Client teaching and physical preparation are the same as for OCG (see p. 618).

➤ Inform the client that the dye is administered IV instead of orally and that the study can take up to 4 hours.

➤ Advise the client that a sensation of warmth and nausea can be experienced and, although temporary, it should be reported to the physician.

➤ Initiate an IV line if ordered for administration of the contrast medium.

➤ Administer an ordered antihistamine or steroid before the study, as toxic reaction to the dye is more likely in this procedure than in OCG.[81]

The Procedure

The client is placed on the x-ray table in a supine position and a plain abdominal film of the URQ is taken. The IV line is initiated, if not already in place, and the iodinated contrast material is administered over a 30-minute period. This time allows the dye to be excreted into the bile ducts by the liver. Films are taken every 15 to 30 minutes in the prone, side-lying, and erect positions. When the gallbladder is filled with dye, usually in 2 to 4 hours, additional films are taken of the gallbladder biliary system. Filming can continue at intervals until the common bile duct is visualized. Tomographic evaluation can be performed after visualization of the ducts.[82]

Nursing Care After the Procedure

Care and assessment after the procedure are the same as for OCG (see p. 619).

➤ Assess the venipuncture site for inflammation and bruising.

➤ Inform the client that some discomfort during urination can be experienced as the dye is excreted.

➤ Monitor for a delayed reaction to the dye for 24 hours and remind the client to report nausea.

➤ *Phlebitis at injection site:* Note and report pain, swelling, and redness at the site. Elevate and position arm on a pillow. Apply warm compress.

➤ *Inflammation of bile duct:* Note and report chills, fever, and abdominal pain. Administer ordered antipyretic and antibiotic therapy. Monitor temperature and vital signs.

T-TUBE CHOLANGIOGRAPHY

The T-tube cholangiogram is performed approximately 7 to 10 days after gallbladder surgery to assess the patency of the common bile duct and to detect any remaining stones. It can, however, be performed during surgery after placement of the tube to ensure that all stones have been removed. For this study, an iodinated contrast medium such as diatrizoate meglumine-diatrizoate sodium (Hypaque) is injected directly into the T-tube, followed by x-ray and fluoroscopic examination.[83] T-tubes are placed during surgical exploration of the common bile duct (Fig. 17–7). The end of the T-tube exits from the abdomen

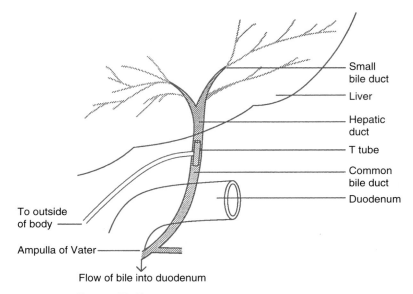

Figure 17−7   Placement of T tube in common bile duct.

through a stab wound and is connected to gravity drainage. T-tube cholangiograms are performed before removal of such tubes if no stones are visualized and bile is flowing freely into the duodenum.

Reference Values

Normal biliary ducts; no stones, strictures, fistula, or neoplasms

Interfering Factors

➤ Barium in the gastrointestinal tract
➤ Failure to follow dietary restrictions before the procedure
➤ Air injected into the biliary tract

Indications for T-Tube Cholangiography

➤ Evaluation of biliary duct patency before T-tube removal
➤ Detection of stones remaining in the biliary tract after gallbladder surgery
➤ Detection of fistula caused by surgical injury to the duct
➤ Detection of strictures and neoplasms of the biliary tract

Contraindications

➤ Pregnancy, unless benefits of performing the procedure greatly outweigh the risks to the fetus
➤ Allergy to iodine or history of allergy to contrast medium
➤ Postoperative wound sepsis

>> Nursing Alert

- A client scheduled for barium studies should have T-tube cholangiography first to prevent any interference in visualization.
- A client scheduled for studies such as thyroid studies to measure iodinated compounds should have T-tube cholangiography after these procedures.
- Assessment and observation for allergic reactions to iodinated contrast media should be made on all clients (see Table 17–1, p. 588).

Nursing Care Before the Procedure

Client teaching and physical preparation are the same as for IVC (see p. 621).
- Inform the client that the dye is injected into the T-tube, that the tube is clamped before the filming, and that it remains clamped during the study.
- Bowel preparation may not be included before this study.

The Procedure

The T-tube is clamped the day before the scheduled study. The client is placed on the x-ray table in a supine position and the area around the T-tube draped for privacy concerns. The end of the T-tube is cleansed with an antiseptic and held straight in a vertical position. A needle that is attached to a tube is inserted into the open end of the T-tube and the clamp is removed. The contrast material is injected into the T-tube, and fluoroscopy is performed to visualize the dye moving through the duct system. Inform the client that a feeling of slight pressure or fullness can be experienced as the dye is injected, and instruct the client to report any sensations of warmth and nausea after the dye is injected. The tube is clamped and films are taken of the URQ in different positions, such as prone, side-lying, and erect. An additional film can be taken 15 minutes later to visualize the passage of the contrast medium into the duodenum.[84]

The procedure is performed as early as 8 hours or as late as 7 to 10 days after cholecystectomy to determine whether the duct is patent and whether the T-tube should be removed or left in place. The total procedure is usually completed within 30 minutes, depending on biliary tree visualization.

Nursing Care After the Procedure

Care and assessment after the procedure are the same as for IVC (see p. 621).
- Monitor the T-tube insertion site for pain, swelling, or redness. If the tube is left in place, apply a skin protector ointment and sterile dressing taped in place around the T-tube.
- Unclamp the tube and attach to a sterile closed drainage system.

OPERATIVE CHOLANGIOGRAPHY

The operative cholangiogram is performed during gallbladder surgery to visualize the biliary ducts and assess for the presence of gallstones, strictures, or tumors that can affect the patency of these structures.[85] For this study, an iodinated contrast medium, usually diatrizoate meglumine-diatrizoate sodium, is injected directly into the cystic or common bile duct with a needle or catheter. It allows the surgeon to view the ducts by x-ray examination to correct abnormalities and ensure that no injury to the ducts has occurred before the surgical procedure has been completed.

Reference Values

Normal biliary tract; no stones, strictures, or tumor to obstruct flow of bile

Interfering Factors

➤ Instruments or other metal objects within the x-ray field

Indications for Operative Cholangiography

➤ Evaluation of biliary ducts for anatomic abnormalities such as tumors, strictures, or stones that prevent flow of bile during the cholecystectomy surgery
➤ Detection of stones in the cystic duct during surgery[86]
➤ Detection of trauma to the bile duct during exploration at the time of surgery
➤ Suspected pancreatitis
➤ Presence of jaundice and increase in hepatic enzymes

Contraindications

➤ Allergy to iodine or history of allergy to contrast medium

Nursing Care Before the Procedure

There are no client teaching and physical preparations other than those already carried out for the cholecystectomy because the procedure is performed during surgery.

The Procedure

During the cholecystectomy procedure, the common bile and cystic ducts are explored. A catheter is inserted into the common bile duct and the dye injected into the catheter. X-rays are taken, developed immediately, and viewed by the surgeon for the presence of abnormal structure, obstructive lesions, or stones in the ducts. Exploration of the ducts can be performed, based on the findings of stones in the ducts and stone removal to ensure patency for normal flow of bile into the duodenum.

Nursing Care After the Procedure

Care and assessment after the procedure include routine postoperative care.
➤ Monitor the client for delayed adverse effects of the contrast medium and for signs and symptoms of an infectious process caused by injection of the material into the ducts.

PERCUTANEOUS TRANSHEPATIC CHOLANGIOGRAPHY (PTHC)

The percutaneous transhepatic cholangiogram (PTHC) allows visualization of the intrahepatic, extrahepatic, and biliary ducts, as well as the gallbladder, to determine obstruction to biliary flow caused by stones, tumor, stricture, congen-

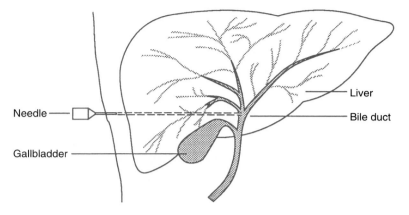

Figure 17–8 Placement of needle in the bile duct in the liver.

ital anomalies, or anatomic abnormalities.[87] It is most commonly performed on clients with jaundice to determine whether or not the cause can be attributed to obstruction of the ducts. For this study, the iodinated contrast medium is administered through a long, fine needle inserted into the liver and, with the aid of fluoroscopy, into a bile duct (Fig. 17–8). Fluoroscopic examination of the ducts is made and spot films taken in various positions.

Reference Values

Normal biliary ducts; no obstruction or deviation of the common bile duct; no anatomic abnormalities or dilated ducts

Interfering Factors

➤ Inability of client to remain still and maintain the position required to perform puncture
➤ Barium in the gastrointestinal tract
➤ Obesity
➤ Failure to follow dietary restrictions before the procedure
➤ Metal objects within the field

Indications for Percutaneous Transhepatic Cholangiography (PTHC)

➤ Evaluation of URQ after cholecystectomy
➤ Differentiation between obstructive and nonobstructive cause of jaundice
➤ Determination of the cause of obstruction of the ducts, such as stones, tumor, cysts, or strictures and whether the obstruction is partial or complete
➤ Diagnosis of biliary sclerosis or sclerosing cholangitis
➤ Determination of congenital or anatomic abnormalities of the ducts that can be the cause of an obstruction
➤ Determination of biliary duct abnormalities in clients with previous gastrointestinal surgery that results in endoscopic inaccessibility
➤ Performing liver biopsy, if ducts are patent, when hepatitis or cirrhosis of the liver is suspected as the cause of jaundice

Contraindications

➤ Pregnancy, unless benefits of performing the procedure greatly outweigh the risks to the fetus

➤ Client unable to cooperate

➤ Allergy to iodine or history of allergy to iodinated contrast material

➤ Severe ascites, cholangitis

➤ Uncontrolled coagulopathy with prolonged clotting time, prothrombin time (PT), and abnormal coagulation factors panel

---

➤➤ Nursing Alert

• Assess and observe for intra-abdominal bleeding or bile leakage as a result of accidental puncture of a large vessel. Symptoms include abdominal pain, distention, and rigidity associated with peritonitis; hypotension; rapid, thready pulse; and cold, clammy skin associated with hypovolemic shock.[88]

Nursing Care Before the Procedure

Client teaching and physical preparation are the same as for oral cholecystography (see p. 618).

➤ Advise the client that the study takes 30 minutes to 1 hour.

➤ Inform the client that the site is anesthetized by a local injection and that some pain is experienced when the liver is punctured.

➤ Include the results of a complete blood count (CBC), clotting time, PT or partial thromboplastin time (PTT), and blood typing and cross-matching in the preprocedure history and assessment.

➤ Advise the client to refrain from using any aspirin products.

➤ Administer ordered vitamin K based on an increased PT.

➤ Administer an ordered antibiotic and antihistamine to prevent infection and reaction to the contrast medium. Administer an ordered intramuscular (IM) sedative and analgesic such as diazepam (Valium) or meperidine (Demerol) for anxiety and pain control.

The Procedure

The client is placed on the x-ray table in a supine position with straps in place to prevent falling when the table is tilted. The right upper abdomen is exposed and the skin cleansed with an antiseptic solution. The area is draped and the insertion site injected with a local anesthetic, usually lidocaine. The insertion site is chosen between the eighth and ninth intercostal space at the midaxillary line to avoid lung puncture and to place the needle near the hilus of the liver. An IV line is initiated at this time and a sedative administered with care so that the client is not oversedated and is able to cooperate when needed. A long, fine (21-gauge, 20-cm) needle is inserted at the site and advanced in a smooth motion into the liver under fluoroscopic guidance. The client is requested to hold the breath during insertion of the needle. When the needle attains its desired position in the bile duct, the stylet is removed and a syringe and tubing are connected to the needle hub. Placement in a duct is evidenced by the flow of bile, and the dye is injected. The client is informed that a sensation of fullness or pressure can be felt. Any nausea, flushing, or sweating after dye injection should be reported to the physician immediately. The contrast material fills the branching tubular structures as noted with the fluoroscopic procedure. Biliary pressure can be measured at this time. To reduce the risk of septicemia, only enough contrast material should be injected to enable proper viewing and diagnosis.[89] Spot films are taken and the table tilted for a side-lying and an erect view for further filming. The needle is then removed and a sterile dressing taped in place over the puncture site. A catheter can be left in the biliary tract if an obstruction is discovered so that the tract can be drained and decompressed.[90]

Nursing Care After the Procedure

➤ Have the client rest for 6 hours in a right side-lying position to relieve pressure on the injection site.

➤ Inform the client that some pain can be experienced in the abdomen and right shoulder.

➤ Monitor vital signs until stable and compare with baseline readings and monitor for changes indicating intra-abdominal bleeding.

➤ Assess for possible peritonitis caused by bile leaking into the abdominal cavity.

➤ If a catheter is placed in the tract, attach to a sterile closed drainage system.

➤ Assess site for swelling, pain, and drainage because some bleeding and drainage usually occur.

➤ Resume food intake in 5 to 8 hours if condition remains stable and no complications have developed.

➤ Administer an ordered mild analgesic if it will not mask more serious signs and symptoms of infection.

➤ *Reaction to iodinated contrast medium:* Note and report anxiety, feeling of warmth or flushing, itching, urticaria, sweating, nausea or vomiting, tachycardia, or hyperpnea. Administer ordered antihistamine or steroid. Initiate resuscitation procedure as needed.

➤ *Peritonitis and septicemia:* Note and report temperature elevation, chills, and abdominal pain, distention, and rigidity. Administer ordered antipyretics and antibiotics. Initiate IV line. Monitor vital signs. Prepare for surgery if needed.

➤ *Intra-abdominal hemorrhage:* Note and report hypotension; rapid, thready pulse; cold, clammy skin; abdominal distention. Obtain CBC and typing and cross-matching. Administer blood transfusion. Prepare for surgery if needed.

ANTEGRADE PYELOGRAPHY

The antegrade pyelogram allows visualization of the kidney's collecting system. It is performed if the kidneys are unable to excrete dye administered for intravenous pyelography (IVP), if ureteral obstruction is present, or if a cystoscopy procedure is contraindicated.[91] For this study, a fine percutaneous needle is inserted into the renal pelvis and the iodinated contrast medium, diatrizoate sodium-diatrizoate meglumine (Renografin), is injected through a tubing connected to the needle. Placement of the needle and injection of the contrast material are accomplished under the guidance of fluoroscopy or ultrasonography. The pressure within the kidney can be measured via a manometer connected to the tubing, and a collection of urine for cytologic examination can be obtained during the procedure.

Reference Values

Normal outline of the urinary collecting system; normal size and position of the ureters and urinary bladder

Interfering Factors

➤ Inability of client to remain still and maintain position required for the procedure
➤ Failure to restrict foods or to drink fluids to dilate the collecting system before the procedure
➤ Metal objects within the x-ray field

Indications for Antegrade Pyelography

➤ Evaluating the kidneys and ureters for obstruction and degree of resulting dilatation
➤ Detecting the cause of an obstruction such as tumor, stone, or stricture
➤ Determining the patency of the upper collecting system when an obstruction prevents a retrograde ureteropyelography from being performed or when it has been unsuccessfully performed
➤ Examining the upper collecting system to evaluate an obstruction in a ureter when a cystoscopy is contraindicated
➤ Determining ureteral obstruction after a surgical urinary diversion procedure or other ureteral surgery
➤ Evaluating hydronephrosis in children, caused by ureteral anomaly or abnormality at the junction of the ureter with the kidney
➤ Placement of a nephrostomy tube for drainage
➤ Measuring intrarenal pressure for increases indicating obstruction

Contraindications

➤ Pregnancy, unless benefits of performing the procedure greatly outweigh the risks to the fetus
➤ Inability of client to cooperate during the procedure
➤ Allergy to iodine or history of allergy to contrast medium
➤ Obesity that prevents needle placement
➤ Uncontrolled coagulopathy with prolonged clotting time, PT, PTT, and abnormal coagulation factors panel

➤➤ Nursing Alert

• Assess and observe for accidental puncture of adjacent organs, leading to pneumothorax or extravasation of the contrast medium into the surrounding area.

Nursing Care Before the Procedure

Client teaching and physical preparation are the same as for percutaneous trans-hepatic cholangiography (PTHC) (see p. 626).

➤ Inform the client that the procedure takes 1 hour.

➤ The history and assessment should include the results of blood urea nitrogen (BUN) and creatinine.

➤ Advise the client of fluid intake before the study, according to agency and physician preference.

The Procedure

The client is placed on the x-ray table in a prone position and the injection site is exposed and draped. The skin is cleansed with an antiseptic solution and injected with a local anesthetic, usually lidocaine. The client is informed that some pain is experienced when the local anesthetic is injected. The client is requested to hold the breath. While fluoroscopy or ultrasonography is being used, a 21-gauge percutaneous needle is inserted at the level of the second lumbar vertebra below the ribs in the direction of the kidney. A smaller needle with a stylet is then advanced through the needle and into the renal midpelvis. Flexible tubing is attached to the needle and a syringe is attached to the tubing to aspirate urine from the kidney.[92] A urine specimen can be obtained and a manometer can be connected to the tubing at this time to measure intrarenal pressure as an indication of obstruction. The dye is then injected via the needle after the urine has been aspirated to prevent overdistention of the pelvis. Inform the client to report any nausea, flushing, or sweating when the dye is injected. Several views are taken, including PA, AP, and oblique. After the injection of the dye, which fills the collecting system, fluoroscopy can reveal ureteral peristalsis and the point of obstruction as the contrast material outlines the organs. If a nephrostomy tube is to be inserted, it takes place at this time to treat renal dilatation caused by intrarenal reflux that leads to nephrosis.[93] The tube is self-retaining and provides continuous drainage of the renal pelvis. The needle is then removed and a sterile dressing applied over the puncture site or nephrostomy tube and taped in place.

Nursing Care After the Procedure

➤ Place the client at rest in a position of comfort, preferably avoiding the side on which the injection was performed.

➤ Monitor vital signs and compare with baseline readings until the client is stable, paying special attention to indications of bleeding.

➤ Assess the site for bleeding and leakage of urine.

➤ Monitor intake and output (I&O) for the first 24 hours for hematuria.

➤ Inform the client to increase fluid intake to 2000 to 3000 mL per day, unless contraindicated.

➤ If a nephrostomy tube is in place, monitor for patency, gravity drainage, and drainage characteristics.

➤ Administer a mild analgesic for any discomfort and antibiotic therapy, if ordered, to prevent infection.

➤ *Reaction to iodinated contrast medium:* Note and report anxiety, warmth or flushing, itching, urticaria, sweating, nausea, or vomiting. Administer ordered antihistamines or steroids. Initiate resuscitation procedure as needed.

➤ *Hemorrhage:* Note and report flank pain, hypotension, or rapid pulse. Administer blood transfusion, if ordered. Prepare for surgery to correct problem.

➤ *Septicemia:* Note and report elevated temperature, chills, and vital sign changes. Administer ordered antipyretic and antibiotic therapy.

➤ *Puncture of organs:* Note and report respiratory changes for possible pneumothorax; note abdominal or flank pain. Administer ordered medications. Assist with chest tube insertion. Prepare for surgery to correct organ damage.

RETROGRADE URETHROGRAPHY

A retrograde urethrogram allows visualization of the male urethral membranous, bulbar, and penile areas or of the female urethra, if diverticula are suspected. It is most commonly performed on men postoperatively to evaluate urethral repair and to assist in the diagnosis of urethral abnormalities and congenital anomalies. For this study, the iodinated contrast medium is instilled into a catheter and inserted into the meatus. Films are made while a portion is injected and again while the remaining portion is instilled. A combination of films and fluoroscopy can be performed to visualize possible trauma to the urethra.[94]

Reference Values

Normal size and shape of the urethra; no deviations or diverticula, fistula, stones, or strictures

Interfering Factors

➤ None

Indications for Retrograde Urethrography

➤ Evaluation of the urethra in male children for congenital anomalies such as hypospadias, inappropriate passages
➤ Detection of stones, urethral stricture, or meatal stenosis causing obstruction
➤ Detection of lesions, lacerations, diverticula, or fistula of the urethra
➤ Evaluation of the male urethra for obstruction at the neck of the bladder caused by hypertrophy of the prostate gland
➤ Preparation for balloon dilatation of the prostatic urethra
➤ Suspected urethral diverticula in females
➤ Determination of the status of the male urethra after surgical correction or repair

Contraindications

➤ Inability of client to assume and maintain the position to perform the procedure
➤ Urinary tract infection (UTI) unless the study is performed with caution
➤ Extensive injury or trauma to the urethra

Nursing Care Before the Procedure

Explain to the client:
➤ That there are no food or fluid restrictions
➤ That a sedative can be administered before the study to promote relaxation
➤ That a catheter will be inserted to administer the contrast medium and that moderate discomfort will be experienced when the material is injected

Prepare for the procedure:
➤ Obtain a history to ascertain the date of the last menstrual period and the possibility of pregnancy, allergy to iodine, known or suspected urinary disorders, and results of associated tests and procedures.
➤ Administer a sedative or analgesic, or both, such as meperidine IM or subcutaneously (SC) 30 minutes before the study to promote comfort and relaxation.
➤ Have client void.

The Procedure

The client is placed on the x-ray table in a supine position, and an AP film is taken to view for stones in the bladder or urethra. The client is draped for privacy with the genitalia exposed. The meatus is cleansed with an antiseptic solution. After the catheter is filled with the contrast medium, the tip is moistened with water and inserted until the balloon part of the catheter is within the urethra just past the meatus. The balloon is then inflated with water and the client placed in a right oblique posterior position. The right leg is flexed at a right angle and, if the client is male, the penis is positioned on the right thigh with the left leg straight. Contrast material is injected into the catheter and a spot film is taken. Additional films are taken while the remaining material is injected into the catheter. If the client is female, a double balloon catheter is used to anchor the catheter above and below the meatus. Fluoroscopic examination can be performed to reveal trauma to the urethra. On completion of the films, the water is removed from the balloon and the catheter is removed.

Nursing Care After the Procedure

Monitor vital signs and compare with baselines until stable.
➤ Monitor I&O for at least 24 hours, with special attention given to the first voiding and urine characteristics.
➤ Assess for suprapubic pain or absence of urination. Inform the client to increase fluid intake to promote hydration, to remove the dye from the urethra, and to prevent dysuria.

RETROGRADE CYSTOGRAPHY

A retrograde cystogram is performed to visualize and evaluate possible rupture and pathology of the urinary bladder. Air or an iodinated contrast medium is instilled into the bladder via a catheter, the catheter is clamped, and several views are taken, depending on the extent of the examination needed and the client's condition. Filming the bladder and urethra after the catheter is unclamped and during emptying is known as a voiding cystourethrogram.[95]

Reference Values

Normal size, shape, and structure of the urinary bladder; no tumor, fistula, diverticula, or perforation of the bladder

Interfering Factors

➤ Barium, feces, or gas in the LGI tract

Indications for Retrograde Cystography

➤ Examination of the bladder when excretory urography has not provided adequate visualization of the bladder or when cystoscopy is contraindicated
➤ Suspected neurogenic bladder, that is, hypotonic or hypertonic bladder
➤ Suspected primary pathology of the bladder including tumor, fistula, or diverticula[96]
➤ Abnormal bladder function and filling defects caused by vesicoureteral reflux and revealed by backflow of dye into the ureters from the bladder
➤ Determination of rupture or perforated bladder revealed by extravasation of the contrast medium
➤ Persistent, recurrent UTIs in children

Contraindications

➤ Acute UTI
➤ Injury to the bladder or urethra
➤ Obstruction of the urethra or other urethral abnormalities affecting the insertion of the catheter into the bladder

Nursing Care Before the Procedure

Client teaching and physical preparation are the same as for retrograde urethrography (see p. 631).
➤ Inform the client that clear liquids are allowed, depending on agency and physician preference.
➤ Insert a Foley catheter, if one has been ordered.

The Procedure

The client is placed on the x-ray table in a supine position and an abdominal flat plate (KUB) film is taken to determine whether stones or calcifications are present in the urinary tract or whether barium or gas is present in the gastrointestinal tract. These substances can interfere with visualization. The client is draped with the genitalia exposed. A Foley catheter is inserted, and urine is drained until the bladder is completely empty. About 300 mL (less for an infant or child) of the contrast medium is instilled into the bladder via the catheter by gravity or a little pressure. Instruct the client to report any nausea, flushing, or sweating when the dye is injected. The catheter is then clamped and an AP view is taken. Additional oblique and lateral views are taken after position changes of the client. A protective shield is placed over the male testes to prevent irradiation; a shield over a woman's abdomen would interfere with visualization of the bladder.[97] A PA view can also be taken if the client is able to assume the jack-knife position. To improve visualization, it is possible for air to be injected into the bladder after removal of the dye. This procedure is known as the double-contrast study. After the filming, the dye is drained from the bladder and the catheter is removed if the client is able to void.

Nursing Care After the Procedure

Care and assessment after the procedure are the same as for retrograde ure-thrography (see p. 631).

➤ Monitor urinary characteristics and pattern and instruct the client to report persistent hematuria caused by the trauma of the procedure or UTI.

➤ If the catheter is left in place, attach to a sterile closed drainage system.

➤ *Reaction to iodinated contrast medium:* Note and report anxiety, warmth, flushing, itching, urticaria, sweating, nausea, or vomiting. Administer ordered antihistamines or steroids. Initiate resuscitation procedure as needed.

➤ *UTI:* Note and report dysuria, urgency, frequency, or cloudy and foul-smelling urine. Administer ordered antimicrobial therapy. Obtain urine specimen for culture and sensitivity (C&S).

RETROGRADE URETEROPYELOGRAPHY

The retrograde ureteropyelogram, also known as a retrograde pyelogram, involves the x-ray filming of the ureters and the renal collecting system. It is used when an IVP does not provide satisfactory visualization of the kidneys or when previous IVP findings must be confirmed.[98] Because the dye is not readily absorbed by the ureters, this study is preferred in clients who are allergic to an iodinated contrast medium when administered IV, as in the IVP. The contrast medium diatrizoate sodium is injected via ureteral catheters inserted by cystoscopy. Various views are filmed with the catheters in place and during and after their removal.

Reference Values

Normal size and shape of the ureters and kidneys; no stones, tumor, strictures, or other abnormalities causing actual or risk of obstruction

Interfering Factors

➤ Barium, feces, or gas in the gastrointestinal tract

Indications for Retrograde Ureteropyelography

➤ Determining presence and location of a stone in the ureter or kidney when this condition has not been established with other diagnostic studies

➤ Diagnosing renal conditions such as impaired renal function or decreased kidney perfusion resulting from vascular disorders or congenital anomaly that could not be identified by excretory urography (IVP)

➤ Determining tumors, strictures, scarring, and compression against the ureter with displacement, causing partial or complete obstruction[99]

➤ Determining whether kidney disease, especially in cases with one kidney involved, is caused by ureteral obstruction

Contraindications

➤ Allergy to the contrast medium (Very little is absorbed through the mucous membranes of the ureter, however.)

➤ Pregnancy, unless benefits of performing the procedure greatly outweigh the risks to the fetus

Nursing Care Before the Procedure

Client teaching and physical preparation are generally the same as for retrograde urethrography (see p. 631).

➤ Inform the client that the procedure takes 60 to 90 minutes and involves the insertion of an instrument into the bladder, which causes some discomfort.

➤ Foods and fluid are restricted for 8 to 12 hours before the study if general anesthesia is used, but a clear liquid diet can be given the morning of the study if a local anesthetic is used.

➤ A laxative, suppository, or enema, or a combination of these measures, should be administered the evening before the study.

➤ Initiate an IV line and administer IM or SC meperidine for relaxation and comfort and atropine sulfate to reduce secretions 1 hour before the study, if ordered.

➤ Kidney function laboratory tests (BUN, creatinine) should be assessed for levels indicating renal impairment.

The Procedure

The client is placed on the x-ray table in the lithotomy position with the legs and feet in stirrups and a drape for privacy concerns. General anesthesia is administered or local anesthetic is inserted into the urethra in the form of a jelly. Oral or IV medications to promote relaxation and comfort can be administered with the local anesthetic. A cystoscope is inserted into the bladder and the organ visualized to observe the size, shape, and presence of abnormalities such as tumor, lesions, or stones. This step is followed by the insertion of opaque catheters through the cystoscope and into the ureters up to the level of the pelves of the kidneys. Placement is verified by x-ray of the opaque catheters. The urine is drained from the kidneys and a small amount of the dye is injected through the ureteral catheters. Instruct the client to report any nausea, flushing, or sweating after the dye is injected. An AP film is taken and an additional amount of dye is injected and lateral and oblique views taken. Films of the ureters are taken while the catheters are withdrawn and small amounts of dye are injected. In some instances, delayed filming is performed 10 to 15 minutes after complete removal of the catheters to determine urinary retention.[100] At the conclusion, the catheters can be left in place and allowed to drain to ensure the return of urinary flow. Otherwise, they are removed.

Nursing Care After the Procedure

Care and assessment after the procedure are the same as for retrograde urethrography (see p. 631).

➤ If the catheters are left in place, connect to a sterile closed drainage system and establish flow by gravity.

➤ Anchor and protect the catheters to prevent backflow and dislodgement.

➤ Assess the catheters for patency and drainage characteristics (pink-tinged color is not unusual because of instrumentation) as well as the first urination if catheters are not in place.

➤ Inform the client to report absence of urination, bright red blood, or clots in the urine.

➤ *UTI:* Note and report dysuria; urgency; frequency; or cloudy, foul-smelling urine. Administer ordered antimicrobial therapy. Obtain urine specimen for C&S.

INTRAVENOUS PYELOGRAM (IVP)

The intravenous pyelogram (IVP), also known as the excretory urogram (EUG), is most frequently performed to evaluate the calyces and pelves of the kidneys, ureters, and urinary bladder when abnormalities of these organs are suspected.[101] An abdominal flat plate (KUB) film is taken, an iodinated contrast medium such as diatrizoate sodium or diatrizoate meglumine is injected, and then serial filming is performed. The study can include a nephrogram as the material concentrates in the renal tubules. Serial nephrotomography can also be performed to delineate kidneys for mass thickness without interference from surrounding tissues.

Reference Values

Normal structure, size, and shape of the kidneys, ureters, and bladder; no tumor, mucosal abnormalities, or impaired renal function

Interfering Factors

➤ Barium, feces, or gas in the gastrointestinal tract
➤ Impaired renal function causing inability of the kidneys to excrete the dye

Indications for Intravenous Pyelogram (IVP)

➤ Suspected diseases or abnormalities of the kidneys, ureters, or bladder as a result of structural defects or tumors
➤ Determination of tumors, stones, or strictures causing partial or complete obstruction[102]
➤ Determination of glomerular disorders revealed by the rate of dye excretion
➤ Diagnosis of renal artery obstruction as shown by the failure of the dye to reach a kidney and the resultant inability to visualize the urinary system
➤ Determination of changes in the size, shape, and position of the kidneys, caused by pathology
➤ Determination of the results of trauma on the urinary organs, such as hematoma or lacerations
➤ Diagnosis of congenital abnormalities such as absence of one kidney, abnormal connection of the two kidneys in the shape of a horseshoe, displaced kidneys in the abdomen, or double ureters[103]
➤ Suspected urinary residual in the bladder
➤ Determination of the cause of renal hypertrophy, such as hydronephrosis or polycystic kidney disease

Contraindications

➤ Allergy to iodine or iodinated contrast media (Antihistamine and steroid therapy should be administered in this case.)
➤ Actual or potential dehydration, especially in children or elderly clients
➤ Abnormal renal function with increases in creatinine and BUN level greater than 40 mg/dL

Nursing Care Before the Procedure

Client teaching and physical preparation are the same as for retrograde ureteropyelography (see p. 631).

➤ Assess laboratory tests and report BUN levels of greater than 40 mg/dL.

➤ Provide bowel preparation according to institution and physician requirements.

➤ Although food is restricted, allow clear fluids the morning of the study.

The Procedure

The client is placed on the x-ray table in a supine position and draped for privacy. An abdominal flat plate (KUB) film is taken to determine the presence of stones, feces, gas, or barium, which can interfere with visualization. An IV line is initiated and the dye is injected; the amount of dye depends on the age of the client. Have the client report any nausea, flushing, or sweating after injection of the dye. While the client remains in the same position, films are taken at intervals of 1, 5, 10, 15, 20, and 30 minutes or as long as it takes the contrast medium to reach the bladder. Within 5 minutes the material concentrates in the renal tubules and a nephrogram can be obtained.[104] After the filming, the client is requested to void and another film is taken to visualize the bladder and determine whether residual urine is present. If filming of the ureters is desired, a rubber bladder is placed around the abdomen and inflated to trap the contrast medium in the upper ureters, and an x-ray is taken. The tube is then deflated and the filming of the lower ureters and bladder continues.

Nephrotomography can be performed as an adjunct to the IVP for better visualization of tumors or occupying lesions. It requires additional films that delineate layers or slices of the kidneys for mass thickness without interference in the views from the surrounding tissue. Serial tomograms are made 10 minutes after the injection of the contrast medium as the x-ray tube and film cassette move in opposite directions.[105,106] This study can be made without IVP after the same procedure.

Nursing Care After the Procedure

Care and assessment are the same as for retrograde urethrography (see p. 631).

➤ Continue IV fluids or provide oral fluids to promote hydration.

➤ Monitor IV site for hematoma or infiltration, and discontinue or change site, if appropriate.

➤ *Reaction to iodinated contrast medium:* Note and report anxiety, warmth, flushing, itching, urticaria, sweating, nausea, or vomiting. Administer ordered antihistamines or steroids. Initiate resuscitation procedure as needed.

➤ *Renal failure:* Note and report anuria, oliguria, increased BUN and creatinine, and fluid intake. Initiate ordered IV and administer fluids and medications. Prepare for dialysis, if appropriate.

VOIDING CYSTOURETHROGRAPHY

The voiding cystourethrogram is performed to visualize the filling and emptying of the urinary bladder. A catheter is inserted into the bladder and an iodinated contrast medium is instilled. Filming is performed to view the filling process and then during voiding to demonstrate the emptying process. The study can be performed in conjunction with retrograde cystography or as a single procedure.

Reference Values

Normal size, shape, and structure of the urinary bladder; no abnormality in bladder function or emptying

Interfering Factors

➤ Barium, feces, or gas in the LGI tract
➤ Trauma or embarrassment that prevents voiding when requested to do so

Indications for Voiding Cystourethrography

➤ Suspected or known neurogenic bladder (hypotonic or hypertonic bladder) causing incontinence
➤ Determination of vesicoureteral reflux in adults and children (Corrective surgery may be required.)
➤ Determination of strictures, urethral stenosis, diverticula, ureteroceles, prostatic enlargement that interferes with bladder function
➤ Evaluation of abnormal bladder function to determine whether surgery is indicated
➤ Diagnosis of the cause of chronic UTIs
➤ Identification of congenital anomalies in infants

Contraindications

➤ Pregnancy, unless benefits of performing the procedure greatly outweigh the risks to the fetus
➤ Acute urethral or bladder infection
➤ Injury to the bladder or urethra

Nursing Care Before the Procedure

Client teaching and physical preparation are the same as for retrograde cystography (p. 632).

The Procedure

The client is placed on the x-ray table in a supine position and draped for privacy. A Foley catheter is inserted, and the contrast medium is injected into the bladder via the catheter. The catheter can then be clamped and films taken in the supine, lateral, and oblique positions. The catheter is then unclamped and removed. The client is requested to void, and films are taken of the bladder and urethra during voiding. If the client has difficulty voiding, a standing position can be assumed while the films are taken. When this procedure is performed on children, they are anesthetized and urine is expressed from the bladder.[107] A protective shield is placed over the male testes to prevent irradiation. Female clients cannot be shielded without interfering with visualization of the bladder.

Nursing Care After the Procedure

Care and assessment after the procedure are the same as for retrograde cystography (see p. 633).

SIALOGRAPHY

The sialogram involves the x-ray examination of the salivary ducts, that is, sublingual, submaxillary, submandibular, and parotid ducts. Filming follows the injection of an iodinated contrast medium into the duct to be studied. Views are taken with the client in various positions to identify pathology in the ducts.

Reference Values

Normal function of salivary glands and ducts; no stones, strictures, tumors, or other abnormalities

Interfering Factors

➤ Stone in a duct that prevents the dye from entering

Indications for Sialography

➤ Evaluation of persistent pain and edema in the salivary gland areas[108]
➤ Suspected stones, tumors, or strictures that obstruct the salivary ducts
➤ Suspected inflammation of the salivary glands

Contraindications

➤ Mouth infection and inflammatory conditions

Nursing Care Before the Procedure

Client teaching and physical preparation are the same as for any plain x-ray procedure (see p. 590).
➤ Client should brush teeth and rinse mouth with mouthwash.

The Procedure

The client is placed on the x-ray table in a supine position, and a plain x-ray is taken to determine whether a stone is present in the duct. A catheter is inserted into the duct and the dye injected into the catheter. Various views of the duct are filmed. The client is then given a sour drink to encourage salivation. Additional views are taken to film ductal drainage and evaluate function and patency.[109]

Nursing Care After the Procedure

➤ Monitor vital signs and compare with baseline readings.
➤ Encourage fluid intake to assist in elimination of the dye.
➤ Monitor the injection site for pain and swelling, and administer a mild analgesic if ordered.
➤ Provide mouth care for comfort and for reduction of the possibility of infection at the injection site.
➤ *Reaction to iodinated contrast medium:* Note and report feeling of warmth, flushing, urticaria, itching, nausea, or vomiting. Administer ordered antihistamine.

ARTHROGRAPHY

The arthrogram involves a series of x-rays to examine the joint as well as soft tissues surrounding the joint, including the meniscus, cartilage, ligaments, and structures of the joint capsule (rotator cuff, subacromial bursa).[110] The procedure usually follows chronic, persistent, and unexplained pain in a joint. The knee and shoulder are the most common sites for the procedure, but other joints (hip, wrist, ankle) can also be examined by arthrography. Various views are taken of a joint site after it has been anesthetized and injected with a contrast medium.

Reference Values

Normal joint structures including articular cartilage, bursae, meniscus, ligaments, and joint space; no fracture, tears, disruptions, or lesions of the joint

Interfering Factors

➤ Inability of client to cooperate in the procedure
➤ Synovial fluid affecting the concentration of the contrast medium

Indications for Arthrography

➤ Determining the cause of persistent, unexplained knee or shoulder pain
➤ Evaluating and differentiating between acute and chronic conditions of the knee or shoulder
➤ Determining traumatic ligament disorders such as tears and lacerations
➤ Evaluating meniscal tears, lacerations, fractures, and extrameniscal lesions such as osteochondritis or chondromalacia[111]
➤ Evaluating chronic shoulder dislocations and resulting joint damage
➤ Determining abnormalities of the synovial membrane, such as synovitis, tumors, or cysts
➤ Evaluating damage to the cartilage and other joint structures caused by arthritis
➤ Detecting shoulder abnormalities such as rotator cuff tear, capsule derangement, capsulitis, or capsule rupture
➤ Diagnosing conditions of the bursa such as bursitis or tears
➤ Performing surgical procedures on the joint to correct minor conditions

Contraindications

➤ Pregnancy, unless benefits of performing the procedure greatly outweigh the risks to the fetus
➤ Infectious process of the joint
➤ Infectious process of the joint
➤ Acute exacerbation of arthritis

Nursing Care Before the Procedure

Client teaching and physical preparation are the same as for percutaneous transhepatic cholangiography (PTHC) (see p. 626) or for any study involving the insertion of the contrast medium directly into the examination site.

➤ The study takes 30 to 45 minutes, fluid and food are not restricted, and no sedation is administered before the procedure.
➤ The procedure is performed under a local anesthetic injected into the examination site.

The Procedure

The client is placed on the x-ray table in a supine position with the shoulder, knee, or other joint exposed. The site is cleansed with an antiseptic solution and draped for a sterile procedure. A local injection of lidocaine is given to anesthetize the skin. A needle is inserted into the joint space and synovial fluid is aspirated. The fluid can be sent to the laboratory for analysis. The syringe is disconnected and another syringe containing a soluble dye is attached after needle placement has been confirmed by fluoroscopic examination. Gas and water as well as the iodinated dye can also be used as a contrast agent. The dye is instilled and the joint is manipulated as in a range-of-motion exercise or the client is requested to walk to distribute the dye throughout the joint space. The client is informed that discomfort is experienced when the dye is injected and movement of the joint takes place. Films are taken with the joint manipulated into several positions. After the x-ray filming, the knee or other joint is bandaged and wrapped with an elastic bandage.

Nursing Care After the Procedure

➤ Assist the client from the x-ray table and place the joint at rest for at least 12 hours.

➤ Monitor vital signs and compare with baseline readings.

➤ Apply ice to the site and administer an ordered mild analgesic.

➤ Inform the client that a crepitant noise in the joint can last for 1 to 2 days, and instruct to report pain and swelling that does not subside.

➤ Advise the client to minimize weight bearing, to avoid strenuous activities if a knee joint was examined, and to maintain the elastic bandage over the joint until the physician recommends its removal.

➤ *Reaction to iodinated contrast medium:* Note and report warmth, flushing, itching, nausea, or changes in breathing pattern. Administer ordered antihistamines and steroids. Have resuscitation equipment on hand.

BRONCHOGRAPHY

The bronchogram involves x-ray examination to visualize the tracheobronchial tree after injection of an iodinated oil contrast medium via a catheter inserted into the trachea and bronchi.[112] The lining of the tracheobronchial tree becomes coated and films are then taken with the client in various positions. Bronchography has been generally replaced as a diagnostic procedure by bronchoscopy, a study that provides direct visualization of the area. Bronchography can be performed to assist with or in conjunction with bronchoscopy or chest tomography. The major advantage of bronchography is provision of permanent films for future reference.

Reference Values

Normal structure of the tracheobronchial airways; no bronchiectasis, airway obstruction, tumors, cysts, or congenital abnormalities

Interfering Factors

➤ Excessive secretions in the tracheobronchial space

➤ Coughing that prevents coating of the airways with the contrast medium

Indications for Bronchography

➤ Detecting obstructions in the bronchi caused by tumor, cyst, or foreign object
➤ Determining the cause of persistent hemoptysis and recurring pneumonia
➤ Diagnosing bronchiectasis, tumors, cysts, or cavities in the pulmonary system
➤ Evaluating tracheobronchial tree before anticipated surgery
➤ Placing bronchoscope for direct visualization of the airways when done in conjunction with bronchoscopy
➤ Diagnosing hyaline membrane disease and transient tachypnea in infants
➤ Detecting congenital malformation of the tracheobronchial tree in infants[113]
➤ Providing a permanent record of films that outline pathology of the tracheobronchial tree

Contraindications

➤ Pregnancy, unless benefits of performing the procedure greatly outweigh the risks to the fetus
➤ Respiratory infection
➤ Excessive coughing and mucus production
➤ Condition causing respiratory insufficiency or possible failure

---

➤➤ Nursing Alert

• Special precautions should be taken in clients with chronic obstructive pulmonary disease (COPD) while contrast medium is injected, as it can exacerbate laryngeal or bronchial spasms or dyspnea, or both.[114]

Nursing Care Before the Procedure

Client teaching and physical preparation are the same as for bronchoscopy (see pp. 537 to 538).

➤ Inform the client that postural drainage or other breathing treatments are performed 1 to 3 days before the study to remove secretions.[115]
➤ An expectorant can be administered if a cough is present; oral care can be recommended, with teeth brushing and mouthwash, to promote cleanliness and prevent introduction of microorganisms into the airways and lungs.
➤ Take a history that includes last menstrual period date to determine possibility of pregnancy; allergy to iodine, iodinated contrast medium, or local anesthetic; or known or suspected pulmonary conditions.
➤ Request that the client remove all jewelry, dentures, and glasses.
➤ Provide pulmonary toilet and mouth care the evening and morning before the study.
➤ Administer IM or SC diazepam for sedation and relaxation, atropine sulfate for reduction of secretions and gag reflex, and expectorant 30 minutes before the procedure for productive cough, if present.

The Procedure

The client is placed on the x-ray table in a sitting position. The throat and nose are sprayed with a local anesthetic and the client placed in a supine position. The client is requested to avoid swallowing the anesthetic. A child or client who is unable to remain still during the procedure is given a general anesthetic. A catheter or a bronchoscope is inserted into the trachea, and an anesthetic is injected into the airway to include the pharynx, larynx, and bronchi. Administration of the anesthetic is followed by injection of the iodinated contrast medium via the catheter or scope. At this time the client is instructed to increase breathing to keep from coughing up the contrast medium.[116] The client is placed in different positions to spread the contrast medium into the areas of the bronchi to be viewed. Films are taken in these positions.

Nursing Care After the Procedure

➤ Perform postural drainage techniques to remove the contrast medium from the tracheobronchial tree. Encourage coughing to assist in this removal.

➤ When the gag reflex returns, resume food and fluid intake (usually in 2 to 4 hours).

➤ Monitor for laryngospasm or bronchospasm and respiratory changes that result from those complications.

➤ After the gag reflex returns, administer throat lozenges and warm fluid gargle for throat soreness or irritation caused by the catheter, taking care to prevent aspiration.

➤ Provide for follow-up x-rays to ensure that all the contrast medium has been removed to prevent pneumonia.

➤ *Reaction to iodinated contrast medium:* Note and report warmth, flushing, itching, and nausea. Administer ordered antihistamine and steroids. Have resuscitation equipment on hand.

➤ *Pneumonia:* Note and report dyspnea, rales, rhonchi, temperature elevation, change in sputum color to yellowish green. Administer ordered antibiotic and oxygen therapy.

HYSTEROSALPINGOGRAPHY

The hysterosalpingogram involves the visualization of the uterine cavity and the fallopian tubes after the injection of a water-soluble or oil-based iodinated contrast medium via a cannula inserted into the cervix. The flow of the material is viewed fluoroscopically and x-ray films are taken.[117] The study is performed to identify abnormalities of the female reproductive organs.

Reference Values

Normal uterus and fallopian tube structure and patency; no tumors, adhesions, fistula, or foreign bodies

Interfering Factors

➤ Feces or gas in the LGI tract

➤ Spasms of the fallopian tubes that can appear as a stricture of the tubes

➤ Excessive traction on the tubes that can appear as normal when the traction displaces adhesions[118]

Indications for Hysterosalpingography

➤ Evaluating tubal patency that cannot be determined by ultrasonography
➤ Detecting foreign bodies such as displaced or dislodged intrauterine device (IUD) or tubal pregnancy
➤ Determining tubal obstruction caused by tumors, scarring, adhesions, kinking, or mucus plugs
➤ Correcting suspected adhesions, mucus plugs, or kinking by therapeutic clearing of these obstructive conditions as an adjunct to fertility studies
➤ Confirming possible fertility difficulties
➤ Diagnosing uterine tumor, fistula, trauma, or congenital abnormalities
➤ Evaluating tubal ligation or tubal reanastomosis procedures
➤ Determining the cause of repeated spontaneous abortions

Contraindications

➤ Pregnancy or suspected pregnancy
➤ Infection of the cervix, vagina, endometrium, or fallopian tubes
➤ Pelvic inflammatory disease
➤ Vaginal bleeding or menstruation

Nursing Care Before the Procedure

Client teaching and physical preparation are the same as for retrograde urethrography (see p. 631).

➤ The history should include assurance of completion of a menstrual period 10 days before the study.
➤ Depending on agency policy and physician preference, administer a laxative the night before and an enema, suppository, and douche before the study.
➤ Administer an ordered sedative such as diazepam to reduce anxiety, promote relaxation, and prevent spasms of the fallopian tubes.

The Procedure

The client is placed on the x-ray table in the lithotomy position with the legs and feet supported by stirrups and draped for privacy. An abdominal flat plate (KUB) film is taken to ensure that nothing exists in the lower bowel to interfere with visualization. A vaginal speculum is inserted and the cervix is cleansed with an antiseptic. A catheter is then inserted into the cervix and, while it is being viewed by fluoroscopy, the dye is injected into the uterus and fallopian tubes until they are filled. The client is informed that some lower abdominal cramping or shoulder pain will be experienced as the dye reaches the peritoneal cavity. The client is also requested to report any nausea, flushing, or sweating after the dye is injected. X-ray films are taken and the client's position is changed to obtain an oblique view. At completion of the filming, the catheter is removed.

Nursing Care After the Procedure

➤ Monitor vital signs and compare with baseline readings.
➤ Provide a pad for vaginal discharge and monitor the drainage for bleeding.
➤ Inform the client that some bloody discharge can be expected for 2 days after the study.
➤ Assess for cramping and dizziness, and remind the client to report any delayed reaction to the dye or possible infection.

➤ *Reaction to iodinated contrast medium:* Note and report anxiety, warmth, flushing, urticaria, itching, nausea, and vomiting. Administer ordered antihistamines and steroids. Have resuscitation equipment on hand.

➤ *Infection:* Note and report temperature, abdominal pain, malaise, and vaginal discharge characteristics. Administer ordered analgesic and antibiotic therapy.

➤ *Perforation:* Note and report abdominal pain, profuse vaginal bleeding, and signs and symptoms of peritonitis. Administer ordered antibiotic therapy. Prepare client for possible surgical repair of uterus.

MYELOGRAPHY

The myelogram allows visualization of the spinal subarachnoid space or the spinal canal to determine abnormalities. A contrast medium is injected into the spinal canal via a lumbar puncture. Fluoroscopy provides a view of the flow toward the head as the table is tilted. X-rays are taken at the same time. A cisternal puncture can be performed if a lumbar puncture is contraindicated.[119]

Reference Values

Normal structure of the subarachnoid spaces of the spinal column; no spinal abnormalities or obstructions

Interfering Factors

➤ Inability of client to remain still during the procedure
➤ Spinal curvatures or other abnormalities that prevent lumbar or cervical puncture for dye injection
➤ Inaccurate needle placement in the spinal column
➤ Metal objects within the field

Indications for Myelography

➤ Suspected congenital abnormalities or injuries that place pressure on the spinal posterior fossa of the skull or on the nerve roots[120]
➤ Detection of lesions of the spinal column such as cord or meningeal tumors, cysts, or ruptured intervertebral disks
➤ Detection of changes in bone structure of the spinal column caused by arthritis and ankylosing spondylosis
➤ Determination of the cause of chronic, unrelieved back pain and pain that radiates down the leg with associated footdrop
➤ Diagnosis of conditions affecting the subarachnoid space or spinal cord in the presence of neurological signs and symptoms that suggest an injury or loss of neuromuscular function
➤ Confirmation of diagnosis or pathology before anticipated or scheduled surgical procedure

Contraindications

➤ Pregnancy, unless benefits of performing the procedure greatly outweigh the risks to the fetus
➤ Known allergy to iodine or iodinated contrast media
➤ Suspected or confirmed increase in intracranial pressure

➤ Infection at the puncture site
➤ Chronic neurological disease such as multiple sclerosis

Nursing Care Before the Procedure

Client teaching and physical preparation are the same as for retrograde urethrography (see p. 631).

➤ The history should include known or suspected neuromuscular disorders that could be exacerbated or worsened by this procedure and medication regimens that include phenothiazines to treat seizure disorders.
➤ Food and fluids are restricted for 8 to 12 hours before the study.
➤ Administer a laxative or enema before the study to clear the bowel of feces or gas.
➤ Shave the puncture area if it is necessary.
➤ Administer an IM or SC sedative such as diazepam to promote relaxation and an anticholinergic such as atropine sulfate to reduce secretions.
➤ Advise the client that the site will be anesthetized by local injection and a lumbar puncture performed to inject the dye into the spinal column to facilitate visualization.

The Procedure

The client is placed at the edge of a tilted x-ray table in a side-lying position. The lumbar or cervical puncture site, depending on the suspected pathology, is cleansed with an antiseptic solution and draped to provide a sterile field. The site is then injected with a local anesthetic. The client is requested to flex the knees and bend the head downward if a lumbar puncture is performed. If a lumbar puncture is contraindicated, a cisternal puncture is performed. Placement of the needle is verified by fluoroscopy, and some cerebrospinal fluid (CSF) can be collected for laboratory examination. The client is then placed in a prone position with straps and shoulder and foot braces to prevent movement or falling. Contrast medium in the same amount as the removed CSF, usually 15 mL, is injected via the needle in the spinal canal. The client is informed that a burning sensation will be experienced when the dye is injected. The client is asked to report a warm, flushed feeling or unusual pain during injection of the dye. An iodinated water-soluble contrast medium (metrizoate sodium) is most commonly used, but an oil-based medium or air contrast can also be injected. Air contrast studies are performed to avoid side effects from other media.[121] The table is tilted to distribute the flow of dye and fluoroscopy is used to follow the dye in a cephalad direction.[122] Spot films are taken and obstructions, if present, are identified. Various views can also be taken with position changes. After conclusion of the filming, the oil-based medium, if used, is aspirated and the needle removed. The site is bandaged and taped in place. CT scanning can be performed during or after the myelogram to identify lesions that are difficult to diagnose. The specimen, if obtained, is properly labeled and sent to the laboratory for examination.

Nursing Care After the Procedure

➤ Inform the client that a headache can occur.
➤ Elevate the head of the bed to a semi-Fowler's position (45 degrees) if a water-soluble medium was used.

➤ Place the client's head in a position lower than the body if air was used.

➤ Keep client in a prone position for 2 hours, followed by a supine position for 2 to 4 hours if an oil-contrast medium was used. If the oil was not withdrawn, elevate the head to prevent the oil from reaching the brain.

➤ Monitor vital signs and compare with baseline readings.

➤ Encourage fluid intake to assist in the removal of the dye and replacement of CSF; monitor voiding pattern.

➤ Perform neurological checks for presence of headache, photophobia, stiff neck, or seizure activity caused by meningeal irritation.

➤ If nausea or vomiting is present, administer an ordered antiemetic other than a phenothiazine.

➤ *Reaction to iodinated contrast medium:* Note and report warmth, flushing, nausea, vomiting, or itching. Administer ordered antihistamine and steroids. Have resuscitation equipment on hand.

➤ *Meningitis:* Note and report severe headache, stiff neck, irritability, seizure activity, or fever. Administer ordered medications. Carry out seizure precautions. Provide a quiet, darkened environment. Monitor temperature and vital signs.

Student Name _____ Class _____

Instructor _____ Date _____

CASE STUDY AND CRITICAL THINKING EXERCISE

Mr. Smith, age 55, has a diagnosis of rectal polyps. He is scheduled to have a barium enema tomorrow.

   a. Why is this test ordered in this case?

   b. What postprocedure information do you need to give Mr. Smith regarding his stool pattern?

References

1. Squire, LF: Fundamentals of Radiology, ed 3. Harvard University Press, Cambridge, Mass, 1982, pp 2–3.
2. Ibid, p 3.
3. Ibid, p 3.
4. Ibid, pp 4, 210.
5. Fischbach, FT: A Manual of Laboratory and Diagnostic Tests, ed 4. JB Lippincott, Philadelphia, 1992, p 632.
6. Ibid, pp 636-639.
7. Ibid, p 639.
8. Springhouse Corporation: Nurse's Reference Library: Diagnostics, ed 2. Springhouse Corporation, Springhouse, Pa, 1986, pp 774–745.
9. Ibid, p 754.
10. Ibid, p 754.
11. Fischbach, op cit, p 642.
12. Miller, WT: Radiologic examination of the chest. In Fishman, AP: Pulmonary Diseases and Disorders, ed 2, vol I. McGraw-Hill, NY, 1988, p 525.
13. Nurse's Reference Library, op cit, p 652.
14. Squire, op cit, p 28.
15. Nurse's Reference Library, op cit, p 652.
16. Miller, op cit, p 479.
17. Nurse's Reference Library, op cit, p 653.
18. Miller, op cit, p 479.
19. Nurse's Reference Library, op cit, p 653.
20. Miller, op cit, p 480.
21. Squire, op cit, p 16.
22. Nurse's Reference Library, op cit, p 657.
23. Umali, CB, and Smith, EH: The chest radiographic examination. In Reppe, JM, et al: Intensive Care Medicine. Little, Brown & Co, Boston, 1985, pp 484–485.
24. Nurse's Reference Library, op cit, p 956.
25. Fischbach, op cit, p 646.
26. Ibid, p 646.
27. Nurse's Reference Library, op cit, p 955.
28. Squire, op cit, pp 168–171.
29. Pagana, KD, and Pagana, TJ: Mosby's Diagnostic and Laboratory Test Reference. Mosby–Year Book, St Louis, 1992, pp 527–528.
30. Ibid, pp 527–528.
31. Pagana and Pagana, op cit, p 549.
32. Ibid, p 549.
33. Ibid, p 550.
34. Ibid, p 550.
35. Ibid, p 681.
36. Ibid, p 681.
37. Corbett, JV: Laboratory Tests and Diagnostic Procedures with Nursing Diagnoses, ed 3. Appleton & Lange, Norwalk, Conn, 1992, p 519.
38. Fischbach, op cit, pp 643–644.
39. Fischbach, op cit, p 643.
40. Nurse's Reference Library, op cit, p 874.
41. Fischbach, op cit, p 644.
42. Nurse's Reference Library, op cit, p 874.
43. Pagana and Pagana, op cit, pp 172–173.
44. Nurse's Reference Library, op cit, pp 657–658.
45. Fischbach, op cit, pp 641-642.
46. Ibid, p 642.
47. Ibid, p 668.
48. Kee, JL: Handbook of Laboratory and Diagnostic Tests with Nursing Implications, ed 3. Appleton & Lange, Norwalk, Conn, 1997, p 400.
49. Fischbach, op cit, pp 670–671.
50. Nurse's Reference Library, op cit, p 731.
51. Fischbach, op cit, p 671.
52. Ibid, p 669.
53. Nurse's Reference Library, op cit, p 731.
54. Fischbach, op cit, pp 670–671.
55. Amberg, JR, and Juhl, JH: The pharynx and esophagus. In Juhl, JH, and Crummy, AB: Paul and Juhl's Essentials of Radiologic Imaging, ed 5. JB Lippincott, Philadelphia, 1987, p 521.
56. Ibid, p 515.
57. Ibid, p 514.
58. Ibid, p 515.
59. Nurse's Reference Library, op cit, p 818.
60. Amberg, JR, and Juhl, JH: The stomach and duodenum. In Juhl, JH, and Crummy, AB: Paul and Juhl's Essentials of Radiologic Imaging, ed 5. JB Lippincott, Philadelphia, 1987, p 525.
61. Pagana and Pagana, op cit, p 672.
62. Nurse's Reference Library, op cit, p 821
63. Fischbach, op cit, p 653.
64. Pagana and Pagana, op cit, p 82.
65. Nurse's Reference Library, op cit, p 824.
66. Fischbach, op cit, p 653.
67. Pagana and Pagana, op cit, p 83.
68. Fischbach, op cit, p 653.
69. Amberg, JR, and Juhl, JH: The gallbladder and biliary ducts. In Juhl, JH, and Crummy, AB: Paul and Juhl's Essentials of Radiologic Imaging, ed 5. JB Lippincott, Philadelphia, 1987, p 496.
70. Nurse's Reference Library, op cit, p 827.
71. Amberg and Juhl, The gallbladder and biliary ducts, op cit, p 492.
72. Fischbach, op cit, p 654.
73. Nurse's Reference Library, op cit, p 828.
74. Amberg and Juhl, The gallbladder and biliary ducts, op cit, p 492.
75. Ibid, p 492.
76. Ibid, pp 502–503.
77. Pagana and Pagana, op cit, p 188.
78. Fischbach, op cit, p 655.
79. Pagana and Pagana, op cit, p 183.
80. Ibid, p 187.
81. Ibid, p 184.

82. Fischbach, op cit, p 656.
83. Ibid, p 656.
84. Nurse's Reference Library, op cit, p 833.
85. Pagana and Pagana, op cit, p 697.
86. Ibid, p 697.
87. Ibid, p 551.
88. Nurse's Reference Library, op cit, p 831.
89. Wojtowycz, M: Interventional Radiology and Angiography. Year Book Medical Publishers, Chicago, 1990, pp 313–314.
90. Pagana and Pagana, op cit, p 553.
91. Nurse's Reference Library, op cit, p 969.
92. Ibid, p 50.
93. Ibid, p 964.
94. Ibid, pp 963–964.
95. Pagana and Pagana, op cit, p 257.
96. Ibid, p 256.
97. Ibid, p 257.
98. Fischbach, op cit, p 664.
99. Ibid, p 646.
100. Nurse's Reference Library, op cit, p 967.
101. Ibid, p 971.
102. Pagana and Pagana, op cit, p 432.

103. Ibid, p 433.
104. Berkow, R (ed): The Merck Manual, ed 16. Merck Sharp and Dohme Research Laboratories, Rahway, NJ, 1992, p 1658.
105. Pagana and Pagana, op cit, p 435.
106. Nurse's Reference Library, op cit, pp 956–957.
107. Ibid, pp 989–990.
108. Pagana and Pagana, op cit, p 661.
109. Ibid, p 662.
110. Nurse's Reference Library, op cit, p 674.
111. Nurse's Reference Library, op cit, p 676.
112. Kee, op cit, p 351.
113. Pagana and Pagana, op cit, pp 126.
114. Nurse's Reference Library, op cit, p 659.
115. Pagana and Pagana, op cit, p 127.
116. Ibid, p 127.
117. Kee, op cit, p 394.
118. Pagana and Pagana, op cit, pp 424–425.
119. Pagana and Pagana, op cit, pp 515–516.
120. Nurse's Reference Library, op cit, p 781.
121. Pagana and Pagana, op cit, pp 513–514.
122. Ibid, p 516.

Bibliography

Amplatz, K: Atlas of Endourology. Mosby–Year Book, St Louis, 1991.

Bassett, LW, and Gold, RH (eds): Breast Cancer Detection: Mammography and Other Methods in Breast Imaging, ed 2. WB Saunders, Philadelphia, 1987.

Bell, G, and Finlay, D: Basic Radiographic Positioning and Anatomy. WB Saunders, Philadelphia, 1984.

Black, JM, and Matassarin-Jacobs, E: Luckmann and Sorensen's Medical-Surgical Nursing: A Psychophysiologic Approach, ed 4. WB Saunders, Philadelphia, 1993.

Brower, AC: Arthritis in Black and White, Vol 2, ed 2. WB Saunders, Philadelphia, 1996.

Chernecky, CC, and Berger, BJ; Cullen, BN (ed): Laboratory Tests and Diagnostic Procedures, ed 2. WB Saunders, Philadelphia, 1996.

Davidson, AJ, and Hartman, DS: Radiology of the Kidney and Urinary Tract, ed 2. WB Saunders, Philadelphia, 1993.

Ell, SR: Handbook of Gastrointestinal and Genitourinary Radiology, Vol 4. Mosby–Year Book, St Louis, 1991.

Forrester, DM, and Brown, JC: The Radiology of Joint Disease, Vol 2, ed 3. WB Saunders, Philadelphia, 1987.

Gehweiler, JA, Osborne, RL, and Becker, RF: The Radiology of Vertebral Trauma. WB Saunders, Philadelphia, 1980.

George, NJR, and Sambrook, P: Diagnostic Picture Tests in Urology. Mosby–Year Book, St Louis, 1991.

Greenfield, GB: Radiology of Bone Diseases, ed 5. Lippincott-Raven, Philadelphia, 1990.

Gyll, C, and Black, NS: Pediatric Diagnostic Imaging. Wiley, NY, 1986.

Heitzman, ER, and Groskin, SA: The Lung: Radiologic-Pathologic Correlations, ed 3. Mosby–Year Book, St Louis, 1993.

Helms, CA: Fundamentals of Skeletal Radiology, ed 2. WB Saunders, Philadelphia, 1994.

Herlinger, H, and Maglinte, D: Clinical Radiology of the Small Intestine. WB Saunders, Philadelphia, 1989.

Johnson, CD: Alimentary Tract Imaging: A Teaching File. Mosby–Year Book, St Louis, 1993.

Laufer, I, and Levine, MS: Double Contrast Gastrointestinal Radiology, ed 2. WB Saunders, Philadelphia, 1992.

Levine, MS: Radiology of the Esophagus. WB Saunders, Philadelphia, 1989.

Ogden, JA: Skeletal Injury in the Child, ed 2. WB Saunders, Philadelphia, 1990.

O'Reilly, PH, George, NJR, and Weiss, RM (eds): Diagnostic Techniques in Urology. WB Saunders, Philadelphia, 1990.

Ozonoff, MB: Pediatric Orthopedic Radiology, ed 2. WB Saunders, Philadelphia, 1991.

Pagana, KD, and Pagana, TJ: Diagnostic Testing and Nursing Implications: A Case Study Approach, ed 4. Mosby – Year Book, St Louis, 1993.

Porth, CM: Pathophysiology: Concepts of Altered Health States, ed 4. JB Lippincott, Philadelphia, 1993.

Potchen, J, et al: Screening Mammography: Breast Cancer Diagnosis in Asymptomatic Women. Mosby – Year Book, St Louis, 1992.

Redman, HC, et al: Emergency Radiology. WB Saunders, Philadelphia, 1992.

Reed, JC: Chest Radiology: Plain Film Patterns and Differential Diagnosis, ed 4. Mosby – Year Book, St Louis, 1996.

Renton, P: Orthopedic Radiology. Mosby – Year Book, St Louis, 1990.

Ruben, CM, and Ruben, S: Diagnostic Pictures Tests in Ophthalmology. Mosby – Year Book, St Louis, 1989.

Silverman, FN (ed): Caffey's Pediatric X-Ray Diagnosis: An Integrated Imaging Approach, ed 9. Mosby – Year Book, St Louis, 1992.

Springhouse Corporation: Diagnostic Tests. Springhouse, Springhouse, Pa, 1991.

Stimac, GK: Introduction to Radiology. WB Saunders, Philadelphia, 1992.

Tilkian, SM: Clinical and Nursing Implications of Laboratory Tests, ed 5. Mosby – Year Book, St Louis, 1995.

Thompson, WM: Common Problems in Gastrointestinal Radiology. Mosby – Year Book, St Louis, 1989.

Whaley, LF: Nursing Care of Infants and Children, ed 4. Mosby – Year Book, St Louis, 1991.

Radiologic
Angiography Studies

> **PROCEDURES COVERED**
>
> Cardiac Angiography, *654*
> Adrenal Angiography, *659*
> Cerebral Angiography, *661*
> Pulmonary Angiography, *663*
> Hepatic and Portal Angiography, *665*
>
> Renal Angiography, *667*
> Mesenteric Angiography, *669*
> Fluorescein Angiography (FA), *671*
> Lymphangiography, *673*
> Upper Extremity Angiography, *675*
> Lower Extremity Angiography, *677*

INTRODUCTION

Angiograms are serial radiographs (x-rays) of blood vessels to evaluate the patency, size, and shape of the veins (venograms); arteries (arteriograms) of organs and tissues; or lymph vessels and nodes (lymphograms). They are films taken in rapid sequence after the injection of an iodinated contrast medium into the vessel or vascular system to be examined.[1]

The contrast medium can be hand-injected into a peripheral vessel via a needle or into a major vessel via a needle and catheter, or it can be power-injected via a catheter placed directly into a heart chamber and vessels (cardiac catheterization with angiography) to visualize the chambers, great vessels, and coronary arteries. Successful visualization of any organ or vessel depends on the position of the client and catheter, size and type of the catheter or needle lumen, and the amount and rate of the injection of the contrast medium into the vessel.[2]

Various types and shapes of catheters are available for angiography, depending on the tip and length of needle required for the selected vessel to be catheterized (Fig. 18-1). Catheters vary in diameter and length and are made of polyethylene, nylon, polyurethane, and teflon to accommodate ease of handling, insertion, and injection rates.[3] Injection rates vary with blood flow of the vessel to be injected with the contrast medium and range from 2 to 3 mL per second to a high of 20 to 30 mL per second and a duration range of 2 seconds to 10 or 15 seconds.[4]

The iodinated contrast media that render the vessels radiopaque for visualization have been until recently ionic agents such as diatrizoate and iothalamate, but these media are now being replaced by low-osmolality agents such as iohexol and iopamidol when the additional expense of these newer agents is warranted. The low-osmolality agents cause less pain and fewer adverse reactions and allergic responses than do the conventional ionic agents. Fatality rates

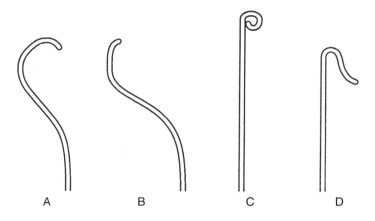

A   B   C   D

Figure 18–1   Catheters used in angiography with selected tips for particular area or vessel to be catheterized. (*A*) Cobra type: renal and mesenteric arteries. (*B*) Headhunter type: femoral artery approach to brachiocephalic vessels. (*C*) Pigtail type: aortography. (*D*) Simmons type: aortic and brachiocephalic arteries. (Adapted from Wojtowycz, M: Angiography and Interventional Procedures, Mosby-Year Book, St. Louis, 1990, p 11.)

have also been reduced with these agents. In rare instances, carbon dioxide can replace the iodinated contrast medium in clients with poor renal function or potentially life-threatening reactions to the other media.[5] Because severe allergic reactions to iodinated contrast media can result in laryngospasms, anaphylactic shock, and cardiac arrest, emergency equipment should be available for treatment and resuscitative measures that can be instituted immediately.

Arterial access for arteriography is achieved by insertion of a catheter through puncture or cutdown into a femoral, axillary, or brachial artery and advancement into the specific artery or vascular system to be examined. Peripheral arteriography can also be achieved by a direct injection of the medium into the target artery, as in the femoral artery.

Venous access for venography is achieved by a direct injection of the contrast medium via venipuncture or cutdown to expose the vein to visualize and evaluate the blood flow of an area. It can also be achieved by injection of the dye into a catheter that has been threaded into the venous system of an organ, as in arteriography, to visualize and evaluate the venous supply to an area.[6] Both peripheral and central veins are studied with venography.

Angiographic procedures are considered invasive, and a signed informed consent is required. Client preparation is similar to that for a minor surgical procedure, with local anesthesia usually administered for an adult and general anesthesia given to a child or an adult who is unable to cooperate. Cardiopulmonary resuscitation equipment should be available during all angiographic studies. The procedures are performed in a special angiography laboratory or treatment room by a physician with special education and expertise in such procedures. All angiographic procedures are performed under strict sterile conditions and use Standard Precautions and transmission-based isolation procedures.

CONVENTIONAL FILM ANGIOGRAPHY

Angiographic films are obtained in rapid succession by special magazines and film changers containing continuous rolls that allow six films per second to be taken. Spot films can also be taken, but they may not produce the desired fine detail. Exposures are made at a rate and for a duration related to the problem being studied. These films have the advantage of a large field of view, a high spatial resolution, and the opportunity to use different filming techniques.[7] The studies are developed and reviewed before the procedure is concluded.

DIGITAL SUBTRACTION ANGIOGRAPHY

Digital subtraction angiography (DSA) is a radiologic method of visualizing details of the vascular system after the intra-arterial injection of a contrast medium, usually in lower amounts than with conventional filming. Its greatest advantage is the removal of images of the surrounding tissue (bone and soft tissue) that interfere with the view of the vessels to be studied. The technique uses a computer to subtract images in real time and store them electronically on a videocassette. This technique allows immediate review of the angiogram on a television monitor. More simply stated, the process involves fluoroscopic images taken before and after injection of the medium with the C-arm of the machine rotated into a lateral projection that provides a visual field. The images taken before the medium is injected are subtracted from the images taken after the medium is contained in the vascular system. This type of study is particularly useful in the detection of carotid and cerebral conditions that cause blood-flow abnormalities. Other vessels such as the aorta and renal, abdominal, and peripheral (ankle and foot) arteries are also studied using this technique.[8] A disadvantage of this method is that the client must be able to remain still and cooperate for the length of time it takes to obtain the films. If such cooperation is not possible, conventional filming is indicated.

ANGIOGRAPHY RISKS

All angiographic studies carry some risk to the client. The risk of injury can be direct or indirect. Direct injuries involve bleeding at the puncture site, resulting in hematoma, and can be serious enough to require transfusion or surgical repair. Indirect injuries are the result of arterial dissection; rupture of an aneurysm; vasovagal reactions; and renal, cardiac, and neurological complications.

Reaction to the contrast medium is also a risk and can range from sneezing, nausea, and urticaria to respiratory changes to cardiac collapse and death. Premedication with antihistamines such as diphenhydramine (Benadryl) and steroids such as methylprednisolone (Medrol) can be administered to reduce the risk of a reaction, especially in those with a history of sensitivity to the contrast medium (iodine) or to shellfish.

Nephrotoxicity is a possible risk that can lead to renal failure if contrast medium is administered to clients who have renal insufficiency, diabetes, or multiple myeloma or who are dehydrated (contrast medium produces diuresis). Special precautions are taken to protect the client who has these conditions by administering a lower dose of the dye, ensuring adequate hydration via the IV or oral route, and, in some, administering osmotic diuretics such as mannitol (Osmitrol) and loop diuretics such as furosemide (Lasix) to ensure renal flow.[9]

Clients receiving anticoagulant therapy should have the medication discontinued or reduced before the procedure to prevent excessive bleeding or possible hemorrhage. Prothrombin time (PT) or partial thromboplastin time (PTT) can be performed to determine whether the risk for emergency angiography is too high or whether medications should be given to counteract the prolonged PT or PTT, such as fresh frozen plasma if warfarin (Coumadin) is the drug taken orally and protamine sulfate if heparin is the drug given intravenously (IV) or subcutaneously (SC).[10]

ANGIOGRAPHIC PROCEDURES

Angiographic procedures are named for the type of vessel to be studied and the method or route of the injection. Among the vessels are arteries (coronary, aorta), veins (peripheral, deep central), or lymphatics. Also included are the vascular system of organs such as the brain, heart, lungs, bronchi, adrenal glands, liver, pancreas, retina, and kidneys, and parts of the body such as the extremities.

CARDIAC ANGIOGRAPHY

Cardiac and thoracic angiography involves the examination of the heart, great vessels, and coronary arteries (Fig. 18–2). A cardiac catheterization is performed with a catheter inserted into a vein or artery and guided through the vascular system into the left or the right side of the heart. The femoral or the brachial artery is the insertion site usually used for left cardiac catheterization and the femoral or the antecubital vein is used for right cardiac catheterization. Films that allow for visualization of the heart structures and activity by cineangiography during and after injection of the dye are taken at a variety of angles as the table is tilted. The client can watch the procedure on a screen, if desired.

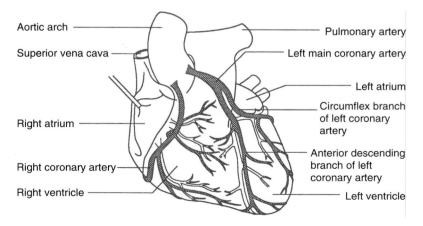

Figure 18–2   Coronary arteries and large vessels.

A variety of disorders can be diagnosed, depending on which side of the heart is catheterized and studied. Pulmonary artery abnormalities are identified with right heart examination; coronary artery and thoracic aorta abnormalities are identified with left heart examination. The procedure can be performed for therapeutic reasons as well as diagnostic purposes. Special attention is needed and given to provide support and allay the anxiety associated with procedures involving the heart.

Many additional studies of heart structure and function can also be performed during the procedure (see Chap. 24, "Cardiac Catheterization Study" section).

Reference Values

Normal patent coronary arteries and great vessels; no evidence of coronary artery obstruction and aortic aneurysm, trauma, or other abnormalities

Interfering Factors

➤ Inability of client to cooperate in the procedure when local anesthesia is used
➤ Catheter occlusion caused by stagnant blood
➤ Atherosclerotic lesions of the vessel to be cannulated, preventing passage of the catheter
➤ Selection of improper catheter and tip or use of incorrect technique

Indications for Cardiac Angiography

➤ Chest pain, especially in clients with cholesterol levels above normal range
➤ Coronary artery disease (CAD), especially in clients with a family history of heart disease
➤ Identification of abnormalities after questionable results from resting or exercise electrocardiographic (ECG) studies
➤ Evaluation of angina with frequent and severe episodes of chest pain
➤ Detection of abnormal coronary circulation and degree of occlusion of the arteries that indicate atherosclerotic disease
➤ Detection of the extent of heart damage in heart disease
➤ Identification of myocardial infarction site and performance of infusion procedure of streptokinase or other thrombolytic agent into the occluded vessel[11]
➤ Evaluation of cardiac status in preparation for cardiac bypass surgery or angioplasty when a decreased coronary perfusion is demonstrated
➤ Evaluation of cardiac function and vessel patency after surgery or angioplasty
➤ Persistent symptoms (e.g., chest pain) after cardiac revascularization
➤ Location and determination of the extent of aortic aneurysm and the presence of atherosclerosis of the arch of this great vessel
➤ Diagnosis of aortic abnormalities by left heart examination such as tumor, diverticula, aortitis, and trauma that create tears or other disruption of the vessel
➤ Evaluation of progress or decline in condition to enable adjustment of existing medical regimen

Contraindications

➤ Pregnancy, unless the benefits of performing the procedure greatly outweigh the risks to the fetus
➤ Allergy to radiopaque contrast medium, unless prophylactic medications are administered before the procedure
➤ Severe cardiomegaly
➤ Poor or severely impaired renal function
➤ Poor surgical risk or refusal to undergo surgery if recommended after the procedure

Nursing Care Before the Procedure

Explain to the client:
➤ That a physician will explain and perform the procedure
➤ That the time required to complete the procedure varies with the type of examination performed for diagnostic or therapeutic purposes but that it can be 1 to 3 hours
➤ That foods and fluids are withheld for 4 to 8 hours before the procedure
➤ That some medications can be withheld for 8 hours before the procedure, depending on the client and the reason for medications taken; that anticoagulants will be withheld or dosage reduced to prevent excessive bleeding; and that aspirin products are withheld for at least a week before the procedure
➤ That an analgesic, sedative, or antianxiety agent can be administered by injection before the procedure to promote relaxation and alleviate discomfort (physician-dependent)
➤ That the client is requested to lie still throughout the procedure
➤ That an IV line is initiated before the procedure to provide access for the administration of fluids and medications when needed
➤ That the catheter insertion site will be anesthetized by local injection
➤ That the client may experience some pressure as the catheter is introduced into the vessel and a feeling of warmth and possible palpitations when the dye is injected, but that this lasts only about 30 seconds
➤ That cough, nausea, and headache may be experienced during the procedure or that chest pain may develop during the injection or during exercises that are part of the examination and that medications are given if these side effects occur
➤ That continuous monitoring by ECG and vital signs is performed during and after the procedure
➤ That bed rest is required for about 8 to 12 hours after the procedure to monitor the insertion site and vital signs and to observe the client for signs of complications, although complications are rare

Prepare for the procedure:
➤ Ensure that dietary, fluid, and medication restrictions have been followed before the procedure.
➤ Obtain a history of allergies or sensitivities to the anesthetics or contrast medium; existing heart, lung, or renal condition; and date of last menstrual period in women of childbearing age to determine the possibility of pregnancy.

➤ Ensure that hematologic status and blood clotting ability have been assessed to include complete blood count (CBC), platelet count, PT, PTT, clotting time, and bleeding time as well as routine urinalysis (UA) and electrolytes. Note and record results of ECG and chest x-ray.

➤ Remove all metallic objects, but allow client to wear dentures, hearing aids, or both.

➤ Obtain and record baseline vital signs, using peripheral pulses on the appropriate extremity. Mark these sites on the skin to ensure that the same location is used to monitor and compare readings to assess circulatory status after the procedure.

➤ Shave and cleanse insertion site if needed.

➤ Have client void.

➤ Administer premedication SC or intramuscularly (IM) as ordered. (Premedication can include an analgesic such as meperidine [Demerol], a sedative such as diazepam [Valium], or an antihistamine such as diphenhydramine to prevent an allergic reaction in those with a history of sensitivity to iodine.)

The Procedure

The client is placed on a tilting type x-ray table in a supine position with straps in place to prevent falling and to keep the client very still during the procedure. Cardiopulmonary resuscitation equipment, defibrillator, pacemaker, and cardiac medications should be on hand during and after the procedure.[12] The operating room is notified of the procedure in the event that emergency cardiac surgery is necessary.

The leads from the ECG machine are attached to the chest for continuous monitoring. An IV access line is initiated to keep the vein open (KVO) for the administration of fluids and drugs when needed. The site is cleansed and draped to prepare a sterile field. A local anesthetic is injected at the site, and a small incision is made. The room is darkened, and a needle with a guide wire is inserted. When the needle and guide wire are placed in the desired site in the heart and coronary vessels or great vessels, the needle only is removed, and the catheter is threaded onto the wire and advanced into the vessel under the guidance of fluoroscopy. The guide wire is then removed, and the catheter is flushed with heparinized saline solution to remove any stagnant blood, a procedure that is repeated every 3 minutes throughout the study.[13] The catheter is advanced through the selected vein to the inferior vena cava and then to the right atrium and ventricle if the right side is being catheterized or through the selected artery to the aorta and into the coronary arteries if the left side is being catheterized. The coronary arteries can be catheterized singly to evaluate patency. After correct placement and flushing of the catheter, the iodinated contrast medium is injected and controlled at a rate determined by the studies to be performed. A rapid series of x-rays are taken during and after the injection.

During the procedure, the client can be requested to deep-breathe or cough to counteract nausea and to ease catheter placement into the pulmonary artery as well as to move the diaphragm in a downward position to allow for clearer visualization of the heart.[14] Filming takes place with the table tilted in different positions, and the client is turned from side to side to obtain views of the heart at a variety of angles. Vital signs and heart activity are monitored continuously to observe for dysrhythmias that can occur during the procedure. The procedure is terminated if severe chest pain, cardiac dysrhythmias, or symptoms of cerebral accident are noted. When the procedure is completed, protamine sulfate is administered to counteract the effect of the heparin and to prevent excessive bleeding. The catheter is removed, the incision site sutured, and a bandage applied and taped in place.

Nursing Care After the Procedure

➤ Remove the client from the x-ray table and place him or her at rest for 8 to 12 hours after the procedure to prevent bleeding from the puncture site.

➤ Time at rest should depend on pressure at the insertion site (venous or arterial) and whether more than one site was used.

➤ Elevate the head of the bed to 45 degrees and extend the extremity used for the insertion site.

➤ Immobilize the extremity with a sandbag, 8 hours for a leg and 3 hours for an arm.

➤ Inspect the insertion site for bleeding or hematoma formation, and change the pressure dressing as needed.

➤ Apply ice to the site to relieve discomfort and edema by promoting vasoconstriction of the vessels at the site.

➤ A mild analgesic can be administered for site pain.

➤ Assess skin color, sensation, and temperature of the extremity to determine circulation status. Take peripheral pulses of the extremity used and compare with preprocedure pulses and pulses of the other extremity.

➤ Perform this assessment every 15 minutes for the first hour, then every 30 minutes for the next 2 hours, and then every hour for the next 8 hours or more if needed.

➤ Take vital signs and apical pulse at the same frequency.

➤ Encourage movement in bed from side to side to exercise uninvolved body parts.

➤ To prevent dehydration and promote excretion of the dye, encourage fluids, first via the IV line and then orally, when client is able.

➤ Sutures, if used, are removed in a week.

➤ *Reaction to anesthetic agent or contrast medium:* Note and report tachycardia, dyspnea, hyperpnea, or delayed feeling of itching (urticaria, rash). Administer antihistamines and steroids. Initiate oxygen and resuscitation procedure if needed.

➤ *Dysrhythmias, cardiac tamponade:* Note and report irregular pulse, postprocedural ECG changes, or signs and symptoms of cardiac tamponade such as anxiety, tachypnea, muffled heart sounds, distended neck veins, or narrowing pulse pressures. Administer ordered cardiac medications. Monitor vital signs and cardiac activity via ECG.

➤ *Thrombophlebitis:* Note and report pain, redness, swelling at the site, or changes in the peripheral pulses. Monitor site for changes. Apply ordered warm compresses.

➤ *Infection at the insertion site:* Note and report pain, swelling, or drainage. Administer ordered analgesic and antibiotic therapy. Apply heat treatments.

➤ *Bleeding, hematoma:* Note and report excessive bleeding from the insertion site or presence of a hematoma. Apply pressure for 15 minutes after the procedure. Apply ice bag and pressure dressing.

ADRENAL ANGIOGRAPHY

Adrenal angiography allows x-ray visualization of the arteries or veins of the adrenal glands. For both arteries and veins, an iodinated contrast medium is injected via the femoral artery or through vein catheterization, depending on whether an arteriogram or a venogram procedure is to be performed. Fluoroscopy provides viewing during the advancement of the catheter to ensure proper placement in an artery or vein. Adrenal arteriography is performed to determine the presence of a tumor or hyperplasia of one or both of the glands, and venography is performed to obtain blood samples from the glands for laboratory analysis. Adrenal complications depend on the type of vessel used and the effect of the pressure placed on the gland tissue by the dye. The presence of a pheochromocytoma can lead to a severe hypertensive crisis and death. α- and β-Adrenergic blockers are administered for several days before the procedure to prevent this life-threatening condition if a tumor is suspected.[15]

Reference Values

Normal arteries and veins of the adrenal glands; no evidence of tumor, abnormal hormones, or abnormal catecholamine levels

Interfering Factors

➤ Inability of client to cooperate and lie still during the procedure when it is performed under local anesthesia
➤ Atherosclerotic lesions causing obstruction or narrowing of the vessel to be cannulated, preventing passage of the catheter
➤ Incorrect catheter lumen size and tip

Indications for Adrenal Angiography

➤ Suspected benign or malignant adrenal tumor such as pheochromocytoma, adenoma, or carcinoma diagnosed by arteriography
➤ Diagnosis of adrenal hyperplasia in both glands by arteriography
➤ Differentiation among adrenal tumor types and, by arteriography and venography of both glands, determination of unilateral or bilateral tumor
➤ Securing of a blood sample from the adrenal vein of each gland for analysis of cortisol levels to diagnose Cushing's syndrome, with an elevation from one gland indicating a tumor and from both glands indicating hyperplasia
➤ Securing of a blood sample from the adrenal vein for analysis of catecholamines to determine the presence of a unilateral or bilateral pheochromocytoma, with an elevation from one gland indicating the tumor on that side, elevation from both glands indicating the tumor on both sides, and absence of elevated level from either side but presence of elevated level in a peripheral venous blood sample indicating a tumor external to the gland[16]

➤ Evaluation of adrenal venous blood for other hormones and substances such as androgen or aldosterone[17]

Contraindications

➤ Pregnancy, unless the benefits of performing the procedure greatly outweigh the risks to the fetus

➤ Allergy to iodinated contrast medium, unless prophylactic medications are administered or nonionic contrast medium is used

➤ Presence of bleeding disorder

Nursing Care Before the Procedure

Client teaching and physical preparation are the same as for any angiographic procedure (see pp. 656 to 657).

➤ Assess the client suspected of having a pheochromocytoma for administration of α- and β-adrenergic blockers (propranolol [Inderal] and phenoxybenzamine [Dibenzyline]) several days before the procedure to avoid the risk of a hypertensive crisis.

The Procedure

The client is placed on the x-ray table in a supine position. The groin is cleansed and draped to prepare a sterile field for the procedure. The site is anesthetized with a local injection, and a catheter is inserted into the femoral vein for venography and into the femoral artery for arteriography. The client should be informed that some pain is experienced at the puncture site when the catheter is inserted. For arteriography, the catheter is advanced into the aorta and then into the inferior adrenal artery via the renal artery. For venography, the catheter is advanced into the adrenal vein. Both are guided and placed into position with the assistance of fluoroscopic visualization. Dye is injected into the catheter; then x-ray films are taken for arteriographic studies and blood is obtained for laboratory examination with venographic studies. At the conclusion of the study the catheter is removed, and a pressure dressing is applied to the insertion site and taped in place.

Nursing Care After the Procedure

Care and assessment after the procedure are the same as for any angiographic procedure (see p. 658).

➤ ECG monitoring is not necessary, but electronic monitoring of blood pressure should be performed every 15 minutes to intervene in or offset an imminent hypertensive crisis.

➤ *Complications and precautions:* With the exception of dysrhythmias, these measures are the same as for any angiographic procedure (see p. 658), with the following additions:

• *Hemorrhage at gland site:* Note and report signs and symptoms of adrenal insufficiency such as hypotension, muscle weakness, fatigue, nausea, or sodium and potassium imbalance if gland function has been affected. Administer replacement therapy as ordered.

• *Hypertensive crisis:* Note and report blood pressure elevations, tachycardia, anxiety, or sweating. Administer ordered antihypertensives or sympathetic inhibitors. Ensure that α- and β-adrenergic blockers have been administered before the procedure.

CEREBRAL ANGIOGRAPHY

Cerebral angiography involves x-ray visualization of the cerebral vessels and the carotid and vertebral arteries (Fig. 18–3). After the injection of an iodinated contrast medium via catheterization of the femoral (most common site), the carotid, or the brachial artery, a series of films are taken to obtain views with the client in various positions. The femoral site allows visualization of any vascular area in the brain or in the carotid or vertebral arteries in which an abnormality is suspected, whereas the other sites are more area- and vessel-specific.

Cerebrovascular abnormalities can be diagnosed by the changes in the size of the vessel lumina or by vessel occlusion. Tumor detection, whether vascular or nonvascular, can be diagnosed by vessel displacement indicating the position and type of tumor. Vascular displacement can also be identified in conditions such as abscess, hematoma, and edema.[18,19]

Reference Values

Normal structure and patency of cerebral vessels and carotid and vertebral arteries; no evidence of cerebral aneurysm, plaques, or spasms; thrombosis; fistulae; tumor; arteriovenous (A-V) malformation; or hematoma

Interfering Factors

➤ Inability of client to lie still and keep head immobilized during the procedure
➤ Atherosclerotic lesions causing narrowing or obstruction of the vessel to be cannulated and difficulty in passage of the catheter

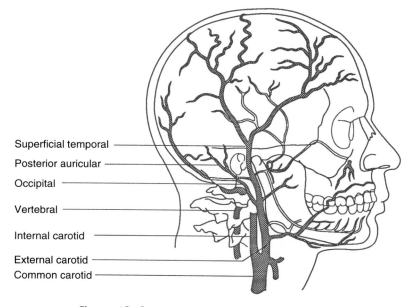

Superficial temporal
Posterior auricular
Occipital
Vertebral
Internal carotid
External carotid
Common carotid

Figure 18–3 Carotid, vertebral, and cerebral vessels.

Indications for Cerebral Angiography

> ➤ Detecting vascular or nonvascular tumor by vessel displacement
> ➤ Detecting spasms, abscess, edema, or hematoma by vascular distortion, displacement, or both
> ➤ Detecting abnormalities or interruptions in cerebral circulation through the narrowing or occlusion of vessels caused by thrombosis or detecting A-V malformation
> ➤ Detecting vessel wall changes caused by aneurysm
> ➤ Detecting atherosclerosis and degree of occlusion of the carotid arteries
> ➤ Diagnosing hydrocephalus in an infant or young child
> ➤ Determining increased intracranial pressure and possible cause
> ➤ Evaluating postoperative placement and status of shunts or clips to vessels

Contraindications

> ➤ Pregnancy, unless the benefits of performing the procedure greatly outweigh the risks to the fetus
> ➤ Allergy to iodinated contrast medium, unless prophylactic medications are administered or nonionic dye is used for those suspected of iodine sensitivity
> ➤ Presence of a bleeding disorder
> ➤ Acute or severe renal or hepatic disease

Nursing Care Before the Procedure

Client teaching and physical preparation are the same as for any angiographic procedure (see pp. 656 to 657).

The Procedure

The client is placed on the x-ray table in a supine position. The arms are placed at the sides, and the head is immobilized with sandbags. The groin (femoral), arm (brachial), or neck (carotid) site is cleansed and draped to prepare a sterile field for the procedure. Site selection depends on previous problems with arterial structure or patency. General anesthesia is administered if the study is to be performed on a child; otherwise, the selected site is anesthetized by local injection. The catheter is advanced under fluoroscopic guidance, and the dye is injected for visualization of the carotid and vertebral arteries, large vessels of the circle of Willis, and the cerebrovascular system, including the arterial branches and venous and capillary blood flow. The catheter is flushed with heparinized normal saline during the procedure to prevent stagnation of blood. A series of x-ray films are taken in sequence to reveal the complete vascular circulation of the brain in anterior-posterior (AP) and lateral views. Neurological checks are made and vital signs are monitored during the study. Depending on the results, another timed series of filming can follow, with additional dye injected. At the conclusion of the procedure, the catheter is removed and pressure is applied to the site for 10 to 15 minutes. A dressing is then applied at the insertion site and taped in place.

Nursing Care After the Procedure

Care and assessment after the procedure are the same as for any angiographic procedure (see p. 658).

➤ Continue neurological checks and vital sign monitoring during the period of bed rest every hour for the first 4 hours and then every 4 hours for 24 hours for changes in breathing pattern or orientation, especially if the carotid site was used.

➤ If the carotid site was used, elevate the head slightly and assess the client for visual, facial, and speech changes resulting from transient ischemic attacks (TIAs) or breathing and swallowing changes caused by neck edema.[20]

➤ *Complications and precautions:* With the exception of dysrhythmias, complications and precautions are the same as for any angiographic procedure (see p. 658), with the following addition:
- *Embolism if atherosclerotic plaque is dislodged by catheter:* Note and report change in vital signs or signs of neurological impairment. Prepare for emergency intervention.

PULMONARY ANGIOGRAPHY

Pulmonary angiography involves x-ray examination of the pulmonary vessels after the injection of an iodinated contrast medium into the pulmonary artery or a branch of this great vessel. The procedure is considered the definitive standard for the diagnosis of acute pulmonary embolism, but it can also be used to identify the presence of other arterial and venous abnormalities. Chest x-ray and radionuclide scan are performed before angiography if pulmonary embolism is suspected in order to rule out the presence of the abnormality or to direct the study to the location of a disease or perfusion abnormality that will provide a diagnosis.[21]

Bronchial-intercostal arteriography involves the examination of the bronchial and intercostal arteries to determine the cause of recurrent or severe hemoptysis and to identify the site of the bleeding.

Cineangiography and digital subtraction angiography techniques can be used in clients if the advantages outweigh the disadvantages of these alternatives, such as higher radiation dose, smaller field size, and risk of a reaction to the contrast medium.[22]

Reference Values

Normal structure and patency of the pulmonary circulation vessels; no evidence of pulmonary embolism, tumor, aneurysm, stenosis, or A-V malformation

Interfering Factors

➤ Inability of client to cooperate and remain still during the procedure
➤ Catheter occlusion caused by stagnant blood
➤ Atherosclerotic lesions causing narrowing or obstruction of the vessel to be cannulated and difficulty in the passage of the catheter

Indications for Pulmonary Angiography

➤ Evaluation of vascular changes in pulmonary circulation
➤ Detection of filling defects caused by acute pulmonary embolism when lung perfusion and ventilation scanning have not provided a definitive diagnosis
➤ Diagnosis of chronic pulmonary embolism
➤ Detection of perfusion defects caused by aneurysms, arterial hypoplasia or stenosis, or thrombi

➤ Detection of vessel displacement caused by pulmonary tumor
➤ Detection of vascular obstruction caused by tumor or inflammatory disease, both for diagnosis and after treatment regimen
➤ Recurrent or massive bleeding caused by tuberculosis, bronchiectasis, sarcoidosis, or aspergilloma[23]
➤ Locatation of bleeding site before embolotherapy by performing bronchial and intercostal angiography
➤ Detection and location of pulmonary embolism before performing an embolectomy in a life-threatening situation
➤ Planning of treatment or surgical procedure for congenital heart disease in children
➤ Evaluation of pulmonary vascular changes associated with emphysema, blebs, and bullae
➤ Suspected aortic laceration after trauma
➤ Diagnosis and evaluation of atherosclerotic aneurysm of the aorta
➤ Evaluation of aortic masses such as invading tumor or diverticulum
➤ Evaluation of aortic aneurysm and dissection before surgery

Contraindications

➤ Pregnancy, unless the benefits of performing the procedure greatly outweigh the risks to the fetus
➤ Allergy to the iodinated contrast medium, unless prophylactic medications are administered or nonionic dye is used
➤ Presence of a bleeding disorder

Nursing Care Before the Procedure

Client teaching and physical preparation are the same as for any angiographic procedure (see pp. 656 to 657).

The Procedure

The client is placed on the x-ray table in a supine position. The leads from the ECG machine are attached to the chest to provide continuous monitoring of the heart's activity to identify dysrhythmias during the procedure. The site is cleansed and draped to prepare a sterile field for the procedure. A local anesthetic is injected at the site, and a small incision is made or a needle inserted. The catheter is inserted into the femoral, brachial, or jugular vein and threaded into the inferior vena cava, then into the right side of the heart under fluoroscopic guidance. From the right ventricle, the catheter is placed in the pulmonary artery and the dye is injected. If aortography is to be performed, the femoral artery is the site of insertion, and the catheter is placed near the aortic valve before injection of the dye. Injection rate is dependent on the area to be examined. If bronchial angiography is to be performed, the catheter is advanced into the descending thoracic aorta and then into the right intercostobronchial trunk and one or two left bronchial arteries before the dye is injected.[24] Serial films are taken during the injection of the dye to visualize pulmonary circulation. Rapid sequence films with at least two views of each lung are obtained after the dye injection.

When the procedure is completed, the catheter is removed, and pressure is applied at the site. A pressure dressing is then applied and taped in place.

Nursing Care After the Procedure

Care and assessment after the procedure are the same as for any angiographic procedure (see p. 658).

HEPATIC AND PORTAL ANGIOGRAPHY

Hepatic angiography allows x-ray visualization of the hepatic arterial and venous systems after injection of a contrast medium in an amount and at a rate based on the vessel and the suspected liver abnormality. Normally, the liver blood circulation is supplied by the hepatic artery and the portal vein. Figure 18–4 portrays the hepatic arterial and venous anatomy involved in this procedure.

Portal venography is performed to assess the patency and size of the portal, splenic, and mesenteric veins. The direction of blood flow and collateral vessel development can also be evaluated. Abnormalities involving the hepatic artery are revealed if a malignant tumor is present. Venous invasion is revealed in hepatocellular carcinoma resulting from hepatitis and cirrhosis.[25]

Reference Values

Normal structure and patency of hepatic artery and portal vein; no evidence of tumors, vascular obstruction, or other liver abnormalities

Interfering Factors

➤ Inability of client to cooperate and remain still during the procedure
➤ Atherosclerotic lesions causing narrowing or obstruction of the vessel to be cannulated and difficulty in passage of the catheter

Indications for Hepatic and Portal Angiography

➤ Diagnosis of malignant liver tumor when other diagnostic procedures such as ultrasonography, computerized scanning, magnetic resonance imaging (MRI), or needle biopsy fail to provide a definitive diagnosis (*Note:* Malignant tumors are supplied by the hepatic artery only, whereas the normal liver is diffused by both arteries and veins.)

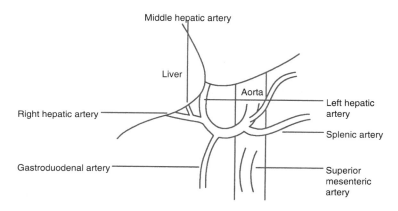

Figure 18–4 Hepatic arterial vessels.

➤ Determination of the location, number of nodes, and vascular invasion of a hepatic malignant tumor before surgery
➤ Determination of the advisability of arterial infusion of chemotherapy to treat a malignant tumor
➤ Determination of the stage of cirrhosis of the liver, which is known to cause a reversal of portal venous blood flow
➤ Evaluation of liver trauma after injury (*Note:* Diagnostic value of the procedure is questionable for this condition.[26])
➤ Definition and determination of hepatic anatomy and blood flow before hepatic transplantation or shunt placement
➤ Postoperative evaluation of the surgical placement of a portosystemic shunt
➤ Evaluation of portal vein patency and size after hepatic transplantation
➤ Diagnosis of nodular hyperplasia or Budd-Chiari syndrome, which causes hepatic venous flow obstruction
➤ Evaluation of tumors of the pancreas or other intra-abdominal masses before surgery to determine advisability of resection
➤ Suspected mesenteric venous thrombosis or varices of the colon or small bowel
➤ Determination of portal vein pressure to diagnose portal hypertension as well as other liver diseases that produce venous obstruction[27]

Contraindications

➤ Pregnancy, unless the benefits of performing the procedure greatly outweigh the risks to the fetus
➤ Allergy to iodinated contrast medium, unless prophylactic medications are administered before the procedure or a nonionic dye is used
➤ Bleeding disorder or severely impaired liver or renal function
➤ Presence of ascites

Nursing Care Before the Procedure

Client teaching and physical preparation are the same as for any angiographic procedure (see pp. 656 to 657).
➤ ECG monitoring of heart activity is not necessary for this procedure unless the client's cardiovascular status is at risk.

The Procedure

The client is placed on the x-ray table in a supine position. The site—usually the femoral for the indirect approach or the upper right quadrant (URQ) for the direct approach—is cleansed and draped to prepare a sterile field for the procedure. The site is anesthetized by local injection. Portal angiography requires a direct approach that involves transhepatic or transplenic insertion of a needle through the skin, as in percutaneous transhepatic cholangiography (PTHC), into the splenic or superior mesenteric vein followed by the injection of the contrast material. Portal venous pressure can be taken with this procedure before x-ray filming by the insertion of the catheter into the hepatic vein until it occludes blood outflow from the vein.[28] In the indirect approach used for hepatic arteriography or venography, the femoral site is used. The catheter is inserted into the femoral artery and advanced to the common hepatic artery via the superior mesenteric artery or gastric artery in arteriography. The catheter is inserted into the femoral vein and advanced into the major hepatic vein for venography. All catheter or needle placements are guided by fluoroscopic viewing.

Dye injection rates depend on the flow rates within the vessels and the projected length of times needed for filming. Filming after dye injection is rapid for a few seconds and then slowed for about 30 seconds to include parenchymal and venous phases of hepatic arteriography and portography. When the procedure is completed, the catheter or needle is removed and pressure is applied to the site. A pressure dressing is then applied and taped in place.

Nursing Care After the Procedure

Care and assessment after the procedure are the same as for any angiographic procedure (see p. 658).

➤ *Liver or splenic hemorrhage:* Note and report changes in vital signs, such as tachycardia, hypotension, or abdominal pain. Administer ordered blood transfusion. Prepare for possible splenectomy in extreme cases.

RENAL ANGIOGRAPHY

Renal angiography allows x-ray visualization of the large and small arteries of the renal vasculature and parenchyma or of the renal veins and their branches, depending on the studies to be performed. It can be done to determine the vascularity, arterial supply, and extent of venous invasion in the evaluation of renal tumors as well as to identify other abnormalities and to study prospective renal donors.[29]

The study is performed by catheterization of the femoral artery or vein, with the advancement of the catheter through the iliac artery and aorta into the renal artery or into the inferior vena cava and renal vein. Imaging for caval patency followed by imaging to study the renal arterial, parenchymal, and venous phases can be performed with the catheter in the inferior vena cava. Depending on the results, insertion of an arterial catheter can follow, including aortography with subsequent arterial examination.

Reference Values

Normal structure, function, and patency of renal vessels; no evidence of obstruction, malformations, cysts, tumors, or variations in number and size of vessels and organs

Interfering Factors

➤ Inability of client to cooperate and remain still during the procedure
➤ Failure to withhold sodium in the diet or medications that interfere with the accurate analysis of a blood sample taken for renin in renal venography
➤ Presence of gas or feces in the gastrointestinal tract or barium left in the tract from recent radiologic studies

Indications for Renal Angiography

➤ Persistent hematuria of unresolved cause
➤ Detection of renal tumors by the arterial supply, extent of venous invasion, and tumor vascularity
➤ Differentiation between tumors and renal cysts for operative planning

➤ Detection of nonmalignant tumors before surgical resection
➤ Evaluation of renovascular hypertension caused by the atherosclerotic lesions that result in the narrowing or occlusion of arteries and renal insufficiency
➤ Suspected renal artery stenosis causing vessel dilation, collateral vessel formation, or increased renovascular pressure
➤ Suspected arterial occlusion caused by transection of the renal artery as a result of trauma or penetrating injury
➤ Detection of abscess or inflammatory conditions, aneurysm, or A-V abnormalities revealed by renal arteriography
➤ Definition of arterial anatomy to evaluate the vascularity of a tumor before surgery or embolization
➤ Evaluation of anatomy of renal vascular system of prospective kidney donors to detect unsuspected renal disease before surgery[30]
➤ Evaluation of postoperative renal transplantation for function or organ rejection
➤ Diagnosis of thrombosis revealed by renal venography
➤ Detection of small kidney or absence of a kidney
➤ Determination of relationship of the renal arterial vasculature to the aorta
➤ Determination of renal function in chronic renal failure, end-stage renal disease, or hydronephrosis
➤ Collection of a sample of blood from the renal vein for renin analysis in the diagnosis of renovascular hypertension[31]

Contraindications

➤ Pregnancy, unless the benefits of performing the procedure greatly outweigh the risks to the fetus
➤ Allergy to iodinated contrast medium, unless prophylactic medications are administered before the study
➤ Bleeding disorder
➤ End-stage renal failure or severe thrombosis of the inferior vena cava or renal vein[32]

Nursing Care Before the Procedure

Client teaching and physical preparation are the same as for any angiographic procedure (see pp. 656 to 657).

➤ Advise the client to eat a special salt-free diet and, if venography is planned to obtain a blood sample for renin level, restrict current medications that include antihypertensives, diuretics, or hormones before the procedure.
➤ Administer a laxative the day before or an enema the day of the study to clear the bowel of feces or barium if ordered.

The Procedure

The client is placed on the x-ray table in a supine position. The site, usually femoral, is cleansed and draped to provide a sterile field for the procedure. The site is injected with a local anesthetic, and the artery (renal arteriography) or vein (renal venography) is punctured and the guide wire inserted. The catheter is inserted over the guide wire and advanced into the aorta and then into the renal artery for arteriography or into the inferior vena cava and then the renal vein for venography. Catheter advancement and placement are achieved under the guidance of fluoroscopic viewing. Blood samples can be obtained from each renal vein for analysis in venography. The contrast medium is injected, and a series of rapid x-rays are taken during and after the filling of the vessels to be examined. Filming can also take place after the dye injection for additional delayed studies or for filming the venous phase of the procedure. At the conclusion of the study, the catheter is removed and pressure is applied to the site. A pressure dressing is then applied and taped in place.

Nursing Care After the Procedure

Care and assessment after the procedure are the same as for any angiographic procedure (see p. 658).

➤ Renal function tests such as blood urea nitrogen (BUN) and creatinine are performed if compromised renal function as a result of the test is suspected.

MESENTERIC ANGIOGRAPHY

Mesenteric angiography involves the x-ray examination of the gastrointestinal vasculature after the injection of an iodinated contrast medium. Serial films that include arterial, capillary, and venous perfusion are taken of the abdominal vasculature. The catheter is inserted into the femoral artery with the advancement into the aorta followed by placement into the superior or inferior mesenteric artery or the celiac artery (Fig. 18–5).[33]

The study can include therapeutic as well as diagnostic angiographic procedures involving the abdominal aorta to identify abnormalities and the stomach, pancreas, and small and large intestines to identify an acute bleeding source and perform perfusion or embolization to control the hemorrhage.

Reference Values

Normal vascular structure and patency; no bleeding activity or ischemia in the blood vessels of the gastrointestinal organs

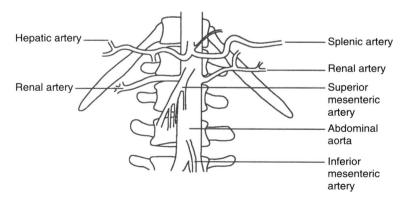

Hepatic artery —
Renal artery —
Splenic artery
Renal artery
Superior mesenteric artery
Abdominal aorta
Inferior mesenteric artery

Figure 18–5   Abdominal aorta, superior and inferior mesenteric arterial vessels.

Interfering Factors

➤ Inability of client to cooperate and remain still during the procedure

➤ Atherosclerotic lesions in the vessel to be cannulated, preventing passage of the catheter

➤ Presence of gas or feces in the gastrointestinal tract or barium remaining from radiologic studies

Indications for Mesenteric Angiography

➤ Diagnosing colonic diverticula, angiodysplasia, Meckel's diverticulum, or inflammatory bowel disease, all of which could become a source of internal bleeding

➤ Determining the source and cause of stomach, pancreas, or small- or large-bowel bleeding when other diagnostic procedures such as endoscopy, radionuclide scan, or barium studies have failed to reveal or resolve the problem

➤ Identifying bleeding site in the tract before surgery or treatment to control hemorrhage

➤ Determining the status of mesenteric circulation or the condition of the iliac or common femoral arteries before surgery to correct and perform graft for abdominal aortic aneurysm

➤ Infusing arterial vasopressin (Pitressin) or performing arterial embolization therapy with a gelatin sponge (Gelfoam) when other measures have failed to control bleeding

➤ Detecting portal or mesenteric venous thrombosis during venous phase of study

➤ Diagnosing acute mesenteric ischemia in the presence of thrombus, embolus, or venous occlusion

➤ Evaluating the extent of a suspected abdominal aortic aneurysm

➤ Detecting islet cell tumor of the pancreas not diagnosed by other studies such as ultrasonography or computerized scanning[34]

➤ Evaluating suspected aortoenteric fistula of intestinal angina[35]

➤ Detecting type (splenic or hepatic) and extent of rupture or injury from trauma that affects major vessels

Contraindications

➤ Pregnancy, unless the benefits of performing the procedure greatly outweigh the risks to the fetus

➤ Allergy to iodinated contrast medium, unless prophylactic medications are administered before the study

➤ Bleeding or coagulation disorder

Nursing Care Before the Procedure

Client teaching and physical preparation are the same as for any angiographic procedure (see pp. 656 to 657).

➤ Administer a laxative the day before or an enema the day of the study to clear the bowel of feces or barium if ordered.

The Procedure

The client is placed on the x-ray table in a supine position. An abdominal flat plate film can be taken at this time. The puncture site, usually the femoral artery, is cleansed and draped to prepare a sterile field for the procedure. The site is anesthetized by local injection, and the catheter is inserted and advanced into the abdominal aorta under fluoroscopic viewing. Dye is injected for filming of the aortic structure and patency. After filming of the abdominal aorta, the catheter is advanced into the celiac superior or inferior mesenteric artery. The injection of the dye is adjusted to match the blood flow of these vessels, and a series of rapid filming are made. The catheter can then be further advanced into the branches of the major artery, and rapid sequence films can be made during and after the dye injection. The filming can then be slowed for capillary and venous phases to complete the study. At the conclusion of the study, the catheter is removed, and pressure is applied to the site. A pressure dressing is then applied and taped in place.

Nursing Care After the Procedure

Care and assessment after the procedure are the same as for any angiographic procedure (see p. 658).

➤ Assess and monitor vital signs if therapeutic procedures were performed to control bleeding in order to determine whether bleeding is persisting.

FLUORESCEIN ANGIOGRAPHY (FA)

Fluorescein angiography (FA) is the rapid filming in color of the retinal vasculature and circulation after the IV injection of a contrast medium known as sodium fluorescein. The study is performed to diagnose eye abnormalities caused by changes in the retinal vasculature. The dye is rapidly injected into the antecubital space (vein) and within 12 to 15 seconds fills the arteries, capillaries, and veins of the retina.[36]

A special camera is used for this study instead of the conventional radiologic equipment. The images taken in sequence and manipulated by a computer can provide views of abnormalities during any of the stages involved in the filling and emptying of the dye in the retinal vessels.

Reference Values

Normal retina and retinal and choroidal vessels; no evidence of vascular abnormalities such as hemorrhage, retinopathy, aneurysm, or obstruction as a result of stenosis

Interfering Factors

➤ Inability of client to keep eyelids open and eyes in a fixed position
➤ Presence of cataracts
➤ Improper dilation of pupils

Indications for Fluorescein Angiography (FA)

➤ Detecting vascular disorders that affect visual acuity
➤ Detecting tumors, retinal edema, or inflammation by the degree or patterns of fluorescence during the study
➤ Diagnosing past reduced flow or patency of the vascular circulation of the retina by presence of neovascularization

➤ Diagnosing macular degeneration in elderly persons and any associated hemorrhage that might be present

➤ Diagnosing diabetic retinopathy caused by long-term diabetes mellitus

➤ Detecting microaneurysms caused by hypertensive retinopathy

➤ Detecting collateral circulation resulting from arterial or venous occlusion caused by stenosis with a reduced, delayed, or absent flow of the dye through the vessels or possible leakage of the dye from the vessel[37]

Contraindications

➤ Allergy to iodinated contrast medium, unless medications are administered before the study

Nursing Care Before the Procedure

Explain to the client:

➤ That the time required to complete the procedure is about 1 hour

➤ That there are no food or fluid restrictions but that eye medications should be withheld on the day of the procedure

➤ That eyedrops to dilate the pupils will be instilled before the procedure

➤ That the client will be exposed to bright light and will be requested to remain still and fixate the eyes during the procedure

➤ That the contrast medium is injected into a vein in the arm, which will cause some nausea or feeling of warmth for a short time

➤ That the dye can cause skin and urine to appear yellow for 1 to 2 days after the study

Prepare for the procedure:

➤ Ensure that restriction of eye medications has been followed.

➤ Obtain a history of allergy to iodine or other sensitivities, visual problems, and known or suspected eye conditions.

➤ Remove constricting clothing from the waist up and provide client with a hospital gown, if needed.

➤ Have client void.

➤ Obtain and record baseline vital signs for later comparison readings.

➤ Administer ordered mydriatics for pupil dilation, usually every 5 minutes for 30 minutes.

The Procedure

The client is seated in a chair that faces the camera. The eyes are checked to ensure that dilation has been achieved. Films are taken by the photographic camera instead of conventional x-ray before any dye is injected. An IV line is initiated in the brachial vein to administer the dye. The client is requested to place the chin and forehead in position and the head is immobilized. The client is then requested to open the eyes wide and look straight ahead. The fluorescein dye is then injected into the vein, and a rapid sequence of photos is taken and repeated after the dye has reached the retinal vascular system. Follow-up photographs are then taken in 20 to 30 minutes.[38] At the conclusion of the procedure, the IV needle is removed and a Band-Aid is applied to the site.

Nursing Care After the Procedure

➤ Care and assessment after the procedure include taking vital signs and comparing them with the baseline readings.

➤ Inform the client that visual acuity and responses to light can temporarily change and that dark glasses can be worn if the client so desires.

➤ Inform the client that driving is restricted for 4 hours after the study or until the pupils return to normal.

➤ Inform the client that the skin and urine may develop a yellowish cast for up to 2 days, but it will then disappear.

➤ *Reaction to fluorescein dye:* Note and report delayed feeling of faintness, increased salivation, dry mouth, urticaria, sneezing, and changes in breathing pattern. Administer antihistamine and steroid therapy as ordered.

LYMPHANGIOGRAPHY

Lymphangiography involves x-ray examination of the lymphatic flow and nodal patterns. The lymphatic vessels in the foot or hand are injected with an iodinated oil-based contrast medium such as Lipiodol or Ethiodol and vital dye such as methylene blue or isosulfan blue. Films in different positions to provide various views are made of the abdomen and chest to reveal the lymphatic channels and any displacement or collateral formation. The same films are taken in 24 hours to assess the lymph nodes, making this a 2-day study to formulate a diagnosis of neoplastic disease.[39] Abnormal findings include pathological nodes identified by enlargement or filling defects and presence of obstructed lymphatic flow patterns. In addition to this procedure, ultrasonography, computerized scan, and node biopsy can be performed to substantiate malignancies.

Reference Values

Normal structure and patency of lymphatic system and nodes; no filling defects, obstruction, or hyperplasia

Interfering Factors

➤ None

Indications for Lymphangiography

➤ Suspected pathology of the lymphatics, such as lymphoma or tumor metastasis to lymph nodes, revealed by node size and filling defects

➤ Determination of the stage of lymphoma between stage I and stage IV to identify extent of involvement ranging from a single node to diffuse metastasis, especially in Hodgkin's lymphoma[40]

➤ Diagnosis of testicular tumor, prostatic carcinoma, and cervical carcinoma when performed in association with ultrasonography, computerized scanning, and node biopsy procedures[41]

➤ Differentiation between primary and secondary lymphedema in an extremity

➤ Evaluation of nodal involvement before treatment regimen and possible surgical intervention

➤ Evaluation of effectiveness of therapy (chemotherapy or radiation) or progression of the disease

Contraindications

➤ Pregnancy, unless benefits of performing the procedure outweigh the risks to the fetus

➤ Allergy to the contrast medium, unless prophylactic medications are administered before the study

➤ Poor or severely impaired pulmonary, cardiac, renal, or hepatic function

Nursing Care Before the Procedure

Client teaching and physical preparation are the same as for any angiographic procedure (see pp. 656 to 657).

➤ Inform the client that the procedure can take as long as 3 hours.

➤ Inform the client that food and fluids are not restricted and that a temporary blue tinge in the skin will appear at the entry site and in the urine and feces after the study because of the dye injection.

The Procedure

The client is placed on the x-ray table in a supine position. Injections of Evans blue or methylene blue dye are administered intradermally into the webs between the first three toes or into the medial and lateral webs. The client is requested to walk at this time to enhance visualization of the lymphatics of the feet. The feet are then cleansed and draped to provide a sterile field for the procedure. A local anesthetic is injected over the dorsum of the foot after a vessel is selected. The client is informed that this injection causes slight pain. An incision is made over the selected lymphatic vessel, which is carefully dissected and then cannulated with a needle connected to tubing filled with the contrast medium, usually an ethiodized oil. The dye is slowly injected into the channel of both feet, and x-ray films are taken to confirm the filling of the lymphatics. After completion of the study, the needles are removed and the incisions are sutured. Dressings are then applied and taped in place.

The filming that follows includes AP and oblique views of the pelvis and abdomen. A lateral view of the abdomen and AP view of the chest can also be filmed.[42] These views provide visualization of the thoracic and supraclavicular as well as the iliac and aortic nodes. The same procedure performed on the hands provides visualization of the axillary and supraclavicular nodes.[43] Additional films are taken in 24 hours and can be repeated for up to 1 year after the procedure because the oil can remain in the nodes for that length of time.

Nursing Care After the Procedure

Care and assessment after the procedure are the same as for any angiographic procedure (see p. 658).

➤ Monitor the extremity for sensation changes and the site for possible infection.

➤ Apply warm compresses to the sites if ordered for discomfort.

➤ Remind the client to return in 24 hours for more films.

➤ Inform the client that the skin, urine, and feces can be blue-tinged for about 2 days.

➤ *Pulmonary emboli, lipid pneumonia:* Note and report dyspnea, chest pain, or hypotension. Monitor vital signs, respiratory pattern, and breath sounds. Administer ordered oxygen and medications.

UPPER EXTREMITY ANGIOGRAPHY

Upper extremity angiography, not performed as frequently as lower extremity angiography, involves x-ray visualization of the arterial or venous system of the hand and arm after injection of an iodinated contrast medium (Fig. 18–6). Low-osmolar agents and digital subtraction angiographic techniques have reduced the pain associated with the injection of the material to perform this procedure. Catheterization and injection sites are dependent on the extent of the arm or hand, or arm and hand, to be examined and the presenting signs and symptoms indicating obstruction, ischemia, vasospasms, lesions, or trauma. Both diagnostic and therapeutic procedures can be performed.

Reference Values

Normal structure and patency of the hand and arm vascular system; no thrombosis or obstruction in the veins and no claudication, aneurysms, or embolization of the arteries

Interfering Factors

➤ Cold environmental temperature that affects the vascular tone and blood flow in the digits
➤ Vasospasms that affect the filling of the digital vessels with dye

Indications for Upper Extremity Angiography

➤ Diagnosis of Raynaud's phenomenon with or without a fixed vascular occlusion

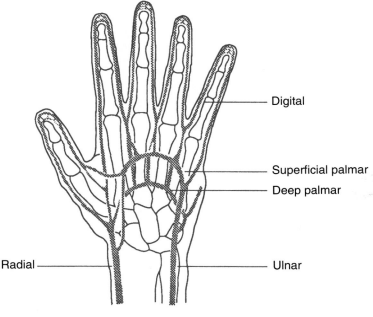

Digital

Superficial palmar
Deep palmar

Radial

Ulnar

Figure 18–6 Hand and wrist arterial vessels.

➤ Determination of unilateral or bilateral Raynaud's phenomenon in the diagnosis of an underlying arterial condition

➤ Differentiation between atherosclerosis and thromboangiitis obliterans by the involvement of proximal or distal vessels, respectively[44]

➤ Claudication to determine the extent of arterial involvement

➤ Determination of the cause of embolization, such as atherosclerosis or aneurysms

➤ Diagnosis of thoracic outlet syndrome by venous obstruction and thrombosis or arterial compression

➤ Diagnosis of arterial or venous insufficiency caused by repeated trauma or other injuries such as thermal or electric shock to the extremity[45]

➤ Determination of a treatment plan based on study findings for thrombolysis in arterial or venous thrombosis or balloon angioplasty for subclavian arterial stenosis

Contraindications

➤ Pregnancy, if filming other than the hand and arm is planned

➤ Allergy to iodinated contrast medium, unless prophylactic medications are administered before the procedure

➤ Edema of the extremity

Nursing Care Before the Procedure

Client teaching and physical preparation are the same as for any angiographic procedure (see pp. 656 to 657).

The Procedure

The client is placed on the x-ray table in a supine position. The groin is cleansed and draped to prepare a sterile field for a femoral arterial approach. In cases of proximal disease or atherosclerosis, the axillary or brachial artery can be used as a site for cannulation. The site is anesthetized by local injection, and the catheter is inserted and advanced through the intrathoracic arteries and into the axillary artery for distal injection of the dye and down into the distal brachial artery if the hand is to be studied. The dye is then injected, and the filming is performed. Digital subtraction angiography can also be performed to reduce the pain associated with the procedure.

To enhance filling of the vessels, spasms can be counteracted by the administration of tolazoline (Priscoline) or phentolamine (Regitine) injected intra-arterially with immediate filming performed. The extremity can be warmed with a heating pad combined with the injection to produce optimal vascular tone and blood flow for the best filming of hand angiography.[46]

At the completion of the procedure, the catheter is removed and pressure is applied to the site. A pressure dressing is then applied and taped in place.

Nursing Care After the Procedure

Care and assessment after the procedure are the same as for any angiographic procedure (p. 658).

LOWER EXTREMITY ANGIOGRAPHY

Lower extremity angiography allows x-ray visualization of the arteries or veins of the leg or foot after the injection of an iodinated contrast medium (Fig. 18–7). Abdominal aortography to evaluate aneurysms preoperatively and pelvic angiography to evaluate mesenteric circulation can also be performed with these studies.[47] In addition to the diagnostic aspects of the procedure, it can be performed for therapeutic reasons. Catheterization or injection sites, or both, are chosen according to the areas and vessels to be examined. Abnormal results include filling defects, vasospasms, lesions, stenosis, and occlusion associated with aortic, arterial, or venous disease.

Reference Values

Normal structure and patency of the leg and foot vascular system; no arterial occlusion, embolus, inflammation, or claudication; no venous thrombosis or incompetence

Interfering Factors

➤ Inability of client to remain still during the procedure
➤ Improper tourniquet or dye injection technique

Indications for Lower Extremity Angiography

➤ Determining the presence of a tumor compressing the arterial or venous system, causing obstruction

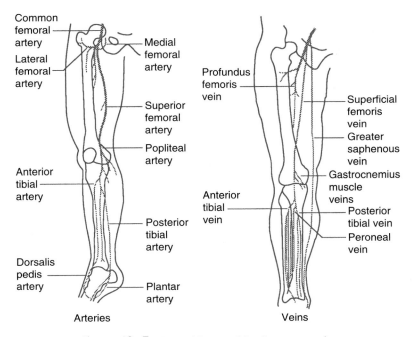

Figure 18–7 Leg and foot arterial and venous vessels.

➤ Diagnosing athero-occlusive disease in clients with diabetes mellitus or peripheral arterial embolus

➤ Determining the effect of thromboangiitis obliterans on the small and medium-sized vessels of the extremity

➤ Determining the cause of claudication or thrombosis such as popliteal entrapment syndrome, cystic adventitial disease, or atherosclerotic disease

➤ Evaluating A-V malformation or other congenital abnormality

➤ Suspected vascular injury to extremity, penetrating and nonpenetrating, that disrupts or occludes arteries or veins or both

➤ Determining the level of limb amputation caused by vascular occlusion after frostbite or electrical injury

➤ Administering thrombolytic agents such as urokinase (Abbokinase)

➤ Identifying and evaluating veins considered for use in bypass graft surgery[48]

➤ Evaluating known or unknown deep venous thrombosis of lower extremity by a defect in intraluminal filling when ascending venography is performed

➤ Evaluating deep venous insufficiency or varicose vein status before vein ligation or stripping

➤ Suspected venous valvular incompetence by descending venography in the presence of venous stasis symptoms

Contraindications

➤ Allergy to iodinated contrast medium, unless prophylactic medications are administered before the study

➤ Edema of the extremity if access to the vessel is not possible

➤ Impaired renal function or bleeding disorder

➤ Poorly controlled hypertension

Nursing Care Before the Procedure

Client teaching and physical preparation are the same as for any angiographic procedure (see pp. 656 to 657).

The Procedure

For arterial studies, the client is placed on the x-ray table in the supine position. The femoral arterial site is used for abdominal aortography and lower extremity arteriography unless occlusive disease prevents its use. Alternative sites are the axillary or the brachial artery. The site is anesthetized by local injection, and the catheter is advanced into the distal abdominal aorta under fluoroscopic guidance. A specified amount of contrast medium is injected at a calculated rate and period of time. Step-table filming is performed that includes three films at the level of the pelvis, then two films at the level of the thighs, four films of the knees, and then six films at the level of the calf. Further filming of the distal vessels of the ankle and foot can be performed in clients with diabetes mellitus, ulcers, or gangrene. This method of filming can be complemented with digital subtraction angiography to perform complete lower extremity studies by filling in areas of special interest or to examine lower extremities separately in obese clients. Warming of the feet and legs by application of external heat, use of an occlusive cuff on the thigh, and intra-arterial injection of a vasodilator such as tolazoline (Priscoline) or dilute nitroglycerin can be administered immediately before the filming to enhance distal vascular opacification.[49]

Ascending phlebography or descending venography can be performed for deep venous thrombosis or venous incompetence as a basis for the study. For lower limb ascending phlebography, the client is placed on a tilting table in a supine position. The dorsum of the foot of the extremity to be examined is cleansed and the table tilted in a semiupright position that allows more complete filling of the vein. Weight bearing is allowed on the foot not being examined to allow for optimal relaxation of the extremity that is prepared for the study. A superficial vein is catheterized and the contrast material is injected slowly after preparation of the site. The flow is monitored by fluoroscopic visualization. A tourniquet can be placed above the ankle and the knee to encourage the dye to flow into the deeper veins, if policy allows this technique. After the injection, spot films are taken in various views over the thigh, calf, knee, and also the foot, if a study of this area is desired. Supine venography can be performed in clients who cannot be maintained in the semiupright position. This position requires that tourniquets be used and that contrast medium be administered by continuous infusion rather than by manual injection. In either position, a cutdown to expose a vein for cannulation can be performed if one cannot be used for a superficial injection of the dye.[50]

For lower limb descending venography, the client is placed on the x-ray table in a supine position. The site can be an arm vein or a femoral vein from the side opposite the one to be examined. After preparation of the site, the vein is cannulated and the contrast medium is injected. The dye can also be injected directly into the femoral vein of the side to be examined via a needle or catheter. After the injection, the reflux of the dye is viewed by fluoroscopy and graded from 0 to 5, indicating absence of reflux to reflux at the level of the ankle. The examination is performed with the table tilted to the upright position or in the horizontal position while the client performs Valsalva's maneuver. At the conclusion of the study, the client is returned to the horizontal position.[51]

At the completion of any of the procedures, the needle or catheter is removed, and pressure is applied to the site. A pressure dressing is applied and taped in place.

Nursing Care After the Procedure

Care and assessment after the procedure are the same as for any angiographic procedure (see p. 658).

➤ If a cutdown is performed, inform the client of the need and the time to have the sutures removed and to report any redness, swelling, or pain at the site.

(Case Study follows on page 681)

Student Name _____ Class _____

Instructor _____ Date _____

CASE STUDY AND CRITICAL THINKING EXERCISE

Ms. White, age 35, is admitted to the clinic for evaluation of hypertension. In the last 3 months, her blood pressure readings have been 140/84, 165/84, and 170/90. Today the reading is 190/110. You also note an abdominal bruit. She had no history of hypertension until 3 months ago and her family history is negative for hypertension. A renal angiogram is ordered.

a. What is the probable diagnosis in this case?

b. How does hypertension occur in this case?

c. What might renal angiography confirm?

References

1. Thomas, CL (ed): Taber's Cyclopedic Medical Dictionary, ed 18. FA Davis, Philadelphia, 1997, p 106.
2. Berkow, R: The Merck Manual, ed 16. Merck Sharp and Dohme Research Laboratory, Rahway, NJ, 1992, p 407.
3. Wojtowycz, M: Interventional Radiology and Angiography. Year Book Medical Publishers, Chicago, 1990, p 10.
4. Ibid, pp 12–13.
5. Ibid, pp 15–16.
6. Corbett, JV: Laboratory Tests and Diagnostic Procedures with Nursing Diagnoses, ed 3. Appleton & Lange, Norwalk, Conn, 1992, p 528.
7. Wojtowycz, op cit, pp 12–13.
8. Fischbach, FT: A Manual of Laboratory and Diagnostic Tests, ed 4. JB Lippincott, Philadelphia, 1992, pp 678–679.
9. Wojtowycz, op cit, pp 19–20.
10. Ibid, p 18.
11. Pagana, KD, and Pagana, TJ: Mosby's Diagnostic and Laboratory Test Reference. Mosby–Year Book, St Louis, 1992, p 153.
12. Fischbach, op cit, p 901.
13. Wojtowycz, op cit, pp 2, 10.
14. Springhouse Corporation: Nurse's Reference Library: Diagnostics, ed 2. Springhouse, Springhouse, Pa, 1986, p 927.
15. Pagana and Pagana, op cit, p 5.
16. Ibid, pp 5, 8.
17. Ibid, pp 5–10.
18. Ibid, p 166.
19. Nurse's Reference Library, op cit, p 927.
20. Corbett, op cit, pp 527–528.
21. Wojtowycz, op cit, pp 241–242.
22. Ibid, pp 242–245.
23. Ibid, p 128.
24. Ibid, p 128.
25. Ibid, p 83.
26. Ibid, pp 65–66.
27. Ibid, pp 65–66, 77, 83–84.
28. Ibid, pp 66, 88–91.
29. Ibid, pp 49–50.
30. Ibid, pp 49–50.
31. Nurse's Reference Library, op cit, p 979.
32. Ibid, pp 976–980.
33. Ibid, p 840.
34. Wojtowycz, op cit, pp 109–112.
35. Ibid, p 101.
36. Ibid, p 571.
37. Nurse's Reference Library, op cit, p 573.
38. Fischbach, op cit, pp 878–879.
39. Wojtowycz, op cit, pp 267–268.
40. Ibid, p 265.
41. Ibid, pp 266–267.
42. Ibid, p 268.
43. Fischbach, op cit, p 666.
44. Wojtowycz, op cit, pp 133–134, 138.
45. Ibid, pp 134–135.
46. Ibid, p 135.
47. Ibid, p 25.
48. Ibid, pp 26, 227.
49. Ibid, p 135.
50. Ibid, pp 228–232.
51. Ibid, p 235.

Bibliography

Bernstein, EF (ed): Vascular Diagnosis, ed 4. Mosby–Year Book, St Louis, 1993.

Black, JM, and Matassarin-Jacobs, M: Luckmann and Sorensen's Medical-Surgical Nursing: A Psychophysiologic Approach, ed 4. WB Saunders, Philadelphia, 1993.

Chernecky, CC, and Berger, BJ; Cullen, BN (ed): Laboratory Tests and Diagnostic Procedures, ed 2. WB Saunders, Philadelphia, 1996.

Clement, DL, and Shepherd, J: Vascular Diseases of the Limbs: Mechanisms and Principles of Treatment. Mosby–Year Book, St Louis, 1993.

Friedman, AC, and Dachman, A: Radiology of Liver, Biliary Tract, and Pancreas. Mosby–Year Book, St Louis, 1993.

Harney, B, et al: Color Atlas of Fluorescein Angiography. Mosby–Year Book, St Louis, 1993.

Kadir, S: Atlas of Normal and Variant Angiographic Anatomy. WB Saunders, Philadelphia, 1990.

Kadir, S: Diagnostic Angiography: Monographs in Clinical Radiology. WB Saunders, Philadelphia, 1986.

Kapp, JP, and Schmidek, HH: The Cerebral Venous System and Its Disorders. WB Saunders, Philadelphia, 1984.

Kee, JL: Handbook of Laboratory and Diagnostic Tests with Nursing Implications, ed 3. Appleton & Lange, Norwalk, Conn, 1997.

Kern, MJ (ed): The Cardiac Catheterization Handbook, ed 2. Mosby–Year Book, St Louis, 1994.

Kim, D, and Orron, DE: Peripheral Vascular Imaging and Intervention. Mosby–Year Book, St Louis, 1992.

Pagana, KD, and Pagana, TJ: Diagnostic Testing and Nursing Implications: A Case Study Approach, ed 4. Mosby–Year Book, St Louis, 1993.

Porth, CM: Pathophysiology: Concepts of Altered Health States, ed 4. JB Lippincott, Philadelphia, 1993.

Reuter, SR, et al: Gastrointestinal Angiography, ed 3. WB Saunders, Philadelphia, 1986.

Springhouse Corporation: Nurse's Reference Library: Diagnostic Tests. Springhouse, Springhouse, Pa, 1991.

Tilkian, SM: Clinical and Nursing Implications of Laboratory Tests, ed 5. Mosby–Year Book, St Louis, 1995.

Tonken, ILD: Pediatric Cardiovascular Imaging. WB Saunders, Philadelphia, 1991.

Whaley, LF: Nursing Care of Infants and Children, ed 4. Mosby–Year Book, St Louis, 1991.

19

Ultrasound Studies

➤ **PROCEDURES COVERED**

Echocardiography, *688*
Echoencephalography, *691*
Transesophageal
 Echocardiography, *692*
Ocular Ultrasonography, *693*
Thyroid/Parathyroid
 Ultrasonography, *695*
Thoracic Ultrasonography, *696*
Lymph Nodes/Retroperitoneal
 Ultrasonography, *697*
Abdominal/Aortic
 Ultrasonography, *698*
Spleen Ultrasonography, *700*
Pancreatic Ultrasonography, *702*
Liver/Biliary System
 Ultrasonography, *703*

Kidney Ultrasonography, *705*
Bladder Ultrasonography, *706*
Prostate Ultrasonography, *707*
Scrotal Ultrasonography, *708*
Breast Ultrasonography, *709*
Pelvic Ultrasonography, *711*
Obstetric Ultrasonography, *712*
Arterial Doppler Extremity
 Studies, *715*
Arterial Doppler Carotid
 Studies, *717*
Arterial Doppler Transcranial
 Studies, *719*
Venous Doppler Extremity
 Studies, *720*

INTRODUCTION

Ultrasound is a noninvasive instrumentation procedure that uses sound waves in the frequency range of 20,000 to 10 billion cycles per second, a sound range beyond that audible to the human ear, to obtain diagnostic information or to perform therapeutic protocols.[1] One cycle per second is equal to 1 hertz (Hz), the unit of measure used to identify the frequency of sound waves. These high-frequency waves are directed into internal tissues of the body and reflected back to a transducer. They are then electronically processed and appear as images on a display screen or oscilloscope for immediate visualization; they are also transformed into audible sounds. The speed of the waves depends on the density and elasticity of the structures as the waves pass through, resulting in differences that depend on tissue abnormalities. The time it takes sound waves to reach the tissue and return to the transducer is recorded on film, moving chart, videotape, or digital recording medium for a permanent record of the study.[2] The recording is known as an echogram or sonogram; these terms are used interchangeably with ultrasound studies.

Techniques to display the echo wave image include A and B modes. The A mode presents the information in a graphic form as in echocardiogram or echoencephalogram. The B mode presents the information in varying intensities of brightness by the use of dots that coalesce to form an anatomic outline as in fetal, pancreatic, kidney, spleen, and bladder sonograms. Real-time scanning uses a multiple transducer to display rapid sequencing of motion that resembles a movie. It allows imaging of a moving fetus, the motion of the heart, and the movement involved with larger blood vessels.[3] The presence of fluid provides an excellent medium for transmission of the waves to organs or other area to be visualized.

The diagnostic value of ultrasound studies is in the ability of the sound waves of varying intensities to outline the shape and position of organs and tissue of the body and the ability to detect pathology such as masses, edema, stones, and displacement of adjacent tissues. These abilities are possible because abnormal tissue is of a different density and elasticity than is the normal tissue in the same area. Because ultrasonography can be performed quickly, it is frequently used when time is important. It is limited as a useful diagnostic method in studies of bones or of air- or gas-filled organs such as the lungs or intestines. Because of this limitation, portions of the body with these organs situated between the beam and the study site render the ultrasound procedure ineffective and inconclusive.[4] Depending on pathological findings revealed with ultrasound, more invasive studies such as radiology or radionuclide scanning can follow to further clarify and diagnose abnormalities.

Ultrasound studies are performed on inpatients and outpatients in the hospital, physician's office, or medical imaging agency in a specially equipped room. A skilled technician usually performs the procedure to ensure satisfactory studies, and a radiologist with special education and expertise interprets the findings. No anesthesia is needed because no pain is experienced during ultrasonography. Signed informed consent forms are not required for these studies unless accompanied by fine-needle biopsy.

The ultrasound procedure is also used therapeutically in frequencies at least 20 times higher than those used for diagnostic studies. They are delivered in a continuous manner when performing the therapy and generate heat that treats the pain associated with low back pain syndrome and that destroys malignant tumor cells.[5]

DOPPLER ULTRASOUND TECHNIQUE

The Doppler method encompasses techniques that transform sound waves into audible sounds heard with the use of earphones. The sound waves are produced when the ultrasound beam is passed through an area of moving blood or fluid to a receiving transducer that amplifies the sounds heard as pulsations (Fig. 19–1). Varying frequencies result from the effect of the sound waves on the different movements of blood or fluid. These pulsating structures can also be displayed as wave motion or forms on a screen and recorded. The technique allows assessment of blood flow through arteries and veins by the monitoring of pulses or sounds in clients with chronic perfusion problems. The sounds vary with the patency of the vessel being examined.

The Doppler technique combined with real-time imaging is known as duplex scanning. It provides flow imaging (Doppler) and vessel function (real-time) to diagnose the presence of aneurysms, plaque formation in arteries, and thromboses in veins or to evaluate the rejection of a kidney transplant.[6] The Doppler ultrasound also allows assessment of blood flow through heart valves as in Doppler echocardiography and for the evaluation of patency of recent ar-

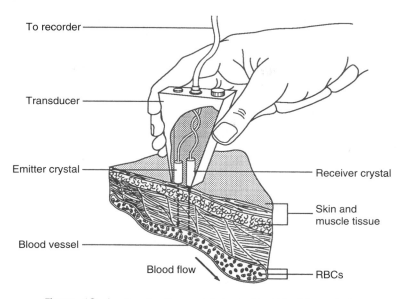

To recorder

Transducer

Emitter crystal

Receiver crystal

Skin and muscle tissue

Blood vessel

Blood flow

RBCs

Figure 19–1 Doppler ultrasound device to detect blood flow velocity.

terial grafts. In critical situations, the techniques can be used to monitor shock states by obtaining serial blood readings when accurate audible readings are not possible. Doppler ultrasound studies on extremities require a normal extremity to use for comparison readings and calculation of the pressure index.

The monitoring of fetal heart tones can be accomplished with the Doppler stethoscope, and the monitoring of the fetus during labor and birth can be accomplished with a technique that uses a transducer and a Doppler instrument. This technique is also used to obtain and monitor blood pressure readings in infants and small children who are acutely ill. This is made possible by the instrument's ability to translate changes in ultrasound frequencies to audible sounds via a transducer in the blood pressure cuff.

Color-flow Doppler imaging uses the colors red and blue to assist in the detection of blood-flow direction and characteristics of blood-flow velocity of specific vessels such as fetal, heart, peripheral, abdominal, and cerebral.[7] The use of color is also effective in accentuating the imaging of blood shunting found in congenital heart defects or in visualizing valvular regurgitation.

Doppler procedures are easily performed on hospitalized clients in an ultrasound vascular room or at the bedside with portable instruments to monitor circulatory competency or to diagnose abnormalities in those too ill to be transported to the laboratory. They are also performed on an outpatient basis in hospitals or medical imaging centers.

ULTRASOUND RISKS

There is no evidence at this time to indicate that ultrasound is harmful if given at the appropriate low-intensity doses. It is a noninvasive procedure unrelated to x-ray studies; thus, there is no exposure to radiation or use of contrast-mediated materials. The greatest known risks to tissues associated with these studies are the production of heat that occurs when the level of waves exceeds the maximum frequency recommended for diagnostic procedures. These higher frequencies are reserved for the therapeutic destruction of bacteria or tumor cells and require an ultrasound instrument designed to deliver this level for a calculated period. Ultrasound diagnostic equipment is designed to deliver a safe level of energy that prevents this known risk. The use of Doppler monitoring of a fetus has been an acceptable practice, but the use of the ultrasound technique for arterial studies produces some heat in tissues and is considered to be damaging to a fetus.[8]

ULTRASOUND PROCEDURES

Ultrasound procedures are named for the organ or region of the body to be examined. Among them are the liver, pancreas, heart, brain, and almost all other organs; vessels such as the aorta; or an entire region consisting of several organs, such as the abdomen or pelvis. Depending on the region or organ to be studied, the transducer or probe is placed in various positions, angles, and rotations. Client position also varies with the site to be studied and includes supine, prone, sitting, semierect, left lateral, and right or left oblique. Scanning is performed in two planes before any images are taken, and all films are made in at least two scanning planes. The planes available for scanning include the sagittal, transverse, and coronal.[9]

ECHOCARDIOGRAPHY

Echocardiography is an ultrasound study performed to assist in the diagnosis of cardiovascular disorders. It allows visualization of the internal cardiac structures for size, shape, position, and movement. All four valves, both ventricles, and the left atrium, as well as the velocity of the blood flow, can be examined during the movement of the transducer over the chest.[10] Electrocardiography (ECG) and phonocardiography can be conducted simultaneously to correlate the findings with the cardiac cycle.[11]

Included in the study are the M-mode method, which produces a linear tracing of timed motions of the heart and its structures, and the two-dimensional method, which produces a cross-section of the structures of the heart and their relationship to one another as well as changes in the coronary vasculature. Another method, used to detect blood-flow pattern and velocity in the heart valves and great vessels, is color-flow Doppler imaging. The differences in blue and red hues are photographed to identify the blood-flow directions and velocities.[12] A combination of these methods is used to obtain a complete study of the heart and its structures.

An important consideration in performing echocardiography is using it in combination with other noninvasive tests in the diagnosis of heart disorders rather than resorting to invasive procedures such as cardiac catheterization and angiography in higher-risk clients.

Reference Values

Normal appearance of the size, structures, position, and movements of the heart valves; normal heart muscle walls of both ventricles, septum, and left atrium, with adequate blood filling

Established values for the measurement of heart activities vary according to physician, equipment, and agency.

Interfering Factors

➤ Inability of client to remain still during the procedure

➤ Obesity, chest thickness, deformity, or other abnormality or trauma that can increase the space between the heart and the transducer, which can affect transmission of waves to and from the chest

➤ Chronic obstructive pulmonary disease (COPD) or use of mechanical ventilation that can increase the air between the heart and chest wall (hyperinflation), which attenuates the ultrasound waves

➤ Dysrhythmias that can affect the test results

➤ Incorrect placement and movement of the transducer over the proper sites or lack of skill in performing the procedure

Indications for Echocardiography

➤ Detecting and determining the severity of mitral valve abnormalities such as torn chordae, stenosis, prolapse, regurgitation, or failure of valve closure revealed by restriction of valve leaflet motion or displacement of a valve leaflet

➤ Detecting and determining the severity of aortic valve abnormalities such as stenosis or failure of valve closure revealed by regurgitation and valve thickening

➤ Diagnosing subaortic stenosis revealed by the displacement of the anterior atrial leaflet and a reduction in aortic valve flow based on the obstruction

➤ Diagnosing pulmonary hypertension and pulmonary valve stenosis revealed by echo changes at the pulmonary valve site

➤ Diagnosing cardiomyopathy associated with cardiac chamber wall defects revealed by large- or small-sized chamber internal dimensions and wall thickness measurements that are less or more than should be expected

➤ Diagnosing cardiac tumors revealed by echoes in the vicinity of the mitral or tricuspid valves

➤ Determining the presence of pericardial effusion revealed by an absence of echoes between the left ventricular epicardium and pericardium and caused by fluid between these membranes

➤ Determining the extent of coronary artery disease (CAD) revealed by the absence of or abnormal ventricular wall movements resulting from infarction or ischemia

➤ Detecting ventricular or atrial mural thrombi and evaluating wall motion after myocardial infarction

➤ In infants and children, diagnosing congenital heart defects such as ventricular or atrial septal defect, pulmonary or aortic stenosis, coarctation of the aorta, patent ductus arteriosus, transposition of the great vessels,

hypoplastic ventricles, tetralogy of Fallot, truncus arteriosus, and other cardiac malpositions and anomalies
➤ Determining congestive heart failure (CHF) revealed by an enlarged chamber size
➤ Detecting changes in valve motion after rheumatic fever exacerbations in children
➤ Detecting direction of blood flow and changes in velocity of the flow (Doppler echocardiography) by imaging of the great vessels and right-to-left shunting of blood in children with congenital heart defects
➤ Determining the dimensions for the root of the aorta to detect the true and false lumens in aortic dissection
➤ Determining the cause of unexplained chest pain, ECG changes, and abnormal chest x-ray (enlarged cardiac silhouette)
➤ Evaluating or monitoring prosthetic valve function[13]

Contraindications

➤ None

Nursing Care Before the Procedure

Explain to the client:
➤ That the procedure takes about 30 to 45 minutes
➤ That there are no food or fluid restrictions before the study
➤ That the client will be placed in appropriate positions and requested to remain still, turn, or sit up during the procedure
➤ That a gel substance will be applied to the skin of the area to be viewed and a device placed and rotated over the area
➤ That a picture is produced on a screen that the client can see, if desired
➤ That no pain or risk of complications is associated with the procedure
Prepare for the procedure:
➤ Obtain a history of previous or existing cardiac conditions, therapeutic regimen, and results of related laboratory tests and procedures.
➤ Assist client to remove clothing from the waist up and provide a hospital gown if client is an outpatient; otherwise, ensure that a hospital gown is worn with the opening in front.
➤ Obtain vital signs for later comparison readings.
➤ Offer the client an opportunity to void before the procedure for comfort.

The Procedure

The client is placed on the examination table in a supine position. A portion of the chest is exposed and ECG leads are attached to the chest for simultaneous recording of heart activity during ultrasound. The client should receive explanations for the use of ECG. A conductive gel is applied to the chest slightly to the left of the sternum. The transducer is placed on the surface of the chest along the left sternal border, subxiphoid area, suprasternal notch, or supraclavicular areas to obtain views and tracings of portions of the heart. The area is scanned by systematic movement of the probe in a perpendicular position to direct the ultrasound waves to each part of the heart. The returning echoes are amplified and displayed on the screen and recorded on a moving chart strip, film, or videotape.[14] To obtain different views or information about heart function, the client is placed on the left side and in sitting positions and requested to breathe slowly, hold the breath, or perform Valsalva's maneuver during the procedure. If the client is requested to inhale a vasodilator such as amyl nitrite (Vaporole) to identify changes in function of the heart, assessment is made for side effects such as dizziness or tachycardia. When the study is completed, the leads and gel are removed from the chest.

Nursing Care After the Procedure

Tell the client when the physician will have and reveal the results, usually 1 to 2 days after the study.

ECHOENCEPHALOGRAPHY

Echoencephalography is an ultrasound study performed to assist in the diagnosis of abnormalities of the midline cerebral structures that are associated with pathology, especially the shift of a ventricle. The procedure has generally been replaced by computed tomography (CT) in adults and children because the ultrasound beam is unable to penetrate the skull bone and is known to attenuate the echo reverberations within the skull. It is, however, still an effective diagnostic study performed on infants and children under 2 years of age because the skull has not yet fused into solid bone mass. Depending on the findings, echoencephalography can be followed by CT and radionuclide scanning.[15]

Reference Values

Normal position and size of cerebral midline structures; no third ventricle deviation or abnormal anatomic position of the right and left lateral ventricles

Interfering Factors

➤ Inability of client to remain still and maintain the head in position, especially if client is a child
➤ Thick hair growth at the test site
➤ Incorrect placement and movement of the transducer over the temporal area of the skull
➤ Jewelry on the neck or ears

Indications for Echoencephalography

➤ Determining the rate of blood flow in an area revealed by changes in intracranial pulsations, distribution patterns, and contours
➤ Suspected cerebral edema, subdural or extradural hemorrhage revealed by a shift of midline structures of 3 mm or more
➤ Suspected lesions such as tumor or abscess in children revealed by enlarged third ventricle of 7 mm or more; 10 mm or more in adults
➤ Monitoring hydrocephalus status in infants

Contraindications

➤ None

Nursing Care Before the Procedure

Client teaching and physical preparation are the same as for any ultrasound procedure (see p. 690).

➤ Remove any jewelry and obtain a history that includes neurological conditions and therapy.

➤ Perform baseline neurological checks for later comparisons.

The Procedure

The client is placed on the examination table in a supine position. The head is positioned to the side on a foam pillow and conductive gel is applied to the temporoparietal area. Heavy hair growth can be cut before the study with client or caregiver permission. The client is requested to lie still during the procedure and, if the client is a small child, the head can be held in place by an assistant. The transducer is placed over the area and an ultrasound beam is directed to the internal structures. As the beam is converted to impulses, the waveforms that are produced are visualized on the screen and recorded for later viewing. When the study is completed, the gel is removed from the head.

Nursing Care After the Procedure

Care and assessment after the procedure are the same as for any ultrasound procedure (see p. 691).

➤ Perform neurological checks and compare with baselines if an underlying pathological condition is known.

➤ Provide a hair shampoo to remove the gel.

TRANSESOPHAGEAL ECHOCARDIOGRAPHY

Transesophageal echocardiography is an invasive study performed to assist in the diagnosis of cardiovascular disorders when the noninvasive echocardiography procedure does not reveal the information necessary to make or confirm a diagnosis. The procedure is usually reserved for use during surgery or for clients with conditions that can affect transmission of the waves to and from the chest.[16] It is performed with a small transducer attached to a gastroscope inserted into the esophagus. The transducer and the ultrasound instrument allow the beam to be directed to the back of the heart, and the echoes are amplified and recorded on a screen for visualization and permanent filming or on a moving chart paper. A signed informed consent form is required for this study.

Reference Values

Normal size, position, structures, and movement of the heart valves, muscle walls, and chamber blood filling

Interfering Factors

➤ Client agitation or inability to remain still during the procedure

➤ Incorrect placement and manipulation of the transducer in the esophagus at the level of the heart

Indications for Transesophageal Echocardiography

➤ Determining cardiac valve and chamber abnormalities when conventional echocardiography does not produce a clear image, as in obesity, trauma to the chest or deformity of the chest wall (barrel chest), and hyperinflation associated with COPD

➤ Confirming diagnosis if conventional echocardiography does not explain or correlate with other clinical or procedural findings

➤ Monitoring cardiac function during open heart surgery

➤ Diagnosis of esophageal pathology (e.g., varices)

Contraindications

➤ None, except that the procedure is not performed on infants or children.

Nursing Care Before the Procedure

Client teaching is the same as for esophagogastroduodenoscopy (EGD) (see pp. 546 to 547).

➤ Inform the client that the scope is positioned at the proper position behind the heart instead of inserted into the other gastrointestinal organs.

The Procedure

The client is placed on the examination table in a left side-lying position. The pharyngeal site is anesthetized, and a bite device is placed in the mouth to prevent damage to the scope if the client bites down. The endoscope with the ultrasound device attached to its tip is inserted 30 to 50 cm to the posterior portion of the heart as in any esophagoscopy procedure (see p. 547). The depth is determined to achieve the position behind the heart. The client is requested to swallow to facilitate placement of the tube as the scope is inserted. When the transducer is in place, the scope is manipulated by controls on the handle to obtain various views of the heart structure. Scanning is provided in real-time images of heart motion and recordings of the images for viewing. Actual scanning is usually limited to 15 minutes or until the desired number of image planes are obtained at different depths of the scope.[17] When the study is completed, the scope is removed and the client is placed in the semi-Fowler's position to prevent aspiration until the gag reflex returns.

Nursing Care After the Procedure

Care and assessment after the procedure are the same as for EGD (see p. 547).

OCULAR ULTRASONOGRAPHY

Ocular ultrasonography is a study performed to assist in the diagnosis of abnormalities of the eye and orbital structures. It is especially useful in identifying pathology in the presence of opacities of the cornea and lens. The study uses both A- and B-mode techniques. The A mode converts the echoes into waveforms that represent the position of different structures, and the B mode converts the echoes into a dot pattern that represents a two-dimensional image of the ocular structures.[18] A hand-held B-mode scanner is now available for eye ultrasound that can be performed in the ophthalmologist's office.

Reference Values

Normal ocular tissues and structures; no tumors, lesions, hemorrhage, or retinal or corneal abnormalities

Interfering Factors

➤ Inability of client to remain still during the procedure, which can result in an injury
➤ Vitreous humor that has been replaced by gas
➤ Incorrect placement of the transducer on the eye

Indications for Ocular Ultrasonography

➤ Diagnosing and identifying type, size, shape, texture, and location of tumors such as melanoma, hemangioma, glioma, neurofibroma, meningioma, metastic lymphoma
➤ Detecting cystic conditions such as mucoid or dermoid and differentiating these from solid tumors
➤ Determining the effect of thyroid disease (Graves' disease) on eye tissues revealed by inflammatory changes and extraocular thickening
➤ Diagnosing orbital lesions and differentiating these from intraocular lesions
➤ Identifying and locating intraocular foreign bodies
➤ Diagnosing the extent of retinal or choroidal detachment
➤ Determining vitreous abnormalities such as opacities, vitreous bands, or hemorrhage revealed by density in image appearance
➤ Evaluating the fundus that is clouded by a cataract and measuring the length of the eye before surgery for insertion of a lens implant after removal of a cataract
➤ Evaluating the eyes for keratoprosthesis
➤ Evaluating the vitreous cavity for abnormalities before vitrectomy[19]

Contraindications

➤ None

Nursing Care Before the Procedure

Client teaching and physical preparation are the same as for any ultrasound procedure (see p. 690).
➤ Obtain a history that includes known or suspected eye trauma or abnormalities and therapy or surgery for an eye disorder.
➤ Inform the client that eyedrops will be instilled to anesthetize the eye for examination and that some temporary eye blurring will be experienced after the procedure.

The Procedure

The client is placed on the examination table in a supine position. Drops to anesthetize the eye are instilled according to ordered dosage and frequency before the study. The client is requested to close the eye and a conductive gel is applied to the eyelid. The transducer is placed on the gel, and sound waves are transmitted into the eye. The waves produce echoes that are viewed on a screen and photographed for future comparison and evaluation. This provides a B scan to diagnose eye abnormalities. An A scan is performed by placing a cup over the eyeball, applying gel to the cup, and gently moving the transducer over the cup or gently manipulating the transducer directly on the corneal surface. The A scan measures the axial length of the eye and assists in diagnosing abnormal lesions. The client can be requested to change the gaze of the eye being examined to obtain orbital echo patterns that can be differentiated from abnormal patterns. When the study is completed, the gel and cup are removed from the eye or eyelid.

Nursing Care After the Procedure

Care and assessment after the procedure are the same as for any ultrasound procedure (see p. 691).

➤ Remind the client that vision may be blurred for a short period and that rubbing the eye should be avoided until the anesthetic has worn off (about 3 to 4 hours) to prevent injury to the eye.

THYROID/PARATHYROID ULTRASONOGRAPHY

Thyroid and parathyroid ultrasonography is a study performed to detect the presence of masses and to determine the size and weight of the thyroid gland as well as any enlargement of the parathyroid glands as a result of pathological processes. It is especially useful in diagnosing thyroid conditions in pregnant women because it does not require the use of radioactive iodine, a substance that can harm the fetus, to perform other thyroid diagnostic procedures. The use of the study for parathyroid abnormalities is limited because the echo patterns are lower in amplitude and smaller in size than for thyroid tissue and are normally indistinguishable from the echo patterns of the nearby neurovascular bundle.[20]

Reference Values

Normal size, position, and structure of the thyroid and parathyroid glands, with uniform echo patterns throughout the glands; no enlargement, tumor, cysts, or nodules in the glands

Interfering Factors

➤ Inability of client to remain still during the study
➤ Incorrect placement and movement of the transducer over the desired test site

Indications for Thyroid/ Parathyroid Ultrasonography

➤ Diagnosing tumor or solid mass such as benign adenoma, carcinoma revealed by an irregular border, shadowing at the distal edge, and peripheral echoes or high- and low-amplitude echoes
➤ Diagnosing cysts revealed by a smoothly outlined echo-free amplitude except at the far border of the mass
➤ Differentiating between a nodule and a solid tumor or a fluid-filled cyst, although small nodules and lesions can escape detection and diagnosis
➤ Diagnosing parathyroid enlargement of a tumor or hyperplasia revealed by echo pattern of lower amplitude than for thyroid tumor
➤ Determining the size and weight of a mass or the thyroid gland (Graves' disease) to evaluate the effectiveness of a therapeutic regimen
➤ Evaluating thyroid abnormalities during pregnancy, as the procedure does not harm the fetus

➤ Determining the need for thyroid biopsy of a tumor or needle biopsy of a cyst

Contraindications

➤ None

Nursing Care Before the Procedure

Client teaching and physical preparation are the same as for any ultrasound procedure (see p. 690).
➤ Obtain a history that includes the presence of a palpable mass and therapy or surgery for a thyroid disorder.

The Procedure

The client is placed on the examination table in a supine position. The neck is hyperextended, and a pillow is placed under the shoulders to maintain the position and provide comfort. A conductive gel or oil is applied to the neck and a transducer is placed on the area and rotated over the entire thyroid site, including both sides of the trachea. Images are projected on the screen and photographed for immediate and future viewing and interpretation or comparison. For visualization of the anterior thyroid, a short-focused transducer is used.[21] When the studies are completed, the gel is removed from the neck and the pillow is removed from under the shoulders.

Another technique is the placement of a bag of water hung over the neck area to serve as a transmitter of the waves from the transducer to the thyroid as the device is positioned over the water bag.[22]

Nursing Care After the Procedure

Care and assessment after the procedure are the same as for any ultrasound procedure (see p. 691).

THORACIC ULTRASONOGRAPHY

Thoracic ultrasonography is a study performed to assist in the diagnosis of lung abnormalities, especially when other diagnostic procedures are inconclusive in providing information. Because the waves do not penetrate air, these studies are not considered useful except when performed to identify conditions associated with fluid accumulation in the chest. It is also useful when combined with CT and Doppler technique to determine the presence of pulmonary embolism.[23] A signed informed consent form is required if needle aspiration or biopsy is planned.

Reference Values

Normal pulmonary and diaphragm position and structures; no fluid, lesion, emboli, or infection in the lungs

Interfering Factors

➤ Inability of client to remain still during the procedure
➤ Incorrect placement and movement of the transducer over the desired test sites

Indications for Thoracic Ultrasonography

➤ Determining the presence of pleural effusion
➤ Diagnosing a lesion or abscess if fluid accumulation or consolidation in the lung is revealed by chest x-ray studies
➤ Determining the cause of acute chest pain
➤ Determining abnormal or malposition of the diaphragm as a result of a lung disorder
➤ Detecting emboli revealed by echo changes that indicate anatomic changes in the lung
➤ Guiding needle placement for a pulmonary fine-needle aspiration biopsy in those who are not candidates for bronchoscopy or who have had a negative bronchogram

Contraindications

➤ None

Nursing Care Before the Procedure

Client teaching and physical preparation are the same as for any ultrasound procedure (see p. 690).
➤ Obtain a history that includes chronic pulmonary conditions, therapy, and results of tests and procedures performed for pulmonary disorders.

The Procedure

The client is placed on the examination table in a supine position. The chest is exposed and a conductive gel applied to the area to be scanned. The transducer is manipulated over the entire lung area to obtain views of the lung(s). Areas that are not filled with air appear on the screen to reveal lung pathology. When the study is completed, the gel is removed from the chest.

Nursing Care After the Procedure

Care and assessment after the procedure are the same as for any ultrasound procedure (see p. 691).
➤ *Needle aspiration site:* Note and report changes in respirations, breath sounds, pneumothorax, redness, swelling, and pain every hour for 4 hours, then every 4 hours for 24 hours. Position for comfort. Change dressing as needed. Administer analgesic and antibiotic therapy.

LYMPH NODES/RETROPERITONEAL ULTRASONOGRAPHY

Lymph nodes and retroperitoneal ultrasonography are studies performed to detect retroperitoneal pathology, usually lymph node enlargement. It is the preferred diagnostic method because this area is inaccessible for conventional radiology in the diagnosis of lymphadenopathy. It can, however, be performed in combination with lymphangiography to confirm a diagnosis.

Reference Values

Retroperitoneal and intrapelvic nodes not visible or less than 1.5 cm in diameter

Interfering Factors

➤ Inability of client to remain still during the study

➤ Incorrect placement and movement of the transducer over the desired test site

➤ Gas or feces in the bowel that attenuate the sound waves

Indications for Lymph Nodes/Retroperitoneal Ultrasonography

➤ Suspected lymphoma to diagnose and locate enlarged aortic and iliac lymph nodes

➤ Determination of visibility and enlargement of nodes in retroperitoneal solid tumor or infection

➤ Determination of the location of enlarged nodes to plan radiation and other therapy[24]

➤ Evaluation of changes in the size of nodes or tumors during and after therapy revealed by a shrinkage of the mass or nodes

Contraindications

➤ None

Nursing Care Before the Procedure

Client teaching and physical preparation are the same as for any ultrasound procedure (see p. 690).

➤ Inform the client that food is restricted for 12 hours before the study to minimize bowel motility but that water is permitted.

➤ Obtain a history that includes known or suspected lymphoma and therapy received to reduce the size of a retroperitoneal mass or lymph nodes.

The Procedure

The client is placed on the examination table in a supine position. The abdomen is exposed from the umbilicus down and draped for privacy. A conductive gel is applied to the flank and abdominal areas to be scanned. The transducer is manipulated over the area, and transverse and longitudinal scans are taken. Sound waves are echoed to the transducer to reflect different densities of tissues. These impulses are displayed on a screen and photographed for immediate or future viewing and interpretation or comparison. When the study is completed, the gel is removed from the area.

Nursing Care After the Procedure

Care and assessment after the procedure are the same as for any ultrasound procedure (see p. 691). Inform the client to resume food intake after the study.

ABDOMINAL/AORTIC ULTRASONOGRAPHY

Abdominal/aortic ultrasonography is a study performed to assist in the diagnosis of aortic aneurysm and to determine its size by display of constriction or dilation of the vessel. Because it is a safe procedure, it can be repeated as often as every 6 months to monitor changes in the size of this great vessel. Ultrasound is performed alone or in combination with Doppler techniques to identify the vessel lumen and associated clot formation within an abdominal aortic aneurysm.[25] The area scanned includes the complete abdomen from the umbilicus to the xiphoid process and includes adjacent organs.

Reference Values

Normal structure of the abdominal organs; normal contour and normal diameter of the abdominal aorta of 1.5 to 2.5 cm at various sections of the vessel

Interfering Factors

➤ Inability of client to remain still during the procedure
➤ Incorrect placement and movement of the transducer over the desired sites
➤ Gas, feces, or barium in the bowel that attenuates the sound waves
➤ Increased bowel motility that affects sound waves
➤ Obesity that increases space between the organs and the transducer, affecting the transmission of waves to and from the abdomen
➤ Scar tissue from previous surgery that prevents transmission of waves through the skin to the abdominal organs

Indications for Abdominal/Aortic Ultrasonography

➤ Detecting and measuring an aortic aneurysm within the abdomen for deviations from the normal diameters at various sections of the vessel
➤ Monitoring aortic aneurysm expansion periodically to prevent rupture revealed by measurements of 7 cm or more in diameter or rapid increases in size
➤ Determining changes in small aortic aneurysms before and after abdominal surgical procedures
➤ Differentiating between the vessel lumen and a clot within an aortic aneurysm with the use of Doppler technique in combination with ultrasonography
➤ Diagnosing pathology of intra-abdominal organs such as the liver, spleen, pancreas, gallbladder, and kidneys, singly or in groups
➤ Determining patency and function of vessels and ducts such as the portal vein, splenic vein, renal arteries and veins, superior and inferior mesenteric veins, and biliary and pancreatic ducts
➤ Determining ascites fluid status and the best site for a diagnostic paracentesis
➤ Diagnosing abdominal pathology during pregnancy, as the fetus is not at risk during ultrasound

Contraindications

➤ None

➤➤ Nursing Alert

- Sudden changes in vital signs and continuous abdominal or back pain can indicate an expanding aneurysm, and sudden onset of severe pain, hypotension, tachycardia, and diaphoresis indicate aneurysm rupture. Both require immediate reporting and interventions.[26]

Nursing Care Before the Procedure

Client teaching and physical preparation are the same as for any ultrasound procedure (see p. 690).

➤ Obtain a history that includes a suspected or existing abdominal aortic aneurysm and the results of the last measurement of aneurysm diameter to use as a comparison.

➤ Inform the client that food is restricted for 12 hours before the study, but encourage fluids to provide a full bladder that pushes the bowel out of the pelvis for scanning.

➤ Administer an enema to remove feces and barium, and administer simethicone (Mylicon) to reduce gas from the bowel if ordered.

The Procedure

The client is placed on the examination table in a supine position. The abdomen is exposed and draped for privacy. The client can be requested to lie on either side or assume a sitting position during the scanning. A conductive gel is applied to the abdominal scanning sites. The transducer is rotated and manipulated over the abdomen, avoiding any scar tissue, from the xiphoid process to the aortic bifurcation and to the left and right of the midline. This process provides scanning of the aorta and other sites of the abdominal organs and vessels. Impulses are transmitted from the device to a screen for visual display and are photographed for future viewing and comparisons. When the studies are completed, the gel is removed from the abdomen.

Nursing Care After the Procedure

Care and assessment after the procedure are the same as for any ultrasound procedure (see p. 691).

➤ Inform the client that food intake can be resumed.

➤ *Increasing size of aneurysm:* Note abdominal or back pain, hypotension, tachycardia, or diaphoresis. Report to physician immediately. Prepare client for possible surgical intervention.

SPLEEN ULTRASONOGRAPHY

Spleen ultrasonography is a study performed to assist in the diagnosis of pathology or trauma of this organ and the surrounding abdominal organs. It allows a view of the size, shape, and position of the organ in the upper left quadrant (ULQ) of the abdomen. Total splenic volume can also be determined by integrating the cross-sectional areas of ultrasound scans that are obtained at 1-cm intervals.[27] Spleen ultrasonography is often performed in association with CT to obtain diagnostic information.

Reference Values

Normal size, position, and contour of the spleen; no splenomegaly, trauma, or masses

Interfering Factors

➤ Inability of client to remain still during the procedure

➤ Incorrect placement and movement of the transducer over the test site

➤ Ribs and an aerated left lung that attenuate the sound waves
➤ Masses near the testing site that displace the spleen, causing confusion with a splenomegaly diagnosis[28]

Indications for Spleen Ultrasonography

➤ Determining the size and volume of the spleen in splenomegaly
➤ Detecting splenic cysts and differentiating them from solid tumors and determining whether they are intrasplenic or extrasplenic when the procedure is combined with CT
➤ Detecting subphrenic abscess after splenectomy
➤ Evaluating extent of abdominal trauma and spleen enlargement or rupture after a recent accident
➤ Differentiating spleen trauma from blood or fluid accumulation between the splenic capsule and parenchyma
➤ Evaluating the spleen before splenectomy performed for thrombocytopenic purpura
➤ Determining late-stage sickle cell disease revealed by decreased spleen size[29]
➤ Evaluating the effect of therapy on the progression or resolution of splenic disease such as with chemotherapy that should reduce spleen size

Contraindications

➤ None

➤➤ Nursing Alert

• Presence of acute pain resulting from trauma to the spleen causes intolerance to the discomfort of the transducer's being manipulated over the area, and comfort measures should be taken to allow performance of the study.

Nursing Care Before the Procedure

Client teaching and physical preparation are the same as for any ultrasound procedure (see p. 690).
➤ Obtain a history that includes any suspected or existing diseases or trauma involving the spleen and any therapy administered to treat splenic disorders.
➤ *Acute pain:* Note and report type, location, and severity of pain. Administer analgesic ordered before the procedure to enhance comfort during the manipulation of the transducer over the abdomen.

The Procedure

The client is placed on the examination table in a supine position. The abdomen and chest are exposed and draped for privacy. A conductive gel is applied to the upper left quadrant (ULQ) of the abdomen, and the transducer is manipulated over the area. Echoes are received, amplified, and converted into images on a screen for viewing. The views can be photographed for future comparisons to evaluate changes in the size of the organ. When the studies are completed, the gel is removed from the abdomen.

Nursing Care After the Procedure

Care and assessment after the procedure are the same as for any ultrasound procedure (see p. 691).

PANCREATIC ULTRASONOGRAPHY

Pancreatic ultrasonography is a study performed to assist in the diagnosis of pathology that affects the size, shape, and position of this organ. Anatomic abnormalities are identified by echo patterns that vary with densities in the tissue examined. The procedure can be performed in combination with a radionuclide scan of the organ for better visualization, or it can be followed by CT and biopsy for confirmation of a diagnosis. A signed informed consent form is required if needle biopsy is planned.

Reference Values

Normal size, contour, and texture of the pancreas; patency of the pancreatic duct; no inflammation, masses, or duct obstruction

Interfering Factors

➤ Inability of client to remain still during the procedure
➤ Incorrect placement of the transducer over the test site
➤ Gas or barium in the bowel or stomach that attenuates the waves
➤ Obesity that increases the space between the organ and transducer, affecting transmission of the waves to and from the abdomen

Indications for Pancreatic Ultrasonography

➤ Diagnosing pancreatitis revealed by enlargement and increase in echoes
➤ Diagnosing pancreatic malignancy revealed by a poorly defined mass in the pancreas that obstructs the pancreatic duct
➤ Diagnosing pseudocysts revealed by a well-defined mass and absence of echoes from the interior
➤ Detecting anatomic abnormalities as a consequence of pancreatitis
➤ Monitoring the response to therapeutic regimen administered for tumor
➤ Providing guidance for needle insertion in percutaneous aspiration and needle biopsy of the pancreas[30]

Contraindications

➤ None

Nursing Care Before the Procedure

Client teaching and physical preparation are the same as for any ultrasound procedure (see p. 690).
➤ Obtain a history that includes suspected or existing disorders of the pancreas, results of diagnostic tests and procedures, and therapy to treat tumor or inflammation.
➤ Inform the client of food restrictions, which can vary with the agency or with physician preference.

The Procedure

The client is placed on the examination table in a supine position, although the position can be changed during the study. A conductive gel is applied to the epigastric region of the abdomen. A transducer is manipulated over the area and the echoes are converted to electrical impulses that are displayed on a screen. During the procedure, the client can be requested to regulate breathing patterns, hold the breath, or drink water to enhance the outline of the abdominal organs and improve visualization of the pancreas.[31] The views are photographed for future comparisons and evaluation. When the study is completed, the gel is removed from the abdomen.

Nursing Care After the Procedure

Care and assessment after the procedure are the same as for any ultrasound procedure (see p. 691). Inform the client that food intake can be resumed.

➤ *Needle aspiration/biopsy site:* Note and report redness, swelling, bleeding, pain at site, and symptoms of peritonitis. Change dressing as needed. Administer analgesic and antibiotic therapy.

LIVER/BILIARY SYSTEM ULTRASONOGRAPHY

Liver and biliary system ultrasonography are studies performed to determine the size, shape, and position of the liver and the gallbladder, located in the upper right quadrant (URQ) of the abdomen. Gallbladder ultrasonography is especially helpful when performed in clients whose gallbladder is unable to opacify gallstones with oral or intravenous (IV) radiologic studies. Liver ultrasonography can be performed in combination with a radionuclide scan (gallium) to obtain information about liver function as well as about density differences obtained by ultrasound.[32] Other diagnostic studies such as CT and liver biopsy can confirm ultrasound findings. A signed informed consent form is required if catheter insertion or needle aspiration or biopsy is planned.

Reference Values

Normal size, position, and shape of the liver and gallbladder; patency of the cystic and common bile ducts; no hepatic cysts, tumors, or duct dilation; no gallbladder constriction, cysts, tumor, stones, or cystic/common bile duct dilation

Interfering Factors

➤ Inability of client to remain still during the procedure
➤ Incorrect placement of the transducer over the test site
➤ Gas or barium in the bowel or stomach that attenuates the sound waves, affecting the imaging of the liver, gallbladder, and biliary system
➤ Ribs that attenuate the sound waves and affect imaging of the right lobe of the liver

Indications for Liver/Biliary System Ultrasonography

➤ Determining the cause of URQ pain
➤ Diagnosing hepatic lesions such as tumor, cyst, abscess, or cirrhosis revealed by differences in density and echo pattern changes

➤ Determining the patency and diameter of the hepatic duct for dilation or obstruction

➤ Determining metastasis to the liver from a primary lesion in the breast, colon or rectum, or other abdominal organs

➤ Differentiating between obstructive and nonobstructive jaundice by identifying the cause

➤ Determining the cause of unexplained hepatomegaly (mass, trauma) and abnormal liver function tests (increased alkaline phosphatase)

➤ Diagnosing acute or chronic cholecystitis revealed by an enlarged gallbladder with wall thickening

➤ Determining gallstones within the gallbladder or biliary ducts revealed by dilation or obstruction, or both, of the biliary tree or ducts and increased bilirubin level

➤ Diagnosing gallbladder stones or inflammation if oral cholecystography is inconclusive

➤ Diagnosing cysts, polyps, or solid tumor of the gallbladder revealed by echoes specific to tissue density and sharply or poorly defined masses

➤ Evaluating therapy for tumor revealed by a decrease in size of the organ

➤ Guiding catheter placement into the gallbladder for stone dissolution and gallbladder fragmentation

Contraindications

➤ None

Nursing Care Before the Procedure

Client teaching and physical preparation are the same as for any ultrasound procedure (see p. 690).

➤ Obtain a history that includes liver or gallbladder disorders and therapy to treat a tumor or obstruction.

➤ Administer an enema before the study, if ordered, to remove feces or barium that can interfere with imaging.

The Procedure

The client is placed on the examination table in a supine position, although the prone or side-lying positions can also be used during the study. The abdomen is exposed and draped for privacy. The conductive gel is applied to the skin of the URQ and the transducer manipulated over the area. During the procedure, the client is requested to hold the breath on inspiration as patterns are displayed on a screen and photographed for future viewing. Several planes of scanning are obtained. Each lobe and border of the liver and border of the gallbladder are examined. The cystic and common bile ducts are examined for patency. Gallbladder contractibility to expel the bile stored within it can be achieved with the administration of a fatty substance (Lipomul) to allow examination of the organ's function.[33] When the studies are completed, the gel is removed from the abdomen.

Nursing Care After the Procedure

Care and assessment after the procedure are the same as for any ultrasound procedure (see p. 691). Inform the client that food intake can be resumed.

➤ *Catheter/needle insertion site:* Note and report pain, redness, and swelling every hour for 4 hours, then every 4 hours for 24 hours. Position on right side. Change dressing as needed. Administer analgesic and antibiotic therapy.

KIDNEY ULTRASONOGRAPHY

Kidney ultrasonography is a study performed to assist in the diagnosis of abnormalities that can be identified by changes in size, structure, or position of either or both organs. The procedure is especially valuable in clients with renal failure because the study does not rely on renal function and in clients with hypersensitivity to iodinated contrast media because none is needed in this diagnostic method. The study can be performed in combination with other urologic tests such as a radionuclide scan to provide a diagnosis. It can also be performed after intravenous pyelography (IVP) to provide a differential diagnosis in the presence of renal masses.[34] A signed informed consent form is required if tube insertion or needle biopsy is planned.

Reference Values

Normal size, position, shape, and structure of the kidneys; no masses, calculi, inflammation, or hydronephrosis

Interfering Factors

➤ Inability of client to remain still during the procedure
➤ Incorrect placement of the transducer over the test sites
➤ Barium remaining in the tract after x-ray studies

Indications for Kidney Ultrasonography

➤ Detecting the size and location of a renal mass in those who are unable to have an IVP because of poor renal function or allergy to iodinated contrast media
➤ Detecting masses and differentiating between cysts and solid tumor revealed by the specific sound waveform patterns or absence of sound waves
➤ Diagnosing the presence and location of renal or ureteral calculi and obstruction
➤ Determining the size, shape, and position of a nonfunctioning kidney
➤ Determining an accumulation of fluid in the kidney, resulting from a backflow of urine, hemorrhage, or perirenal fluid or blood collection
➤ Diagnosing hydronephrosis in one or both kidneys, polycystic kidneys, or other congenital anomalies of the organs in children
➤ Monitoring children for changes in the size of the kidneys as a congenital renal disease progresses
➤ Diagnosing effect of chronic glomerulonephritis and end-stage chronic renal failure on the kidneys, such as a progressive decrease in size
➤ Evaluating renal transplantation for changes in kidney size
➤ Locating the site and guiding percutaneous renal biopsy, aspiration needle or nephrostomy tube insertion
➤ Evaluating or planning therapy for renal tumor such as radiation or chemotherapy

Contraindications

➤ None

Nursing Care Before the Procedure

Client teaching and physical preparation are the same as for any ultrasound procedure (see p. 690).

➤ Obtain a history that includes suspected and existing renal disease, therapy received to treat a tumor, or other condition.

The Procedure

The client is placed on the examination table in a supine position, although a side-lying position can be used. A child can be held in the proper position, if necessary. The area is draped and a conductive gel applied. The transducer is rotated and manipulated over the area as the sound waves are transmitted to the organ, bounced back to the transducer, and projected onto a screen for viewing. The client can be requested to breathe as deeply as possible to obtain views of the upper portions of the kidneys. When the studies are completed, the gel is removed from the area.

Nursing Care After the Procedure

Care and assessment after the study are the same as for any ultrasound procedure (see p. 691).

➤ *Tube or needle biopsy/aspiration site:* Note and report redness, swelling, pain at site, and patency of tube, if inserted; position for comfort; change dressing as needed; administer analgesic and antibiotic therapy.

BLADDER ULTRASONOGRAPHY

Bladder ultrasonography is a study performed to visualize the size and contour of the bladder by providing an outline of the organ while it is full of urine. Abnormal contour changes or distortion of bladder position is an indication of pathology of the pelvic organs or bladder wall. The procedure can be performed with ultrasonography of the kidneys, ureters, bladder, urethra, and gonads to diagnose renal/urologic disorders.[35]

Reference Values

Normal size, position, and contour of the urinary bladder; no masses or urinary residual

Interfering Factors

➤ Inability of client to remain still during the procedure
➤ Incorrect placement of the transducer over the test site
➤ Barium or gas in the bowel or small amount of residual urine in the bladder

Indications for Bladder Ultrasonography

➤ Assessing residual urine after voiding to diagnose urinary tract obstruction
➤ Detecting tumor of the bladder wall or pelvis revealed by distortion in position or change in contour of the bladder

> Determining bladder malignancy resulting from an extension of a primary tumor of the ovary or other pelvic organs

Contraindications

> None

Nursing Care Before the Procedure

Client teaching and physical preparation are the same as for any ultrasound procedure (see p. 690).

> Obtain a history that includes any disease or dysfunction of the urinary bladder, therapy received, and results of tests and procedures associated with the urinary bladder.

> Encourage fluid intake to ensure a full bladder to enhance imaging of the organs or have client void immediately before the procedure if residual volume is to be measured.

The Procedure

The client is placed on the examination table in a supine position. The lower abdomen is exposed and draped for privacy. The bladder is palpated to ensure that it is full of urine and a conductive gel is applied to the area. A transducer is manipulated over the bladder and pelvic sites, and sound waves are projected onto the screen and photographed for immediate and future viewing. If the client is to be examined for residual urine volume, the bladder is emptied, the procedure repeated, and the volume calculated. When the study is completed, the gel is removed from the abdominal sites.

Nursing Care After the Procedure

Care and assessment after the study are the same as for any ultrasound procedure (see p. 691).

PROSTATE ULTRASONOGRAPHY

Prostate or transrectal ultrasonography is a study performed to assist in the diagnosis of prostatic malignancy. The procedure is performed in combination with a digital rectal examination. In addition to the prostate gland, the seminal vesicles and periprostate structures are examined. Because of the high incidence of prostate cancer in men over 55 years of age, this study is undertaken frequently to identify and locate early-stage small tumors in this population.[36]

Reference Values

Normal size, shape, and structure of the prostate gland; no abnormal urinary pattern, gland tumor, or hypertrophy

Interfering Factors

> Inability of client to remain still during the procedure
> Incorrect placement of the transducer or rectal probe at the test site
> Feces or barium in the rectum

Indications for Prostate Ultrasonography

➤ Diagnosing prostate abnormalities such as prostatitis, prostatic hypertrophy, or nodules that have been palpated

➤ Detecting tumor at an early stage revealed by difference in tissue densities

➤ Assessing location of tumor and direct placement of radioactive seeds in the treatment of carcinoma

➤ Locating site and serving as a guide for prostate biopsy

➤ Evaluating results of therapy such as radiation and chemotherapy revealed by a reduction in tumor size

➤ Evaluating voiding disorders and changes in patterns after treatment

Contraindications

➤ None

Nursing Care Before the Procedure

Client teaching and physical preparation are the same as for any ultrasound procedure (see p. 690).

➤ Obtain a history that includes suspected and known prostate and urinary elimination conditions, results of tests and procedures associated with these disorders, and therapy received for tumor, enlargement, or micturition abnormalities.

➤ Administer an enema, if ordered, to remove feces or barium from the rectum to ensure clear imaging.

The Procedure

The client is placed on the examination table in a left side-lying position. The knees are flexed and the rectal area is exposed and draped for privacy. A manual rectal examination is performed and a lubricated rectal probe transducer is inserted into the rectum along the anterior wall at the level of the prostate gland. The condom covering the probe is filled with water to provide the necessary medium between the probe and the prostate gland to allow transmission of the sound waves. The client is informed that some discomfort is experienced when the water-filled probe is inserted. Scanning is performed as the rectal probe transducer is rotated and manipulated to obtain the desired views. In some studies, the bladder is filled with fluid to assist in exposing the prostate to the sound waves.[37] When the study is completed, the probe is removed and the anus cleansed of the gel and patted dry.

Nursing Care After the Procedure

Care and assessment after the study are the same as for any ultrasound procedure (see p. 691).

➤ *Needle biopsy site:* Note and report redness, swelling, and pain at the site. Change dressing as needed. Administer analgesic and antibiotic therapy.

SCROTAL ULTRASONOGRAPHY

Scrotal ultrasonography is a study performed to assist in the diagnosis of scrotal pathology and anatomic abnormalities. If indicated in the presence of scrotal edema, it can be performed in combination with or after radionuclide scan studies for further clarification of a testicular mass.[38]

Reference Values

Normal scrotum and normal size, shape, and structure of the testes; no tumor, abscess, or other abnormality

Interfering Factors

➤ Inability of client to remain still during the procedure
➤ Incorrect placement of the transducer over the test site

Indications for Scrotal Ultrasonography

➤ Determining the cause of chronic scrotal swelling
➤ Clarifying a diagnosis of scrotal or testicular abnormality or pathology after questionable results from a radionuclide scan
➤ Diagnosing a mass and differentiating it from cyst, solid tumor, or abscess revealed by specific image patterns
➤ Diagnosing a chronic inflammatory condition such as epididymitis
➤ Determining the existence of a hydrocele, spermatocele, or scrotal hernia before surgery for repair
➤ Diagnosing torsion and associated testicular infarction

Contraindications

➤ None

Nursing Care Before the Procedure

Client teaching and physical preparation are the same as for any ultrasound procedure (see p. 690).
➤ Obtain a history that includes any suspected or known disorders of the scrotum or testes and any therapy or surgery to treat abnormalities or pathology.

The Procedure

The client is placed on the examination table in a supine position. The scrotal area is exposed and draped for privacy. The penis is lifted upward and gently taped to the lower part of the abdomen. Special sensitivity should be displayed for the client and possible embarrassment during this part of the procedure. The conductive gel is applied to the skin of the scrotum and the transducer is manipulated over all areas. The waves received are converted to images on the screen to be viewed and photographed. When the procedure is completed, the gel is removed from the area and the penis untaped and returned to its normal position.

Nursing Care After the Procedure

Care and assessment after the study are the same as for any ultrasound procedure (see p. 691).

BREAST ULTRASONOGRAPHY

Breast ultrasonography is a study performed to visualize and record palpable and nonpalpable masses. It is especially useful in clients with dense or fibrocystic breasts and those with silicone prostheses because the beam easily penetrates this material. For these clients, the procedure allows routine examination that cannot be performed with x-ray mammography. Ultrasonography can also be performed as an adjunct to or in place of mammography in those who refuse or should not be exposed to x-ray diagnostic studies, such as pregnant women.

Reference Values

Normal subcutaneous, mammary, and retromammary layers of tissue in both breasts; no pathologic lesions in either breast

Interfering Factors

➤ Inability of client to remain in or assume the necessary positions during the procedure

➤ Incorrect placement and movement of the transducer over the breasts or a particular site on a breast

➤ Largeness of breasts that cannot be accommodated by selected methods of ultrasound examination

Indications for Breast Ultrasonogrphy

➤ Monitoring changes in nonpalpable abnormalities viewed on mammography of fibrocystic breast tissue

➤ Differentiating among breast masses such as cysts, solid tumor, or other lesions

➤ Early detection of very small tumors in combination with mammography for diagnostic validation

➤ Assessing palpable masses in pregnant women to avoid exposure to the radiation of x-ray mammography

➤ Evaluating breast abnormalities in women who refuse or should not be exposed to mammography

➤ Evaluating breasts of women who have breast augmentation with silicone prostheses, as more accurate examination can be achieved with ultrasound as opposed to x-ray beams, which are absorbed by the implant

Contraindications

➤ None

Nursing Care Before the Procedure

Client teaching and physical preparation are the same as for any ultrasound procedure (see p. 690).

➤ Obtain a history that includes suspected or known breast abnormalities or surgeries, risk status for breast tumor, presence of prostheses, last menstrual period dates, and past therapy for breast abnormalities.

➤ Inform the client to avoid use of lotions, bath powder, or other substances on the skin of the chest and breasts.

➤ Administer an analgesic before the study if procedure is painful to breasts.

The Procedure

The client is placed on the examination table in a supine position. The chest is exposed and draped for privacy. A warmed conductive gel is applied to the breasts and the transducer is manipulated over the skin of one or both breasts. Sound waves are received and displayed on a screen and photographed. If the procedure is performed using a tank of warm, chemically prepared water, the client is placed in a prone position, and each breast is immersed in the tank. The transducer placed at the bottom of the tank transmits waves through the water. The waves are reflected from both breasts, producing echoes that are displayed as waveforms on a screen and photographed for future viewing.[39] When the study in completed, the gel is removed and the breasts are dried.

Nursing Care After the Procedure

Care and assessment after the study are the same as for any ultrasound procedure (see p. 691).

PELVIC ULTRASONOGRAPHY

Pelvic ultrasonography is a study performed to determine the presence of masses; their sizes and structure; and the location of other abnormalities of the ovaries, fallopian tubes, uterus, cervix, and vagina. The procedure can be performed transabdominally or transvaginally, depending on the information needed. The transabdominal approach provides a view of the pelvic organs posterior to the bladder, and the transvaginal approach provides a method of monitoring ovulation over a period of days in clients undergoing fertility assessment.[40]

Reference Values

Normal size, position, location, and structure of the ovaries, fallopian tubes, uterus, and vagina; no masses or inflammatory disease; intrauterine device (IUD) located in the proper position within the uterine cavity

Interfering Factors

➤ Inability of client to remain still during the procedure
➤ Incorrect placement of the transducer over the pelvic area or of the probe within the vagina for proper examination
➤ Gas in the bowel
➤ Bladder that is not full and does not push the bowel from the pelvis and the uterus from the symphysis pubis as needed to view the pelvic organs

Indications for Pelvic Ultrasonography

➤ Determining masses in the pelvis and differentiating them from cysts or solid tumors revealed by differences in sound patterns
➤ Determining the mobility of a pelvic mass and metastasis of a pelvic or other lesion
➤ Detecting ovarian cysts and determining possible type revealed by the size, outline, and change in the position of other pelvic organs
➤ Diagnosing pelvic inflammatory disease when performed in combination with other laboratory tests
➤ Detecting uterine masses such as fibroids or adnexal tumor without differentiating between the two or confirming a diagnosis
➤ Evaluating or planning therapy, including radiation or chemotherapy, of a tumor revealed by a reduction in mass size
➤ Diagnosing pelvic abscess or peritonitis as a result of a ruptured appendix or diverticulitis

➤ Determining bleeding into the pelvis as a result of trauma to the area or fluid (ascites) accumulation associated with tumor metastasis

➤ Evaluating pathology associated with postmenopausal bleeding

➤ Determining the type and ascertaining the location of an IUD and determining whether the device is in its proper position within the uterus or whether it has perforated the uterus

➤ Monitoring follicular size in association with fertility studies, to locate follicles and determine readiness to remove follicles for in vitro transplantation[41]

Contraindications

➤ None

Nursing Care Before the Procedure

Client teaching and physical preparation are the same as for any ultrasound procedure (see p. 690).

➤ Obtain a history that includes gynecologic disorders and therapy received for them

➤ Encourage fluids to ensure a full bladder if a transabdominal approach is planned.

➤ Inform the client of a planned procedure using a transvaginal approach.

The Procedure

The client is placed on the examination table in a supine position. The lower abdomen is exposed and draped for privacy. A conductive gel is applied to the area and a transducer is manipulated over the skin while the bladder is distended (transabdominally). The full bladder permits the transmission of the beam and pushes the uterus and bowel out of their positions to provide a better view of the structures posterior to the bladder. The sound waves are received and displayed on a screen and photographed. If a transvaginal approach is performed, a covered, lubricated probe is inserted into the vagina and manipulated as the sound waves are received and imaged on the screen. This approach is used in obese clients, as the additional tissue causes a greater distance between organs and transducer, or in clients with retroversion of the uterus, as sound waves are better able to reach the organ from the vaginal site. A full bladder is not necessary for performing the transvaginal procedure. When the study is completed, the gel is removed from the skin or the probe from the vagina and the area is cleansed and patted dry, if needed.

Nursing Care After the Procedure

Care and assessment after the procedure are the same as for any ultrasound procedure (see p. 691).

OBSTETRIC ULTRASONOGRAPHY

Obstetric ultrasonography is a study performed to visualize the fetus and placenta and can be performed as early as the 5th week of gestation. It is the safest method of examination to determine fetal size, growth, and position as well as fetal structural abnormalities. The procedure can also be used in combination with Doppler monitoring of the fetal heart or respiratory movements in the detection of high-risk pregnancy. Because the pregnant uterus is filled with amniotic fluid, ultrasonography is an ideal method of evaluating the fetus and placenta and is safer than procedures with more potential danger such as radiologic and radionuclide studies.

Uses of obstetric ultrasonography to secure information regarding the fetus vary with the trimester in which the procedure is performed. The methods of scanning include the transvaginal technique, which is used during the first trimester, and the transabdominal technique, which is used during the second trimester.[42]

Reference Values

Normal fetal age, size, viability, position, and functional capacities; normal placental size, position, and structure with adequate volume of amniotic fluid

Interfering Factors

➤ Incorrect placement or angulation of the transducer over the test site, depending on the determinations to be made
➤ Air or barium in the bowel
➤ Inability of the sound beam to penetrate to the site because of client size
➤ Bladder that is not full enough to push the uterus from the pubic area to provide a better view of the pregnant uterus

Indications for Obstetric Ultrasonography

➤ Determining and confirming pregnancy or multiple pregnancies with the number of gestational sacs in the first trimester, usually by the 4th or 5th week
➤ Determining fetal heart and body movements and detecting high-risk pregnancy via fetal heart and respiratory movements in combination with Doppler ultrasound or real-time scanning, usually by the 6th or 7th week for real-time or the 12th week for Doppler
➤ Measuring gestational age and evaluating umbilical artery, uterine artery, and fetal aorta by Doppler examination to determine intrauterine fetal growth rate (IUGR) for retardation[43]
➤ Determining gestational age by uterine size and measurements of crown-rump length, biparietal diameter, extremities, head, and other parts of the anatomy at different phases of fetal development
➤ Determining structural anomalies of the fetus such as hydrocephalus, myelomeningocele, skeletal defects, renal abnormalities, intestinal atresias, cardiac defects, and other congenital conditions, usually at 20th week or later
➤ Detecting fetal death revealed by an absence of movement and fetal heart tones
➤ Determining the cause of bleeding, as in placenta previa or abruptio placentae
➤ Possibly determining gender of fetus
➤ Determining placental size, location, and site of implantation
➤ Monitoring placental growth and amniotic fluid volume
➤ Diagnosing fetal abnormalities to prepare for surgical correction or pregnancy termination

➤ Determining position of the fetus before birth, such as breech or transverse presentations

➤ Determining effect of Rh incompatibility on the fetus, as in fetal hydrops

➤ Guiding the needle during amniocentesis and fetal transfusion

Contraindications

➤ None

Nursing Care Before the Procedure

Client teaching and physical preparation are the same as for any ultrasound procedure (see p. 690).

➤ Obtain a history that includes menstrual dates; medications taken for fertility, birth control, or other reasons; previous pregnancies and complications; treatments received for high-risk-status pregnancy; and results of tests and procedures associated with pregnancy.

➤ Encourage fluids or provide fluids 1 hour before the study to retain a full bladder.

➤ Reassure the client that this study is not harmful to the fetus because it does not involve radiation.

➤ Provide special support for anxiety that arises about concern for a normal fetus.

➤ Inform the client that the screen will be in full view and explanations will be given about the fetus as it appears. Inform the client if a transvaginal approach is planned.

The Procedure

The client is placed on the examination table in a supine position. Attention is given to a hypotensive and faintness response from pressure on the vena cava in this position, and the client is repositioned on the left side to relieve this pressure. The lower abdomen is exposed and draped for privacy. The conductive gel is applied to the abdomen and the transducer is manipulated over the entire abdomen or lower abdomen, depending on the size of the uterus. The examination uses both A- and B-mode techniques that convert echoes into waveforms that represent the positions of structures, and two-dimensional or cross-sectional images are displayed on the screen and photographed for future viewing. Real-time imaging reveals the fetus in motion on the screen. The scanning is performed while the bladder is full for visualization of the uterus and its contents. If a transvaginal approach is used, a full bladder is not needed, and this method is not used past the first trimester (see "Pelvic Ultrasonography"). When the study is completed, the gel is removed from the skin or the probe is removed from the vagina and the area cleansed and patted dry, if needed.

Nursing Care After the Procedure

Care and assessment after the procedure are the same as for any ultrasound procedure (see p. 691).

➤ Provide the client with an opportunity to void.

➤ *Abnormal procedure results, complications, and precautions:* Provide special support and sensitivity to the expectant mother's feelings and her ability to deal with findings that reveal fetal abnormalities.

DOPPLER PROCEDURES

Doppler ultrasound techniques are described in the beginning of this chapter. Aside from their main focus of identifying and locating peripheral venous and arterial occlusive disease, specific Doppler techniques are also valuable in the study of blood vessels of the cerebrovascular system (Table 19–1). These techniques detect extracranial cerebrovascular disease in clients with diabetes, hypertension with a risk for stroke, or a cardiac condition. They are also used to study abdominal and fetal blood vessels. The testing method most commonly used is duplex scanning, which permits measurement of blood-flow direction and velocity by combining real-time imaging with Doppler flow spectrum analyses. This and other types of noninvasive arterial and venous diagnostic procedures are performed before an invasive procedure such as angiography, which provides information regarding vascular patency.[44] Plethysmography is a technique that uses blood pressure cuffs and a pulse volume recorder and can be performed instead of or after Doppler ultrasound to diagnose arterial and venous occlusion or obstruction (see p. 839). There are no contraindications to these diagnostic studies or complications associated with their use.

ARTERIAL DOPPLER EXTREMITY STUDIES

Arterial Doppler ultrasound is a technique performed to obtain diagnostic information about the arterial vasculature of the upper and lower extremities. The swishing, pulsatile, and multiphasic sounds produced by an artery are audible with earphones. Changes in these sounds indicate an abnormal flow and vessel patency alteration and assist in determining partial or complete obstruction of arterial circulation in an extremity. Tests conducted in association with the Doppler technique to detect peripheral arterial disease include the treadmill exercise study to measure ankle pressure before and after exercise, the reactive hyperemia study to measure ankle pressure before and after application of a thigh cuff, duplex scanning to measure blood-flow direction and arterial patency through imaging and waveform analysis, the limb pressure index study to measure leg and arm pressures for comparison (ankle-brachial index), and the examination of extremities for multiphasic signals to assist in identification of the presence, location, and extent of disease. The measurement of ankle-brachial index is the most common study performed to evaluate lower extremity arterial circulation.[45] Plethysmography can also be performed to determine volume changes in digital arteries revealed by decreased pressure in a toe or finger when compared with the ankle (see pp. 839 to 840).

Table 19–1 ➤ OVERVIEW OF DOPPLER ULTRASOUND STUDIES

Area Examined	Method/Modalities	Findings
Peripheral arterial vessels	Duplex scanning	Arterial stenosis and occlusion
	Doppler examination	Peripheral arteriosclerotic occlusive disease
Peripheral venous vessels	Duplex scanning	Venous obstruction
Intracranial vessels	Doppler examination	Arterial spasms or stenosis, arteriovenous (A-V) malformation
Carotid vessels	Duplex scanning	Plaques or stenosis and occlusion

Reference Values

Normal Doppler signals and pressure readings; no partial or complete arterial occlusion

Interfering Factors

➤ Inability of client to remain still during the procedure
➤ Incorrect placement of the transducer over the desired test sites
➤ Smoking before the procedure, which can constrict vessels
➤ Arterial occlusion proximal to the test site that affects blood flow to the area

Indications for Arterial Doppler Extremity Studies

➤ Detecting arterial stenosis causing occlusion in an extremity
➤ Diagnosing arteriosclerosis obliterans and monitoring degree of arterial insufficiency and tissue ischemia, graded as mild, moderate, or severe
➤ Detecting arterial spasms present in Raynaud's phenomenon
➤ Determining arterial occlusive disease of the small arteries in diabetes mellitus
➤ Determining whether an occlusion is the result of an embolism
➤ Determining arterial damage after trauma to a site
➤ Determining the presence or absence of collateral circulation
➤ Diagnosing abdominal aortic aneurysm
➤ Determining the presence and size of aneurysms or dilations in an extremity
➤ Assessing initial and continuing patency of an arterial graft
➤ Assessing abdominal arteries after renal transplantation in determining possible rejection
➤ Monitoring effectiveness of therapeutic interventions revealed by progression or maintenance of the status of an arterial disease graded as deteriorated, improved, or maintained
➤ Determining whether further diagnostic procedures such as angiography are needed to confirm a diagnosis

Contraindications

➤ None

➤➤ Nursing Alert

• The procedure cannot be performed successfully on an extremity that appears pale, waxen, or cyanotic and is cold to the touch because these signs indicate severely impaired circulation.[46]

Nursing Care Before the Procedure

Client teaching and physical preparation are the same as for any ultrasound procedure (see p. 690).
➤ Obtain a history that includes vascular signs and symptoms, known or suspected vascular disorders, and procedures or therapy, or both, administered for vascular conditions.

➤ Advise the client to refrain from smoking for at least 30 minutes before the study.

➤ Advise the client that blood pressure cuffs are placed at various sites on the arms or legs to perform the study.

➤ Administer an ordered analgesic to clients experiencing pain from severe ischemia.

The Procedure

The client is placed on the examination table in a supine position. The arms and legs are positioned and exposed, depending on the limbs to be studied. The client is reminded to remain very still to ensure accurate measurements during the procedure.

Blood pressure cuffs are applied to the calf and ankle and the systolic pressure is measured by noting the first sound with the Doppler transducer and comparing it with the brachial pressure. This comparison determines the presence and location of peripheral arteriosclerotic occlusive disease because a decrease in blood pressure of more than 20 mm Hg in the arm as compared with the leg indicates an occlusion proximal to the tested site in the leg. Also, the ankle pressure divided by the brachial pressure equals the ankle-to-brachial-pressure index, indicating arterial obstruction if the index is less than 0.96.[47]

To perform the study, blood pressure cuffs are placed at the thigh, calf, and ankle of a lower extremity or at the forearm and upper arm of an upper extremity. A conductive gel is applied to the arterial sites distal to the cuffs, i.e., femoral, popliteal, tibial, or dorsalis pedis arteries of the legs or brachial, radial, ulnar, or digital arteries of the arms.[48] The most proximal cuff is inflated to a level higher than the systolic reading noted in the normal limb, and the Doppler transducer is placed in contact with the conductive gel distal to the cuff. The procedure requires a normal extremity for comparison. The cuff is then slowly released while the examiner notes the highest pressure at which the characteristic swishing sound of the blood flow is heard. This reading is recorded as the blood pressure of that artery. The study continues with recordings of the blood pressure of the arteries at each level.[49] The studies performed on the upper extremity are made with the client in a sitting or supine position and the arm in hyperextension and hyperabduction to determine whether compression affects blood flow.[50] When the studies are completed, the cuffs and conductive gel are removed from the extremities.

Nursing Care After the Procedure

Care and assessment after the procedure are the same as for any ultrasound procedure (see p. 691).

➤ *Gangrene or ulcerations:* Note and report pain level, tissue breakdown, and condition of skin on extremities. Administer ordered analgesics. Change dressings as needed. Protect limb from trauma or pressure. Avoid leg elevation, and support limb during movement.[51]

ARTERIAL DOPPLER CAROTID STUDIES

Arterial Doppler carotid ultrasound is a technique performed to obtain information about the carotid arteries using duplex scanning. It provides measurement of the amplitude and waveform of the carotid pulse with a two-dimensional image of the artery. The result is visualization of the artery to diagnose stenosis or atherosclerotic occlusion affecting the flow of blood to the brain.[52] Depending on the degree of stenosis causing a reduction in vessel diameter, oculoplethysmography (OPG), a pressure measurement, can be performed to determine the effect of stenosis on the hemodynamic status of the artery (see pp. 843 to 845).[53]

Reference Values

Normal blood flow through carotid arteries; no plaque or stenosis indicating occlusive disease

Interfering Factors

➤ Inability of client to remain still during the procedure
➤ Incorrect placement of the transducer over the desired test site
➤ Abnormally large neck that makes direct examination difficult

Indications for Arterial Doppler Carotid Studies

➤ Detecting plaque or stenosis of carotid artery revealed by turbulent blood flow or changes in Doppler signals, indicating occlusion
➤ Detecting irregularities in the structure of the carotid arteries
➤ Diagnosing carotid artery occlusive disease revealed by visualization of blood flow disruption

Contraindications

➤ None

Nursing Care Before the Procedure

Client teaching and physical preparation are the same as for arterial Doppler extremity studies (see pp. 716 to 717).

The Procedure

The client is placed on the examination table in a supine position. The neck is exposed and the head supported to prevent movement. The client is reminded to remain very still during the procedure and to not turn the head. A conductive gel is applied to the skin of the neck at the carotid artery site. The transducer is placed over the site and moved slowly in the area of the common carotid artery to the bifurcation and then to areas of the internal and external carotids. Duplex scanning provides images of the blood flow and measurement of the waveform of the carotid pulse. A reduction in vessel diameter of more than 16 percent indicates stenosis. When the studies are completed, the gel is removed from the sites.

Nursing Care After the Procedure

Care and assessment after the procedure are the same as for any ultrasound procedure (see p. 690).
➤ *Transient ischemic attack (TIA):* Note and report neurological symptoms such as dizziness, syncope, or blurred vision. Protect from injury if symptoms occur. Administer or resume ordered medication regimen.

ARTERIAL DOPPLER TRANSCRANIAL STUDIES

Arterial Doppler transcranial ultrasound is a technique performed to obtain information about cerebral vessel patency and blood viscosity. The study measures and records the velocity of blood traveling through a vessel via a transducer that transmits waves through a section of the cranium that is thin or that contains a gap or opening. The procedure provides valuable information that once could be obtained only by the more invasive angiography procedure to assist in the diagnosis and treatment of neurological and cerebrovascular disorders.[54]

Reference Values

Normal blood flow through cranial arteries; no stenosis, hyperemia, arteriovenous (A-V) malformation, or increased intracranial pressure

Interfering Factors

➤ Inability of client to remain still and maintain the head position during the procedure
➤ Incorrect placement of the transducer over the site of the skull

Indications for Arterial Doppler Transcranial Studies

➤ Detecting arterial stenosis or A-V malformation in the cerebrovascular system revealed by low wave pulsations caused by low flow resistance
➤ Determining the presence of intracranial collateral pathways
➤ Diagnosing hyperemia caused by head injury or congestion in the tissue surrounding an ischemic area revealed by a higher velocity and wave pulsations
➤ Determining vertebral or basilar arterial insufficiency
➤ Monitoring increased intracranial pressure revealed by high wave pulsations
➤ Monitoring vasospasms revealed by changes in cerebral blood flow
➤ Confirming brain death[55]

Contraindications

➤ None

Nursing Care Before the Procedure

Client teaching and physical preparation are the same as for arterial Doppler extremity studies (see pp. 716 to 717).

The Procedure

The client is placed on the examination table in a supine position. The head is positioned to expose the site and supported to prevent movement. These sites include the transtemporal (at the temporal site) to view the middle, anterior, or posterior cerebral arteries and the circle of Willis; the transorbital (over the eye) to view the circle of Willis; and the transoccipital (at the foramen magnum) to view the vertebral and basilar arteries. The client is reminded to remain still and to not move the head.

A conductive gel is applied to the skin of the site and the transducer placed over it and gently manipulated around the area. Sound waves are transmitted through the transducer to the site and bounced off the cerebral vessel back to the probe; the waves are then bounced back to the monitor to be displayed as a wave on a screen and permanently recorded by computer. Normal velocity ranges are 30 to 50 cm per second in posterior arteries and 40 to 70 cm per second in middle and anterior arteries.[56] When the studies are completed, the gel is removed from the site.

Nursing Care After the Procedure

Care and assessment after the procedure are the same as for any ultrasound procedure (see p. 691).

➤ Perform vital signs and neurological checks to compare with baseline as needed.

➤ *Neurological changes:* Note and report dizziness, headache, syncope, or visual disturbances. Assist client to position of comfort. Monitor vital signs and neurological status for changes from baselines. Administer or resume ordered medication regimen.

VENOUS DOPPLER EXTREMITY STUDIES

Venous Doppler ultrasound is a technique performed to obtain information about the patency of the venous vasculature in the upper and lower extremities. The sounds produced by the movement of the red blood cells in a vein are of a swishing quality that occurs with spontaneous respirations. Changes in these sounds during respiration indicate a possible abnormal venous flow in the presence of occlusive disease; an absence of sounds indicates complete obstruction. Plethysmography can be performed to determine the filling time of calf veins in the diagnosis of a thrombotic disorder of a major vein and to identify incompetent valves in the venous system (see pp. 839 to 840).[57]

Reference Values

Normal venous blood flow; no venous occlusion or obstruction, vascular insufficiency, or vascular injury

Interfering Factors

➤ Inability of client to remain still during the procedure
➤ Incorrect placement of the transducer over the desired test sites
➤ Cold extremities resulting in vasoconstriction
➤ Occlusion proximal to the site, affecting blood flow to the test area

Indications for Venous Doppler Extremity Studies

➤ Detecting chronic venous insufficiency revealed by a reverse blood flow, indicating incompetent valves
➤ Diagnosing superficial or deep venous thrombosis that leads to venous occlusion or obstruction revealed by the absence of flow, variations in flow during respiration, or the absence of flow upon compression of the extremity
➤ Determining source of emboli when pulmonary embolism is suspected or diagnosed
➤ Determining venous damage after trauma to the area

➤ Differentiating between primary and secondary varicose veins
➤ Determining whether further diagnostic procedures such as angiography are needed to make or confirm a diagnosis
➤ Monitoring effectiveness of therapeutic interventions (medical and surgical) in the treatment of venous abnormalities

Contraindications

➤ None

Nursing Care Before the Procedure

Client teaching and physical preparation are the same as for arterial Doppler extremity studies (see pp. 716 to 717).

The Procedure

The client is placed on the examination table in a supine position. The arms or legs are exposed, depending on the limbs to be tested. The client is reminded to remain very still during the procedure and to breathe normally.

A conductive gel is applied to the skin at the vein sites. Sites include the femoral, popliteal, and tibial veins of the legs and the jugular, axillary, and brachial veins of the neck or arms.[58] The transducer is placed over the venous site and the waveforms visualized and recorded with variations in respirations. Recordings are also made after limb compression performed proximally or distally to an obstruction or proximally to the transducer to obtain information about venous occlusion or obstruction. Normally, the distal compression or release of proximal limb compression increases the speed of blood flow.[59] The procedure can be performed for both arms and legs to obtain bilateral blood flow determinations. When the studies are completed, the conductive gel is removed from the test sites.

Nursing Care After the Procedure

Care and assessment after the procedure are the same as for any ultrasound procedure (see p. 691).

➤ *Venous stasis or ulcer:* Note and report any lesion that is open or draining, skin discolorations, or other abnormalities. Maintain clean, dry dressings to ulcer. Protect limb from trauma. Avoid allowing transducer to be placed on ulcer site.

(Case Study follows on page 723)

Student Name _____ Class _____

Instructor _____ Date _____

CASE STUDY AND CRITICAL THINKING EXERCISE

Mr. Brown, age 76, is seen at the clinic for his regular checkup. He has a 22-year history of hypertension that has been managed with medication. Your assessment findings are: T98°F (36.6°C), P 82, R 16, and BP 148/84. Pulses are palpable and strong. You detect a carotid bruit on the right side.

a. What is the significance of the presence of a carotid bruit in this patient?

b. What specific noninvasive test may be ordered?

c. What is a probable treatment option?

References

1. Thomas, CL (ed): Taber's Cyclopedic Medical Dictionary, ed 18. FA Davis, Philadelphia, 1997, p 2025.
2. Fischbach, FT: A Manual of Laboratory and Diagnostic Tests, ed 4. JB Lippincott, Philadelphia, 1992, pp 767–768.
3. Corbett, JV: Laboratory Tests and Diagnostic Procedures with Nursing Diagnoses, ed 3. Appleton & Lange, Norwalk, Conn, 1992, p 575.
4. Fischbach, op cit, p 768.
5. Corbett, op cit, p 574.
6. Ibid, pp 576–577.
7. Fischbach, op cit, p 768.
8. Corbett, op cit, p 576.
9. Tempkin, BB: Ultrasound Scanning: Principles and Protocols. WB Saunders, Philadelphia, 1993, pp 3, 12–15.
10. Berkow, R (ed): The Merck Manual, ed 16. Merck Sharp and Dohme Research Laboratories, Rahway, NJ, 1992, p 388.
11. Corbett, op cit, p 581.
12. Pagana, KD, and Pagana, TJ: Mosby's Diagnostic and Laboratory Test Reference. Mosby–Year Book, St Louis, 1992, p 281.
13. Berkow, op cit, p 389.
14. Ibid, p 369.
15. Fischbach, op cit, p 906.
16. Berkow, op cit, p 1390.
17. Fischbach, op cit, p 906.
18. Springhouse Corporation: Nurse's Reference Library: Diagnostics, ed 2. Springhouse, Springhouse, Pa, 1986, p 577.
19. Ibid, pp 795–796.
20. Springhouse Corporation: Nurse's Ready Reference: Diagnostic Tests. Springhouse, Springhouse, Pa, 1991, p 486.
21. Nurse's Reference Library, op cit, p 541.
22. Fischbach, op cit, p 791.
23. Corbett, op cit, p 583.
24. Nurse's Ready Reference, op cit, p 479.
25. Berkow, op cit, p 569.
26. Ibid, p 474.
27. Ibid, p 1261.
28. Nurse's Reference Library, op cit, p 860.
29. Fischbach, op cit, p 790.
30. Ibid, p 784.
31. Ibid, p 784.
32. Ibid, p 870.
33. Ibid, p 787.
34. Ibid, p 782.
35. Berkow, op cit, p 1659.
36. Nurse's Ready Reference, op cit, p 488.
37. Ibid, p 488.
38. Fischbach, op cit, p 800.
39. Ibid, p 799.
40. Ibid, pp 779–780.
41. Ibid, p 779.
42. Ibid, pp 773–775.
43. Ibid, p 776.
44. Ibid, pp 907–909.
45. Ibid, pp 909–910.
46. Ibid, p 911.
47. Pagana and Pagana, op cit, p 278.
48. Nurse's Reference Library, op cit, p 914.
49. Pagana and Pagana, op cit, p 279.
50. Nurse's Reference Library, op cit, p 915.
51. Fischbach, op cit, p 912.
52. Pagana and Pagana, op cit, p. 164.
53. Fischbach, op cit, p 916.
54. Nurse's Ready Reference, op cit, p 487.
55. Ibid, p 487.
56. Ibid, p 487.
57. Fischbach, op cit, p 913.
58. Nurse's Reference Library, op cit, pp 913–915.
59. Fischbach, op cit, p 908.

Bibliography

Athey, PA, and Hadlock, FP: Ultrasound in Obstetrics and Gynecology, ed 2. Mosby–Year Book, St Louis, 1985.

Bisset, RAL, and Khan, AN: Differential Diagnosis in Abdominal Ultrasound. WB Saunders, Philadelphia, 1990.

Black, JM, and Matassarin-Jacobs, E: Luckmann and Sorensen's Medical-Surgical Nursing: A Psychophysiologic Approach, ed 4. WB Saunders, Philadelphia, 1993.

Bowerman, RA: Atlas of Normal Fetal Ultrasonographic Anatomy, ed 2. Mosby–Year Book, St Louis, 1992.

Chernecky, CC, and Berger, BJ; Cullen, BN (ed): Laboratory Tests and Diagnostic Procedures, ed 2. WB Saunders, Philadelphia, 1996.

Cranley, JJ, et al: Atlas of Duplex Scanning: Carotid Arteries. WB Saunders, Philadelphia, 1989.

Fleischer, AC, and Kepple, DM: Diagnostic Sonography: Principles and Clinical Applications, ed 2. WB Saunders, Philadelphia, 1995.

Goldberg, BB, and Kurtz, A: Atlas of Ultrasound Measurement. Mosby–Year Book, St Louis, 1990.

Gosink, BB: Diagnostic Ultrasound, ed 2. WB Saunders, Philadelphia, 1981.

Hagen-Ansert, SL: Textbook of Diagnostic Ultrasonography, ed 3. Mosby–Year Book, St Louis, 1989.

Kee, JL: Handbook of Laboratory and

Diagnostic Tests with Nursing Implications, ed 3. Appleton & Lange, Norwalk, Conn, 1997.

Kremkau, FW; Allen, A (ed): Diagnostic Ultrasound: Principles, Instruments, and Exercises, ed 5. WB Saunders, Philadelphia, 1998.

Kremkau, FW: Doppler Ultrasound: Principles and Instruments, ed 2. WB Saunders, Philadelphia, 1994.

Nyberg, D: Ultrasound of Fetal Anomalies. Mosby–Year Book, St Louis, 1994.

Nyberg, D, et al: Transvaginal Ultrasound. Mosby–Year Book, St Louis, 1992.

Pagana, KD, and Pagana, TJ: Diagnostic Testing and Nursing Implications: A Case Study Approach, ed 4. Mosby–Year Book, St Louis, 1993.

Porth, CM: Pathophysiology: Concepts of Altered Health States, ed 4. JB Lippincott, Philadelphia, 1993.

Resnick, MI: Prostatic Ultrasonography. Mosby–Year Book, St Louis, 1990.

Rumack, CM, Wilson, SR, and Charboneau, JW: Diagnostic Ultrasound. Mosby–Year Book, St Louis, 1991.

Salcedo, E: Atlas of Echocardiography, ed 2. WB Saunders, Philadelphia, 1985.

Teele, RL, and Share, C: Ultrasonography of Infants and Children. WB Saunders, Philadelphia, 1991.

Tempkin, BB: Ultrasound Scanning: Principles and Protocols. WB Saunders, Philadelphia, 1992.

van Holsbeek, M: Musculoskeletal Ultrasound. Mosby–Year Book, St Louis, 1990.

Wechsler, LR, and Babikian, VL: Transcranial Doppler Ultrasonography. Mosby–Year Book, St Louis, 1992.

Whaley, LF: Nursing Care of Infants and Children, ed 4. Mosby–Year Book, St Louis, 1991.

Williamson, MR, and Williamson, S: Gamuts in Ultrasound. WB Saunders, Philadelphia, 1992.

Zwiebel, WJ: Introduction to Vascular Ultrasonography, ed 3. WB Saunders, Philadelphia, 1992.

20

Nuclear Scan and Laboratory Studies

▶ **PROCEDURES COVERED**

Brain Scanning, *733*

Cerebrospinal Fluid (CSF) Flow
   Scanning, *735*

Parotid/Salivary Gland Scanning, *737*

Bone and Joint Scanning, *738*

Bone Marrow Scanning, *740*

Adrenal Scanning, *741*

Pheochromocytoma Scanning, *743*

Cardiac Scanning, *744*

Lung Scanning (Ventilation-
   Perfusion [V/Q] Scanning), *749*

Thyroid Scanning, *752*

Parathyroid Scanning, *754*

Abscess/Inflammatory Scanning, *755*

Gastric Emptying Scanning, *756*

Gastrointestinal Reflux Scanning, *758*

Gastrointestinal Bleeding
   Scanning, *760*

Meckel's Diverticulum Scanning, *761*

Pancreas Scanning, *762*

Liver Scanning, *763*

Spleen Scanning, *765*

Deep Vein Scanning, *766*

Gallbladder/Biliary System
   Scanning, *768*

Kidney/Renography Scanning, *769*

Scrotal Scanning, *772*

Gallium 67 (^{67}Ga) Scanning, *773*

Iodine 131 (^{131}I) Scanning, *775*

Positron Emission Tomography
   (PET), *776*

Total Blood Volume Study, *778*

Red Blood Cell (RBC) Survival Time
   Study, *781*

Platelet Survival Time Study, *784*

Radioactive Iodine Uptake (RAIU)
   Study, *786*

Thyroid-Stimulating Hormone (TSH)
   Study, *788*

Thyroid Cytomel/Perchlorate
   Suppression Studies, *790*

Schilling Test, *792*

INTRODUCTION

Nuclear scan studies are procedures that use radiopharmaceuticals (radionuclides in compounds that permit entry into body tissues), radiation detectors with imaging devices, and computers to visualize organs and study the dynamic processes that differentiate normal from pathological tissues. They are commonly referred to as computed tomography (CT) scanning; however, there are CT scans that do not use radiopharmaceuticals (see Chap. 21). These diagnostic studies provide more physiological information than the structural types of information gained from radiologic studies. They can be used to complement x-ray procedures or can be used exclusively to study an organ such as the thyroid gland that has no comparable x-ray procedure.[1] Nuclear studies do provide clinical information with a much lower dose of radiation than x-ray procedures and are much less expensive than other imaging procedures, such as magnetic resonance imaging (MRI). Although nuclear scans are primarily diagnostic studies, the radionuclides are also administered in therapeutic doses to treat pathologic conditions.

Radionuclide scanning studies involve the administration of a radiopharmaceutical intravenously (IV) or orally, depending on the radioactive material selected and the organ to be studied, followed by the measurement of the radiation emitted. The radionuclide is an element that has a nucleus that has been made radioactive and that emits radiation as it decays or disintegrates. Alpha (α), beta (β), and gamma (γ) rays can be emitted by the radionuclides used in diagnostic studies. γ-Rays are the least ionizing type, and the electromagnetic radiation that is emitted is readily detected with the modern equipment used in the scanning procedure. Each radionuclide decays at a specific rate (half-life) and has a specific spectrum of γ-ray energies that allows its identification in tissues. A small amount of produced radiation can be detected and is known as a tracer dose. This small dose eliminates the risk of physical and chemical toxicity and allows the studies to be performed on clients with sensitivities to diagnostic materials such as iodine 123 (^{123}I), which is known to cause an allergic reaction in some people.

The dose used for diagnostic studies is measured in microcuries (μCi) or millicuries (mCi) to identify the units of radioactivity. These measurements are now being replaced by the becquerel (Bq). Radiation doses used for therapy are measured in rads (radiation absorbed doses) to identify the amount of radiation energy absorbed by the tissues. The incorporation and distribution of a radionuclide into organ tissues depend on the physiological and biochemical properties of an organ and the specific radiopharmaceutical used.[2] This tissue specificity allows distribution of material in specific organs and differentiation between diseased and normal tissue by its activity (Table 20-1).

After the administration of the radiopharmaceutical, the amount and changing levels of the substance are detected by scanning with a scintillation camera. This camera is capable of monitoring the levels of radioactivity in an area and provides imaging and count rate information. The device detects the location and energy of γ-rays in an organ and feeds the readings into a computer that converts them into a two-dimensional scan or picture for immediate viewing. The computers also store the data for later viewing, analysis, and comparison. The time between the administration of a radiopharmaceutical and the scanning procedure varies from immediately to hours or days, depending on the radionuclide and the organ to be examined.

The image or scan is printed on a gray scale that reveals varying shades of gray to identify the distribution of the radionuclide in parts of an organ and is interpreted by a nuclear medicine physician. Dark spots are known as "hot spots" and indicate a greater concentration in the area. Spots that do not take up the radionuclide are identified by light shaded areas and are known as "cold spots."[3] The images can also be recorded in color.

The therapeutic use of ionizing radiation derives from its ability to kill cells by penetrating the targeted cells and depositing energy within them, thereby inhibiting their division and growth. The specific rad is calculated according to the half-life, type, and energies of the radioactive emissions; volume and density of the target organ to be exposed to the radiation; and the half-life

Table 20–1 ➤ RADIONUCLIDES/RADIOPHARMACEUTICALS AND DIAGNOSTIC SCANNING USES*

Radionuclide / Radiopharmaceutical	Organ/Study
Technetium 99m (Tc 99m or ^{99m}Tc)	
Technetium Tc 99m pertechnetate	Brain—delayed imaging
	Cardiac gated blood pool imaging
	Thyroid gland
	Parathyroid gland
	Parotid and salivary glands
	Scrotum and contents
	Meckel's diverticulum
Technetium Tc 99m stannous pyrophosphate	Cardiac infarction
	Cardiac gated blood pool imaging
Technetium Tc 99m diethylenetriamine pentaacetic acid (DTPA)	Brain—early imaging
	Cerebrospinal fluid (CSF) flow imaging
	Renal glomerular filtration rate (GFR) and blood flow imaging
Technetium Tc 99m RBC or albumin	Gastrointestinal bleeding
Technetium Tc 99m sulfur colloid	Gastrointestinal bleeding
	Gastric emptying
	Gastroesophageal reflux
	Esophageal motility
	Liver and spleen
	Bone marrow
Technetium Tc 99m glucoheptonate	Brain—early imaging
	Renal structural defects
Technetium Tc 99m hydroxyethylene disphosphonate (HEDP)	Bone and joint
Technetium Tc 99m methylene diphosphonate (MDP)	Bone and joint
Technetium Tc 99m albumin (MAA or HAM)	Lung perfusion
Technetium Tc 99m diisopropyl (IDA)	Gallbladder and biliary systems
Technetium Tc 99m dimercaptosuccinic acid (DMSA)	Renal excretion
Indium 111 (^{111}In)	
Indium In 111 diethylenetriamine pentaacetic acid (DTPA)	CSF flow imaging
Indium In 111 chloride	Bone marrow
	Gastric emptying
Indium In 111 WBC	Abscess and inflammatory areas
Iodine 131, 123, 125 (^{131}I, ^{123}I, ^{125}I)	
Metaiodobenzylguanidine (MIBG) I 131	Thyroid malignancy total body scanning
	Pheochromocytoma
Norcholestenol iodomethyl I 131	Adrenal gland
Orthoiodohippurate (OIH) I 131	Renal function
Iodide I 123	Thyroid gland function
Iofetamine I 123	Brain scanning
Fibrinogen I 125	Deep venous thrombosis (DVT)
Thallium 201 (^{201}Tl)	
Thallium chloride Tl 201	Cardiac perfusion
	Parathyroid gland
Selenium 75 (^{75}Se)	
Selenomethionine Se 75	Pancreas
Gallium 67 (^{67}Ga)	
Gallium citrate Ga 67	Body imaging for tumor or inflammatory process

continued on page 730

Table 20–1 ➤ **RADIONUCLIDES/RADIOPHARMACEUTICALS AND DIAGNOSTIC SCANNING USES***—(*Continued*)

Radionuclide / Radiopharmaceutical	Organ/Study
Xenon 133 (^{133}Xe)	
Xenon Xe 133 gas	Lung ventilation
Krypton 81m (^{81m}Kr)	
Krypton Kr 81m gas	Lung ventilation
Radionuclides and PET and SPECT Diagnostic Scanning	
Oxygen 15 (^{15}O), nitrogen 13 (^{13}N), carbon 11 (^{11}C), fluorine 18 (^{18}F)	PET scanning
Gallium 67 (67Ga), thallium 201 (^{201}Tl), technetium 99m (^{99m}Tc)	SPECT scanning
Radionuclides/Radiopharmaceuticals and Laboratory Diagnostic Testing	
Chromium 51 (^{51}Cr)	
Chromated Cr 51 sodium	RBC volume and survival time
Chromated Cr 51 albumin	Gastrointestinal protein loss
Cobalt 57 (^{57}Co)	
Cyanocobalamin Co 57	Pernicious anemia
Iodine 131, 123, 125 (^{131}I, ^{123}I, ^{125}I)	
^{131}I or ^{123}I	Thyroid gland function
^{125}I	Radioassays
	Total blood volume
Iodinated I 125 albumin	Plasma volume

*In this table, radionuclides appear in bold italic type and radiopharmaceuticals appear in regular type. For convention throughout the table and this chapter, radionuclides (i.e., radioactive isotopes) appear as the name of the element and the isotope number, abbreviated after initial mention (e.g., iodine 131 initially, ^{131}I thereafter). Radiopharmaceuticals appear as the name of the drug containing the radionuclide followed by the element symbol, the isotope number, and the carrier agent, if one is used. This table includes the most commonly used pharmaceuticals and does not preclude the use of others for specific studies or laboratory tests.

of the radionuclide while within the organ.[4] The most common therapeutic uses are in the treatment of malignancies of the thyroid, chest, and abdomen and in hyperthyroid and polycythemia vera conditions.

Nuclear studies can be considered invasive or noninvasive procedures, and therefore a signed informed consent is required for scanning procedures involving the administration of a radiopharmaceutical according to agency and nuclear department policies. Laboratory tests that use radiolabeled materials do not usually require a signed consent. Client preparation is similar for all nuclear studies and focuses on anxiety reduction caused by the beliefs about the effects of radiation. An explanation of the benefits and risks of performing the study and of the process of elimination of the radioactive substance by dissipation and via feces and urine can allay this anxiety. The studies are performed in a special department by physicians specializing in nuclear medicine and assisted by trained technicians.

POSITRON EMISSION TOMOGRAPHY (PET)

Positron emission tomography (PET), also known as emission computed tomography (ECT), is a noninvasive procedure that combines the tomographic capabilities of computed tomography scanning with the use of radiopharmaceuticals to provide clinical information about physiological organ function and structure.[5] The physiological organ activities that are studied include tissue metabolism; structure or density; and body fluid volume or flow, or both.

These studies involve the IV administration of tracers tagged with a radioactive isotope designed to measure biochemical activities. This isotope emits positrons (positive electrons) as it deteriorates or decays; the positrons combine with electrons (negative electrons) normally found in specific tissue cells. The combination then emits γ-rays that can be detected by a PET scanner or camera that transmits the information to a computer.[6] The computer determines the location and distribution of the radioactivity and translates the emissions as color-coded images on a screen. The images can be viewed immediately, and the information and images are stored for future use.

The radionuclides used for PET are produced by a cyclotron and are different from those produced by a nuclear reactor used in conventional scanning. They have a short half-life and are free of contaminants.[7] Only institutions that have access to this capability and have a team of professionals and a facility to accommodate this technology can perform PET studies because the radionuclide must be used immediately after its production. The isotopes used are oxygen 15 (^{15}O), nitrogen 13 (^{13}N), fluorine 18 (^{18}F), and carbon 11 (^{11}C), which are the main body constituents.

Although PET is more expensive than are conventional nuclear scans, it is becoming a widely used diagnostic method, especially for brain and heart pathology, staging of disease, and effectiveness of therapy protocols.[8] It also has diagnostic value in the study of the function of other regions or organs of the body through its ability to obtain physiological and biochemical information not possible with other scanning methods.

SINGLE-PHOTON EMISSION COMPUTED TOMOGRAPHY

Single-photon emission computed tomography (SPECT) is another imaging method used to scan organs. It does not need a positron-emitting isotope as used in PET, but it uses the same isotopes as conventional nuclear scans, such as gallium 67 (^{67}Ga), thallium 201 (^{201}Tl), and technetium 99m (Tc 99m, or ^{99m}Tc).[9] The procedure allows more sensitive and specific imaging to obtain diagnostic information because it uses a more advanced gamma camera. This camera reveals an additional third dimension of the tissue segment for viewing. Organs commonly studied by SPECT are the brain, lungs, heart, spleen, liver, and bones and joints, depending on the suspected pathology.[10]

RADIONUCLIDE LABORATORY STUDIES

Radionuclides can be administered in very small doses orally or IV and, at a later time, detected in the body by laboratory testing of blood, urine, and other body fluids. These tests determine the ability of the body to absorb the radionuclide by measurement of the concentration of radioactivity. Glands such as the thyroid can also be examined for the concentration of radioactivity by determining the ability of the body to localize the radionuclide as in the use of iodine radionuclide in thyroid testing. Radionuclides and laboratory tests are listed in Table 20–1 (see pp. 729–730). Scanning is performed in combination with laboratory testing for some studies.[11] Depending on the test to be conducted, the laboratory, the department of nuclear medicine, and the client or the hospital staff share responsibility in performing these studies.

A wide variety of substances can be measured by radioimmunoassay (RIA) studies included in the laboratory section of this book. They include hormones, proteins, immunoglobulins, carcinogens, antibodies, vitamins, and drugs that are antigenic or that can be made so by adding them to an antigenic substance. These tests involve the administration of a labeled compound that is produced by chemically binding the radionuclide to another molecule. They can be labeled to antigens or antibodies because the assay is based on an antigen-antibody reaction to detect and measure a substance. This method of testing provides a high level of sensitivity and specificity in substance detection. Easily measured isotopes such as iodine 25 (^{25}I), carbon 14 (^{14}C), or cobalt 57 (^{57}Co) are labeled and used in this method. Some substances are measured in the blood by the tagging of proteins with radionuclides. Protein-binding properties are the basis for estimating the amount of substances such as cortisol, folate, thyroxine, and vitamin B_{12} as the radionuclide-labeled compound competes with existing compounds for these binding sites. This competition permits the measurement of the substances that are bound to the protein, even in minute amounts.[12,13]

NUCLEAR SCANNING RISKS

The risk of radiation from the diagnostic use of radionuclides is very small because of the low dosage and short half-life of the materials used. Most radionuclides leave the body in 6 to 24 hours; others can take as long as 8 days. The radiation dose is actually less than that received in x-ray studies. The use of radionuclides for diagnostic studies does not require that personnel and others be protected from the presence of radiation in the client. Specific precautions, however, are required to protect others from the radiation in the client if therapeutic doses are administered, as these doses are much higher and the radiation that results is about 1000 times more than that from a diagnostic dose. Agencies that are approved to use radioactive materials for diagnosis, therapy, or research are provided with standards and guidelines from the government regulating commissions. These guidelines include directions to be followed in the handling, storage, and disposal of radiopharmaceuticals with short and long half-lives. Also provided are guidelines and requirements for the care and handling of specimens collected for testing, procedures to follow to protect the client and others from radiation, and procedures for the disposal of body excretions.

Because of the potential effect of radiation on cell growth if a fetus is exposed to radionuclide material, pregnant women are not considered candidates for nuclear scanning procedures. Mothers who are breast-feeding their babies are generally excluded as well, but they can be considered for this method of diagnostic testing with dosages calculated to provide the maximum results while using a minimum amount of the radionuclide.[14] Children are another group that are not generally considered candidates for nuclear testing unless dosage is carefully calculated, although there are instances when frequent scanning is performed, such as in bone cancer. The decision to perform nuclear studies on these groups varies with diagnosis and physicians as they compare the benefits and risks of using the very low doses for scanning against more invasive diagnostic procedures.

RADIONUCLIDE-MEDIATED SCANNING STUDIES

Radionuclide-mediated scanning studies, known as an "in vivo" diagnostic method, are performed to measure the amount of a specific radionuclide distributed in the body or specific organs by scanning and imaging. The studies are named for the organ or region of the body to be examined or imaged. The radiopharmaceutical and route used, as well as the time involved to perform the study, are specific to the organ studied. A list of commonly used radiopharmaceuticals and their tissue sites are found in Table 20–1 (see pp. 729–730). The scanning procedure provides a picture of the location, shape, size, and functional disturbances of an organ. Almost all organs can be scanned for diagnostic information related to the presence of tumors or other abnormalities.

BRAIN SCANNING

Brain scanning is a nuclear study performed to assist in diagnosing abnormalities of the brain and cerebral blood flow that are characteristic of pathology. The radionuclide ^{99m}Tc is administered IV as technetium Tc 99m pertechnetate, which requires a delayed imaging, as technetium Tc 99m diethylenetriamine pentaacetic acid (DTPA) (technetium Tc 99m DTPA), or as technetium Tc 99m gluceptate, which allows earlier imaging and increased sensitivity.[15] These substances do not cross the blood-brain barrier to enter the brain because this complex system prevents materials from being transported from the blood into the neural tissue. The presence of disease that can cause a breakdown or disruption in this protective barrier allows the radionuclide to cross into and become concentrated in the abnormal parts of the brain. Scanning provides the location, size, and shape of an abnormality. Newer lipid-soluble radionuclides that are able to cross an intact blood-brain barrier are now used to scan and study the distribution of a tracer dose to evaluate cerebral perfusion over a period of time. These newer materials allow imaging of the entire brain instead of areas involving pathology only.[16]

Brain scanning has generally been replaced by diagnostic studies such as MRI and CT scanning, neither of which requires the use of a radionuclide.

Reference Values

Blood-brain barrier intact with no uptake in flow and static views revealed; no intracranial pathology indicating a demyelinating disease, infection or inflammatory disease, atherosclerosis or stenosis, hemorrhage, aneurysm, tumors, or arteriovenous (A-V) malformation

Interfering Factors

➤ Inability of client to remain still during the procedure, especially if the client is a child
➤ Environmental stimuli such as noise or bright lights that can affect the distribution of radionuclide used in PET or SPECT

Indications for Brain Scanning

➤ Frequent headache, seizure activity, or neurosensory or neuromuscular complaints or symptoms of unknown etiology

➤ Determination of the cause of cerebrovascular disease with or without a stroke, such as atherosclerosis, thrombosis, hemorrhage, or stenosis revealed by decreased uptake of radionuclide

➤ Identification of sites of cerebral ischemia or infarction with known presence of atherosclerotic disease

➤ Detection of intracranial masses such as gliomas, meningiomas, neuromas, cystic lesions, pituitary adenoma, malignant primary or metastatic tumors revealed by an increased uptake and irregular distribution of the radionuclide

➤ Diagnosis of the cause of intracranial bleeding as in a ruptured aneurysm, subdural hematoma resulting from trauma, or an A-V malformation

➤ Diagnosis of infectious diseases such as encephalitis and brain abscess

➤ Diagnosis of demyelinating diseases such as multiple sclerosis

➤ Determination of whether hydrocephalus in children is surgically treatable or evaluation of shunt patency postoperatively

➤ Visualization of suture lines in children

➤ Detection of cerebral edema, hematoma, or contusion after head trauma

➤ Diagnosis of neurological disorders with presenting deficits or symptoms as in dementia, epilepsy, Parkinson's disease, Huntington's chorea, and Alzheimer's diseases when studied by PET

➤ Evaluation of the effect of radiation or chemotherapy on malignant brain tumor

➤ Determination of brain death revealed by an absence of uptake in the sinus or brain vascular system

Contraindications

➤ Pregnancy, unless benefits of performing the procedure greatly outweigh the risks to the fetus

Nursing Care Before the Procedure

Explain to the client:

➤ That the procedure takes about 1 hour unless delayed scanning is planned within hours, requiring the client to return to the department

➤ That a sedative can be administered before the study to promote relaxation

➤ That a minute amount of radioactive material will be administered by IV injection and that this does not cause harm to the client or those in contact with him or her

➤ That the radioactive material is excreted by the body, usually in the urine

➤ That scanning will take place immediately after the injection or at a later time, depending on the material used, with a machine that moves over the area to be examined

➤ That a medication to enhance scanning can be administered before the procedure

➤ That the only discomfort experienced is the injection of the radiopharmaceutical

Prepare for the procedure:

➤ Obtain a history to ascertain last menstrual period date and possible pregnancy in women of childbearing age, known and suspected cerebral disorders, allergy to iodine, assessment information of neurological system, tests and procedures conducted and results, or therapeutic interventions performed.

➤ Administer any ordered medications such as potassium iodine to block thyroid uptake of the radionuclide or potassium chloride to block choroid plexus uptake if a radionuclide other than ^{99m}Tc is used.[17]

➤ Have the client void before the study to prevent discomfort or interruption.

The Procedure

The client is placed on the examining table in a supine position. If the client is a young child and unable to lie still, a general anesthetic can be administered. The radiopharmaceutical is administered IV, and scanning is performed with the scanner moved back and forth over the head for immediate computer images. If a SPECT study is performed, the images are obtained with the client in a supine position and the scanner rotated around the head. The client is reminded to lie very still while the scanner is operating. Scanning can be delayed and performed 30 minutes after the injection, depending on the radionuclide used. The client's position is changed to lateral and prone to obtain anterior, lateral, and posterior projections. Blood pool images and flow studies through the arterial, venous, and capillary phases are anatomically displayed, based on counts determined from the radioactivity of the radionuclide. In some instances, initial normal scans can appear abnormal at a later time. Later delayed images are obtained in 3 to 4 hours in the anterior, posterior, lateral, and vertex positions with the head in flexion. These static views can reveal abnormally increased uptake in the cortex to identify pathological tissue.

Nursing Care After the Procedure

➤ Advise the client of the time to return for additional imaging, if appropriate.

➤ Inform the client that the radioactive substance is eliminated from the body within 6 to 24 hours and that fluid intake should be increased to encourage this process.

➤ *Phlebitis:* Note and report redness, pain, and swelling at the IV site. Elevate arm, and apply warm compress to the site.

CEREBROSPINAL FLUID (CSF) FLOW SCANNING

Cerebrospinal fluid (CSF) flow scanning is a nuclear study performed to evaluate patency and filling of the CSF pathways and the reabsorption or leakage of CSF. It is most commonly used to diagnose surgically treatable hydrocephalus and to evaluate shunt patency postoperatively. A radiopharmaceutical is administered by injection into the spinal column via a lumbar puncture. Radionuclides used are ^{99m}Tc or indium 111 (^{111}In) administered as technetium Tc 99m DTPA or indium In 111 DTPA, which flow with CSF. Imaging is performed in 1 hour and periodically up to 72 hours after the injection.

Reference Values

Reflux of CSF into the ventricles; no obstruction of or increase in CSF volume or pressure

Interfering Factors

➤ Inability of client to remain still during the procedure, expecially if the client is a child

Indications for Cerebrospinal Fluid (CSF) Flow Scanning

➤ Diagnosing and differentiating between communicating nonobstructive hydrocephalus or noncommunicating obstructive hydrocephalus in infants as revealed by reflux into ventricles or absence of reflux into ventricles, respectively

➤ Evaluating the size of the ventricles with CSF reflux if an obstruction is present or evaluating the ability to reabsorb the fluid revealed by an increased uptake of the radionuclide in the ventricles

➤ Determining spinal masses or lesions

➤ Evaluating preoperatively for shunt type and placement and postoperatively for shunt patency and effectiveness

Contraindications

➤ Pregnancy, unless benefits of performing the procedure greatly outweigh the risks to the fetus

Nursing Care Before the Procedure

Client teaching and physical preparation are the same as for brain scanning (see pp. 734 to 735).

➤ Additional teaching should include information about the route of the radiopharmaceutical administration (lumbar puncture) and an explanation of the procedure.

➤ Inform that the schedule of delayed studies may continue up to 3 days and that no medications are administered before the procedure.

➤ Maintain the client in a supine position after the lumbar puncture.

The Procedure

The client is placed flat on the examining table in a supine position 1 hour after injection of the radiopharmaceutical into the spinal column. A head-down position is also sometimes used. The client is reminded to lie very still while the scanner is operating. The scanner is moved over the head for imaging of ventricular flow. Subsequent imaging takes place in 4, 6, 24, 48, and 72 hours, depending on persistent reflux. Anterior, posterior, vertex, and lateral views are made, with client position changed as needed for the desired projections.

Nursing Care After the Procedure

Care and assessment after the procedure are the same as for brain scanning (see p. 735).

➤ Assess the puncture site for leakage and apply a small dressing.

➤ Return the client to the hospital room in a prone position.

➤ Have the client maintain a prone or supine position for 4 to 8 hours after the study.

➤ *Lumbar puncture:* Note and report changes in neurological status, increased blood pressure or temperature, sensory changes in extremities (tingling, numbness), irritability, or headache. Administer ordered analgesic for headache. Perform neurological checks every 2 to 4 hours for possible infection or brain or cord damage.

Parotid/Salivary Gland Scanning

Parotid or salivary gland scanning is a nuclear study performed to assist in diagnosing abnormalities of secretory function and duct patency of either or both glands. The radionuclide ^{99m}Tc as technetium Tc 99m pertechnetate is administered IV, and the immediate imaging of blood flow, uptake, and secreting capability is performed. This study is not made, however, to provide a definitive diagnosis before surgery.[18]

Reference Values

Normal size, shape, and position of the glands; no masses or duct obstruction

Interfering Factors

➤ Inability of client to remain still during the procedure

Indications for Parotid/Salivary Gland Scanning

➤ Determining the cause of pain and swelling in the gland area
➤ Detecting tumors of the parotid or salivary glands, such as oncocytoma, Warthin's tumor, or mucoepidermoid tumor, revealed by "hot" nodule surrounded by radionuclide uptake
➤ Detecting tumors, cysts, or abscesses and differentiating between them and malignant tumors revealed by smooth or ragged outlines of the respective masses
➤ Determining duct obstruction commonly seen in sialadenitis or Sjögren's syndrome revealed by decreased uptake of the radionuclide
➤ Diagnosing acute parotitis and other inflammatory processes of the glands revealed by an increased uptake of the radionuclide[19]

Contraindications

➤ Pregnancy, unless benefits of performing the procedure greatly outweigh the risks to the fetus

Nursing Care Before the Procedure

Client teaching and physical preparation are the same as for any nuclear scan study (see pp. 734 to 735).
➤ No medications are administered before the study.
➤ Teaching should include informing the client that the time to complete the study is usually 1 hour and that the scanner is positioned over the neck.
➤ Obtain a history of glandular disorders.

The Procedure

The client is placed in a sitting position and the radiopharmaceutical is administered IV. The client is reminded to remain very still during the scanning. Immediate scanning is performed for 30 minutes in anterior, posterior, and oblique views for blood flow and uptake studies. If secretory function of the glands is desired, the client is requested to suck on a lemon about three fourths of the way through the study to increase gland secretion and cause the gland to empty.

Nursing Care After the Procedure

Care and assessment after the procedure are the same as for brain scanning (see p. 735).

BONE AND JOINT SCANNING

Bone and joint scanning is a nuclear study performed to assist in diagnosing pathological conditions as well as complications of bone disease. The advantage of bone scanning over other bone diagnostic procedures is that abnormalities, or "hot spots," appear 3 to 6 months before x-ray reveals any pathology. Total body scanning is performed if metastatic disease to the bone is suspected. Total body scanning is important because all of the skeleton can reveal different locations of the metastases, such as the skull, long bones, pelvis, vertebrae, ribs, and sternum.[20]

The study is performed after the IV administration of the radionuclide ^{99m}Tc as technetium Tc 99m hydroxyethylene diphosphonate (HEDP) or technetium Tc 99m methylene diphosphonate (MDP), with scanning, flow studies, and blood pool studies undertaken immediately or delayed to allow concentration of the radionuclide in the bones and joints. Concentration depends on bone metabolism, which determines the amount of uptake of the substance, and the blood flow, which increases the deposition of the material as the flow is increased. A decrease or absence of blood flow produces "cold" bone defects. It is the increase of radionuclide uptake and activity (chemisorption) on the scan that represents an abnormality as it becomes concentrated at a higher or lower rate than does normal bone tissue. There are, however, normal areas of increased activity in adults, such as the sternum and the sacroiliac, clavicular, and scapular joints. In children, normal areas of increased activity are growth centers and cranial sutures.[21] Gallium (^{67}Ga) scanning after the administration of gallium citrate Ga 67 can follow a bone scan to obtain a more definitive study if acute inflammatory conditions such as osteomyelitis or septic arthritis are suspected (see p. 773).

Reference Values

Normal uptake by chemisorption of radionuclide by the bone; no tumors, infection or inflammation, fracture, or joint derangement or joint inflammation

Interfering Factors

➤ Inability of client to remain still during the procedure, especially if the client is a child
➤ Multiple myeloma or thyroid malignancy causing false-negative scan for bone abnormalities

Indications for Bone and Joint Scanning

➤ Determining the cause of unexplained bone or joint pain
➤ Diagnosing degenerative joint changes or septic arthritis that occurs in arthritic conditions revealed by increased uptake of radionuclide

➤ Confirming a diagnosis of temporomandibular joint derangement by SPECT studies

➤ Diagnosing primary malignant bone tumors such as osteogenic sarcoma, chondrosarcoma, and Ewing's sarcoma

➤ Determining metastatic malignant tumor from primary sites such as breast, lung, thyroid, prostate, or kidney revealed by an increased uptake of radionuclide

➤ Diagnosing benign tumors or cysts revealed by minimal or normal uptake, with the exception of osteoid osteoma, which is revealed by increased uptake and blood pool activity

➤ Diagnosing osteomyelitis, usually in the femur, tibia, fibula, and humerus

➤ Determining acute osteomyelitis when performed with a ^{67}Ga scan

➤ Detecting fractures (traumatic and stress) and evaluating healing after a fracture, especially when an underlying bone disease is present

➤ Diagnosing metabolic bone disease and differentiating among osteoporosis, osteomalacia, Paget's disease, and bone disorders secondary to hyperparathyroidism

➤ Detecting Legg-Calvé-Perthes disease and determining the phase of the disease in children, revealed by changes in uptake activity in each phase

➤ Evaluating prosthetic joints for infection, loosening, dislocation, or breakage revealed by increased uptake around the prosthesis

➤ Evaluating tumor response to radiation or chemotherapy

➤ Identifying appropriate site for bone biopsy

Contraindications

➤ Pregnancy, unless benefits of performing the procedure greatly outweigh the risks to the fetus

Nursing Care Before the Procedure

Client teaching and physical preparation are the same as for any nuclear scan study (see pp. 734 to 735).

➤ Inform the client of the scanning schedule, which begins 2 to 4 hours after the injection and then takes 1 hour to complete.

➤ A history should include assessment information about the musculoskeletal system and known and suspected bone diseases.

➤ Request that the client remove all clothing and provide him or her with a hospital gown if a full body scan is to be performed.

The Procedure

The client is placed on the examining table in a supine position with the site to be scanned exposed. To conduct a flow study, the radiopharmaceutical is injected IV, and images are obtained in sequence every 3 seconds for 1 minute. The client is reminded or assisted to remain very still during the procedure. A blood pool image is then obtained over the area. To improve tumor imaging by allowing the radionuclide to be taken up by the bones, a 2- to 3-hour delay takes place before static images are made. The client is requested to drink fluids during this time and is allowed to walk around or sit and read. Also, request that the client void before the delayed imaging to prevent interference with examination of the pelvic bones. After the delay, multiple images are obtained over the complete skeleton. A large-field-of-view camera is used to cover the entire area. Sacral lesions can be imaged by positioning the client on the hands and knees and using a tail on the detector.[22] After 24 hours, additional views can be taken of a specific area, which can be useful in evaluating a fracture for repair processes. Total body imaging is performed primarily to determine metastatic sites that can be detected long before they are seen with x-ray radiography. If a SPECT study is performed for bone and joint imaging, the scanner is rotated around the client, with various views taken.

Nursing Care After the Procedure

Care and assessment after the procedure are the same as for any nuclear scan study (see p. 735).

BONE MARROW SCANNING

Bone marrow scanning is a nuclear study performed to assist in diagnosing pathological conditions of active bone marrow in the axial skeleton in adults and in the full length of extremities in infants, with a gradual retraction in children until 10 years of age. The marrow moves peripherally in the long bones as red blood cell production requirements increase, and this distribution can be detected on the scan. The degree of bone marrow activity and bone marrow distribution revealed provides the clinical information related to pathological processes.[23] The abnormalities seen on the scan include focal defects, increased size of the liver and spleen, decrease in the central marrow, peripheral extension, and increased uptake outside of normal areas (extramedullary hematopoiesis). Depending on the suspected pathology, ^{99m}Tc administered as technetium Tc 99m sulfur colloid is used when imaging the entire body about 1 hour after injection, or ^{111}In as indium In 111 chloride is used when imaging the entire body 48 hours after injection.

Reference Values

Normal distribution of active marrow in the axial skeleton; no avascular necrosis, extramedullary hematopoiesis, bone marrow infarcts or hemolytic anemia, metastatic bone tumor, or diffuse hematologic disorders

Interfering Factors

➤ Inability of client to remain still during the procedure

Indications for Bone Marrow Scanning

➤ Diagnosing avascular necrosis in hip studies revealed by the absence or decrease of uptake activity
➤ Determining extramedullary hematopoiesis sites such as the liver, spleen, lymph nodes, lungs, kidneys, breasts, or adrenal glands
➤ Diagnosing thalassemia, sickle cell anemia, hereditary spherocytosis, and myeloproliferative disorders revealed by an increased uptake of radionuclide
➤ Diagnosing bone marrow infarcts common in sickle cell anemia and thalassemia revealed by "cold" areas with increased uptake in the surrounding active bone marrow

➤ Detecting metastases of malignant tumor to bone revealed by focal defects

➤ Diagnosing and determining the stage of diffuse hematologic disorders such as polycythemia vera, leukemia, hemolytic anemia, aplastic anemia, myelofibrosis, Hodgkin's and non-Hodgkin's lymphoma revealed by a decrease or absence of radionuclide uptake

➤ Evaluating a disparity between marrow histology and blood smear results to determine errors in marrow sampling

➤ Determining splenic erythrocytosis before splenectomy and determining whether enough active bone marrow is present to allow removal of the spleen[24]

➤ Determining bone marrow depression during or after chemotherapy or radiation therapy

Contraindications

➤ Pregnancy, unless benefits of performing the procedure greatly outweigh the risks to the fetus

Nursing Care Before the Procedure

Client teaching and physical preparation are the same as for any nuclear scan study (see pp. 734 to 735).

➤ Inform the client of the scanning schedule and explain that the study takes 1 hour.

➤ Obtain a history to include information about known or suspected hematologic disorders and other associated tests and procedures performed.

The Procedure

The client is placed on the examining table in a supine position and reminded to remain very still during the scanning procedure. The radiopharmaceutical technetium Tc 99m sulfur colloid is injected IV, and imaging is begun after 30 minutes to 1 hour. Scanning of the entire body, both anteriorly and posteriorly, is performed. Technetium Tc 99m sulfur colloid is used to examine for avascular necrosis, bone marrow infarct and hemolytic anemias, metastatic tumors, and diffuse hematologic disorders. If indium In 111 chloride is injected, imaging is started in 48 hours, and scanning of the entire body is performed. This agent is used to examine the client for extramedullary hematopoiesis and sites of occurrence.

Nursing Care After the Procedure

Care and assessment after the procedure are the same as for any nuclear scan study (see p. 735).

ADRENAL SCANNING

Scanning of the adrenal glands is a nuclear study performed to assist in diagnosing pathology based on the secretory function of the adrenal cortex. This function is controlled primarily by the anterior pituitary through the adrenocorticotropic hormone (ACTH) that stimulates the adrenal cortex to produce cortisone as well as to secrete aldosterone. High concentrations of cholesterol, the precursor in the synthesis of adrenocorticosteroids including aldosterone, are stored in the adrenal cortex. This storage allows the radiopharmaceutical nor-cholestenol iodomethyl I 131 to be used in identifying pathology. The uptake of this substance occurs gradually and imaging reveals increased uptake, unilateral or bilateral uptake, or absence of uptake in the detection of pathological processes. Suppression studies can be performed to differentiate the presence of a tumor from hyperplasia of the glands, followed by prescanning treatment with corticosteroids.[25]

Reference Values

Normal bilateral secretory function of the adrenal cortex with the uptake of the radionuclide; no tumors, infection, or secretory suppression

Interfering Factors

➤ Inability of client to remain still during the procedure

Indications for Adrenal Scanning

➤ Diagnosing Cushing's syndrome revealed by increased symmetrical uptake, indicating bilateral hyperplasia, or asymmetric uptake, indicating unilateral hyperplasia or adenoma
➤ Determining aldosteronism revealed by asymmetric uptake
➤ Differentiating between asymmetric hyperplasia and asymmetry from aldosteronism with dexamethasone suppression test
➤ Determining adrenal suppressibility with prescan administration of corticosteroid to diagnose and localize adrenal adenoma, aldosteronomas, androgen excess, or low-renin hypertension
➤ Diagnosing glandular tissue destruction caused by infection, infarction, neoplasm, or suppression

Contraindications

➤ Pregnancy, unless benefits of performing the procedure greatly outweigh the risks to the fetus

Nursing Care Before the Procedure

Client teaching and physical preparation are the same as for any nuclear scan study (see pp. 734 to 735).
➤ Inform the client that there will be a prolonged scanning schedule over a period of days and that the time to complete each scan is 30 minutes.
➤ Administer supersaturated potassium iodide (SSKI) 24 hours before the study to prevent thyroid uptake of the free iodine.
➤ Obtain a history to include information about the endocrine system, allergy to iodine, laboratory results for cortisol, and urinary adrenal function tests.

The Procedure

The client is placed on the examining table in a supine or sitting position. The radiopharmaceutical is injected IV and the client is returned to the hospital room or requested to return to the department in 24 hours, when the scanning procedure will begin. The client is requested to remain very still in the prone position and the imaging then takes place for posterior views for at least 20 minutes. Scanning is then performed each day for 3 to 5 days after this first scan. If a suppression test is to be performed, 4 mg of dexamethasone is administered for 7 days before the scanning procedure.

Nursing Care After the Procedure

Care and assessment after the procedure are the same as for any nuclear scan study (see p. 735).

➤ Administer supersaturated potassium iodide 10 days after the injection of the radiopharmaceutical to ensure that the iodine is not taken up by the thyroid gland until the material is entirely excreted.

PHEOCHROMOCYTOMA SCANNING

Pheochromocytoma scanning is a nuclear study performed to identify the presence of this tumor in the body. The tumor arises from the chromaffin cells of the sympathetic adrenal system, with 90 percent occurring within the adrenal medulla and 10 percent in extra-adrenal sites. A higher percentage of the extra-medullary tumor sites occur in children. The defining characteristic of pheochromocytomas is the production of excessive catecholamines (epinephrine, norepinephrine) with epinephrine-secreting tumors found in the intra-adrenal site and norepinephrine-secreting tumors found in the intra-adrenal or extra-adrenal sites. About 10 percent are malignant, with an increased incidence in the extra-adrenal sites.[26]

The study involves a total body scanning after the IV injection of iodine 131 (^{131}I) administered as metaiodobenzylguanidine (MIBG) I 131, composed of bretylium and guanethidine, which localizes sympathetic tissue. Imaging is performed primarily to localize the tumor site rather than to formulate a diagnosis; the site is revealed by an abnormal uptake of the radionuclide at the intra-adrenal or extra-adrenal sites. Laboratory measurements of catecholamines in the urine and blood are performed to determine an increased secretion of these substances and, combined with CT and ultrasonography, provide definitive diagnostic information. Once diagnosed, surgical removal of the tumor is the most effective treatment.[27]

Reference Values

Normal uptake of radionuclide in all areas of the body: liver, spleen, urinary bladder, salivary glands, heart, and adrenal glands; no adrenergic tumor

Interfering Factors

➤ Inability of client to remain still during the procedure
➤ Barium in the gastrointestinal tract from previous diagnostic procedures

Indications for Pheochromocytoma Scanning

➤ Confirming a diagnosis and localizing an adrenergic tumor when CT has not provided a definitive diagnosis
➤ Identifying extra-adrenal sites of a tumor such as the organ of Zuckerkandl revealed by increased uptake
➤ Confirming a suspected tumor in the area of the adrenal glands revealed by an abnormal uptake of the radionuclide

➤ Identifying and localizing related tumors such as neuroblastomas, carcinoid tumors, and paraganglionomas (tumors found outside of the adrenal medulla)

➤ Diagnosing medullary cancer of the thyroid gland

Contraindications

➤ Pregnancy, unless benefits of performing the procedure greatly outweigh the risks to the fetus

Nursing Care Before the Procedure

Client teaching and physical preparation are the same as for any nuclear scan study (see pp. 734 to 735).

➤ Assess for iodine allergy, and note the results of catecholamine measurement in blood and urine laboratory tests.

The Procedure

The client is placed on the examining table in a supine or sitting position. The radiopharmaceutical is injected IV and the client is returned to the hospital room or requested to return to the department in 24 hours. The client is requested to remain very still during the procedure, and imaging of the whole body is performed at that time and then again in 48 and 72 hours as the radionuclide localizes in the sympathetic tissues of the body. Renal scanning is also performed to outline the kidneys. In some instances, an additional scan takes place 4 days after the injection. The daily scanning is necessary because the tumor can be visualized on a specific day or on all days.

Nursing Care After the Procedure

Care and assessment after the procedure are the same as for any nuclear scan study (see p. 735).

➤ Administer supersaturated potassium iodide 10 days after the injection of the radiopharmaceutical.

CARDIAC SCANNING

Cardiac scanning is a nuclear study that includes several categories of procedures depending on the radionuclide used and the suspected pathology. The various studies can reveal clinical information about wall motion (contractions), ejection fraction, coronary blood flow, ventricular size and function, valvular regurgitation, and cardiac blood shunting. Contractions are performed by wall motion of the left ventricle and the movements are graded from 3+ (normal) to 0 (akinesis). Blood ejection is performed by movements of the right ventricle. The ejection fraction is calculated from the end-diastolic volume and end-systolic volume in the left ventricle and equals the percentage of the end-diastolic volume pumped per beat or contraction. Coronary blood flow is greatest during diastole because the vessels are not constricted by a contracting cardiac muscle at this time; however, the blood flow is increased with exercise.

Thallium chloride (Tl 201) rest or stress studies are performed to assist in diagnosing ischemic cardiac disease, risk for coronary artery disease (CAD), and myocardial infarct. The radiopharmaceutical is used because it is an analogue of potassium, an element that is normally taken up by heart muscle and distributed in the myocardium, depending on the blood flow in the muscle. The narrowing of the coronary vessels affects the blood flow and uptake of the radionuclide and, because the flow increases with exercise, significant narrowing can be detected during stress testing. A reduction in the uptake is an indication of pathology and appears as "cold spots" on the image. This procedure is best suited for clients who are suspected of having CAD or angina pectoris or who need physiological information about cardiac function but are not able to undergo invasive procedures such as angiography or cardiac catheterization.

If stress testing cannot be performed by exercising, dipyridamole (Persantine) can be administered orally or IV. The drug is a coronary vasodilator and is administered before thallium chloride Tl 201 and the scanning procedure. It increases the blood flow in normal coronary arteries 2 to 3 times without exercise and reveals perfusion defects when blood flow is compromised by vessel pathology. This study is reserved for clients with lung disease (COPD), neurological disorders (multiple sclerosis or spinal cord injury [SCI]), and orthopedic disorders (arthritis or amputation) who are unable to participate in treadmill, bicycle, or handgrip activities for stress testing.[28] There is a risk of angina or coronary infarction during this study.

Technetium Tc 99m pyrophosphate studies are performed to diagnose the presence and location of myocardial infarction. The study is usually made in combination with electrocardiography (ECG) and laboratory cardiac enzyme blood tests to provide a diagnosis. This test depends on the uptake and concentration of the radionuclide, depending on blood flow, because the material must reach the damaged tissue to be taken up. This uptake is found in abnormal areas of the myocardium, most commonly the left ventricle. The earliest uptake occurs 4 hours after coronary artery occlusion, the peak uptake in 48 hours, and a continuing diminished uptake for 5 to 7 days, depending on the size and extension of the infarct. Abnormalities are based on an increased uptake by the myocardium, and activity is graded from 4+ (activity greater than bone) to 0 (activity less than bone). A wide range of conditions causes uptake of the radionuclide, and the delay in producing a definitive myocardial infarction diagnosis limits this procedure as a useful tool. Imaging with labeled monoclonal antibodies achieves a more accurate identification and localization of an infarct site.

Gated blood pool imaging is performed to assist in diagnosing cardiac abnormalities. The radiopharmaceuticals used for this study are technetium Tc 99m pyrophosphate labeled with red blood cells (RBCs) for multiple gated studies and technetium Tc 99m sulfur colloid for first-pass studies. Information gained from this study includes wall motion abnormalities at rest or with exercise, ejection fraction, ventricular dilation, unequal stroke volumes, and cardiac output. ECG is performed and synchronized with the imager and computer and is termed gated. Multiple gated acquisition imaging (MUGA) is the scanning of the heart in motion during the cardiac cycle to obtain multiple images of the heart in contraction and relaxation.[29] The MUGA procedure is also performed after administration of nitroglycerin sublingually to determine its effect on ventricular function. These studies are less risky to the client than cardiac catheterization in obtaining information about heart function.

Reference Values

Normal wall motion, ejection fraction, coronary blood flow, and ventricular size and function; no cardiac ischemia, myocardial infarction, cardiac hypertrophy, akinesia or dyskinesia (wall motion), or heart chamber disorder

Interfering Factors

➤ Inability of client to remain still or to assume different positions during the procedure, especially if the client is a child
➤ Exhaustion that prevents reaching maximum heart rate
➤ Excessive eating or exercising between initial and redistribution imaging 4 hours later
➤ Other nuclear scan, such as bone, thyroid, or lung, performed on the same days as the stress or gated scans with thallium chloride Tl 201 or technetium Tc 99m pyrophosphate labeled with RBCs
➤ Drug therapy that includes sustained-release nitrates for angina, as such therapy affects cardiac performance
➤ Chest wall or cardiac trauma, angina that is difficult to control, significant cardiac dysrhythmias, or recent cardioversion procedure

Indications for Cardiac Scanning

➤ Rest or stress scan with thallium chloride Tl 201
  • Determination of risk for or diagnosis of CAD revealed by a decrease or absence of radionuclide uptake
  • Evaluation of the extent of CAD with the number of vessels involved and the functional significance of these abnormalities
  • Evaluation of site of an old infarction for obstruction of cardiac muscle perfusion
  • Assessment of function of collateral coronary arteries
  • Determination of rest defects and reperfusion with delayed imaging in unstable angina
  • Evaluation of bypass graft patency after surgery revealed by normal flow studies when compared with abnormal studies before surgery
  • Evaluation of effectiveness of medication regimen and effect of balloon angioplasty on narrowed coronary arteries
➤ Cardiac myocardial imaging with technetium Tc 99m pyrophosphate
  • Diagnosis in the absence of a diagnosis from ECG and tests for enzyme elevation
  • Diagnosis or confirmation and location of acute myocardial infarction revealed by an increased uptake of the radionuclide in the infarcted cells
  • Evaluation of possible reinfarction or extension of the infarct
  • Differentiation between recent and past infarction
  • Obtaining of baseline information about infarction before open heart surgery
  • Diagnosis of perioperative myocardial infarction
  • Detection of possible cardiac toxicity, myocardial contusion or trauma, and pericarditis or myocarditis
➤ Gated blood pool imaging with technetium Tc 99m pyrophosphate labeled with RBCs or technetium Tc 99m sulfur colloid

- Diagnosis of ischemic CAD revealed by wall motion abnormalities and fall in ejection fraction during exercise
- Diagnosis of myocardial infarction revealed by regional wall motion abnormalities
- Diagnosis of true or false ventricular aneurysm revealed by paradoxical wall motion, bulge in the shape of the left ventricle, and site of the defect
- Evaluation of ventricular size and function after an acute episode or in chronic heart disease
- Diagnosis of valvular heart disease and determination of the optimal time for valve replacement surgery revealed by the degree of regurgitation
- Quantification of cardiac output (CO) by calculating ejection fraction
- Determination of cardiomyopathy revealed by diffuse wall motion abnormalities, decreased ejection fraction, and dilated left ventricle
- Differentiation between COPD and left ventricular failure revealed by an enlarged right ventricle, decreased ejection fraction in the right ventricle, and diffuse hypokinesis
- Determination of doxorubicin (Adriamycin) cardiotoxicity to discontinue the therapy before congestive heart failure (CHF) develops, revealed by a reduced ejection fraction and dilated left ventricle
- Detection of left-to-right shunts and determination of the pulmonary-to-systemic blood-flow ratios, especially in children[30]

Contraindications

➤ Pregnancy, unless benefits of performing the procedure greatly outweigh the risks to the fetus

➤ Stress test not performed in presence of left ventricular hypertrophy, right and left bundle branch block, or hypokalemia, or in those receiving cardiotonic therapy[31]

➤ Dipyridamole testing not performed in presence of anginal pain at rest or severe atherosclerotic coronary vessels

---

>> Nursing Alert

- Stress testing is terminated if the client develops angina, severe dyspnea, fall in blood pressure, exhaustion, or if significant ischemia or cardiac dysrhythmias are revealed by ECG.
- The use of dipyridamole in testing can precipitate myocardial infarction or angina. IV aminophylline should be on hand to reverse the effects of the drug if needed.

Nursing Care Before the Procedure

Client teaching and physical preparation are the same as for any nuclear scan study (see pp. 734 to 735).

➤ Inform the client of the scanning schedule and explain that the study takes about 30 minutes.

➤ Advise the client that food and fluids are restricted for 2 to 4 hours, smoking for 4 to 6 hours, and medications such as theophylline for 24 hours before the study.

➤ Inform the client that exercising is often performed during a stress test and that medications may be administered before or during the test to evaluate heart function but that medications are not part of the routine preparation.

➤ If an ECG is to be performed during the test, inform the client that electrodes will be attached to the chest.

➤ Include cardiovascular assessment information and the client's medication regimen in the history.

The Procedure

Rest or Stress Cardiac Scan. For the rest study, the client is placed in an upright position for 15 minutes to reduce pulmonary flow before and during the injection of the radiopharmaceutical. The client is then placed in a supine position and requested to remain very still. Imaging by a scanner placed above the chest begins 20 minutes after the injection to allow maximum concentration because of a delay at rest that is caused by slower blood clearance. Scanning is performed to obtain anterior, left anterior-oblique, and lateral views. For the stress study, electrodes are applied to the chest, and ECG monitoring is begun; a blood pressure cuff is applied to the arm to monitor changes during the test. An IV line is initiated on the arm without the blood pressure cuff to allow access during the exercising. Exercise is carried out on a treadmill to a maximum heart rate. Alternatives to the treadmill for those unable to use it are the bicycle ergometer, isometric handgrip, or cold pressor (immersion of hand in ice water) tests. To allow distribution during stress, the radiopharmaceutical is injected into the line about 60 to 90 seconds before the exercise is to be terminated. With the client in a supine position as in the rest study, imaging takes place as soon as possible after exercising, and a computer analysis of the images is performed. Redistribution imaging can take place 4 hours after the injection to differentiate between ischemia (heart function returns to normal) and infarction (heart function remains abnormal). For clients unable to exercise, dipyridamole can be administered orally or IV 4 minutes before the injection of thallium chloride Tl 201.

Cardiac Myocardial Imaging. The client is placed on the examining table in a supine position and the radiopharmaceutical injected IV. Scanning is performed 2 to 4 hours later to obtain anterior left, left anterior-oblique, and left lateral views.

Gated Blood Pool Imaging. For MUGA studies, the client is placed at rest in a supine position and the ECG is attached for use as a reference point of electric and diastole and end systole. The reference points are to be synchronized with the data collection in frames that are recorded throughout the cardiac cycle by the computer. The client is requested to remain still during the scanning. The radiopharmaceutical is administered IV, and scanning is performed to obtain anterior, left anterior-oblique, posterior-oblique, and left lateral views. As many as 12 to 64 consecutive frames can be recorded, and the data from each beat of each cardiac cycle are added to the counts stored in the frame. Exercise imaging is also possible by taking the client through graded exercises on a bicycle in a recumbent position and imaging at each exercise level and after the exercise. For first-pass studies, scanning is performed immediately after the injection as the material passes through the right heart, to the lungs, and then to the left ventricle. Anterior or right anterior-oblique views are taken. If nitroglycerin is given after a resting multiple gated study, a scan is performed and another dose of the medication is given, with scanning to follow until the desired blood pressure level is obtained.

Heart Shunt Imaging. The client is placed on the examining table in a supine position with the head slightly elevated. The radiopharmaceutical is injected into the external jugular vein and immediate scanning is performed. This procedure is performed in conjunction with a resting multiple gated acquisition study to obtain the ejection fraction.[32]

PET or SPECT Imaging. This specialized three-dimensional study can be performed if the radiopharmaceutical and a positron camera are available for PET. SPECT studies can be performed to provide short axis, vertical long axis, and horizontal long axis views to obtain a more sensitive study of heart function.[33]

Nursing Care After the Procedure

Care and assessment after the procedures are the same as for any nuclear scan study (see p. 735).

➤ Monitor ECG and blood pressure until baselines have been achieved and maintained.

➤ Remove the electrodes from the sites and cleanse the areas as needed.

➤ Inform the client of the schedule for prescribed follow-up exercise plan.

➤ *Phlebitis:* Note and report redness or swelling at the IV site. Elevate the arm and apply warm compresses to the site.

➤ *Exercise reactions:* Note and report angina, dyspnea, nausea, headache, or exhaustion during the stress study. Also note and report a fall in blood pressure, ECG change indicating ischemia or dysrhythmias, or confusion, pallor, clammy skin, or unsteady gait. Terminate test early if symptoms appear.

➤ *Dipyridamole administration:* This medication is administered by the physician in attendance for a stress study, while aminophylline is administered IV to reverse any occurrence of ischemia, which could cause angina.

LUNG SCANNING (VENTILATION-PERFUSION [V/Q] SCANNING)

Lung scanning, or ventilation-perfusion [V/Q] scanning, is a nuclear study performed to assist in diagnosing acute and chronic pulmonary conditions. These diseases cause decreased pulmonary blood flow and hamper air flow and gas exchange, resulting in a ventilation-perfusion imbalance. A radiopharmaceutical is injected IV or inhaled; scanning is performed to obtain views of the lungs and evaluate blood flow or perfusion (perfusion scan) and patency of the pulmonary airways or ventilation (ventilation scan). One or both scans are performed to obtain clinical information that assists in differentiating among the many possible pathological conditions revealed by the procedure. The scan results are correlated with other diagnostic studies such as pulmonary function, chest x-ray, pulmonary angiography, and arterial blood gases (ABGs).

Lung perfusion scanning is performed primarily to diagnose pulmonary embolism, especially when the chest x-ray is normal. Because blood flow is restricted in the area of an embolus, perfusion defects or areas of decrease or absence of activity are visualized by scanning. The radionuclide ^{99m}Tc as technetium Tc 99m macroaggregated albumin (MAA) or technetium Tc 99m human albumin microspheres (HAM) is injected IV and distributed throughout the pulmonary vasculature, depending on the gravitational effects of perfusion. Normally, gravity causes an uneven distribution of blood flow with a 3 to 5 times greater flow volume in the lower than in the upper regions of the lungs. Many diseases decrease the pulmonary blood flow, and the multiple views of areas of visible activity of the radionuclide assist in the differentiation of these diseases based on these gravitational effects.[34]

Lung ventilation scanning is performed with perfusion scans to provide specific information about perfusion abnormalities by differentiating between pulmonary embolism and other pulmonary diseases. Ventilation also is not uniform in the lungs because of gravity, causing a 1 to 2 times greater intrapleural pressure in the apex than in the base of the lungs. Abnormalities are visualized by imaging areas of decreased activity in the lungs after inhalation of a radionuclide as xenon Xe 133 gas or krypton Kr 81m gas. The compound is distributed through the airways with the inspired air. Defects in regional ventilation are identified as areas not normally well ventilated with regular breathing, based on the gravitational effect on ventilation. The areas of decreased activity indicate that the total lung volume is not ventilated. Diagnosis of COPD and pulmonary embolism is confirmed by perfusion and ventilation studies that reveal a match or mismatch between perfusion and ventilation. COPD causes a match of perfusion and ventilation (abnormal ventilation in an area of a perfusion defect), and pulmonary embolism causes a mismatch of perfusion and ventilation (normal ventilation in an area of diminished perfusion).[35]

Reference Values

Normal perfusion and ventilation of lungs and ventilation-perfusion ratio; no pulmonary embolism, COPD, tumors, pneumonia, atelectasis, or pulmonary hypertension

Interfering Factors

➤ Inability of client to remain still during the procedure or to breathe through a mask for the ventilation study
➤ Improper positioning during the inhalation of the radiopharmaceutical, because gravity affects the distribution of the material in the lungs
➤ Other nuclear scans performed on the same day, which would affect the distribution of the radionuclide
➤ Conditions that can simulate a perfusion defect similar to pulmonary embolism, such as emphysema, effusion, or infection, as these conditions affect perfusion or ventilation[36]

Indications for Lung Scanning (Ventilation-Perfusion [V/Q] Scanning)

Perfusion Study

➤ Diagnosing pulmonary embolism when the chest x-ray is normal (Pulmonary embolism is revealed by areas of decreased activity.)

➤ Differentiating between pulmonary embolism and other pulmonary disease such as pneumonia, pulmonary effusion, atelectasis, asthma, bronchitis, tumors, and emphysema revealed by a perfusion defect matching an abnormal area on the chest x-ray

➤ Evaluating perfusion changes associated with CHF and pulmonary hypertension

➤ Detecting lung displacement by fluid or chest mass

➤ Detecting malignant tumor of the lung revealed by perfusion defects resulting from bronchial obstruction

➤ Evaluating pulmonary function preoperatively in clients with pulmonary disease

Ventilation Study

➤ Diagnosing COPD revealed by areas of abnormal ventilation, with washout images and decreased activity representing defects in regional ventilation in single-breath images

➤ Differentiating between COPD (abnormal ventilation in an area of perfusion defect) and pulmonary embolism (normal ventilation in an area of decreased perfusion)

➤ Evaluating pneumonectomy when performed with a perfusion study to determine the potential for pulmonary insufficiency

➤ Determining smoke inhalation injury that could lead to edema, infection, or atelectasis

Contraindications

➤ Pregnancy, unless benefits of performing the procedure greatly outweigh the risks to the fetus

Nursing Care Before the Procedure

Client teaching and physical preparation are the same as for any nuclear scan study (see pp. 734 to 735).

➤ Inform the client of the scanning schedule and explain that the study takes 30 minutes.

➤ Inform the client that a breathing mask is used to administer the radiopharmaceutical for the ventilation study, and allay anxiety associated with this procedure.

➤ History should include information about the pulmonary status, recent x-ray results, and the determination of whether the client can lie flat or needs to elevate the head on pillows to facilitate breathing during the procedure.

The Procedure

Perfusion Study. The client is placed on the examining table in a supine position. The syringe containing the radiopharmaceutical is shaken to resuspend the particles, and the material is administered IV. The client is requested to remain still during the scanning, and imaging is performed immediately to obtain anterior, posterior, both lateral, and both oblique views. Multiple views are the best confirmation of perfusion defects within the lung vasculature.

Ventilation Study. The client is placed in an upright position with the camera positioned posteriorly. The client is requested to remain still during the scanning. The mask is positioned over the nose and the gas containing the radiopharmaceutical is injected into the intake port of the mask as the client takes a deep inspiration. Single-breath images are obtained. After this imaging, the client rebreathes the gas containing the radiopharmaceutical in a closed spirometry system for 4 minutes, allowing the gas to enter the abnormal lung areas. Images are obtained during and at the end of this procedure. Valves are then readjusted to allow the client to breathe room air that washes out the gas. Washout images are obtained for 6 minutes at 30- to 60-second intervals. After these images, additional scanning can be performed in the oblique positions to allow location of abnormal anteroposterior areas.[37] Ventilation scanning can be performed using krypton Kr 81m gas on clients unable to perform breathing techniques needed for the study. These images can be obtained regardless of the timing of perfusion studies; otherwise, ventilation studies are performed before perfusion studies.

Nursing Care After the Procedure

Care and assessment after the procedures are the same as for any nuclear scan study (see p. 735).

➤ Ensure ease of breathing by elevating the client's head on pillows, if needed.

THYROID SCANNING

Thyroid scanning is a nuclear study performed to assist in diagnosing thyroid dysfunction and benign or malignant thyroid tumor. Normally, the thyroid reveals a homogeneous uptake of the radionuclide; an absent or diminished uptake is an indication of pathology. The most frequent indication for thyroid scanning is the presence of a nodule or enlarged thyroid gland.

The procedure is performed after an IV injection of ^{99m}Tc administered as technetium Tc 99m pertechnetate and imaging in 20 minutes or an oral ingestion of ^{123}I as iodide I 123 and imaging in 4 or 24 hours. Iodide I 123 is the most commonly used radiopharmaceutical because of its short half-life and lower radiation exposure. Iodine 131 (^{131}I) administered as metaiodobenzylguanidine (MIBG) I 131 is used in scanning for thyroid cancer and therapy.

The classification of "cold" nodules results from a decrease or absence of radioactivity in the gland and suggests a malignant tumor. "Hot" nodules result from an increase or normal activity in the gland, and this finding suggests a benign tumor or thyrotoxicosis.[38,39] Thyroid scanning with iodide I 123 is usually performed in combination with a radioactive iodine uptake study on the same day. Thyroxine (T_4) level is also obtained to diagnose thyroiditis and thyroid function tests to diagnose Graves' disease. Thyroid ultrasound and nodal biopsy can be performed to confirm a diagnosis.

Reference Values

Normal size, shape, weight, position, and function of the thyroid gland with a homogeneous uptake of the radiopharmaceutical; no thyroiditis, Graves' disease, or benign or malignant tumor

Interfering Factors

➤ Inability of client to remain still during the procedure
➤ Other recent nuclear scans or radiologic studies using iodinated media that can affect uptake of the radionuclide
➤ Dietary intake deficient in iodine content, as this increases uptake, or intake of foods containing iodine, as this decreases uptake
➤ Vomiting or diarrhea, or both, that can decrease uptake of the radionuclide
➤ Medications such as thyroid drugs, multivitamins, steroids, cough medications, thyroid hormone antagonists, or phenothiazines

Indications for Thyroid Scanning

➤ Assessing palpable nodules and differentiating these from benign tumor cyst (uptake of radionuclide) and malignant tumor (absence of uptake)
➤ Determining the cause of neck or substernal masses
➤ Differentiating between Graves' disease with a diffuse and enlarged thyroid and Plummer's disease with a nodular thyroid, both resulting in hyperthyroidism
➤ Evaluating thyroid function in hyperthyroidism and hypothyroidism when analyzed with laboratory thyroid function tests, thyroxine (T_4), triiodothyronine (T_3), and thyroid uptake tests
➤ Diagnosing thyroiditis conditions such as acute or chronic Hashimoto's thyroiditis revealed by uptake below or above normal, depending on disease stage
➤ Determining thyroid gland as a primary site in clients with metastatic tumors

Contraindications

➤ Pregnancy, unless benefits of performing the procedure greatly outweigh the risks to the fetus

Nursing Care Before the Procedure

Client teaching and physical preparation are the same as for any nuclear scan study (see pp. 734 to 735).
➤ Instruct the client to restrict iodine-containing foods for 2 to 3 weeks before the procedure.
➤ Inform the client of the scanning schedule and explain that the procedure takes 30 minutes.
➤ Restrict food and fluids for 2 to 4 hours before the study, according to policy and physician preference.
➤ History should include medications taken or withheld before the procedure, previous scans or radiologic studies, results of laboratory tests, and foods or medications containing iodine ingested before the study.

The Procedure

The client is given iodide I 123 by mouth in a capsule or technetium Tc 99m pertechnetate by IV injection, depending on which has been ordered. The client is placed on the examining table in a supine position, and imaging is performed 20 minutes after an IV injection or 2 to 4 hours after an oral dose. The client is requested to remain still and the scanning camera is moved over the neck. Additional scanning after the oral dose can be performed in 24 hours. Counts per minute are obtained and the percentage of uptake is calculated, using the dose administered and the decay factor.[40]

Nursing Care After the Procedure

Care and assessment after the procedure are the same as for any nuclear scan study (see p. 735).

➤ Resume withheld food, fluid, and medications after the study.

PARATHYROID SCANNING

Parathyroid scanning is a nuclear study performed to assist in diagnosing tumors or hyperplasia of the glands. The main function of the glands is to synthesize, secrete, and store parathyroid hormone (PTH), which regulates the level of calcium and phosphorus in the blood. Change in these levels indicates hyperparathyroidism. The radionuclide ^{201}Tl as thallium chloride Tl 201 is administered IV, and scanning is performed in 20 minutes. This is followed by the administration of ^{99m}Tc as technetium Tc 99m pertechnetate, and additional scanning is performed. Computer subtraction of images is performed to complete the study and determine the amount of the radionuclide concentrated in the parathyroid glands as opposed to the thyroid gland (thallium chloride Tl 201 is taken up by normal thyroid tissue).[41]

Reference Values

Normal size, position, number, weight, and function of the parathyroid glands with normal uptake of the radionuclide in the parathyroid and thyroid glands, no hyperplasia or adenoma of the parathyroids

Interfering Factors

➤ Inability of client to remain still during the procedure
➤ Recent intake of iodine-containing foods or medications, or recent tests and procedures using iodinated contrast media

Indications for Parathyroid Scanning

➤ Differentiating between parathyroid hyperplasia and adenoma revealed by a larger-sized gland in adenoma
➤ Identifying and locating ectopic glands to prevent missing a tumor during surgical excision

Contraindications

➤ Pregnancy, unless benefits of performing the procedure greatly outweigh the risks to the fetus

Nursing Care Before the Procedure

Client teaching and physical preparation are the same as for any thyroid nuclear scan study (see pp. 734 to 735).

The Procedure

The client is placed on the examining table in a supine position with the neck slightly hyperextended. The client is requested to remain still during the scanning, and thallium chloride Tl 201 is administered IV. Scanning is performed in 5 to 30 minutes for mediastinal and neck views. Technetium Tc 99m pertechnetate is then injected, and scanning is performed for the same views. Computer subtraction of images is performed by the subtraction of the ^{99m}Tc imaged in the thyroid from the ^{201}Tl uptake in the parathyroid glands.

Nursing Care After the Procedure

Care and assessment after the procedure are the same as for any nuclear scan study (see p. 735).

ABSCESS/INFLAMMATORY SCANNING

Abscess or inflammatory scanning, also known as leukocyte imaging, is a nuclear study performed to assist in the diagnosis of inflammatory lesions indicating an infectious process. Abscess detection by nuclear scanning is performed on clients suspected of having an abscess but with no localized signs of infection. Abnormalities are identified by scanning 24 hours after the IV injection of ^{111}In administered as indium In 111 oxine–labeled leukocytes (WBCs) that are separated from other components of the blood. This is followed by the injection of ^{99m}Tc administered as technetium Tc 99m sulfur colloid and the performance of a liver and spleen scan to compare with the indium In 111 oxine–labeled WBC scan. Diagnosis is based on the intensity of uptake outside of normal organs as compared with the liver. CT and ultrasonography are performed to provide a diagnosis in a client with localized signs of an abscess.[42]

Reference Values

Absence of uptake of radionuclide outside of normal organs; no inflammation in the abdomen, lungs, or gastrointestinal tract

Interfering Factors

➤ Inability of client to remain still during the procedure
➤ Gastrointestinal bleeding caused by ulcers, diverticula, or tumors
➤ Other sites that take up the radionuclide, such as colostomies, hematomas, postoperative wounds, or IV catheters
➤ Long-term therapies, such as hemodialysis, hyperalimentation, or steroidal or antibiotic therapy, which affect the function of the WBCs

Indications for Abscess/Inflammatory Scanning

➤ Diagnosing abdominal abscess revealed by focal area of increased uptake that is greater or equal to the liver
➤ Diagnosing lung infections revealed by focal or diffuse uptake of the radionuclide (although uptake can be caused by CHF, aspiration, atelectasis, or pulmonary emboli)

➤ Determining whether an infection is causing an elevated temperature of unknown origin

➤ Diagnosing infectious disorders of the gastrointestinal tract, such as necrotic bowel, inflammatory bowel disease, or pseudomembranous colitis, which are revealed by a greater intensity of uptake

➤ Diagnosing inflammatory processes in the extremities, such as osteomyelitis

Contraindications

➤ Pregnancy, unless the benefits of performing the study greatly outweigh the risks to the fetus

Nursing Care Before the Procedure

Client teaching and physical preparation are the same as for any nuclear scan study (see pp. 734 to 735).

➤ Inform the client of the scanning schedule and explain that scanning for each radionuclide administered takes about 1 hour.

➤ History should include signs and symptoms of any infectious process in any area of the body and results of recent diagnostic laboratory tests and procedures.

The Procedure

The client is placed on the examining table in a supine position and requested to remain still during the scanning. The indium In 111 oxine–labeled WBC is injected IV. The client is returned to or requested to return to the department in 24 hours for imaging of the liver, followed by posterior and anterior imaging of the abdomen, pelvis, and chest. Extremities can also be imaged, but they require a longer time to scan. After abscess inflammatory scanning, technetium Tc 99m sulfur colloid is injected, and a standard liver scan is obtained. These scans are compared to determine areas outside the liver and spleen that concentrate the radionuclide. This concentration indicates an abnormality and reveals a 90 percent accuracy for identifying an abscess/inflammatory site.

The procedure for labeling the WBCs with indium In 111 oxine is performed on a sample of the client's blood or a donor's blood if the client's WBC is low. The WBCs are separated from the blood and labeled and reinjected into the client. This process can take up to 3 hours, and the client can wait or be requested to return for administration of the radiopharmaceutical.

Nursing Care After the Procedure

Care and assessment after the procedure are the same as for any nuclear scan study (see p. 735).

Gastric Emptying Scanning

Gastric emptying scanning is a nuclear study performed to determine the time it takes for the stomach to empty itself of foods or fluids. Normally, solids are emptied by reduction to allow passage through the pylorus by antral contractions, and liquids are emptied primarily by gravity. Thus, solids are more sensitive for use in the detection of abnormal gastric emptying. The radionuclide ^{99m}Tc as technetium Tc 99m sulfur colloid mixed with cooked liver made into a pâté or mixed with egg white (test meal of 300 g) or ^{111}In as indium In 111 chloride mixed with orange juice is administered orally to the client. Scanning is performed after the meal, and an analysis of the delayed emptying curve (the percent of food retained compared with the time) provides the diagnostic information.[43]

The study can include the administration of metoclopromide (Reglan) to evaluate the effect of the drug on gastric motility, providing that no obstruction is present.[44]

Reference Values

Normal gastric emptying of standard test meal; no abnormal gastric function or mechanical obstruction

Interfering Factors

➤ Inability of client to remain still during the procedure
➤ Food intake during the fasting period before the study, which would affect emptying time
➤ Medications such as anticholinergics or narcotics that affect motility

Indications for Gastric Emptying Scanning

➤ Determining the existence of mechanical obstruction caused by gastric tumor or ulcer disease revealed by delayed emptying time
➤ Evaluating gastric function or absence of function revealed by delayed emptying in diabetic neuropathy or gastroparesis
➤ Determining the cause, after surgery, of delayed gastric emptying caused by a nonfunctioning anastomosis
➤ Determining the cause of delayed gastric emptying in conditions such as anorexia, diabetes, scleroderma, or amyloidosis
➤ Evaluating the effects of medication regimens

Contraindications

➤ Pregnancy, unless benefits of performing the procedure greatly outweigh the risks to the fetus

Nursing Care Before the Procedure

Client teaching and physical preparation are the same as for any nuclear scan study (see pp. 734 to 735).

➤ Instruct the client to withhold food and medications that can decrease motility for 8 hours before the study; also specify whether fluid intake is allowed.
➤ Inform the client of the scanning schedule and explain that the study takes 1 hour or longer, depending on the time it takes the stomach to empty.
➤ History should include information about gastrointestinal status and known or suspected abnormal conditions, as well as results of associated diagnostic tests and procedures.

The Procedure

The client is requested to ingest the test meal containing the radiopharmaceutical as quickly as possible. Using a standardized test meal allows accurate determination of gastric emptying because the rate of emptying varies with meal size and caloric content. The client is maintained in a sitting position; after the ingestion of the test meal, the images are obtained at 10- and 20-minute intervals in anterior and posterior views. Imaging is then performed over the stomach with the client in a supine position until the stomach empties (normally 1 to 1½ hours). Emptying time is calculated based on data obtained from the computer system as well as on the percentage of counts obtained, decay time of the radionuclide, and depth variables. An emptying curve is determined by calculating the percentage of retention versus the time. These results are interpreted by the nuclear medicine physician at the completion of the procedure. In general, a longer time indicates impaired gastric emptying and a shorter time indicates gastric hypermotility.

Nursing Care After the Procedure

Care and assessment after the procedure are the same as for any nuclear scan study (see p. 735).

GASTROINTESTINAL REFLUX SCANNING

Gastrointestinal reflux scanning is a nuclear study performed to assist in diagnosing esophageal reflux in clients complaining of heartburn and regurgitation. This disorder is common in the adult population, but it also occurs in infants and children, causing significant complications such as esophagitis, stricture, aspiration pneumonia, and failure to thrive.[45] Lung scanning can be performed if aspiration of gastric contents into the lungs is suspected. The study can be combined with the gastric emptying study because reflux is known to be associated with a delay in emptying. The radionuclide ^{99m}Tc as technetium Tc 99m sulfur colloid is mixed with orange juice or other acidic fluid and administered orally. Scanning is performed over the gastroesophageal area and later over the lungs, if aspiration is suspected. This study is more sensitive for this condition than is endoscopy, fluoroscopy, or manometry to measure esophageal sphincter pressure.

Esophageal motility studies are performed to diagnose achalasia and esophageal spasms. The technetium Tc 99m sulfur colloid is mixed with water and administered to the client, followed by scanning. A significant reduction in esophageal activity indicates the presence of abnormalities. This test is more sensitive than esophageal manometry in clients with complaints of dysphagia.[46]

Reference Values

Normal passage of fluid through the esophagus into the stomach; no reflux into the esophagus from the stomach

Interfering Factors

➤ Inability of client to remain still during the procedure
➤ Any condition that prevents application of the compression binder during the procedure

Indications for Gastroesophageal Reflux Scanning

➤ Unexplained persistent heartburn, dysphagia, or regurgitation that occurs frequently and regularly
➤ Evaluating esophageal function and detecting the presence of reflux with more accuracy than is possible with endoscopic or radiologic studies
➤ Diagnosing esophageal motility disorders, such as spasms; achalasia is revealed by a prolonged transit time
➤ Differentiating between significant and insignificant reflux in infants
➤ Detecting aspiration of gastric contents into the lungs (aspiration scan)
➤ Diagnosing reflux when performed with the gastric emptying study, as the condition is linked to delayed gastric emptying
➤ Evaluating the effectiveness of surgical or medical interventions for gastroesophageal reflux

Contraindications

➤ Pregnancy, unless benefits of performing the procedure greatly outweigh the risks to the fetus

Nursing Care Before the Procedure

Client teaching and physical preparation are the same as for any nuclear scan study (see pp. 734 to 735).
➤ Instruct the client to restrict food or ingest a meal before the study, depending on the policy of the nuclear medicine department.
➤ Inform the client of the scanning schedule and explain that the study takes 30 minutes.
➤ History should include information about gastrointestinal status and complaints resulting from an abnormality.

The Procedure

The client is given the radiopharmaceutical in 300 mL of orange juice and is then placed in an upright position for scanning. The client is requested to remain still, and imaging is performed in 10 to 15 minutes over the esophageal area. Imaging is also performed in other positions to determine whether reflux occurs in a specific position. After this initial imaging, an abdominal compression binder is applied to sequentially lower esophageal sphincter pressure 5 mm Hg at a time. Images are recorded on the computer at each pressure level, and the reflux is calculated for each pressure level. Esophageal motility or transient time can be determined by the presence of radionuclide in the esophagus. If an infant is scanned, the radiopharmaceutical is administered in the formula or instilled via a gastrointestinal tube, and imaging is performed at intervals for 1 hour.

If an aspiration scan is performed, the radiopharmaceutical is given to the client in the evening meal before the study. The client remains in the supine position until morning, and scanning is performed over the lungs to note uptake of the radionuclide, indicating aspiration.

Nursing Care After the Procedure

Care and assessment after the procedure are the same as for any nuclear scan study (see p. 735).

GASTROINTESTINAL BLEEDING SCANNING

Gastrointestinal bleeding scanning is a nuclear study performed to assist in locating bleeding sites in the upper tract proximal to the ligament of Treitz or in the lower tract distal to the ligament of Treitz. This study is much more sensitive than is endoscopy, barium-mediated radiography, or angiography in locating a bleeding site in the lower gastrointestinal (LGI) tract, although very slight rectal hemorrhages can be missed. Only the site of the bleeding is revealed, not the cause of it. The radionuclide ^{99m}Tc as technetium Tc 99m sulfur colloid or technetium Tc 99m RBC is injected IV, and scanning of the abdominal quadrants is performed. Abnormal flow and static studies reveal a focal area of increased intensity of activity during initial scanning with technetium Tc 99m sulfur colloid. The same abnormalities are revealed to locate slow or intermittent bleeding during delayed scanning of up to 24 hours with technetium Tc 99m RBC. Surgical intervention is usually required to correct a persistent bleeding problem.

Reference Values

No active bleeding at any gastrointestinal tract site

Interfering Factors

➤ Inability of client to remain still during the procedure
➤ Barium in the tract from previous radiologic studies

Indications for Gastrointestinal Bleeding Scanning

➤ Detecting and localizing recent or active bleeding sites before medical or surgical treatments
➤ Identifying and localizing small sites of bleeding in the lower tract caused by tumor, diverticula, angiodysplasia, or inflammatory bowel disease; sites are revealed by focal area of increased activity
➤ Detecting and localizing upper tract hemorrhage caused by medications such as heparin, warfarin, aspirin, or corticosteroids or conditions such as gastritis, ulcer, or varices (gastric or duodenal)
➤ Detecting bleeding from stress ulcer in severely stressed clients
➤ Diagnosing and detecting bleeding sites in children with intussusception, Meckel's diverticulum, or juvenile polyps
➤ Determining bleeding in the tract from unknown source revealed by increased focal area of activity in flow and static images

Contraindications

➤ Pregnancy, unless benefits of performing the procedure greatly outweigh the risks to the fetus
➤ Hemodynamic instability that presents a risk because of the prolonged time needed for the study

Nursing Care Before the Procedure

Client teaching and physical preparation are the same as for any nuclear scan study (see pp. 734 to 735).
➤ Inform the client of the scanning schedule for immediate and delayed imaging, and explain that each test takes 30 minutes.

➤ Take baseline vital signs and monitor if their stability is questionable.
➤ History should include information about conditions and medication regimen that can lead to hemorrhage.

The Procedure

The client is placed on the examining table in a supine position. The client is requested to remain still during the study, and the radiopharmaceutical is administered IV. Imaging for flow studies is performed immediately every 5 seconds for 60 seconds. Static imaging is performed every 1 to 2 minutes for 30 minutes, then at 45 minutes, and at 1 hour. Lateral and oblique views of the upper abdomen are taken to obtain an image of a higher bleeding site if the lower portion is negative (reveals no focal increase activity of the radionuclide). A longer imaging time is required to detect slow bleeding rate, and the technetium Tc 99m RBC allows intermittent imaging for 24 hours without reinjection.[47]

Nursing Care After the Procedure

Care and assessment after the procedure are the same as for any nuclear scan study (see p. 735).
➤ Continue monitoring vital signs if bleeding is present.
➤ *Hemorrhage/shock state:* Note and report upper gastrointestinal (UGI) or LGI blood loss and amount (vomiting, feces), decreasing blood pressure, increased pulse, and pallor and coolness of skin. Monitor vital signs. Prepare for ordered blood transfusion, surgery, or both, to control bleeding.

MECKEL'S DIVERTICULUM SCANNING

Meckel's diverticulum scanning is a nuclear study performed to assist in diagnosing the presence and size of this congenital anomaly of the gastrointestinal tract. The condition can become symptomatic in children and adults, causing bleeding, diverticulitis, volvulus, or intussusception. The radionuclide ^{99m}Tc as technetium Tc 99m pertechnetate is administered IV, and immediate and delayed imaging are performed of the abdominal lower right quadrant (LRQ). The radionuclide is taken up and concentrated by gastric mucosa, a type of tissue found in Meckel's diverticulum, and a focal increase in activity is associated with an abnormality.

Reference Values

Normal distribution of radionuclide by gastric mucosa at normal sites; no ectopic gastric mucosa revealed by uptake activity in abnormal structures

Interfering Factors

➤ Inability of client to remain still during the procedure
➤ Barium in the bowel from previous radiologic studies

Indications for Meckel's Diverticulum Scanning

➤ Unexplained abdominal pain and gastrointestinal bleeding in adults and children as a result of hydrochloric acid and pepsin secretions by ectopic gastric mucosa causing ulceration of nearby mucosa[48]
➤ Detecting sites of ectopic gastric mucosa revealed by focal increased activity in areas other than normal structures

Contraindications

➤ Pregnancy, unless benefits of performing the procedure greatly outweigh the risks to the fetus

Nursing Care Before the Procedure

Client teaching and physical preparation are the same as for any nuclear scan study (see pp. 734 to 735).

➤ Inform the client of the scanning schedule and explain that the study takes 1 hour.

➤ Instruct the client to restrict food for 6 to 8 hours and to restrict water and medications according to agency policy or physician preference.

➤ Advise that a nasogastric (NG) tube can be inserted and medications administered during the procedure to enhance imaging.

➤ A histamine H_2 antagonist, cimetidine (Tagamet), in doses of 300 mg 4 times per day, is administered 2 days before the scan to block acid secretion and to keep the radionuclide from gastric mucosa. This practice improves the lesion-background ratio in the scan.[49]

➤ History should include information about signs, symptoms, and conditions associated with Meckel's diverticulum, such as pain, bleeding, intussusception, volvulus, and diverticulitis, and results of diagnostic tests and procedures.

The Procedure

The client is placed on the examining table in a supine position and the radio-pharmaceutical is administered IV. Initial anterior abdominal images are obtained for 1 minute to screen for a vascular lesion that could cause bleeding. The client is requested to remain still during the scanning and is informed that positions are changed to obtain different views. Delayed imaging of the left upper portion of the abdomen to obtain stomach views and of a lower field of view of the bladder is performed. Imaging takes place every 5 minutes for 1 hour in anterior, oblique, and lateral views, including a postvoiding view. Modifications can be made to facilitate the study, such as positioning the client on the left side with the table tilted 45 to 90 degrees to decrease emptying of the radiopharmaceutical from the stomach into the bowel. Another modification is insertion of an NG tube into the stomach to decrease peristalsis and emptying of the radiopharmaceutical from the stomach into the bowel. Also, glucagon or pentagastrin, or both, can be administered to control uptake of the radionuclide.[50]

Nursing Care After the Procedure

Care and assessment after the procedure are the same as for any nuclear scan study (see p. 735).

PANCREAS SCANNING

Pancreas scanning is a nuclear study performed to assist in the diagnosis of pancreatic disease resulting from abnormalities of the exocrine portion of the organ. Focal lesions are identified by the absence of uptake of the radionuclide selenium 75 (^{75}Se) during scanning, which indicates the presence of a tumor or inflammatory process when the procedure is performed in combination with ultrasonography and evaluation of laboratory enzyme levels. Other processes that impede the secretory ability leading to the stimulation of pancreatic enzyme formation and secretion into the bowel are vagotomy, acute peptic ulcer, ascites, cancer, starvation, and gastroenterostomy. Enzyme production decreases the radionuclide uptake and determines the diagnosis of pancreas pathology.[51]

Reference Values

Normal function and anatomically intact pancreas; no decreased radionuclide uptake indicating pancreatic disease

Interfering Factors

➤ Inability of client to remain still during the procedure

Indications for Pancreas Scanning

➤ Determining pancreatic functional process affecting enzyme formation and secretion revealed by a diffuse decrease in radionuclide uptake
➤ Detecting tumors or chronic inflammation, although diagnostic value is limited, revealed by focal lesion that decreases the uptake of the radionuclide

Contraindications

➤ Pregnancy, unless benefits of performing the procedure greatly outweigh the risks to the fetus

Nursing Care Before the Procedure

Client teaching and physical preparation are the same as for any nuclear scan study (see pp. 734 to 735).
➤ Inform the client of the scanning schedule and explain that the study takes 30 minutes.
➤ History should include a gastrointestinal assessment and medications affecting pancreatic function, as well as results of diagnostic tests and procedures.

The Procedure

The client is placed on the examining table in a supine position. He or she is then requested to remain still during the scanning, and selenomethionine Se 75 is administered IV. Scanning over the abdominal area is performed and images are obtained and compared with other studies to determine abnormalities that the scan alone cannot detect.

Nursing Care After the Procedure

Care and assessment after the procedure are the same as for any nuclear scan study (see p. 735).

LIVER SCANNING

Liver scanning is a nuclear study performed to assist in diagnosing abnormalities in the structure and function of that organ. It can be performed simultaneously with spleen scanning or in combination with lung scanning to assist in the diagnosis of masses or inflammation in the diaphragmatic area. The radionu-clide ^{99m}Tc as technetium Tc 99m sulfur colloid is injected IV and taken up by the Kupffer cells that normally function to remove particulate matter, including radioactive colloids, in the liver. Early or delayed and increased or decreased uptake indicate pathology when flow studies are performed (dynamic scintigra-phy). Static imaging reveals abnormalities in size and shape of the liver in the presence of pathology.[52]

Liver scans are evaluated with liver function laboratory studies and can complement ultrasonography and CT in confirming a diagnosis. Scanning is also performed to confirm catheter placement for chemotherapy and to deter-mine whether a tumor is being infused and the normal parenchyma bypassed. This procedure is accomplished by imaging after the slow IV infusion of ^{99m}Tc administered as technetium Tc 99m MAA and later imaging after an injection of technetium Tc 99m sulfur colloid and computer subtraction.[53]

Reference Values

Normal size, shape, position, and function of the liver; no tumors, cysts, inflam-mation, trauma, or infiltrative disease

Interfering Factors

➤ Inability of client to remain still during the procedure
➤ Barium in the gastrointestinal tract from previous radiography
➤ Other nuclear scans performed on the same day

Indications for Liver Scanning

➤ Diagnosing primary or metastatic tumor and differentiating between them as revealed by uptake that appears as a filling defect or by solitary or multiple focal "cold" defects
➤ Diagnosing diffuse hepatocellular disease, such as hepatitis, cirrhosis (early and advanced), or hepatomegaly; shunting to spleen or bone marrow revealed by patchy, decreased uptake in hepatitis or atrophy; and shunting to spleen or bone marrow and decreased or absent uptake in cirrhosis
➤ Diagnosing benign tumors such as adenoma or cavernous hemangiomas as revealed by hepatomegaly or solitary "cold" defect
➤ Detecting bacterial abscess revealed by solitary or multiple "cold" defects, especially after gastrointestinal surgery
➤ Detecting amebic abscess revealed by solitary defect, especially after amebiasis
➤ Diagnosing cystic focal disease revealed by "cold" defects
➤ Determining the effect of traumatic lesions such as lacerations or hematomas
➤ Detecting infiltrative processes of the liver such as sarcoidosis or amyloidosis
➤ Evaluating palpable abdominal masses and differentiating between splenomegaly and hepatomegaly
➤ Determining superior vena cava obstruction or Budd-Chiari syndrome revealed by increased uptake of the radionuclide, or "hot spots"
➤ Evaluating liver damage caused by radiation therapy or hepatotoxic drug therapy

Contraindications

➤ Pregnancy, unless benefits of performing the procedure greatly outweigh the risks to the fetus

Nursing Care Before the Procedure

Client teaching and physical preparation are the same as for any nuclear scan study (see pp. 734 to 735).

➤ Inform the client of the scanning schedule and explain that the study takes 1 hour.

➤ History should include hepatic disorders and any signs and symptoms associated with the liver as well as past medical and surgical treatment or regimens.

The Procedure

The client is placed on the examining table in a supine position. The client is then requested to remain still during the scanning and the radiopharmaceutical is administered IV. Scanning follows in 1 to 2 seconds and continues for 30 minutes to 1 hour to perform flow studies. A 1-minute blood pool image can also be performed. This image is followed by static imaging in the anterior, posterior, laterals, anterior-oblique, and posterior-oblique views to determine the size and shape of the liver. Defects that fail to take up the radionuclide (normally concentrated in the Kupffer cells in the liver) are known as "cold spots." Normal indentations in the liver can be confused for focal diseases of the liver. SPECT imaging, a three-dimensional study, can be performed to obtain more specific views of the liver. The liver scan is performed in combination with a lung scan when a systemic tumor or infection is suspected in the upper abdomen or below the diaphragm.

Nursing Care After the Procedure

Care and assessment after the procedure are the same as for any nuclear scan study (see p. 735).

SPLEEN SCANNING

Spleen scanning is a nuclear study performed to assist in diagnosing abnormal structure or function of this organ. It is often performed to differentiate between splenomegaly and hepatomegaly, and it is performed in combination with liver scanning because the radionuclide is distributed in both organs at the same time (86 percent in the liver and 6 percent in the spleen). The radionuclide ^{99m}Tc administered as technetium Tc 99m sulfur colloid is injected IV, followed by scanning. The appearance or absence of "cold" defects or the appearance of multiple "cold" defects, resulting from the presence of the radionuclide on the images, determines splenic pathology.

Reference Values

Normal size, length, perfusion, and function of the spleen; no infarction, hematoma, tumor, abscess, or cysts

Interfering Factors

➤ Inability of client to remain still during the procedure
➤ Barium in the gastrointestinal tract from prior radiography

Indications for Spleen Scanning

➤ Determining splenic arterial obstruction or pathological infiltration resulting from splenic inflammation or infarction as revealed by a marked decrease in radionuclide compared with liver intake
➤ Determining splenic involvement in diseases such as leukemia, lymphoma, or melanoma as revealed by splenic enlargement and focal changes
➤ Determining splenic rupture or hematoma after abdominal trauma as revealed by splenomegaly and diffuse diminished radionuclide uptake

Contraindications

➤ Pregnancy, unless benefits of performing the procedure greatly outweigh the risks to the fetus

Nursing Care Before the Procedure

Client teaching and physical preparation are the same as for any nuclear study, such as the liver scan (see p. 765).

The Procedure

The procedure is the same as for liver scanning (see p. 765). To obtain flow studies, imaging for 1 minute begins 30 minutes after injection of the radiopharmaceutical. Static imaging is performed to determine the size (anterior view), length (posterior view), and shape (lateral and anterior views) of the organ.

Nursing Care After the Procedure

Care and assessment after the procedure are the same as for any nuclear scan study (see p. 735).

DEEP VEIN SCANNING

Deep vein scanning, or fibrinogen uptake study (FUT), is a nuclear study performed to assist in diagnosing thrombi in the lower extremity veins. It allows detection of newly formed as well as old clots. The radionuclide iodine 125 (^{125}I) as fibrinogen I 125 is administered IV followed by immediate and delayed scanning. Increased uptake of the radionuclide indicates an abnormality because fibrinogen is involved in blood clotting and appears at the clot site. This study can be continued on a daily basis for up to 1 week after the injection in clients at risk for formation of deep venous thrombosis (DVT), that is, in postoperative, postpartum, and immobile clients.[54]

Reference Values

Normal structure of veins of lower extremities and venous patency; no formation or presence of DVT

Interfering Factors

➤ Inability of client to remain still during the procedure

➤ Other abnormalities in the extremity, such as infection, edema, or phlebitis, that cause fibrinogen concentration

Indications for Deep Vein Scanning

➤ Detecting DVT in its earliest stages, especially in immobilized clients, as revealed by steadily increased counts over 1 to 2 weeks

➤ Diagnosing and identifying the area of clot formation revealed by increased counts when compared with the opposite extremity

➤ Diagnosing DVT in clients who are too ill for radiographic venography or who are sensitive to the contrast media used

Contraindications

➤ Allergy to iodine, unless a steroid or antihistamine is administered before the study

➤ Need for diagnosis of DVT immediately or sooner than 24 hours

➤ Lymphedema, cellulitis, superficial phlebitis, or active arthritis[55]

Nursing Care Before the Procedure

Client teaching and physical preparation are the same as for any nuclear scan study (see pp. 734 to 735).

➤ Inform the client that a radiation Geiger-type detector is the device used for scanning and that the study takes 1 hour.

➤ Administer potassium iodide before and during the procedure to prevent uptake of the radionuclide by the thyroid gland, which would affect uptake in the areas to be examined.

➤ History should include chronic disorders of the vascular system of the extremities; allergies to iodine; and signs, symptoms, and risks for DVT.

The Procedure

The areas on the extremity to be scanned are marked and the radiopharmaceutical is administered IV. The client is requested to remain still, and the marked areas (calf and thigh) are scanned 10 minutes after the injection. A Geiger-type device is used to detect and count radiation levels. This provides a baseline for later comparisons when scanning is performed in 24 hours. In some cases, scanning is performed daily for 7 or more days after the injection of the radiopharmaceutical because it takes that long for the radionuclide to concentrate in possible thrombi. Subsequent scanning of the marked areas in 24 hours is compared with the amount of uptake in the opposite extremity. A reading of 15 times greater than the baseline or the opposite extremity reading indicates DVT.[56]

Nursing Care After the Procedure

Care and assessment after the procedure are the same as for any nuclear scan study (see p. 735).

GALLBLADDER/BILIARY SYSTEM SCANNING

Gallbladder and biliary system scanning is a nuclear study performed to assist in diagnosing gallbladder disease and duct obstruction. The radionuclide ^{99m}Tc as Tc 99m diisopropyl iminodiacetic acid (DISIDA) is administered IV followed by serial imaging. Biliary and duct concentrations are achieved by the liver excretion of the radionuclide into the bile. Failure of the substance to enter the gallbladder demonstrates duct obstruction, and the organ and ducts will not be visualized. The ejection capabilities of the gallbladder can also be calculated to evaluate gallbladder functional disorders.[57]

Compared with ultrasonography, this study demonstrates a higher sensitivity in providing diagnostic information. It is also preferred for clients with sensitivities to contrast media used in oral cholecystography or IV cholangiography, and it provides information about clients with bilirubinemia, information not obtainable with cholangiography.

Reference Values

Normal size, shape, and function of the gallbladder with patent cystic and common bile ducts; no inflammation of the gallbladder or obstruction of ducts

Interfering Factors

➤ Inability of client to remain still during the procedure
➤ Absence of food ingestion for longer than 24 hours as in fasting, total parenteral nutrition (TPN), or alcoholism
➤ Bilirubin levels of greater than 30 mg/dL depending on the radionuclide used, as increased bilirubin decreases hepatic uptake

Indications for Gallbladder/Biliary System Scanning

➤ Suspected gallbladder disorders such as inflammation, perforation, or calculi as revealed by decreased or absent radionuclide flow to the gallbladder or into the peritoneal cavity
➤ Diagnosing acute cholecystitis revealed by nonvisualization in 1 hour after the injection of the radiopharmaceutical
➤ Diagnosing chronic cholecystitis revealed by a delayed visualization caused by fibrosis, calculi, or viscous bile
➤ Determining common duct obstruction caused by tumor or cholelithiasis revealed by a dilated duct; nonvisualization of the common bile duct, gallbladder, and duodenum; or visualization of the common bile duct or gallbladder with absence of flow into the duodenum
➤ Evaluating biliary enteric bypass patency after surgery as revealed by delayed bowel visualization
➤ Assessing obstructive jaundice when the procedure is performed in conjunction with radiography or ultrasonography

Contraindications

➤ Pregnancy, unless benefits of performing the procedure greatly outweigh the risks to the fetus

Nursing Care Before the Procedure

Client teaching and physical preparation are the same as for any nuclear scan study (see pp. 734 to 735).

➤ Instruct the client to restrict food and fluid for 4 to 6 hours before the study.
➤ Explain the scanning schedule and that the study takes 1 to 4 hours.
➤ Inform the client that a fatty meal or medication may be given during the study for special additional tests.
➤ History should include hepatic and gallbladder conditions and laboratory function tests and signs and symptoms of biliary system abnormalities.

The Procedure

The client is placed on the examining table in a supine position. The client is then requested to remain very still during the imaging, and the radiopharmaceutical is administered IV. Scanning begins immediately, with images taken every 5 minutes for the first 30 minutes and every 10 minutes for the next 30 minutes. Delayed views are taken in 2, 4, and 24 hours if the gallbladder is not visualized to differentiate acute from chronic cholecystitis or to detect the degree of obstruction. Instruct the client to restrict fats during the 24 hours before returning to the department for further scanning. The drug sincalide is given by some departments before the study to promote release of cholecystokinin (CCK), which causes the gallbladder to contract and empty. Also, if the organ is not visualized within 1 hour after injection of the radiopharmaceutical, morphine sulfate can be administered to initiate spasms of the sphincter of Oddi, forcing the radionuclide into the gallbladder. Imaging is then performed 20 to 50 minutes after the morphine to determine delayed visualization or nonvisualization related to cystic duct patency.[58]

Nursing Care After the Procedure

Care and assessment after the procedure are the same as for any nuclear scan study (see p. 735).
➤ Resume food and fluids after the study, and monitor for mentation effects of morphine sulfate, if it was administered.

KIDNEY/RENOGRAPHY SCANNING

Kidney scanning is a nuclear study performed to assist in diagnosing abnormal blood flow, collecting system defects, and excretory function of the organs. It can also provide information about the size and shape of the kidneys. Flow studies, excretion studies, determination of glomerular filtration rate (GFR), and static imaging reveal the presence of the different types of pathology. Such pathology includes vascular disease, inflammation or infection, obstructive uropathy, masses, congenital anomalies, acute or chronic renal failure, and the effects of trauma or injury. Renography involves the times of uptake and excretion of the radionuclide by the kidneys, which is plotted out on a graph and compared with normal parameters of organ function.[59]

Several radiopharmaceuticals administered IV are used in kidney scanning, depending on their distribution in the organs. Technetium 99m (^{99m}Tc) administered as technetium Tc 99m DTPA is used to study blood flow and GFR, and technetium Tc 99m dimercaptosuccinic acid (DMSA) or technetium Tc 99m gluceptate is used to assess the parenchyma for structural defects with static imaging; technetium Tc 99m glucoheptonate is the agent of choice for children. Iodine 131 (^{131}I) as orthoiodohippurate (OIH) I 131 is administered to study renal plasma flow and tubular secretion. Time schedule for scanning varies with the radiopharmaceutical administered and the information to be obtained. Abnormalities are identified by a delayed, diminished, or absent flow to the affected kidney. A triple renal study can be performed with the administration of two IV injections of radiopharmaceuticals to obtain perfusion, excretion, and structural information.

Another study performed on the genitourinary system involves imaging of the valve action at the ureterovesicular junction to assist in the diagnosis of vesicoureteral reflux. It is performed on adults and children using technetium Tc 99m DTPA instilled into the bladder. This procedure is preferred over voiding cystourethrography because it has a very low radiation exposure to the bladder and surrounding organs.[60]

Reference Values

Normal size, shape, position, symmetry, perfusion, and function of the kidneys; no renal vascular disease, trauma, infection or inflammation, obstructive uropathy, masses, congenital anomalies, or renal failure

Interfering Factors

➤ Inability of client to remain still during the procedure, especially if the client is a child
➤ Antihypertensives taken within 24 hours of the study

Indications for Kidney/Renography Scanning

➤ Diagnosing renal artery stenosis resulting from dysplasia or atherosclerosis and causing arterial hypertension and reduced glomerular filtration revealed by a diminished flow to the affected kidney
➤ Diagnosing renal vein thrombosis resulting from dehydration in infants or obstruction of blood flow resulting from tumors in adults revealed by enlarged kidney and decreased flow
➤ Diagnosing renal artery embolism or renal infarction causing obstruction as revealed by absent flow and function
➤ Determining effect of renal trauma such as arterial injury, renal contusion, hematoma, rupture, A-V fistula, or urinary extravasation as revealed by decreased or absent flow and an abnormal renal outline
➤ Detecting renal infection or inflammatory disease such as acute or chronic pyelonephritis, renal abscess, or nephritis as revealed by decreased perfusion in the affected area, decreased kidney size, and scarring
➤ Determining and locating the cause of obstructive uropathy such as calculi, neoplasm, inflammation, or congenital disorders as revealed by delayed or reduced blood flow to the affected kidney; determining and locating the cause of nonvisualization of the bladder in complete obstruction and nonvisualization of the kidney if the obstruction is of long standing
➤ Detecting cystic disease such as simple cysts, polycystic disease in children or adults, or medullary sponge kidney or cystic disease in adults as revealed by abnormal renal size and shape, single or multiple cysts, or unperfused or perfused areas, depending on the type of cyst
➤ Detecting type, position, and number of congenital anomalies such as ectopic kidney, horseshoe kidney, supernumerary kidneys, or agenesis of left kidney as revealed by changes in size, shape, or position of kidney(s)

➤ Evaluating acute and chronic renal failure as revealed by a reduction in uptake, depending on renal function, and by an absence of uptake in renal insufficiency, indicating a poor prognosis

➤ Evaluating kidney transplant for acute or chronic rejection as revealed by decreased flow and function early in rejection, acute tubular necrosis (ATN) within 24 hours of rejection with absence of excretion from the kidney, acute rejection within 5 days postoperatively, and chronic rejection revealed by ongoing decreased flow and function

➤ Determining vesicoureteral reflux in children as revealed by reflux during bladder filling or micturition, or both, during or after voiding, and calculating the amount of reflux[61]

Contraindications

➤ Pregnancy, unless benefits of performing the procedure greatly outweigh the risks to the fetus

Nursing Care Before the Procedure

Client teaching and physical preparation are the same as for any nuclear scan study (see pp. 734 to 735).

➤ Inform the client of the scanning schedule, and explain that the study takes 30 to 60 minutes initially but that an additional 4 hours are needed if special imaging or renogram is to be performed.

➤ Ensure that the client has had adequate fluid intake before the study and provide 2 glasses of fluids to drink immediately before the study.

➤ Advise the client to withhold antihypertensive medications 24 to 48 hours before the test.

➤ Administer ordered Lugol's solution before the study to reduce uptake of the radionuclide by the thyroid gland.

➤ Inform the client that additional medications may be administered during the study.

➤ History should include information about renal-urinary status and results of renal function laboratory tests (blood-urea-nitrogen [BUN], creatinine).

The Procedure

The client is placed on the examining table in a prone, supine, or sitting position depending on the study to be performed. Positions can be changed during the imaging. The client is requested to remain still during the scanning procedure. The radiopharmaceutical for flow studies is administered IV and sequential imaging is performed every 2 seconds for 30 to 60 seconds. Blood pool imaging can also be obtained at this time. Excretion studies are performed after the administration of the appropriate radiopharmaceutical, and one image every minute for 3 minutes at 30-minute intervals is obtained. There is an immediate uptake for flow and excretory studies, with a peak at 3 to 5 minutes, followed by a decline. Renal pelvis and bladder activities can be seen in 3 to 6 minutes. Excretion studies are best performed on the hydrated client, unless the study is performed for hypertension. These are followed by static imaging to reveal the collecting system and delayed static imaging 2 to 3 hours later to reveal cortex abnormalities. In some cases, imaging can be performed 24 hours later, especially in clients with renal failure, as this condition slows the uptake of the radionuclide. All information obtained is stored in a computer for further interpretation and computation. During the flow and static imaging, a loop diuretic such as furosemide (Lasix) can be administered IV to encourage large urinary output, which is then followed by imaging.[62]

Renogram curves can be plotted concurrently with flow studies in which blood flow is imaged and recorded as it occurs. Information is displayed and a chart recording is made. A curve is plotted based on the amount of radionuclide uptake over a period of time, which results in curve shapes with diagnostic value. The graphed data provide information about vascular, tubular, and excretory phases of radionuclide uptake and removal by the kidneys. Urine and blood laboratory studies are performed after the renogram to correlate findings before diagnosis.[63]

For a vesicoureteral reflux procedure, the client is requested to void and a catheter is inserted into the bladder. The radiopharmaceutical is instilled into the bladder, and multiple images are obtained during bladder filling. The client is then requested to void after catheter removal or the bladder is emptied with the catheter in place, depending on department policy. Imaging continues during voiding and after voiding is completed. Reflux is determined by calculating the urine volume and counts obtained by imaging. This study is preferred for children who require repeated studies for long-term care for vesicoureteral reflux to avoid the high gonadal radiation exposure that results from x-ray contrast cystourethrography.

Nursing Care After the Procedure

Care and assessment after the procedure are the same as for any nuclear scan study (see p. 735).

SCROTAL SCANNING

Scrotal scanning is a nuclear procedure performed to assist in diagnosing diseases and disorders of the testis, epididymis, spermatic cord, and other contents of the scrotal sac. An IV injection of ^{99m}Tc as technetium Tc 99m pertechnetate is administered, and perfusion and tissue studies are conducted. Based on an increased radionuclide activity and flow, arterial and venous supply, torsion, infections, and tumor abnormalities can be imaged.

Reference Values

Normal blood flow and structures of scrotal contents; no tumor, hematoma, infection or inflammation, or torsion

Interfering Factors

➤ Inability of client to remain still during the procedure, as with a child

Indications for Scrotal Scanning

➤ Unexplained testicular pain and swelling to determine the cause
➤ Determining infectious processes and differentiating between epididymitis and orchitis as revealed by increased flow and focal increase of the radionuclide
➤ Diagnosing hydrocele or varicocele as revealed by radionuclide concentration, depending on the size

➤ Diagnosing torsion abnormalities as revealed by absence of perfusion on the affected side and decreased activity of the radionuclide in the tissue of the affected side when compared with the unaffected side

➤ Evaluating the effects of trauma such as hematoma or hematocele as revealed by diffuse increase of flow

➤ Determining the existence and placement of inguinal hernia as revealed by intake extending from the inguinal region to the scrotum

➤ Diagnosing benign and malignant tumors of the testes as revealed by diffuse increased uptake with some decreased areas

Contraindications

➤ None

Nursing Care Before the Procedure

Client teaching and physical preparation are the same as for any nuclear scan study (see pp. 734 to 735).

➤ Inform the client that the study takes 30 to 60 minutes. A child should be accompanied by the parent of the child's choice.

➤ History should include information about the reproductive system and signs and symptoms associated with disorders of the scrotum and its contents.

The Procedure

The client is placed on the examining table in a supine position. Potassium perchlorate is administered orally to block thyroid uptake of the radionuclide. The penis is taped in a position over the pubis. If needed, a sling or towel is used to support the scrotum and the scrotum is positioned in the field of the scanner. The client is requested to remain still during the scanning. Imaging is performed initially without a lead shield; then a lead shield is positioned and imaging is repeated. The radiopharmaceutical is administered IV and flow study imaging is performed for 60 seconds at 3- to 6-second intervals. Delayed imaging is then performed to scan the scrotum and activity of the sac contents.[64]

Nursing Care After the Procedure

Care and assessment after the procedure are the same as for any nuclear scan study (see p. 735).

GALLIUM 67 (⁶⁷GA) SCANNING

Gallium 67 (⁶⁷Ga) body scanning is a nuclear study performed to assist in diagnosing neoplasm and inflammatory activity in any body tissue or organ. To identify the presence and location of these abnormalities, the radionuclide ⁶⁷Ga as gallium citrate Ga 67 is administered IV, followed by a total body scanning procedure. This radionuclide is readily distributed throughout the plasma and body tissues with a 90 percent sensitivity for inflammatory disease. It binds to transferrin receptors on cell surfaces, which is useful in identifying the presence of tumors, and to lactoferrin in neutrophils, useful in identifying inflammatory lesions.

Reference Values

Normal organ systems in the body; no tumors or infectious processes in the body tissues.

Interfering Factors

➤ Inability of client to remain still during the procedure

➤ Antineoplastic drug therapy affecting the results of the study

Indications for Gallium 67 (^{67}Ga) Scanning

➤ Detecting infections or inflammatory diseases such as amebic and perinephric abscess, pyelonephritis, osteomyelitis, septic arthritis, and *Pneumocystis carinii* pneumonia as revealed by increased uptake of the radionuclide in the affected organ

➤ Detecting primary and metastatic tumor in the lung, bone, brain, liver, head and neck, or gastrointestinal and genitourinary tracts as revealed by uptake of the radionuclide, depending on the organ system involved

➤ Diagnosing and determining the stage of lymphomas, especially in Hodgkin's disease, and bronchogenic cancer as revealed by uptake in lymph nodes or extranodal locations

➤ Detecting primary hepatoma, sarcoma, melanoma, or sarcoidosis as revealed by an abnormal uptake of the radionuclide in related organs

➤ Differentiating between benign and malignant tumors and detecting recurrent tumors when performed in combination with other studies such as CT and ultrasonography

➤ Screening for abnormalities when performed with other nuclear scan studies using ^{99m}Tc or ^{111}In

➤ Determining effectiveness of chemotherapy or radiation therapy

Contraindications

➤ Pregnancy, unless benefits of performing the procedure greatly outweigh the risks to the fetus

Nursing Care Before the Procedure

Client teaching and physical preparation are the same as for any nuclear scan study (see pp. 734 to 735).

➤ Inform the client that the scanning schedule can extend over 3 days and that each scanning procedure takes 1 to 2 hours.

➤ Administer an ordered suppository or tap water enema, or both, before the study.

➤ History should include information about the physical examination of all systems and results of any previous diagnostic tests and procedures.

The Procedure

The client is placed on the examining table in a supine position. The radiopharmaceutical is administered IV, with the amount dependent on whether tumor or inflammation imaging is to be performed. The client is requested to remain still during the scanning. Because of slow blood clearance, scanning is performed in 6, 24, 48, or 72 hours, or at more than one or at all of these times, for infectious or inflammatory identification. Scanning is performed in 24 and 48 hours, with delayed imaging up to 120 hours possible for tumor identification. Soft tissue activity is present on 6- and 24-hour scans, and this activity decreases for scans performed after the initial 24 hours because of slow blood clearance. Depending on the reason for the scan, anterior and posterior views of the head, neck, chest, and abdomen and anterior views of the extremities are performed in whole body scanning. Lateral and oblique views can also be performed.

Nursing Care After the Procedure

Care and assessment after the procedure are the same as for any nuclear scan study (see p. 735).

IODINE 131 (^{131}I) SCANNING

Iodine 131 (^{131}I) body scanning is a nuclear study performed to assist in diagnosing metastatic thyroid cancer anywhere in the body or in detecting extrathyroid tissue or residual thyroid tissue after a total thyroidectomy. The radionuclide ^{131}I as MIBG I 131 is administered orally, followed by scanning to reveal concentrations in the neck, lungs, or bones, indicating metastatic activity.

Reference Values

Absence of thyroid gland tissue outside of the thyroid gland; no metastatic tumor from a primary thyroid malignancy

Interfering Factors

➤ Inability of client to remain still during the procedure
➤ Other nuclear scans performed before or on the same day as the body scan

Indications for Iodine 131(^{131}I) Scanning

➤ Determination of remaining thyroid tissue anywhere outside of the normal thyroid gland after thyroidectomy
➤ Determination of metastasis from a diagnosed primary thyroid malignancy
➤ After administration of ^{131}I therapy for thyroid cancer

Contraindications

➤ Pregnancy, unless benefits of performing the procedure greatly outweigh the risks to the fetus

Nursing Care Before the Procedure

Client teaching and physical preparation are the same as for any nuclear scan study (see pp. 734 to 735).
➤ Inform the client of the scanning schedule and explain that imaging takes 2 to 3 hours.
➤ Ensure that changes in thyroid medication regimen and administration of other medications have been implemented before the study.
➤ History should include thyroidectomy, postoperative treatments, medication regimen, and results of other diagnostic tests and procedures.

The Procedure

The client is given an oral dose of the radiopharmaceutical in a capsule and returned to or requested to return to the department 24 to 72 hours later. The client is then placed on the examining table in a supine position and requested to remain still while full body scanning is performed. Thyroid-stimulating hormone (TSH) can be administered IV before the radiopharmaceutical to stimulate any residual tissue to take up the radionuclide, if this is the reason for the study. A higher level of TSH also increases uptake by metastatic tumors.

Nursing Care After the Procedure

Care and assessment after the procedure are the same as for any nuclear scan study (see p. 735).

POSITRON EMISSION TOMOGRAPHY (PET)

Positron emission tomography (PET) scanning, as described in the introduction of this chapter, is a nuclear study performed to assist in diagnosing central nervous system (CNS), cardiac, pulmonary, and breast disorders. Although these particular organ systems are the usual ones examined for pathological processes, this procedure can be performed to examine any part of the body to obtain clinical information regarding diseases and effects of therapeutic interventions.

A radionuclide prepared for use in this study, usually ^{15}O, ^{13}N, ^{11}C, or ^{18}F, capable of emitting a positron, is administered by IV injection or via inhalation. PET scanning follows after the radionuclide becomes concentrated in the organ to be studied. The time required for radionuclide concentration varies with the organ system. As the positron combines with negative electrons, the specialized PET scanner translates the emission from the radioactivity into color-coded images for viewing and analysis. Scanning is conducted over a period of time to allow repetition or sequencing of three-dimensional images. The expense of the study limits its use, even though it is more sensitive than are traditional nuclear scanning and SPECT scanning.

Reference Values

Normal blood flow and metabolism in body tissues; no patterns that reveal organ abnormalities

Interfering Factors

➤ Inability of client to remain still during the procedure
➤ High anxiety levels that can affect study for brain function
➤ Use of alcohol, tobacco, or caffeine-containing beverages at least 24 hours before the study
➤ Tranquilizers that alter mentation or insulin that alters glucose metabolism

Indications for Positron Emission Tomography (PET)

➤ Identifying seizure foci in clients with focal seizures as revealed by decreases in metabolism between seizures and increases in the ictal state
➤ Diagnosing Alzheimer's disease and differentiating it from other causes of dementia as revealed by a decreased cerebral blood flow and metabolism and a change in receptor chemistry
➤ Determining cerebrovascular accident (CVA) or aneurysm as revealed by decreased blood flow and oxygen utilization

➤ Diagnosing Parkinson's disease or Huntington's chorea as revealed by decreased metabolism and changes in receptor chemistry

➤ Evaluating cranial tumors preoperatively to determine the stage and appropriate treatment or procedure

➤ Determining physiological changes in psychosis and schizophrenia as revealed by decreased metabolic activity

➤ Determining the effect of drug therapy as revealed by biochemical activity of normal and abnormal tissues

➤ Diagnosing breast tumor, lung infection, and chronic pulmonary edema, depending on the radionuclide used and the concentrations at the sites

➤ Determining the presence of and the extent of myocardial infarction and the size of the infarct as revealed by regional metabolic activity in the heart

➤ Determining CAD as revealed by metabolic state of the myocardium during ischemia and after anginal pain

Contraindications

➤ Pregnancy, unless benefits of performing the procedure greatly outweigh the risks to the fetus

Nursing Care Before the Procedure

Client teaching and physical preparation are the same as for any nuclear scan study (see pp. 734 to 735).

➤ Inform the client that the study takes 30 to 60 minutes, depending on the organ to be examined.

➤ Instruct the client to restrict smoking and intake of alcohol or caffeine-containing beverages for 24 hours before the study.

➤ Client should be instructed also to restrict medications except for a long-acting insulin that should be administered before a meal 3 to 4 hours before the study.

➤ Advise the client that a blindfold and earplugs are used to reduce stimuli during the study if the brain is being examined.

➤ History should include information about the system being studied, signs and symptoms that determined the need for the study, and results of other diagnostic tests and procedures.

The Procedure

Brain Study. The client is placed on a reclining bed in a semiupright position. An IV line is initiated in each arm. The radionuclide is injected into one line and serial blood samples are taken from the second line. The client is requested to perform deep breathing to reduce anxiety. Earplugs and blindfold are applied to reduce external stimuli. The client is requested to remain still during the study. Scanning of the brain begins 45 minutes after the injection, and the client is requested to read, perform letter-recognition activities, or recite a familiar quotation, depending on whether speech, reasoning, or memory is to be tested.

Heart, Lung, or Breast Study. The client is placed on the examining table in a supine position. The two IV lines are initiated as for a brain study. Scanning over the chest is performed 45 minutes after the injection of the radionuclide.

The scanning takes place for 1 hour as the detectors record the radiation and establish its source in the body. A computer transforms the rays into a visual display on a screen for viewing.

Nursing Care After the Procedure

Care and assessment after the procedure are the same as for any nuclear scan study (see p. 735).

➤ Advise the client to assume a standing position slowly to prevent postural hypotension.

RADIONUCLIDE-MEDIATED LABORATORY STUDIES

Radionuclide-mediated laboratory studies are known as "in vitro" diagnostic testing, and they are performed to measure the amount of a specific radionuclide in body fluid (blood or urine) samples by laboratory analysis. Feces can also be tested for radionuclide concentration. The studies include procedures that determine the ability of the body to absorb a radionuclide or the ability of the body to localize the radionuclide.[65] Some of the studies include scanning procedures to obtain immediate or delayed images of an organ or area of the body. A list of commonly used radionuclides and their tissue sites can be found in Table 20–1 (see pp. 729–730).

TOTAL BLOOD VOLUME STUDY

The total blood volume study is a nuclear laboratory test performed to determine the amount of circulating blood volume in the body. It includes a combination of tests for plasma volume and RBC volume that make up the total volume, although the tests can be performed individually, depending on the reason for the study and the needed diagnostic information. The total blood volume is estimated in milliliters (mL) per kilogram (kg) because of the variations in individual body weight and frame. Normally, the blood constitutes 6 to 8 percent of the total body weight. It consists of blood cells suspended in plasma. Plasma forms 45 to 60 percent of the total blood volume and the RBCs constitute most of the remaining volume.[66]

The test involves the IV administration of the client's own RBCs labeled with chromated Cr 51 sodium for RBC volume or human serum albumin labeled with ^{125}I for plasma volume. After the preparation and reinjection of the radiopharmaceutical, blood samples are periodically drawn and the volumes calculated. RBC is calculated using the following formula: counting standard expressed as counts per minute per milliliter $\times$ 1000 $\times$ 5, ÷counts per minute per milliliter in the blood sample. Plasma volume is calculated using the following formula: counting standard expressed as counts per minute $\times$ 1000, ÷counts per minute in the blood sample. When findings in RBC volume exceed 36 mL/kg in male clients and 32 mL/kg in female clients, polycythemia vera is diagnosed, whereas a normal or reduced RBC volume indicates stress polycythemia. Normal or mild changes in plasma volume indicate polycythemia vera, and a reduced plasma volume indicates stress polycythemia.[67]

Reference Values

Total blood volume	80–85 mL/kg
Red blood cell (RBC) volume	
Men	25–35 mL/kg
Women	20–30 mL/kg
Plasma volume	
Men and women	30–45 mL/kg

Interfering Factors

➤ IV administration of fluid or blood replacement before the study
➤ Dehydration, overhydration, or excessive blood loss

Indications for Total Blood Volume Study

➤ Evaluating blood and fluid losses resulting from hemorrhage, burns, surgery, or dehydration:
  * Responses include hypotension, increased pulse, oliguria, or dry skin, leading to shock state or fluid imbalance.
  * A sudden reduction in the total blood volume can lead to shock, whereas a gradual loss can lead to an increasing plasma volume and decreasing RBC volume.
➤ Differentiating between stress polycythemia and polycythemia vera:
  * RBC volume remains at a normal or reduced level in stress polycythemia and increases in polycythemia vera.
  * Increased RBC volume in combination with increased WBCs and platelets that occur in polycythemia lead to stroke, hemorrhage, myocardial infarction, and venous thrombosis as the blood becomes more viscous.[68]
  * Plasma volume is reduced and hematocrit is elevated with a normal level of RBC volume in stress polycythemia, and it remains at a normal or slightly increased or decreased level in polycythemia vera.
➤ Determining replacement therapy:
  * In hemorrhage or loss caused by surgery, gastrointestinal bleeding, or trauma, whole blood is usually administered.
  * In reduced RBC volume caused by bleeding or cell destruction, packed RBC is administered.
  * In reduced plasma volume caused by bleeding, burns, or trauma, plasma volume expander is administered.
  * In dehydration state, IV fluids of normal saline or distilled water with or without glucose are administered.
  * This test is used before surgical procedures to anticipate need for replacement therapy and type of replacement needed.
➤ Monitoring response to replacement therapy

Contraindications

➤ Pregnancy, unless benefits of performing the test greatly outweigh the risks to the fetus

Nursing Care Before the Procedure

Client preparation is the same as for any study involving the collection of a peripheral blood sample (see Appendix I).

➤ Inform the client of the injection of a radiopharmaceutical and explain that a minute amount of the material is administered and excreted from the body within 24 hours without causing any harmful effects.

➤ Inform the client of the schedule for blood samples and explain that the venipunctures are the only discomfort experienced.

➤ Obtain and record client's height and weight, because values are calculated and expressed in milliliters per kilogram.

➤ History should include hematologic system information, assessment of vital signs, and potential causes of fluctuations.

The Procedure

Red Blood Cell Volume. The client is placed on the examining table in a supine position for 30 minutes. The prepared dose (5 mL) of the labeled radiopharmaceutical is injected into the vein of one arm. Blood samples (5 mL) are drawn from a vein in the opposite arm in 10 and 40 minutes after the injection. Normally, these samples are equal in counts, but if there is a delay in equal readings caused by splenomegaly or polycythemia, the reading at 40 minutes is the more accurate. A 2-mL sample is taken from the 5-mL sample and counted. A microhematocrit is performed to assist in a polycythemia diagnosis. The blood samples are counted to determine the concentration of the radionuclide and compared with the amount administered to obtain the volume of RBCs.

Plasma Volume. The client is placed on the examining table in a supine position for 30 minutes. A blood sample (5 mL) is drawn and centrifuged, and 2 mL is removed to perform a count and establish a standard. The radiopharmaceutical is injected into one arm, and in 10 minutes a blood sample is drawn from the opposite arm. The sample is centrifuged, and 2 mL of plasma is removed and counted. Plasma volume is determined by comparing the counts from the sample with the established count standard.

Nursing Care After the Procedure

Care and assessment after the test are the same as for any study involving a venipuncture for injection or collection of a peripheral blood sample (see Appendix I).

➤ Assess vital signs and compare them with pretest readings. Continue to monitor if total blood volume falls below 80 mL/kg.

➤ Monitor ordered replacement therapy such as blood or blood component transfusion or IV fluids.

➤ Monitor intake and output (I&O) to prevent or assist in controlling blood or fluid loss or overload, or both.

➤ Provide support when diagnostic findings are revealed, especially if continuing treatment is necessary, as in polycythemia vera (phlebotomy every 2 to 3 months, myelosuppressive drug therapy to reduce bone marrow activity).

RED BLOOD CELL (RBC) SURVIVAL TIME STUDY

Red blood cell (RBC) survival time study is a nuclear laboratory test performed to determine whether an anemic state is caused by a decrease in the survival of RBCs. Normally, RBCs have a life span of 120 days, with 0.8 percent loss per day and a half-time of 60 days. The normal half-time, which serves as a basis for determining the rate of survival or destruction in this study, is 25 to 35 days for this test because of an additional loss of tagging from RBCs.[69] When the RBCs are destroyed or sequestered in the spleen, the life span of the cells is reduced and a diagnosis of hemolysis can be made as a cause of anemia. The study is performed in combination with RBC volume and iron studies (see Chap. 1).

The test involves two stages. The first stage provides laboratory testing of blood after the injection of a specially prepared radiopharmaceutical. The client's own blood is drawn and labeled with chromated Cr 51 sodium and reinjected. Scheduled blood samples are drawn daily to test for blood levels of radioactivity in the circulation. The second stage provides for a scanning of the spleen to determine whether the reduced life span of the RBCs is caused by splenic sequestration. The liver and pericardium are also scanned to determine pathogenic mechanisms. Counts are made for each area and a ratio is established for spleen to liver and spleen to pericardium to determine splenic abnormalities, as a rising ratio indicates sequestration significant to RBC destruction.

Reference Values

> Survival Time
> Normal life span of RBCs = 120 days, with a normal loss of 0.8% per day
> Normal half-time of RBCs = 60 days
> Normal half-time of labeled RBCs = 25–35 days
> Splenic Sequestration
> Spleen-to-liver ratio = 1 : 1
> Spleen-to-pericardium ratio = 2 : 1 or less

Interfering Factors

➤ Recent transfusion or hemorrhage falsely decreases RBC survival.
➤ High WBC and platelet counts falsely decrease RBC survival time.

Indications for Red Blood Cell (RBC) Survival Time Study

➤ Known or suspected hemolytic anemia conditions causing a decreased survival value:
  • Intrinsic or extrinsic defects listed in Table 20–2
  • Identification of the need for further studies to confirm diagnosis of intrinsic or extrinsic defects causing the anemia
➤ Known or suspected disorders causing an increased survival of RBCs as revealed by more than a 35-day survival value:

Table 20–2 ➤ CLASSIFICATION OF HEMOLYTIC ANEMIAS

Intrinsic Defects
Hereditary defects
  Abnormalities of the red blood cell membrane
    Hereditary spherocytosis
    Hereditary elliptocytosis
    Hereditary pyropoikilocytosis
    Hereditary stomatocytosis and xerocytosis
  Inherited erythrocyte enzyme disorders
    Glucose-6-phosphate dehydrogenase (G-6-PD) deficiency
    Other enzyme deficiencies
      Pyruvate kinase (PK) deficiency
      Pyrimidine-5′-nucleotidase deficiency
  Disorders of hemoglobin production
    Hemoglobinopathies
    Sickle cell syndromes
      Sickle cell disease
      Sickle cell trait
      HbS β-thalassemia syndrome
      Hemoglobin C disease
      Hemoglobin SC disease
    Methemoglobins/hemoglobin M
    Unstable hemoglobin
    Thalassemia syndromes
      α-Thalassemia
      Homozygous β-thalassemia
      Heterozygous β-thalassemia
      Thalassemia heterozygotes with other hemoglobinopathies
Acquired defects
  Paroxysmal nocturnal hemoglobinuria

Extrinsic Defects
Nonimmune destruction
  Microangiopathic and macroangiopathic hemolytic anemia
  Chemical and toxic agents
  Infections causing hemolysis
  Hypersplenism
  Systemic disorders
Immune hemolytic anemias
  Primary
  Secondary (associated with chronic lymphocytic leukemia, lymphomas, and carcinomas)
  Drug-induced
  Infections

Note: From Sacher, RA, and McPherson, RA: Widmann's Clinical Interpretation of Laboratory Tests, ed 10. FA Davis, Philadelphia, 1991, p 94, with permission.

- Erythrocytosis caused by primary or secondary polycythemia or thalassemia minor
- Chronic hypoxia, respiratory or cardiovascular disease, high altitudes, hypoventilation syndromes, and renal disorders, which can stimulate production of RBCs
➤ Determination of RBC sequestration in the spleen as revealed by a spleen-to-liver or spleen-to-pericardium ratio:
  - Differentiation between splenomegaly, as revealed by an increased spleen-to-liver ratio with a normal spleen-to-pericardium ratio, and

sequestration, as revealed by an increased spleen-to-liver ratio of 2 : 1 to 4 : 1 over the entire study period or a spleen-to-pericardium ratio of more than 2 : 1[70]

- Provision of guidance for treatment (splenectomy) that removes the source of RBC destruction, resulting in a prolonged RBC survival

Contraindications

➤ Pregnancy, unless benefits of performing the study greatly outweigh the risks to the fetus
➤ Excessive bleeding or clotting abnormality

Nursing Care Before the Procedure

Client preparation is the same as for any study involving the collection of a peripheral blood sample (see Appendix I) and any nuclear laboratory study (see p. 967).

➤ Instruct the client in collection and testing of a stool specimen for occult blood if this part of the test is ordered.
➤ History should include a hematologic system assessment, vital signs, and results of hemoglobin, hematocrit, platelet, WBC, and reticulocyte counts.

The Procedure

Phase 1. A blood specimen of 10 mL is drawn from the client and centrifuged to remove the plasma. The remaining cells are labeled and reinjected. A blood sample is drawn 24 hours after the injection and then every other day for 3 weeks. Each specimen is analyzed for counts per minute of the radionuclide and plotted out on graph paper to determine the RBC survival half-time. The rate at which the labeled cells disappear during the timed testing indicates the progression of cell destruction.

Phase 2. Scanning of the spleen, liver, and pericardium is performed on the same schedule as for phase 1 in conjunction with the RBC survival study. Splenic sequestration is determined by the concentration of the radionuclide at the site of cell damage. To determine splenic abnormalities, counts are performed for each area and a ratio is established for spleen to liver and spleen to pericardium.

Nursing Care After the Procedure

Care and assessment after the tests are the same as for any study involving a venipuncture for injection or collection of a peripheral blood sample (see Appendix I).

If scanning is performed, care and assessment are the same as for any nuclear scan study (see p. 735).

➤ Monitor vital signs and compare them with pretest readings.
➤ Monitor ordered replacement therapy in severe anemic state (packed RBC, IV fluids).
➤ Assess for fatigue or activity intolerance when RBC survival is decreasing, and provide rest and measures to preserve energy.
➤ Assess for jaundice, adequate hydration, and pain in anemic state when RBC survival is decreasing.

➤ Assess for hypoxic states when RBC survival rate is increasing and provide oxygen, if needed.

➤ Assess for ability to follow instructions for return to the laboratory for blood tests and scanning. Provide a written schedule.

➤ Provide support when diagnostic findings are revealed, especially if a congenital or chronic disorder is diagnosed, and assist in coping with the chronicity or life-threatening risk associated with an increase or decrease in RBC survival rate.

PLATELET SURVIVAL TIME STUDY

Platelet survival time study is a nuclear laboratory test performed to measure the life span of circulating platelets to assist in the diagnosis of conditions involving vascular integrity and hemostasis. Platelets are formed in the bone marrow and have a normal life span of 9 days. Disappearance of the platelets from the circulating blood depends on their destruction by the reticuloendothelial system (RES). If the platelet survival time is decreased, there is generally a proportional decrease in the platelet count. Within the few days of continuing platelet destruction, platelet production can increase 2 to 8 times their normal rate. If the production rate does not compensate for the increased rate of destruction, thrombocytopenia will persist. Many conditions reflect a diminished platelet survival time, most commonly, diabetes, vascular disorders, cirrhosis, and idiopathic thrombocytopenic purpura (ITP).

The test involves the labeling of the client's own platelets with chromated Cr 51 or indium In 111 chloride. The labeled material is reinjected IV and blood samples are drawn over a period of days. The number of platelets and their progressive reduction in numbers are determined by testing the samples and formulating a curve over the scheduled testing days. Nonlinear curve shapes indicate a pathological condition causing destruction of the platelets. Scanning can also be performed to diagnose vascular abnormalities such as thrombosis or embolism.

Interfering Factors

➤ IV administration of fluid or volume expanders before the study

➤ Large emboli that obstruct an artery and prevent the emboli from being exposed to the radionuclide in the blood

➤ Heparin, which can prevent visualization of an embolus

➤ Therapy with drugs known to alter platelet survival, unless the test is performed to evaluate the effects of such drugs

Indications for Platelet Survival Time Study

➤ Disorders that increase or decrease levels by reduced production or increased destruction of platelets (see Table 2–6, p. 62).

➤ Non-immune-mediated disorders associated with reduced platelet survival:
• Disseminated intravascular coagulation (DIC) associated with shock, severe crush and burn injuries, surgical trauma, tissue infarction, overwhelming sepsis, and the obstetric complication of abruptio placentae
• Consumptive coagulopathy associated with vascular injury such as thrombotic thrombocytopenic purpura, hemolytic-uremic syndrome, and vasculitis[71]

- Prosthetic heart valves
- Arterial grafts
- Renal transplantation
- Peripheral vascular disease
- Hepatic cirrhosis
- Post-transfusion purpura or use of extracorporeal circulation during surgery

➤ Immune-mediated disorders associated with reduced platelet survival:
  - ITP, as revealed by extremely short platelet survival measured in minutes to hours, chronic lymphocytic leukemia, lymphomas, systemic lupus erythematosus (SLE), and isoimmune neonatal thrombocytopenia
  - Drug sensitivity reactions from heparin, quinine, sulfonamide derivatives, gold salts, digitoxin, or thiazides
  - Diagnosis and location of DVT revealed via imaging
  - Diagnosis of pulmonary embolism revealed by visualization through imaging of the adherence of the radionuclide to the emboli, although not a very sensitive test for older thrombi in the lung because adherence is reduced with aging[72]

Contraindications

➤ Pregnancy, unless benefits of performing the study greatly outweigh the risks to the fetus

Nursing Care Before the Procedure

Client preparation is the same as for any study involving the collection of peripheral blood samples (see Appendix I) and nuclear laboratory tests (see pp. 734 to 735).

➤ History should include information about the hematologic status, assessment of vital signs, and results of reticulocytes, WBC, platelet counts, and hemoglobin level.

The Procedure

A blood specimen is drawn from the client and centrifuged to produce platelets containing plasma. The platelets are labeled with the radioactive substance and reinjected into the client's other arm. Blood samples are drawn in 48 hours and daily thereafter for 7 to 8 days. The amount of radionuclide is measured as it disappears from the circulation; this process is related to age-destruction of the platelets. A graph is plotted using the number and time of platelet destruction over a period of scheduled testing days (Fig. 20–1). Imaging for DVT and pulmonary embolism can take place immediately or can be delayed to determine the degree of uptake in the affected areas.[73] The scanning phase is reserved for these conditions and is not to determine platelet destruction.

Nursing Care After the Procedure

Care and assessment after the test are the same as for any study involving a venipuncture for injection or collection of a peripheral blood sample (see Appendix I).

If scanning is performed, care and assessment are the same as for any nuclear scan study (see p. 735).

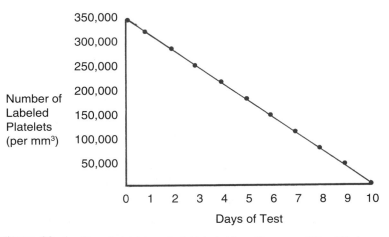

Figure 20–1   Normal platelet survival. (Adapted from Thompson, AR and Harker, LA: Manual of Hemostasis and Thrombosis, ed 3. FA Davis, Philadelphia, p 18, 1983.)

➤ Immediately report platelet count of less than 20,000 per µL, considered a critical level, if this laboratory test is performed.

➤ Assess for bleeding and blood loss from mucous membranes, skin (petechiae, ecchymoses, epistaxis, feces, hematuria, hematemesis, or hemoptysis) with thrombocytopenia.

➤ Provide measures to prevent bleeding with thrombocytopenia (gentle handling, trauma protection, soft toothbrush, or electric razor).

➤ Monitor ordered platelet infusion for treatment of thrombocytopenia.

➤ Monitor ordered anticoagulant therapy if thrombosis or embolus is diagnosed.

➤ Resume ordered administration of corticosteroid therapy for thrombocytopenia.

➤ Provide a written schedule for return to the laboratory and nuclear medicine department for testing or scanning, or both.

➤ Provide support when diagnostic findings are revealed, and assist client to cope with chronicity of a disease and the need for repeated testing and long-term therapy.

RADIOACTIVE IODINE UPTAKE (RAIU) STUDY

Radioactive iodine uptake (RAIU) study is a nuclear laboratory test performed to evaluate thyroid function. Its primary value is in its ability to assist in diagnosing hyperthyroidism, because the radionuclide is readily concentrated in the thyroid gland. The radionuclide ^{123}I is administered orally, followed by scanning of the thyroid area. Clients with hyperthyroid conditions reveal an increased uptake of the radionuclide. The test is not as effective in the diagnosis of hypothyroidism. Uptake is expressed in percentages of radionuclide absorbed in a specific amount of time. This percentage is calculated by dividing the amount of uptake by the amount or dose administered. An increase of more than 35 percent in 24 hours indicates hyperthyroidism.[74] The test is usually performed in combination with thyroid hormone tests when other thyroid function studies do not provide a definitive diagnosis.

Reference Values

2-hr absorption	1–13% of radionuclide
6-hr absorption	6–15% of radionuclide
24-hr absorption	8–30% of radionuclide

Interfering Factors

➤ Recent use of iodinated contrast media for radiographic studies, which would decrease the uptake of the radionuclide
➤ Ingestion of foods containing iodine or medications containing iodine, such as cough syrup, potassium iodide, vitamins, Lugol's solution, or thyroid replacement therapy, which would decrease the uptake of the radionuclide
➤ Medications such as propylthiouracil, corticosteroids, warfarin, antihistamines, sulfonamides, nitrates, tolbutamide (Orinase), or isoniazid, which would decrease the uptake of the radionuclide
➤ Severe diarrhea, which would affect absorption of the radionuclide dose
➤ Lithium, estrogen, TSH, barbiturates, and phenothiazines, which would increase the uptake of the radionuclide
➤ Iodine-deficient conditions, cirrhosis, or renal failure, which would increase the uptake of the radionuclide

Indications for Radioactive Iodine Uptake (RAIU) Study

➤ Evaluating thyroid function:
  * A response of increased uptake of 20 percent absorption in 1 hour, 25 percent in 6 hours, and 45 percent in 24 hours indicates hyperthyroidism.[75]
  * A response of decreased uptake of 0 to 10 percent over a 24-hour period indicates a hypothyroid state but not necessarily hypothyroidism because of the many interfering factors reducing the uptake.
➤ Monitoring response to therapy for thyroid dysfunctional states

Contraindications

➤ Pregnancy, unless benefits of performing the study greatly outweigh the risks to the fetus
➤ Sensitivity to iodine in foods or medications

Nursing Care Before the Procedure

Client preparation is the same as for any nuclear laboratory test (see p. 778) and nuclear scan study (see pp. 734 to 735).
➤ Inform the client of the scanning schedule and explain that the study can take 24 hours.
➤ Instruct the client to restrict any iodine-containing foods and medications for at least 1 week before the study.

➤ Withhold all foods and fluids for 8 to 12 hours before the study, according to department policy.

➤ History should include previous thyroid studies, allergies to iodine, medication regimen, and results of thyroid hormone tests.

The Procedure

The client is given the radionuclide orally, unless a 2-hour scan is to be performed, which requires IV administration. The client is placed on the examining table in a supine position with the neck slightly hyperextended on a small pillow. The client is then requested to remain still during the procedure. The scanning is performed with a detector over the neck in 30 minutes to determine the gland's ability to take up the radionuclide, in 6 hours to determine the gland's ability to bind iodine, and in 24 hours to determine the gland's total uptake of the radionuclide. Subsequent imaging can be performed for information about the gland's ability to release the radionuclide.[76] Determination of the percentage of uptake is calculated using the amount of the dose and the amount absorbed in a specific time period.

Nursing Care After the Procedure

Care and assessment after the procedure are the same as for any nuclear scan study (see p. 735) and venipuncture for injection of the radionuclide (see Appendix I).

➤ Assess for fatigue, nervousness, increased appetite, increased sweating, or weight loss common in hyperthyroidism and caused by increased metabolic activity.

➤ Resume normal dietary intake and thyroid replacement therapy.

➤ Resume medication regimen if iodine-containing drugs have been withheld before the study.

➤ Provide a written schedule for the client's return to the department for scanning.

THYROID-STIMULATING HORMONE (TSH) STUDY

Thyroid-stimulating hormone (TSH) study is a nuclear laboratory test performed to measure thyroid gland response to the administration of a dose of TSH. The test involves the administration of TSH intramuscularly (IM) followed by an IV injection of iodide I 123 and scanning to determine the effect of TSH on thyroid gland uptake of the radionuclide.[77] It is performed in combination with the radioactive iodine uptake study to differentiate between primary and secondary hypothyroidism. TSH, also known as thyrotropin, is produced by the basophil cells of the adenohypophysis in response to stimulation by its hypothalamic releasing factor, thyrotropin-releasing hormone (TRH). Primary hypothyroidism that results from thyroid pathology does not respond to the TSH dose, whereas secondary hypothyroidism, resulting from an abnormally reduced stimulation by the pituitary gland secreting the TSH, causes a positive response to the TSH dose. Thyroid and pituitary glands therefore can both be evaluated with this test.

Reference Values

> Less than 10μU/mL of thyroid-stimulating hormone (TSH)
> Increase in TSH levels, thyroxine (T_4), and radioactive iodine
> uptake by 8 hr after administration of TSH

Interfering Factors

➤ Recent radionuclide scanning, which can affect uptake
➤ Foods or medications containing iodine, which can decrease uptake of iodine
➤ Aspirin, heparin, dopamine, or corticosteroids, which can decrease levels of TSH

Indications for Thyroid-Stimulating Hormone (TSH) Study

➤ Evaluating thyroid function to differentiate between primary and secondary hypothyroidism:
  • TSH level decreased in secondary hypothyroidism (hypothalamic or pituitary gland source) as revealed by near 0 levels with a low T_4 level because TSH cannot be secreted
  • TSH level increased in primary hypothyroidism (Hashimoto's thyroiditis, congenital disorders, thyroidectomy, radioactive therapy) as revealed by TSH level greater than 3 times the normal range and T_4 level decreased, causing a compensatory rise in TSH
  • Diminished uptake of the radionuclide in RAIU study at all intervals in hypothyroidism
➤ Monitoring response to thyroid hormone therapy

Contraindications

  • Pregnancy, unless benefits of performing the procedure greatly outweigh the risks to the fetus

Nursing Care Before the Procedure

Client preparation is the same as for any nuclear laboratory (see p. 778) and nuclear scan (see pp. 734 to 735) studies.
➤ Inform the client of the scanning schedule and explain that the hormone is administered IM by the physician twice during the study.
➤ Inform the client that a counterscanner is placed over the region of the thyroid gland each time in the series that the test is performed.

The Procedure

The client is given 10 units of TSH by IM injection by the physician and placed on the examining table in a supine position with the head slightly hyperextended on a small pillow. Counts are taken over the thyroid gland, followed by the IM injection of another 10 units of TSH and the oral administration of the radionuclide for the RAIU scan. An uptake and scan are performed in 2 to 6 hours and again 24 hours later. Refer to the radioactive iodine uptake scan procedure (see p. 786) and thyroxine laboratory test (see pp. 238 to 240) for further information about this test.

Nursing Care After the Procedure

Care and assessment after the procedure are the same as for any nuclear scan study (see p. 735) and venipuncture for injection of the radionuclide (see Appendix I).

THYROID CYTOMEL/PERCHLORATE SUPPRESSION STUDIES

Thyroid Cytomel (liothyronine) and perchlorate suppression studies are nuclear laboratory tests performed to determine thyroid function. Cytomel suppression is performed to assist in diagnosing goiter disease and borderline hyperthyroidism. It involves the administration of triiodothyronine followed by scanning for ^{123}I or ^{131}I uptake, revealing the effect of suppression or the absence of suppression. Normally, uptake decreases more than 60 percent when compared with an initial scan. Hyperthyroidism evaluated in this test is caused by Graves' disease (toxic goiter), an autoimmune disease causing antibodies to bind to thyroid cells, resulting in glandular hypertrophy and the secretion of thyroid hormone. It can also be caused by Plummer's disease (multinodular goiter), resulting in an increased gland size and progressively developing hyperthyroidism or a solitary hyperfunctional adenoma (toxic adenoma) that is multinodular and produces hyperthyroidism. This test has generally been replaced by the thyrotropin-releasing hormone (TRH) stimulation test.

Perchlorate suppression is performed to assist in diagnosing organification defects responsible for hypothyroidism, a term used to indicate a hypometabolic state caused by deficient thyroid secretions. The test involves measurement of thyroid gland activity after scanning for ^{131}I uptake and subsequent admission of potassium perchlorate. Abnormal findings reveal a fall in uptake in 2 hours when compared with uptake after the perchlorate intake. The counts and timing of the uptake are displayed on a graph from which thyroid activity is calculated.[78]

Reference Values

> Cytomel suppression: 50% depression of thyroid uptake after liothynonine (T_3) administration
> Perchlorate suppression: Absence of change in thyroid uptake after perchlorate administration

Interfering Factors

➤ Foods and medications containing iodine taken before the study

Indications for Thyroid Cytomel/Perchlorate Suppression Studies

Cytomel Suppression

➤ Evaluation of the effect of T_3 on thyroid uptake of the radionuclide in the diagnosis of thyroid function:
  • Uptake is increased initially and decreases after Cytomel in thyroiditis, deficient iodine, or other hormone abnormality. Decrease can be more than half of the baseline level.

- Uptake is increased initially, and no change is demonstrated after Cytomel in Graves' disease, Plummer's disease, and toxic adenoma. Suppression is absent in borderline hyperthyroidism.
➤ Diagnosis of thyroid pathology that causes changes in uptake after Cytomel and subsequent suppression:
  - Suppression is absent if nodules are present.
  - Slight suppression is absent if thyroid malignancy is present.
➤ Absence of changes in uptake after thyroid therapy that causes destruction of tissue

Perchlorate Suppression

➤ Diagnosis of thyroid disorders that reveal changes in the organification process that causes decreases in uptake of the radionuclide:
  - Congenital hypothyroidism in infants with a decrease of at least 15 percent in uptake after perchlorate indicates a congenital enzyme deficiency (peroxidase) within the gland as perchlorate removes unbound iodine and prevents further uptake.
  - Decrease in uptake after perchlorate in Hashimoto's thyroiditis is commonly found in autoimmune diseases such as lupus erythematosus and rheumatoid arthritis, as well as pernicious anemia and Addison's disease, as iodine is prevented from being concentrated by the thyroid and unbound iodide is prevented from being released.

Contraindications

➤ Pregnancy, unless benefits of performing the procedure greatly outweigh the risks to the fetus

Nursing Care Before the Procedure

Client preparation is the same as for any nuclear scan study (pp. 734 to 735).

Cytomel Suppression. Instruct the client to take ordered 25 μg of Cytomel every 8 hours for 5 to 10 days, explain the schedule, and ask the client to return to the department for the scanning.
➤ Inform the client that foods and medications containing iodine should be restricted before the test.
➤ Explain that a radionuclide is administered IV and that some discomfort will be experienced at that time but that this is the only discomfort experienced during the test.
➤ History should include previous thyroid tests, allergies to iodine, medication regimen, and other therapy.

Perchlorate Suppression. Preparation is the same as for Cytomel suppression except that food and fluids are withheld 8 to 12 hours before the test and foods and medications containing iodine are withheld for at least 1 week before the test. The client can be given a list of foods and medications to avoid. Inform the client that the radionuclide is administered orally instead of IV and that the per-chlorate is given orally during the test.

The Procedure

The procedure for radioactive iodine uptake is found on p. 789.

Cytomel Suppression. The client comes to the nuclear medicine department 1 day before the last dose of Cytomel. Scanning is performed at that time and residual uptake is recorded. The radionuclide ^{123}I or ^{131}I is administered, and scanning is then performed 2 and 6 hours later.

The client is requested to return to the department after the last dose of Cytomel and an additional uptake scan is performed. Uptakes are compared, and increases or other changes are determined, based on the dose of the radionuclide, the timing of the medications, and scanning.

Perchlorate Suppression. Scanning is performed to determine whether any residual radionuclide is present. The radionuclide is administered orally, and scanning for uptake is performed in 1 and 2 hours. After the 2-hour measurement, 1 g of perchlorate is given orally, as this dose is trapped by the thyroid and displaces the iodide that has not been organified. Uptakes obtained by scanning are then performed every 15 minutes for 90 minutes. Additional scanning can be performed every 30 minutes for the next 2 hours. Uptakes after the perchlorate and those performed 2 hours before the perchlorate are compared and results graphed, based on time of uptakes, amount of the radionuclide concentrated in the thyroid gland, or absence of it in the gland.

Nursing Care After the Procedure

Care and assessment after the procedures are the same as for any nuclear scan study (see p. 735).

➤ Resume normal dietary intake and medication regimen.
➤ Provide a written schedule for return to the department for scanning and test completion.

SCHILLING TEST

The Schilling test is used to determine the cause of a vitamin B_{12} deficiency, which can result from lack of intrinsic or extrinsic factors or malabsorption in the ileum. Absorption of this vitamin requires that it be bound to intrinsic factor, a glycoprotein secreted by the gastric mucosa. Pernicious anemia, the most common and severest form of vitamin B_{12} deficiency, involves a deficiency of intrinsic factor, which reduces absorption of the vitamin in the ileum. Intestinal malabsorption syndrome, pancreatic disorders, and medications can also cause this vitamin deficiency.

The test involves the oral administration of a capsule of vitamin B_{12} labeled with the radioactive substance cobalt as cyanocobalamin Co 57 to determine gastrointestinal absorption of the vitamin. An injection of a nonradioactive vitamin B_{12} can be given in addition to the oral dose to enhance saturation of binding sites, intestinal absorption, and renal excretion of the radionuclide. A 24-hour urine specimen is then collected. Test results are expressed as the percentage of radionuclide excreted in the urine in relation to the amount administered. If less than 5 to 15 percent of the radionuclide is excreted, a two-stage test is indicated. For the second phase, an oral dose of intrinsic factor is given in addition to the labeled and unlabeled doses of the vitamin. If subsequent excretion of vitamin B_{12} reaches normal levels, pernicious anemia is confirmed; if not, malabsorption syndrome is present.[79]

Reference Values

Normally, 15–40% of a 0.5-μg dose and 5–40% of a 1.0-μg dose of radioactive vitamin B_{12} excreted

Less than 7% of the smaller dose and 0–3% of the larger dose excreted in impaired absorption states

Interfering Factors

➤ Recent diagnostic tests with radioactive materials
➤ Incomplete collection of the timed urine sample
➤ Laxatives before the test that impair intestinal absorption of the vitamin B_{12}

Indications for Schilling Test

➤ Identification of deficiency of vitamin B_{12} absorption (one-stage test)
➤ Determination of the cause of vitamin B_{12} deficiency by differentiating between pernicious anemia and gastrointestinal malabsorption problems:
  • In pernicious anemia, urinary excretion of B_{12} approaches normal levels when intrinsic factor is administered as part of the study (two-stage test).
  • In gastrointestinal malabsorption, urinary excretion of B_{12} is decreased.

➤➤ Nursing Alert

• Urine collection time can be prolonged to 48 to 72 hours in clients with severe renal disease. The normal percentage of the labeled vitamin B_{12} will eventually be excreted, however, as long as the client does not have impaired vitamin B_{12} absorption.

Contraindications

➤ Pregnancy, unless benefits of performing the procedure greatly outweigh the risks to the fetus

Nursing Care Before the Procedure

Client preparation is the same as for any nuclear laboratory study (see p. 780).

➤ Inform the client that a radioactive vitamin B_{12} is administered orally and a nonradioactive vitamin B_{12} is administered IM for the test and that the substances are eliminated from the body without harmful effects.
➤ Advise the client that food and fluid are withheld for 8 hours and that laxatives should be avoided for at least 2 days before the study.
➤ Provide a schedule for both administrations of the B_{12} and for urine collection, and provide a container to collect the urine.
➤ Inform and instruct the client in the collection of the urine specimen, including the length of time (usually 24 hours), care of the special container, **importance of saving all the urine,** and avoidance of contamination with feces or toilet tissue (see Appendix II).

➤ History should include information about hematologic and gastrointestinal status, results of folate, total binding capacity, B_{12} blood tests, and signs and symptoms of anemia or malabsorption.

The Procedure

One-Stage Test. The client voids and the urine is discarded. If a radionuclide study has been performed recently, a sample of the urine to be discarded can be sent to the laboratory for radioactivity residual. A 0.5- to 1.0-µg capsule of labeled vitamin B_{12} is administered orally. This dose is followed by an IM dose of 1000 µg of unlabeled B_{12} 1 to 2 hours later (depending on laboratory preference). Foods and fluids can be resumed after the IM injection. All urine is collected for 24 hours in a container without a preservative (48 to 72 hours in those with renal disease) and sent to the laboratory for analysis (see Appendix II). When absorption is normal, vitamin B_{12} in excess of body needs is excreted by the kidneys. If absorption is impaired, the vitamin either does not appear in the urine or is found in only limited amounts. The unabsorbed B_{12} is excreted in the feces.

Two-Stage Test. The client voids and the urine is discarded. If the test is performed on the day after a one-stage test, a specimen from the first morning voiding should be checked by the laboratory for persistent radioactivity. A 0.5- to 1.0-µg capsule of labeled vitamin B_{12} is administered orally. The client can then eat breakfast, after which a 60-µg dose of intrinsic factor is administered orally. In 1 to 2 hours, an IM dose of 1000 µg of unlabeled vitamin B_{12} is administered ("flushing dose"). This dose competes with the absorbed radioactive material for binding sites and allows excretion of the radioactive B_{12} in the urine. All urine is collected for 24 hours in a container as in the one-stage test. Findings are based on the amount of B_{12} excreted in the urine over a specific period.

Nursing Care After the Procedure

Care and assessment after the test are the same as for any nuclear laboratory test (see p. 780).
➤ Resume normal dietary intake.
➤ Assess for fatigue, weakness, sore tongue, anorexia, vomiting, or abdominal pain indicating pernicious anemia.

Student Name _____ Class _____

Instructor _____ Date _____

CASE STUDY AND CRITICAL THINKING EXERCISE

Mr. Jones, age 73, is admitted to the ER. He complains of dyspnea and chest pain every time he breathes. He is moderately overweight and reports a sedentary lifestyle. Physical exam reveals VS: T 98°F (36.6°C), P 84, R 28, BP 164/84. He has poor skin turgor and dry mucous membranes. Lung fields are clear and he has a nonproductive cough. A lung scan is ordered.

a. What is the probable diagnosis?

b. What are the risk factors associated with this diagnosis?

c. What is the probable treatment plan?

References

1. Berkow, R (ed): The Merck Manual, ed 16. Merck Sharp and Dohme Research Laboratory, Rahway, NJ, 1992, p 2548.
2. Ibid, pp 2548–2549.
3. Corbett, JV: Laboratory Tests and Diagnostic Procedures with Nursing Diagnoses, ed 3. Appleton & Lange, Norwalk, Conn, 1992, p 552.
4. Berkow, op cit, p 2164.
5. Ibid, p 2549.
6. Pagana, KD, and Pagana, TJ: Mosby's Diagnostic and Laboratory Test Reference. Mosby–Year Book, St Louis, 1992, p 575.
7. Fischbach, FT: A Manual of Laboratory and Diagnostic Tests, ed 4. JB Lippincott, Philadelphia, 1992, p 609.
8. Ibid, p 622.
9. Corbett, op cit, p 543.
10. Fischbach, op cit, pp 569–570.
11. Ibid, p 609.
12. Ibid, p 569.
13. Berkow, op cit, p 2550.
14. Corbett, op cit, p 556.
15. Datz, FL: Nuclear Medicine. Mosby–Year Book, St Louis, 1988, p 51.
16. Pollycove, M: Nuclear Medicine Manual. San Francisco General Hospital, San Francisco, 1990.
17. Pagana and Pagana, op cit, p 124.
18. Fischbach, op cit, p 579.
19. Ibid, p 579.
20. Datz, op cit, pp 82–83.
21. Ibid, pp 76–78.
22. Ibid, pp 78–79.
23. Ibid, pp 284–285.
24. Ibid, pp 289–296.
25. Ibid, pp 42–43.
26. Ibid, pp 38–39.
27. Ibid, pp 39–40.
28. Pagana and Pagana, op cit, p 161.
29. Fischbach, op cit, p 583.
30. Ibid, pp 256, 263–269.
31. Ibid, p 586.
32. Ibid, p 584.
33. Datz, op cit, p 243.
34. Ibid, p 108.
35. Ibid, p 122.
36. Pagana and Pagana, op cit, p 489.
37. Datz, op cit, p 115.
38. Ibid, pp 5–6, 132.
39. Berkow, op cit, p 2550.
40. Ibid, p 8.
41. Datz, op cit, p 36.
42. Ibid, pp 274–277.
43. Ibid, pp 161–164.
44. Corbett, op cit, p 562.
45. Datz, op cit, p 170.
46. Ibid, pp 168–169.
47. Ibid, pp 172–173.
48. Ibid, p 165.
49. Ibid, p 165.
50. Ibid, p 165.
51. Berkow, op cit, pp 801, 2551.
52. Datz, op cit, pp 138–139.
53. Ibid, pp 152–153.
54. Pagana and Pagana, op cit, pp 351–352.
55. Ibid, p 352.
56. Ibid, pp 352–353.
57. Ibid, p 358.
58. Datz, op cit, p 155.
59. Corbett, op cit, p 565.
60. Datz, op cit, pp 216–218.
61. Ibid, pp 200–217.
62. Pagana and Pagana, op cit, p 636.
63. Springhouse Corporation: Nurse's Reference Library, Diagnostics, ed 2. Springhouse, Springhouse, Pa, 1986.
64. Datz, op cit, p 225.
65. Fischbach, op cit, p 609.
66. Sacher, RA, and McPherson, RA: Widmann's Clinical Interpretation of Laboratory Tests, ed 10. FA Davis, Philadelphia, 1991, p 21.
67. Datz, op cit, pp 303–04.
68. Ibid, p 301.
69. Ibid, p 300.
70. Pagana and Pagana, op cit, p 624.
71. Sacher and McPherson, op cit, pp 224–226.
72. Datz, op cit, p 283.
73. Ibid, pp 280–283.
74. Corbett, op cit, p 567.
75. Fischbach, op cit, p 616.
76. Pagana and Pagana, op cit, p 612.
77. Fischbach, op cit, pp 617–618.
78. Datz, op cit, pp 9–10.
79. Sacher and McPherson, op cit, p 40.

Bibliography

Armstrong, P, et al: Imaging of Diseases of the Chest. Mosby–Year Book, St Louis, 1989.

Bernier, DR, et al: Nuclear Medicine: Technology and Techniques, ed 4. Mosby–Year Book, St Louis, 1997.

Black, JM, and Matassarin-Jacobs, E: Luckmann and Sorensen's Medical-Surgical Nursing: A Psychophysiologic Approach, ed 4. WB Saunders, Philadelphia, 1993.

Chernecky, CC, and Berger, BJ; Cullen, BN (ed): Laboratory Tests and Diagnostic Procedures, ed 2. WB Saunders, Philadelphia, 1996.

Datz, FL (ed): Nuclear Medicine: A Teaching

File. Mosby – Year Book, St Louis, 1992.

Fogelman, E, et al: An Atlas of Clinical Nuclear Medicine, ed 2. Mosby – Year Book, St Louis, 1993.

Freeman, LM (ed): Johnson's Clinical Radionuclide Imaging, ed 3. WB Saunders, Philadelphia, 1986.

Freeman, LM, and Blaufox, MD (eds): Seminars in Nuclear Medicine. WB Saunders, Philadelphia, 1992.

Goodman, LR, and Putnam, CE: Critical Care Imaging, ed 3. WB Saunders, Philadelphia, 1992.

Gossman, ZD, and Rosebrough, SF: Clinical Radioimmunoimaging. WB Saunders, Philadelphia, 1988.

Hoffer, PB, et al: Year Book of Nuclear Medicine. Mosby – Year Book, St Louis, 1995.

Hubner, K, et al: Clinical Positron Emission Tomography. Mosby – Year Book, St Louis, 1992.

Iskandrian, AS: Nuclear Cardiac Imaging: Principles and Applications, ed 2. FA Davis, Philadelphia, 1996.

Kee, JL: Handbook of Laboratory and Diagnostic Tests with Nursing Implications, ed 3. Appleton & Lange, Norwalk, Conn, 1997.

Kricun, ME: Imaging Modalities in Spinal Disorders. WB Saunders, Philadelphia, 1988.

Maisey, MN, et al (eds): Clinical Nuclear Medicine. WB Saunders, Philadelphia, 1983.

Mazziotta, JC, and Gilman, S: Clinical Brain Imaging: Principles and Applications. FA Davis, Philadelphia, 1992.

Mettler, FA, Jr, and Guiberteau, MJ: Essentials of Nuclear Medicine Imaging, ed 3. WB Saunders, Philadelphia, 1990.

Pagana, KD, and Pagana, TJ: Diagnostic Testing and Nursing Implications: A Case Study Approach, ed 4. Mosby – Year Book, St Louis, 1993.

Porth, CM: Pathophysiology: Concepts of Altered Health States, ed 4. JB Lippincott, Philadelphia, 1993.

Ryo, UY, et al: Atlas of Nuclear Medicine Artifacts and Variants, ed 2. Mosby – Year Book, St Louis, 1990.

Sorenson, JA, and Phelps, ME: Physics in Nuclear Medicine, ed 2. WB Saunders, Philadelphia, 1986.

Thomas, CL (ed): Taber's Cyclopedic Medical Dictionary, ed 18. FA Davis, Philadelphia, 1997.

Tilkian, SM: Clinical and Nursing Implications of Laboratory Tests, ed 5. Mosby – Year Book, St Louis, 1995.

Whaley, LF: Nursing Care of Infants and Children, ed 4. Mosby – Year Book, St Louis, 1991.

Zaret, BL, and Beller, GA: Nuclear Cardiology: The State of the Art and Future Directions. Mosby – Year Book, St Louis, 1992.

21

Non-Nuclear Scan Studies

➤ **PROCEDURES COVERED**

Body Scanning (CT, CAT, CTT), *801*
Head and Intracranial Scanning, *804*
Neck and Spinal Scanning, *806*
Thoracic Scanning, *808*
Abdominal Scanning, *810*
Pelvic Scanning, *811*
Body Magnetic Resonance Imaging (MRI, NMR), *813*
Angiography Magnetic Resonance Imaging (MRI), *816*

Abdominal Magnetic Resonance Imaging (MRI), *817*
Head and Intracranial Magnetic Resonance Imaging (MRI), *819*
Heart and Chest Magnetic Resonance Imaging (MRI), *820*
Musculoskeletal Magnetic Resonance Imaging (MRI), *822*

INTRODUCTION

Non-nuclear scan studies include computed tomography (CT) and magnetic resonance imaging (MRI), neither of which uses radiopharmaceuticals and the detectors or devices that are needed to count or image the uptake of these substances by body tissues. Each procedure uses a special machine and scanning system. Both use computer-generated images on a screen for viewing and recording.

Non-nuclear scan procedures are not considered invasive and a signed informed consent form is not required for diagnostic CT unless a contrast medium is used. A signed consent is required for MRI procedures. The studies are performed by physicians or trained technicians on inpatients or outpatients in a specially equipped room in or near the radiology department in a hospital. The results are interpreted by physicians with special education and expertise in such procedures.

COMPUTED TOMOGRAPHY (CT)

Computed tomography (CT), also known as computed axial tomography (CAT) or computed transaxial tomography (CTT), is a noninvasive procedure that uses tomographic radiography (x-ray) combined with a special scanning machine, detectors that determine the amount of radiographic beams absorbed by tissues, and a computer that processes these readings and reconstructs a body region by calculating the differences in tissue absorption of the radiographic beams. It produces a series of three-dimensional, cross-sectional anatomic views of the tissue structure of solid organs as well as differences between soft tissue and water. Imaging can also reproduce sagittal, horizontal, and coronal planes of tissue for viewing. The procedure was originally developed to identify brain abnormalities but has now advanced to include scans of the entire body, a body region, and specific body organs. Its most recent use is imaging of the heart movements and blood flow to the brain.[1] It is primarily performed to assist in the diagnosis of tumors and inflammatory disorders, although the CT scan study can produce views of many types of tissue pathology by allowing differentiation from normal tissue.

The CT scanner uses varying motions and techniques as the beam sweeps across the region to be imaged and records measurements of the radiation that is transmitted. The recordings are converted into digital form and entered into the computer, where they are processed, displayed on the screen, and stored on disks for future review. Displays on the screen provide a view of an area that is divided into slices that allow a clear picture of the relationships of the structures shown in the slices.[2] Identification is made of tissues on the screen based on higher or lower densities, which appear on the screen as patterns of shading; for example, bone appears as white, air appears as black, and soft tissue appears as shades of gray.

Iodinated or barium contrast media can be administered before and during the procedure to further clarify or enhance unusual findings, that is, tissue density, differentiation of a specific organ from other structures, or identification of small tumors.[3] Special contrast preparations made for CT scanning (that contain less iodine, are water-soluble, and contain lower-density barium in a solution) are administered for examination of specific regions or organs of the body.

The advantage of CT, even though it is more costly than other types of diagnostic studies, is that it provides an excellent, clear, and detailed image of structures not visible with other studies. This allows earlier diagnosis and treatment and more efficient follow-up of treatments and postoperative complications. It can also eliminate the need for more invasive procedures such as angiography. A disadvantage of performing CT studies is higher cost, especially if adequate results can be obtained by less expensive procedures. Another disadvantage is the length of time the client is exposed to radiation, even though more recent CT equipment has reduced the amount of radiation required for the study or allows the study to be completed in less time. Risks are also involved with the use of contrast media in clients with sensitivities to the materials and in pregnant women, because radiation can have an adverse effect on the developing fetus.

MAGNETIC RESONANCE IMAGING (MRI, NMR)

Magnetic resonance imaging (MRI), also known as nuclear magnetic resonance (NMR), is a noninvasive procedure that uses a magnet, radio waves to create a field of energy, and a computer that allows visualization of a body region. The use of the word "nuclear" has been generally excluded to reduce the anxiety provoked by the term that is often present in clients needing this study.[4] The study produces cross-sectional, multiplanar images of the entire body, a body part, and specific body organs. It is primarily used to assist in the diagnosis of conditions affecting blood flow and in the detection of tumors, infections, and any other types of tissue pathology because of its ability to produce images through bone tissue and fluid-filled soft tissues. It also allows the study of tissue concentrations of chemicals (proton spectroscopy) such as sodium, water, fat, inorganic phosphate, hydrogen ions (determines pH), and lactate.[5]

The MRI machine contains a huge magnet in the scanner that is capable of creating a magnetic field that causes the nuclei of ions, particularly hydrogen, in tissues to align themselves in an organized fashion. Hydrogen is the atom measured because it is found in all tissues of the body and has a high sensitivity to the MRI machine. Radio-frequency energy is directed to the nuclei, causing the alignment to become disorganized when the machine is turned on and then allowing the nuclei to realign themselves again when the machine is turned off. The radio signals emitted, which are determined by the nuclei density, type of specific tissue, and the realignment time, are processed by the computer. A computer-generated image is then displayed on a screen or a magnetic tape for immediate and later viewing on a video monitor.

The greatest advantage of MRI is its ability to obtain an excellent detailed image of the region studied without the use of radiopharmaceuticals, radiologic beams, or administration of a contrast medium. Its disadvantages are the cost of the study, the fact that all institutions do not provide this service, and the need for immobilization for long periods to perform the study. Although the study is considered low risk, pregnant women are not scanned with MRI, unless the benefits of performing the study outweigh the unknown risks to the fetus.

COMPUTED TOMOGRAPHY (CT) SCANNING STUDIES

Computed tomography (CT) scanning studies are imaging procedures of body parts. The studies are performed to view tissue characteristics and structures of solid organs. They have many uses and are named for the organ, as in ocular or renal studies; a region of the body, as in pelvic or abdominal studies; and body studies, which include the abdomen, chest, and pelvis, depending on the reason for the study and the type of diagnostic information needed. The multiple number of images produced provides a series of detailed views of tissue density and depth used to determine the presence, location, and extent of pathology; to identify and locate lesions for guidance of percutaneous fine-needle biopsies; to determine the presence of foreign bodies and other abnormalities; and to evaluate the effectiveness of treatments administered to eliminate or ameliorate disease states.

BODY SCANNING (CT, CAT, CTT)

Body scanning is a CT study performed to assist in diagnosing abnormalities in any part of the body other than the head, such as the neck, chest, abdomen, pelvis, spine, and extremities. It can reveal malignant and benign masses; lymph node enlargement or pathology; and abnormal fluid, blood, or fat accumulation in organs or cavities. A contrast medium is administered by mouth, by injection (intravenously [IV]), or by enema, depending on the need for initial or additional views to ensure clear images of specific organs (see the specific body region scans that follow).[6]

Scanning provides an immediate image of all internal parts on a screen as the machine rotates around the body. All or selected images can be photographed and preserved for future viewing. The images define the contours of organs and display contrast differences as the scanning is performed in various planes to produce three-dimensional pictures on a monitor screen.

Reference Values

Normal size and contour of body structures and organs; no pathology such as masses or abnormal accumulation of body fluids or substances

Interfering Factors

➤ Inability of client to remain still during the procedure
➤ Metallic objects within the examination field, such as watches or jewelry
➤ Feces, barium, or gas in the gastrointestinal tract

Indications for Body Scanning (CT, CAT, CTT)

➤ Diagnosing benign and malignant tumors and metastasis to other organs such as bone or liver as revealed by alterations in normal densities in the various body tissues; that is, reduced density is darker and increased density is lighter
➤ Diagnosing cysts or nodules in organs, such as in liver cirrhosis, pancreatic pseudocyst, or renal cystic disease, revealed by water density in the presence of cysts
➤ Determining enlargement of lymph nodes and retroperitoneal lymphadenopathy in diagnosing lymphoma
➤ Detecting aortic or abdominal aneurysms
➤ Detecting infections and inflammatory processes, that is, appendicitis, diverticulosis, pancreatitis, pneumonitis, inflammatory nodules, abscess of the liver or other soft tissue
➤ Assessing mediastinum, hilum, and pleura of the chest to assist in early diagnosis of conditions affecting these areas
➤ Detecting accumulation of fluid or blood, such as in ascites, fatty liver, pleural effusion, or hemorrhage
➤ Determining hepatobiliary duct dilation and determining whether obstruction is present
➤ Determining obstruction of the renal system in the presence of calculi
➤ Diagnosing congenital anomalies of the renal and gastrointestinal systems
➤ Measuring bone density in menopausal women for estrogen replacement in osteoporosis revealed by an increased density based on calcium levels
➤ Verifying the precise location of a lesion for a CT-guided fine-needle biopsy of a mass to eliminate the need for a surgical procedure to obtain a specimen
➤ Evaluating the effect of medical or surgical interventions on any pathology

Contraindications

➤ Pregnancy, unless the benefits of performing the study greatly outweigh the risks to the fetus
➤ Allergy to iodine, if an iodinated contrast medium is to be used
➤ Extreme obesity

➤ Unstable medical status, including vital signs, vomiting, increased peristalsis

➤ Extreme claustrophobic response that prevents client from remaining still while enclosed in the scanner, unless medications are given before the study

Nursing Care Before the Procedure

Explain to the client:

➤ That the procedure requires from 45 minutes to 2 hours, depending on the extent of the imaging and whether a contrast medium is used

➤ That foods and fluids are withheld for 4 hours before the procedure if a contrast medium is used; otherwise there are no food or fluid restrictions

➤ That medications can be continued, insulin can be administered, diet can be followed, and study scheduled around this need

➤ That clothing, including belts, jewelry, and all metallic objects, are removed and a hospital gown without snaps or other metallic closures will be worn

➤ That a contrast medium can be given IV or orally before the study if better visualization of an area is desired

➤ That, if a contrast medium is given, nausea, flushing, and sweating experienced after administration should be reported to the physician

➤ That the client is encircled by the scanning camera during the study while the pictures are taken and that claustrophobia is not uncommon

➤ That the only discomfort experienced is undergoing the venipuncture to administer the contrast medium and lying in one position on the hard table for a long period

Prepare for the procedure:

➤ Administer ordered medications for sedation and anxiety, such as diazepam (Valium) for claustrophobia, steroids, or antihistamines such as diphenhydramine (Benadryl) or prednisone (Deltasone) for known allergies to the contrast medium before the study.

➤ Have the client void.

➤ If the procedure is closed, known claustrophobia should be reported to the physician before the study.

The Procedure

The client is placed in a supine position on a flat table within the scanning apparatus after IV or oral administration of a contrast medium, if this position is appropriate for the views to be obtained. The client is requested to remain very still because movement results in blurring of the picture. A series of images are taken while the table is manipulated and scanning of various levels of the body is performed. Instructions to hold the breath during the scanning are given by the technician via an intercommunication system. In some instances, scanning is performed and the contrast medium administered with further scanning taking place to enhance visualization of specific areas. The client is advised to report nausea after the administration of contrast medium and is instructed to take deep breaths if nausea occurs. An emesis basin can be made available if needed.

As the scanning takes place, images are immediately portrayed on the screen and recorded on permanent film. Tissue density and composition of the organs are demonstrated in white, black, or gray shades and interpreted by the radiologist.

If the study is being performed on an infant, a child under 3 years of age, or an uncooperative adult, sedation can be given to ensure immobilization. Children and adults can usually be taught the importance of remaining very still, and, if claustrophobia is present, an antianxiety agent can be administered. Diversional interventions, such as music via earphones, have been used to allay anxiety in adults.

Nursing Care After the Procedure

➤ Care and assessment after the procedure include the return of clothing and personal items. Advise the client to resume food intake and to increase fluid intake to eliminate the contrast medium, if one was used.

➤ *Adverse reaction to contrast medium:* Note and report nausea, skin rash, sweating, palpitations, respiratory changes, and changes in vital signs. Administer ordered antihistamines if needed. Have resuscitation equipment on hand.

➤ *Phlebitis:* Note and report redness and swelling at the IV site. Apply ordered warm compress to site and elevate arm.

HEAD AND INTRACRANIAL SCANNING

Head and intracranial or brain scanning is a CT study performed to assist in diagnosing abnormalities of brain tissue and blood circulation and their effects, such as tumors, infarctions, aneurysms, infections and inflammations, congenital brain anomalies, and injury or trauma to the head and orbital structures. The procedure provides a faster and safer diagnosis of brain pathology for adults and children because it eliminates the need for more invasive studies such as cerebral angiography and pneumoencephalography. It also provides diagnostic information that once could be obtained only by craniotomy. An iodinated contrast medium, possibly iothalamate meglumine, can be administered IV for image enhancement when tumor or other pathology causing the destruction of the blood-brain barrier is suspected.[7] The circulating iodine leaks through the damaged barrier, the solid portion of the tumor is visualized, and the size and extent of the mass are defined.

The CT scanning provides images of internal structures of the head, brain tissues, and the cerebrospinal fluid (CSF) taken from the top of the head looking downward. The density and composition calculations made by the computer are different for different types of tissue. Differences in tumor from normal soft tissue, clotted blood from normal blood, and spaces containing air from those containing CSF are identified. Detailed images are portrayed on a screen, photographed, and interpreted for abnormalities in the shape, size, position, symmetry, and tissue densities of intracranial structures. Other studies conducted by CT scanning of the head are for the purpose of detecting abnormalities involving the eye, ear, and pituitary gland. Various planes are used in the scanning process for the specific tissues or organs to be viewed.[8]

Reference Values

Normal size, shape, and position of intracranial contents; no tumor, hemorrhage, aneurysm, infarction, infection, ventricular or tissue displacement, enlargement, or congenital abnormalities

Interfering Factors

➤ Inability of client to maintain the head in an immobilized position during the procedure

➤ Metal objects such as jewelry, hairpins or barrette, dentures, or hearing aid within the examination field

Indications for Head and Intracranial Scanning

➤ Early diagnosis of multiple sclerosis revealed by detection of sclerotic plaques as small as 3 to 4 mm in diameter

➤ Determination of the cause of increased intracranial pressure (ICP)

➤ Diagnosis of intracranial benign and malignant tumors; diagnosis of cyst formation revealed by changes in tissue densities, such as white with increased density and darker areas with decreased density

➤ Determination of the size and location of a lesion causing a stroke, such as infarct or hemorrhage

➤ Detection of ventricular enlargement or displacement by CSF increases and type of hemorrhage in infants and children experiencing signs and symptoms of intracranial trauma or congenital conditions such as hydrocephalus and arteriovenous (A-V) malformations

➤ Differentiation between cerebral infarction and hemorrhage

➤ Detection of the presence of brain infection or inflammatory condition such as abscess or necrosis revealed by decreased density

➤ Differentiation among hematoma locations after trauma, such as subdural, epidural, and cerebral, and determination of the extent of edema resulting from injury, revealed by higher densities of blood compared with normal tissue

➤ Evaluation of the effectiveness of treatment and the course of a disease

➤ Diagnosis of abnormalities of the optic nerve, detection of foreign body in the eye, evaluation of orbital bone fracture or destruction, and determination of the cause of unilateral exophthalmos[9]

➤ Diagnosis of abnormalities of the middle ear ossicles and auditory nerve

Contraindications

➤ Pregnancy, unless the benefits of performing the study greatly outweigh the risks to the fetus

➤ Allergy to iodine, if a contrast medium is to be used

➤ Extreme claustrophobia that prevents the client from lying still, unless medications are given before the study

➤ Unstable medical status, that is, vital signs or dehydration

Nursing Care Before the Procedure

Client teaching and physical preparation are the same as for any CT scanning study (see p. 803).

➤ Inform the client that the head is placed in a stabilized holder with the face uncovered and that the holder is then placed in a frame that revolves around the head while the pictures are taken.

➤ Inform the client that the study takes 30 minutes to 1 hour.

➤ Obtain baseline vital signs and neurological checks for later comparisons.

> Obtain a history and assessment of the neurological system, known or suspected neurological disorders, and results of associated laboratory tests and other diagnostic procedures.

The Procedure

The client is placed on a flat table in a supine position with the head on an apparatus that fits into a frame that revolves around the head in a 180-degree arc from one side to the other. Imaging is performed at each degree during this rotation. Additional images can be taken in other planes as the scanner is moved to different positions.[10] The face is left exposed during the imaging to allow the client to see at all times. The client is requested to lie very still during the procedure because movement causes blurring of the pictures. An IV administration of an iodinated contrast medium can be given before the imaging or the images can be taken first and then the medium injected to enhance any unusual findings. The client is advised of the possibility of nausea and feeling of warmth after the injection and is instructed to take deep, slow breaths if nausea occurs. An emesis basin should be made available, if it is needed. All images are portrayed on the screen immediately for viewing and photographs are made of selected views for future use.

If the study is being performed on an infant, a child under 3 years of age, or an uncooperative adult, sedation can be given to ensure immobilization. Most children and adults can be taught and relied on to lie still during the scanning. An antianxiety agent can be administered if claustrophobia is present.

Nursing Care After the Procedure

Care and assessment after the procedure are the same as for any CT scan study (see p. 804).

> Perform vital signs and neurological checks and compare with baselines if indicated.

NECK AND SPINAL SCANNING

Neck and spinal CT scanning is a study performed to assist in diagnosing abnormalities of these areas and resulting consequences, such as structural and degenerative changes or malformations, tumors, vascular malformations, and congenital spinal malformations. The procedure provides detailed cross-sectional images of selected areas of the cervical, thoracic, or lumbar spine suspected of lesions or abnormalities. Varying planes are used in the scanning process to produce images of a specific location or the entire spinal column and its contents.

Reference Values

Normal tissues and structures of the spinal column and contents; no herniated disks, tumors, degenerative disease, or stenosis

Interfering Factors

> Inability of client to remain still during the procedure
> Metallic objects such as jewelry within the examination field
> Barium, feces, or gas in the lower gastrointestinal (LGI) tract, if lumbar spine is to be imaged

Indications for Neck and Spinal Scanning

➤ Diagnosing benign, primary, and metastatic tumors of the spine and their location, revealed by altered density in the areas of pathology as differentiated normal tissue densities

➤ Detecting the presence and location of herniated disks, usually in the cervical or lumbar spine, with unilateral or bilateral nerve root compression

➤ Diagnosing or evaluating stenosis of the lumbar spine with hypertrophy, causing compression of the cord as the space within the column is decreased

➤ Detecting cervical spondylosis with cord compression, caused by structural changes resulting from bone hypertrophy

➤ Diagnosing fluid-filled cysts revealed by increased density

➤ Detecting vascular malformations in adults and congenital spinal malformations, that is, meningocele, myelocele, or myelomeningocele, in infants[11]

➤ Monitoring the effectiveness of therapeutic regimen and spinal surgical procedure

Contraindications

➤ Pregnancy, unless the benefits of performing the study greatly outweigh the risks to the fetus

➤ Allergy to iodine, if an iodinated contrast medium is to be used

➤ Extreme obesity

➤ Extreme claustrophobic response that prevents the client from remaining still during the procedure, unless medications are given before the study

Nursing Care Before the Procedure

Client teaching and physical preparation are the same as for head and intracranial CT scanning study (see pp. 805 to 806).

➤ Inform the client about a lumbar puncture if an air CT is to be performed (see Chap. 8).

The Procedure

The client is placed in a supine position on a flat table, which is then placed into the scanner, which covers the whole body except for the head. The scanner revolves around the client's body at different angles, and images are portrayed on the screen. Selected images are photographed for future viewing. The client is requested to lie very still during the scanning procedure to prevent blurring of the pictures. An IV administration of an iodinated contrast medium can be given before the study or after the initial imaging to further enhance any unusual findings and to allow further accentuation of the spinal vasculature and tissue. The table is removed from the scanner to administer the contrast medium to the client; the table is then returned to the scanner 30 minutes after the client's IV line has been established. The client is advised of the possibility of nausea and feeling of warmth after the injection of the contrast medium and is instructed to take deep, slow breaths if nausea occurs.

If an air CT is to be performed, a lumbar puncture is made and a small amount of CSF fluid is replaced with air; the table is returned to the scanner for client imaging. This procedure provides enhanced visualization of the area be-

tween the subarachnoid space and surrounding tissue. The IV injection of an iodinated contrast medium enhances visualization of very slight differences in tissue density, providing more accurate diagnostic information. Images are portrayed according to density, with the bones or vertebrae appearing as white,
CSF as black, and soft tissue as shades of gray.[12]

As with other CT scans of an infant, child, or uncooperative adult, sedation can be given before the procedure to ensure immobilization. An antianxiety
agent can also be given to those clients who suffer from claustrophobia.

Nursing Care After the Procedure

Care and assessment after the procedure are the same as for any CT scan study
(see p. 803).

➤ Perform vital signs and neurological checks and compare with baselines, if
   indicated.
➤ Maintain the client in a prone or supine position for 4 to 8 hours, and assess
   the site for leakage if a lumbar puncture has been performed.
➤ *Lumbar puncture:* Note and report changes in neurological status, increase
   in blood pressure or temperature, sensory changes in extremities (tingling,
   numbness), irritability, or headache. Administer analgesic for headache.
   Perform neurological checks every 2 to 4 hours for possible infection or
   brain or spinal cord damage.

THORACIC SCANNING

Thoracic or chest scanning is a CT study performed to assist in diagnosing abnormalities of the heart chambers and great vessels, lungs, and lymph nodes;
examples are masses, aneurysms, lymphoma with mediastinal lymph node involvement, inflammation and infection, hiatal hernia, and pleural effusion. A
newer, rapid method of CT scanning called *cine scan* can take moving images
of the heart.[13] The study provides a cross-sectional view of the chest and its
contents and has the ability to produce a more detailed display of tissues than
do the conventional x-ray procedures. As different tissues absorb different
amounts of radiation from the x-rays, density differences of the tissue type are
revealed, based on a predetermined value that is converted by the computer into
black, white, or gray shades. The sections of the anatomic area are photographed and displayed on a screen for viewing.

Reference Values

Normal size, position, and shape of chest organ tissue and structures; no tumors, cysts, infection or inflammation, aneurysm, enlarged lymph nodes, or
fluid accumulation

Interfering Factors

➤ Inability of client to remain still during the procedure
➤ Metal objects such as jewelry within the examination field

Indications for Thoracic Scanning

➤ Diagnosing pulmonary, esophageal, or mediastinal tumors (primary and
   metastatic) revealed by the differences in tissue densities that can go
   undetected in routine studies because of small size

➤ Diagnosing a benign tumor, such as a granuloma, and differentiating it from a malignant tumor, revealed by a sharply defined contour as opposed to an irregular edge in malignant lesions

➤ Detecting mediastinal and hilar lymphadenopathy in the diagnosis of lymphoma, especially Hodgkin's disease

➤ Differentiating tumors or masses from coin-sized calcified lesions such as those found in tuberculosis

➤ Detecting tumor extension of a neck mass to the thoracic area

➤ Detecting bronchial abnormalities such as stenosis, dilation, or tumor

➤ Detecting aortic aneurysm and differentiating it from tumors near the aorta

➤ Determining infectious or inflammatory processes such as abscess, nodules, or pneumonitis

➤ Determining fluid, blood, or fat accumulation in tissues, vessels, or pleuritic space

➤ Evaluating cardiac chambers and pulmonary vessels

➤ Monitoring or evaluating effectiveness of a medical or surgical therapeutic regimen

Contraindications

➤ Pregnancy, unless the benefits of performing the study greatly outweigh the risks to the fetus

➤ Allergy to iodine, if an iodinated contrast medium is to be used

➤ Extreme obesity

➤ Unstable medical status, that is, vital signs or dehydration

➤ Extreme claustrophobic response that prevents the client from remaining still during the procedure, unless medications are given before the study

Nursing Care Before the Procedure

Client teaching and physical preparation are the same as for any CT scanning study (see p. 803).

➤ Inform the client that the study takes about 30 minutes to 1 hour.

➤ Obtain a history that includes cardiac and pulmonary assessment findings, known or suspected pulmonary conditions, and results of associated laboratory tests and diagnostic procedures.

The Procedure

The procedure is the same as for a body CT scanning study. The scanner takes images at different levels and angles of the chest region, from the neck to the waist instead of the whole body (see p. 803). Contrast-enhanced studies are performed by the IV administration of an iodinated contrast medium for blood vessel evaluation or by oral administration of a contrast medium for esophageal evaluation.[14]

Nursing Care After the Procedure

Care and assessment after the procedure are the same as for any CT scan study (see p. 804).

➤ Monitor vital signs if the client has an acute or chronic cardiac or pulmonary condition.

ABDOMINAL SCANNING

Abdominal scanning is a CT study performed to assist in diagnosing abnormalities of the liver, spleen, pancreas, large and small bowel, biliary system, kidneys, adrenals, aorta, and lymph nodes. Identifiable pathology includes tumors, cysts, inflammation and infection, trauma and injury, aneurysm, hemorrhage, calculi, duct or lymph node enlargement, congenital anomalies, and fluid accumulation in the abdominal cavity. As in other CT studies, organ contour and contrast differences are displayed by the variations in densities of soft tissue based on their composition.

Reference Values

Normal size and contour of abdominal structures and organs; no pathology such as masses, inflammation or infection, duct dilation or obstruction, bleeding, congenital abnormalities, or accumulations of fluids or blood in body organs or cavities

Interfering Factors

➤ Inability of client to remain still during the procedure
➤ Metal objects such as jewelry and watches within the examination field
➤ Feces, gas, or barium in the gastrointestinal tract

Indications for Abdominal Scanning

➤ Diagnosing and locating benign and malignant tumors and metastasis to other organs, that is, intrahepatic, pancreatic, gallbladder, kidneys, spleen, adrenal glands, and small and large bowel as revealed by changes in tissue density, depending on the organ
➤ Determining pancreatic abnormalities such as pancreatitis, pseudocysts, bleeding, or abscess revealed by enlargement, changes in shape, and decreased tissue density
➤ Detecting dilatation or obstruction, or both, of the bile or pancreatic ducts with or without calcification or gallstones to differentiate between obstructive and nonobstructive jaundice
➤ Diagnosing liver abnormalities such as hepatic abscess, intrahepatic hematomas, cysts, cirrhosis with ascites, or fatty liver as revealed by an increased density compared with the surrounding organs
➤ Diagnosing spleen abnormalities such as tumor, venous thrombosis, or trauma that results in hematoma, laceration, or rupture
➤ Evaluating the retroperitoneum for tumor or infections, revealed by enlarged lymph nodes of more than 2 cm, or evaluating previously diagnosed lymphadenopathy[15]
➤ Determining the presence and type of adrenal tumor, that is, benign adenoma, malignancy, or pheochromocytoma
➤ Detecting bleeding or hyperplasia of the adrenal glands
➤ Diagnosing kidney pathology and congenital anomaly, that is, tumor, cysts, polycystic disease, calculi and obstructions, horseshoe kidney, absence of one kidney, or kidney displacement
➤ Determining the spread of a tumor or the invasion of nearby retroperitoneal organs

➤ Detecting infectious or inflammatory conditions of the bowel and mesentery, that is, appendicitis, diverticulitis, or Crohn's disease

➤ Detecting abdominal aortic aneurysm and evaluating the amount of dilation and presence of intramural thrombi

➤ Defining and locating a lesion site for fine-needle biopsy and verifying that the needle is in the proper position

➤ Evaluating the effectiveness of the medical or surgical regimen

Contraindications

➤ Contraindications are the same as for thoracic scanning study (see p. 809).

Nursing Care Before the Procedure

Client teaching and physical preparation are the same as for any CT scanning study (see p. 803).

➤ Inform the client that it takes an additional 30 minutes to complete each abdominal and retroperitoneal study.

➤ Obtain a history that includes gastrointestinal tract, hepatobiliary, and renal assessment findings; known or suspected conditions; and results of associated laboratory tests and diagnostic procedures.

The Procedure

The procedure is the same as for body CT scanning. The scanner is directed at the abdominal region from the waist to the pelvis instead of at the whole body (see p. 803). Anatomic image enhancement can be obtained by the administration of an oral contrast medium for small- and large-bowel imaging and an IV administration of iodinated contrast medium for the other abdominal and retroperitoneal organs.

Nursing Care After the Procedure

Care and assessment after the procedure are the same as for any CT scan study (see p. 804).

➤ Monitor vital signs and intake and output (I&O) if the client has a renal disorder.

➤ *Impaired renal function:* Note and report change in urinary output or hypertension after iodinated contrast medium administration. Promote adequate fluid intake before the study.

PELVIC SCANNING

Pelvic scanning is a CT study performed to assist in diagnosing abnormalities of the uterus, fallopian tubes, ovaries, rectum, prostate, urinary bladder, and lymph nodes. Pathology of these organs that can be identified are tumors, cysts, infections and inflammations, and hypertrophy. CT of the pelvis is performed primarily to identify urinary bladder pathology, because the other pelvic organs can effectively be studied by ultrasonography and other procedures. The CT scan of the pelvic organs, however, is used after ultrasonography to determine the extent of the pathology once it has been identified. The study is based on the same principles of anatomic identification of organs as the abdominal CT scan and also includes the use of contrast enhancement for a more detailed imaging of the organs (see "Abdominal Scanning").

Reference Values

Normal size and shape of pelvic organ tissue and structures; no tumors, cysts, infections, or lymph node pathology

Interfering Factors

➤ Inability of client to remain still during the procedure
➤ Metal objects such as jewelry within the examination field
➤ Barium, feces, or gas in the LGI tract

Indications for Pelvic Scanning

➤ Detecting the extent of tumors, cysts, abscess, or other abnormalities of the ovaries, fallopian tubes, and uterus after a diagnosis has been obtained by other studies such as ultrasonography or radiography
➤ Determining prostate hypertrophy or tumors revealed by enlargement of glandular tissue
➤ Determining the stage of urinary bladder malignant tumor revealed by its invasion through the bladder wall and extension to pelvic organs and lymph nodes
➤ Monitoring effectiveness of the medical or surgical regimen

Contraindications

Contraindications are the same as for thoracic scan (see p. 809).

Nursing Care Before the Procedure

Client teaching and physical preparation are the same as for any CT scan study (see p. 803).
➤ Inform the client of the possibility of barium enema administration before the study.
➤ Inform female clients that a vaginal tampon will be inserted.
➤ Inform the client that the procedure takes from 30 minutes to 1 hour.
➤ Obtain a history that includes assessment of the reproductive system of male and female clients, known and suspected disorders, and results of associated laboratory tests and diagnostic procedures.

The Procedure

The procedure is the same as for body CT scanning. The scanner takes images of the pelvic region instead of the whole body. In addition to IV administration of an iodinated contrast medium, a barium contrast medium enema can be given before the study. A vaginal tampon is inserted immediately before the study in female clients.[16]

Nursing Care After the Procedure

Care and assessment after the procedure are the same as for any CT scan study (see p. 804).

MAGNETIC RESONANCE IMAGING (MRI, NMR)

Magnetic resonance imaging (MRI, NMR) scanning studies are imaging procedures of body parts. The studies are performed to view characteristics and structures of organs, primarily the heart, brain, bones and joints, spinal cord, blood vessels, and soft tissue. MRIs are performed after or in place of CT. Although almost any organ can be imaged, MRI is used most commonly to evaluate the nervous and musculoskeletal systems. Of the MRI procedures performed today, 40 percent are of the head, 30 percent are of the back, 20 percent are of the joints, and 10 percent are of the rest of the body.[17] The MRI is performed to determine specific organ pathology (brain, liver) or to diagnose a specific condition (multiple sclerosis). Some consider the procedure overused because it provides multiple, detailed views without radiation risk.

Different measurements are made in MRI, depending on the density of soft tissues; the prolonged relaxation times of certain organs such as brain, liver, muscle, and spinal cord; the blood flow and perfusion rates in blood vessels; and the results of spectroscopy to obtain information about chemical constituents and metabolic changes.[18] A new paramagnetic contrast medium has been developed for MRI called gadopentetate dimeglumine (Magnevist), which can be administered IV to enhance contrast differences between normal and abnormal organ tissues.[19] MRI imaging is most useful for tissue density and blood-flow scanning abnormalities for specific organ or disease diagnoses; however, it is believed that its use will be expanded to include more diagnostic information about more organs, sports injuries, and ailments common to the aging population. At this time, its use is determined by cost-benefit considerations rather than by risk considerations.

Body Magnetic Resonance Imaging (MRI, NMR)

Body magnetic resonance imaging (MRI, NMR) scanning is a study performed to assist in diagnosing abnormalities in any region of the body other than the head, that is, chest, abdomen, spinal cord, pelvis, and extremities. It can reveal tumors and other soft tissue pathology; bone, joint, and surrounding tissue disorders; vascular abnormalities (congenital and noncongenital); and infections. A special paramagnetic contrast medium can be administered IV to enhance differences between normal and abnormal tissues, that is, lesions as opposed to normal parenchyma.

Scanning provides images based on the water content of the body, after computer analysis of the data provided by the scanning apparatus. The pictures are projected onto a screen, and all or selected images can be taped for later viewing. Blood-flow scanning data are computed in milliliters per minute, pictures are projected onto a screen, and a printout is made for evaluation. Information for imaging and blood flow studies is permanently recorded and stored for future diagnostic reference.

Reference Values

Normal anatomic structures and soft tissue density, biochemical constituents of body tissues, and flow and perfusion rates; no pathology such as masses, lesions, infarcts, hemorrhage, infections, malformations, or metabolic abnormalities

Interfering Factors

➤ Inability of client to remain still during the procedure
➤ Metallic objects within the examination field that cause artifacts in the image, such as jewelry; watches; infusion pumps; metallic or other implants such as heart valves, cochlear or orthopedic prostheses, rods or screws, or dentures; hairpins or hair clips; pacemaker; or ferromagnetic aneurysm clips

Indications for Body Magnetic Resonance Imaging (MRI, NMR)

➤ Diagnosis of renal diseases, that is, hydronephrosis, glomerulonephritis, acute tubular necrosis, renal vein thrombosis, abscesses, and focal or diffuse pyelonephritis
➤ Differentiation between renal cysts and lymphocele
➤ Determination of adrenal hemorrhage revealed by blood characteristics and calcification of the gland
➤ Acute rejection of kidney transplant
➤ Detection of prostate malignancy and extension of the tumor with local staging preoperatively
➤ Evaluation of prostate gland for postbiopsy complications
➤ Evaluation of seminal vesicle abnormalities, such as hypoplastic, nonsecreting, atrophic, and testicular metabolism
➤ Localization of leiomyomas and other tumors of the uterus preoperatively
➤ Detection of A-V malformations of the vascular tree and organs such as the spinal cord
➤ Detection and determination of the stage of malignant tumors of the urinary bladder wall
➤ Diagnosis of benign, primary, and metastatic tumors in any body organ
➤ Diagnosis of diffuse bone marrow disease such as leukemia, polycythemia, and bone marrow changes in Gaucher's disease
➤ Detection of spinal cord lesions, tumors, and intramedullary A-V abnormalities
➤ Viewing of breast implant for separation, leakage, and other abnormalities
➤ Detection of abnormalities of the vessels and blood flow of the extremities, that is, thrombus, embolism, or atherosclerosis
➤ Determination of blood flow in differentiating between ischemia and infarction of vessels
➤ Determination of chemical constituent changes by spectroscopy in the diagnosis of malignancies, ischemia, and infarction of organs and in the diagnosis of metabolic disorders
➤ Evaluation of the effects of chemotherapy and radiation therapy on tumors

Contraindications

➤ Pregnancy, unless the benefits of performing the study greatly outweigh the possible risks to the fetus
➤ Extreme obesity
➤ Unstable medical status, including confusion or combative demeanor, monitoring of vital signs, use of cardiopulmonary or other monitoring or assistive life-support equipment, and use of neurological or musculoskeletal stimulators

➤ Extreme claustrophobic response that prevents the client from remaining still while enclosed in the scanner, unless medications are given before the study

➤ Presence of cardiac pacemaker that can be deactivated by MRI, metallic clips or prostheses, or heart valves that can be displaced and cause injury to the client during MRI

Nursing Care Before the Procedure

Explain to the client:

➤ That the procedure requires 30 to 90 minutes, depending on the region to be examined

➤ That alcohol, caffeine-containing beverages, and smoking are restricted for at least 2 hours and that food is withheld for at least 1 hour before the procedure, especially if blood-flow studies are being performed

➤ That the usual medication regimen can be continued except for those medications containing iron, as they will interfere with imaging

➤ That clothing, jewelry, and all metallic objects including credit cards are removed and that a hospital gown without snaps or other metallic closures will be supplied

➤ That a special contrast medium may be given IV before the study to enhance tissue imaging

➤ That the client is placed into the scanner and that a steady clanging noise is heard during the procedure; that earplugs are available, if desired, to block out the noise

➤ That claustrophobia is not uncommon and that an antianxiety medication can be administered to allay this feeling; if the client is a child, a sedative can be given to ensure immobilization during the study unless blood-flow studies are to be performed or if the caregiver can talk or read to the child during the procedure

➤ That there is no discomfort during the procedure except for a venipuncture if a contrast medium is administered

Prepare for the procedure:

➤ Ensure that dietary, fluid, and other restrictions have been followed.

➤ Obtain a history of allergies or sensitivities to contrast media, last menstrual period to ascertain possible pregnancy, and known or suspected pathology.

➤ Inquire about the presence of devices or prostheses in any part of the body, results of laboratory tests and diagnostic procedures, and presence of claustrophobia.

➤ Provide a hospital gown and ensure that all metallic objects have been removed from the client and safely stored with clothing.

➤ Administer ordered medications for anxiety or sedation, or both, and known sensitivity to iodine (antihistamine or steroid).

➤ Have client void.

The Procedure

The client is placed on a narrow, flat table in a supine position. The table is placed into a cylindrical structure (the scanner) in a special room to ensure that imaging can be performed without outside interference from radio signals. The client is requested to lie very still throughout the entire procedure. The face remains uncovered to allow the client to see out. Varying radio energy waves are directed at the area(s) to be imaged. Local surface antennae are attached to specific areas if improved resolution is desired.[20] If a contrast medium is used for the study, a specially prepared MRI material is administered IV before the procedure. The client is advised that he or she can speak to the technician during the study if desired. The client is also advised to keep the eyes closed to promote relaxation and prevent a closed-in feeling common to those undergoing this procedure. If nausea is experienced because of claustrophobia, the client is told to take deep breaths.

If the study is performed on a child, sedation can be given or the caregiver can read or talk to the child, as there is no radiation risk involved in this procedure. If necessary, judicious use of soft restraints can be used to immobilize parts of the body.

Nursing Care After the Procedure

➤ Care and assessment after the procedure include returning the client's clothing and personal items removed for the study.

➤ Advise the client to resume usual food, fluid, and medication intake, if applicable.

➤ *Phlebitis:* Note and report redness and swelling at the IV site. Apply ordered warm compress to site and elevate arm.

ANGIOGRAPHY MAGNETIC RESONANCE IMAGING (MRI)

Angiography magnetic resonance imaging (MRI) scanning is a study performed to assist in diagnosing abnormalities of the vascular system. It produces images like those obtained with conventional angiography without the use of a contrast medium. It is used to provide quantitative, functional, and morphologic views of the large and peripheral blood vessels, as well as blood flow and characteristics. Areas included in the study are the vasculature (arteries or veins, or both) of the neck, thorax, abdomen, extremities, and intracranial contents. Various methods are used, depending on the type of information needed to make a diagnosis, that is, echo-planar flow imaging, real-time imaging, phase-sensitive flow imaging, time-of-flight flow imaging, fast imaging, and diffusion and perfusion imaging.

Reference Values

Normal blood flow, diffusion and perfusion rate, and blood vessel anatomic structure; no vascular malformations, aneurysms, thrombosis, vascular stenosis or obstruction, hemorrhage, embolus, or arteriosclerosis

Interfering Factors

➤ Inability of client to remain still during the procedure

➤ Metal objects within the examination field, such as jewelry, infusion pumps, metallic or other implants or prostheses, hairpins or hair clips of any kind, pacemaker, orthopedic prostheses, rods or screws, dentures, or heart valve replacement, which cause artifacts in the image

Indications for Angiography Magnetic Resonance Imaging (MRI)

➤ Detecting cranial blood vessel and blood-flow abnormalities, that is, vascular malformations, aneurysms, thrombosis and occlusion, or hemorrhage

➤ Determining arteriosclerotic plaque and stenosis of the carotid arteries and evaluating endarterectomy postoperatively

➤ Detecting thoracic aortic aneurysm and diagnosing aortic dissection

➤ Diagnosing pulmonary artery and vein abnormalities such as emboli and anatomic malformations

➤ Detecting coronary occlusion and evaluating bypass grafts and the angioplasty procedure postoperatively

➤ Determining lower extremity blood vessel and blood-flow abnormalities, that is, atherosclerosis, thrombus, embolus, or vascular malformations

➤ Determining abnormal venous blood flow in the abdomen and pelvis such as that found in thrombosis or occlusion

Contraindications

➤ Contraindications are the same as for any MRI scanning study (see pp. 814 to 815).

Nursing Care Before the Procedure

Client teaching and physical preparation are the same as for any MRI scanning study (see p. 815).

➤ Obtain a history that includes known and suspected vascular disorders and assessment findings related to this system and results of associated laboratory tests and diagnostic procedures, including surgical interventions.

The Procedure

The procedure is the same as for any MRI scanning study except that the scanner is directed at the area suspected of an abnormality (see pp. 815 to 816). If an extremity is to be studied, it is placed on the table after sites are marked for examination and stored in the computer. The limb is moved in and out of the scanner after examination of the ankle, knee, and hip, with fingertips, wrist, and elbow studies afterward, if all extremities are to be scanned. A blood vessel or complete extremity can be scanned and flow data rate obtained in milliliters per minute for each 100 cm of tissue.[21] Measurement of limb circumference is obtained during the study to reconcile limb size with blood-flow measurement.

Nursing Care After the Procedure

Care and assessment after the procedure are the same as for any MRI scan study (see p. 816).

ABDOMINAL MAGNETIC RESONANCE IMAGING (MRI)

Abdominal magnetic resonance imaging (MRI) scanning is a study performed to assist in diagnosing abnormalities of the abdominal and pelvic organs. CT is considered to be superior to MRI in abdominal imaging, except in the assessment of liver pathology, because it can distinguish organs from one another. It is performed alone or as part of a body MRI scan to identify tumor metastasis and other lesions or soft tissue abnormalities. Contrast enhancement for liver, spleen, pancreas, stomach, and proximal duodenum have been developed and used in MRI imaging of these abdominal organs. As in other MRI studies, abdominal scans provide cross-sectional images in the transverse, sagittal, and coronal planes without any interference from bone tissue. Images are portrayed on a screen and taped for viewing and analysis.

Reference Values

Normal anatomic structures, soft tissue density, and biochemical constituents of body tissues; no pathology such as masses, lesions, infections, or inflammations of abdominal organs

Interfering Factors

➤ Interfering factors are the same as for any MRI scanning study (see p. 814)
➤ Chest and abdominal movements during respiration will impair clear imaging

Indications for Abdominal Magnetic Resonance Imaging (MRI)

➤ Determining vascular complications of pancreatitis, such as venous thrombosis or pseudoaneurysm
➤ Diagnosing chronic pancreatitis and pancreatic malignancy, and determining stage of disease when CT information is insufficient to produce a satisfactory conclusion
➤ Diagnosing primary or metastatic malignant tumors of the liver
➤ Detecting liver cysts and cavernous hemangiomas and differentiating them from malignant tumors
➤ Diagnosing hepatic amebic abscess in combination with CT scanning
➤ Evaluating effectiveness of medical and surgical interventions and course of a disease

Contraindications

➤ Contraindications are the same as for any MRI scan study (see pp. 814 to 815).

Nursing Care Before the Procedure

Client teaching and physical preparation are the same as for any MRI scanning study (see p. 815).
➤ Inform the client about the use of paramagnetic contrast media and other medications that enhance the imaging of specific abdominal organs by reducing peristalsis.
➤ Obtain a history that includes assessment findings about the liver, pancreas, and LGI tract and known or suspected disorders, previous tests, diagnostic procedures, and medical and surgical interventions associated with these organs.

The Procedure

The procedure is the same as for any MRI scan except that the scanner is directed at the abdominal organs to be examined (see pp. 815 to 816). A special paramagnetic contrast medium such as gadopentate dimeglumine or a super-paramagnetic medium such as ferrite iron oxide used for spleen, liver, and pancreas imaging is administered IV before the procedure. Glucagon can be administered to improve visualization of the pancreas by removing artifacts resulting from stomach and bowel peristalsis. Ferric ammonium citrate (Geritol) and gadopentate dimeglumine are the media used for stomach and bowel imaging to decrease the lumen signal intensity resulting from bowel peristalsis.[22]

Nursing Care After the Procedure

Care and assessment after the procedure are the same as for any MRI scan study (see p. 816).

HEAD AND INTRACRANIAL MAGNETIC RESONANCE IMAGING (MRI)

Head and intracranial magnetic resonance imaging (MRI) scanning is a study performed to assist in diagnosing abnormalities of the brain and face. It can reveal tumors and other soft tissue lesions, infarctions, aneurysms, hematomas, nerve demyelination, A-V malformations, and other vessel pathology such as atherosclerosis. The study provides cross-sectional images in multiple planes for viewing as they are projected onto a screen. Fluid appears as gray and blood appears dark on the screen. Tissue changes are revealed by measurements of density and relaxation time changes.

Reference Values

Normal anatomic structures; soft tissue density; and blood-flow rate of head, face, nasopharynx, neck, tongue, and brain; no pathology such as masses, lesions, infarcts, hemorrhage, aneurysms, hematomas, edema, or demyelinization of nerve fibers

Interfering Factors

➤ Interfering factors are the same as for any MRI scanning study (see p. 814).

Indications for Head and Intracranial Magnetic Resonance Imaging (MRI)

➤ Diagnosing and locating brain tumors, that is, primary and metastatic malignancy, acoustic neuroma, optic nerve tumor, pituitary microadenoma, lipoma, or benign meningioma
➤ Determining vascular disorders of the brain, that is, aneurysm, infarcts, intraparenchymal hematoma or hemorrhage, A-V malformations
➤ Detecting areas of nerve fiber demyelination in the definitive diagnosis of multiple sclerosis (MS)
➤ Determining the cause of cerebrovascular accident (CVA), cerebral infarct, or hemorrhage
➤ Determining cranial bone or face, throat, and neck soft tissue lesions, such as spread of tumor or infections

➤ Diagnosing intracranial infections, that is, pyogenic abscess, ventriculitis, subdural empyema, toxoplasmosis associated with acquired immunodeficiency syndrome (AIDS), or tuberculosis, when procedure is performed in combination with or in place of CT

➤ Determining the cause of seizures, that is, intracranial infection or edema or increased intracranial pressure

➤ Assessing intracranial vascular integrity in evaluating the predisposition to cerebral atherosclerosis

➤ Determining cerebral changes associated with dementia

➤ Evaluating effectiveness of chemotherapy or radiation therapy in tumor treatment

➤ Evaluating postoperative shunt placement and function performed for hydrocephalus in infants

Contraindications

➤ Contraindications are the same as for any MRI scanning study (see pp. 814 to 815).

Nursing Care Before the Procedure

Client teaching and physical preparation are the same as for any MRI scan study (see p. 815).

➤ Inform the client about the round-shaped apparatus placed around the head during the scanning procedure.

➤ Obtain a history that includes the assessment of the neurological system, known or suspected neurological disorders, associated laboratory tests and diagnostic procedures, medical and surgical interventions, and presence of any ferrous metal clips or prostheses, implants, or any other interferences to the study.

The Procedure

The procedure is the same as for any MRI scan study (see pp. 815 to 816). The scanner is directed at the client's head after the application of a plastic apparatus around the head. This apparatus contains an antenna to receive the radio waves from the scanning machine. A special paramagnetic contrast medium, Gd-DTPA, which has the ability to cross the blood-brain barrier, can be administered IV to enhance imaging of the brain tissue.

Nursing Care After the Procedure

Care and assessment after the procedure are the same as for any MRI scan study (see p. 816).

➤ Monitor vital signs and neurological checks to ensure stability.

HEART AND CHEST MAGNETIC RESONANCE IMAGING (MRI)

Heart and chest magnetic resonance imaging (MRI) scanning is a study performed to assist in diagnosing abnormalities of the cardiovascular and pulmonary structures and circulation. It involves the evaluation of the anatomy and function of all the areas of the chest, including all acquired and congenital diseases of the heart and great vessels except coronary artery disease (CAD); that is, it assists in diagnosing and evaluating thoracic aortic disease; pericardial disease; cardiac, paracardiac, and intracardiac masses; and congenital diseases, which include pulmonary atresia, aortic coarctation, and single ventricle with transportation of the great vessels. Although ventricular function and valvular regurgitation are usually assessed by cardiac nuclear scan studies (see p. 744), cine MRI can also provide quantitation of ventricular function.[23]

There are two techniques for MRI imaging of the cardiovascular structures. One is the electrocardiograph (ECG) gated multislice spin echo sequence that is used to diagnose heart and aortic anatomic abnormalities, and the other is the ECG referenced gradient refocused sequence that is used to diagnose heart function and analysis of blood-flow patterns. Because of MRI's ability to provide accurate quantitative information, it is useful in monitoring medication and other medical regimens in the treatment of heart failure and hypertension.[24]

Reference Values

Normal heart structure, soft tissue, and function, including blood-flow rate; no atherosclerosis, coronary infarction, or congenital anomalies; no thoracic aortic stenosis, occlusion, dissection, or pericardial or pulmonary effusion

Interfering Factors

➤ Interfering factors are the same as for any MRI scanning study (see p. 814).
➤ Movement of chest with respirations causes artifacts in the imaging.

Indications for Heart and Chest Magnetic Resonance Imaging (MRI)

➤ Diagnosing thoracic aortic diseases, that is, aortic dissection preoperatively; monitoring after treatment; and diagnosing intramural or periaortic hematoma
➤ Determining pericardial abnormalities, such as increased pericardial thickness indicating constrictive pericarditis or signal pattern indicating hematoma and pericardial effusion
➤ Confirming suspected cardiac and paracardiac masses, including mediastinal masses after echocardiography
➤ Identifying congenital heart diseases, that is, pulmonary atresia, absence or agenesis of a pulmonary artery, aortic coarctation, and transportation of the great vessels with a single ventricle[25]
➤ Determining cardiac ventricular function by measurement of right and left volume and wall thickness, valvular stenosis, or regurgitation by turbulent blood flow
➤ Diagnosing myocardial infarct and ischemic conditions of the cardiac muscle
➤ Detecting pleural effusion and fluid within the lung parenchyma and differentiating this fluid from hemorrhage fluid
➤ Evaluating bypass grafts and angioplasty postoperatively

Contraindications

➤ Contraindications are the same as for any MRI scan study (see pp. 814 to 815).

Nursing Care Before the Procedure

Client teaching and physical preparation are the same as for any MRI scan study (see p. 815).

➤ Inform the client about the ECG performed during the study.

➤ Obtain a history that includes assessment of the heart and great vessels and pulmonary systems, known or suspected cardiac or lung disorders, associated laboratory tests and diagnostic procedures, and medical and surgical interventions.

The Procedure

The procedure is the same as for any MRI scan study, with the scanner directed at the chest (see pp. 815 to 816). If an ECG is to be performed in conjunction with the scan, the electrodes are applied to the appropriate sites and the machine is readied to produce the ECG strips when needed.

Nursing Care After the Procedure

Care and assessment after the procedure are the same as for any MRI scan study (see p. 816).

➤ Monitor vital signs for stability.

MUSCULOSKELETAL MAGNETIC RESONANCE IMAGING (MRI)

Musculoskeletal magnetic resonance imaging (MRI) scanning is a study performed to assist in diagnosing abnormalities of bones and joints and surrounding soft tissue structures of cartilage, synovia, ligaments, and tendons. Its multiplanar imaging capability can reveal articular disorders, such as arthritis and temporomandibular joint detachment; bone marrow disorders, such as primary tumors, anemias, and avascular necrosis of bone; and tumors, such as sarcoma, osteochondroma, hemangioma, and metastatic tumors of the bone, as well as infection and trauma. MRI provides a more sensitive diagnostic study than CT and x-ray examination of musculoskeletal conditions. If it is not performed as an initial procedure, it is performed when a diagnosis is uncertain or when the need for surgery must be ascertained.

As with other MRI studies, the scanner, with its magnetic field and energy specific for the tissue to be examined, is directed at the area to be examined; it produces images based on the water content of the body. The area could be any large joint (usually the knee, wrist, hip, shoulder, temporomandibular joint, or spine) or some or all of the bones (usually the pelvis, long bones, patella, and femoral neck). Images are projected on a screen after a computer analysis of the data provided by the scanning. The images are also taped at the same time for later viewing.

Reference Values

Normal bones, joints, and surrounding tissue structures; no articular disease; no bone marrow disorders; no tumors; no infection; no trauma to the bones, joints, and muscles

Interfering Factors

➤ Interfering factors are the same as for any MRI scanning study (see p. 814).

➤ Casted limbs can cause difficulty in placement in the scanner if the cast is too large.

Indications for Musculoskeletal Magnetic Resonance Imaging (MRI)

➤ Determining new or recurrent herniated disk of the spine and differentiating this from spinal degenerative disease

➤ Diagnosing degenerative spinal diseases such as spondylosis and arthritis

➤ Determining postoperative changes such as hematoma, fibrosis, and scar formation in the diagnosis of spinal stenosis

➤ Determining the cause of low back syndrome pain, such as disk herniation or lesions

➤ Diagnosing avascular necrosis (osteonecrosis) of the femoral head or knee

➤ Detecting bone infarcts in the epiphyseal and diaphyseal sites

➤ Diagnosing bone infections such as osteomyelitis

➤ Evaluating arthritides by identification of erosions and lesions; synovial inflammation producing edema; and effusions causing cartilage, bone, ligament, tendon, and joint capsule destruction[26]

➤ Evaluating progression or improvement of synovitis after treatment

➤ Diagnosing primary or secondary malignant tumor process of the bone marrow, that is, leukemia or myeloma

➤ Determining bone marrow changes characteristic of Gaucher's disease, aplastic anemia, sickle cell disease, and polycythemia

➤ Detecting tears or degeneration of ligaments, tendons, and meniscus resulting from trauma or pathology

➤ Differentiating between stress fractures and neoplasms of the bone

➤ Evaluating meniscal detachment of the temporomandibular joint and functional derangement of the masticatory muscles, such as fibrosis and contracture, or osseous abnormalities such as fusion or sclerosis[27]

➤ Diagnosing benign and malignant tumors and cysts of bones and soft tissues, that is, osteogenic sarcoma, fibrosarcoma, osteochondroma, muscular and osseous hemangioma, liposarcoma, aneurysmal cysts, and other cysts

Contraindications

➤ Contraindications are the same as for any MRI scan study (see pp. 814 to 815).

Nursing Care Before the Procedure

Client teaching and physical preparation are the same as for any MRI scan study (see p. 815).

➤ Obtain a history that includes musculoskeletal system assessment findings, known or suspected musculoskeletal disorders, associated laboratory tests, diagnostic procedures, and medical and surgical interventions.

The Procedure

The procedure is the same as for any MRI scan study (see pp. 815 to 816). The scanner is directed at the body area to be examined, which determines the planes of imaging and the size and configuration of surface coils used to transmit or receive the magnetic radiation. A paramagnetic medium can be used as a contrast enhancement to define the vascularity of a lesion and its boundary with adjacent muscle.[28]

Nursing Care After the Procedure

Care and assessment after the procedure are the same as for any MRI scan study (see p. 816).

➤ *Bone and soft tissue pain:* Note and report pain severity. Administer ordered analgesic as needed for comfort before or after the procedure.

Student Name _____ Class _____

Instructor _____ Date _____

CASE STUDY AND CRITICAL THINKING EXERCISE

Mrs. Brown is an overweight 71-year-old woman. On admission to the ER, she presents with slurred speech, right hand weakness, and asymmetry of her facial expression. VS: T 98°F (36.6°C), P 108, R 18, BP 174/92. LP was negative.

a. What is this client's probable diagnosis?

b. A CT scan of the bran is ordered. Define this test and its purpose. How does it differ from an MRI and cerebral angiography?

c. Heparin is ordered for Mrs. Brown. What specific problem does Mrs. Brown have?

References

1. Corbett, JV: Laboratory Tests and Diagnostic Procedures with Nursing Diagnoses, ed 3. Appleton & Lange, Norwalk, Conn, 1992, p 541.
2. Berkow, R: The Merck Manual, ed 16. Merck Sharp and Dohme Research Laboratory, Rahway, NJ, 1992, p 2005.
3. Fischbach, FT: A Manual of Laboratory Diagnostic Tests, ed 4. JB Lippincott, Philadelphia, 1992, p 676.
4. Corbett, op cit, p 544.
5. Fischbach, op cit, p 916.
6. Ibid, pp 676–677.
7. Pagana, KD, and Pagana, TJ: Mosby's Diagnostic and Laboratory Test Reference. Mosby–Year Book, St Louis, 1992, p 220.
8. Fischbach, op cit, pp 672-673.
9. Springhouse Corporation: Nurse's Reference Library: Diagnostics, ed 2. Springhouse, Springhouse, Pa, 1986, p 575.
10. Pagana and Pagana, op cit, p 222.
11. Nurse's Reference Library, op cit, p 761.
12. Ibid, pp 760–761.
13. Corbett, op cit, p 541.
14. Pagana and Pagana, op cit, p 223.
15. Ibid, p 213.
16. Fischbach, op cit, p 677.
17. Margulis, AR, and Gooding, CA (eds): Diagnostic Radiology 1989. JB Lippincott, Philadelphia, 1989, p 27.
18. Ibid, p 105.
19. Ibid, p. 35.
20. Fischbach, op cit, p 918.
21. Ibid, p 918.
22. Margulis, op cit, p 35.
23. Ibid, p 228.
24. Ibid, pp 227, 229.
25. Ibid, p 228.
26. Ibid, p 228.
27. Ibid, p 383.
28. Ibid, pp 413, 418.

Bibliography

Black, JM, and Matassarin-Jacobs, E: Luckmann and Sorensen's Medical-Surgical Nursing: A Psychophysiologic Approach, ed 4. WB Saunders, Philadelphia, 1993.

Chernecky, CC, and Berger, BJ; Cullen, BN (ed): Laboratory Tests and Diagnostic Procedures, ed 2. WB Saunders, Philadelphia, 1996.

Christoforidis, AJ: Atlas of Axial, Sagittal, and Coronal Anatomy with CT and MRI. WB Saunders, Philadelphia, 1988.

Cohen, M, and Edwards, MK: Magnetic Resonance Imaging of Children. Mosby–Year Book, St Louis, 1990.

Edelman, RR, and Hesselink, JR: Clinical Magnetic Resonance Imaging, ed 2. WB Saunders, Philadelphia, 1996.

Firooznia, H, et al: MRI and CT of the Musculoskeletal System. Mosby–Year Book, St Louis, 1991.

Freidman, AC, et al: Clinical Pelvic Imaging: CT, Ultrasound, and MRI. Mosby–Year Book, St Louis, 1990.

Gedgaudas-McClees, RK (ed): Essentials of Body Computed Tomography. WB Saunders, Philadelphia, 1987.

Gutierrez, FR, Brown, JJ, and Mirowitz, S: Cardiovascular Magnetic Resonance Imaging. Mosby–Year Book, St Louis, 1992.

Haaga, A, et al: Computed Tomography and Magnetic Resonance Imaging, ed 3. Mosby–Year Book, St Louis, 1994.

Hayman, LA, and Hinch, VC: Clinical Brain Imaging: Normal Structure and Functional Anatomy. Mosby–Year Book, St Louis, 1992.

Kang, HS, and Resnick, D: MRI of the Extremities: An Anatomic Atlas. WB Saunders, Philadelphia, 1991.

Kee, JL: Handbook of Laboratory and Diagnostic Tests with Nursing Implications, ed 3. Appleton & Lange, Norwalk, Conn, 1997.

Latchaw, RE: MRI and CT Imaging of the Head, Neck, and Spine, ed 2. Mosby–Year Book, St Louis, 1991.

Lufkin, RB: The MRI Manual. Mosby–Year Book, St Louis, 1990.

Mitchell, DG, and Stark, DD: Hepatobiliary Magnetic Resonance Imaging. Mosby–Year Book, St Louis, 1992.

Pagana, KD, and Pagana, TJ: Diagnostic Testing and Nursing Implications: A Case Study Approach, ed 4. Mosby–Year Book, St Louis, 1993.

Potchen, JE, and Gottschalk, A: MRI Angiography. Mosby–Year Book, St Louis, 1993.

Shapiro, R, et al: Magnetic Resonance Imaging in Neuro-Ophthalmology. Mosby–Year Book, St Louis, 1992.

Springhouse Corporation: Diagnostic Tests. Springhouse, Springhouse, Pa, 1991.

Thomas, CL (ed): Taber's Cyclopedic Medical Dictionary, ed 18. FA Davis, Philadelphia, 1997.

Toombs, BD, and Sandler, CM: Computed Tomography in Trauma. Mosby–Year Book, St Louis, 1987.

Weinreb, JC, and Redman, HC: Magnetic Resonance Imaging of the Body. WB Saunders, Philadelphia, 1987.

Whaley, LF: Nursing Care of Infants and Children, ed 4. Mosby–Year Book, St Louis, 1991.

Yock, DH: Magnetic Resonance Imaging of CNS Disease: A Teaching File. Mosby–Year Book, St Louis, 1994.

22

Manometric Studies

➤ **TESTS COVERED**

Cystometry (CMG), *830*

Uroflowmetry, *833*

Urethral Pressure Profile, *835*

Esophageal Manometry, *836*

Arterial Plethysmography, *839*

Venous Plethysmography, *840*

Body Plethysmography, *841*

Oculoplethysmography, *843*

Contraction Stress Test, *845*

INTRODUCTION

Manometry is the measurement of liquid or gas pressures expressed in millimeters of mercury (mm Hg), or torr, or in centimeters of water (cm H_2O).[1] The types of liquids measured are blood in the arteries and veins, spinal fluid in the spinal column, and stomach contents in the esophagus. The type of gas measured is the lung air volume. Special devices are used for measurement, depending on the organ to be examined and the liquid or gas to be measured: a calibrated tube for spinal fluid pressure; a transducer for blood volume changes; a transducer attached to gastric tubes for sphincter competency; a cystometer attached to a urinary catheter for bladder capacity and pressure and urethra competency; or a transducer attached to a mouthpiece for lung gas volume, resistance, and compliance.

Plethysmography is a technique that uses different types of transducers, such as air, water, impedance, and photoelectric transducers, to determine and record volume and pressure changes of a body organ or extremity.[2]

A signed informed consent form is required for manometric procedures and for oculoplethysmography, which are considered invasive. No consent form is required for other types of plethysmography. The examinations are performed alone or in association with other diagnostic procedures by physicians or technicians in specially equipped rooms.

URODYNAMIC STUDIES

Urodynamic studies involve the measurement of urinary bladder function. They include neuromuscular function (cystometry), urinary flow rate (uroflowmetry), and urethral pressure and closing ability (urethral pressure profile). Among the aspects of bladder function studied are the changes in bladder, urethral, and intra-abdominal pressures; the characteristics of the urinary flow; and the external sphincter and pelvic floor muscle competency. The studies are usually performed to determine the cause of abnormal voiding patterns, bladder pathology, and the effect of therapeutic regimens on bladder function. One or more of the studies can be performed in conjunction with other urologic procedures, such as excretory urography and cystourethrography (regular and voiding). The most common complication resulting from these studies is urinary bladder infection.

Physiologically, micturition is facilitated or inhibited by neurological centers. Motor function of the detrusor muscle and the internal sphincter is controlled by the parasympathetic nervous system with cell bodies located in the lower spinal cord (S2 to S4). The cell bodies communicate with the bladder through the pelvic nerve. In the brain, detrusor muscle activity and external sphincter activity are controlled by the center in the brainstem, and the conscious control of micturition is controlled by the center in the brain cortex. Abnormalities of bladder function and structure can result from an interruption at any level of sensory or motor innervation or both. Other abnormalities can result from diseases (neuropathies from diabetes or multiple sclerosis) involving the neurons that supply the bladder and interrupt sensory or motor pathways or both.[3] Trauma and injury to the spinal cord or spinal roots, cerebral and cerebrovascular disorders, radical pelvic surgery, neuropathies, and advanced age are known causes of neurogenic bladder manifestations.

CYSTOMETRY (CMG)

Cystometry (CMG) is a manometric study performed to assist in diagnosing motor and sensory abnormalities (neurogenic bladder), obstructive abnormalities (prostatic hypertrophy, urethral stenosis), or infectious disorders (recurrent cystitis) that affect urinary bladder structure and function. The study measures bladder pressure during the filling and emptying phases in cm H_2O and provides information about uninhibited bladder contractions, sensations of bladder fullness and need to void, and ability to inhibit voiding. These abnormalities cause incontinence and other signs and symptoms associated with impaired patterns of micturition. Neuromuscular function of the bladder is determined by measurement of detrusor muscle competency, intravesical pressure and capacity, and response to thermal stimulation.[4]

The types and effects of neurogenic bladder dysfunction can be diagnosed with this study (Table 22–1). In addition to lesions and trauma of the spinal cord, the effects of other neurological disorders such as neuropathies, congenital anomalies, neurectomy, tumors, and cerebrovascular conditions on urinary patterns and vesical function can be evaluated. CMG can be performed in association with cystoscopy (see pp. 559 to 563) and sphincter electromyography (see p. 863).

Reference Values

➤ Normal sensory perception of bladder fullness, desire to void, ability to inhibit urination, and response to temperature (hot and cold)
➤ Normal bladder capacity: 350 to 750 mL for men and 250 to 550 mL for women
➤ Normal functioning bladder pressure: 8 to 15 cm H_2O
➤ Normal sensation of fullness: 40 to 100 cm H_2O
➤ Normal bladder pressure during voiding: 30 to 40 cm H_2O

Table 22–1 ➤ TYPES AND EFFECTS OF NEUROGENIC BLADDER		
Type/Site of Damage	**Characteristics**	**Causes**
Detrusor muscle hyperreflexia (above the level of voiding reflex)	Uninhibited or mild spastic incomplete/reflex spastic complete neurogenic bladder	Parkinson's disease, cerbrovascular accident (CVA), spinal cord injury (SCI), aging process
Detrusor muscle areflexia (level of sacral voiding reflex)	Autonomous or flaccid, nonreflexive, incomplete/sensory paralytic or motor paralytic neurogenic bladder	Diabetes mellitus, spinal cord tumor, SCI, congenital spinal cord defects, multiple sclerosis (MS)
External sphincter muscle	Impaired relaxation	Local irritation or inflammation, anxiety or depression
Brainstem	Loss of perception and control of bladder	Brain tumor, brain injury

➤ Normal detrusor pressure: less than 10 cm H_2O
➤ Urethral pressure that is higher than bladder pressure to ensure continence

Interfering Factors

➤ Inability of client to understand and carry out instructions during the procedure
➤ Inability of client to void in a supine position; straining at voiding during the study
➤ High level of client anxiety or embarrassment
➤ Administration of drugs such as muscle relaxants or antihistamines that affect bladder function

Indications for Cystometry (CMG)

➤ Determining the cause of bladder dysfunction and pathology: neurological, obstructive, or infectious disorders, for example
➤ Evaluating signs and symptoms of urinary elimination pattern dysfunction: dysuria, frequency, hesitancy, nocturia, urgency, retention, and incontinence
➤ Diagnosing the type of incontinence: functional (involuntary and unpredictable), reflex (involuntary when a specific volume is reached), stress (weak pelvic muscles), total (continuous and unpredictable), urge (involuntary when urgency is sensed), or psychological (dementia, confusion affecting awareness)
➤ Determining type of neurogenic bladder and effect on urination and determining bladder function and structure based on cause and level of abnormality or innervation interruption
➤ Evaluating the usefulness of drug therapy on the detrusor muscle and internal and external sphincters in controlling urinary bladder function
➤ Determining cause of urinary retention: urethral obstruction, prostatic hypertrophy, meatal stenosis, sexually transmitted infections that produce strictures, and so on
➤ Detecting urinary abnormalities resulting from congenital defects such as spina bifida, myelomeningocele, or vesicoureteral reflux

➤ Determining the cause of recurrent urinary tract infections (UTIs)
➤ Evaluating the management of neurological bladder before surgical interventions: sphincterectomy or reconstruction of the sphincter, urinary diversion, nerve resection, or transurethral prostatectomy

Contraindications

➤ *Acute UTI:* Study can cause infection to spread to kidneys.

➤➤ Nursing Alert

- The procedure should be performed using strict sterile technique to prevent infection.
- Clients with spinal cord injury (SCI) should be transported on a stretcher, and the study should be performed without transferring the client from the stretcher.

Nursing Care Before the Procedure

Explain to the client:
➤ That the procedure requires 30 to 45 minutes unless further studies are to be made
➤ That there are no food or fluid restrictions
➤ That all clothing or clothing from the waist down is removed and a hospital gown worn
➤ That the client will be draped appropriately and privacy protected
➤ That the client will be requested to refrain from straining at urination and to stand or walk during the study
➤ That a catheter is inserted into the bladder and solutions or gas are instilled while urethral and bladder pressures are measured
➤ That the client should report pain, sweating, nausea, headache, and urge to void experienced during the study
➤ That the only discomfort is the insertion of the urethral catheter
Prepare for the procedure:
➤ Obtain a history of signs and symptoms of impaired urinary function, known or suspected disorders leading to urinary dysfunction, associated diagnostic tests and procedures, medications, and medical and surgical interventions.
➤ Have client void.

The Procedure

The client is placed on the examination table in a supine or lithotomy position or remains on a stretcher in a supine position if SCI is present. Privacy is ensured and embarrassment prevented with proper draping while in position. The client is requested to void and lie still during the procedure. During the voiding, characteristics are assessed such as the time started, force and continuity of the stream, volume voided, and presence of dribbling, straining, or hesitancy.[5] A catheter is inserted into the bladder using sterile technique and the residual urine is measured and recorded. A test for sensory response to temperature is then performed: 30 mL of room temperature sterile water and then 30 mL of warm sterile water are instilled into the bladder, and the client's sensations are assessed and recorded. The fluid is removed from the bladder and the catheter is connected to a cystometer, which measures the pressures. Sterile normal saline, distilled water, or carbon dioxide gas in controlled amounts are instilled into the bladder. When the client indicates the urge to void, the bladder is considered full and amounts and times are recorded. Pressure and volume readings are also recorded and graphed for response to heat, fullness of bladder, urge to void, and ability to inhibit voiding. The client is requested to void without straining, and pressures are taken and recorded during this activity. After completion of voiding, the bladder is emptied of any other fluid and the catheter is withdrawn unless further testing is planned.

If further testing is performed to determine whether abnormal bladder function is caused by muscle incompetency or interrupted innervation, an anticholinergic such as atropine or cholinergic medication such as bethanechol (Urecholine) can be injected and the study repeated in 20 or 30 minutes.[6]

Nursing Care After the Procedure

➤ Advise the client to increase fluid intake and report any changes in voiding pattern or urine characteristics such as hematuria, cloudy and foul-smelling urine, inability to void or incontinence, dysuria, frequency, and urgency.

➤ Provide a warm tub bath to relieve discomfort at the urethral site.

➤ If indicated, monitor intake and output (I&O) for 24 to 48 hours.

➤ *Urinary bladder infection:* Note and report positive urine culture, burning, frequency, or urgency. Monitor culture results. Administer ordered antimicrobial as ordered. Offer sitz bath for comfort.

➤ *Autonomic reflexia:* Note and report sweating, flushing, bradycardia, hypertension, and severe headache. Administer propantheline bromide (Pro-Banthine) as ordered.

➤ *Sepsis:* Note and report temperature elevation, chills, or hematuria after third voiding. Monitor temperature and vital signs. Administer ordered antimicrobial and antipyretic drugs.

UROFLOWMETRY

Uroflowmetry is a manometric study performed to measure the urinary flow rate during the process of urination over a period of time. It is performed to assist in diagnosing abnormalities of the urinary pattern. It includes the recording and plotting of urinary volume flow over a period of time to determine the presence of external sphincter dysfunction, obstruction, and detrusor muscle hypotonia, any of which can lead to incontinence or urinary bladder infection. The study uses a system that includes a device called a uroflowmeter, a container to hold the urine, a transducer, start and flow cables, and a recorder. Evaluation of the test results is based on the volume of urine in milliliters, with output measured in milliliters per second or per minute, and on the client's age and gender.[7] This test has generally been replaced by the urethral pressure profile unless the insertion of a urinary bladder catheter is contraindicated.

Reference Values

<table>
<tr><td colspan="3" align="center">**Normal Urinary Flow Rate by Age and Gender**</td></tr>
<tr><td></td><td align="center">**Male**</td><td align="center">**Female**</td></tr>
<tr><td>Child</td><td>100 mL/10–12 sec</td><td>100 mL/10–15 sec</td></tr>
<tr><td>Adult</td><td>200 mL/12–21 sec</td><td>200 mL/15–18 sec</td></tr>
<tr><td>Older adult</td><td>200 mL/9 sec</td><td>200 mL/10 sec</td></tr>
<tr><td colspan="3">*Note:* No external sphincter dysfunction, obstruction, or hypotonia of the detrusor muscle.</td></tr>
</table>

Interfering Factors

➤ Inability of client to remain still and carry out instructions during the study
➤ Toilet tissue or other material that alters study findings
➤ Administration of drugs such as anticholinergics or muscle relaxants that affect bladder and sphincter function
➤ Room temperature changes that can affect transducer measurements

Indications for Uroflowmetry

➤ Determining abnormal urinary flow patterns in the evaluation of incontinence and recurrent urinary bladder infections
➤ Diagnosing external sphincter dysfunction revealed by an increased flow rate
➤ Determining the cause of abnormal urinary flow patterns (detrusor muscle hypotonia, outflow obstruction) revealed by a decrease in flow rate

Nursing Care Before the Procedure

Client teaching and physical preparation are the same as for any urodynamic study (see p. 832), except that a catheter is not inserted for this procedure.

➤ Inform the client that the study is completed in about 15 minutes, that it is performed while seated on a commode (women) or in a standing position (men), and that the pressures are measured during the process of voiding.

The Procedure

The client is placed in a sitting position on a commode (women) or in a standing position next to the commode (men). Privacy is ensured by draping or covering the client from the waist down. A weight-recording device (gravimetric uroflowmeter) is placed at the bottom of the commode. This unit weighs the urine as it flows, and weight changes are recorded electronically by converting weight to milliliters and recording time frames in seconds or minutes. The client is requested to void without straining during the procedure. Volume and times are recorded on a graph from the beginning of voiding to the end. The characteristics of the peaks of the curve on the graph indicate incontinence (high peak flow), detrusor muscle abnormality (many peaks), or obstruction (low peak flow).[8]

Nursing Care After the Procedure

Care and assessment after the procedure are the same as for any urodynamic study (see p. 833).

URETHRAL PRESSURE PROFILE

Urethral pressure profile is a manometric study performed to measure pressure changes along the urethra while the bladder is at rest. It is performed to assist in the diagnosis of urethral sphincter function abnormalities and to evaluate the effectiveness of surgical correction of sphincter abnormalities. Urethral pressures are evaluated by the client's age and gender and are measured in cm H_2O.

Reference Values

Normal Urethral Pressures for Age and Gender		
	Male	**Female**
Young adult	37–126 cm H_2O	55–103 cm H_2O
Middle adult	35–123 cm H_2O	31–115 cm H_2O
Older adult	35–105 cm H_2O	35–75 cm H_2O

Note: No obstruction or incontinence.

Interfering Factors

➤ Interfering factors are the same as for any urodynamic study (see p. 831).

Indications for Urethral Pressure Profile

➤ Determining external urethral sphincter competency in the presence of incontinence or abnormal urinary elimination pattern

➤ Detecting cause of stress incontinence in women, resulting from weakened pelvic floor muscle

➤ Determining obstruction of urinary flow caused by hypertrophic prostate gland and evaluating incontinence after prostatectomy

➤ Evaluating drug therapy regimen for urethral sphincter muscle control

➤ Evaluating function and management of postoperative procedures after sphincterectomy or artificial urethral device implantation

Contraindications

➤ *Acute UTI:* Study can cause infection to spread to the upper urinary tract and kidneys.

Nursing Care Before the Procedure

Client teaching and physical preparation are the same as for any urodynamic study (see p. 832).

➤ Inform the client that it takes 15 minutes to complete the study and that it has no adverse effects.

The Procedure

The client is placed on the examination table in a supine or a lithotomy position. The client is draped for privacy and prevention of embarrassment and is requested to remain very still during the procedure. A double-lumen catheter connected to a transducer is inserted into the bladder, and fluid or gas is constantly infused by a pumping apparatus. Urethral pressures are measured along the urethra while the catheter is withdrawn. When the study is completed, the catheter is removed. Pressure readings are recorded and analyzed for abnormalities based on the age and gender of the client.

Nursing Care After the Procedure

Care and assessment after the procedure are the same as for any urodynamic study (p. 833).

ESOPHAGEAL STUDIES

Esophageal studies involve the measurement of esophageal sphincter pressure, peristalsis and contraction, and acidity through the use of esophageal manometry, esophageal acid reflux and clearing, and acid perfusion (Bernstein) tests. Manometry is usually performed to detect the cause of pyrosis and dysphagia by determining esophageal sphincter competency and the effectiveness and coordination of esophageal movements during swallowing. The acid reflux test measures backflow or reflux of acid from the stomach into the esophagus, the acid clearing test measures motility in the esophagus, and the acid perfusion test confirms and evaluates esophageal reflux.[9] One or more of the tests can be performed, depending on the client's symptoms, and a definitive diagnosis can be obtained by radiologic (barium swallow) or endoscopic (esophagogastroduodenoscopy [EGD]) studies.

The esophagus is a tubelike organ that receives food from the pharynx and moves it into the stomach by peristaltic contractions. The upper and lower parts of the esophagus act as sphincters to control passage of the food from the pharynx and into the stomach. Failure of the lower sphincter to relax (sphincter hypertension) can cause achalasia as food passage into the stomach is slowed. This condition can result in aspiration of esophageal contents into the lungs. Reflux of stomach contents containing gastric acid into the esophagus at the lower sphincter (sphincter hypotension) can result in inflammation and cause associated pyrosis and pain. In time, inflammation results in edema and erosion of the esophageal lumina, forming thickness and scar tissue and causing associated dysphagia.[10]

ESOPHAGEAL MANOMETRY

Esophageal manometry and associated tests are manometric studies performed to assist in evaluating esophageal muscle function and diagnosing structure abnormalities. The studies measure esophageal pressure and the presence or effects of gastric acid in the esophagus. Abnormalities cause dysphagia, regurgitation, and pyrosis, indicating possible spasms, achalasia, chalasia in children, gastroesophageal reflux, esophagitis, and esophageal scleroderma.

Esophageal manometry measures lower esophageal sphincter pressure and motility patterns that result during swallowing. The acid reflux test measures the presence of gastric acid in the lower esophagus. The acid clearing test measures the motility by the number of swallows it takes to clear hydrochloric acid from the esophagus. The acid perfusion test measures or evaluates the effect of hydrochloric acid on the esophagus to confirm that symptoms of pain are caused by esophagitis and not some other condition that can cause chest or epigastric pain.

Reference Values

Normal Esophageal Structure and Function	
Esophageal sphincter pressure	10–20 mm Hg
Esophageal secretions	pH 5.0–6.0
Acid reflux	No regurgitation into the esophagus
Acid clearing	10 swallows or less
Acid perfusion	No gastroesophageal reflux

Note: No gastroesophageal reflux, esophagitis, achalasia, spasms, or chalasia.

Interfering Factors

➤ Inability of client to understand or follow instructions during the study
➤ Intake of food or fluids within 6 hours before the study
➤ Administration of medications such as sedatives, antacids, anticholinergics, cholinergics, or corticosteroids, which can change pH or relax the sphincter muscle

Indications for Esophageal Manometry

➤ Diagnosis of pyrosis and dysphagia to determine whether the cause is gastroesophageal reflux or esophagitis
➤ Diagnosis of chronic gastroesophageal reflux revealed by low pressures in manometry, decrease in pH in acidity test, and pain during acid reflux and acid perfusion tests
➤ Diagnosis of esophagitis revealed by decreased motility requiring more than 10 swallows to clear acid from the esophagus in the acid clearing test
➤ Diagnosis of achalasia revealed by failure of the lower sphincter to relax when swallowing and by spasms, causing increased pressure in manometry
➤ Diagnosis of chalasia in children, revealed by relaxed esophageal sphincter causing low pressures in manometry
➤ Suspected esophageal scleroderma revealed by impaired sphincter and abnormal contractions causing low pressures in manometry
➤ Differentiation between cardiac condition and epigastric pain resulting from esophagitis as revealed by introduction of acid in the acid perfusion test

Contraindications

➤ *Unstable medical condition:* vital signs, esophageal varices or bleeding, infection, cardiac condition

Nursing Care Before the Procedure

Client teaching and physical preparation are as follows:
➤ Foods and fluids are withheld for 6 to 8 hours and medications for 24 hours before the study.
➤ For the client with diabetes, make special arrangements for insulin administration, meals, and time for the study to be performed.
➤ Inform the client that one or more tubes are inserted into the mouth or nose and positioned into the esophagus and that some gagging and discomfort are experienced during insertion and placement.

➤ Take baseline vital signs for later comparisons.
➤ Obtain a history that includes signs and symptoms of gastrointestinal distress, known or suspected gastrointestinal disorders or hiatal hernia, treatments, and medication regimens.

The Procedure

The client is placed in a high-Fowler's or a sitting position initially while the tubes are inserted. After placement of the tube, the client is placed on the examination table in a supine position.

Esophageal Manometry. One or more small tubes are inserted into the esophagus via the mouth. A small transducer is attached to the ends of the tubes to measure the lower esophageal sphincter and intraluminal pressures and the regularity and duration of peristaltic contractions to determine motility abnormalities. The tubes are allowed to pass into the stomach and then pulled backward into the lower esophagus. Pressures are taken and recorded. The client is requested to swallow, and the motility pattern is recorded on a graph. Lower esophageal sphincter pressure of 0 to 5 mm Hg is considered incompetent and indicative of gastroesophageal reflux. A pressure of 50 mm Hg is indicative of achalasia. This test can also be performed during esophagoscopy via the endoscope to measure lower esophageal sphincter pressure.

Esophageal Acid and Clearing. With the tubes in place in the esophagus, a pH electrode probe is inserted into the esophagus. The client can be requested to lift both legs or perform Valsalva's maneuver to stimulate reflux of stomach contents into the esophagus. If acid reflux is absent, 100 mL of 0.1 percent hydrochloric acid (HCl) is instilled into the stomach over a period of 3 minutes and the pH measurement repeated. If reflux is present, the pH probe indicates a drop to between 1.0 and 3.0 as the acid is regurgitated into the esophagus. To determine acid clearing, HCl is instilled into the esophagus and the client is requested to swallow while the probe measures pH. The number of swallows it takes to clear the acid from the esophagus based on the pH probe readings determines the esophageal motility capabilities in clearing the acid from the esophagus.

Acid Perfusion. A catheter is inserted through the nose into the esophagus. The client is requested to inform the technician when pain is experienced. Normal saline solution is allowed to drip into the catheter at about 10 mL per minute. Then HCl is allowed to drip into the catheter. Pain experienced when HCl is instilled determines the presence of an esophageal abnormality. If no pain is experienced, the client's symptoms are the result of some other condition.

Nursing Care After the Procedure

➤ Inform the client that some irritation of the nose and throat is common for 24 hours after the study and that discomfort can be reduced by gargling with warm water.
➤ Monitor vital signs, compare with baseline readings, and monitor bleeding from the nose or mouth.
➤ Resume food, fluid, and medications after the study.
➤ *Aspiration of contents into lungs:* Note and report any change in respirations (dyspnea, tachypnea, adventitious sounds). Suction mouth,

pharynx, and trachea. Administer ordered oxygen. Have resuscitation
equipment on hand.

PLETHYSMOGRAPHY

Plethysmography is a noninvasive diagnostic technique used to measure changes
in the size of blood vessels by determining changes in the volume of blood in
the vessels of the eye, extremities, or neck or changes in gas volume in the
lungs. Various transducers and instruments are used to determine arterial, venous, or lung abnormalities: body box, impedance plethysmograph, pulse volume recorder, and others. Plethysmography is usually performed instead of or
after Doppler examination in vascular studies and in conjunction with pulmonary function testing in lung studies. There are no complications associated
with plethysmography.

ARTERIAL PLETHYSMOGRAPHY

Arterial plethysmography is a manometric study that measures toe or finger
volume changes after Doppler ultrasonography when ankle, thigh, and arm
pressures are elevated. Normal toe pressure should equal or exceed ankle pressure, and normal finger pressure should equal or exceed wrist pressure.[11] This
assessment of arterial circulation in the upper or lower limbs can assist in the
diagnosis of lower extremity occlusive diseases and upper extremity arteriosclerotic disease. The study requires very little cooperation from the client
and can be performed at the bedside for those who cannot be moved to the vascular laboratory.

Reference Values

Normal arterial pulse wave	Steep upslope and less steep downslope, with narrow, pointed peaks
Normal pressure	<20 mm Hg in the systolic difference between the lower and upper extremities; toe pressure 80% or more of ankle pressure; finger pressure 80% or more of wrist pressure[12]

Interfering Factors

➤ Smoking 2 hours before the study constricts the arteries.
➤ Environmental temperatures (hot or cold) can affect peripheral circulation.
➤ Arterial occlusion proximal to the extremity to be examined can prevent
blood flow to the limb.

Indications for Arterial Plethysmography

➤ Suspected arterial occlusive disease revealed by a decreased pulse wave
amplitude and a pressure difference of greater than 20 mm Hg
➤ Determination of changes in toe or finger pressures when ankle pressures
are elevated, as a result of calcifications in arteries
➤ Determination of the effect of trauma on the arteries in an extremity

➤ Determination of peripheral small artery changes (ischemia) caused by diabetes and differentiation of these changes from other neuropathy

➤ Diagnosis of vascular changes associated with Raynaud's phenomenon

➤ Determination of degree and location of arterial atherosclerotic obstruction and vessel patency in peripheral atherosclerotic disease

➤ Determination of inflammatory changes causing obliteration in the vessels in thromboangiitis obliterans

➤ Confirmation of suspected acute arterial embolization

Contraindications

➤ An extremity that is cold to the touch, cyanotic, or pale in color, indicating a compromised blood flow to the limb

Nursing Care Before the Procedure

Explain to the client:

➤ That the procedure requires about 30 minutes

➤ That foods and fluids are allowed but that smoking is restricted for at least 2 hours before the study

➤ That all clothing is removed from the extremities that are to be examined

➤ That some cuffs are applied to the extremity to measure the blood flow

➤ That no pain is associated with the study

Prepare for the procedure:

➤ Obtain a history of signs and symptoms of vascular disorders, known or suspected peripheral vascular disease, associated diagnostic tests and procedures, and medication regimen.

➤ Ensure that the client has refrained from smoking for 2 hours before the study.

➤ Obtain baseline vital signs for later comparison.

➤ Administer an ordered analgesic to control pain, if pain is present.

➤ Have client void.

The Procedure

The client is placed on the examination table or in a bed in a semi-Fowler's position. The client is requested to lie very still during the procedure. Three cuffs are applied to the extremity and attached to a pulse volume recorder, which displays the amplitude of each pulse wave on a paper called the *plethysmogram*. The cuffs are inflated to 65 mm Hg, and the pulse waves of each cuff are measured. These measurements when compared with a normal limb determine the presence of arterial occlusive disease.[13]

Nursing Care After the Procedure

➤ Help the client dress, if help is needed.

➤ Handle the extremity gently if severe ischemia, ulcers, and pain are present.

VENOUS PLETHYSMOGRAPHY

Venous plethysmography is a manometric study that measures changes in venous capacity and outflow (volume and rate of outflow). It is usually performed to assist in the diagnosis of a thrombotic condition that causes obstruction of the major veins of the extremities. The study is performed on the leg and uses two blood pressure cuffs, one occluding circulation and one containing a plethysmography recorder. The study can be performed in conjunction with Doppler ultrasonography. Suspected deep venous thrombosis (DVT) that is not confirmed by plethysmography can require venography studies. The study can be performed at the bedside for those clients who cannot be transported to the vascular laboratory.

Reference Values

Normal venous blood flow in extremities; no incompetent valves, thrombosis, or thrombotic obstruction in the major veins of the extremities; venous filling time should be greater than 20 seconds.

Interfering Factors

➤ Cold air or cold extremity, constricting the vessels
➤ High level of anxiety, causing a tenseness of muscles
➤ Venous occlusion at the proximal part of the extremity to be examined, affecting blood flow to the extremity

Indications for Venous Plethysmography

➤ Diagnosing partial or total venous thrombotic obstruction revealed by an absence of an increase in leg volume as venous outflow is obstructed
➤ Determining valve competency in conjunction with Doppler ultrasonography in the diagnosis of varicose veins

Nursing Care Before the Procedure

Client teaching and physical preparation are the same as for any vascular plethysmography study (see p. 840).

The Procedure

The client is placed on the examination table or in a bed in a semi-Fowler's position. Two cuffs are applied to the extremity, with one cuff attached to a pulse volume recorder. One cuff is placed on the proximal part of the extremity (occlusion cuff), and the second cuff is placed on the distal part of the extremity (recorder cuff). The recorder cuff is inflated at the level of 10 mm Hg, and the effects of respiration on the volume in the veins are evaluated. Absence of changes during respirations indicates the presence of venous occlusion. Next, the occlusion cuff is inflated to the level of 50 mm Hg to record the venous volume on the pulse monitor. The occlusion cuff is deflated after the highest volume is recorded in the recorder cuff. A delay in the return to preocclusion volume indicates venous thrombotic occlusion.[14]

Nursing Care After the Procedure

Care and assessment after the procedure are the same as for any vascular plethysmography study (see p. 840).

BODY PLETHYSMOGRAPHY

Body plethysmography is a manometric study that measures the total amount of air within the thorax (volume), both in and out of ventilatory communication with the lung; the elasticity (compliance) of the lungs; and the resistance to air flow in the respiratory tree. Values are based on the height, weight, and gender of the client. The volume is calculated in milliliters by multiplying the pressure by the volume obtained during the test. Compliance is calculated in liters per centimeter of H_2O by dividing the volume change by the pressure change. Airway resistance is calculated in centimeters of H_2O per liter per second by dividing the pressure change by the flow change. The diagnosis of pulmonary disease is determined from increases in volume, compliance, and resistance, indicating obstructive lung disorders, and from decreases in compliance, indicating restrictive lung disorders, infection, or atelectasis.[15]

Body plethysmography can be performed in conjunction with pulmonary stress testing and pulmonary function tests.

Reference Values

Normal Thoracic Gas Volume, Compliance, and Airway Resistance	
Thoracic gas volume	2400 mL
Compliance	0.2 L/cm H_2O
Airway resistance	0.6–2.5 cm H_2O/L per sec

Note: No obstructive or restrictive lung disease, infection, or atelectasis.

Interfering Factors

➤ Inability of client to follow breathing instructions during the procedure

Indications for Body Plethysmography

➤ Determining the status of obstructive pulmonary disease (emphysema, asthma, chronic bronchitis) revealed by an increased gas volume, compliance, and airway resistance
➤ Determining the status of restrictive pulmonary disease such as fibrosis revealed by a decrease in compliance, resulting from lung stiffness
➤ Detecting acute pulmonary disorders such as atelectasis and pneumonia by changes in compliance caused by congestion
➤ Differentiating between obstructive and restrictive pulmonary pathology
➤ Evaluating pulmonary status before pulmonary rehabilitation to determine the baselines and possible benefits from the therapy

Contraindications

➤ Extreme claustrophia that prevents enclosure in the box

Nursing Care Before the Procedure

Client teaching and physical preparation are the same as for any plethysmography procedure (see p. 840).
➤ Inform the client that the test is performed in an enclosed box while the client is seated on a chair; a soft clip is placed on the nose to assist in breathing through a mouthpiece.
➤ Obtain and record client's weight, height, gender, and history including known or suspected pulmonary conditions, associated diagnostic tests and procedures, and treatment or medication regimen.

The Procedure

The client is placed in a sitting position on a chair in the body box. A nose clip is positioned to prevent breathing through the nose and a mouthpiece is placed in the mouth. The client is requested to breathe through the mouthpiece, which is connected to the transducer and the recorder device. The door to the box is closed, and time is given for the pressure in the box to stabilize before the test is started. The client is informed to notify the technician if claustrophobia or breathing difficulties occur when the client is requested to change breathing patterns. At the beginning of the study, the client is requested to pant without allowing the glottis to close. The box and mouth pressures are recorded, and this information is used to calculate the thoracic gas volume. The client is then requested to breathe in a rapid, shallow pattern; the box pressure is recorded and compared with the pressures recorded on the screen and used to calculate airway resistance. If compliance is tested, a double-lumen catheter is inserted into the esophagus via the nose, and the bag is inflated with air. Intraesophageal pressure is recorded during normal breathing to determine intrapleural pressure, which is considered to be similar. The changes in the intraesophageal pressure provide the information needed to determine lung compliance.[16]

Nursing Care After the Procedure

Care and assessment after the procedure are the same as for any plethysmography study (see p. 840). Allow the client time to resume a normal breathing pattern.

OCULOPLETHYSMOGRAPHY

Oculoplethysmography is a manometric study to measure blood flow in the ipsilateral orbit of the eye in diagnosing carotid artery disease. The blood flow in one eye is compared with that in the other eye to determine decreases indicating pathology. The blood flow of the carotid artery and circulation in the brain are reflected by the blood flow of the ophthalmic artery because of its connection to the internal carotid artery.

The study can be performed in conjunction with duplex scanning of the carotid arteries and followed by cerebral angiography to diagnose blood flow patterns to the brain from the carotid arteries.

Reference Values

Normal blood flow in the carotid arteries; no atherosclerotic occlusive disease

Interfering Factors

➤ Inability of client to prevent blinking during the procedure

Indications for Oculoplethysmography

➤ Determining the cause of transient ischemic attacks (TIAs) and symptoms of neurological disorders, such as syncope and ataxia
➤ Diagnosing carotid atherosclerotic stenosis or occlusive disease revealed by a reduced rate of blood flow in the ophthalmic artery
➤ Determining the extent of carotid stenosis
➤ Evaluating carotid artery patency before or after endarterectomy[17]

Contraindications

> ➤ Eye surgery as recent as 2 to 6 months before the study
> ➤ Clients with cataracts or lens implants
> ➤ Clients who have had retinal detachment in the past
> ➤ Allergy to the local anesthetic used in the study

Nursing Care Before the Procedure

Client teaching and physical preparation are the same as for any plethysmography procedure (see p. 840).

> ➤ Inform the client that the usual medications and eyedrops are not restricted but that additional eyedrops that cause a slight burning sensation will be administered to anesthetize the eyes.
> ➤ Remove contact lenses and store in a safe place.
> ➤ Obtain baseline blood pressure in both arms.
> ➤ Attach electrodes for ECG, if one is ordered.
> ➤ Obtain a history that includes cardiovascular and neurological status, known or suspected disorders associated with the carotid artery, and results of associated diagnostic tests and procedures.

The Procedure

The client is placed on the examination table in a supine position. The electrodes are connected and the ECG machine is turned on to monitor for arrhythmias when the study begins. After the eyedrops have been administered in the amounts and frequency ordered to anesthetize both eyes, small photoelectric detectors are attached to both earlobes. Pulsations from blood flow to the ears via the external carotid arteries are detected, compared, and recorded. Small suction cups are then attached to both eyeballs and held in place with 40 to 50 mm Hg of suction.[18] Blood flow within each eye causes pulsations that are detected and recorded. Blood flow to each eye is interrupted temporarily by the application of increased pressure to the eyeball. When blood flow is resumed, pulsations are recorded to determine whether the flow is simultaneous for both eyes. Blood flow to the eye is delayed if carotid occlusive disease is present. The difference in the timing of pulsations is measured in milliseconds. The study results are evaluated based on a comparison of pulsations in one eye with those in the other or of pulsations in one ear with those in the other, or in some cases, of pulsations of one eye with those of the ear on the opposite side. The delay in blood flow measures the degree of carotid artery disease as mild, moderate, or severe.

Nursing Care After the Procedure

> ➤ Care and assessment after the procedure include advising the client to refrain from rubbing the eyes for 2 hours and to gently blot tearing with a soft tissue.
> ➤ Inform the client that contact lenses should not be replaced for 2 hours and that sunglasses can be worn if temporary photophobia is experienced.
> ➤ Explain that the eyes can appear bloodshot after the study and that, if the eyes are irritated, drops of artificial tears should be instilled.

➤ Remind the client that the anesthetic wears off in about 30 minutes.

➤ *Corneal abrasion:* Note and report eye pain or vision changes. Apply an ordered lubricant and an eye bandage.

➤ *Conjunctival irritations and hemorrhage:* Note and report redness of conjunctiva and complaints of pain. Apply ordered medications and treatments. Cover the eye with a bandage.

FETOPLACENTAL ADEQUACY STUDIES

Fetoplacental studies involve the measurement of placental blood flow to determine the adequacy of placental reserve oxygen. They are performed to detect high-risk pregnancies by identification of intrauterine asphyxia as well as the effect of maternal diabetes, hypertension, Rh factor sensitization, and other conditions on fetal status.

Two tests can be performed to determine intrauterine hypoxia and to evaluate fetal well-being—the contraction stress test and the nonstress test. The nonstress test provides information about fetal status based on fetal heart rate (FHR) acceleration during fetal movement in the absence of uterine contractions. A fetal monitor is attached to the mother and the FHR is monitored to obtain a reactive pattern, that is, two or more accelerations in a 10-minute period. Fewer than two accelerations are rated as equivocal, and an absence of accelerations is rated as nonreactive. The nonstress test can be performed by a nurse, with the FHR strip interpreted by the nurse or physician. The stress test can follow the nonstress test when the nonstress test is rated as nonreactive. The stress test provides information about fetal status based on FHR during the stress of uterine contractions, evaluating placental reserve adequacy that allows the fetus to receive adequate oxygen during uterine contractions. The results are considered to be useful for a week in the late stages of pregnancy or before labor.

Because nonstress tests are performed routinely, only the contraction stress test procedure is fully developed in this section.

CONTRACTION STRESS TEST

Contraction stress test, also known as the oxytocin (Pitocin) challenge test, is a manometric study performed to measure the adequacy of the placenta to provide oxygen to the fetus during the stress of oxytocin-induced uterine contractions. Uterine contractions normally produce a decrease in placental blood flow, and in the later stages of pregnancy (at least 34 weeks' gestation) this study can predict whether a fetus might be at risk for intrauterine asphyxia. The test can be repeated weekly until the onset of labor and delivery if the fetus is at risk for intrauterine hypoxia. An adequate placental reserve, in which the blood flow is not compromised and the FHR is within the normal range, indicates a negative test, meaning that the fetus is not in jeopardy and can tolerate the stress of labor. A positive result is determined by consistent late deceleration of the FHR during two or more contractions and indicates an inadequate oxygen supply to the fetus and a risk for uterine asphyxia. If the late decelerations are not consistent, the test is considered equivocal and is repeated in 24 hours.[19] Only specially trained personnel can administer and monitor this test.

Reference Values

Negative; no late deceleration in the FHR after a contraction

Interfering Factors

➤ Maternal hypotension, which can cause an inaccurate positive result

Indications for Contraction Stress Test

➤ Evaluation of the fetus at risk for hypoxia or the effects of hypoxia and possible in utero or postpartum respiratory distress or death
➤ Determination of the effects of maternal diabetes, hypertension with toxemia on fetoplacental adequacy, and fetal well-being
➤ Past history of stillbirth, postmaturity birth, intrauterine growth retardation, low estriol levels, and Rh factor sensitization
➤ A nonreactive result from a nonstress test to determine the ability of the fetus to withstand uterine contractions before labor begins
➤ Assessment of possible impact of cesarean birth on the fetus
➤ Assessment of the need to terminate the pregnancy by labor inducement and early birth (in conjunction with other diagnostic procedures such as ultrasonography and amniocentesis)

Contraindications

➤ Conditions that may increase the possibility of early labor and birth or other danger to mother or fetus:
   • Prematurely ruptured membranes
   • Multiple pregnancy
   • Previous transverse or classic cesarean birth or other surgical hysterotomy
   • Previous premature labor
   • Abnormalities such as abruptio placentae or placenta previa
   • Gestation of less than 34 weeks[20]

Nursing Care Before the Procedure

Explain to the client:
➤ That the procedure requires 2 hours
➤ That food and fluid are withheld for 4 to 8 hours before the study to prepare for possible premature labor (This requirement is determined by agency policy.)
➤ That breathing and relaxation techniques will be used during the study to allay the mild contractions that are induced to perform the test (Teach these techniques to the client if she has not attended childbirth class, and allow her to practice.)
➤ That a monitor is placed on the abdomen to check FHR, another monitor is placed on the lower abdomen to check uterine contractions, and blood pressure is monitored during the study
➤ That uterine contractions are induced by the intravenous (IV) administration of the hormone oxytocin
➤ That mild contractions are the only discomfort experienced during the study
Prepare for the procedure:
➤ Ensure that food and fluid restrictions have been followed.

➤ Obtain blood pressure and FHR for baselines to use as a comparison during or after the study.
➤ Have client void.
➤ Obtain a history of past pregnancies, known and suspected medical conditions, known and suspected risks to the fetus and mother, previous diagnostic tests and procedures, and medical treatments for chronic disorders and those associated with the pregnancy.

The Procedure

The client is placed on the examination table or bed in a semi-Fowler's slightly side-lying position. The client is draped for privacy. The blood pressure is taken and the cuff is left on the arm to monitor the pressure every 10 minutes during the procedure, as a drop in blood pressure can affect the placental blood flow and produce inaccurate results. The fetal monitor is placed on the abdomen and a tocodynamometer is placed on the lower abdomen to monitor contractions. A baseline recording is made of fetal heart tones and uterine contractions. Continuous monitoring takes place for 20 minutes, and a recording of the FHR and uterine movement is obtained. A recording of FHR during spontaneous uterine contractions should be obtained, but if no contractions occur, IV oxytocin should be administered in the dilution and rate ordered by the physician, with the rate regulated by an infusion pump. The rate is increased until three contractions per minute are noted. FHR and contractions are then monitored and recorded and the infusion discontinued to determine the FHR response to the stress of the contractions. The client is advised to use the deep-breathing exercises learned in childbirth class to control any discomfort from the contractions. Monitoring of the FHR is continued for 30 minutes (the time it takes to metabolize the oxytocin) as the uterine movements return to normal.

Another procedure to stimulate oxytocin for the contraction stress test in clients after 26 weeks' gestation is the breast stimulation test. This test releases oxytocin by stimulation of the nipples instead of IV administration of the drug. The stimulation creates nerve impulses to the hypothalamus, causing the release of oxytocin into the bloodstream, which results in uterine contractions. The same monitoring and recording are performed when sufficient contractions have been obtained.[21]

Nursing Care After the Procedure

➤ Help the client dress, if help is needed. Monitor the blood pressure and FHR and compare with baseline values.
➤ Remove the IV catheter.
➤ Assess the site for pain, swelling, redness, and bleeding; apply a dressing.
➤ *Premature labor:* Note and record frequency, strength, and continuation of contractions. Prepare for first stage of labor or cesarean birth.

(Case Study follows on page 849)

Student Name _____ Class _____

Instructor _____ Date _____

CASE STUDY AND CRITICAL THINKING EXERCISE

Mike, age 17, is admitted to the ER with a suspected spinal cord injury (SCI). After stabilization, cystometry is ordered. Results are: volume 600 mL, bladder pressure 20 cm H_2O, detrussor pressure 15 cm H_2O.

a. What complication of SCI is Mike experiencing?

b. What interventions may be ordered during this phase?

References

1. Thomas, CL (ed): Taber's Cyclopedic Medical Dictionary, ed 18. FA Davis, Philadelphia, 1997, p 1160.
2. Fischbach, FT: A Manual of Laboratory Diagnostic Tests, ed 4. JB Lippincott, Philadelphia, 1992, p 909.
3. Porth, CM: Pathophysiology: Concepts of Altered Health States, ed 4. JB Lippincott, Philadelphia, 1994, pp 511–512.
4. Pagana, KD, and Pagana, TJ: Mosby's Diagnostic and Laboratory Test Reference. Mosby–Year Book, St Louis, 1992, p 258.
5. Ibid, p 259.
6. Ibid, p 260.
7. Springhouse Corporation: Nurse's Reference Library: Diagnostics, ed 2.

Springhouse, Springhouse, Pa, 1986, pp 981–982.
8. Ibid, p 982.
9. Pagana and Pagana, op cit, p 317.
10. Porth, op cit, p 671.
11. Fischbach, op cit, p 910.
12. Ibid, p 910.
13. Pagana and Pagana, op cit, p 567.
14. Ibid, p 569.
15. Ibid, pp 832–833.
16. Fischbach, op cit, p 833.
17. Pagana and Pagana, op cit, p 530.
18. Nurse's Reference Library, op cit, p 764.
19. Pagana and Pagana, op cit, p 229.
20. Ibid, p 230.
21. Ibid, p 232.

Bibliography

Berkow, R (ed): The Merck Manual, ed 16. Merck Sharp and Dohme Research Laboratory, Rahway, NJ, 1992.

Black, JM, and Matassarin-Jacobs, E: Luckmann and Sorensen's Medical-Surgical Nursing: A Psychophysiologic Approach, ed 4. WB Saunders, Philadelphia, 1993.

Brumfitt, W, and Hamilton-Miller, JMC: Urinary Tract Infections. Mosby–Year Book, St Louis, 1992.

Chernecky, CC, and Berger, BJ; Cullen, BN (ed): Laboratory Tests and Diagnostic Procedures, ed 2. WB Saunders, Philadelphia, 1996.

Corbett, JV: Laboratory Tests and Diagnostic Procedures with Nursing Diagnoses, ed 4. Appleton & Lange, Norwalk, Conn, 1995.

Jamieson, GG, and Duranceau, A: Gastroesophageal Reflux. WB Saunders, Philadelphia, 1988.

Kee, JL: Handbook of Laboratory and Diagnostic Tests with Nursing Implications,

ed 3. Appleton & Lange, Norwalk, Conn, 1997.

Lowell, RK, et al: Bladder Reconstruction and Continent Urinary Diversion, ed 2. Mosby–Year Book, St Louis, 1991.

O'Reilly, PH, George, NJR, and Weiss, RM: Diagnostic Techniques in Urology. WB Saunders, Philadelphia, 1990.

Pagana, KD, and Pagana, TJ: Diagnostic Testing and Nursing Implications: A Case Study Approach, ed 4. Mosby–Year Book, St Louis, 1993.

Springhouse Corporation: Diagnostic Tests. Springhouse, Springhouse, Pa, 1991.

Tilkian, SM: Clinical and Nursing Implications of Laboratory Tests, ed 5. Mosby–Year Book, St Louis, 1991.

Wein, AJ, and Barrett, DM: Voiding Function and Dysfunction. Mosby–Year Book, St Louis, 1988.

23

Electrophysiologic Studies

➤ **TESTS COVERED**

Electrocardiography (ECG), *852*
Holter Electrocardiography
  (ECG), *856*
Phonocardiography, *858*
Exercise Electrocardiography
  (ECG), *860*
Signal-Averaged
  Electrocardiography (SAE), *862*

Pelvic Floor Sphincter
  Electromyography, *863*
Electromyography (EMG), *865*
Electroneurography, *867*
Electroencephalography (EEG), *869*
Evoked Brain Potentials, *871*
Electronystagmography (ENG), *874*
Electroretinography (ERG), *876*
Electro-oculography (EOG), *878*

INTRODUCTION

Electrophysiologic studies are procedures that use electric and electronic devices in the diagnosis of tissue and organ pathology. They measure electric events for indirect assessment of the structure and function of an organ. Assessment is based on a determination of the effects of electric stimulation on tissues, the production of electric currents by organs and tissues, and the results of the therapeutic use of electric currents.[1] Electrodes are attached to a portion of the body to measure the current or activity produced by the examined organ or tissue to identify pathology. The studies produce an electrogram, a graphic display or recording of electric activities produced by tissues or organs, for analysis and diagnostic information.

The studies are most commonly used in the investigation of heart, muscle, and nerve abnormalities. They are performed on inpatients or outpatients in specially equipped rooms; in a physician's office; or, for some studies, at the bedside by a physician or a technician, depending on the procedure. All except electromyography (EMG) and studies that use needle insertions are considered noninvasive procedures with little or no risk to the client and do not require a signed informed consent form.

ELECTRODIAGNOSTIC STUDIES

Electrodiagnostic procedures are named for the organ or region of the body to be examined, including the heart, brain, eye, and muscle. Depending on the organ or region to be studied, electrodes are placed and positioned on the skin over the area containing the organ or directly on the organ. The studies are performed to support and extend information obtained from other diagnostic procedures in diagnosing or evaluating congenital and acquired diseases of the involved organs, that is, physical assessment and history, ultrasonography, radiography, angiography, and computerized scanning.

ELECTROCARDIOGRAPHY (ECG)

Electrocardiography (ECG) is an electrophysiologic study that measures the electric currents or impulses that are generated by the heart during a cardiac cycle. The heart has the ability to produce impulses and contractions, and these impulses and contractions are able to conduct electric currents that flow throughout the body. The electric activity is recorded in waveforms and complexes by an ECG and are analyzed with time intervals and segments. Continuous tracing of all the activities of each cardiac cycle is captured as heart cells are electrically stimulated, causing depolarizations and movement of the activity through the cells of the myocardium. The electric impulses that are generated are conducted via the fluid-containing tissues of the body to the surface and to the electrodes that are positioned in strategic places on the chest and extremities.[2] Analysis of the tracings obtained reveals varied diagnostic information about cardiac function.

The components of the cardiac cycle that are displayed and recorded and that serve as a basis for analysis of the ECG are the P, Q, R, S, T, and U waves (Fig. 23–1). The Q, R, and S waves are grouped and represent the QRS complex. Measurements are made in seconds or numbers of blocks on the tracing paper.

1. P waves record atrial depolarization as the impulse from the sinoatrial (SA) node spreads through the atria to produce an atrial contraction. When present and normal in amplitude and width, the waves confirm that the impulse originated in the SA node and not in an area outside the node.
2. QRS complex waves record ventricular depolarization associated with a

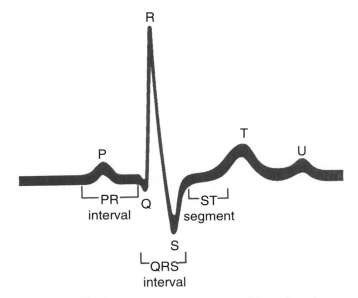

Figure 23–1   Wave, interval, and segment of the cardic cycle.

ventricular contraction. On the tracing in sequence, the Q wave is a small, downward or negative deflection; the R wave is a large, pointed, upward or positive deflection; and the S wave is a small, downward deflection. Any abnormal widening of this complex indicates a prolonged ventricular depolarization time.[3]

3. T waves record a period of ventricular repolarization with no electric activity after the QRS complex and they appear before another cardiac cycle begins.

4. PR interval is the time it takes for the impulse from the SA node to travel to the ventricle or atrioventricular (AV) node. It is the measured time between atrial depolarization (P wave begins) and onset of ventricular depolarization (QRS complex begins). A prolonged time indicates a delay in conduction activity.

5. QT or QRS interval is the time it takes for ventricular depolarization (Q wave begins) and repolarization (S wave ends).

6. ST segment is the period between the end of depolarization and the beginning of repolarization of the ventricular contraction.

7. PR segment is the period from the end of the P wave to the beginning of the QRS complex.

The ECG study is performed using 10 leads (electrodes) attached to the skin surface to obtain the total electric activity of the heart. Each lead records the electric potential between the limbs or between the heart and the limbs. The tracings are recorded on graph paper with vertical and horizontal lines for analysis. Time calculations are measured by the vertical lines (1 mm apart and 0.04 seconds per line), and voltage is measured by the horizontal lines (1 mm apart and 0.5 mV per 5 squares).[4] Pulse rate can be determined from the ECG strip by counting the number of large squares between each QRS complex and multiplying this number by 0.20 seconds (1 large square). To obtain the beats per minute, divide the result into 60 (the number of seconds in a minute).[5]

Vectorcardiography is another form of ECG; it has the ability to portray a three-dimensional display of the heart's activity as opposed to the two-dimensional display of the conventional ECG. The ECG records activity in the frontal and horizontal planes, and vectorcardiography records activity in the frontal, horizontal, and sagittal planes. The instrument displays three loops (P, QRS, and T) on the screen for each complete cardiac cycle, which correspond to the same waves on the ECG. These loop configurations can be recorded or photographed for analysis. This procedure is considered to be more sensitive and more specific in diagnosing such diseases as myocardial infarct and ventricular hypertrophy.[6]

Apexcardiography is a study that can be performed simultaneously with ECG or phonocardiography to record chest movements resulting from cardiac impulses. This study uses a transducer placed at the apical site that converts the impulses into waveforms recorded on an apexcardiogram.[7] The recording can be accompanied by tracings from the ECG and other procedures on the apexcardiogram and can provide additional information about the cardiac cycle in diagnosing ventricular abnormalities.

Reference Values

➤ Normal heart rate according to age, 60 to 100 beats per minute in adults

➤ Normal regular rhythm and wave deflections with normal measurement ranges of cycle components and height, depth, and duration of complexes

- P wave: 0.12 seconds, or three small blocks, with amplitude of 2.5 mm
- Q wave: less than 0.04 seconds
- R wave: amplitude range of 5 to 27 mm, depending on lead
- T wave: amplitude range of 1 to 13 mm, depending on lead
- QRS complex: 0.12 seconds, or three small blocks
- PR interval: 0.2 seconds, or five small blocks
- ST segment: 1 mm

➤ No arrhythmias, myocardial infarction, electrolyte imbalances, myocardial ischemia, chamber hypertrophy, or conduction abnormalities

➤ No myocardial infarction or ventricular hypertrophy with vectorcardiography

➤ No ventricular or heart sound abnormalities with apexcardiography

Interfering Factors

➤ Improper placement of electrodes, especially in conjunction with abnormal chest configuration or heart location within chest cavity; inadequate contact between skin and electrodes by ineffective conductive jelly or seal

➤ ECG machine malfunction or interference from electromagnetic rays in the vicinity

➤ Inability of client to remain still during the procedure

➤ Strenuous exercise before the procedure

➤ High level of anxiety and deep respirations or hyperventilation

➤ High intake of carbohydrates; electrolyte imbalances of potassium or calcium

➤ Distortions in cardiac cycle caused by age and gender, especially if the client is an infant or a woman

➤ Obesity, ascites, and pregnancy

➤ Medications such as barbiturates and digitalis preparations

Indications for Electrocardiography (ECG)

➤ Identification and diagnosis of cause of arrhythmias as revealed by abnormal wave deflections

➤ Determination of heart rate

➤ Determination of conduction defects or diseases revealed by delay of electric impulses, with abnormal time duration and amplitude of waves and intervals recorded on the strip

➤ Determination of the site and extent of myocardial or pulmonary infarction and myocardial ischemia revealed by abnormal wave and interval times and amplitudes

➤ Determination of hypertrophy of chambers of the heart (atrial and ventricular) or heart hypertrophy

➤ Determination of the position of the heart in the thoracic cavity

➤ Diagnosis of pericarditis and Wolff-Parkinson-White syndrome revealed by ventricular pre-excitation caused by accelerated AV conduction and changes in the QRS complex

➤ Suspected electrolyte imbalances of potassium, calcium, and magnesium and their effect on the heart

➤ Evaluation of drugs such as digitalis preparations and antiarrhythmics, vasodilators, and antihypertensives

➤ Evaluation of cardiac pacemaker function
➤ Monitoring of myocardial infarction during recovery
➤ Differentiation between possible causes of intraventricular conduction abnormalities and ventricular hypertrophy by vectorcardiography
➤ Suspected ventricular abnormalities

Contraindications

➤ None

➤➤ Nursing Alert

• If the ECG changes indicate severe ischemia or necrosis associated with myocardial infarction, immediate interventions should be carried out, such as administration of oxygen, sedation, antiarrhythmics, vasodilators, and other medications to control coronary artery spasms and tachycardia.

Nursing Care Before the Procedure

Explain to the client:
➤ That the procedure requires 15 minutes
➤ That there are no food or fluid restrictions but that smoking may be disallowed before the test
➤ That electrodes are attached to the skin of the chest, arms, and legs with a paste or pads and connected to the wires and ECG machine
➤ That the electric impulses from the heart are transmitted from the body and that no electricity is delivered to the body
➤ That no discomfort is associated with the procedure

Prepare for the procedure:
➤ Obtain a history of known or suspected cardiac disorders and present cardiovascular status, medication regimen, and associated diagnostic laboratory tests and procedures.
➤ Ensure that assessment of the cardiovascular system has been performed for use in interpretation of the study.

The Procedure

The client is placed on an examination table or in a bed in a supine position. The chest, arms, and legs are exposed and proper draping is done for privacy. A 5-minute rest period is allowed before the procedure. The sites for electrode placement are cleansed with alcohol. Excessive hair on the skin can be shaved, if necessary. The skin sites are dried and electrode paste is applied to provide conduction between the skin and the electrode. The electrodes are strapped in place on the extremities and placed in proper positions on the chest. Some newer electrodes do not need paste applied to the skin, as the backing is prepared with an adhesive electropaste that provides the conduction. The electrodes are color-coded for placement sites (chest, right and left arm, and right and left leg) and matched to coded lead wires with the sites labeled. The wires are connected to the matched electrodes and the ECG machine.

Ten leads are used in ECG to obtain and record the flow of electric impulses in different planes. Six unipolar precordial leads are placed on the chest: V_1 at the fourth intercostal space at the border of the right sternum, V_2 at the fourth intercostal space at the border of the left sternum, V_3 between V_2 and V_4, V_4 at the fifth intercostal space at the midclavicular line, V_5 at the level of V_4 horizontally and at the left axillary line, V_6 at the level of V_4 horizontally and at the left midaxillary line.[8] Three bipolar limb leads (two electrodes combined for each) are placed on the arms and legs. Lead I is the combination of two arm electrodes, lead II is the combination of right arm and left leg electrodes, and lead III is the combination of left arm and left leg electrodes.[9]

The client is reminded to lie still and to refrain from tensing muscles after electrode placement. The machine is set and turned on after the electrodes, grounding, connections, and paper supply are checked. The ECG machine records and marks the 10 leads on the strip in proper sequence, usually 6 inches of the strip for each lead.

The procedure is the same for vectorcardiography. Apexcardiography, which can be performed in conjunction with ECG or vectorcardiography, is performed by the placement of a transducer with electropaste over the apex of the heart or at the point of maximal impulse (PMI). The client is placed in the left side-lying position and is requested to perform different exercises such as breathing slowly, holding the breath, and using handgrips to determine the effect of these activities on ventricular function. The pulsations that are obtained by the transducer are converted to electric energy and recorded as waveforms that are identified as periods of systole and diastole on the paper strip.[10]

Nursing Care After the Procedure

➤ Remove the electrodes from the skin sites and cleanse the paste from the skin.
➤ Monitor the heart rate, rhythm, and pulse deficit for possible arrhythmias or in instances of chest pain experienced and noted on the strip during the procedure.
➤ *Decreased cardiac output (CO):* Note and report peripheral pulses, skin color, capillary refill time, dyspnea, abnormal heart sounds, angina, or decreased urinary output. Administer ordered oxygen and cardiac medications.
➤ *Arrhythmias:* Note and report cardiac rhythm abnormalities on the strip. Administer ordered oxygen, vasodilators, and antiarrhythmics if infarction or ischemia, life-threatening arrhythmias, or ventricular tachycardia is revealed.

HOLTER ELECTROCARDIOGRAPHY (ECG)

Holter electrocardiography (ECG), also known as ambulatory ECG monitoring, is an electrophysiologic study performed to record cardiac activity on a continuous basis for 24 to 48 hours. It is performed to identify rhythm abnormalities, to relate them with symptoms experienced by the client, and to evaluate the effectiveness of medication regimen and pacemaker function. The study includes the use of a portable device worn around the waist or over the shoulder that records cardiac electric impulses on a magnetic tape. The recorder has a clock that allows accurate time markings on the tape. When the client pushes a button indicating that symptoms (pain, palpitations, dyspnea, or syncope) have occurred, an event marker is placed on the tape for later evaluation. The study monitors heart activities during different types of daily activities engaged in by the client, such as sleeping, resting, walking, and working. Tapes are played back, interpreted, and summarized by a computer. The results can also be compared with data collected from documentation by the client in a journal and with the event markers on the tape, either of which can indicate the symptoms experienced during the monitoring period.

Reference Values

Normal sinus rhythm; no arrhythmias such as premature ventricular contractions, bradyarrhythmias, or tachyarrhythmias

Interfering Factors

➤ Improper placement of the electrodes or movement of the electrodes
➤ Failure of client to maintain a daily log of symptoms or to push the button to produce a mark on the strip when experiencing a symptom

Indications for Holter Electrocardiography (ECG)

➤ Detecting arrhythmias that occur during normal daily activities and correlating them with symptoms to determine whether they are caused by cardiac rhythm abnormalities
➤ Evaluating antiarrhythmic medications
➤ Monitoring for ischemia and arrhythmias after myocardial infarct or cardiac surgery
➤ Evaluating cardiac rehabilitation and other therapy regimens
➤ Evaluating pacemaker function

Contraindications

➤ Clients who are unable or unwilling to maintain the electrodes and ECG apparatus and the daily log of activities and symptoms

Nursing Care Before the Procedure

Client teaching and physical preparation are the same as for electrocardiography (see p. 855).
➤ Inform the client that the wires from the electrodes on the chest are connected to a portable ECG machine that is worn over the shoulder or on a belt at the waist for 24 to 48 hours.
➤ Instruct the client to avoid contact with electric devices such as shavers and toothbrushes, tight-fitting clothing over the electrodes, bathing, and disturbing or disconnecting the electrodes or wires.
➤ Instruct the client to maintain a log noting normal activities such as walking, sleeping, climbing stairs, sexual activity, cigarette smoking, and bowel or urinary elimination.
➤ Instruct the client to enter any symptoms experienced, such as chest pain, dizziness, fatigue, dyspnea, syncope, palpitations, or emotional upsets and to push the button on the monitor when these symptoms occur.

➤ Advise the client to return to the laboratory with the log to have the machine and strip removed and interpreted.

➤ Reassure the client that no electricity is delivered to the body during this procedure and that no discomfort is experienced during the monitoring process.

➤ Obtain a history that includes known or suspected cardiac disorders, cardiac medication regimen, and previous diagnostic tests and procedures.

The Procedure

The client is placed on the examination table in a supine position. The chest is exposed and the skin sites thoroughly cleansed with alcohol and rubbed until red in color. Excessive hair on the skin can be shaved. The electropaste is applied to the skin sites to provide conduction between the skin and the electrodes. Disk electrodes that are prelubricated and disposable can also be applied. The electrodes are applied over bony prominences rather than muscular areas, two on the manubrium (negative electrodes) and two in the V_1 (fourth intercostal space at the border of the right sternum) and V_5 (fifth intercostal space at the midclavicular line, horizontally and at the left axillary line) positions (positive electrodes).[11] A ground electrode is also placed and secured to the skin of the chest or abdomen. Check that the electrodes are secure; then attach the electrode cable to the monitor and the lead wires to the electrodes. The monitor is checked for paper supply and battery, the tape is inserted, and the recorder turned on. All wires are taped to the chest, and the belt or shoulder strap is placed in the proper position.

Nursing Care After the Procedure

➤ Care and assessment after the study include removing the tape and electrodes and cleansing the electropaste from the skin sites.

➤ Remove the monitor and retrieve the tape for analysis by the physician.

PHONOCARDIOGRAPHY

Phonocardiography is an electrophysiologic study performed to identify, amplify, and record heart sounds and murmurs. The sounds of blood flowing through the heart and great vessels are recorded from sites on the chest by a microphone containing a transducer that converts the sounds into electric impulses. Selected high- and low-frequency events are recorded on a graph. This recording is performed simultaneously with the ECG, and monitoring of the respiratory cycle and external cardiovascular impulse such as the carotid pulse, jugular venous pulse, and apexcardiography. They provide an accurate timing of the heart sounds and events for the detailed analysis of heart sounds, murmurs, and impulses that is not possible by bedside examination with a stethoscope. The phonogram allows visualization of the total duration of the cardiac cycle and valvular events when performed alone or in conjunction with the carotid or jugular pulse or with apexcardiography. Information is provided about the fourth heart sound (S_4), first heart sound (S_1), mitral valve closure, tricuspid valve closure, pulmonic valve closure, tricuspid valve opening, mitral valve opening, opening snap, third heart sound (S_3), and systolic time intervals.[12] Abnormalities in any of these events assist in the diagnosis of valvular heart disease and cardiomyopathies.

Reference Values

Normal heart sounds; no cardiac valvular disease

Interfering Factors

➤ Improper placement of the microphone on the chest, background noises, or other interferences

➤ The same factors that affect accurate results of ECG (see p. 854)

Indications for Phonocardiography

➤ Detecting valvular defects revealed by abnormal heart sounds: increased intensity of the first sound (S_1), heard in tricuspid or mitral stenosis, or lower frequency of the fourth sound (S_4), heard in aortic stenosis

➤ Differentiating between mitral and tricuspid opening snaps from the third sound (S_3) as revealed by a higher frequency of the snaps in phonocardiography

➤ Differentiating among early, mid, and late systolic murmurs

➤ Diagnosing hypertrophic cardiomyopathies and pulmonary hypertension revealed by the presence of the fourth sound (S_4) and murmurs

➤ Diagnosing abnormal left ventricular function revealed by changes in systolic time interval ratio, that is, left ventricular ejection and pre-ejection time

Nursing Care Before the Procedure

Client teaching and physical preparation are the same as for electrocardiography (see p. 855).

➤ Provide the client with additional information about the microphone strapped to the chest, position changes, and the need to perform several activities during the ECG procedure.

➤ Inform the client that other tests may be conducted during the procedure, such as carotid pulse and respiration recordings, and that the total study time is about 30 minutes.

The Procedure

The client is placed on the examination table in a supine position with the head elevated on a pillow in a quiet room. The ECG leads are placed on the appropriate skin sites and the monitors for the pulse, using a cuff around the neck and respiration recordings, are prepared. The microphones are then placed over the apex and pulmonary region and strapped in place. The client is requested to inhale and then exhale, while stopping the expiration as the recording is obtained. The microphone is moved from the pulmonary region to the aortic region and the procedure is repeated to obtain the recording. These recordings are followed by recordings made with the cuff removed from the neck and the recorder placed at the V_2 position (fourth intercostal space at the border of the left sternum) while the client is requested to hold the breath after exhaling.[13] Heart sounds can also be recorded with the client in a different position (left side-lying) and while breathing slowly or performing exercises.

Nursing Care After the Procedure

Care and assessment after the procedure are the same as for electrocardiography (see p. 856).

EXERCISE ELECTROCARDIOGRAPHY (ECG)

Exercise electrocardiography (ECG), also known as the stress test, is an electrophysiologic study performed to measure cardiac function during physical stress. It is performed to assist in diagnosing coronary artery disease (CAD) and to evaluate the safe level of activity or activity tolerance for work or cardiac rehabilitation. The physical stress is provided by walking on a treadmill, climbing stairs, or pedaling an exercise bicycle, with the treadmill most commonly used. The heart, pulse, and blood pressure are monitored continuously during the procedure by ECG, pulse, and blood pressure devices. The client exercises to 80 to 90 percent of the maximal heart rate determined by age and gender. This rate is known as the target heart rate.[14] Changes in the ECG (arrhythmias), blood pressure (hypotension), pulse (tachycardia), respirations (dyspnea), and symptoms such as chest pain and extreme fatigue during the procedure indicate a reduction in cardiac efficiency and presence of or risk for heart disease. The test is discontinued if these abnormalities occur. The risks involved in the procedure are possible myocardial infarct and death in those experiencing frequent anginal episodes before the test.

Although useful, this procedure is not as accurate in diagnosing CAD as are the nuclear scans, thallium 201 (^{201}Tl) cardiac stress studies (see pp. 744 to 749) or multiple gated cardiac stress studies using technetium 99m (^{99m}Tc) labeled with red blood cells (see pp. 745 to 746). Exercise ECG is primarily useful in determining the extent of coronary artery occlusion by the heart's ability to meet the need for additional oxygen in response to the stress of exercising.

Reference Values

Normal heart rate during physical exercise; no cardiac abnormalities on the ECG or presence of associated symptoms at 80 to 90 percent of maximal heart rate based on client age and gender

Interfering Factors

- Improper placement of electrodes, improper conduction, or improper ECG machine function
- High food intake or smoking before the testing
- Medications such as β-blockers, cardiac glycosides, calcium channel blockers, and coronary vasodilators
- Cardiac conditions such as hypertension, valvular heart defects, left bundle branch block, left ventricular hypertrophy, and other conditions such as anemia, hypoxia, and chronic obstructive pulmonary disease (COPD)[15]

Indications for Exercise Electrocardiography (ECG)

- Suspected CAD in the presence of chest pain and other symptoms
- Screening for CAD in the absence of pain and other symptoms in those who are at risk
- Diagnosis of heart abnormalities such as tachycardia, bradycardia, and arrhythmias during exercising as revealed by ECG changes
- Evaluation of cardiac function after myocardial infarction or cardiac surgery in order to determine safe cardiac rehabilitation exercise and work limitations
- Determination of hypertension as a result of exercise

➤ Detection of peripheral arterial occlusive disease (intermittent claudication) revealed by leg pain or cramping during exercise

➤ Evaluation of effectiveness of medication regimens: antianginals or antiarrhythmics

Contraindications

➤ Frequent anginal episodes or presence of chest pain

➤ Myocardial infarction unless limitations are placed on testing activities

➤ Uncontrolled arrhythmias, dissecting aortic aneurysm, aortic valvular disease, or inflammatory conditions of the cardiac muscles

➤ Inability of client to walk or pedal because of motor disability or impaired lung function

Nursing Care Before the Procedure

Client teaching and physical preparation are the same as for the electrocardiography procedures (see p. 855).

➤ Food, fluids, and smoking are avoided for at least 4 hours before the test (see p. 860).

➤ Instruct the client to wear comfortable shoes and clothing for the exercises and inform the client that fatigue, sweating, and breathlessness can occur during the test as the speed is increased.

➤ Inform the client that a total time of 45 to 90 minutes is needed to complete the procedure. Provide assurance that the test has very few risks and that exercising can be terminated if extreme symptoms occur.

➤ Instruct the client to discontinue specific medications that interfere with test results before the study.

➤ Obtain baseline vital signs and ECG to use as a comparison in evaluating the study.

The Procedure

The skin sites are cleansed with alcohol and rubbed until red and the electrodes are placed in the appropriate positions. Clothing from the waist up is removed from a male client, and a hospital gown that opens in the front can be worn by a female client. A physician is in attendance during this study. A blood pressure cuff is applied to the arm and connected to a monitoring device. Oxygen consumption using a mouthpiece can also be monitored continuously by blood pressure and ECG. A baseline ECG tracing and a blood pressure reading are obtained. Heart sounds are auscultated and recorded if the physician requests or performs this physical assessment. The client is requested to walk on a treadmill (most commonly used) or pedal a bicycle after the setting of the apparatus to stages of increased grade and miles per hour. As the stress is increased, the client is requested to report any symptoms such as chest or leg pain, dyspnea, or fatigue. The stress is increased until the client's maximal heart rate is reached. The client is reminded that symptoms such as dizziness or nausea can be experienced and are normal. The test is terminated if pain or fatigue is severe or when maximum heart rate under stress is attained. A 3- to 10-minute rest period in a sitting position follows the exercise period, during which time the ECG, blood pressure, and heart rate are monitored. The results are read and interpreted by the physician.

Nursing Care After the Procedure

➤ Provide a period of rest and monitor vital signs and ECG in 3-, 10-, and 30-minute intervals.

➤ Remove the electrodes and paste and cleanse the skin sites.

➤ *Cardiac arrhythmias:* Note and report abnormal ECG cardiac cycle impulses. Terminate test and administer ordered medication (antiarrythmics).

➤ *Myocardial infarction:* Note and report chest pain and abnormal ECG recordings, pallor, skin mottling, and diaphoresis. Terminate test and administer ordered oxygen and medications (morphine sulfate).

➤ *Anginal pain:* Note and report chest pain, fatigue, and cyanosis. Terminate test and administer ordered oxygen and medications (vasodilators).

➤ *Dizziness or fainting:* Note and report extreme faintness, confusion, and dizziness. Terminate test and allow the client to sit on a chair. Administer an ordered stimulant.

SIGNAL-AVERAGED ELECTROCARDIOGRAPHY (SAE)

Signal-averaged electrocardiography (SAE) is an electrophysiologic study performed to determine the risk for ventricular arrhythmias in those clients who have experienced myocardial infarction. It is similar to conventional ECG except that the electrodes are placed at different sites and a computer is used to supply signal averaging, amplification, and electric potentials. These readings are analyzed to provide diagnostic information about late potentials (signals produced by the myocardium) based on the averaging of a large number of heartbeats. The late potentials then are evaluated in the diagnosis of myocardial pathology and sustained ventricular tachycardia that can place a client at risk for sudden death. The study can be followed with the His bundle electrophysiology study by cardiac catheterization if findings are not definitive for ventricular tachycardia (see p. 886).[16]

Reference Values

Normal complex (QRS) and segment (ST); no ventricular arrhythmias or risk for arrhythmias

Interfering Factors

➤ Improper placement of electrodes or inadequate contact between the skin and the electrodes

➤ Inability of client to remain quiet during the procedure

➤ Electrical equipment in the vicinity

➤ Conditions such as ventricular tachycardia and bundle branch block, which affect obtaining late potentials and impulse averaging

➤ Insufficient time to obtain heartbeats if the rate is slow or if ectopic beats are present[17]

Indications for Signal-Averaged Electrocardiography (SAE)

➤ Screening of high-risk clients for arrhythmias, especially individuals with postmyocardial infarct and those in need of His bundle study to diagnose ventricular tachycardia

➤ Unexplained symptoms such as syncope that could be caused by ventricular tachycardia

➤ Diagnosis of CAD as revealed by late potentials

➤ Determination of sustained ventricular tachycardia and potential for sudden death, which are associated with late potentials

➤ Diagnosis of delayed conduction in the myocardium in conditions such as infarction, hypertrophic cardiomyopathy, ventricular aneurysm, and congenital ventricular defects

Nursing Care Before the Procedure

Client teaching and physical preparation are the same as for electrocardiography (see p. 855).

➤ Inform the client that electrodes will also be placed on the abdomen and on the front and back of the chest and that the study takes 20 to 30 minutes.

The Procedure

The client is prepared in the same way as for ECG (see p. 855). The electrodes are placed on the abdomen and on the anterior and posterior areas of the chest. The high-frequency, low-amplitude signals from the cardiac myocardium are converted into digital signals, which are compared with normal cardiac cycle signals, mainly the QRS complex. A number of heartbeats are averaged to obtain late potentials, which are indicative of ventricular tachycardia, other ventricular abnormalities, or myocardial infarction.

Nursing Care After the Procedure

Care and assessment after the procedure are the same as for electrocardiography (see p. 856).

➤ *Arrhythmias:* Note and report cardiac rhythm abnormalities on the strip. Administer ordered oxygen, vasodilators, and antiarrhythmics if infarction or ischemia, life-threatening arrhythmias, or ventricular tachycardia is revealed.

PELVIC FLOOR SPHINCTER ELECTROMYOGRAPHY

Pelvic floor sphincter electromyography, also known as rectal electromyography, is an electrophysiologic study performed to measure and record the adequacy of urinary or anal sphincter muscle function. Rectal muscle pressure is usually performed to measure abdominal pressure. Urethral muscle pressure is performed to evaluate the neuromuscular function of the external sphincter during urination to determine the flow rate and other urinary pattern disturbances. The external sphincter muscle surrounds the urethra distal to the bladder base and functions to terminate urination while it occurs and to maintain continence when bladder pressure increases as the bladder fills with urine. Muscles located on the pelvic floor support the bladder and also contribute to continence.[18] Electrodes are placed on the surface of or within the muscle to be tested and recordings are made of muscle activity before and during the process of voiding. The recordings are evaluated for changes that indicate neurogenic bladder or other urinary dysfunctions such as incontinence. The study can be performed in combination with manometric urodynamic studies such as cystometry (see p. 830), uroflowmetry (see p. 833), or urethral pressure profile (see p. 835).

Reference Values

Normal urinary and anal sphincter muscle function; increased electromyographic signals during the filling of the urinary bladder and at the conclusion of voiding; absence of signals during the actual voiding; no incontinence

Interfering Factors

➤ Inability of client to remain still or to cooperate with requests for movement during the procedure

➤ Improper placement of surface or needle electrodes

Indications for Pelvic Floor Sphincter Electromyography (EMG)

➤ Evaluation of lower urinary sphincter muscle function during voiding to diagnose neuromuscular dysfunction

➤ Evaluation of voluntary sphincter muscle activity and pelvic floor muscles in the presence of incontinence or other urinary problems

➤ Suspected detrusor hyperreflexia in neuromuscular dysfunction

➤ Ruling out of psychological factors in urinary dysfunction

Nursing Care Before the Procedure

Explain to the client:

➤ That the procedure requires 30 minutes

➤ That there are no food, fluid, or other restrictions before the study

➤ That electrodes are placed on the perineal area and the leg or that needles are inserted into the muscle and that recordings are made during the procedure

➤ That discomfort is minimal from the insertion of the catheter and the testing of muscle activity

Prepare for the procedure:

➤ Obtain a history of neuromuscular and genitourinary status, medical treatment and medication regimens, and previous tests and procedures performed for urinary function.

➤ Have client void immediately before the study.

The Procedure

The client is placed on the examination table in a supine position and draped to expose the perineal area. Two skin electrodes are positioned at the perianal area slightly to the left and right of the anterior portion, and a grounding electrode is placed on the thigh. If needle electrodes are used, they are inserted into the muscle surrounding the urethra. Muscle activity signals are recorded as waves that are interpreted for numbers and configurations in diagnosing urinary abnormalities. The client is reminded to lie quietly and relax. A Foley catheter is inserted and the bulbocavernous reflex is tested by asking the client to cough while the catheter is carefully tugged. Then voluntary control is tested by asking the client to contract and relax the muscle. Electric activity is recorded during this period of relaxation with the bladder empty. The bladder is filled with 100 mL of sterile water per minute while the electric activity during filling is recorded. The catheter is then removed; the client is placed in a position to void and is requested to urinate to empty the full bladder. This voluntary urination is then recorded until completed. The complete test includes recordings of electric signals before, during, and at the end of urination.[19]

Nursing Care After the Procedure

➤ Care and assessment after the study include removal of the electrodes and cleansing of the sites.

➤ Monitor the sites for pain, redness, swelling, and hematoma if needle electrodes are used.

➤ *Inflammation from needle electrodes:* Note and report pain, swelling, and redness at the insertion sites. Administer an ordered analgesic. Apply warm compresses.

ELECTROMYOGRAPHY (EMG)

Electromyography (EMG) is an electrophysiologic study performed to determine the electric activity of specific muscles to assist in the diagnosis of muscular diseases and the effects of other diseases on muscles. Skeletal muscle activity is measured during rest, voluntary contraction, and electric stimulation. Comparison and analysis of the amplitude, duration, number, and configuration of the muscle activity provide diagnostic information about the extent of nerve and muscle involvement in neuromuscular disorders. Responses of a relaxed muscle are electrically silent, but fibrillation and fasciculations can be detected in a relaxed denervated muscle. Muscle action potentials are detected with minimal or maximal muscle contractions. The differences in the size and numbers of activity potentials during voluntary contractions determine whether the muscle weakness is myogenic or neurogenic.[20] A signed informed consent form is required for this study.

Nerve conduction studies or electroneurography (see p. 874) is commonly performed in conjunction with electromyography and the combination of the procedures is known as electromyoneurography. This study is performed to assist in diagnosing diseases of and damage to the peripheral nerves. It can test both motor and sensory nerve abnormalities.

Reference Values

Normal muscle electric activity during rest and contraction states; no neuromuscular disorders or primary muscle diseases

Interfering Factors

➤ Inability of client to remain still and to cooperate with instructions during the procedure

➤ Hemorrhage, edema, excessive subcutaneous fat, and pain

➤ Increased age

➤ Medications such as muscle relaxants, cholinergics, and anticholinergics

Indications for Electromyography (EMG)

➤ Diagnosing primary muscle diseases affecting striated muscle fibers or cell membrane: muscular dystrophy or myasthenia gravis

➤ Diagnosing secondary muscle disorders caused by polymyositis, sarcoidosis, hypocalcemia, thyroid toxicity, tetanus, and other disorders

- Diagnosing neuromuscular disorders such as peripheral neuropathy caused by diabetes or alcoholism
- Diagnosing muscle disorders caused by diseases of the lower motor neurons involving the motor neurons on the anterior horn of the spinal cord: anterior poliomyelitis, amyotrophic lateral sclerosis, amyotonia, or tumors
- Diagnosing muscle disorders caused by diseases of the lower motor neuron involving the nerve root: Guillain-Barré syndrome, herniated disk, or spinal stenosis
- Differentiating between primary and secondary muscle disorders or neuropathy and myopathy as revealed by differences in the amplitude, duration, number, and configurations of the electric activity
- Determining whether a muscle abnormality is caused by drugs (antibiotics, chemotherapy) or toxins (botulism, snake venom, heavy metals)
- Monitoring and evaluating myopathies or neuropathies[21]

Contraindications

- Medication regimen that includes anticoagulant therapy
- Infection near or at the sites of electrode placement

Nursing Care Before the Procedure

Client teaching and physical preparation are the same as for pelvic floor sphincter EMG (see p. 864).

- Inform the client that the study takes about 1 to 3 hours, depending on the extent of the problem and the areas to be studied.
- Advise the client to avoid cigarette smoking and caffeine beverages 3 hours before the study.
- Inform the client that the sites of needle insertion are the areas to be studied, usually the muscles of an extremity.
- Administer an ordered analgesic or, if the client is a child, a sedative.
- Obtain a history and assessment of neuromuscular and neurosensory status, diseases or conditions that affect muscle function, level of muscular function and range of motion, traumatic events, and previous diagnostic tests and procedures associated with the neuromuscular system.

The Procedure

The client is placed on the examination table in a supine position or on a chair in a sitting position, depending on the location of the muscles to be tested. The area or room is protected from noise or metallic interferences, which can affect test results. An electrode is applied to the skin to ground the client. A 24-gauge needle containing a fine wire electrode is inserted into the muscle. The electric potentials of the muscle are amplified, fed into a loudspeaker, displayed on a screen in waveforms, and recorded on a magnetic tape all at the same time. As many as 10 needle electrodes can be inserted to detect the electricity in the muscle. The client is forewarned of the pain caused by the needle insertions. During the test, the muscle activity is tested at rest, during incremental needle insertion, and during varying degrees of muscle contraction. This testing is accomplished by requesting that the client maintain a relaxed muscle state or perform progressive muscle contractions while the potentials are being measured. A muscle in the relaxed state is usually electrically silent, but fibrillations and fasciculations are detected in a relaxed denervated muscle. Minimal and maximal contractions reveal single action or fused patterns of muscle potentials. A reduction in size or amplitude of the electric waveforms indicates muscle abnormality.[22]

Nerve conduction studies (electroneurography) that are conducted in conjunction with EMG are usually performed before muscle potential testing (see p. 867).

Nursing Care After the Procedure

➤ Remove the electrodes from the sites and cleanse the skin.
➤ Assess the sites for hematoma or inflammation, and administer an ordered analgesic for pain as needed.
➤ Provide time for the client to rest if needed.
➤ *Inflammation at electrode sites:* Note and report pain, swelling, and redness at the insertion sites. Administer ordered analgesic. Apply warm compresses.
➤ *Hematoma at electrode sites:* Note and report hematoma formation. Administer ordered medication and treatments. Provide rest, immobilize part, and position for comfort.

ELECTRONEUROGRAPHY

Electroneurography, or nerve conduction study, is an electrophysiologic study performed to determine peripheral nerve disease or injury by the measurement of nerve conduction velocity. It is performed to provide diagnostic information about the location and nature of peripheral nerve abnormalities. Both motor and sensory nerves can be tested by using electrodes placed on the skin surface, recording the electric stimuli to a peripheral nerve and the muscle contraction response, and then analyzing the time and velocities between the two. Nerve conduction velocities remain normal in the presence of muscle disease, but conduction velocity is slowed in diseases that affect peripheral nerves, with the extent depending on the pathology.

The presence of a muscular disease requires that conduction studies for peripheral nerve abnormalities be performed after the evaluation of a decreased velocity that can be caused by the muscle pathology. This evaluation can be accomplished by determining the time required for stimulation of the distal end of the nerve to produce muscle contraction (distal latency), followed by stimulation of the proximal part of the nerve. This variable is included in the calculation of conduction velocity by dividing the distance in meters by the difference between the total and distal latency.[23]

Reference Values

Normal nerve conduction velocity rates; no peripheral or axial nerve damage or disease

Interfering Factors

➤ Nerve conduction decreases with age and this should be considered when test results are analyzed.

➤ Severe pain can affect test performance.
➤ Inability of client to remain still or to cooperate during the study.

Indications for Electroneurography

➤ Suspected peripheral nerve degenerative diseases
➤ Evaluation of peripheral neuropathies resulting from diabetes, as revealed by a reduced conduction velocity rate
➤ Evaluation of nerve damage or transection as in carpal tunnel syndrome
➤ Suspected damage to peripheral nerves by toxic substances such as solvents, heavy metals, and antimicrobials
➤ Differentiation between muscle disease and peripheral nerve disease revealed by normal as opposed to reduced conduction velocity

Nursing Care Before the Procedure

Client teaching and physical preparation are the same as for electromyography (see p. 866).

➤ Inform the client that, instead of needle electrodes, surface-stimulating electrodes with electropaste are applied and taped to the nerve site (leg, arm, or face).
➤ Inform the client that an electric current is passed through the electrode and that a mild sensation is experienced for the length of time the current is applied.

The Procedure

The client is placed on the examination table in a position that allows exposure of the areas to be studied. The surface-stimulating electrode is placed over the nerve to be studied near the placement of the recording electrode. The electrodes are prepared with electropaste to ensure proper contact with the skin. A device produces the shock, and movement of the stimulating electrode along the nerve assists in determining the location of nerve damage. The client is reminded that a shock is felt each time stimulation is administered. Time is measured from stimulation to muscle activation or response between two stimulating sites (distal latency). The time for the stimulation to travel from the site to muscle activity (total latency) reveals the velocity of nerve conduction; this time is recorded in milliseconds (ms). Distances between the stimulation and recording electrodes are measured in centimeters (cm). The conduction velocity is calculated by dividing the distance by the difference between total latency and distal latency and is recorded in meters per second.[24]

Results from the studies indicate the presence of abnormalities based on nerve conduction velocities. If the velocities remain normal, the weakness is caused by muscle weakness, although muscle action potentials during repeated stimulation of a nerve can reveal disorders of the neuromuscular junction. If the velocities are slowed, diseases affecting the peripheral nerves are suspected.[25]

Nursing Care After the Procedure

Aftercare and nursing observations after the study are the same as for electromyography (see p. 867).

ELECTROENCEPHALOGRAPHY (EEG)

Electroencephalography (EEG) is an electrophysiologic study performed to measure the electric activity of the brain cells. It is conducted to assist in diagnosing and evaluating the course of structural abnormalities involving the brain. Electrodes are placed at 8 to 16 sites or at pairs of sites on the scalp and connected to an amplifier. Recordings of waveforms on a moving paper strip during sleep and waking periods reveal patterns characteristic of specific disorders. Guidelines for electrode placement and the use of a uniform lettering and numbering system to obtain the recordings are standardized for each client and allow comparison of repeated studies on a single client.[26]

The study can be performed at the bedside in the comatose client, although this environment cannot be controlled in a way necessary to obtain diagnostic information. Evoked brain potentials can also be obtained during EEG to measure nerve tract activity by stimulation of the sensory system (see p. 871).

Another study, known as brain mapping, is similar to EEG in procedure. It produces and displays a color-coded map of computer-analyzed EEG signals for amplitude and distribution of alpha, beta, theta, and delta frequencies. It can also map evoked potential responses in determining latency increases and cognitive function abnormalities. It is undertaken to specifically locate a problem site in the brain in a general area of deficit revealed by conventional EEG. It is useful in obtaining diagnostic information about headaches, seizure activity, dementia and its possible causes, and psychiatric abnormalities.[27]

Reference Values

Normal brain structure and function; electric activity characteristics with waveforms that indicate normal EEG signals in frequency and amplitude

Interfering Factors

➤ Inability of client to remain still and to refrain from moving facial muscles, mouth, head, or eyes during the study
➤ Medications such as sedatives, anticonvulsants, antiaxolytics, or alcohol
➤ Caffeine-containing beverages or other stimulants
➤ Hypoglycemia or hypothermia
➤ Hair that is dirty, oily, or has had hairspray or other preparations applied can affect electrode placement and contact

Indications for Electroencephalography (EEG)

➤ Diagnosis and evaluation of epilepsy and seizure activity
➤ Suspected intracranial cerebrovascular lesions such as hemorrhages and infarcts
➤ Suspected intracranial lesions such as tumors (glioblastoma) or abscesses
➤ Suspected metabolic disorders or inflammatory process (encephalitis)
➤ Suspected increased intracranial pressure caused by trauma or disease
➤ Mapping of area of abnormality in dementia, especially Alzheimer's disease, or of focal irritation in migraine headaches and psychiatric disorders such as schizophrenia or psychosis
➤ Evaluation of sleep disorders such as apnea and narcolepsy
➤ Evaluation of the effect of drug intoxication on the brain

➤ Detection of cerebral ischemia during endarterectomy
➤ Determination of brain death in nonresponsive clients

Nursing Care Before the Procedure

Explain to the client:
➤ That the procedure requires 1 to 2 hours
➤ That a meal should be eaten before the test to prevent a hypoglycemic state but that caffeine-containing beverages should be avoided for 8 hours before the test
➤ That some medications are discontinued before the study but that anticonvulsants should be taken unless the physician temporarily discontinues them before the test
➤ That the hair should be shampooed the night before the test and hair preparations should not be applied
➤ That sleep time the night before the test should be limited to 5 hours for an adult and 7 hours for a child; young children and infants should not be allowed to nap before the test
➤ That small electrodes are attached to the scalp with a paste substance and connected to wires attached to a machine that records the brain waves
➤ That electricity flows from the body and not into the body during the study
➤ That the test reveals only brain activity—not thoughts, feelings, or intelligence
➤ That no pain is associated with the study
Prepare for the procedure:
➤ Obtain a history and assessment of the neurological system, known or suspected seizure activity, intracranial abnormalities, sleep disorders, associated diagnostic laboratory tests and procedures, and medication regimen.
➤ Ensure that caffeine-containing beverages and medications have been withheld and that a meal has been ingested before the study.
➤ Ensure that the client is able to relax. Report any extreme anxiety or restlessness.
➤ Ensure that the hair is clean and free of hair sprays, gels, or lotions.

The Procedure

The client is placed on a bed in a supine position or on a recliner in a semi-Fowler's position in a special room protected from any noise or electric interferences that could affect the tracings. A window in the room allows the technician to observe the client for movements or other interferences during the study. The client is reminded to relax and not to move any muscles or parts of the face or head. The electrodes are prepared with paste and applied to the scalp to provide conduction of the electric activity between the skin and the electrode. Electrodes are small metal disks connected to the amplifier by wires and positioned on the scalp after standards for placement. As many as 16 locations over the frontal, temporal, parietal, and occipital areas of both sides of the head can be used. Electrodes are attached to each earlobe as grounders. At this time, a baseline recording can be made with the client at rest.

As the test begins, recordings are made with the client at rest with the eyes closed. Recordings are also made during drowsy and sleep periods, depending on the client's clinical condition and symptoms. A period in which the recording is stopped and movement is allowed during the test is provided about every 5 minutes. In certain instances, procedures are undertaken to bring out abnormal patterns: hyperventilation for 3 minutes to produce a state of alkalosis, which could record a seizure pattern or other abnormalities; stroboscopic light stimulation to record seizure activity produced by photic stimulation; or sleep induction by administration of a sedative to detect abnormalities that occur only during sleep through recording of activity while falling asleep, during sleep, and during waking. Observations for seizure activity are carried out during the study and a description and the time of the activity are noted by the technician. Frequencies and sites of alpha, beta, delta, and theta waves are recorded and compared with normal values in analyzing the EEG results.

Brain mapping or computed tomography is performed in the same manner as an EEG study except that 42 electrodes are placed on the scalp and the study is performed while the client is awake and at rest. The skin on the scalp is prepared by cleansing with an omniprep solution before the electrodes are attached to the skin with an adhesive paste. The client is requested to keep the eyes closed and to remain very still during the complete study. The color map of the brain's electric activity is displayed for analysis. Comparisons are made with normal reference values for amplitude, and distribution of the different frequencies is recorded.[28]

Nursing Care After the Procedure

➤ Care and assessment after the study include removing the electrodes and paste from the scalp and hair with acetone.

➤ Provide a shampoo to remove the substance from the hair.

➤ Inform the client to resume medications that were withheld before the study.

➤ Allow clients who received sedatives sufficient time to rest and provide safety precautions to prevent injury: side rails for bedridden clients or assistance with transportation for outpatients.

➤ Perform neurological checks and provide seizure precautions if the client's condition is not stable.

➤ Inform the client that normal activity can be resumed after the rest period.

➤ *Seizure activity:* Note and report time and observations of seizure. Perform seizure precautions to prevent injury. Administer anticonvulsive after the study if it has been withheld.

EVOKED BRAIN POTENTIALS

Evoked brain potentials, also known as cortical evoked responses, are electrophysiologic studies performed to measure the electric responses in brain waves when stimulated by various sensory stimuli or skin electrodes. They include the visual evoked response (VER), auditory brainstem evoked response (ABR), and somatosensory evoked response (SER). The stimuli activate the nerve tracts that connect the stimulated area (receptor area) with the cortical (visual and somatosensory) or midbrain (auditory) sensory area. A series of stimuli are given, electronically displayed in waveforms, and recorded. Abnormalities are determined by a delay in time between the stimulus and the response, also known as an increased latency, and measured in milliseconds (ms). The latency factor used to diagnose these abnormalities is influenced by client size; area of stimulation; number of synapses; speed of axons at the location studied, whether the nerves are located in the cortex or in the brainstem; and effects of pathological processes on the central nervous system (CNS).[29] Evoked brain potential studies are performed to assist in determining structural and functional abnormalities of organs and providing diagnostic information about neurological diseases or surgical procedures that cause changes in the sensory pathways.

The studies are especially useful in clients with behavior problems and those unable to speak or respond to instructions during the test, because their voluntary cooperation or participation in the activity is not required. This benefit allows objective diagnostic information about visual or auditory disorders affecting infants and children and differentiation between organic brain and psychological disorders in adults.

Another study, known as event-related potential (ERP), can be performed using the same methodology as for the auditory response study to measure mental function in the presence of neurological disorders that cause cognitive changes or abnormalities. Abnormalities are revealed by the ability of cognitive function to process a specific tone (P_3), evidenced by the latency increases resulting from dementia disorders or decreased mental functioning. Because P_3 increases normally with age, the latency is compared with the normal age-matched value in evaluating test results for dementia. As with the other evoked potential studies, this test has the advantage of objectivity and can be performed on clients who are unable or unwilling to cooperate or participate in differentiating between organic brain disorder and cognitive function abnormality.[30]

Reference Values

Normal latency in recorded cortical and brainstem waveforms, depending on age, gender, and stature; no neurological lesions or sensory disorders associated with the CNS

Interfering Factors

➤ Inability of client to understand instructions or to cooperate with requests made during the study
➤ Improper placement of electrodes

Indications for Evoked Brain Potentials

Visual Evoked Potentials
➤ Diagnosis of neurological disorders such as Parkinson's disease, Huntington's chorea, and multiple sclerosis (MS) as revealed by abnormal bilateral latency resulting from the demyelination of nerve fibers
➤ Diagnosis of cryptic or past retrobulbar neuritis revealed by abnormal latency or lengthened conduction time along optic pathways
➤ Determination of optic pathway lesions and visual cortex defects revealed by abnormal latency
➤ Diagnosis of lesions of the eye or optic nerves revealed by an extended latency
➤ Evaluation of binocularity in infants

Auditory Evoked Potentials
➤ Detection of abnormalities or lesions in the brainstem or auditory nerves that cannot be diagnosed by other diagnostic methods
➤ Suspected hearing loss (peripheral) and screening or evaluation of low-birth-weight neonates, infants, children, and adults for auditory problems
➤ Early detection of brainstem tumors and acoustic neuromas, revealed by abnormal latency responses

Somatosensory Evoked Potentials
➤ Evaluation of spinal cord and brain injury and function
➤ Diagnosis of sensorimotor neuropathies and cervical pathology revealed by abnormal latencies in the upper limb studies
➤ Diagnosis of MS and Guillain-Barré syndrome as revealed by abnormal latencies in the lower limb studies
➤ Monitoring of sensory potentials to determine spinal cord function during a surgical procedure or medical regimen

Nursing Care Before the Procedure

Client teaching and physical preparation are the same as for electroencephalography (see p. 870).
➤ Inform the client that the electrodes are placed in specific positions on the scalp and stimuli are provided, depending on which study is being performed.
➤ Inform the client that there are no food, fluid, or medication restrictions and that the study takes about 30 minutes.
➤ Obtain a history that includes known and suspected neurological conditions, changes in sensory perception, and traumatic incidents to the head or spinal cord.

The Procedure

Visual Evoked Potentials. The client is placed in a comfortable position at a specific distance from the stimulation source. The electrodes are attached to the occipital and vertex lobes, and a reference electrode is attached to the ear. A light-emitting stimulation or a checkerboard pattern is projected on a screen at a regulated speed. This procedure is performed for each eye as the client is requested to look at a dot on the screen with one eye covered while the stimuli are delivered. A computer interprets the brain's responses to the stimuli and records them in waveforms.

Auditory Evoked Potentials. The client is placed in a comfortable position and the electrodes are positioned on the scalp at the vertex lobe and on each earlobe. Earphones are placed in the client's ears, and a clicking stimulus is delivered into one ear while a continuous tone is delivered to the opposite ear. The response to the stimuli is recorded as waveforms for analysis.

Somatosensory Evoked Potentials. The client is placed in a comfortable position and the electrodes are positioned at the nerve sites of the wrist, knee, and ankle and on the scalp at the sensory cortex of the hemisphere on the opposite side (the electrode that picks up the response and delivers it to the recorder).

Additional electrodes can be positioned at the cervical or lumbar vertebrae for upper or lower limb stimulation. The rate at which the electric shock stimulus is delivered to the nerve electrodes and travels to the brain is measured, interpreted by a computer, and recorded in waveforms for analysis. Both sides can be tested by switching the electrodes and repeating the procedure.[31]

Nursing Care After the Procedure

Aftercare and nursing observations after the study include removing the electrodes and paste and cleansing the scalp, hair, and skin sites.

ELECTRONYSTAGMOGRAPHY (ENG)

Electronystagmography (ENG) is an electrophysiologic study performed to measure the direction and degree of nystagmus. Nystagmus is the involuntary back-and-forth eye movement resulting from initiation of the vestibulo-ocular reflex, which maintains visual fixation when the head's position is changed. The vestibular system also maintains body balance through postural reflexes. This study evaluates the vestibulo-ocular reflex, which is the relationship between the vestibular system and the muscles that control eye movements. It is performed by measurement of electric responses of and around the eye at rest and to various stimuli applied to the eye to elicit nystagmus: positioning, caloric stimulation, gaze change, and pendulum movement.[32]

The duration and velocity of the eye movements recorded are compared with normal values, with prolonged nystagmus indicating an abnormality in the vestibular or ocular system. Abnormalities of the vestibular system are characterized by vertigo and manifestations such as nausea, vomiting, and perspiration. Tinnitus and hearing impairment can also result from abnormal nystagmus. Nystagmus that is controlled by the vestibular system is known as the slow phase, in which the eyes move in opposite directions to maintain a fixation point in the visual field. Nystagmus that is controlled by the CNS is known as the fast phase, in which an eye correction takes place to obtain a new fixation point (saccadic return) if the head is rotated beyond the range of lateral eye movement. The described slow-fast phases of nystagmus are the result of sensory organ or vestibular nerve function. Nystagmus that involves equal rates in the direction of eye movements (vertical, horizontal, rotary, mixed) is the result of CNS pathology.[33]

Reference Values

Normal nystagmic response during the turning of the head and normal oculo-vestibular reflex; no hearing loss or lesions of the ocular or vestibular systems

Interfering Factors

➤ Inability of client to understand or to cooperate by refraining from blinking the eyes
➤ Improper placement of electrodes around the eyes
➤ Visual impairment that prevents the ability to cooperate
➤ Medications such as sedatives, stimulants, depressants, and antivertiginics, which can prevent the client from cooperating in the test, suppress nystagmus, or produce other eye movements

Indications for Electronystagmography (ENG)

➤ Dizziness, vertigo, or tinnitus
➤ Suspected lesions of the CNS (brainstem and cerebellum)
➤ Location of an abnormality: tumors, cerebral brain damage, circulatory disorders, or demyelinating diseases[34]
➤ Suspected lesions of the peripheral system (end organ or vestibular branch of the eighth cranial nerve): tumors, middle ear infection, ototoxicity from drugs, food allergies, head trauma, balance instability, Ménière's disease, or changes caused by advancing age
➤ Differentiation between nystagmus caused by the peripheral nervous system and that caused by the CNS
➤ Diagnosis of congenital disorders in infants
➤ Determination of cause of hearing loss

Contraindications

➤ Perforated eardrum if water calorics test is to be performed, unless the test is modified by placing a fingercot in the canal
➤ Presence of a pacemaker because the test can interfere with its function
➤ Disorders of the neck that prevent position changes of the head during the tests

Nursing Care Before the Procedure

Client teaching and physical preparation are the same as for electroencephalography (see p. 870).
➤ Inform the client that electrodes are placed on the face around the eye.
➤ Inform the client that the study takes about 1 hour; instruct the client to avoid applying makeup to the face, to eat a light meal before the study, and to avoid smoking and caffeine-containing beverages for 48 hours before the study.
➤ Instruct the client to withhold stimulants, depressants, or antivertiginous drugs for 5 days before the study.
➤ Assess ear canals to determine the presence of wax in the ears; obtain a history and assessment of the neurological system for symptoms such as tinnitus, hearing loss, vertigo, dizziness, or ear pain or drainage; obtain a history of the medication regimen, diagnostic laboratory tests, and procedures.

The Procedure

The client is placed on the examination table in a supine or seated position in a darkened room. The client is informed that some discomfort is associated with some of the tests and that someone will be in attendance to assist if dizziness or other symptoms such as nausea and vomiting occur. Cerumen in the ears is removed, and the skin at the electrode sites is cleansed and dried. The five electrodes, prepared with paste to ensure proper conduction, are positioned at the outer canthus of each eye to test horizontal nystagmus, above and below the eye center for vertical nystagmus, and, at the center of the forehead, a ground electrode is placed. The electrodes pick up the potentials as the eyes move in a horizontal or vertical direction and a recorder amplifies the signals and charts them with a pen writer.[35] The client is reminded that instructions will be given for activities and position changes to be performed during the test. Several tests can be performed to examine the nystagmic response to the different procedures:

➤ *Gaze nystagmus:* Request the client to close the eyes. Spontaneous eye movements are recorded while the client concentrates on a mental task. Center gaze is recorded by having eyes fix on a center light; right gaze, by moving the eyes to the right; and left gaze, by moving the eyes to the left. A recording is made with eyes closed after each directional change, with timing of each gaze change and closed-eyes period.

➤ *Pendulum tracking:* Request that the client follow a pendulum or light. Body and eye movements are recorded.

➤ *Positional changes:* Request that the client change the head position as follows: eyes looking straight ahead and closed, head turning to the right and then to the center, head turning to the left and then to the center, lying to sitting position, sitting to lying position, lying in supine to both right and left side-lying position, head hanging over the edge from lying to sitting and after sitting position, and head hanging over the edge to the right and left positions.

➤ *Water caloric:* While the client is in a supine position with the head elevated to a semi-Fowler's position, water of a specific temperature is instilled into the ear canals for 30 seconds. The irrigation return is collected in a basin placed under the ear. Recordings are made during the study as the client is requested to perform mental tasks, open and fix the eyes on an object, and then close the eyes. Stimulation by different water temperatures is performed, cold water in some instances, and the response is recorded; air of different temperatures as an alternative to water can be introduced into each ear to obtain the same information.[36]

The results of these tests are recorded on charts and portions are analyzed for abnormalities by comparing them with the established values. They are noted as normal, borderline, or abnormal.

Nursing Care After the Procedure

➤ Care and assessment after the study include removal of the electrodes and cleansing of the skin.

➤ Allow a period of rest and assess for complaints of nausea, dizziness, or fatigue.

➤ Instruct the client to remain at rest for as long as weakness or dizziness is present.

➤ *Nausea and dizziness:* Note and report symptoms if they persist. Provide bed rest. Resume ordered medication regimen. Assist with transportation home, if it is needed.

ELECTRORETINOGRAPHY (ERG)

Electroretinography (ERG) is an electrophysiologic study performed to measure the electric activity of the retina in response to a flash of light stimulus. Electrodes are placed in a corneal contact lens and on the forehead of the client, and electric activity changes are recorded and displayed on a screen for viewing and analysis. The study allows diagnostic information in evaluation of retinal function and viability in those with opaque lens, corneal opacity, or vitreous body.

The retina is the inner layer of the posterior two thirds of the eyeball; it contains the neural receptors for vision. It is at this portion of the eye that light is converted to activity potentials and transmitted to visual centers in the brain via its connection to the optic nerve. Two types of photoreceptors are present: rods, which discriminate black and white, and cones, which discriminate color. Light energy causes nerve excitation, allowing the test to assist in diagnosing congenital and acquired retinal diseases and retinal blood vessel abnormalities.

Reference Values

Normal electric responses to light (alpha and beta waveforms); no acquired or inherited retinal conditions

Interfering Factors

➤ Inability of client to remain still during the procedure
➤ Improper placement of the electrode on the cornea

Indications for Electroretinography (ERG)

➤ Suspected retinal detachment or degeneration in the presence of opacities of the ocular contents or parts
➤ Suspected retinal damage caused by drugs as revealed by decreased response
➤ Evaluation of color blindness and night blindness revealed by a reduced response
➤ Suspected congenital disorders such as mucopolysaccharidosis revealed by the effect on the lens of the cornea, causing a reduced response
➤ Diagnosis of retinitis pigmentosa when performed with electro-oculography (EOG)
➤ Detection of retinopathy or vascular ischemia and other blood vessel abnormalities resulting from diabetes, atherosclerosis, and aging changes, revealed by a reduced response[37]
➤ Evaluation of retinal status before surgery or other treatment such as laser

Nursing Care Before the Procedure

Client teaching and physical preparation are the same as for electronystagmography (see p. 875).
➤ Administer ordered eyedrops to anesthetize the eye and a sedative if the client is a child.
➤ Prepare a child or infant for general anesthesia if it is to be administered.
➤ Inform the client that a light is used to perform the test and that little or no discomfort is experienced during the procedure.
➤ Obtain a history of known or suspected congenital or acquired eye disorders or diseases that predispose to eye abnormalities, signs and symptoms of eye condition, and previous associated diagnostic tests and procedures.

The Procedure

The client is placed on the examination table in a supine position or on a chair in a sitting position in a room that allows light adjustments. The eyes are anesthetized and then propped open with a retractor. Electrodes saturated with saline are placed on the cornea to receive the light stimuli that record and display electric changes on a screen. A recording is made in ordinary room light, in a dark room with a flash of white light delivered after the eye has had a chance to accommodate to the dark, and a flash of a very bright light if vitreous opacity is present.[38] Normal values are established, depending on the intensity of the wavelengths of light, which determine the expected electric response (usually increased in proportion to the intensity).

Nursing Care After the Procedure

➤ Assess the eyes for irritation after the removal of the electrodes.
➤ Inform the client that the anesthetic dissipates in about 20 minutes but that the eyes should not be rubbed or touched for at least 1 hour to prevent any injury.
➤ Allow time for the client to rest if needed.
➤ *Corneal abrasion:* Note and report eye pain or visual impairment complaints. Restrain or instruct the client to refrain from rubbing or touching the eyes after the procedure. Administer eye medications as ordered and apply sterile eye pad dressing.

ELECTRO-OCULOGRAPHY (EOG)

Electro-oculography (EOG) is an electrophysiologic study performed to measure electric potentials between the front of the eye and the retina in the back of the eye. The study determines changes in the potentials in dark and light environments with the eye at rest. Abnormalities are based on increases in electric potentials in relation to increased light. Electrodes are placed in specific areas of the canthi and the electric potentials are recorded on a graph for viewing and analysis.[39] The EOG study can be followed by fluorescein angiography (see p. 671) to diagnose vascular disorders of the retina or in conjunction with ERG (see p. 876) to diagnose congenital disorders of the retina.

Reference Values

Normal retinal function with an electric potential of 1.80 to 2, depending on testing methods used; no inherited or acquired retinal pathology

Interfering Factors

➤ Inability to understand or to to cooperate in instructions for eye movement during the procedure
➤ Improper placement of the electrodes around the eyes

Indications for Electro-oculography (EOG)

➤ Evaluation of retinal functional status in retinitis pigmentosa (degeneration of the outer pigmented layer) when performed in conjunction with ERG as revealed by a decrease in the electric potential
➤ Suspected retinopathy caused by antimalarial or other toxic drugs, revealed by abnormally reduced potentials
➤ Evaluation of retinal damage in albinism or irideremia revealed by an abnormal increase in potentials
➤ Diagnosis of congenital macular degeneration in the younger population as revealed by abnormal decrease in electric potentials[40]

Nursing Care Before the Procedure

Client teaching and physical preparation are the same as for electronystagmography (see p. 875).

➤ Obtain a history of known or suspected congenital or acquired eye disorders or diseases that predispose to eye abnormalities, signs and symptoms of an eye condition, and previous eye diagnostic tests and procedures.

➤ Determine whether ERG or fluorescein angiography is to be performed on the same day, the proper succession of the tests, and the waiting periods between them.

The Procedure

The client is placed on a chair in a sitting position. The electrodes are applied to the skin at the inner and outer canthi sites of the eye. The electrodes receive the stimulus, and the responses are recorded on a chart. The first recording is made of measurements of electric potentials of the eye at rest and during specific movements in a dark room. Then a light stimulus is provided and measurements of the eye potentials are recorded at rest and during the same movements as in the first recording. The normal recordings should reflect an increase in potentials between the front and back of the eye when light is applied, with increases proportional to increases in the light stimulus.[41]

Nursing Care After the Procedure

➤ Care and assessment after the study include assessment of the eyes and removal of the electrodes and cleansing of the skin sites.

➤ Help clients with impaired vision to return home or to their room in the hospital. Allow the client to rest and proceed with teaching and physical preparation if another procedure is to follow, such as fluorescein angiography.

(Case Study follows on page 881)

Student Name _____ Class _____

Instructor _____ Date _____

CASE STUDY AND CRITICAL THINKING EXERCISE

Mr. Smith, age 55, is recovering from a myocardial infarction. You are assessing his latest ECG strip, which reveals the following: R 86 bpm, P waves present (not all followed by a QRS complex), PR interval 0.24–0.32, QRS interval <0.12, T waves normal.

a. What problem has Mr. Smith developed as a result of his myocardial infarction?

b. What further complication can develop from this problem?

References

1. Thomas, CL (ed): Taber's Cyclopedic Medical Dictionary, ed 18. FA Davis, Philadelphia, 1997, p 617.
2. Fischbach, FT: A Manual of Laboratory Diagnostic Tests, ed 4. JB Lippincott, Philadelphia, 1992, pp 884–885.
3. Pagana, KD, and Pagana, TJ: Mosby's Diagnostic and Laboratory Test Reference. Mosby–Year Book, St Louis, 1992, p 285.
4. Ibid, pp 284–285.
5. Corbett, JV: Laboratory Tests and Diagnostic Procedures with Nursing Diagnoses, ed 3. Appleton & Lange, Norwalk, Conn, 1992, p 594.
6. Fischbach, op cit, p 886.
7. Springhouse Corporation: Nurse's Reference Library: Diagnostics, ed 2. Springhouse, Springhouse, Pa, 1986, p 895.
8. Pagana and Pagana, op cit, pp 286–287.
9. Corbett, op cit, p 590.
10. Nurse's Reference Library, op cit, p 895.
11. Fischbach, op cit, p 892.
12. Ibid, p 893.
13. Ibid, p 894.
14. Pagana and Pagana, op cit, p 333.
15. Ibid, p 334.
16. Fischbach, op cit, pp 889–890.
17. Ibid, p 890.
18. Porth, CM: Pathophysiology: Concepts of Altered Health States, ed 4. JB Lippincott, Philadelphia, 1993, p 509.
19. Pagana and Pagana, op cit, p 548.
20. Berkow, R: The Merck Manual, ed 16. Merck Sharp and Dohme Research Laboratory, Rahway, NJ, 1992, p 1392.
21. Ibid, p 1392.
22. Fischbach, op cit, p 872.
23. Pagana and Pagana, op cit, pp 295-296.
24. Nurse's Reference Library, op cit, p 774.
25. Berkow, op cit, p 1392.
26. Ibid, p 1391.
27. Fischbach, op cit, p 869.
28. Ibid, p 869.
29. Pagana and Pagana, op cit, p 330.
30. Fischbach, op cit, p 868.
31. Nurse's Reference Library, op cit, p 757.
32. Ibid, p 614.
33. Porth, op cit, p 819.
34. Berkow, op cit, p 2325.
35. Nurse's Reference Library, op cit, p 617.
36. Ibid, pp. 617–619, 624.
37. Porth, op cit, p 795.
38. Fischbach, op cit, pp 877–878.
39. Ibid, p 875.
40. Ibid, p 876.
41. Ibid, p 876.

Bibliography

Black, JM, and Matassarin-Jacobs, E: Luckmann and Sorensen's Medical-Surgical Nursing: A Psychophysiologic Approach, ed 4. WB Saunders, Philadelphia, 1993.

Brooks, HL: Electrocardiography: 100 Diagnostic Criteria. Mosby–Year Book, St Louis, 1987.

Chernecky, CC, and Berger, BJ; Cullen, BN (ed): Laboratory Tests and Diagnostic Procedures, ed 2. WB Saunders, Philadelphia, 1996.

Conover, MB: Understanding Electrocardiography. Mosby–Year Book, St Louis, 1995.

Davis, D: Differential Diagnosis of Arrhythmias. WB Saunders, Philadelphia, 1992.

Froelicher, VF, and Marcondes, GD: Manual of Exercise Testing. Mosby–Year Book, St Louis, 1989.

Gillette, PC, and Garson, A, Jr: Pediatric Arrhythmias: Electrophysiology and Pacing. WB Saunders, Philadelphia, 1990.

Goldberger, AL: Clinical Electrocardiography: A Simplified Approach, ed 5. Mosby–Year Book, St Louis, 1994.

Heckenlively, JR, and Arden, G (eds): Principles and Practice of Clinical Electrophysiology of Vision. Mosby–Year Book, St Louis, 1991.

Holmes, GL: Diagnosis and Management of Seizures in Children. WB Saunders, Philadelphia, 1987.

Jimeniz-Sierra, JM, et al: Inherited Retinal Diseases: A Diagnostic Guide. Mosby–Year Book, St Louis, 1989.

Johnson, RA, and Schwartz, MH: A Simplified Approach to Electrocardiography. WB Saunders, Philadelphia, 1986.

Jones, KM, and Ochs, GM: Interpretation of the Electrocardiogram, ed 2. Appleton & Lange, Norwalk, Conn, 1990.

Kee, JL: Handbook of Laboratory and Diagnostic Tests with Nursing Implications, ed 3. Appleton & Lange, Norwalk, Conn, 1997.

Owen, JH, and Davis, H (eds): Evoked Potential Testing: Clinical Applications. WB Saunders, Philadelphia, 1985.

Owen JH, and Donohoe, CD (eds): Clinical Atlas of Auditory Evoked Potentials. WB Saunders, Philadelphia, 1987.

Pagana, KD, and Pagana, TJ: Diagnostic Testing and Nursing Implications: A Case Study Approach, ed 4. Mosby–Year Book, St Louis, 1993.

Park, MK, and Guntheroth, WG: How to Read Pediatric ECGs, ed 3. Mosby–Year Book, St Louis, 1992.

Ramaiah, LS, and Chou, TC; Zorab, R (ed): Electrocardiography in Clinical Practice, ed 4. WB Saunders, Philadelphia, 1996.

Regenbogen, LS, and Coscas, GJ: Oculo-Auditory Syndromes. Mosby–Year Book, St Louis, 1985.

Seelig, CB: Simplified EKG Analysis: A Sequential Guide to Interpretation. Mosby–Year Book, St Louis, 1992.

Springhouse Corporation: Diagnostic Tests. Springhouse, Springhouse, Pa, 1991.

Tilkian, SM: Clinical and Nursing Implications of Laboratory Tests, ed 5. Mosby–Year Book, St Louis, 1995.

Wellens, HJJ, and Conover, M: The ECG in Emergency Decision Making. WB Saunders, Philadelphia, 1991.

Wiederhold, R: Electrocardiography: The Monitoring Lead. WB Saunders, Philadelphia, 1989.

24

Studies of Specific Organs or Systems

➤ **TESTS COVERED**

Cardiac Catheterization Study, *886*
Pulmonary Artery Catheterization Study, *891*
His Bundle (EP) Study, *894*
Cold Stimulation Test, *897*
Pulmonary Function Study, *899*
Exercise Pulmonary Function Study, *905*
Oximetry, *906*
Sweat Test, *908*
Spinal Nerve Root Thermography, *910*
Tensilon Test, *912*
Hearing Loss Audiometry, *914*

Hearing Loss Tuning Fork Tests, *917*
Acoustic Admittance Tests, *919*
Otoneurological Tests, *922*
Otoneural Lesion Site Tests, *924*
Spondee Speech Reception Threshold (SRT) Test, *927*
Visual Acuity Tests, *928*
Visual Field Tests, *930*
Color Perception Tests, *933*
Tonometry, *934*
Refraction, *936*
Slit-Lamp Biomicroscopy, *938*
Schirmer Tearing Test, *939*
Corneal Staining Test, *940*

INTRODUCTION

This chapter provides information about invasive and noninvasive diagnostic tests related to organs or body systems. These tests can be performed to determine abnormal patterns and functions, deficits, or pathology of a particular organ or system. The tests or studies of the cardiovascular, pulmonary, and neurological systems that have been placed in this chapter fail to meet the criteria for inclusion in the other chapters of this book. Note that some of the tests or studies in this chapter contain more than one procedure that can be used to obtain different types of information about an organ system or to differentiate between the types of pathology affecting an organ.

CARDIOVASCULAR SYSTEM

Cardiovascular system studies include procedures to obtain diagnostic information about the heart's chambers, coronary artery patency, and conduction disturbances and to correctly place catheters to measure pulmonary artery pressures. These studies are performed to support and extend information obtained by other procedures such as echocardiography, radiography, and radionuclide computerized scanning in diagnosing and evaluating the heart and the coronary and great vessels. Also included in this section is the test performed to determine peripheral vascular alterations associated with Raynaud's syndrome.

Cardiovascular procedures are performed by a cardiologist in a special cardiac laboratory room, except for pulmonary artery catheter monitoring, which can be performed at the bedside as well. Local anesthesia and strict sterile technique are used for cardiovascular procedures. A signed informed consent is required unless otherwise specified.

CARDIAC CATHETERIZATION STUDY

Cardiac catheterization is an invasive study that provides diagnostic information about the heart chambers and valves, coronary arteries, and the great vessels. In general, it is usually reserved for use when noninvasive procedures have not provided a definitive diagnosis, when more exact knowledge of the extent and severity of a heart condition is needed, or when the medical regimen is no longer effective and surgical intervention is advised. The study is performed by the insertion and passage of a flexible catheter into the heart chambers, the pulmonary artery, and the coronary vessels under the guidance of fluoroscopy. Catheter insertion is followed by the injection of a dye or contrast medium into the heart chambers or great vessels, which allows instant visualization and filming of heart activity or measurement of pulmonary artery pressures (angiography). Injection into the coronary arteries allows visualization and filming of vessel abnormalities (coronary arteriography). A right or left heart catheterization, or both, with different types of tests can be performed during the procedure, based on a client's history and signs and symptoms.

Left heart catheterization to obtain information about the left side of the circulation involves the retrograde insertion of the catheter via a cutdown in the right brachial artery, via a percutaneous puncture of the right femoral artery (most common site), or via a transseptal technique. The catheter is advanced into the aorta and left heart or into the coronary arteries in the retrograde technique (Fig. 24–1). It is advanced into the right atrium and right septum, then into the left atrium and across the mitral valve into the left ventricle in the transseptal technique. The transseptal technique is used when aortic valve

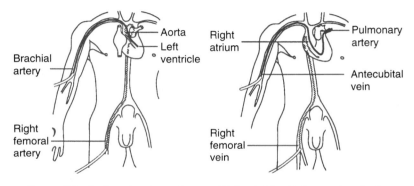

Figure 24–1 Insertion sites and routes of left and right side heart catheterization.

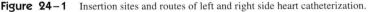

stenosis prevents passage of the catheter into the left side of the heart via the retrograde technique.[1] This technique permits examination of left heart activity and, after the injection of a contrast medium, evaluation of aortic and mitral valve abnormalities and patency of coronary arteries. Left heart catheterization and coronary artery cannulation with a special balloon catheter can be performed by forcefully inflating the balloon to dilate specific stenotic or obstructed areas in the coronary vessels. This is known as percutaneous transluminal coronary angioplasty (PTCA).

Right heart catheterization to obtain information about the right side of the circulation involves the insertion of the catheter via a cutdown in the antecubital vein or via a puncture of the femoral vein. The catheter is advanced into the inferior vena cava, the right atrium, and then the right ventricle, across the pulmonary valve, and into the pulmonary arteries (see Fig. 24–1). This procedure permits examination of the right heart activity and measures the pressures of the right atrium, ventricle, and pulmonary artery as the catheter is advanced through these parts of the heart. Pulmonary artery pressure (PAP) and pulmonary artery wedge pressure (PAWP) are also measured during this procedure, as these measurements reflect changes that occur in left atrium pressure. Blood samples for blood gases can be obtained, primarily oxygen content of blood at different levels within the heart and great vessels, to evaluate the shunting of blood and its characteristics within the heart. The function of the tricuspid and pulmonary valves can be evaluated after the injection of a contrast medium in right heart catheterization.[2]

Cardiac output (CO) and related blood volume studies can be calculated from findings obtained from cardiac catheterization. Cardiac output is the volume of blood ejected by the heart in 1 minute. It can be calculated by the Fick technique, by which the oxygen content of expired air is measured and subtracted from the oxygen content of room air. The difference is divided by the arteriovenous (A-V) oxygen difference obtained from both arterial and venous blood samples. Another technique is the dye dilution technique, usually performed in association with cardiac catheterization. This technique involves the injection of a predetermined amount of indocyanine green or Evans blue dye into the venous system while arterial blood is withdrawn, with the concentration of the dye measured and recorded as a curve. Cardiac output is calculated from the curve using the appearance time, the buildup time, and the disappearance time segments. Both methods are based on the total uptake or release of a substance by an organ, depending on blood flow to the organ and the artery and on venous concentration differences of a substance.[3]

Equipment that provides visualization includes an image intensifier, a television system, and an instant replay recording of the fluoroscopic images. Special equipment for measurement of pressures of the heart and vessels and other procedures and emergency events is available in a catheterization laboratory to accommodate this study.

Reference Values

Normal heart chambers and great vessel size, structure, function, direction of blood flow, and valves; normal pressures of heart chambers and pulmonary artery, cardiac output, ejection fraction, blood volume and oxygenation, and patency of the cardiac vascular system

Pressures	
Left ventricular systolic	90–140 mm Hg
Left ventricular end-diastolic	4–12 mm Hg
Central venous pressure (CVP)	2–14 cm H_2O
Left atrium	2–12 mm Hg
Pulmonary artery systolic/end-diastolic	17–32/4–13 mm Hg
Pulmonary wedge pressure	6–13 mm Hg
Cardiac Output	3–6 L/min
Ejection Fraction	60–70%

Note: No coronary artery disease (CAD), congenital or acquired anatomic abnormalities or septal defects, valvular abnormalities, aneurysm, pulmonary embolism, or hypertension.

Interfering Factors

➤ Anxiety level can affect cardiac rate, which affects pressures in the chambers.

➤ Inability of client to remain still or to understand the need to cooperate during the study.

➤ Improper placement of the catheter or other failures in technique.

Indications for Cardiac Catheterization Study

➤ Diagnosis and determination of the severity of cardiac and great vessel diseases when other noninvasive studies have not produced a definitive diagnosis

➤ Chest pain in clients at risk for heart disease or in those with known angina or abnormal electrocardiography (ECG)

➤ Determination and location of partial or complete coronary artery occlusion in the diagnosis of CAD or confirmation of the need for cardiac bypass surgery revealed by narrowing of the lumen of coronary arteries and lack of coronary perfusion

➤ Diagnosis of acquired and congenital valvular disease (stenosis, insufficiency, regurgitation) and determination of the severity as revealed by abnormal pressures and blood flow at the valve site

➤ Confirmation or evaluation of acquired and congenital atrial and ventricular septal defects or shunting of blood, extent of the abnormality, and direction and volume of the shunting, as revealed by abnormal blood oxygen content at different levels of the right and left sides of the heart and great vessels

➤ Determination of the presence and severity of congenital cardiac abnormalities in infants, that is, patent ductus arteriosus, transposition of the great vessels, and need for corrective surgery

➤ Determination of left ventricular hypertrophy or ventricular aneurysm as revealed by abnormal chamber size, cardiac muscle or wall motion, and ejection fraction

➤ Diagnosis and determination of the extent of aortic atherosclerosis or aneurysm as revealed by abnormal pressure in the aortic artery

➤ Diagnosis of pulmonary venous return abnormalities and determination of the presence of pulmonary hypertension or embolism

➤ Monitoring of PAP, PAWP, and blood volumes after insertion of a Swan-Ganz catheter in acutely ill clients

➤ Acute myocardial infarction to infuse a thrombolytic medication into the occluded coronary arteries to relieve obstruction caused by blood clot

➤ Performance of PTCA to relieve occluded or stenotic coronary arteries

➤ Evaluation of the success of cardiac surgery or PTCA procedures, as revealed by improved blood flow to the myocardium

➤ Measuring of cardiac output and calculating ejection fraction based on end-diastolic and systolic volumes and stroke volume findings in cardiac monitoring of acutely ill clients

➤ Obtaining of blood samples from the chambers or by the dye dilution technique for oxygen content and saturation analysis in determining cardiac abnormalities, especially cardiac output

Contraindications

➤ Allergy to the contrast medium used in the angiography portion of the study

➤ Pregnancy, unless the benefits of performing the study greatly outweigh the risks to the fetus

➤ Clients who will not allow cardiac surgery to be performed to correct pathology diagnosed by the study

➤ Medical conditions such as severe infection, irreversible brain damage, or congestive heart failure (CHF), which are considered relative to their extent, emergency status, and potential benefit as opposed to the risk

---

➤➤ Nursing Alert

• The following equipment and associated supplies should be on hand when performing cardiac catheterization to treat ventricular arrhythmias or other complications: resuscitation bag; oxygen; suction; oximetric device; endotracheal tube; airway; defibrillator; monitor for pulse and blood pressure; ECG; external temporary pacemaker; and medications such as lidocaine (Xylocaine), bretylium (Bretylol), epinephrine (Adrenalin), atropine, morphine, and isoproterenol (Isuprel).

Nursing Care Before the Procedure

Explain to the client:

➤ That the procedure is performed in a special cardiac laboratory equipped with monitors and supplies to minimize the risk of complications

➤ That the procedure is performed by a physician (cardiologist) and takes about 1 to 3 hours, depending on the tests to be performed

➤ That food and fluids are withheld for at least 4 to 6 hours before the study

➤ That some routine medications are withheld according to physician instruction, especially anticoagulant therapy, which is discontinued before the study

➤ That the site is shaved, cleansed, and anesthetized with a local anesthetic, that the catheter is inserted into a vein or artery as appropriate for the tests to be performed, and that children are given general anesthesia for this procedure

➤ That a feeling of pressure is experienced as the catheter is inserted and that a sensation is experienced as the catheter is advanced

➤ That a sedative, analgesic, or other medication to allay anxiety and promote comfort is given 1 hour before the study
➤ That ECG activity, pulse, and blood pressure are monitored during the procedure because a temporary increase in pulse or arrhythmia can occur during the advancement of the catheter
➤ That a contrast medium can be injected into the heart and vessels and cause a warm feeling or metallic taste but that it lasts only a few minutes
➤ That the client can be requested to cough or breathe deeply during the study to enhance the blood flow through the heart

Prepare for the procedure:

➤ Obtain the client's height and weight, which will be used to determine dye administration.
➤ Ensure that dietary and fluid restrictions have been followed.
➤ Ensure that routine medications are restricted or allowed per physician order and that anticoagulants have been discontinued.
➤ Provide a hospital gown without metallic closures. Allow the client to retain dentures, glasses, or hearing aids, as they do not interfere with the study.
➤ Ensure that medications to reduce allergic response to the contrast medium are administered, that is, antihistamine or corticosteroid.
➤ Obtain baseline pulse, blood pressure, ECG, and peripheral pulses, and mark the sites of peripheral pulses for comparison after the study.
➤ Administer a sedative or antianxiety agent such as diazepam (Valium), or both types of medication, and an analgesic such as meperidine (Demerol) as ordered before the procedure (30 minutes to 1 hour).
➤ Initiate an intravenous (IV) line to administer fluids and medications as needed during the procedure.
➤ Have the client void before the procedure.
➤ Obtain a history of suspected or known cardiac conditions, cardiovascular status, cardiac medications, allergies to iodine, and previous tests and procedures.

The Procedure

The client is placed in a supine position on the examining table. Straps secure the client in place on the table in the event of tilting. An IV infusion of D_5W is initiated to keep the vein open for medication administration. ECG leads are positioned and attached to the client. Blood pressure, pulse, and respiration equipment is used for continuous monitoring of heart activity and vital signs. The catheterization site is shaved if necessary, cleansed, and draped to establish a sterile field. All aspects of the study are carried out using sterile technique. A local anesthetic is injected at the insertion or cutdown site, and general anesthesia via gas or rectal suppository is administered to young children. The site selected depends on whether the right or left side of the heart is to be catheterized, that is, femoral or antecubital vein for the right side and brachial or femoral artery for the left side. The vein or artery is punctured with a needle and a wire inserted through the needle. The catheter is then passed over the wire and into the vessel after the needle is removed. Guided by fluoroscopy in a darkened room, the physician advances the wire and catheter into the right atrium, through the tricuspid valve, into the right ventricle, through the pulmonary valve, and into the pulmonary arteries for right side catheterization and into the aorta, through the aortic valve, and into the left ventricle or coronary arteries for left side catheterization.[4] Cardiac pressures, volume readings, and blood gas levels are obtained. The contrast medium is injected into the chamber to visualize heart size and activity, aneurysms or stenosis, and ventricular abnormalities and into each coronary artery to determine patency. X-ray films are taken in rapid sequence at all angles as the client's position is changed. The client can be requested to cough or perform exercises during the study to measure heart activity during stress.

The catheter is removed with one smooth movement after the completion of the study. The site is sutured if a cutdown was performed, and a sterile pressure dressing is applied.

Nursing Care After the Procedure

➤ Care and assessment after the study include monitoring vital signs every 15 minutes for 1 hour, every 30 minutes for the next hour, and every hour if stable, taking peripheral pulses and assessing skin for color and temperature on both extremities of the site and comparing for circulatory alterations.

➤ Maintain bed rest for 6 to 8 hours, depending on the procedure (for femoral artery puncture; less if the right heart was catheterized via the femoral vein).

➤ Extend the extremity used and immobilize it with sandbags.

➤ Encourage movement of the unaffected extremities.

➤ Resume food, fluids, and medications, and encourage additional fluids to offset the diuretic effect of the contrast medium.

➤ Schedule postprocedure ECG and future suture removal from the insertion site.

➤ *Reaction to iodinated contrast medium:* Note and report pruritus, urticaria, rash, breathing changes, or pulse changes. Administer antihistamines and corticosteroids. Have resuscitation equipment and supplies on hand.

➤ *Thrombophlebitis/infection/bleeding at site:* Note and report excessive bleeding, hematoma formation, pain, skin color, swelling, or drainage at site. Administer ordered antibiotics, monitor vital signs and peripheral pulses, and apply ice or warm compresses to the site as appropriate.

➤ *Arrhythmias:* Note and report ventricular cardiac rhythm abnormalities on the ECG strip. Monitor vital signs. Administer ordered antiarrhythmics, oxygen, or other treatments.

➤ *Cardiac tamponade:* Note and report reduced cardiac output and associated anxiety, tachypnea, distended neck veins, narrowing pulse pressure, muffled heart sounds, paradoxic pulse, or changes in vital signs. Have resuscitation equipment and supplies and pericardiocentesis supplies on hand.

➤ *Systemic or pulmonary emboli:* Note and report dyspnea, tachypnea, chest pain, or increase in pulse rate. Position the client in a sitting or high-Fowler's position. Administer oxygen and monitor vital signs.

PULMONARY ARTERY CATHETERIZATION STUDY

Pulmonary artery catheterization is an invasive study that provides information about the pumping ability of the heart by measurement of the pulmonary artery pressure (PAP) and the pulmonary artery wedge pressure, or pulmonary capillary wedge pressure (PAWP). It is performed in acutely ill clients to monitor left atrial and ventricular end-diastolic pressure and other hemodynamic parameters, that is, central venous pressure (CVP) and cardiac output. Measurement is achieved by obtaining readings of the pulmonary capillary pressures in the pulmonary artery because they are the same as pressures in the left side of the heart during diastole. A multiluminal, flow-directed, balloon-tipped Swan-Ganz catheter is inserted into a peripheral vein (cephalic, subclavian, femoral) and advanced into a position in the pulmonary artery that allows pressure readings. The catheters are available in two, three, or four lumens of varying lengths. A balloon lumen is used for the inflation of air to measure PAWP and to advance the catheter into the desired position; a distal lumen is used to measure PAP and PAWP and to obtain blood samples; a proximal lumen is used to measure right atrial or CVP and to inject ice water for cardiac output determination; and a fourth lumen is equipped with a thermistor probe to measure cardiac output by thermodilution after the injection of ice water.[5]

Reference Values

Normal PAP and PAWP

Pressures	
PAP	<20 mm Hg
PAWP	6–12 mm Hg[6]

Interfering Factors

➤ Improper placement or position of the catheter.
➤ Mechanical ventilation equipment can alter pressure readings as the intrathoracic pressure is increased. Improper functioning or problems with the monitoring or recording equipment, such as air or clot in system, waveform or transducer damage or dampness, balloon overinflation or rupture, leaks resulting from loose connections, or incorrect position of stopcock or monitor calibration.

Indications for Pulmonary Artery Catheterization Study

➤ Monitoring acutely ill clients with sudden respiratory failure or failure of two or more organ systems
➤ Determining right or left ventricular impairment, defects, or failure as revealed by abnormal PAP and PAWP readings
➤ Determining pulmonary hypertension, pulmonary diseases, or pulmonary edema or embolus as revealed by increased PAP and PAWP
➤ Determining atrial or ventricular septal defects causing shunting of blood and increased pulmonary blood flow as revealed by high PAP
➤ Determining pulmonary vascular resistance and ventricular stroke work to diagnose cardiac function abnormalities
➤ Diagnosing pericardial involvement affecting cardiac function, that is, effusion, tamponade, or pericarditis, as revealed by increased right atrial and ventricular pressures
➤ Determining oxygen delivery to tissues by measurement of arterial oxygen content and thermodilution flow, especially if mechanical ventilation is used, as mechanical ventilation can depress cardiac output

➤ Evaluating the composition of mixed venous blood (oxygen tension) obtained from the pulmonary artery to assist in determining a prognosis (Decreases indicate a poor prognosis.)

➤ Measuring cardiac output via thermodilution in the evaluation of myocardial contractility after a myocardial infarction or in the presence of fluid losses

➤ Evaluating or monitoring cardiac, pulmonary, and fluid status after cardiac surgery

➤ Evaluating the effects of inotropic drugs, respiratory therapy, and fluid infusion status

---

➤➤ Nursing Alert

- Troubleshooting interventions to solve potential problems associated with pulmonary artery catheters and monitoring equipment should be carried out in a systematic manner to ensure accurate readings by experienced personnel, and agency policy or written suggested solutions provided by the manufacturer should be followed.

Nursing Care Before the Procedure

Explain to the client:

➤ That the procedure is performed by a physician at the bedside and that it takes about 30 minutes to insert and position the catheter

➤ That a local anesthetic will be injected at the site of the catheter insertion and that this discomfort will be the only pain experienced

➤ That the catheter will remain in place for 3 to 4 days and that no discomfort will be experienced when the catheter is in place or when the tests are performed

➤ That the catheter will be sutured in place at the insertion site and bandaged to prevent movement and infection

Prepare for the procedure:

➤ Obtain a history or assessment of cardiac and pulmonary system status and other known or suspected medical conditions, previous tests and procedures, and medication regimen.

The Procedure

The client is placed in supine position in bed with the selected site exposed and the client draped for privacy. The equipment and supplies, including the Swan-Ganz or the four-lumen pulmonary artery catheter, are prepared per hospital policy or manufacturer direction. The site is shaved if necessary, cleansed, and draped to provide a sterile field. A local anesthetic is injected at the site, the catheter is inspected for defects, and a puncture or cutdown incision is made to access the vein. The catheter is inserted into the peripheral vein and advanced into the superior vena cava and right atrium. The balloon is partially inflated to allow it to move with the blood flow through the tricuspid valve and into the right ventricle and pulmonary artery until it becomes wedged into a smaller distal pulmonary artery. Waveforms are recorded on a screen as the catheter is advanced into the right heart to note any tachycardia caused by catheter irritation and to obtain baseline information. Medications can be administered to prevent arrhythmias or right bundle block if these risks should be present. PAP is obtained while the catheter is positioned in the pulmonary artery. The catheter is advanced into a wedged position in one of the smaller pulmonary arteries and inflated with 1 mL of air to obtain PAWP. After a PAWP reading, the balloon is deflated to prevent pulmonary tissue necrosis; it then moves back into the pulmonary artery. The catheter is observed on the screen for the waveforms indicating its position. Cardiac output is measured with the catheter in the pulmonary artery, not in the wedged position. Ten milliliters of ice water is injected into the proximal lumen, and a temperature-time curve is obtained with the thermistor at the end of the catheter. An x-ray verifies catheter placement, and the catheter is sutured to the skin. Sterile dressings are applied to protect and maintain cleanliness of the insertion site.

Monitoring activities associated with pulmonary artery catheter procedures include vital signs and ECG. Frequency and types of monitoring depend on client status, as do PAP and PAWP measurements. The system is flushed and recalibrated after each PAWP reading. When monitoring via a pulmonary artery catheter is concluded, the balloon is deflated, and the dressing and sutures are removed. The catheter is removed with a slow and smooth motion. Vital signs and ECG monitoring continue, and a sterile dressing is applied to the insertion site.

Nursing Care After the Procedure

➤ Care and assessment after removal of the pulmonary artery catheter include monitoring the insertion site, vital signs, and ECG for complications.

➤ *Abnormal monitoring results, complications, and precautions:* Provide support to the client and report any difficulty in obtaining readings and flushing the system. Troubleshooting activities to correct pressure readings, catheter placement, monitoring device, or transducer problems should be assessed and solved according to the manufacturer's instructions.

➤ *Infection, local/systemic:* Note and report redness, pain, swelling, drainage, or elevated temperature. Administer antibiotic therapy. Apply warm compresses to the site. Use strict aseptic technique during insertion, while obtaining blood samples, and during cardiac output measurement and pressure monitoring.

➤ *Arrhythmias:* Note and report changes in ECG strip and vital signs. Administer ordered antiarrhythmics. Monitor vital signs and ECG.

➤ *Pulmonary emboli/infarction:* Note and report dyspnea, tachypnea, hypoxia, or chest pain. Monitor vital signs. Administer ordered medications and oxygen. Place client in a semi-Fowler's position. Restrict time that the catheter is in a wedge position.

His Bundle (EP) Study

The His bundle evoked potential (EP) study is an invasive electrophysiologic study using cardiac catheterization to insert electrodes that measure and identify defects in the electric conduction activity of the heart. Heart muscle has the ability to generate and conduct electric impulses. It also contains special pacemaker cells that make up the conduction system that controls the rhythm of the heart. Each contraction is initiated by the sinoatrial (SA) node, located in the posterior wall of the right atrium, and passes down to the atrioventricular (AV) node. The AV node connects the conduction systems that control the atrial and ventricular activity. Fibers within the AV node conduct the impulses into the His bundle that extends into the ventricular system. The normal velocity of the conduction system through the atrium and ventricles is necessary for the atrial emptying before ventricular contractions and the proper ejection of blood from the heart by the ventricular system.[7]

The procedure for the study is performed in the same manner as cardiac catheterization, but it uses bipolar or tripolar catheters that contain electrodes instead of the luminal catheters. The catheter is inserted into the femoral vein and advanced into the right atrium, through the tricuspid valve, and into the right ventricle under the guidance of fluoroscopy. The electrode at the end of the catheter measures conduction intervals or times that indicate nodal defects and cardiac arrhythmias. Conduction intervals that are measured include the H-V, which represents the time it takes for the electric activity to pass from the His bundle to the Purkinje fibers of the ventricular system, and the A-H, which represents the time it takes for the atrial node activity to activate the His bundle.[8] The study also can also be performed to induce an abnormal rhythm to evaluate the effectiveness of antiarrhythmics or to determine the need for pacemaker implantation. Intracardiac electrograms are recorded from the electrode on the catheter as it passes the His bundle. Conventional 10-lead ECG monitoring is conducted at the same time to obtain a recording of the total electric activity of the heart.

Reference Values

Normal atrioventricular conduction system intervals, recovery, and refractory times; no arrhythmias and conduction disturbances

Interfering Factors

➤ Improper placement of catheter
➤ Equipment dysfunction or failure
➤ Sedatives and antianxiety agents, which can alter test results

Indications for His Bundle (EP) Study

➤ Providing a cardiac mapping of the entire conduction system to evaluate normal and abnormal pathways of electric activity
➤ Diagnosing and identifying heart conduction defects and sinoatrial (SA) and atrioventricular (AV) nodes as revealed by shortened or delayed intervals
➤ Determining the cause of syncope or cardiac arrest episode
➤ Diagnosing sick sinus syndrome as revealed by prolonged recovery time or heart block as revealed by prolonged conduction time
➤ Determining the site of bundle branch block as revealed by prolonged conduction interval in the His bundle and Purkinje fibers
➤ Diagnosing ventricular arrhythmias and determining appropriate therapy, or pacing the heart and inducing an arrhythmia to evaluate the effectiveness of therapy by determining if the drug prevents the arrhythmia
➤ Determining cardiac pacing abnormalities and need for pacemaker implantation

Contraindications

> ➤ Medical conditions such as coagulation disorder
> ➤ Myocardial infarct, unless time is limited and determination is made that the benefits of performing the study outweigh the risks

---

➤➤ Nursing Alert

- Life-threatening arrhythmias can occur or can be induced during this study, and emergency equipment (defibrillator) and drugs (antiarrhythmics) should be on hand during the procedure.

Nursing Care Before the Procedure

Client teaching and physical preparation are the same as for cardiac catheterization (see pp. 889 to 890).

> ➤ In addition, instruct the client to report any dizziness during the study; inform the client that palpitations can be experienced when the heart is paced and that sedatives or analgesics are not administered before the study as they can influence the accuracy of the results.

The Procedure

The procedure is the same as for cardiac catheterization (see p. 891) of the right side of the heart via a vein, using a solid tubular electrode catheter that is advanced into the right atrium and ventricle. Fluoroscopy is used in guiding the catheter into the chambers of the heart, and monitors allow visualization of the catheter. Electrograms from the catheter and traditional ECG are obtained during the procedure. Baseline ECG readings are obtained, and conduction intervals are recorded and measured as the catheter passes along the ventricle wall and His bundle. Atrial or ventricular pacing can be produced by the catheter to induce arrhythmias for identification and to determine drug therapy effectiveness. Also, drugs can be administered during the study to determine their effectiveness in preventing an induced arrhythmia. Support is given to the client to allay fear during the study when pacing is performed, and the client is reminded to report symptoms such as palpitations or lightheadedness.

Nursing Care After the Procedure

Care and assessment after the procedure are the same as for cardiac catheterization (see p. 891) except that a contrast medium is not used in this study.

> ➤ Continue ECG and vital signs monitoring if drugs are administered during the procedure or if arrhythmias persist.
> ➤ *Thrombophlebitis/infection/bleeding at site:* Note and report excessive bleeding, hematoma formation, pain, swelling, or drainage at the site. Administer ordered antibiotics. Monitor vital signs and peripheral pulses. Apply ice or warm compress to the site as appropriate.

➤ *Adverse reaction to drugs:* Note and report abdominal cramps and hypotension resulting from quinidine, hypotension resulting from procainamide (Pronestyl), or behavior change resulting from phenytoin (Dilantin). Monitor heart activity via ECG. Administer IV fluid infusion.

➤ *Fibrillation/arrhythmias:* Note and report cardiac rhythm abnormalities. Administer ordered antiarrhythmics and other treatments. Monitor ECG. Have emergency fibrillation equipment and supplies on hand for life-threatening arrhythmias.

COLD STIMULATION TEST

The cold stimulation test is a noninvasive peripheral vascular procedure that is performed to provide information to assist in diagnosing Raynaud's syndrome. The test measures temperature changes in the fingers after exposure to cold temperature changes and the time it takes for the finger temperature to return to normal after the cold stimulus has been removed. It is usually performed when chronic arterial occlusive disease has been ruled out as the cause of signs and symptoms that indicate a peripheral vascular disorder.

The cause of Raynaud's syndrome is a functional abnormality resulting from an intense vasospasm of the small arteries and arterioles of the fingers and, in some cases, the toes. The disorder can be classified as Raynaud's disease (primary type), which occurs without any cause other than exposure to cold or extreme stress, or Raynaud's phenomenon (secondary type), which occurs as a result of occupational trauma, arterial occlusive disease, or in association with collagen diseases such as scleroderma and lupus erythematosus. The vasospasms cause ischemia, which changes the skin color from pallor to cyanotic, starting at the fingertips and traveling up the distal portion of the phalanges. Tingling, numbness, and cold sensation are experienced during ischemia. After the ischemia, hyperemia occurs, with a change in skin color to red, and a throbbing sensation is experienced. The cause of Raynaud's disease is unknown but is believed to be associated with local circulatory mechanisms (prostaglandins) and does not affect the anatomic structure of the vessels. Raynaud's phenomenon, however, does involve abnormal changes in the anatomic structure of the vessels.[9]

Reference Values

Normal temperature, blood pressure, and skin color of fingers and toes after exposure to cold temperatures; no Raynaud's disease or phenomenon

Interfering Factors

➤ Extreme environmental temperatures

Indications for Cold Stimulation Test

➤ Diagnosing Raynaud's syndrome, as revealed by inability of digits to return to pretest temperature within a specific length of time, usually 20 minutes

➤ Differentiating between Raynaud's primary disease and Raynaud's phenomenon as a secondary disease associated with connective tissue disorders

Contraindications

➤ Infectious process at the digit sites to be used in the test
➤ Advanced disease in which gangrene of the digits is present and circulation impairment is evident

Nursing Care Before the Procedure

Explain to the client:
➤ That the procedure is performed in the laboratory by a physician or a staff technician and takes about 30 minutes
➤ That there are no food or fluid restrictions before the study
➤ That small devices connected to wires are attached to the fingers, and the hand is immersed in cold water while finger temperature is recorded
➤ That only a slight discomfort may be experienced when the hands are placed in the cold water and that no pain is felt from the devices taped to the digits

Prepare for the procedure:
➤ Have the client void before the procedure.
➤ Obtain a history of known or suspected scleroderma or lupus erythematosus, effects of temperature and stress on digital blood flow, treatments, or previous tests and procedures.

The Procedure

The client is placed in a sitting position in a room with optimal temperature control. A thermistor is attached to each finger above the nail area. Wires are attached to record temperature changes. The temperature is recorded to obtain baseline measurements, and the hands are immersed in ice water for 20 seconds. The hands are removed, and the temperature is again recorded and continues to be recorded every 5 minutes until the baseline level is attained. A delayed return to baseline temperatures of more than 20 minutes indicates Raynaud's syndrome.[10]

Nursing Care After the Procedure

Care and assessment after the study include removing the thermistors and returning the clothing and belongings to the client.

PULMONARY SYSTEM

Pulmonary system studies include procedures to obtain diagnostic information about the lungs and their ability to provide oxygen to and remove carbon dioxide from the body tissues and organ systems. This process is known as gas exchange, and it is dependent on respiratory function that involves ventilation (inspiration and expiration), diffusion (movement of gases across the alveolar capillary membrane), and perfusion (movement of blood through the pulmonary vasculature to body tissues). These studies, along with arterial blood gas (ABG) studies (see pp. 288 to 291), are performed to determine the existence or extent of pulmonary disease or abnormalities to support information obtained by medical history, chest radiography, lung scans, and pulmonary angiography. Also included in this section is the sweat test, performed to determine alterations associated with cystic fibrosis in children because the disease has a major effect on pulmonary function.

Procedures associated with the pulmonary system are usually performed in special laboratories, clinics, or physician's office by a trained technician with a physician present, if warranted. A signed informed consent form is not required for these studies.

PULMONARY FUNCTION STUDY

Pulmonary function is a noninvasive study that provides information about the volume, pattern, and rates of flow involved in respiratory function to assist in the diagnosis of insufficiencies associated with pathophysiological abnormalities such as tumors, infections, and obstructive and restrictive disorders. It can also include tests involving the distribution (pulmonary circulation that facilitates gas exchange) and diffusing capabilities of the lungs (volume of gases that diffuse across a membrane). A complete pulmonary study profile includes the determination of all lung volumes, spirometry, diffusing capacity, maximum voluntary ventilation, flow-volume loop, and maximum expiratory and inspiratory pressures.[11] Other studies include diffusing capacity and small airway volumes. ABGs also reveal the distribution and diffusing capabilities of pulmonary function (see pp. 288 to 291). Some or all of the tests can be performed to obtain the necessary clinical assessment of the pulmonary airways, alveoli, and vascular function, depending on client history and status. Modifications that include only the more common tests can be performed at the bedside or in outpatient settings, but a comprehensive study must be performed in a pulmonary function laboratory and values must be determined by computer.

The process of respiration is the body's means of gas exchange in providing oxygen to and removing carbon dioxide from the tissues; the process consists of ventilation (movement of gases in and out of the lung), perfusion (blood flow within the lung tissue), and diffusion (movement of oxygen and carbon dioxide across the alveolar membranes). It can be divided anatomically into airways of different sizes (nose, trachea, bronchi, bronchioles) that conduct the gases and the tissues (alveoli, pulmonary capillaries) that control gas exchange.

Respiration is controlled by the respiratory center in the medulla of the brain with two groups of neurons, one that is primarily concerned with inspiration and control of the impulses from the lungs and airways that compose the ventilatory response, and a second that is concerned with both inspiration and expiration and control of the spinal motor neurons of the intercostal and abdominal muscles. Breathing control is achieved by automatic regulation of ventilation by chemoreceptors and lung receptors. The chemoreceptors are located in the medulla (central) or in the carotid and aortic bodies (peripheral), and they monitor levels of oxygen, carbon dioxide, and pH in the blood. The chemoreceptors have the ability to adjust ventilation patterns to the body's metabolic requirements. Lung receptors are located in the airways and monitor breathing patterns and lung function by adjusting rate and volume to accommodate changes in lung compliance, airway resistance and pressure, and lung congestion.

Breathing can also be controlled through voluntary regulation, which provides the ability to suspend automatic breathing such as by holding the breath or by integrating breathing with activities such as eating, speaking, and singing. The mechanics of breathing involve the inspiration of air, which increases the volume of the thoracic cavity as the intercostal muscles contract, enlarging the chest; the diaphragm contracts, forcing the abdominal contents down as the chest expands. This process lowers the alveolar pressure below the atmospheric pressure and allows the air to flow into the large and small airways and alveoli. During expiration of air, elasticity of the chest wall and lung recoil cause the lung volume to decrease and the pressure to become greater than the atmospheric pressure, which allows the air to flow out of the lungs. Although expiration is a passive event, intercostal and abdominal muscles can be used if needed to increase this effort.[12]

Pulmonary function studies are classified into lung volumes and capacities, rates of flow, and gas exchange. Except for the gas exchange tests, pulmonary function tests are measured by spirometry, which allows the recording of the amounts of a gas present during inspiration and expiration. Lung volumes and capacities are the amounts of air that are inhaled or exhaled from the lungs compared with normal reference values, using age, height, weight, and gender of the client. The volumes and capacities measured by spirometry without regard to time limits include the following:

Tidal volume (TV): Total amount of air inhaled and exhaled with one breath

Residual volume (RV): Amount of air remaining in the lungs after a maximum expiration effort (not measured by spirometry, but it can be calculated from the functional residual capacity [FRC] minus the expiratory reserve volume [ERV]; indirect measurement can be achieved by body plethysmography [see p. 841])

Inspiratory reserve volume (IRV): Maximum amount of air inhaled at the point of maximum expiration

Expiratory reserve volume (ERV): Maximum amount of air exhaled after a resting expiration; can be calculated by the vital capacity (VC) minus the inspiratory capacity (IC)

Vital capacity (VC): Maximum amount of air exhaled slowly at the point of maximum inspiration; can be calculated by adding the inspiratory capacity (IC) and the expiratory reserve volume (ERV)

Total lung capacity (TLC): Total amount of air that the lungs can hold after maximum inspiration; can be calculated by adding the vital capacity (VC) and the residual volume (RV)

Inspiratory capacity (IC): Maximum amount of air inspired after normal expiration; can be calculated by adding the inspiratory reserve volume (IRV) and the tidal volume (TV)

Functional residual capacity (FRC): Volume of air that remains in the lungs after normal expiration; can be calculated by adding the residual volume (RV) and expiratory reserve volume (ERV)

The pulmonary function studies for lung volumes, capacities, and rates of flow measured by spirometry that involve timing include:

Forced vital capacity (FVC): Maximum amount of air that can be forcefully exhaled after a full inspiration

Forced expiratory volume in 1 second (FEV$_1$): Amount of air exhaled in the first second of forced vital capacity (FVC); can also be determined at 2 or 3 seconds. The percentage of FVC is the amount of air exhaled in seconds expressed in percent (%)

Maximum midexpiratory flow (MMEF): Maximum rate of air flow during a forced expiration

Forced inspiratory flow (FIF) rate: Volume inspired from the residual volume (RV) at a point of measurement; can be expressed as a percentage to identify the corresponding volume pressure and inspired volume

Peak inspiratory flow rate (PIFR): Maximum flow of air during a forced maximum inspiration

Peak expiratory flow rate (PEFR): Maximum flow of air expired during forced vital capacity (FVC)

Flow-volume (F-V) loop: Continuous flow rates and volumes displayed on a screen during forced expiratory and inspiratory vital capacity procedures

Maximum inspiratory/expiratory pressures: Measures the strength of the respiratory muscles in neuromuscular disorders

Maximum volume ventilation (MVV): Maximum volume of air inspired and expired in 1 minute

Other studies for gas exchange capacity, small airway abnormalities, and allergic responses in hyperactive airway disorders can be performed during the conventional pulmonary function study and include:

Diffusing capacity of lungs (D$_L$): Rate of transfer of carbon monoxide through the alveolar and capillary membranes in 1 minute

Closing volume (CV): Measure of the closure of small airways in the lower alveoli by monitoring volume and percent of alveolar nitrogen after inhalation of 100 percent oxygen

Isoflow volume ($_{iso}$V): Flow-volume loop test followed by inhalation of mix of helium and oxygen to determine small airways disease

Body plethysmography: Measures thoracic gas volume, airway resistance, and lung compliance (see p. 841)

Bronchial provocation: Detects airway sensitivities after inhalation of methacholine in those with asthma

Arterial blood gases (ABGs): Measures oxygen and carbon dioxide in arterial blood in the determination of hypoxia (see p. 288 to 291); reveals the perfusion and diffusion capabilities of pulmonary function

The findings or measurements are recorded on a spirogram that is used to diagnose or differentiate between obstructive and restrictive lung diseases. Values are expressed in units of milliliter (mL), percent (%), liter (L), liter per second (L/sec), or liter per minute (L/min), depending on the test performed.

Reference Values

Normal respiratory volume and capacities, gas diffusion, and distribution; no obstructive or restrictive lung disease

Lung Volumes, Capacities, and Flow Rates (values based on age, gender, height, and weight)	
TV	500 mL at rest
RV	1200 mL (approximate)
IRV	3000 mL (approximate)
ERV	1100 mL (approximate)
VC	4600 mL (approximate)
TLC	5800 mL (approximate)
IC	3500 mL (approximate)
FRC	2300 mL (approximate)
FVC	3000–5000 mL (approximate)
FEV_1	81–83%
MMEF	25–75%
FIF	25–75%
MVV	25–35% or 170 L/min
PIFR	300 L/min
PEFR	450 L/min
F-V loop	Normal curve
D_L	25 mL/min/mm Hg (approximate)
CV	10–20% of VC
$_{iso}V$	Based on age formula
Bronchial provocation	No change or less than 20% reduction in FEV_1

Interfering Factors

➤ Client confusion or inability of client to understand instructions or cooperate during the study

➤ The aging process (can cause increases or decreases in values, depending on the study)

➤ Inability of client to put forth the necessary breathing effort

➤ Bronchodilators or narcotic analgesics (can change breathing patterns)

➤ Improper placement of the nose clamp or mouthpiece, allowing leakage

Indications for Pulmonary Function Study

➤ Diagnosis and differentiation between pulmonary obstructive and restrictive disease or a combination of both revealed by abnormal expired or inspired volumes, respectively

➤ Determination of the presence of lung disease when other studies such as x-rays do not provide a definitive diagnosis or determination of the progression and severity of known obstructive and restrictive lung disease

➤ Diagnosis of chronic obstructive pulmonary diseases (COPDs) that affect the peripheral airways (asthma, bronchitis), parenchyma (emphysema), and upper airways (tumors of pharynx, larynx, trachea, infections, or foreign body)

➤ Diagnosis of chronic restrictive pulmonary diseases that affect the chest wall (neuromuscular disorders, kyphosis, scoliosis), interstitium (pneumonitis, fibrosis), pleural conditions (pneumothorax, hemothorax), lesions (tumors, cysts), and other conditions such as obesity, ascites, or peritonitis

➤ Dyspnea with or without exertion, coughing, and wheezing to determine the cause
➤ Determination of the effectiveness of therapy regimens while following the course of a pulmonary disorder and identification of bronchospasm response to long-term administration of bronchodilators
➤ Evaluation of the lungs and respiratory status to determine the ability of the client to tolerate procedures such as surgery or diagnostic studies, especially on the lungs
➤ Screening of high-risk populations for early detection of pulmonary conditions (those who smoke, those whose occupations require exposure to potentially harmful inhalants, and those who have a hereditary predisposition)
➤ Evaluation of a pulmonary function after surgical pneumonectomy, lobectomy, or segmental lobectomy
➤ Evaluation of pulmonary disability for legal or insurance claims
➤ Determination of allergic response to inhalants in those with an airway reactive disorder
➤ Evaluation of lung compliance to determine elasticity as revealed by changes in lung volumes, which are decreased in restrictive disease and increased in obstructive disease and in elderly people
➤ Determination of the diffusing capacity of the lungs in diagnosing CHF, adult respiratory distress syndrome, and collagen vascular disorders[13]

Contraindications

➤ Medical conditions such as cardiac insufficiency or recent myocardial infarct
➤ Presence of chest pain that affects inspiration or expiration ability
➤ Upper respiratory infection such as a cold or acute bronchitis

Nursing Care Before the Procedure

Explain to the client:
➤ That medications such as bronchodilators (oral or inhalant) and smoking should be avoided for at least 4 hours before the study
➤ That the study takes about 1 hour, depending on the number of tests performed
➤ That food and fluids are allowed before the study but that a large meal should be avoided, as it causes pressure against the diaphragm and can affect breathing
➤ That a clamp is placed on the nose and that the client is requested to breathe through the mouth into a tube
➤ That the client is requested to perform various breathing patterns during the study
➤ That no pain is associated with the study

Prepare for the procedure:
➤ Obtain height and weight for use in determining the normal range in interpreting results.
➤ Ensure that medication and smoking restrictions have been followed.
➤ Take vital signs and note any respiratory abnormalities such as dyspnea.
➤ Have client void before the procedure for comfort.

➤ Obtain a history of suspected or known pulmonary conditions, respiratory status and patterns, medications (oral, inhalant, other), and previous tests and procedures.

The Procedure

The client is placed in a sitting position on a chair near the spirometry equipment. A soft clip is placed on the nose to restrict nose breathing, and the client is instructed to breathe through the mouth. The client is allowed to practice breathing rapidly and deeply through the mouth in preparation for the tests. A mouthpiece is placed in the mouth, and the client is requested to close the lips around it to form a seal. The client is then requested to inhale deeply and to quickly exhale as much air as possible into the mouthpiece. Other breathing maneuvers are performed on inspiration and expiration (normal and forced) and holding of the breath, depending on the test that is being performed. The tests can also be timed to obtain information for specific tests. The tubing from the mouthpiece is connected to a cylinder that is connected to a computer that measures and records the values for the tests. Some measurements can be calculated with the values obtained from the computer printout. A bronchodilator can be administered, with the test repeated to determine whether ventilation improves over the predicted value for the client in the diagnosis of pulmonary disease.

The lung diffusing capacity test is performed by having the client take a deep breath of a gas mixture (10 percent helium [He] and 0.3 percent carbon monoxide [CO] and room air) from a bag, holding the breath for 10 seconds, and then exhaling. The measurement of the amount of the functioning capillary bed in contact with the alveoli and the alveoli volume are then calculated. Another method involves breathing from a bag of a gas mixture (0.1 to 0.2 percent CO) for a few minutes, after which the exhaled air in the bag is analyzed for oxygen, carbon dioxide, and carbon monoxide concentrations. ABG analysis is also performed for this method of testing for diffusing capacity.[14]

The bronchial provocation test is performed after the FVC test. Inhalation of 1.25 mg of methacholine is administered, and a repeat FVC is performed after waiting about 5 minutes. A reduction in FEV_1 reveals a positive response for bronchial asthma. If no change is revealed, the dosage of medication is gradually increased and, if the FEV is not reduced after 5 dosage dilutions, the result is considered a negative response. A histamine challenge test can follow if no change in FEV is noted. An inhalant bronchodilator should be on hand to treat any bronchospasms that occur with these tests.[15]

At the conclusion of the tests, the mouthpiece and nose clip are removed, and the client is taken to another room to rest.

Nursing Care After the Procedure

➤ Care and assessment after the study include allowing the client to rest in a comfortable chair because clients with impaired pulmonary function can become fatigued by the procedure.

➤ Resume medications that have been withheld and offer water for a dry mouth.

➤ Monitor respirations for dyspnea or breathlessness in clients with severe pulmonary disease.

➤ *Bronchospasms/respiratory distress:* Note and report dyspnea, tachycardia, or apprehension. Administer ordered inhalant bronchodilators. Monitor vital signs.

EXERCISE PULMONARY FUNCTION STUDY

Exercise pulmonary function is a noninvasive study that evaluates the ability to perform exercises or other activities in clients with obstructive or restrictive lung disorders. It assists in determining the extent or severity of respiratory impairment. Testing identifies the level of tolerance through a display of fatigue and dyspnea on a bicycle ergometer during exercise. Activity causes increased oxygen (O_2) consumption and carbon dioxide (CO_2) production, and this study reveals the ability of the pulmonary system to adapt to increases in exercises. The study includes measurements of O_2 needed to accommodate activities and spirometry measurements of air volume and flow. Blood pressure, pulse, and respiration are also monitored during the study. The exercises are increased in increments until the maximum level is attained. More complex pulmonary exercise tests can be performed, based on abnormal results such as measurements of mixed venous CO_2 tension and ABGs; additional ventilatory tests and ratios can be used to obtain more specific diagnostic information.[16]

Reference Values

Normal pattern of air flow during respirations (inspiration and expiration) during exercising; normal ABGs during exercising; no dyspnea caused by respiratory disease

Interfering Factors

➤ Obesity, which can affect the results because more oxygen is consumed with exercise
➤ Weakness and poor physical condition
➤ Impaired cardiac status
➤ Degree of abnormal gas exchange and ventilation impairment

Indications for Exercise Pulmonary Function Study

➤ Evaluating severity of pulmonary impairment in those with respiratory disease to determine status or progression of disease
➤ Diagnosing psychogenic dyspnea as revealed by absence of abnormal response during the test in those with complaints of shortness of breath
➤ Evaluating activity tolerance in those with known pulmonary impairment before planning and prescribing pulmonary rehabilitation
➤ Diagnosing asthma induced by exercise
➤ Differentiating dyspnea caused by pulmonary or cardiac conditions and determining abnormal states that contribute to a decrease in activity intolerance

Contraindications

➤ Medical conditions such as respiratory failure, epilepsy, pulmonary edema, and acute illnesses
➤ Uncontrolled asthma or hypertension with systolic pressure greater than 250 mm Hg and diastolic pressure greater than 120 mm Hg[17]

Nursing Care Before the Procedure

Explain to the client:
➤ That the client should wear comfortable clothing and shoes
➤ That pulse, respirations, and blood pressure are monitored throughout the procedure
➤ That the client will exercise by pedaling a bicycle with increases in speed as the tests are performed
➤ That the client will be requested to breathe through the mouth into a mouthpiece with the nose clamped
➤ That no pain is associated with the study unless more advanced tests are performed that require arterial blood samples

Prepare for the procedure:
➤ Obtain baseline vital signs and note any breathing pattern abnormalities.
➤ Have the client void before the procedure.
➤ Obtain age, weight, height, and history of suspected or known pulmonary conditions, medications and time of last doses, and previous tests and procedures.

The Procedure

The client is seated on the bicycle adjusted to the proper height, and the feet are strapped to the pedals. A soft clip is placed on the nose to restrict nose breathing, and the client is instructed to breathe through the mouth. A mouthpiece is placed in the mouth, and the client is requested to close the lips around it to form a seal. The client is requested to start pedaling while breathing through the mouthpiece, which is attached to the computerized equipment that measures the pulse, blood pressure, and respiratory rates while the spirometry component measures expiratory air flow and tidal volume for each minute of exercise. Exercising is increased in increments until the client can no longer tolerate the continued pedaling. In some testing, 100 percent oxygen is administered to determine the amount of oxygen therapy needed to improve activity tolerance, if improvement is a possibility. The results are analyzed and recorded by the computer. More extensive testing to obtain additional measurements includes rebreathing maneuvers and ABG analysis, which extends the testing time up to 2 hours.

At the conclusion of the test, the mouthpiece and nose clip are removed, and the client is assisted off the bicycle and to a chair to rest.

Nursing Care After the Procedure

➤ Care and assessment after the study include allowing the client to rest until respirations return to normal.
➤ Resume any medications withheld before the study.
➤ Monitor respirations for continued dyspnea in clients with severe pulmonary impairment.
➤ *Respiratory distress:* Terminate test early if extreme dyspnea, exhaustion, cyanosis, or vital sign changes indicate possible respiratory arrest. Have aminophylline and emergency resuscitation equipment on hand.

OXIMETRY

Oximetry, also known as pulse oximetry, is a noninvasive study that provides continuous readings of arterial blood oxygen saturation (SaO_2) by using a sensor site (earlobe or fingertip). Oxygen is transported in combination with hemo-globin (Hgb) or dissolved in blood plasma, with 99 percent of the oxygen used by the body tissues carried by Hgb. About 95 to 97 percent is carried if the Hgb is saturated with O_2, because a small amount of unoxygenated blood from the bronchial circulation is mixed with the oxygenated blood in the pulmonary veins. The SaO_2 equals the ratio of the amount of O_2 in the Hgb to the maximum amount of Hgb expressed in percent.

This procedure is performed to monitor oxygenation status that compares favorably with oxygen saturation levels obtained by ABG analysis without the need to perform successive arterial punctures. The device is a clip or probe containing a sensor that increases the blood flow to the site and produces a light beam through the tissues at the site. The sensor measures the absorption of the light to determine the oxygen saturation reading, which is recorded on a stationary or portable screen for viewing.[18]

Reference Values

Normal arterial blood oxygen saturation of 95 percent or more

Interfering Factors

➤ Movement of the finger or ear affects the measurement readings.
➤ Anemic conditions with a reduction in Hgb, the oxygen-carrying component in the blood, affect measurement readings.
➤ Vasoconstriction from cool skin temperature, drugs, hypotension, or vessel obstruction causes a decrease in blood flow readings.

Indications for Oximetry

➤ Monitoring of oxygenation of tissues and organs postoperatively and during acute illnesses to determine impaired cardiopulmonary function
➤ Monitoring of oxygenation status in clients on a ventilator
➤ Suspected nocturnal hypoxemia in COPD to measure oxygen saturation during nocturnal oxygen therapy
➤ Monitoring of oxygen saturation during activities such as pulmonary exercise stress testing or during pulmonary rehabilitation exercises to determine optimal tolerance
➤ Determination of effectiveness of pulmonary gas exchange function
➤ Monitoring of response to pulmonary drug regimens, especially bronchodilators, to determine effectiveness in promoting air flow and oxygen content
➤ Monitoring of oxygenation during testing for sleep apnea

Nursing Care Before the Procedure

Explain to the client:
➤ That the test is performed by the nurse, technician, or respiratory therapist, depending on the reason for the monitoring
➤ That a clip will be placed on the upper ear, earlobe, or finger and attached to a monitor that records the oxygen measurements
➤ That the test will last as long as monitoring is needed and can be continuous if done after surgery or for acute pulmonary conditions
➤ That no pain is associated with the test
Prepare for the procedure:

➤ Obtain a history of pulmonary disorders, respiratory and cardiac status, vital signs, reasons for monitoring procedure, and ABG results.

The Procedure

The ear or finger is massaged to increase blood flow to the area. The oximetry probe clip is placed on the site. Blood flow is warmed and increased to the area by the sensor or probe. As a beam of light is passed through the tissue at the site, the sensor measures the amount of light that is absorbed.[19] The reading of this measurement is recorded on a monitor (stationary or portable handheld).

At the conclusion of the test or monitoring, the clip is removed.

Nursing Care After the Procedure

No special care is required after this procedure.

➤ *Hypoxemia:* Note and report measurements of less than 95 percent. Note extreme measurement of 75 percent as a critical value requiring immediate interventions. Monitor oximetry readings and vital signs. Have oxygen, ventilator, and other resuscitation equipment on hand.

SWEAT TEST

The sweat test, also known as the pilocarpine iontophoresis sweat test, is a non-invasive study performed to obtain a definitive diagnosis of cystic fibrosis in children when considered with other test results and physical assessments. Cystic fibrosis is a hereditary disease characterized by elevated sodium chloride (NaCl) in the sweat, chronic lung disease, and pancreatic insufficiency. This test measures the sodium (Na) and chloride (Cl) content in the sweat produced by the sweat glands of the skin after inducement to increase its production by a small electric current carrying the drug pilocarpine. An analysis of the collected sweat is performed to determine sodium and chloride content, with high concentrations indicating the presence of the disease. The newborn is not a candidate for this test because the amount of sweat produced is insufficient for testing.

Screening for cystic fibrosis can be performed with the use of a silver ni-trate test paper and validation of a positive test by pilocarpine iontophoresis.[20] A new battery-operated device that uses patches on the skin that change color when sweat chloride levels are elevated after induction of sweating by pilo-carpine iontophoresis is also used to perform this test.[21]

Reference Values

	Conventional Units	**SI Units**
Sodium concentration in sweat	10–40 mEq/L	10–40 mmol/L
Chloride concentration in sweat	0–35 mEq/L	0–35 mmol/L

Note: No cystic fibrosis values of greater than 70 mEq/L sodium or greater than 50 mEq/L chloride in children.

Interfering Factors

➤ Inadequate amount of sweat to perform test accurately
➤ Improper cleansing of skin or application of gauze pad or paper

➤ Hot environmental temperatures that can reduce sodium chloride or cool environmental temperatures that affect the amount of sweat collected

Indications for Sweat Test

➤ Diagnosis or confirmation of cystic fibrosis in children
➤ Screening for cystic fibrosis in those with a family history of the disease
➤ Suspected cystic fibrosis in failure-to-thrive infants or malabsorption syndrome or recurrent respiratory infections in children

---

➤➤ Nursing Alert

• The test should be terminated if the client complains of burning at the electrode site, and the electrode should then be repositioned before the test is resumed. The site for electrode placement should never include the chest because of the risk for cardiac arrest from the current.

Nursing Care Before the Procedure

➤ Inform the client that an electrode is placed on the forearm, thigh, and possibly the back and that sweat is collected for laboratory analysis of sodium and chloride content.
➤ Assurance should be given that no pain is associated with the test but that a stinging sensation can be experienced at the site and that the electric current causing it is delivered at a very low level.
➤ The history should include the presence of cystic fibrosis in other members of the family, endocrine disorders, failure to thrive, respiratory status, and malabsorption syndrome as well as results of other tests.

The Procedure

The client is placed in a position to allow exposure of the site on the forearm. If the client is a small infant, two sites (back and thigh) can be used to ensure the collection of an adequate amount of sweat. The client should be covered to prevent evaporation caused by cool environmental temperatures, which affect sweat collection. The site is washed with distilled water and dried. A positive electrode is attached to the site and covered with a pad that is saturated with pilocarpine hydrochloride, a drug that stimulates sweating. A negative electrode is covered with a pad that is saturated with bicarbonate solution. Iontophoresis is achieved by supplying a low-level electric current via the electrode for 5 to 12 minutes. Battery-powered equipment is preferred over an electrical outlet to supply the current. The electrodes are removed, revealing redness at the site, and the site is washed with distilled water and dried to remove any possible contaminants on the skin. Disks made of filter paper are weighed, placed on the site with a forceps, and covered with paraffin to prevent any possible evaporation of the sweat collected. The disks are left in place for about 1 hour, the paraffin removed, and the disks placed in a preweighted flask with a forceps. The flask is sent to the laboratory for weighing and analysis for sodium and chloride content.[22] At least 100 mg of sweat is required for testing.

Nursing Care After the Procedure

➤ Care and assessment after the test include washing and drying the site and assessing it for any unusual sensations or redness.

➤ Place the stopper in the flask containing the filter paper and take it to the laboratory immediately.

➤ Assess the site for unusual color or discomfort. Inform the client that the redness at the site will fade out in 2 to 3 hours.

➤ Provide support if necessary when diagnostic findings are revealed and assist the client or caregiver, or both, to cope with long-term implications (effect on organs and systems, early death).

➤ If cystic fibrosis is diagnosed, provide referral for genetic counseling, further education, and possible screening of other members of the family.

NEUROLOGICAL SYSTEM

Neurological system studies primarily include procedures to obtain diagnostic information about otological and ophthalmologic conditions. Emphasis is placed on those procedures that provide assessment data about auditory and visual deficits that lead to diagnosis and treatment regimens to correct sensory impairments. Tests that have commonalities in the data collection or obtained information are grouped under general headings. Neuromuscular tests that are included in this section are spinal nerve root thermography and the Tensilon test.

The procedures can be performed in various settings by a physician, nurse, or trained technician, depending on the test. A signed informed consent form is not needed unless specified.

SPINAL NERVE ROOT THERMOGRAPHY

Spinal nerve root thermography is a noninvasive study that measures and compares the heat emitted from the surface of the skin at two adjacent areas of the spinal column (lumbar, thoracic, cervical). It is performed to detect sensory nerve irritation, which causes distinct heat patterns at the skin sites of peripheral afferent fibers, indicating nerve root injury.[23] Spinal nerves divide into two roots: One is the dorsal root, which carries afferent neuron axons into the central nervous system (CNS), and the other is the ventral root, which carries the axons of the afferent neurons to the periphery. The irritation of these nerve roots by conditions such as a ruptured intervertebral disk or soft tissue injuries produces abnormal heat levels, which are revealed by this study. The most common site tested is the lumbar region to assist in diagnosing the cause of low back syndrome. This study can be performed in conjunction with myelography, electromyography (EMG), and computerized scanning diagnostic procedures.

Reference Values

Normal diffusion of heat patterns of lumbar, thoracic, and cervical spinal nerve areas; no nerve irritation or soft tissue trauma

Interfering Factors

➤ Changes in room temperatures

➤ Smoking before the test, which can affect circulation and change the heat course of a specific dermatome

➤ Leg asymmetry caused by varicose veins, if the legs are scanned

Indications for Spinal Nerve Root Thermography

➤ Diagnosis of herniated intervertebral disk that presses on a nerve root as revealed by an abnormal and asymmetrical heat pattern along the dermatome course

➤ Evaluation of preoperative and postoperative status of a lumbar herniated intervertebral disk as revealed by a change from asymmetrical to symmetrical heat emission in the thighs and a diffusion of heat emission in the lower back region

➤ Chronic or acute back pain to determine the cause, such as nerve root irritation or soft tissue injury

Nursing Care Before the Procedure

Explain to the client:

➤ That the procedure is performed in a specially equipped room in the radiology department by a technologist and that it takes about 60 to 90 minutes

➤ That there are no food or fluid restrictions but that smoking should be restricted for 4 to 6 hours before the test

➤ That no lotions or powders should be applied to the scanning sites before the study

➤ That a device will scan the areas to determine the heat emitted from the skin surfaces

➤ That there is no pain or radiation associated with this study

Prepare for the procedure:

➤ Assist the client in removing clothing from the waist down for lumbar studies and from the waist up for cervical studies, and provide a gown.

➤ Wash the areas of any lotions or powders that might be present and pat dry.

➤ Have client void before the procedure.

➤ Obtain a history of musculoskeletal conditions; severe or chronic pain in a spinal area, legs, or arms; last physical therapy session; and past tests and procedures; note whether EMG has been performed on the day of the study.

The Procedure

The client is placed in a prone position with the lower back, buttocks, and legs exposed and draped or the back of the neck, shoulders, and arms exposed and draped, depending on the area to be scanned. The skin sites are cooled with water at room temperature (68°F [20°C]) or with alcohol in a spray bottle and are blown dry with a hair dryer. The client is requested to lie quietly and relax for 10 minutes. An electronic apparatus containing infrared sensors is placed on two adjacent areas of skin surfaces and scanning is performed over the lower back, buttocks, and both legs for lumbar examination or over the back of the neck and both shoulders and arms for cervical examination. Heat patterns and any changes are measured, and views are photographed for analysis. A difference between the temperature of the surface on one side and that on the other side is considered an abnormality. Local abnormalities indicate soft tissue injury, and an abnormality that follows a specific course indicates sensory nerve irritation.[24]

Nursing Care After the Procedure

No special aftercare is required for this test.

➤ *Chronic pain:* Note and report severity and characteristics of pain. Support positioning of painful areas during and after the study. Administer ordered analgesic.

TENSILON TEST

The Tensilon test is a pharmacological challenge study performed to assist in the diagnosis of myasthenia gravis. The drug used is edrophonium chloride (Tensilon), a short-acting form of the drug used to treat this disorder. The test involves the IV administration of the drug before and during the performance of various muscular movements and the evaluation of these movements for changes in muscle strength. A positive diagnosis is made when the administration of the drug results in an improvement in muscle function. A negative diagnosis is made if muscle fasciculations occur as a result of the drug.

Myasthenia gravis is a disease affecting the neuromuscular junction. It is caused by a deficiency of acetylcholine receptor sites on the muscle side of the junction. It is thought that the reduction in these sites is caused by an autoimmune response that blocks the receptor site and is responsible for receptor destruction. The most prominent symptom of the disease is weakness of the involved muscles, which progresses in severity to all areas of the body.

Reference Values

Absence of muscle fasciculations after injection of edrophonium chloride; no myasthenia gravis revealed, that is, no muscle weakness or autonomic dysfunction

Interfering Factors

➤ Corticosteroids, muscle relaxants, and anticholinergics, which can alter test results by their effect on muscle function or on the action of Tensilon

Indications for Tensilon Test

➤ Diagnosing myasthenia gravis when fatigue and muscle weakness are present, as revealed by an immediate improvement after injection of Tensilon

➤ Monitoring medication regimen of oral anticholinesterase to determine whether increase in dose is advised, as revealed by an improvement in muscle strength after IV Tensilon

➤ Determining whether an overdose is present, which can place the client in cholinergic crisis, as revealed by an exaggeration of muscle weakness after IV Tensilon

Contraindications

➤ Breathing difficulties or apneic conditions, because the disease can cause respiratory difficulties severe enough to require ventilatory support

Nursing Care Before the Procedure

Explain to the client:

➤ That the test is performed by a physician in an examining room equipped with all the necessary supplies and that it takes about 30 minutes

➤ That the nurse will remain with the client during the entire test because the medication can have some side effects

➤ That any side effects from the medication will disappear quickly

➤ That there are no food or fluid restrictions but that some medications that can affect muscle function are withheld before the test

➤ That the medication for the test is administered IV (or intramuscularly [IM] in a child)

➤ That the client is requested to make repeated movements during the test to check muscle function and that several tests can be performed to ensure acceptable results

➤ That no pain is associated with the test

Prepare for the procedure:

➤ Have the client void before the test.

➤ Obtain a history of respiratory/musculoskeletal disorders; drug sensitivities; medication regimen that includes medications that affect muscle function, anticholinesterase therapy, and time and amount of last dose; and previous diagnostic procedures.

The Procedure

The client is placed in a supine or a sitting position on the examining table, with the arm to be used for the IV exposed and supported with an armboard. An infusion of 5 percent glucose in water or normal saline is started, and an initial dose of Tensilon is administered, usually about 2 mg for an adult, with adjustments based on weight in kilograms for children. The client is requested to perform activities to fatigue the muscles, such as holding the arms up or looking up until the arms or eyelids drop. The remaining 8 mg of Tensilon is then administered over a 30-second period to a total dose of 10 mg. The client is then requested to perform muscle movements such as crossing and uncrossing the legs, opening and closing the eyes, and raising and lowering the arms. Observations for muscle strength improvement are made, and a dramatic improvement indicates that the weakness is caused by myasthenia gravis. The test is repeated to ensure accuracy if muscle strength does not improve after the injection. Atropine is administered during the test for those clients with asthma to decrease the side effects of the Tensilon. Oral anticholinesterase medication regimen is evaluated by infusion of 2 mg of Tensilon 1 hour after a dose of the anticholinesterase medication. A brief improvement in muscle strength indicates that an increase in therapy would be beneficial. A decrease in muscle strength indicates that a reduction in therapy is needed. Differentiation between myasthenic and cholinergic crisis is evaluated by the infusion of 1 to 2 mg of Tensilon and the observation for muscle strength improvement or respiratory difficulty. In the absence of muscle strength improvement, another 5 mg can be infused, 1 mg at a time, under close observation for any distress. Resuscitation equipment should be on hand, as well as atropine for treatment of cholinergic crisis and neostigmine for treatment of myasthenic crisis, to be administered IV.[25]

Nursing Care After the Procedure

➤ Care and assessment after the test include discontinuing the IV line and assessing the vital signs and injection site.

➤ Inform the client to resume any medications withheld before the test.

➤ *Cholinergic/myasthenic crisis:* Note and report respiratory distress/muscle activity during Tensilon administration. Provide resuscitation equipment, oxygen, and tracheostomy supplies. Administer ordered 0.5 to 1 mg of atropine IV for cholinergic crisis or 0.5 to 2 mg neostigmine IV for myasthenic crisis.

HEARING LOSS AUDIOMETRY

Hearing loss audiometry involves the quantitative testing for a hearing deficit by using an electronic instrument called an audiometer that measures and records thresholds of hearing by air conduction and bone conduction tests. These results determine whether the hearing loss is conductive, sensorineural, or a composite of both. An elevated air conduction threshold with a normal bone conduction threshold indicates a conductive hearing loss. An equally elevated threshold for both air and bone conduction indicates a sensorineural hearing loss. An elevated threshold of air conduction that is more than an elevated threshold of bone conduction indicates a composite of both types of hearing loss. A conductive hearing loss is caused by an abnormality in the external auditory canal or middle ear; a sensorineural hearing loss is caused by an abnormality in the inner ear or of the auditory (eighth) nerve.[26] Sensorineural hearing loss can be further differentiated clinically by sensory (cochlear) or neural (eighth nerve) lesions. Some common causes of conductive hearing loss include otosclerosis, middle ear infection, and obstruction or infectious process of the external ear. Causes of sensorineural hearing loss include congenital damage or malformations of the inner ear, tumor, trauma to the inner ear, vascular disorders, ototoxic drugs, serious infections, and constant exposure to excessive levels of sound or noise. Comparing and differentiating between conductive and sensorineural hearing loss can further be evaluated by performing hearing loss tuning fork tests (see p. 917).

The test is performed on one ear at a time with the audiometer, which delivers specific frequencies of acoustic stimuli of specific intensities that determine a threshold (lowest intensity level) for each frequency. Air conduction thresholds are obtained using earphones; bone conduction thresholds are determined by an oscillator placed in contact with the head. The hearing loss is measured in decibels; the acoustic powers required to obtain the thresholds are compared with the acoustic powers required to obtain the same thresholds in one with normal hearing. The results are recorded on a graph called an audiogram, which plots the hearing threshold levels in decibels (dB), with the frequencies between 125 or 250 to 8000 hertz (Hz).[27]

Hearing tests to estimate hearing ability can be performed on infants and children using special procedures, depending on the age of the client. This can be performed as part of the general physical assessment or as part of a screening program for hearing deficit identification in the schools, or under both circumstances. In infants under 6 months of age, normal reflexive responses can be observed when sounds are administered with a handheld device. In children between 6 months and 2 years of age, minimal response levels can be determined by behavioral responses to test tones. In children 2 years of age and older, play audiometry that requires the child to perform a task or raise a hand in response to a specific tone is performed. In children 12 years of age and older, response to speech of specific intensities, with the child following directions in identifying objects, can evaluate hearing loss affected by speech frequencies.[28] A simpler, faster screening test, consisting of covering one ear and whispering in the direction of the other ear from 1 to 2 feet away and noting the response of the child, can also be used.

Presbycusis, also known as aging hearing loss, is a sensorineurai hearing loss that is part of the normal aging process. It is a progressive decrease in acuity in which high-frequency tones are affected more than low-frequency tones. Various levels of deficit at different ages can be experienced, with the incidence higher in men than in women.

Reference Values

Normal pure tone average of 0 to 25 dB for adults and 0 to 15 dB for children; ability to detect 1 dB of increased intensity or loudness, with the area of intelligible speech sounds anywhere between 0 and 70 dB and a decrease in hearing loss evident as the number increases; no conductive, sensorineural, or mixed hearing loss

Interfering Factors

➤ Obstruction of the ear canal by cerumen or other material or object, which affects decibel perception

➤ Noisy environment or extraneous movements

➤ Tinnitus or other sensations, which can cause inaccurate responses

➤ Improper earphone fit or audiometer calibration

➤ Inability or refusal of client to cooperate or follow instructions

Indications for Hearing Loss Audiometry

➤ Screening for hearing loss in infants and children and determining the need for a referral to an audiologist

➤ Determining the type and extent of hearing loss (conductive as revealed by a reduced air threshold and unchanged bone threshold, sensorineural as revealed by a reduced air and bone threshold, or mixed as evidenced by abnormal air and bone thresholds) and determining whether further radiologic, audiologic, or vestibular procedures are needed to identify the cause

➤ Evaluating the degree and extent of preoperative and postoperative hearing loss after stapedectomy in clients with otosclerosis

➤ Evaluating communication disabilities and planning for rehabilitation interventions

➤ Determining the need for and type of hearing aid and evaluating its effectiveness

Nursing Care Before the Procedure

Explain to the client:

➤ That the test will be performed in a quiet room by a nurse or an audiologist and that it takes about 20 minutes or less, depending on the test

➤ That each ear will be tested separately by using earphones through which tones of varying intensities are delivered, by using a device placed behind the ear, or by using whispered sounds spoken at a specific distance

➤ That the client will be requested to press a button at the time a tone is heard or to signal when a whisper is heard

➤ That no pain is associated with the test

Prepare for the procedure:

➤ Obtain history of known or suspected hearing loss and cause; use of a hearing aid; complaints of changes in auditory acuity; past auditory testing, procedures, and results; and age of the client.

The Procedure

The client is placed in a sitting position in comfortable proximity of the audiometer in a soundproof room. The audiometer is an electronic device that delivers acoustic stimuli of specific frequencies at specific intensities to determine hearing thresholds for each frequency. An otoscopy examination is performed to ensure that the external ear canal is clear of any obstruction. Testing for closure of the canal by the pressure of earphones is accomplished by compressing the tragus. Tendency for the canal to close (often the case in children and elderly clients) can be corrected by the careful insertion of a small, stiff plastic tube into the anterior canal. The earphones are positioned on the head and over the ear canals. A trial of a tone of 15 to 20 dB above the expected threshold is delivered to an ear for 1 second to familiarize the client with the sounds and to start the test. The client is instructed to press the button each time a tone is heard, no matter how loudly or faintly it is perceived. The test results are plotted on a graph called an audiogram using symbols that indicate the ear tested and responses with earphones (air conduction) or oscillator (bone conduction).

First, air conduction is tested by starting at 1000 Hz and gradually decreasing the intensity 10 dB at a time until the client no longer presses the button, indicating that the tone is no longer heard. The intensity is then increased 5 dB at a time until the tone is heard again. This process is repeated until the same response is achieved two out of three times at the same level. The threshold is derived from the lowest decibel level that achieves a 50 percent response rate. The test is continued for each ear, testing the better ear first, with tones delivered at 1000 Hz, 2000 Hz, 4000 Hz, 8000 Hz, and then 1000 Hz, 500 Hz, and 250 Hz to determine a second threshold. Averaging the air conduction thresholds at 500 Hz, 1000 Hz, and 2000 Hz reveals the degree of hearing loss. Tone averages between 25 and 40 dB indicate a mild loss, 40 and 55 dB indicate a moderate loss, 56 and 90 dB indicate a moderately severe to severe loss, and over 90 dB indicates a profound or total loss.

Bone conduction is then tested by using an oscillator placed on the mastoid process behind the ear(s) after removal of the earphones. The raised and lowered tones are delivered as in air conduction, using 250 Hz, 500 Hz, 1000 Hz, 2000 Hz, and 4000 Hz to determine the thresholds. An analysis of threshold responses for air and bone conduction tones is made to determine the type of hearing loss (conductive, sensorineural, or mixed).[29]

A simpler test of hearing can be performed without the use of an audiometer but it is not as accurate or as comprehensive in determining the type and extent of hearing loss. It involves using a ticking watch or whispering at a specific distance from each ear. The ear not being tested is occluded with a finger, and the tester stands at 15 ft from the client and whispers or speaks words toward the ear to be tested. If the words are not heard, the tester moves closer, to 10 or 5 ft from the client. The second ear is then tested in the same manner. The results are recorded as 15/15 or 10/15, and so on. The test using a ticking watch is similar except that the watch is held next to the ear and then moved away from the ear 1 ft at a time until the ticking is no longer heard. The test is repeated for the second ear, and the results are recorded at the distance when the ticking is no longer heard.

Nursing Care After the Procedure

➤ Care and assessment after this test include informing the client of the schedule for retesting and instruction in the use, cleansing, and storing of a hearing aid, if one is used.

➤ *Crossover tone:* Note and report test tones that cause crossover to the opposite ear during air conduction testing (over 40 dB or 125 to 750 Hz, 50 dB or 1000 to 8000 Hz) or bone conduction testing. Mask the ear that is not being tested.[30] (Present a sound to the ear not being tested to ensure that responses are based on hearing in the ear being tested.)

HEARING LOSS TUNING FORK TESTS

Tuning fork tests are noninvasive assessment procedures that are used to distinguish conduction hearing loss from sensorineural hearing loss. They use a tuning fork of 1024 Hz that is set into a light vibration with a tap on the handle. Three types of tuning fork tests can be performed: the Weber test, the Rinne test, and the Schwabach test. The Weber test is performed to evaluate bone conduction deafness by lateralizing the tuning fork tone to one ear. Placement of the vibrating tuning fork on the head stimulates the inner ears equally, and the bone-conducted sound is heard more loudly and clearly on the side with a conduction deficit. The Rinne test is performed to compare air and bone conduction of sound in both ears. Placement of the vibrating tines near the external auditory meatus (air conduction) and then placement of the stem on the mastoid process (bone conduction) determines whether conduction or sensorineural hearing loss is present. If the sound is louder and longer at the mastoid process than near the front of the ear, a conduction hearing loss is identified. If a reduced sound in both air and bone conduction is present, a sensorineural hearing loss is identified. The Schwabach test is performed by comparing the bone conduction of the client with the normal bone conduction of the examiner.[31]

The tuning fork tests are performed as a part of the physical assessment examination and are followed by hearing loss audiometry for confirmation of questionable or abnormal results.

Reference Values

Normal air and bone conduction in both ears; no hearing loss

Weber test: Same tone loudness heard equally in both ears

Rinne test: Longer and louder tone heard by air conduction (40 seconds) than by bone conduction (20 seconds)

Schwabach test: Same tone loudness heard equally long by the examiner and the client

Interfering Factors

➤ Poor technique in striking the tuning fork or incorrect placement
➤ Inability of client to understand and cooperate in identifying sites
➤ Hearing loss in the examiner, which can affect results in the Schwabach test

Indications for Hearing Loss Tuning Fork Tests

➤ Screening for hearing loss as part of a routine physical examination and determining the need for a referral to an audiologist
➤ Obtaining information about the type of hearing loss (conductive or sensorineural) as revealed by a tone heard on one side, indicating a conductive loss on that side or sensorineural loss on the other side in the Weber test; bone conduction tone heard louder or for a longer time than air conduction tone, indicating a conductive loss; or air conduction tone heard louder, indicating a sensorineural loss in the Rinne test; tone that is heard longer by the client than by the examiner, indicating a conductive loss, and heard for a shorter time, indicating a sensorineural loss in the Schwabach test

Nursing Care Before the Procedure

Explain to the client:
➤ That the test is conducted in a quiet room by the nurse or the physician during a physical or hearing examination and that it takes less than 5 minutes
➤ That there are no restrictions or special preparations before the tests
➤ That the client will be requested to respond verbally or by pushing a button to indicate the tones heard in each ear
➤ That no pain is associated with these tests
➤ Obtain history of known or suspected hearing loss and cause, use of hearing aid, changes in auditory acuity, and other hearing tests and procedures performed and the results.

The Procedure

The client is placed in a comfortable sitting position facing the examiner in a chair or on the examining table in a quiet environment. A tuning fork of 1024 Hz is used because it tests within the range of human speech (400 to 5000 Hz).

Weber Test. Tap the tuning fork on the handle against the hand to start a light vibration. Hold the base of the vibrating tuning fork with the thumb and forefinger of the dominant hand, and place it on the middle of the forehead or at the vertex of the head. Ask the client to determine whether the sound is heard better and longer on one side than on the other. Record as Weber right or left or, if the sound is heard equally, as Weber negative.

Rinne Test. Tap the tuning fork on the handle against the hand to start a light vibration. Have the client move a finger in and out of the canal of the ear not being tested (masking). Hold the base of the vibrating tuning fork with the thumb and forefinger of the dominant hand and place it in contact with the mastoid process. Ask the client to indicate when he or she can no longer hear the sound. Then place the same vibrating tuning fork in front of the ear canal without touching the external part of the ear. Ask the client which of the two has the louder or longer tone. Repeat the test in the other ear. Record as Rinne positive if air conduction is heard longer and as Rinne negative if bone conduction is heard longer.

Schwabach Test. Tap the tuning fork on the handle against the hand to start a light vibration. Hold the base of the tuning fork against the client's mastoid process and ask whether the tone is heard. Have the client mask the other ear by moving a finger in and out of the ear not being tested. Then place the same tuning fork against your own mastoid process of the same side and listen for the tone. Continue to alternate the tuning fork until the sound is no longer heard, and determine whether both cease to hear the tone at the same time. Repeat the procedure on the other ear. If the client hears the tone for a longer or shorter time, count and note this in seconds.[32]

Abnormal test results require further testing by audiometry to confirm findings and detect the type and extent of hearing loss with more specificity.

Nursing Care After the Procedure

There is no special care after these tests.

➤ Refer the client to an audiologist if a hearing loss is detected.

ACOUSTIC ADMITTANCE TESTS

Acoustic admittance tests are procedures used to measure the flow of sound into the ear (admittance) and the resistance to that flow (impedance). Two tests are included to measure acoustic admittance: tympanometry testing, which measures the impedance of the middle ear to acoustic energy, and acoustic reflexes testing, which measures admittance change brought about by reflex contraction of the stapedius muscle. Tympanometry is performed with the use of a source of sound and a microphone that is sealed in the external auditory canal. This instrument measures the acoustic energy that passes through or is reflected by the middle ear. In conductive hearing loss, less sound passes through to the middle ear, and more sound is reflected by the middle ear. Middle ear compliance responds normally to external ear pressure that is equal to atmospheric pressure, and the increase or decrease in the pressure results in various patterns of compliance. The measurement of compliance supplies the diagnostic information needed to determine middle ear abnormalities such as effusion or eustachian tube pathological conditions. It also detects changes in compliance that are produced by reflex contraction of the stapedius muscle to supply diagnostic information about facial (seventh) nerve paralysis by the presence or absence of the reflex and about auditory (eighth) nerve adaptation or fatigue by the presence or absence of the reflex adaptation or decay in neural hearing loss.[33] The results of the tests are recorded and graphed on a tympanogram with curves that are classified according to shape (smooth, flat, peaked), amplitude (increased, decreased, normal), and pressure (positive, negative, normal) and that are correlated with ear abnormalities.

These tests are easily performed on children and older clients who are unable to cooperate during the test, because voluntary participation is not required.

Those clients who do not respond voluntarily to acoustic stimuli are candidates for electrocochleography, a test to measure cochlear response and potentials of the auditory (eighth) nerve, or for evoked response audiometry (see pp. 871 to 874) to measure responses from the brainstem and auditory cortex.

Reference Values

Normal admittance responses by the tympanic membrane and stapedius muscle; no hearing loss; no middle ear or eustachian tube abnormalities; no lesions of the cochlear apparatus or facial (seventh) or auditory (eighth) nerves

Tympanometry: Smooth and symmetrical tympanogram with air pressure range of about 100 decapascals (daPa)

Acoustic reflexes: Trans-brainstem reflex threshold of tones of 70 to 100 dB; ipsilateral thresholds of 3 to 12 dB lower; reflex decay, no more than half of the baseline over 10 seconds[34]

Interfering Factors

➤ Probe that is incorrectly placed, clogged, or moved or failure to obtain and maintain a seal of the probe in the ear canal during the test

➤ Equipment artifacts that can produce inaccurate measurement of the admittance reflex stimuli, which can affect acoustic reflexes testing

➤ Client movement, talking, or swallowing

Indications for Acoustic Admittance Tests

➤ Diagnosing middle ear pathology such as acute otitis media, tumor, or effusion as revealed by changes in the shape, amplitude, and pressure readings on the tympanogram

➤ Determining tympanic membrane abnormalities such as perforation, scarring, or tympanosclerosis affecting auditory acuity, as revealed by large changes in admittance

➤ Determining or confirming the type of lesion in conductive hearing loss, as the middle ear absorbs less sound and reflects more sound in tympanometry

➤ Determining eustachian tube dysfunction caused by obstruction or failure of the tube to open periodically, resulting in a negative air pressure in the middle ear with an accumulation of effusion and edema, as revealed by pressure and amplitude changes and air pressure fluctuations, with respirations recorded in tympanometry

➤ Determining ossicular chain discontinuity or fusion causing conductive hearing loss that results from disorders such as necrosis or dislocation of the incus or stapedial footplate anklyosis, as revealed by changes in admittance

➤ Diagnosing facial (seventh) nerve paralysis, as evidenced by compliance changes produced by reflex contraction of the stapedius muscle

➤ Differentiating among cochlear lesions or abnormalities of the cochlear apparatus (sensory) and acoustic (eighth) nerve brainstem lesions (neural) that cause sensorineural hearing loss by decreasing or distorting the transmission of information to the brain, revealed by reflex adaptation or decay in the acoustic reflex test

➤ Differentiating between acoustic (eighth) nerve and peripheral brainstem lesions from intra-axial brainstem lesions as evidenced by ipsilateral and brainstem determinations and changes in reflex magnitude

➤ Differentiating between sensory and neural hearing loss as revealed by the presence or absence of reflex adaptation or decay below 2000 Hz

➤ Determining or confirming the presence of pseudohypacusis as revealed by confirming voluntary thresholds

Contraindications

➤ Recent surgical procedures on the middle ear to treat chronic otitis media or to correct anatomic abnormalities

Nursing Care Before the Procedure

Explain to the client:

➤ That the tests are performed by the audiologist or physician in a quiet room and that each test takes less than 5 minutes

➤ That there are no restrictions in food, fluid, or activity before the tests

➤ That the introduction of air pressure into the ear can cause dizziness that should be reported but that the dizziness disappears

➤ That a probe is placed into the ear and that some mild discomfort can be experienced at this time

➤ That the tests do not harm the ears when the air and sound stimuli are introduced

Prepare for the procedure:

➤ Obtain a history of known or suspected hearing loss and type and cause, ear conditions with treatment regimens, ear surgery procedures, and other tests and procedures to assess and diagnose auditory deficit.

The Procedure

The client is placed in a sitting position (a child can be held on the lap of the caregiver) in a quiet room. An audiometer can be included in the equipment needed for the test if acoustic reflexes are to be tested. An otoscopy examination is performed to ensure that the external ear canal is clear of any obstruction. The appropriate probe cuff is selected to fit the size and shape of the ear canal. This cuff assists in maintaining a proper seal of the probe. The calibrated probe tip is inserted into the ear canal with the dominant hand while the non-dominant hand pulls the ear upward and backward (adult) or downward (child). The probe tip is equipped with a microphone. The probe is sealed to maintain a negative pressure of 200 daPa, and some silicone putty is used to ensure the seal, if needed, to prevent possible leaks that would cause inaccurate threshold results. The calibrated probe contains an admittance meter, electronic tone generator (sound source), and air pressure manometer and pump used in the delivery of sound and air pressure stimuli. The probe tone level and meter sensitivity are set, and air pressure is delivered to perform the tympanometry. The client is requested to remain very still and to avoid any movement of the face, mouth, and head during the test or upon hearing the sounds. The air pressure is changed, and the admittance is recorded manually or on a strip chart with a recorder. At least six measurements are taken, more if needed to measure extensive admittance changes. A tympanogram that displays no admittance change requires evaluation of probe placement or clogging and repetition of the test.

The acoustic reflex test is performed by the introduction of a pure tone stimulus of 500 to 4000 Hz to one ear via the probe. This stimulus causes a bilateral reflex activation. Changes in admittance in the ear receiving the stimulus (ipsilateral) or in the opposite ear (trans-brainstem) are measured and recorded. The reflex thresholds are determined by the introduction of the sound stimuli in increases of 10 dB and then a decrease of 10 dB when the first reflex occurs. This decrease is followed by increases of 5 dB at a time, with recordings made at the lowest level of stimulus at which a reflex is noted. The reflex decay is then measured in the opposite ear at 500 to 1000 Hz; the sound stimulus is introduced at 10 dB above the reflex threshold for 10 seconds. The reflex magnitude at 5 or 10 seconds is compared with the baseline taken at 1 second to determine reflex decay. Abnormal reflex decay is concluded if the reflex magnitude decreases to less than half of the baseline.[35]

Nursing Care After the Procedure

Care and assessment after these tests include removing the probe from the ear canal and gently cleansing and drying the canal.

OTONEUROLOGICAL TESTS

Otoneurological tests are noninvasive procedures performed in the assessment of cerebellar or vestibular function. They include the falling test, past-pointing test, and Romberg test. The falling test determines dysfunction affecting the entire body through the performance of body maneuvers with the eyes open and closed to note a swaying or falling tendency. The past-pointing test determines dysfunction through performance of finger pointing with the eyes open and closed to note the ability and direction of the past pointing.[36] The Romberg test determines static vestibular dysfunction through the performance of body maneuvers with the eyes open and closed to note arm drift and postural stability. It is also performed as part of the neurological physical examination to evaluate the muscle control of balance and posture (inability to stand with the feet together while the eyes are closed).

The vestibular receptive organs are located in the inner ear and are connected to the CNS, both of which contribute to the reflex activity needed in maintaining body balance, posture, and movement. These vestibular receptors involve nerve fibers that travel in a portion of the acoustic (eighth) nerve to the cerebellum via the medulla and pons. Abnormalities of vestibular function are characterized by vertigo, tinnitus, and hearing loss. They can include peripheral vestibular dysfunction such as motion sickness or Ménière's disease and trauma, infection, or reaction to ototoxic drugs that cause irritation or damage to the vestibular end organs or nerves. Irritation or injury to the system can result in balance disorders reflected by posture instability, dystaxia, and falling. They also can also include central vestibular dysfunction caused by cerebellar tumor compression resulting in vertigo, nystagmus, and dystaxia.[37]

Reference Values

Normal cerebellar and vestibular structure and function; no dizziness, nystagmus, or balance abnormalities

Falling test: Balance maintained with eyes open and closed

Past-pointing test: Ability to touch examiner's index finger with own index finger with eyes open and closed

Romberg test: Ability to stand with feet together and eyes closed

Interfering Factors

➤ Sedatives, antivertiginic agents, stimulants, or depressants that act on the CNS

➤ Alcohol intake before the test, which can affect ability to maintain equilibrium and coordination

➤ Inability of client to understand or perform the body movements needed for the tests

Indications for Otoneurological Tests

➤ Dizziness, nystagmus, or equilibrium dysfunction to determine the cause

➤ Screening for neurological disorders as part of the routine neurological physical examination

➤ Identification of cerebellar or vestibular lesions that affect movements of the entire body or the upper body as revealed by swaying when the eyes are open or closed or by swaying in the direction opposite to nystagmus when the eyes are closed, respectively

➤ Evaluation of posture, balance, and ability to coordinate movements in determining the extent of neurological abnormalities

Nursing Care Before the Procedure

Explain to the client:

➤ That the tests are performed by the nurse or physician during the routine physical examination and that they take about 10 minutes

➤ That there are no restrictions of food or fluids before the tests

➤ That the client is requested to open and close the eyes and perform several movements with the arms and legs during the tests

➤ That no pain is associated with the tests

➤ Obtain a history of known or suspected neurological disorders, signs and symptoms that are related to balance and coordination problems, alcohol and medications taken, and neurological tests and procedures and results.

The Procedure

The client is placed in a sitting position or stands and faces the examiner, depending on the test. The examiner should stand near the client to hold or catch him or her if he or she sways or falls.

Falling Test. Request that the client stand with the arms at the sides and perform the following activities: Stand with the feet together for 20 seconds with eyes open and closed, stand on one foot and then the other for 5 seconds with the eyes open and closed, stand with heel to toe for 20 seconds with eyes open and closed, and walk both forward and backward with the eyes open and closed. Inform the client that he or she will not be allowed to fall. Note and record any swaying or falling by the client, the direction, and closed or open eyes.

Past-Pointing Test. Request that the client sit in a chair. Hold an index finger out and request that the client touch it with the right index finger with the eyes open. Have the client then lower the arm and touch the finger again with the eyes closed. Repeat the procedure using the client's left index finger. Note and record any past pointing, the direction, the side of the finger used, and open or closed eyes.

Romberg Test. Request that the client stand with the feet together with the eyes closed for 20 seconds, and note any swaying or falling and the direction.

Nursing Care After the Procedure

There are no special care or assessment activities after these tests.

➤ *Trauma from a fall:* Stand close to the client if he or she has complained of dizziness. Enlist a second person to help if the client is obese, tall, or disoriented.

OTONEURAL LESION SITE TESTS

Otoneural lesion site tests are procedures performed to localize the site of lesions and to determine the extent of damage to the auditory system. These tests are usually performed when hearing loss audiometry, admittance tests, and presenting signs and symptoms indicate sensorineural hearing loss. They assist in differentiating between sensory (cochlear) and neural (acoustic nerve) hearing loss. A battery of tests is administered that includes Békésy automatic audiometry, tone decay, binaural loudness balance and midplane localization, masking level differences, speech discrimination, and auditory brainstem electric response. Site-of-lesion tests use earphones to present tones of varying intensities that are distinguished from the sensation level. The intensity is the hearing level, and the sensation level is the number of decibels above the threshold for a specific tone. Depending on the test performed, lesions of the cochlear nerve, retrocochlear system, and brainstem and lesions or damage to the cortex, any of which affect hearing acuity, can be located.[38]

Reference Values

Normal auditory system and sensorineural hearing; no lesions of the cochlear apparatus, acoustic (eighth) nerve, or auditory pathways to the brain

Békésy audiometry: Pulsed and continuous tones overlap on the tracings

Tone decay: Tone perceived at 0–10 dB above threshold for 1 min

Binaural loudness balance: Two sounds perceived as being of equal loudness when presented in equal intensity

Binaural midplane localization: One tone heard at the center of the head when two tones of equal intensities are presented

Masking level differences: A threshold difference of 12 dB between homophasic and antiphasic conditions

Auditory brainstem electric response: Acoustic nerve and upper brainstem response wave tracings that follow the same pattern

Interfering Factors

> ➤ Improper electrode placement or poor equipment function
> ➤ Inability of client to understand or cooperate during the test
> ➤ Severe hearing impairment, which can affect the ability of the client to participate in the tests when tones are presented and responses are expected

Indications for Otoneural Lesion Site Tests

> ➤ Dizziness, tinnitus, hearing loss, and other neurological complaints to determine whether they are caused by sensorineural hearing function
> ➤ Determination of the presence and location of lesion sites when conductive hearing loss has been previously tested and ruled out
> ➤ Differentiation between sensory (cochlear) and neural (acoustic nerve) hearing loss; differentiation between cochlear and retrocochlear hearing loss; location of lesions of the retrocochlear system at the acoustic nerve that can be extra-axial or intra-axial brainstem or cortex lesions
> ➤ Determination of the presence, site, and effects of neural lesions of the auditory system
> ➤ Diagnosis of Ménière's disease as revealed by sensory hearing loss

Nursing Care Before the Procedure

Explain to the client:

> ➤ That the tests are performed by an audiologist in a quiet specially equipped room and that they take up to 90 minutes, depending on the number of tests to be conducted
> ➤ That there are no restrictions in foods or fluids or special preparation before the tests
> ➤ That each ear can be tested individually and that earphones are used to transmit sounds that the client responds to verbally or by pushing a button
> ➤ That no pain is associated with the tests

Prepare for the procedure:

> ➤ Obtain history of known or suspected hearing loss and cause; signs and symptoms associated with the auditory system; and past auditory tests, procedures, and results.

The Procedure

The client is placed in a quiet environment in a sitting position. The earphones are placed on the head and secured over both ears.

Békésy Audiometry. The audiometer is set to record at the desired frequencies (one or across all of them, from 100 to 10,000 Hz). The threshold for a pulsing tone and a continuous tone is determined for this test. The client is requested to control the intensity by pressing a response button every time a tone is heard until the tone is no longer heard and then releasing the button. This procedure causes the tone intensity to increase and allows the client to trace back and forth across his or her threshold. The procedure is repeated for 5 minutes and can be increased gradually from 100 to 10,000 Hz. The tracings of the frequencies (broken for the pulsed tone and solid for the continuous tone) are recorded on an audiogram. Tracings reveal movements above and below the client's threshold, and the types of curves on the tracing identify the type of auditory lesions as follows:

Type I: Normal overlapping tracings in which continuous and interrupted tracings are superimposed

Type II: Superimposed tracings up to 1000 Hz with a separation of tracings of 20 dB above this frequency, indicative of cochlear loss or Ménière's disease

Type III: Separation of the tracings at lower frequencies and decline in the threshold for the continuous tone, indicative of retrocochlear pathology (neural lesions such as acoustic neurinoma)

Type IV: Separation of the tracings at all frequencies, indicative of active severe cochlear lesions or early neural lesions

Type V: Separation of the tracings with the threshold of the interrupted tracings greater than the threshold for continuous tracings, indicative of psychogenic hearing loss[39]

Tone Decay Test. A tone is presented at the client's threshold and the client is requested to identify the time at which the tone is audible through the earphones. Tones are increased 5 dB if sounds are inaudible so that a tone can be heard again. The tone is repeated until it is heard continuously for a minute to determine the presence of pathological adaptation that is mildly abnormal in sensory lesions and severely abnormal in neural lesions. In cochlear or retrocochlear lesions a tone is lower or higher than the threshold, respectively.

Binaural Loudness Balance. A tone is presented to one ear and then the other; the tone at one ear is kept at a constant intensity of 90 dB, and then a varied tone is used in the other. The client is requested to respond when the tones sound the same in both ears. This procedure differentiates between cochlear and retrocochlear lesions by the presence of recruitment (abnormal increase in the perception of loudness or hearing of sounds despite a hearing loss) or absence of recruitment, respectively.

Binaural Midplane Localization. A tone is presented to one ear at 90 dB while tones of varied intensities are presented to the other ear. The client is requested to indicate when a single tone is heard at the center of the head. This procedure differentiates between cochlear and retrocochlear lesions by hearing a centered sound or never hearing the centered sound, respectively.

Masking Level Differences. A tone of 500 Hz and a masking noise are presented to both ears at a constant intensity, and the threshold is determined. This determination is followed by a change that cannot be heard by either ear individually to establish another threshold level. This procedure determines acoustic nerve or brainstem lesion if no change is noted at different threshold levels.

Auditory Brainstem Electric Response. Electrodes are placed at the scalp vertex, and the mastoid process of one ear is tested and then the other. The stimuli are presented in rapid tone times of 1 millisecond at 10 per second until a desired number of responses are recorded. The responses are recorded as waves at 1-millisecond intervals at different intensities. Cochlear and retrocochlear lesions are differentiated by normal responses at high intensities or by absent or late responses at high intensities, respectively.[40]

Nursing Care After the Procedure

Care after these tests includes removing the devices from the head.

SPONDEE SPEECH RECEPTION THRESHOLD (SRT) TEST

The spondee speech reception threshold (SRT) test is a noninvasive speech audiometry procedure used to measure hearing loss related to speech. The intensity at which speech is recognized is determined by presenting a list of spondee words, which are familiar words containing two syllables equally accented, for example, "baseball," "birthday," and "railroad." The test represents hearing levels at speech frequencies of 500, 1000, and 2000 Hz. The words are presented at specific intensities, and the intensity at which a client repeats 50 percent of the words correctly reveals the test results. Word recognition tests can also be used to assist in diagnosing high-frequency hearing loss. Those with this type of hearing loss miss consonant sounds that affect the understanding of speech. The test involves the ability to recognize and repeat words such as "pin," "din," "bin," and "sin" that are distinguished by consonants and that are presented at a level above the spondee threshold. Word recognition ability is a different type of hearing loss than that diagnosed by audiometry.[41]

Reference Values

Normal spondee threshold of about 10 dB of the pure tone threshold with 50 percent of the presented words correctly repeated at an appropriate intensity; normal speech recognition with 90 to 100 percent of the presented words correctly repeated at an appropriate intensity

Interfering Factors

➤ Client lack of familiarity with the language the words are presented in or with the words themselves

➤ Improper placement of the earphones and inconsistency in frequency of word presentation

Indications for Spondee Speech Reception Threshold (SRT) Test

➤ Determining the extent of hearing loss related to speech recognition as revealed by the faintest level at which the spondee words are correctly repeated

➤ Differentiating a real hearing loss from pseudohypacusis

➤ Evaluating clarity of speech sounds or speech discrimination as revealed by word recognition at 40 dB above the spondee threshold

Nursing Care Before the Procedure

Explain to the client:

➤ That the test is performed by an audiologist in a specially equipped soundproof booth and that it takes about 5 to 10 minutes

➤ That there are no food or fluid restrictions before the test

➤ That a series of words that change from loud to soft tones will be presented via earphones and that the client will be requested to repeat them

➤ That each ear is tested separately

➤ That no pain is associated with the test

Prepare for the procedure:

➤ Obtain a history of known or suspected hearing disorders and results of pure tone audiometry and other hearing tests, and determine ability to understand English words and sounds.

The Procedure

The client is seated on a chair in a soundproof booth. The earphones are placed on the head and secured over the ears, and the audiometer is set at 20 dB above the known pure tone threshold obtained from audiometry (see p. 914). The client is introduced to the list of spondee words (two-syllable words) to be used in the test, for example, *baseball* or *staircase,* but the list is not used by the client during the test. The spondee words are presented to the ear with the best auditory acuity, first via a speech audiometer with the intensity decreased. The intensity is then increased to the softest sound at which the client is able to hear the words and to respond correctly to 50 percent of them. The procedure is repeated for the other ear.

Speech discrimination is tested by presenting a list of 50 phonetically balanced words such as "pin," "bin," and "kin" at an intensity of 40 dB above the spondee reception threshold. A score is determined from the number of responses. A normal score of 90 to 100 percent indicates a conductive hearing loss, and a reduced score indicates sensorineural hearing loss and acoustic (eighth) nerve impairment.[42]

Nursing Care After the Procedure

There are no special care and assessment activities after this test.

VISUAL ACUITY TESTS

Visual acuity tests are noninvasive procedures performed to evaluate the ability to see and to perceive details. They include the Snellen test, which uses an eye chart to determine distance visual acuity, and the Jaeger test, which uses a card to determine near visual acuity. Both eyes are always tested individually with and without corrective lenses, and the scores are recorded for each eye. Visual acuity that cannot be quantitated by these tests should be tested and noted by the ability of the client to count fingers, detect hand movements, or distinguish light. Visual changes can occur as manifestations of conditions such as lesions or atrophy of the optic (second) nerve, eyelid muscle abnormalities and ptosis, conjunctivitis, trauma or abrasions of the cornea or keratitis, changes in intraocular pressure, cataract, retinal abnormalities or defects, and neurological conditions.

The Snellen test is the most common test and uses a standardized eye chart that consists of lines of block letters that are graded from the largest letters at the top line to the smallest at the bottom line. It tests visual acuity of each eye by the client's ability to read the letters on a chart that is hung on a wall at a distance of 20 ft. Each line has a number that indicates the distance in feet at which an average person can read 50 percent of the letters correctly. The score is derived from this number and the distance and is recorded as a fraction, with the distance (20 ft) over (/) the number of the smallest line read. For example,

20/30 is the distance of 20 ft, and 30 is the number at the lowest line read. A minus number can be added to indicate errors made in reading the numbers on that line, for example, 20/30 − 2. The lower the line of numbers that can be read, the better the visual acuity. The chart numbers can be replaced by figures or other symbols for children and clients who cannot read.

The Jaeger test uses a standardized card that consists of reading material in print that is graded from large to small. Each eye is tested for its ability to read the print while the card is held at a specific distance. Print size is identified based on the ability of a person with normal sight to read the card while it is held at a specific distance. The smallest size of print and the nearest distance for reading the print are noted as a fraction, with the distance of 14 inches/print size able to be read at that distance. This test is usually reserved for those over 40 years of age who have difficulty reading.[43] Visual acuity tests are performed as part of the general physical examination with or without the presence of visual complaints.

Presbyopia is the diminished visual acuity experienced in older people as part of the normal aging process. Presbyopia results in the thickening of the lens, causing its fibers to become less elastic and affecting the range of focus and accommodation.

Reference Values

Normal distance visual acuity of 20/20 and near visual acuity of 14/14

Interfering Factors

➤ Inability of client to cooperate and participate in the tests
➤ Inability of client to recognize and identify the letters or words on the chart or card
➤ Failure of client to bring corrective lenses to be used for testing the corrected vision during the test

Indications for Visual Acuity Tests

➤ Screening for impaired visual acuity in children with no complaints and determination of the need for a referral to an ophthalmologist
➤ Screening for presbyopia and near vision impairment in clients over 40 years of age, with or without complaints, to determine the need for a referral
➤ Eye strain, blurring, difficulty in reading, or other complaints to determine whether the cause is related to visual acuity
➤ Determination of the type of visual impairment, distance or near visual acuity deficit, and the need for corrective lenses
➤ Evaluation of existing visual correction for change in prescription lenses

Nursing Care Before the Procedure

Explain to the client:
➤ That the tests are performed by a physician, technician, or nurse and that they take 5 to 10 minutes
➤ That the client should bring corrective glasses or contact lenses to the test for evaluation
➤ That there are no food or fluid restrictions before the tests
➤ That each eye is tested separately with and without the corrective lenses

➤ That the client is requested to read letters or symbols of different sizes on a chart or words of different-sized print on a card to test vision

➤ That no pain is associated with the tests

Prepare for the procedure:

➤ Obtain a history of known or suspected visual impairment and cause, use of corrective lenses, and age of client.

The Procedure

The client is seated 20 ft away from the Snellen chart to test distance visual acuity. If the client wears glasses or contact lenses, he or she is requested to remove them to first test the vision without correction. The client is requested to occlude the left eye with a hand-held occluder, or the eye is occluded with an eye patch if the client is unable to hold the device to test the right eye (OD). The client is then requested to read the line on the chart with the smallest letters or symbols, which is recorded as the denominator of the fraction, with the numerator indicating the distance of 20 ft. The number of errors on the line with the smallest letters or symbols read can be recorded as a minus next to the denominator, that is, 20/20 − 1. The test is then repeated on the left eye (OS) by occluding the right eye. If the client wears corrective lenses, the same tests are performed on the right and left eyes with the corrective lenses in place to test the effectiveness of the lenses and to determine whether further correction is needed. A pinhole test can be performed if the vision is less than the normal 20/20 to determine whether the abnormal acuity is caused by a refractive error or an organic disorder. The test is conducted by asking the client to look through a pinhole in a card when reading the chart. If vision cannot be quantitated by this test, the client can be requested to count fingers at different distances or to distinguish light by penlight or room light.

Clients who are unable to read the large E at the top of the chart can be tested by asking them to walk toward the chart and stop at the distance at which the E can be visualized. This is recorded as the distance in feet and the line of the large E, that is, 20/200.

The client is seated to read the Jaeger card held at a usual reading distance to test near visual acuity (14 inches). Both eyes are tested as in the Snellen chart without and then with corrective lenses. The results are recorded with the distance as the numerator and the distance needed by those with normal vision to read the same print at a specific distance as the denominator, that is, 14/14 for normal vision and a larger denominator indicating reduced near vision.[44]

Nursing Care After the Procedure

There are no special care and assessment activities after these tests.

Visual Field Tests

Visual field tests are noninvasive procedures performed to detect and locate lesions that cause major defects in the visual fields. These defects occur as a result of damage to the visual pathways or the visual cortex. Tests include perimetry, which records the total extent of the visual field, tangent screen, which records the central visual field from a fixed point, and the confrontation test, which is a simple method to screen the visual field in those who are not candidates for the other tests. Confrontation testing is also performed as a part of the routine neurological physical examination to determine gross abnormalities that, if a defect is detected, should be followed by perimetric or tangent screen testing.[45] Disorders that can interrupt the visual pathways include trauma, tumors, and vascular lesions. Disorders of the visual cortex include damage or pathology in the binocular portion of the primary visual cortex.

The visual field comprises the areas that are visible during the fixation of vision in one direction. The complete visual field is seen by both eyes (binocular) and is divided into the central and peripheral sections. The central section provides the highest visual acuity and focuses on the central fovea, whereas the peripheral section provides the ability to detect objects, stationary or moving. The right and left periphery of the visual field, which is beyond the visual field shared by both eyes, reflects the side of the retina on which the images are seen. When the image reaches the retinas, the visual information is carried to the brain by the optic (second) nerve, which extends from the back of the optic globe through the orbit and optic foramen to the base of the brain. The two optic nerves fuse at the optic chiasm, and the optic tracts contain fibers from both eyes that transmit information from the same visual field. The primary visual cortex is located in the occipital lobe of the brain and functions to add meaning to visual perception, based on past experiences. The circuitry in this area contains specific neurons that respond to shapes, colors, and moving edges of an inclination. Its organization allows separate and multiple representations of a visual field.

Retinal defects also cause visual field defects. Normally, a hole, or scotoma, is present in the visual field because the optic nerve does not contain photoreceptors and the corresponding location in the visual field becomes a blind spot. Retinal damage caused by localized pathology or vascular accidents can produce additional blind spots. The absence of vision in the center of the bilateral visual field is annoying and can be dangerous because part of the visual field disappears, depending on the location of the fixation point.[46] The Amsler grid test is performed to screen for the detection of central scotomas when abnormal vision is present and macular pathology is suspected as the cause. It involves the viewing of squares on a grid with a black dot in the center and evaluating vision for any blurring, distortion, or inability to see the dot.

Reference Values

Normal visual field perception in both eyes; no lesions of the visual pathways or visual cortex

Confrontation test: Correct visualization by each eye of an object moving from the center to the periphery and from the periphery to the center and into four visual quadrants while the client's eye is fixated on the examiner's eye

Tangent screen test: Ability of each eye to visualize an object within the entire central visual field circle, with detection of the blind spot in its correct position in relation to the central fixation point

Perimetry: Visualization by each eye of different-sized test objects as they are moved in all areas of the visual field and disappear and reappear normally at appropriate degrees within the field

Interfering Factors

➤ Severely impaired visual acuity that prevents perception of the moving object within the field

➤ Inability of client to understand or cooperate with the instructions given during the test

Indications for Visual Field Tests

➤ Assessing the monocular vision field of each eye to detect abnormalities as part of the routine neurological examination

➤ Identifying central and peripheral visual field defects to determine lesion sites in the retina, optic pathways, and visual cortex

➤ Evaluating the progression or resolution of ocular disorders such as glaucoma, tumors, trauma, vascular insufficiency, and neurological disorders such as cerebrovascular accident (CVA) or brain tumor

Nursing Care Before the Procedure

Client teaching and physical preparation are the same as for visual acuity tests (see pp. 929 to 930).

➤ Inform the client that the test takes 30 minutes.

➤ Obtain a history of known or suspected eye or neurological disorders, change in visual acuity, treatment regimens, and other tests and procedures performed and the results.

The Procedure

The client is placed in a comfortable sitting position.

Confrontation Test. This test is commonly performed as a part of the routine neurological exam to detect major or large defects in the visual fields. The examiner sits or stands 2 to 3 ft directly in front of the client. The client is requested to cover or close one eye and focus the other eye on the examiner's eye. The examiner slowly moves a finger from the periphery toward the center and from the center toward the periphery through the vertical, horizontal, and oblique areas of the field. The client is requested to respond when the finger becomes visible during each movement. The test is then repeated for the other eye.

Tangent Screen Test. A black screen is placed about 3 ft in front of the client. One eye is covered, and the client is requested to fixate the other eye on a target site on the screen. A test object at the tip of a wand is moved out along the meridians from the central fixation point to 30 degrees. The size of the test object is determined by the client's visual acuity. The client is requested to respond when the test object appears, and the responses are plotted on the screen. The other eye is then covered and the test is repeated. Test objects of various sizes and colors can also be used to outline the field and identify the presence of small holes (scotomas). Results are determined and recorded by comparing the defect with the various sizes of the test objects and the distance between the client and the screen.

Perimetric Test. The client is seated and the head is stabilized by a chin rest while one eye is occluded and the other eye is fixated on a central point directly in front of the eye. A small dot, light, or colored object is moved back and forth in all areas of the visual field. The client is requested to respond to the visibility and color of the object and to signal when the object disappears. Test objects of various sizes are used. The arc is rotated, and another meridian is checked. Standardized movements of the test object are made at 30-degree or lesser intervals to identify the defect. The opposite eye is occluded, and the test is repeated on the other eye. The results are recorded from the plotting on a circular chart of the visual field perceptions with radii at 30-degree intervals.[47]

Nursing Care After the Procedure

There are no special care or assessment activities after the tests.

COLOR PERCEPTION TESTS

Color perception tests are performed to determine the acuity for color discrimination that is most commonly partial but that can be complete. Deficits can be genetic and result from the defective function of one or more of the three cone color systems (blue, green, red), or the deficits can be acquired and result from outer (red, green) or inner (blue) retinal layer pathology. The most common test performed for color discrimination defects uses pseudoisochromatic plates with numbers or letters buried in a matrix of colored dots. Color blindness is determined by the client's misreading of the numbers or letters.

The photoreceptors on the retina include rods, which discriminate black and white, and cones, which discriminate color. The cone receptors are sensitive to different wavelengths of light, which provide for color vision. Three types of cones respond to the red, blue, and green spectrums, depending on the presence of one or more of the color-sensitive molecules that are bound by the visual pigment substance. The amount of involvement of each cone color system determines the hue of a color, and the amount of light received determines the brightness of each hue.[48]

Color perception tests to determine the presence of a deficiency can be part of a routine eye examination or can be initiated after a complaint of difficulty in discriminating between a red and a green traffic light or becoming aware of wearing the wrong combination of colors. Additional tests of retinal function can be performed to determine the extent of an identified deficiency.

Reference Values

Normal visual color discrimination, no difficulty in the identification of color combinations

Interfering Factors

➤ Inability of client to read
➤ Poor visual acuity, failure to wear corrective lenses, poor lighting, or anything that affects the ability to see the test plate
➤ Inability of client to cooperate and participate in the test
➤ Plates that are discolored or damaged

Indications for Color Perception Tests

➤ Detection of deficiencies in color perception

➤ Suspected retinal pathology affecting the cones that are responsible for color discrimination

➤ Family history of color visual deficit, as the deficiency can be inherited

Nursing Care Before the Procedure

Client teaching and physical preparation are the same as for visual acuity tests (see pp. 929 to 930).

➤ Obtain a history of known or suspected color visual impairment in client or family members, importance of color discrimination in work life, or use of corrective lenses.

The Procedure

The client is placed in a sitting position. One eye is covered, and a test book containing pseudoisochromatic plates is held about 12 to 14 inches from the exposed eye. An object that can be used to point is given to the client. Acquaint the client with the plates and the patterns and symbols that will be shown. Advise the client that he or she will be requested to identify the numbers or letters that are buried in a matrix of colored dots or to trace patterns or symbols with the pointed object. As the test is given, record the client responses as the numbers or letters are misread or the patterns are not traced correctly. Repeat the same test on the other eye.

Nursing Care After the Procedure

There are no special care or assessment activities after this test.

TONOMETRY

Tonometry is a noninvasive procedure performed to indirectly measure intraocular pressure to assist in diagnosing glaucoma. Secretion of aqueous humor is continuous, regardless of the pressure of secreted fluid and the rate of production, and it is normally equal to the rate of drainage. An increased intraocular pressure results from an interference with the drainage of the fluid anywhere along the outflow pathway. Glaucoma is a group of eye conditions characterized by a rise in intraocular pressure, which can result in a progressive loss of peripheral vision; later loss of central vision; and, finally, blindness, if left untreated. It can be closed-angle or open-angle glaucoma, depending on the location of the fluid circulation and absorption. It can occur as a primary disease or in association with other conditions of the eye such as inflammation and infection, tumors, or trauma.

Tonometry is performed with an instrument called a tonometer. One type of tonometer (Schiøtz) is placed directly on the anesthetized eye and measures the pressure by the corneal deformation produced by force applied against it. The instrument consists of a plate that rests on the cornea and has a plunger-type apparatus that can apply pressure with an indicator to measure the ocular pressure. Another type is a noncontact tonometer that is mounted on a slit lamp and measures the time needed to flatten an anesthetized area of the cornea with an air blast. The intraocular pressure is read on a dial as the complete flattening is measured electronically. This method is performed by a physician during routine slit-lamp examinations.

Other procedures performed to detect glaucoma are ophthalmoscopy, perimetry, and gonioscopy.

Reference Values

Normal intraocular pressure of 12 to 20 mm Hg, depending on the time of day

Interfering Factors

➤ Corneal surface that inhibits correct placement of the tonometer footplate, which can alter measurement
➤ Flaccid or rigid cornea that prevents proper indentation of the tonometer footplate, which can affect correct measurement
➤ Inability of client to cooperate and remain quiet during the test
➤ Improper technique in the use of the tonometer in performing the measurement

Indications for Tonometry

➤ Screening for glaucoma in clients over the age of 40
➤ Measuring intraocular pressure to assist in the diagnosis of glaucoma or determining whether other tests should be performed to confirm the diagnosis
➤ Monitoring the progression of glaucoma and effectiveness of the treatment regimen

Contraindications

➤ Corneal ulceration or infection that could cause further damage

Nursing Care Before the Procedure

Explain to the client:
➤ That the test is performed by the physician and takes about 1 to 2 minutes
➤ That eyedrops are administered to anesthetize the eyes and that no pain is associated with the test
➤ That corrective lenses (glasses or contacts) are removed before the test and that contacts are not reinserted for 2 hours after the test
Prepare for the procedure:
➤ Obtain a history of known or suspected ocular disorders, changes in visual acuity, eye pain, and other visual tests and procedures performed and the results.

The Procedure

The client is placed in a supine position on the examining table and informed of the importance of lying very still. Ask the client to avoid blinking or tightly closing the eyelids during the test. Instill 1 drop of the topical eye anesthetic in each eye, and request that the client close the eyes to spread the medication over the sclerae. Check the tonometer for a zero reading and a freely moving plunger, and prepare the instrument to measure the pressure using 5.5 g of weight. Instruct the client to look at a spot on the ceiling and to breathe normally. Gently hold the lids of one eye with the thumb and forefinger of the nondominant hand without touching the eyelashes. While holding the tonometer upright with the thumb and forefinger of the dominant hand, place the footplate of the instrument on the apex of the cornea. Avoid any pressure on the cornea by the fingers or any movement of the tonometer, which can cause abrasions. Observe the needle on the calibrated part of the tonometer for a pulsating movement. Record the reading on the scale part of the instrument and the time of day that the procedure was performed. A reading of less than 4 requires that additional weight (7.5 g or more) be applied to obtain a measurement of intraocular pressure. Repeat the procedure to measure the pressure of the other eye.[49]

Nursing Care After the Procedure

➤ Care and assessment after the test include informing the client not to rub the eyes for 30 minutes or to reinsert contact lenses for 2 hours after the procedure until the anesthetic has had time to wear off.

➤ Inform the client that any scratchy feeling is caused by tonometer movement during the test and that this feeling disappears within 24 hours.

➤ *Corneal abrasion:* Note and report complaints of scratchy sensation. Hold tonometer still during the test. Avoid touching the eyelashes, which can cause blinking. Promote relaxation to prevent movement during the procedure. Apply an eye pad for comfort and protection, if needed.

REFRACTION

Refraction is a noninvasive procedure that tests the visual acuity of eyes and determines any abnormalities or refractive errors that need correction. Visual defects such as hyperopia (farsightedness), in which the point of focus lies behind the retina; myopia (nearsightedness), in which the point of focus lies in front of the retina; and astigmatism, in which the refraction is unequal in different curvatures of the eyeball, can be corrected by glasses or contact lenses after this examination. Hyperopia requires a convex lens for correction, myopia requires a concave lens, and astigmatism requires a cylindrical lens.[50]

Usually, pupils are dilated with eyedrops and the eyes are examined with a retinoscope initially to view the brightness, uniformity, and clarity of the light reflection from the instrument. This examination is followed by trying lenses of different powers as the client reads the lines on a Snellen chart to determine the optimal lens to correct the deficit and ensure visual acuity.

This test can be performed during any eye examination, but it is most likely to be performed on those who already wear corrective lenses or complain of a decrease in visual acuity.

Reference Values

Normal refractive power of 44 diopters (distance from the surface at which the rays come into focus, measured in meters) in the cornea and aqueous humor, 10 to 14 diopters in the lens, and overall refractive power of the eye at 58 diopters; no evidence of refractive error[51]

Interfering Factors

➤ Improper pupil dilation, which prevents adequate examination for refractive error

➤ Inability of client to remain still and cooperate during the test

Indications for Refraction

➤ Diagnosing refractive errors in vision
➤ Determining whether an optical defect is present and whether light rays entering the eye focus correctly on the retina (emmetropia), whether the point of focus is behind the retina (hyperopia or farsightedness), whether the point of focus is in front of the retina (myopia or nearsightedness), or whether a nonuniform curvature of the horizontal plane is in contrast with the vertical plane (astigmatism)
➤ Determining the type of corrective lenses needed for refractive errors, that is, biconvex or plus lenses for hyperopia, biconcave or minus lenses for myopia, or compensatory lenses for astigmatism

Contraindications

➤ Pupil dilation in clients with narrow-angle glaucoma
➤ Allergies to medication (mydriatics) used for pupil dilation

Nursing Care Before the Procedure

Explain to the client:
➤ That the examination is performed by a physician in a darkened room and that it takes about 15 to 20 minutes
➤ That eyedrops are administered before the test to dilate the pupils for better viewing of the eyes
➤ That the client is requested to look straight ahead while the eyes are examined with an instrument and while different lenses are tried so that the best corrective lenses can be prescribed
➤ That there is no pain associated with this examination

Prepare for the procedure:
➤ Administer an ordered mydriatic, 1 drop of 5 percent phenylephrine, to each eye, and repeat in 5 to 15 minutes to achieve pupil dilation.
➤ Obtain a history of known or suspected visual impairment, changes in visual acuity, use of glasses or contact lenses, other tests and procedures performed to diagnose eye conditions needing corrective lenses, and results.

The Procedure

The client is placed in a sitting position in the examination chair and the examiner is seated about 2 ft away at eye level with the client. The room light is dimmed, and the retinoscope light is held in the examiner's hand in front of the client's eyes and directed through the dilated pupil. Each eye is examined for the characteristics of the red reflex, which should normally move in the same direction as the light. Lenses of differing strengths are then tried on each eye as the client is requested to read the letters on a Snellen chart posted on a wall 20 ft away. When optimal visual acuity is obtained with the trial lenses in each eye, a prescription for corrective lenses is written.

Nursing Care After the Procedure

There are no care or assessment activities after this examination.
➤ Inform the client that some visual blurring from the dilating medication can be experienced for about 2 hours.

SLIT-LAMP BIOMICROSCOPY

Slit-lamp biomicroscopy is a noninvasive procedure that allows visualization of the anterior portion of the eye and its parts, that is, eyelid and eyelashes, sclera, conjunctiva, cornea, iris, lens, and anterior chamber, to detect pathology of any of these areas. The slit lamp has a binocular microscope and light source that can be adjusted to examine the fluid, tissues, and structures of the eyes. Special attachments to the slit lamp are used for special studies and more detailed views of specific areas.[52]

Reference Values

Normal anterior tissues and structures of the eyes; no corneal, iridic, conjunctival, lens, tearing, or eyelid and eyelash pathology

Interfering Factors

➤ Inability of client to cooperate during the examination
➤ Improper administration of mydriatics

Indications for Slit-Lamp Biomicroscopy

➤ Detection of corneal abrasions, ulcers, or abnormal curvatures (keratoconus) before performing a corneal staining procedure
➤ Detection of lens opacities indicative of cataract formation
➤ Redness, itching, edema, inflammation, ulcerations of the eyelids, eyelashes, sclerae, and conjunctivae to determine the cause, for example, reactions to environmental allergens, infectious process (blepharitis, conjunctivitis, hordeolum, entropion, ectropion, trachoma, scleritis, iritis)
➤ Detection of conjunctival and corneal injuries by foreign bodies and determination of ocular penetration or anterior chamber hemorrhage
➤ Detection of deficiency in tear formation indicative of lacrimal dysfunction, causing dry eye disease, which can lead to corneal erosions or infections
➤ Evaluation of the fit of contact lenses

Contraindications

➤ Pupil dilation in clients with narrow-angle glaucoma
➤ Allergies to mydriatics if used for pupil dilation

Nursing Care Before the Procedure

Explain to the client:
➤ That the examination is performed by a physician and that it takes about 10 minutes
➤ That the client is requested to remain still during the examination and to look straight ahead while the eyes are examined with the slit-lamp instrument to view the eye structures
➤ That eyedrops can be administered to dilate the pupils if the examination is not performed for routine purposes
➤ That there is no pain associated with the examination
Prepare for the procedure:
➤ Administer an ordered mydriatic, 1 drop of 5 percent phenylephrine, in each eye and repeat in 5 to 15 minutes to achieve pupil dilation if the exam is not performed for routine inspection.

➤ Remove contact lenses or glasses before the examination unless the study is being performed to check the fit and effectiveness of the contact lenses.

➤ Obtain a history of external and anterior eye structure conditions and known and suspected eye disorders, signs and symptoms of eye abnormalities, treatment regimens, and previous eye tests and procedures and the results.

The Procedure

The client is seated in a dimmed room in a chair with the feet on the floor, the chin on the rest apparatus, and the forehead against the bar apparatus. The slit lamp is placed in front of the client's eyes in line with the examiner's eyes. The external structures of the eyes are inspected with the special bright light and microscope of the slit lamp. The light is then directed into the client's eyes to inspect the anterior fluids and structures; the light is adjusted for the shape, intensity, and depth needed to visualize these areas. The magnification of the microscope is also adjusted to optimize visualization of the eye structures. To obtain further diagnostic information about the eyes, special attachments and procedures can also be used, such as a camera to photograph specific parts, gonioscopy to determine anterior chamber closure, and cobalt blue filter to detect minute corneal scratches, breaks, or abrasions with corneal staining.

Nursing Care After the Procedure

Care and assessment after the test include informing the client that some blurring of vision can occur and can last about 2 hours if the pupils have been dilated.

SCHIRMER TEARING TEST

The Schirmer tearing test is a noninvasive procedure performed to assess tear formation by the lacrimal glands after stimulation of tearing by the introduction of a foreign object (filter paper) into the lower conjunctival sac of the eyes. Measurement of the moisturized portion of the paper is then made to determine the absence of tears, or "dry eyes." This condition can result in corneal keratinization and ulceration if left undiagnosed and untreated.

Reference Values

Normal amount of moisture in 5 minutes is usually 15 mm of the strip, depending on the client's age. The amount of moisture can be as low as 10 mm in 5 minutes in elderly people.

Interfering Factors

➤ Contact of the strip with the cornea, which can cause reflex tearing
➤ Closing of the eyes during the test, which can increase tearing

Indications for Schirmer Tearing Test

➤ Diagnosis of Sjögren's syndrome, characterized by dryness of the eyes
➤ Detection of tearing deficiency associated with systemic diseases such as rheumatic disorders or systemic lupus erythematosus
➤ Dry or gritty sensation in the eyes, burning, itching, photosensitivity, redness, pain, or inability to move eyelids to diagnose dry eye disorder, especially in elderly people

> Suspected tearing abnormality of the lacrimal apparatus to determine the cause, that is, dacryostenosis, dacryocystitis, or foreign body

Nursing Care Before the Procedure

Explain to the client:
> That the test is performed by the physician and that it takes about 15 minutes
> That both eyes can be anesthetized and tested at the same time and that contact lenses are not reinserted for 2 hours after the test
> That a small strip of paper is gently inserted under the lower lids and left for 5 minutes, removed, and measured for the amount of tearing
> That corrective glasses or contact lenses are removed before the test
> That there is no pain associated with the test

Prepare for the procedure:
> Obtain a history of known or suspected autoimmune systemic diseases; symptoms of eye dryness; and previous eye tests, procedures, and results.

The Procedure

The client is placed in a sitting position. A topical eye anesthetic, 1 drop in each eye, is administered to prevent reflex tearing, and the client is requested to close the lids to spread the medication over the sclerae. The sterile test strips (35- by 5-mm strips of filter paper) are removed from their wrappers after bending the portions to be inserted and cutting the ends to facilitate removal. The client is requested to look upward; the lower lid is gently pulled downward, and the bent end of a strip is inserted into the lower conjunctival sac of one eye, toward the nasal side. The client is requested to remain quiet and not to rub or squeeze the lids closed during the time that the strip is in place. The time of insertion is recorded and the strip is left in place for 5 minutes. The strip is removed, and the tearing response to the irritation of the filter paper strip or the length of the moistened portion is measured, using a millimeter scale. The test is repeated on the other eye. The test results are recorded as a fraction for each eye, with the length in millimeters as the numerator and the time in minutes that the strip was left in place as the denominator, that is, 10 mm/5 min.[53]

Nursing Care After the Procedure

> Care and assessment after the test include instructing the client to avoid rubbing the eyes for 30 minutes or reinserting contact lenses for 2 hours after the test, if the eyes were anesthetized.
> *Corneal abrasion:* Note and report complaints of scratchy sensation or any change in visual acuity. Instruct the client to avoid touching or rubbing the eyes or inserting contact lenses if a topical anesthetic has been instilled, as these activities can damage the cornea.

CORNEAL STAINING TEST

Corneal staining is a noninvasive procedure performed to assist in diagnosing corneal or conjunctival abnormalities. The test uses a sodium fluorescein dye to stain the surface of the eyes, which provides a more detailed view of the anterior portions not ordinarily seen during slit-lamp examination. It allows detection of the depth and pattern of even very small injuries to the eye, which result in definite staining details that can be identified with a special attachment to the slit lamp.[54]

Reference Values

Normal corneal surface; no keratitis, corneal scratches, abrasions, or ulcerations

Interfering Factors

➤ Inability of client to cooperate during the test

Indications for Corneal Staining

➤ Detecting minute abnormalities of the corneal surface made visible by a fluorescein dye and visualizing with a special attachment to the slit lamp
➤ Diagnosing the type of corneal injuries or damage as revealed by predetermined staining patterns or colors

Nursing Care Before the Procedure

Client teaching and physical preparation are the same as for any visual acuity test (see pp. 929 to 930).

➤ Obtain a history of known or suspected eye disorders or injuries; signs and symptoms of eye pain, irritation, or changes in visual acuity; or previous eye tests, procedures, and the results.

The Procedure

The procedure is the same as for slit-lamp biomicroscopy with a special blue filter attached to observe the fluorescence resulting from the dye (see p. 939). Before the slit-lamp examination, the eye surface is stained with the fluorescein dye by touching the tip of a sterile fluorescein strip moistened with sterile saline to the lower conjunctival sac. The client is requested to close the eye to spread the dye over the corneal surface. Defects are recorded depending on the amount of dye absorbed and the color that results, that is, green for breaks, trauma, or chemical injury to the cornea.[55]

Nursing Care After the Procedure

There are no special care and assessment activities after the test.

(Case Study follows on page 943)

Student Name _____ Class _____

Instructor _____ Date _____

CASE STUDY AND CRITICAL THINKING EXERCISE

Ms. Jones, age 24, is seen in the clinic, complaining of double vision and generalized fatigue. A Tensilon test is ordered.

a. What disease is indicated by a positive Tensilon test?

b. What medication therapy is indicated?

References

1. Berkow, R: The Merck Manual, ed 16. Merck Sharp and Dohme Research Laboratory, Rahway, NJ, 1992, p 406.
2. Ibid, pp 396–397.
3. Porth, CM: Pathophysiology: Concepts of Altered Health States, ed 4. JB Lippincott, Philadelphia, 1993, p 271.
4. Corbett, JV: Laboratory Tests and Diagnostic Procedures with Nursing Diagnoses, ed 3. Appleton & Lange, Norwalk, Conn, 1992, p 642.
5. Berkow, op cit, p 396.
6. Springhouse Corporation: Nurse's Reference Library, Diagnostics, ed 2. Springhouse, Springhouse, Pa, 1986, pp 939–940.
7. Porth, op cit, pp 257–258.
8. Nurse's Reference Library, op cit, p 934.
9. Porth, op cit, pp 212–213.
10. Ibid, p 942.
11. Berkow, op cit, pp 607–614.
12. Porth, op cit, pp 339–340, 354–355.
13. Pagana, KD, and Pagana, TJ: Mosby's Diagnostic and Laboratory Test Reference. Mosby–Year Book, St Louis, 1992, p 611.
14. Fischbach, FT: A Manual of Laboratory and Diagnostic Tests, ed 4. JB Lippincott, Philadelphia, 1992, p 826.
15. Ibid, p 834.
16. Ibid, pp 837–838.
17. Ibid, p 838.
18. Pagana and Pagana, op cit, p 537.
19. Ibid, p 537.
20. Ibid, p 693.
21. Porth, op cit, p 383.
22. Ibid, p 693.
23. Nurse's Reference Library, op cit, p 762.
24. Ibid, p 762.
25. Ibid, pp 783–784.
26. Berkow, op cit, p 2319.
27. Ibid, p 1939.
28. Ibid, p 1942.
29. Ibid, p 595.
30. Rambo, BJ (ed): Nursing Skills for Clinical Practice, ed 3. WB Saunders, Philadelphia, 1985, pp 21–22.
31. Nurse's Reference Library, op cit, p 590.
32. Ibid, p 601.
33. Berkow, op cit, p 2321.
34. Ibid, p 600.
35. Ibid, pp 2322–2324.
36. Nurse's Reference Library, op cit, p 613.
37. Porth, op cit, pp 820–821.
38. Nurse's Reference Library, op cit, p 608.
39. Ibid, p 2323.
40. Ibid, pp 608–612.
41. Ibid, pp 602, 604.
42. Ibid, pp 549–550.
43. Ibid, pp 548–549.
44. Berkow, op cit, p 1429.
45. Ibid, p 1429.
46. Porth, op cit, p 797.
47. Nurse's Reference Library, op cit, p 566.
48. Ibid, p 789.
49. Ibid, p 557.
50. Berkow, op cit, p 2363.
51. Ibid, p 562.
52. Nurse's Reference Library, op cit, p 561.
53. Ibid, pp 563–564.
54. Ibid, p 562.
55. Ibid, p 562.

Bibliography

Anderson, DR: Automated Static Perimetry. Mosby–Year Book, St Louis, 1991.

Black, JM, and Matassarin-Jacobs, E: Luckmann and Sorensen's Medical-Surgical Nursing: A Psychophysiologic Approach, ed 4. WB Saunders, Philadelphia, 1993.

Chernecky, CC, and Berger, BJ; Cullen, BN (ed): Laboratory Tests and Diagnostic Procedures, ed 2. WB Saunders, Philadelphia, 1996.

Clausen, JL (ed): Pulmonary Function Testing Guidelines and Controversies: Equipment, Methods, and Normal Values, A Project of the California Thoracic Society. WB Saunders, Philadelphia, 1984.

Darley, FL: Aphasia. WB Saunders, Philadelphia, 1982.

Darley, FL, et al: Motor Speech Disorders. WB Saunders, Philadelphia, 1975.

Hoskins, HD, and Kass, MA: Becker-Shaffer's Diagnosis and Therapy of the Glaucomas, ed 6. Mosby–Year Book, St Louis, 1989.

Huber, MJE: Clinical Tests in Ophthalmology. Mosby–Year Book, St Louis, 1991.

Jones, NL; Fletcher, J (ed): Clinical Exercise Testing, ed 4. WB Saunders, Philadelphia, 1997.

Kee, JL: Handbook of Laboratory and Diagnostic Tests with Nursing Implications, ed 3. Appleton & Lange, Norwalk, Conn, 1997.

Kern, MJ (ed): The Cardiac Catheterization Handbook, ed 2. Mosby–Year Book, St Louis, 1994.

Leibowitz, HM: Corneal Disorders: Clinical Diagnosis and Management. WB Saunders, Philadelphia, 1984.

Ludman, H: Mawson's Diseases of the Ear, ed 5. Mosby–Year Book, St Louis, 1989.

Meyerhoff, WL: Diagnosis and Management of Hearing Loss. WB Saunders, Philadelphia, 1984.

Pagana, KD, and Pagana, TJ: Diagnostic Testing and Nursing Implications: A Case Study Approach, ed 4. Mosby–Year Book, St Louis, 1993.

Roberton, JIS, and Birkanhager, WH (eds): Cardiac Output Measurement. WB Saunders, Philadelphia, 1991.

Springhouse Corporation: Nurse's Reference Library: Diagnostic Tests. Springhouse, Springhouse, Pa, 1991.

Tilkian, SM: Clinical and Nursing Implications of Laboratory Tests, ed 5. Mosby–Year Book, St Louis, 1995.

Whaley, LF: Nursing Care of Infants and Children, ed 4. Mosby–Year Book, St Louis, 1991.

Wilhelmus, KR, and Osato, M: Atlas of Diagnostic Ocular Microbiology. Mosby–Year Book, St Louis, 1992.

25

Skin Tests

➤ **TESTS COVERED**

Scratch Tests for Allergens, *948*
Patch Tests for Allergens, *949*
Intradermal Tests for Allergens, *951*
Tests for Immune Competence, *952*

Tuberculin Tests, *954*
Mumps Test, *957*
Histoplasmosis/Coccidioidomycosis/
Blastomycosis Tests, *958*
Trichinosis/Toxoplasmosis Tests, *960*

INTRODUCTION

Skin tests provide biologic and diagnostic information about hypersensitivity, as in the strength of body reactivity to harmful agents (allergens); about immunity, as in the susceptibility of resistance of the body to harmful agents (infectious disease); and about cell-mediated immune function, as in the presence or absence of a hypersensitive inflammatory response to an antigenic agent (immune competence). The five types of skin testing are the following: (1) scratch, (2) patch, (3) culture, (4) multipuncture, and (5) intradermal injection. Test reliability depends on (1) a faultless injection procedure (intradermal rather than subcutaneous [SC]); (2) scratch, patch, and culture procedures; (3) correct sites and site identification records; (4) correct dilution and measurement of the antigen; and (5) accurate reading, measurement, and recording of skin reactions.

Skin tests are generally considered microbiologic invasive procedures because a break in skin integrity is essential to introduce the allergens, toxins, or antigens to obtain a systemic response to the disease-producing agent. Some tests are performed routinely as screening procedures or specifically when symptomology indicates the need. Some tests are performed primarily on children, some on adults, and some on both. Skin tests can be performed by the physician or a nurse in a hospital, clinic, or physician's office.

TESTS FOR ALLERGENS

Skin tests for allergens are performed to determine unknown and suspected hypersensitivities (allergies) to environmental substances that are inhaled (dust, pollens, animal dander, grasses, molds), foods that are ingested (eggs, wheat, shellfish, citrus fruits), substances that are injected (horse serum, insect venom), or drugs (penicillins) that cause atopic diseases. Provocative food testing can be performed to determine food sensitivities because skin tests are of doubtful clinical significance. Skin tests are performed by patch tests that confirm a contact sensitivity and by scratch and intradermal tests that use allergenic extracts to confirm sensitivity to various substances. An exaggerated response to the substances (antigens) introduced by direct skin testing is considered a positive response if a wheal and flare reaction becomes obvious in 15 to 20 minutes.

The results of skin testing for hypersensitivities lead to various treatment modalities. One method is to avoid the identified allergens; if avoidance is not possible, desensitization (immunotherapy) is attempted to control or relieve the symptoms. Desensitization is accomplished by the year-round SC injection of increased doses of the extract of the allergen. Another treatment is to selectively eliminate specific foods from the diet until symptoms are relieved or to start with a diet that eliminates all potential allergens and gradually add one food at a time until symptoms recur (provocative food testing).[1]

SCRATCH TESTS FOR ALLERGENS

Scratch tests are direct skin tests to detect sensitivities to allergens. They are performed by applying a test solution containing the antigen to shallow scratches in the skin. This type of skin testing is safer than injections because a smaller amount of the antigen is introduced. Scratch tests are often performed before intradermal injection tests for allergens to identify materials that can cause a severe systemic response. They are always performed instead of intradermal tests if the client has a known severe sensitivity to a substance. If a positive wheal and flare (redness and swelling) response measuring 0.5 cm or more is observed, intradermal injection tests should not be performed.

Reference Values

Negative reaction, no evidence of a wheal and flare reaction of 0.5 cm or larger than control test in 15 to 20 minutes after application of test extract

Interfering Factors

➤ Using scratches that are made too deeply, causing bleeding to occur
➤ Touching the skin with the dropper, causing contamination when applying the substance
➤ Using antigens that have expired
➤ Using antihistamines

Indications for Scratch Tests for Allergens

➤ Determining allergic response to various antigens before intradermal testing in clients who have a history of severe sensitivities
➤ Suspected allergic condition to confirm sensitivity to an antigen

Nursing Care Before the Procedure

Explain to the client:
➤ That the tests are performed by a physician or a nurse and that they take 30 to 45 minutes to administer, including reading of the results of the tests
➤ That a series of scratches are made on the lower forearm or back and a drop of a different allergen is introduced into each scratch
➤ That a moderate amount of pain is experienced when the scratches are made

Prepare for the procedure:

➤ Request that the client remove the clothing from the waist up if the back is to be used for testing, and provide a gown to wear with the opening to the back.

➤ Obtain a history of known allergies to substances, desensitization therapy, diseases or conditions known to be caused by allergens, and severity of symptoms when exposed to allergens.

➤ Use distraction techniques in children.

The Procedure

The skin sites on the lower anterior portion of the forearm or the scapular area of the back are cleansed with alcohol or acetone swabs and allowed to air-dry. The sterile lancet is removed from the package and held in the dominant hand. The skin at the sites is held taut with the nondominant hand, and scratches are made 1 cm long and 2.5 cm apart with the sterile lancet or needle. The scratches should be made through the uppermost layer of the skin (epidermis) without causing bleeding. A drop of the concentrated (1:20) test extract is placed on each scratch without touching the skin to avoid contamination of the substance. The tests can also be performed by using commercially produced scarifiers and puncturing the skin through a drop of the test extract. Control tests are performed simultaneously by intradermal injection of the diluent. The tests are read in 15 to 20 minutes for a wheal and flare reaction and, if a wheal is present and the diameter is more than 0.5 cm larger than the control wheal, the test is positive for the test extracts producing it. An intradermal test using histamine (0.01 mg/mL) or morphine (0.1 mg/mL) is performed if the wheal is smaller than 0.5 cm or if no wheal (negative test) results. These control tests produce a wheal that measures 1 cm or less when the scratch tests are negative. They are performed when the client has been taking drugs that block the effect of histamine on blood vessels and inhibit the skin tests (histamine, hy-droxyzine) or drugs that are mast cell degranulators (morphine, meperidine).[2] A record is made of the allergens and their sites for the later identification of substances causing a positive reaction.

Nursing Care After the Procedure

➤ Care and assessment after the tests include assessing the sites and any systemic effects of the tests.

➤ Inform the client that any redness or edema at the sites will disappear within 24 hours.

PATCH TESTS FOR ALLERGENS

Patch tests are direct skin tests to detect and confirm contact sensitization to allergens. Common potentially irritating substances (allergens) are applied to disks of filter paper, cotton squares, or gauze squares and securely taped to the skin. Unknown and suspected allergens can be tested when unexplained contact dermatitis and other skin eruptions are present, although the tests do not produce a definitive cause of the condition. A response of redness or edema at the site of application indicates a contact sensitivity to the substance.[3]

Reference Values

Negative reaction; no evidence of redness or edema at the site after the removal of the patch

Interfering Factors

➤ Corticosteroids (systemic or topical), which can affect test results
➤ Impure or insufficient concentration of the antigen
➤ Improper technique in applying the patch, reactions to the tape on the patch, or incorrect reading of the results
➤ Contamination of the patch during application

Indications for Patch Tests for Allergens

➤ Determination or confirmation of contact sensitivities to substances
➤ Unexplained skin eruptions or dermatitis conditions to determine whether allergic contact is the cause

Contraindications

➤ Areas with skin eruptions or any kind or inflammation should not be used as test sites.

Nursing Care Before the Procedure

Explain to the client:
➤ That the patches are applied by the physician or the nurse and left in place for 48 hours, removed, and read for reactions to the substance
➤ That no pain is associated with the test
Prepare for the procedure:
➤ Ask the client to remove clothing from the waist up if the back is to be used, and provide a gown to wear with the opening to the back.
➤ Obtain a history of skin disorders, suspected or known contact dermatitis disorders, medications taken, or other known or suspected allergies.

The Procedure

The sites on the inner aspect of the lower forearm or the scapular area of the back are cleansed with alcohol or acetone swabs and allowed to air-dry. Remove the cover of each patch from the pad containing the testing substance of common allergens, and apply the pads to the sites by firmly pressing down on the adhesive surrounding the pads. Patch testing can also be performed by placing the potentially irritating substances (diluted to a 1 to 2 percent strength in water or mineral oil) on a small circle of filter papers, covering with plastic, and taping to the sites. A record is made of the allergens and their sites for later use to identify the substances that reveal a positive reaction. Patches are left in place for 48 hours, at which time they are removed and the test sites read immediately and in 30 minutes. Some can be evaluated again 4 days after removal of the patches for any delayed reactions. Positive reactions can range from a slight irritation to redness and edema to vesicle and ulcer formation.[4]

Nursing Care After the Procedure

➤ Care and assessment after the tests include the evaluation of the test results and the application of an ordered topical corticosteroid to relieve severe effects of a positive reaction.

➤ *Severe reaction:* Note and report pain, irritation, or pruritus at the sites. Remove the patch and apply steroid ointment.

INTRADERMAL TESTS FOR ALLERGENS

Intradermal tests are direct skin tests to detect sensitization to allergens that cause clinical conditions such as asthma, rhinitis, anaphylaxis, insect sting reactions, and food and drug reactions manifested by urticaria, angioedema, bronchial or gastrointestinal muscle spasms, or hypotension.[5] A series of common allergen extracts are injected intradermally to determine reactions within a specific period. A wheal and flare reaction of 0.5 cm or larger is considered a positive response and usually correlates with the presenting symptoms.

Reference Values

Negative reaction; no evidence of a wheal reaction of 0.5 cm or larger than the control wheal in 15 minutes after injection of the test extract

Interfering Factors

➤ Improper technique in performing the intradermal injections and injecting the test extract into subcutaneous tissue
➤ Incorrect concentration and measurement of the test extract

Indications for Intradermal Tests for Allergens

➤ Determination or confirmation of allergic sensitivities to specific substances that induce exaggerated reactions in a sensitive host
➤ Unexplained single episode or seasonal or year-round symptoms caused by inhalants, foods, drugs, or injected substances
➤ Determination of the need for desensitization to the allergen

Contraindications

➤ Areas that have skin eruptions or inflammation should not be used as test sites.

Nursing Care Before the Procedure

Explain to the client:
➤ That the physician or nurse performs the test, which takes 15 to 30 minutes, including reading of the the results
➤ That a series of injections are given under the skin to introduce the test extract
➤ That the client waits for 15 minutes after the injections for the test to be read for responses that indicate a sensitivity
➤ That moderate pain and discomfort are experienced when the injections are given
Prepare for the procedure:
➤ Obtain a history of known and suspected allergies, diseases, or conditions known to be caused by allergens, and severity and frequency of symptoms.

The Procedure

The skin sites on the lower anterior area of the forearm are cleansed with alcohol or acetone swabs and allowed to air-dry. The test extract, usually 0.02 mL of a 1:500 or 1:1000 concentration, is drawn up into a tuberculin syringe with a short 26-gauge needle attached. A different syringe is used for each test extract. The skin is held taut with the nondominant hand and, with the bevel up, the needle is inserted into the top level of the skin with the dominant hand holding the syringe almost level with the site. Material that is injected into subcutaneous tissue instead of intradermal tissue will cause invalid test results. The text extract is injected, and, if more than one test is to be performed, the next test extract is injected 2.5 cm from the initial site. This process is repeated until all test materials have been injected. Control tests of the diluent are performed simultaneously for comparison. The sites are examined in 15 minutes for any reactions. A wheal and flare reaction that is more than 0.5 cm larger than the control wheal 15 minutes after the injection is considered to be a positive response. A record of the sites and test extracts is made for identification of substances causing a positive reaction.

Nursing Care After the Procedure

➤ Care and assessment after the tests include assessing the sites and any systemic effects from the test extracts.

➤ Inform the client that any redness or edema at the sites should disappear within 24 to 48 hours.

➤ *Severe systemic response:* Note and report urticaria, dyspnea, or hypotension. Administer ordered antihistamine or epinephrine, depending on the severity of the reaction.

TESTS FOR IMMUNE COMPETENCE

Immune competence tests are performed to determine cell-mediated immune response by skin testing with the intradermal injection of several commonly encountered antigens. The reading of the test results provides information about an intact cell-mediated immune function by a positive, delayed hypersensitivity response at the injection site and indicates a present or past exposure to the antigen used. A negative response indicates no exposure to the antigen or an ineffective immune response to the antigen (anergy). Anergy indicates an impaired immunity and can occur in advanced stages of infectious diseases or in chronic diseases such as lymphoma or sarcoidosis. Tests (and their associated diseases) related to the antigens that commonly cause an immune response are candidin (*Candida albicans*), streptokinase-streptodornase ([SKSD] streptococcal infections), Mantoux ([PPD, or purified protein derivative] tuberculosis), trichophytin (ringworm), and others.

Reference Values

Positive response at the injection site

Candidin: 10 mm or more induration and erythema in 48–72 hr
Streptokinase-streptodornase (SKSD): 10 mm or more induration in 48 hr
Mantoux (PPD): 10 mm or more induration and erythema in 24–72 hr
Trichophytin: 5 mm or more induration in 48–72 hr

Interfering Factors

➤ Improper technique in performing the intradermal injections and injecting the antigen into subcutaneous tissue instead of intradermal tissue

➤ Incorrect dilution or measurement of the amount of antigen administered

➤ Use of expired antigens, contaminated antigens, or improperly stored antigens

➤ Incorrect measurement and timing of the reading of the skin responses to the antigens

➤ Oral contraceptives, corticosteroids, and other immunosuppressive drugs

➤ Age of the client, because infants under 3 months have immature immune systems and elderly people have a decrease in sensitivity with age

Indications for Tests for Immune Competence

➤ Detecting impaired or intact cellular immunity by evaluation of the immune responses to the test antigens

➤ Monitoring chronic diseases such as Hodgkin's disease, sarcoidosis, leprosy, or chronic renal failure to determine the course and prognosis of the disease

➤ Evaluating the effectiveness of immunotherapy after administration of steroids and vaccines such as bacille Calmette-Guérin (BCG)[6]

Contraindications

➤ Sites that have dermatitis, inflammation, or breaks in the skin should not be used for testing.

➤ Hypersensitivity to any antigen to be used in the tests.

Nursing Care Before the Procedure

Explain to the client:

➤ That the physician or the nurse performs the series of skin injections, which take 10 to 30 minutes to administer, depending on the number of antigens injected, and that a reaction should appear in 48 to 72 hours

➤ That the client is requested to come back to have these test reactions read in 48 or 72 hours

➤ That moderate pain may be experienced when the injections are performed

Prepare for the procedure:

➤ Obtain a history of known and suspected diseases and conditions reflected or affected by abnormalities of the immune system, hypersensitivity to the test antigens, other allergies, and past skin tests and responses.

The Procedure

The skin sites on the lower anterior surface of the forearms are cleansed with alcohol or acetone swabs and allowed to dry. Small doses of correctly diluted antigens are prepared in tuberculin syringes with 26- to 27-gauge needles attached. Each antigen is injected intradermally, making a small bleb under the skin (see p. 956 for the procedure), and the site is circled and labeled. The sites are examined with good lighting for the presence of induration and are measured in millimeters with a metric ruler in 48 and then 72 hours. This reaction indicates a positive test result. Absence of induration or erythema indicates a negative test result.

Nursing Care After the Procedure

➤ Care and assessment after the test include evaluating for local and systemic reactions to the antigens for 15 to 30 minutes and informing the client to avoid any scratching of the sites or washing of the marks.

➤ Inform the client of the time to return for a reading and evaluation of the test sites.

➤ *Severe local response:* Note and report pain, edema, itching, or blister formation. Administer ordered corticosteroids. Inform the client that hyperpigmentation can result and can last for up to 2 weeks.

➤ *Anaphylactic shock:* Note and report respiratory distress, hypotension, or tachycardia. Administer ordered epinephrine SC. Have resuscitation equipment and supplies on hand.

TESTS FOR INFECTIOUS DISEASES

Skin tests for infectious diseases are performed to determine past or present exposure to an infectious agent (sensitivity) or susceptibility or resistance to an infectious disease (immunity). The tests involve the administration of the specific antigen prepared for a specific disease by intradermal injection (most common), multipuncture, patch, or scratch techniques. Included in this section are skin tests for infectious microorganisms such as bacteria (tuberculosis, diphtheria, scarlet fever), viruses (mumps), fungi (histoplasmosis, coccidioidomycosis, blastomycosis), and parasites (trichinosis, toxoplasmosis).

TUBERCULIN TESTS

Tuberculin tests are skin tests that use a purified protein derivative (PPD) or old tuberculin (OT) of the tubercle bacillus administered by intradermal injection (Mantoux) or multipuncture technique (Tine) to determine sensitization to the tuberculosis bacillus from a previous exposure, not the actual presence of the disease. Tuberculosis is an infectious disease caused by *Mycobacterium tuberculosis* and is transmitted by droplet nuclei particles harbored in the respiratory tract and in the secretions of those with the active disease. A positive response of induration and erythema that appears at the site in 48 to 72 hours reveals the development of a cell-mediated immunity to the organisms or a delayed hypersensitivity caused by interaction of the sensitized T lymphocytes with the tuberculin antigen. The tests are used on children and adults to screen for or to diagnose active or dormant tuberculosis.

Primary (initial infection) tuberculosis is always asymptomatic, and secondary (subsequent infection) tuberculosis is usually asymptomatic, with the main diagnostic evidence of the disease obtained by a positive skin test and the presence of lesions on the chest x-ray. In the multipuncture technique, PPD (Aplitest, Sclavo Test) or OT (Tine, Mono-Vacc) is used; this test is usually performed to screen for the disease in asymptomatic clients. Verification of a positive response of a multipuncture test is performed with the more definitive Mantoux test (Aplisol, Tubersol), which allows more precise measurement of the antigen. A positive response of the Mantoux is followed by chest radiography and bacteriologic laboratory tests to confirm a diagnosis of tuberculosis.[7]

Reference Values

Negative response or minimal response, with no exposure to tuberculosis

> *Tine test:* Less than 2 mm or absence of induration around one or more of the punctures in 48–72 hr
> *Mantoux test:* Less than 5 mm or absence of induration and erythema in 24–72 hr

Interfering Factors

➤ Improper technique in performing the intradermal injection and injecting the PPD or OT into subcutaneous tissue
➤ Incorrect reading (measurement of the response) or timing of the reading
➤ Incorrect amount or dilution of antigen injected or delay in the injection after drawing the antigen up into the syringe
➤ Improper storage or contamination of the antigen
➤ Recent or present bacterial, viral, or fungal infections
➤ Diseases such as hematologic malignancies or sarcoidosis
➤ Immunosuppressive drugs or steroids, which can alter results

Indications for Tuberculin Tests

➤ Screening of asymptomatic clients for tuberculosis exposure or infection
➤ Routine screening of infants with the Tine test at the time of first immunizations to determine tuberculosis exposure
➤ Recent known or suspected exposure to tuberculosis with or without symptoms to determine whether tuberculosis infection is present
➤ Cough, weight loss, fatigue, hemoptysis, and abnormal x-rays to determine whether the cause is tuberculosis
➤ Medical conditions that place the client at risk for tuberculosis, such as acquired immunodeficiency syndrome (AIDS), lymphoma, or diabetes
➤ Populations at risk for developing tuberculosis, such as nursing home residents, prison inmates, and residents of the inner city living in poor hygienic conditions
➤ Mantoux test to confirm findings of a positive Tine test

Contraindications

➤ History of tuberculosis or previous positive skin test
➤ Rash or other eruptions at the injection site
➤ Hypersensitivity to other skin tests or vaccinations

Nursing Care Before the Procedure

Explain to the client:
➤ That the nurse performs the test by injecting a small amount of medicine under the skin of the forearm and that the test takes about 5 to 10 minutes
➤ That the nurse will inform the client of the time to return to have the skin test read and will provide instructions after the reading
➤ That the area should not be scratched or disturbed from the time of the injection until it is read

➤ That a moderate amount of pain can be experienced when the injection is given

Prepare for the procedure:

➤ Obtain a history of tuberculosis or tuberculosis exposure, signs and symptoms indicating possible tuberculosis, other diagnostic procedures and results, and other skin tests or vaccinations and sensitivities.

The Procedure

The skin site on the lower anterior portion of the forearm is cleansed with alcohol or acetone swabs and allowed to air-dry.

Multipuncture Test. The cap covering the tines is removed, and the skin of the forearm is stretched taut. The device is firmly pressed onto the prepared site and held in place for a second and removed. The four punctures should be visible. The site is recorded, and the client is reminded to return in 48 to 72 hours to have the results read. The diameter of the largest indurated area is measured in a good light with a plastic ruler. A palpable induration of 2 mm or more at one or more of the punctures indicates a positive test result. A Mantoux test is then performed to confirm the positive results unless vesicles appear at the site.

Intradermal Test. The PPD or OT is prepared in a tuberculin syringe with a short 26-gauge needle attached. The appropriate dilution and amount are prepared for the most commonly used intermediate strength (5 tuberculin units in 0.1 mL) or for a first strength, which is usually used for children (1 tuberculin unit in 0.1 mL). The preparation is injected at the prepared site intradermally, that is, within the layers of the skin, as soon as it is drawn up into the syringe, causing a bleb or wheal to form. The site is recorded and the client is reminded to return in 48 to 72 hours to have the test read. The arm is inspected in good light, and the diameter of any induration is measured with a plastic ruler and palpated for thickening of the tissue. A positive result is indicated by a 10-mm or more reaction with erythema and edema. A positive test result is not a definite diagnosis of tuberculosis; however, it does mean that there is a great chance that the disease is present if the client presents symptoms. A positive test result in a well person indicates that the client has had tuberculosis in the past or is infected with a different bacteria.

An induration of 5 to 9 mm is considered doubtful and possibly caused by another infection. This response warrants a repeat test. A higher concentration of the antigen can be administered to those who do not have a reaction from the intermediate dose. Subsequent chest x-rays and culture of the sputum for microorganism identification are performed to confirm a diagnosis of tuberculosis.

Nursing Care After the Procedure

➤ Care and assessment after the test include observation of the site and a reminder to the client not to scratch or rub it after the injection.

➤ Remind the client to return for the reading and explain that the effects from a positive response at the site can remain for up to a week.

➤ *Severe positive reaction:* Note and report ulceration or necrosis developing at the site. Apply cool, wet compresses and topical corticosteroids to the injection site.

MUMPS TEST

The mumps test is a skin test performed to determine the previous exposure to or the active presence of the disease. Mumps, or parotitis, is an infectious disease of the parotid glands caused by a myxovirus and transmitted by direct contact with an infected person or the droplets spread from the saliva of an infected person. The mumps test involves intradermal injections of an antigen from infected animals and of a material made from noninfected animals to serve as a control. The measurement of the response is made in 48 hours, with a positive response of erythema with or without induration indicating varying degrees of protection from or resistance to the mumps virus and a negative response with no reaction indicating susceptibility to the mumps virus. The test is also used as part of the series to determine immune competence.[8]

Reference Values

Negative response or no reaction at the test site or minimal response of erythema measuring less than 10 mm indicates susceptibility to mumps with routine use of mumps vaccine since 1997.

Interfering Factors

➤ Improper technique in performing the skin test or inaccurate time or measurement in reading the reaction

Indications for the Mumps Test

➤ Detecting impaired or intact cellular immunity when used with other test antigens to test immune responses
➤ Determining resistance to or protection against the mumps virus by a positive reaction or susceptibility to mumps by a negative reaction
➤ Evaluating mumps-like diseases and differentiating between them and actual mumps

Nursing Care Before the Procedure

Teaching and physical preparation are the same as for any diagnostic skin test (see p. 953).
➤ The history should include prior exposure to the disease and past immunizations.

The Procedure

The skin sites on both lower anterior portions of the forearms are cleansed with alcohol or acetone swabs and allowed to air-dry. The inactivated vaccine prepared from infected animals and the vaccine prepared from noninfected animals are drawn up into tuberculin syringes with 26-gauge needles attached. Both are injected intradermally, and the site is recorded. The client is reminded to return in 48 hours to have the test read. A positive result consists of erythema with or without induration at least 10 mm in diameter, indicating some protection against mumps. A positive reaction at the onset of a mumps-like disease can rule out mumps as the cause. A delayed positive reaction that occurs several days after the test can indicate the presence of mumps and no previous exposure. The lack of erythema indicates a negative result and lack of resistance to the disease.

Nursing Care After the Procedure

Care and assessment after the test are the same as for any diagnostic skin test (see p. 954).

HISTOPLASMOSIS/COCCIDIOIDOMYCOSIS/ BLASTOMYCOSIS TESTS

Histoplasmosis, coccidioidomycosis, and blastomycosis skin tests are performed to determine exposure to these fungal infections affecting the pulmonary system. Diagnosis of these fungal diseases is made by visualization and identification of the organisms and by measurement of antibodies produced in response to a specific infection.

Histoplasmosis is caused by the fungus *Histoplasma capsulatum* and is transmitted by inhalation of spores in the dust that are released when soil contaminated with bird excreta is disturbed. The manifestations of histoplasmosis are similar to those of tuberculosis. It can be a mild, self-limiting respiratory infection or a chronic disorder that can lead to the progressive destruction of lung tissue. The skin test involves the intradermal injection of an antigen, histoplasmin, prepared from killed fungi obtained by culture. The skin test is read in 48 to 72 hours for a positive response of induration and erythema at the site; response can remain positive after the initial infection has occurred, indicating a past or present origin of the disease. Other tests that provide diagnostic information are the complement fixation and the immunodiffusion tests, which test and measure antibodies produced by exposure. Both tests can become positive after symptoms appear. Cultures of specimens of sputum, urine, oral lesions, or lymph nodes are also obtained to confirm the presence of the disease by visualization and identification of the specific organism.

Coccidioidomycosis is caused by the fungus *Coccidioides immitis* and is transmitted by inhalation of the spores found in the dust from disturbed soil containing the organisms. It occurs as a self-limiting infection manifested as an upper respiratory infection or pneumonia or as a chronic, progressive disseminated disease involving the lungs and spreading to the bones, joints, skin, liver, and brain. The skin test involves the intradermal injection of an antigen, coccidioidin or spherulin, prepared from a culture filtrate of the organism causing the disease. The test is read in 24 to 72 hours, and a positive response is revealed by induration and erythema. A skin reaction appears 10 to 21 days after the infection has occurred and remains positive throughout a lifetime, even though the organisms and disease have been eliminated. Other tests that provide diagnostic information are the complement fixation and tube-precipitin tests as well as the culture of sputum, pleural fluid, pus, skin lesions, and gastric washings to visualize and identify the spherules.

Blastomycosis is caused by the fungus *Blastomyces dermatitidis* and is characterized by an acute infection manifested by lesions of the lungs and skin. The infection can be self-limiting or can progress to involve bone, prostate gland, testes, and oral mucosa. The skin test involves the intradermal injection of an antigen, blastomycin, and it is commonly performed in conjunction with the skin tests for histoplasmosis and coccidioidomycosis. The test is read in 48 hours, and a positive response reveals induration and erythema at the site, indicating a past or present infection. Because the test lacks specificity, it is thought to be of little value in diagnosing the disease. A culture of sputum, pus, or exudate and preparation by the proper fixation and staining to visualize the budding yeasts are done to provide a more definitive diagnosis of the disease.[9]

Reference Values

Histoplasmosis: Negative response of no reaction at the test site or minimal erythema measuring less than 5 mm with an absence of induration, indicating absence of infection
Coccidioidomycosis: Negative response of no reaction at the test site or minimal induration and erythema of less than 5 mm, indicating absence of infection
Blastomycosis: Negative response of no reaction at the test site or minimal erythema measuring less than 5 mm with an absence of induration, indicating absence of infection

Interfering Factors

➤ Improper technique in performing the skin tests, inaccurate recording of sites or time, or inaccurate measurement in reading the reaction

Indications for Histoplasmosis/ Coccidioidomycosis/Blastomycosis Skin Tests

➤ Diagnosing past or present acute or chronic infection by a specific fungal microorganism as evidenced by a positive skin test in histoplasmosis and blastomycosis
➤ Evaluating improvement in a diagnosed blastomycosis infection
➤ Diagnosing an active coccidioidomycosis infection in the presence of symptoms as evidenced by a positive skin test

Nursing Care Before the Procedure

Teaching and physical preparation are the same as for any diagnostic skin test (see p. 953). A history should include exposure to any fungal infective agents or residence in an endemic area.

The Procedure

The skin sites on the lower anterior portion of the forearm are cleansed with alcohol or acetone swabs and allowed to air-dry. Three tuberculin syringes with 26-gauge needles attached are prepared with the antigens histoplasmin, coccidioidin, and blastomycin. Each antigen is injected intradermally, and the sites are labeled and noted for each. The client is reminded to return for the test to be read, 24 to 72 hours for histoplasmosis, 24 to 72 hours for coccidioidomycosis, and 48 hours for blastomycosis. All three tests are usually performed and read at the same time. A positive result for histoplasmosis reveals a measured area of erythema and induration of 5 mm or more, and a negative reaction is an absence of induration and erythema of less than 5 mm. A positive result for coccidioidomycosis reveals a measured induration of 5 mm or more and a negative reaction of less than 5 mm. A positive result for blastomycosis reveals a measured area of erythema and induration of 5 mm or more. A doubtful result is revealed by erythema alone or induration of less than 5 mm, and a negative reaction is an absence of induration and erythema of less than 5 mm. A positive test of any of the fungal infections indicates past or present infection.

Nursing Care After the Procedure

Care and assessment after the test are the same as for any diagnostic skin test (see p. 954).

TRICHINOSIS/TOXOPLASMOSIS TESTS

Trichinosis and toxoplasmosis skin tests are performed to determine exposure to those parasitic diseases. Although the skin tests are discouraged and are considered unreliable, commercially available antigens are available and can be used in conjunction with serologic tests to detect antibodies after the onset of the disease.

Trichinosis is caused by the parasite *Trichinella spiralis* and is transmitted by the ingestion of raw or partially raw pork containing the larvae. The larvae invade the stomach and duodenum and penetrate the duodenal and jejunal mucosa. The disease is manifested by gastrointestinal symptoms followed by edema of the eyelids and eye pain, muscle pain, fever, and chills, among other systemic symptoms. The skin test involves the intradermal injection of an antigen, *T. spiralis*, prepared from the killed larvae. It is read 15 minutes after injection, with a positive response consisting of a wheal and erythema at the site. Other tests performed to obtain diagnostic information include the complement fixation, indirect fluorescent antibody, precipitin, and flocculation tests. Biopsy of muscle tissue later in the infection can reveal the larvae or myositis, indicating the presence of the disease.

Toxoplasmosis is caused by the protozoan parasite *Toxoplasma gondii* and is transmitted transplacentally by the mother's ingestion of raw or partially raw meat containing the cysts or by exposure to the cysts in cat feces. It can also be acquired and can occur as a mild infection, as a disseminated infection in those who are immunodeficient, or as a chronic infection. The skin test involves the intradermal injection of an antigen, toxoplasmin, which is read in 24 to 48 hours, with a positive result producing erythema at the site. The most definitive diagnostic information is obtained by performing tests for IgM antibodies initially and, later in the disease, for IgG antibodies, detected by the indirect fluorescent antibody procedure, complement fixation, and indirect hemagglutination.[10]

Reference Values

Negative response or no reaction at the test sites, indicating absence of a specific infection

Interfering Factors

➤ Improper technique in performing the skin test or inaccurate time or measurement in reading the reaction
➤ Commercially available antigens for the trichinosis test, which are considered unreliable for diagnostic purposes

Indications for Trichinosis/Toxoplasmosis Skin Tests

➤ Diagnostic adjunct for trichinosis in conjunction with serology and muscle biopsy

➤ Diagnostic adjunct for toxoplasmosis in conjunction with serology

Nursing Care Before the Procedure

Teaching and physical preparation are the same as for any diagnostic skin test (see p. 953).

➤ A history should include dietary inclusion of uncooked meats and possible exposure to infected cats, and the results of serologic tests performed to identify the microorganisms causing the diseases.

The Procedure

The skin site on the lower anterior portion of the forearm is cleansed with alcohol or acetone swabs and allowed to air dry. *T. spiralis* antigen or toxoplasmin is prepared in a syringe with a 26-gauge needle attached and injected intradermally for the test to be performed, trichinosis or toxoplasmosis, respectively. The test for trichinosis is read in 15 to 20 minutes. The client is reminded to return in 24 to 48 hours to have the test read for toxoplasmosis. A positive result for trichinosis reveals a wheal with surrounding erythema; it is considered a questionable positive result if the reaction occurs after 24 hours. A positive result for toxoplasmosis reveals a measured erythema of more than 10 mm.

Nursing Care After the Procedure

Care and assessment after the test are the same as for any diagnostic skin test (see p. 954).

(Case Study follows on page 963)

Student Name _____ Class _____

Instructor _____ Date _____

CASE STUDY AND CRITICAL THINKING EXERCISE

Mr. Smith, age 78, is seen at the clinic complaining of fatigue, chest pain, and a productive cough with sputum "sometimes streaked with blood." VS: T 99.5°F (37.5°C), P 104, R 18, BP 166/84.

  a. What tests should be ordered in this case?

  b. What medications may be ordered?

References

1. Berkow, R (ed): The Merck Manual, ed 16. Merck Research Laboratory, Rahway, NJ, 1992, pp 320–321.
2. Ibid, p 320.
3. Springhouse Corporation: Nurse's Reference Library: Diagnostics, ed 2. Springhouse, Springhouse, Pa, 1986, p 1042.
4. Ibid, p 1043.
5. Berkow, op cit, p 320.
6. Ibid, p 1040.
7. Ibid, p 134.
8. Fischbach, FT: A Manual of Laboratory Diagnostic Tests, ed 4. JB Lippincott, Philadelphia, 1992, pp 452–453.
9. Berkow, op cit, p 165.
10. Ibid, p 235.

Bibliography

Aronoff, SC (ed): Advances in Pediatric Infectious Diseases. Mosby – Year Book, St Louis, 1995.

Black, JM, and Matassarin-Jacobs, E: Luckmann and Sorensen's Medical-Surgical Nursing: A Psychophysiologic Approach, ed 4. WB Saunders, Philadelphia, 1993.

Byrne, CJ, et al: Laboratory Tests: Implications for Nursing Care, ed 2. Addison-Wesley, Menlo Park, Calif, 1986.

Chernecky CC, and Berger, BJ; Cullen, BN (ed): Laboratory Tests and Diagnostic Procedures, ed 2. WB Saunders, Philadelphia, 1996.

Corbett, JV: Laboratory Tests and Diagnostic Procedures with Nursing Diagnoses, ed 4. Appleton & Lange, Norwalk, Conn, 1995.

Kee, JL: Handbook of Laboratory and Diagnostic Tests with Nursing Implications, ed 3. Appleton & Lange, Norwalk, Conn, 1997.

Korenblat, PE, and Wedner, HJ: Allergy: Theory and Practice, ed 2. WB Saunders, Philadelphia, 1992.

Porth, CM: Pathophysiology: Concepts of Altered Health States, ed 4. JB Lippincott, Philadelphia, 1993.

Rippon, JW: Medical Mycology, ed 3. WB Saunders, Philadelphia, 1988.

Whaley, LF: Nursing Care of Infants and Children, ed 4. Mosby – Year Book, St Louis, 1991.

Appendices

Obtaining Various Types of Blood Specimens

Most hematology tests, as well as numerous other laboratory tests, require venous blood. Microsamples of capillary blood may be obtained from the fingertips or earlobes of older children and adults and from the heels of infants and neonates. Capillary punctures can also be used instead of venipunctures if the client has poor veins, very small veins, or a limited number of usable veins and if the client is extremely apprehensive about having a venipuncture. When the amount of blood needed is greater than 1.5 mL, however, a venipuncture must be performed.

Blood samples can also be obtained from vascular access devices such as heparin locks, triple-lumen subclavian catheters, and right atrial catheters (RAC). In the sick or high-risk neonate monitored in a neonatal intensive care unit, blood samples can be obtained from an indwelling catheter positioned and secured in an umbilical vein and connected to a heparin lock system to prevent clotting in the needle. Such procedures avoid the necessity of repeated skin punctures and must be performed with strict aseptic technique to avoid contamination of the indwelling device or catheter and to prevent possible septicemia. Special techniques are performed when obtaining samples from indwelling devices or catheters to avoid altered results from drugs and intravascular infusions and, in the neonate, to avoid excessive blood loss resulting from the need for numerous laboratory blood analyses.

Recent advances allow fetal blood samples to be obtained to assess fetal health. The samples are obtained by the physician, when special circumstances warrant it, by percutaneous umbilical cord blood sampling (PUBS), in which blood is aspirated from a 20- or 22-gauge spinal needle inserted into the umbilical vessel under the guidance of ultrasonography. Fetal hematologic and metabolic status, genetic disorder identification, and perinatal infection evaluation are the most common tests performed through PUBS.

Tests requiring arterial blood are arterial blood gas (ABG) analyses and are obtained from the radial or the brachial artery or from arterial lines. The background information and clinical applications data for arterial blood collection are found on pp. 288 to 292.

▶▶ Nursing Alert

- According to the most recent guidelines from the Centers for Disease Control and Prevention, gloves should always be worn when obtaining and handling blood samples.

CLIENT PREPARATION

Client preparation is essentially the same for all sites and for all studies.

Client Teaching

Explain to the client:
- ➤ The purpose of the test
- ➤ The procedure, including the site from which the blood sample is likely to be obtained
- ➤ That momentary discomfort may be experienced when the skin is pierced
- ➤ That food, fluids, and drugs are to be withheld before to the test

For children, a doll may be used as the "patient" for demonstration purposes. A laboratory technician's equipment basket may hold the child's attention during the actual procedure. For all clients, encourage questions and verbalization of concerns about the procedure, and provide a calm, reassuring environment and manner.

Physical Preparation

- ➤ For capillary punctures, the skin is assessed for lesions, edema, and temperature, as the site selected should be warm and free of lesions or edema: application of warm compresses for 3 minutes will dilate capillaries if the skin feels cool or looks pale or cyanotic.
- ➤ For venipunctures, the condition of the veins should be noted, and the use of tortuous, sclerotic veins or those in which phlebitis has previously occurred should be avoided, as should the use of an extremity with an intravenous (IV) site or heparin lock. If the extremity must be used, obtain the sample from a site distal to the IV or heparin lock. (Extremities with functioning hemodialysis access sites should not be used, nor should the arm on the affected side after mastectomy.)
- ➤ The skin is prepared by cleansing with an antiseptic such as povidone-iodine (Betadine) or 70 percent alcohol and is allowed to air dry or is dried with sterile gauze. (Drying prevents dilution of the sample with antiseptic.) For the immunosuppressed patient, povidone-iodine should be used, followed by a 70 percent alcohol pad taped over the site for 10 minutes—the site should be allowed to air-dry or be dried with sterile gauze before the venipuncture.
- ➤ For blood withdrawal from a device or catheter, assess for patency, damage, and type of catheter to determine the need for clot removal, heparinization, or irrigation. If a heparin lock device is in place or attached to an indwelling catheter in the umbilical vein, prepare heparin in saline solution in a syringe with a needle attached. If a right atrial catheter is in place, prepare heparin in saline solution in a syringe with a needle attached or prepare 30 mL saline in a syringe to flush the catheter if blood is to be withdrawn from a Groshong catheter. The injection site is prepared by cleansing the catheter-cap junction or hub with povidone-iodine, followed by swabbing with 70 percent alcohol for 2 minutes, and then allowing it to air-dry before the blood withdrawal.

THE PROCEDURE
Capillary Punctures
(Fingertip, Earlobe, Heel)

The equipment needed is assembled: sterile lancet, skin disinfectant, gauze pads or cotton balls, collection device, bandage, and materials to label the sample. The client is placed in a position of comfort and safety, either sitting or lying down. If an extremity is to be used, it is supported on the bed or on a table. A small pillow or rolled towel or blanket may be used to improve positioning of the extremity or to promote comfort.

The site is selected and the skin prepared as described previously. The area to be used is grasped firmly. The skin is punctured with the sterile lancet using a quick, firm motion to a depth of approximately 2 mm. With one wipe, the first drip of blood is removed. If flow is poor, the site should not be squeezed, as squeezing may produce more tissue fluid than blood. A hand or foot may be held in the dependent position to improve blood flow.

The sample is collected in microhematocrit tubes or pipettes and evacuated into a container holding the proper reagent. For smears, a drop of blood is placed on a clean microscope slide and spread gently with the edge of another slide. Slight pressure is applied to the puncture site with a small, sterile gauze square until bleeding stops.

The sample is labeled with the patient's name and other required identifying information and is sent promptly to the laboratory.

Venipunctures

The equipment needed is assembled: tourniquet; skin disinfectant; gauze pads or cotton balls; syringe and needle or vacuumized tube, holder, and needle; bandage; and materials to label the specimen. A 20-gauge needle is usually used to prevent damage to blood cells. Needles with smaller lumens, such as 21- to 23-gauge, may be used, depending on the age of the client, the size of the vein, and the size of the vacuumized tube. Soft rubber tubing, approximately 1 inch wide, may be used for the tourniquet; however, a rubber tourniquet of the same width with a Velcro closure is preferable.

The vacuumized tubes used in collecting samples of venous blood come in various sizes appropriate to the age of the client or to the type of laboratory analysis equipment and may or may not contain an anticoagulant. The color of the rubber stopper used to seal the tube indicates the presence and type of anticoagulant (Table A–1). Care must be taken to ensure that the correct tube is used for the test to be performed.

A syringe and needle may be used to obtain a venous blood sample if it is felt that the vacuumized tube system will collapse the vein before the volume of needed blood is obtained. In such instances, the sample must be transferred promptly to the appropriate blood tube. To accomplish this transfer, the needle is removed from the syringe and the rubber stopper from the tube, and blood is allowed to flow gently down the inside of the tube. Another approach is to insert the needle into the rubber stopper of the vacuumized tube, allowing the vacuum to draw the blood into the tube. This procedure may be done safely, without hemolysis of blood cells, if the needle is 21-gauge or larger. Most au-

Table A–1 ➤ TYPES OF VACUUMIZED TUBES USED FOR BLOOD TESTS			
Color of Stopper	Substance in Tube	Action of Substance	Tests Used/Not Used for
Red, pink	None	None	Used for tests in which *serum* is required (e.g., many chemistry and serology tests); *serum* is plasma that has been withdrawn from the body and in which the fibrinogen has been used during normal coagulation of the sample Not used for test requiring whole, uncoagulated blood
Lavender, purple	Ethylenediaminetetra-acetic acid (EDTA)	Blocks coagulation by binding calcium Causes minimal distortion of the size and shape of blood cells Prevents platelet aggregation	Used mainly for hematology tests
Light blue	Sodium citrate	Blocks coagulation by binding calcium May result in dilution of the specimen due to volume needed to anticoagulate the sample	Most frequently used in coagulation studies Not used for cell counts or chemistry studies
Green (navy blue, tan)	Sodium heparin	Prevents coagulation by blocking the action of thrombin Does not alter blood cell size May cause a bluish background when blood smears are stained	Used for red blood cell osmotic fragility studies May also be used for selected chemistry and toxicology studies Not use for coagulation studies
Gray	Sodium fluoride and potassium oxalate	Blocks coagulation by binding calcium Blocks action of enzymes in red blood cells, which break down glucose and alcohol May also inactivate cardiac and liver enzymes	Used primarily for blood glucose and alcohol testing Not used for blood glucose tests if the laboratory uses an enzyme testing procedure for determining blood glucose levels Not used for studies of cardiac and liver enzymes

(Continued on page 971)

Color of Stopper	Substance in Tube	Action of Substance	Tests Used/Not Used for
Black	Sodium oxalate	Blocks coagulation by binding calcium May distort blood cells May result in dilution of the specimen due to the volume needed to anticoagulate the sample	Used for coagulation studies Not used for blood smears, cell counts, or chemistry tests
Yellow	Sodium polyanethol sulfonate (SPS)	Blocks coagulation Inactivates white blood cells and antibiotics	Used primarily for blood cultures (blood sample must be added to blood culture bottle containing additional SPS withing 1 hour of obtaining sample)

thorities recommend changing the needle before injecting the rubber stopper. If the sample is for a blood culture, the rubber stopper is cleansed with povidone-iodine before the needle is inserted.

The client is placed in a position of comfort and safety, either sitting or lying down. The extremity to be used is supported on the bed or on a table. A small pillow or rolled towel or blanket may be used to improve positioning of the extremity or to promote comfort.

The tourniquet is applied 1 to 1.5 inches above the site to be used, usually the antecubital area, but the dorsum of a hand or foot can be considered. Tourniquets should be applied tightly enough to cause the veins to enlarge but should never occlude arterial circulation. They should not be kept in place for more than 1 minute before the venipuncture or for more than 2 to 3 minutes for the entire procedure. If a vein in the arm is to be used, the client is asked to open and close the hand a few times and then to clench the fist. If the puncture cannot be made within 1 minute, the tourniquet is removed and then reapplied when the puncture site is definitely located. This practice prevents hemoconcentration, which may alter test results.

The skin is cleansed as described previously (see under "Physical Preparation"). If the vein is palpated after the skin is prepared, the site is recleansed.

The needle cover is removed and the needle inserted into the vein approximately ½ inch below the point at which the needle is expected to enter the vein itself. When the needle is smaller than the vein, it is inserted bevel up at a 15- to 45-degree angle through the skin. When the needle is larger than the vein, it is inserted bevel down and almost parallel to the skin. This technique allows the skin to be punctured first and then the vein; it is a useful approach for entering difficult veins.

If the vacuumized tube system is used, the tube is pushed into the holder until the rubber stopper is punctured and blood flows into the tube. If more than one tube of blood is required, the filled tube is removed from the holder and another inserted until the desired number of samples is obtained. The sequence for obtaining multiple samples using different types of tubes is as follows: (1) blood culture tubes (the rubber stopper must be cleansed before insertion into the holder to prevent contamination of the sample), (2) tubes with no additives, (3) tubes for coagulation studies, and (4) tubes with additives (see Table A–1, pp. 970–971).

If a syringe is used, pull back on the plunger until the desired amount of blood is obtained. The sample is then transferred into the desired blood tubes as described previously (see p. 969).

The tourniquet is released and the client is instructed to unclench the fist. It should be released within 1 minute after the start of blood withdrawal if multiple samples are needed. The needle is removed and pressure is immediately applied to the puncture site with a gauze pad or cotton ball. Pressure should be maintained for 3 minutes to prevent hematoma formation. If the puncture site is on the dorsum of the hand, the hand is elevated while pressure is applied. Pressure is maintained until bleeding has stopped.

The sample is labeled with the client's name and other required identifying information and sent promptly to the laboratory.

Pediatric venous blood sample collections are considered and performed only when a capillary puncture cannot provide the amount of blood needed or when a test is needed that can be performed only on whole blood, blood serum, or plasma. Modifications such as needle lumen, mentioned previously, are made according to the child's age. The site for older children is the same as for adults. The site for infants can be a scalp vein or a superficial vein of the wrist, hand, foot, or arm. The infant and very young child require some restraint, which can be provided by the caregiver or nurse. Venous samples can also be obtained by aspiration from an IV infusion site, depending on the type or components of the fluid being infused. Children have a particular need for reassurance that the blood loss is not a threat to their life and that the body produces blood that replaces the blood withdrawn. Also, a Band-Aid can provide assurance that more blood will not leak out of the body through the puncture site.

Indwelling Devices and Atrial Venous Catheters

Assemble all necessary equipment: disinfectant swabs (povidone-iodine and alcohol), sterile gauze pads, sterile injection cap, 10-mL syringe, blood collection tubes, vial of heparin with syringe and needle or Tubex unit dose of heparin, normal saline in a 50-mL syringe, sterile gloves, and materials to label the specimen.

The client is placed in a position of comfort and safety, usually semi-Fowler's, for blood withdrawal from a right atrial catheter, with the cap or hub exposed at the site of insertion, that is, right upper chest or neck. A sitting or lying position with the extremity supported on a small pillow or towel can be used for blood withdrawal from a heparin lock. If the client is a neonate, the heparin lock system is positioned next to the neonate, taped in place, and connected to a tubing that leads to an indwelling catheter placed in an umbilical vein. It is important to note that frequent removal of blood from the neonate for laboratory testing can deplete blood volume and is the most common indication for transfusion therapy. The development of microtechnology and electronic devices that facilitate in vivo testing and monitoring allows continuous laboratory evaluation with a minimum of blood sampling.

All of the procedures for blood withdrawal from a device or catheter are performed using strict sterile technique. The heparin is prepared in a syringe or the unit dose heparin is placed in a Tubex and the medication allowed to warm to room temperature for better tolerance as it enters the blood flow. The heparin prevents obstruction of the needle or tubing by clotting the blood. Dosage varies for the sick neonate with an umbilical catheter in place. If a Groshong right atrial catheter is in place, irrigation takes place instead of heparinization. For this type of catheter, a syringe is prepared with 30 mL of sterile normal saline to flush the catheter. This irrigation is performed before blood withdrawal and after total parenteral nutrition (TPN). A syringe prepared with 20 mL of sterile normal saline is used after blood withdrawal.

The labeled blood tubes are placed in an upright position in a small glass. The catheter-cap junction or hub is cleansed with a povidone-iodine swab and a 70 percent alcohol swab for 2 minutes. Sterile gloves are donned, the cap is removed, and a 10-mL syringe is attached to the connector. Blood in the catheter can cause inaccurate test results, so 6 mL of blood is withdrawn with the syringe and the catheter is then clamped. Clamping is not necessary if a Groshong catheter is in place because it has a special valve that eliminates the need for clamping. This blood is discarded with the syringe. Another 10-mL syringe is attached, and the needed amount of blood is withdrawn, using only a moderate amount of suction. The appropriate amount of blood is placed in the tubes (usually 7 to 10 mL in each tube), and blood withdrawal is continued until the tubes are filled. Color-coded stoppers are applied to the tubes as they are filled, and specimens that require the blood to be mixed with substances in the tube are gently rotated.

At the conclusion of the blood withdrawal, heparinization of the device or catheter or flushing of the Groshong catheter with saline is performed. Heparinization is performed by inserting the needle into the cap or hub and slowly injecting the prepared syringe of medication into the device or catheter. The catheter is then clamped 2 inches from the cap or hub as the last of the medication is injected. The needle is removed from the cap or hub, and the catheter is unclamped. A new sterile injection cap or hub is attached if the old cap is discarded. To irrigate the Groshong, a solution of 20 to 30 mL of sterile normal saline is gently injected through the injection cap with moderate force. The needle is then removed, but some positive pressure is maintained on the plunger of the syringe during withdrawal to prevent the solution from backing up into the syringe.

The client is left in a comfortable position after the procedures, and the labeled specimens are promptly sent to the laboratory.

NURSING CARE AFTER THE PROCEDURE

➤ After bleeding has stopped, apply an adhesive bandage.
➤ Application of an adhesive bandage on the finger of a child under 6 years of age is not recommended because the child may swallow the bandage and choke on it.

➤ Apply a new dressing to the catheter site using a sterile 2 × 2-inch gauze pad. Coil the catheter on the dressing with the cap or hub directed upward, cover with a transparent dressing, and tape in place.

➤ Rebandage and tape a heparin lock device if necessary.

NURSING OBSERVATIONS AND PROBLEM-SOLVING ACTIVITIES

Before the Test

➤ Assess the client's understanding of the explanations provided.

➤ Assess the client's degree of anxiety about the procedure.

➤ Assess the infant's or child's need for restraint and reassurance.

➤ Ensure that food, fluid, and medication restrictions have been followed.

➤ Fill out the requisition accurately and include all information that is requested on the form.

During the Test

➤ Note the client's response to the procedure and provide support if needed.

➤ Obtain the blood sample using proper technique and standard precautions and transmission-based isolation procedures.

➤ Avoid possible invalid testing caused by prolonged use of a tourniquet; excessive suction on the syringe; vigorous shaking of the specimen in a tube or expulsion from the syringe into a tube; moisture in the syringe or tube; leakage of air into the syringe or tube; contamination of the site, equipment, or blood.

➤ Provide support to the client if the puncture is not successful and another must be performed to obtain the blood sample.

➤ Select appropriate evacuated tubes or syringe, needle, and laboratory tubes, depending on tests to be performed.

➤ Note obstruction of vascular access device or catheter caused by blood clotting, and notify the physician.

After the Test

➤ Apply the necessary pressure to the puncture site until the bleeding stops. If oozing continues, elevate the extremity and apply a pressure type of dressing.

➤ Remain with the client until the bleeding has completely stopped.

➤ If the client is experiencing excessive and lingering pain or syncope, allow the client to lie down and rest.

➤ Assess for extreme anxiety and signs of possible shock state such as tachycardia and hypotension.

➤ Check the venipuncture site in 5 minutes for hematoma formation. If the client is immunosuppressed, check the puncture site every 8 hours for signs and symptoms of infection or septicemia, such as fever, chills, petechiae, and inflamed joints.

➤ Monitor vascular device or catheter insertion site for redness, swelling, pain, and purulent drainage indicating infection and monitor for sepsis caused by contamination during the procedure.

➤ If the specimen cannot be transported to the laboratory within a reasonable time or if analysis is delayed, arrange for proper storage to prevent deterioration or contamination that can cause inaccurate results.

Obtaining Various Types of Urine Specimens

One of the main reasons for invalid results of urine tests is improper specimen collection and maintenance. Therefore the nurse must know how the specimens are collected and how to instruct clients on specimen collection. The various types of specimens are discussed here.

RANDOM SPECIMENS

Random specimens are urine samples that are collected at any time of day in clean containers. Usually 15 to 60 mL of urine is sufficient for tests performed on random samples. Random samples are used for routine screening tests to detect obvious abnormalities. The client is instructed to void directly into the urine container or to void in some other type of clean container, after which the sample is transferred to another type of laboratory container. If the sample is collected by the client at home, it must be transported to the laboratory within 2 hours or test results may be inaccurate.

FIRST MORNING SPECIMENS

First morning specimens are collected upon arising in the morning, when urine is most concentrated. Such samples are ideal for screening purposes, as substances may be detectable in them that are not found in more dilute samples. In addition to routine screening tests, first morning samples are desirable for pregnancy tests and tests for orthostatic proteinuria.

DOUBLE-VOIDED SPECIMENS

Double-voided specimens are used when testing urine for sugar and acetone. The purpose of this approach is to ensure that the urine tested is fresh so that it serves as a valid indicator of current blood glucose and ketone levels. The client is instructed to empty the bladder and, if possible, to drink a glass of water. Approximately 30 minutes later, the client voids again. The second sample is then tested. Some individuals advocate testing the first sample as well, in case the client cannot void a second time. The validity of results on the first sample may be questionable, however. The double-voided specimen is particularly critical for the first urine sample of the day because urine that has accumulated in the bladder overnight is not a valid indicator of current status.

CLEAN-CATCH MIDSTREAM SPECIMENS

Clean-catch midstream specimens are used to avoid contamination of the sample with urethral cells, microorganisms, and mucus. The procedure is as follows: The client is provided with a clean-catch kit containing a sterile specimen container and materials for cleansing the meatus. The male client should cleanse the urinary meatus with the agent provided (or with soap and water), void a few milliliters of urine into the toilet or urinal, and then void directly into the specimen container. Women should cleanse the labia minora and meatal orifice carefully, working from front to back, and then manually keep the labia separated while voiding a few milliliters into the toilet or bedpan. With the labia still separated, the client should then void directly into the collection container. If a woman is menstruating or has a heavy vaginal discharge, she should insert a clean vaginal tampon before beginning the cleansing process. Care must be taken by all clients to avoid touching the inside of the urine container and lid.

Clean-catch midstream urine specimens are used primarily for microbiologic and cytologic analysis of urine. Some individuals also advocate using this method for specimens for routine urinalysis (UA), especially in women, because the sample is less likely to be contaminated with substances that alter results of routine screening tests.

CATHETERIZED SPECIMENS

Urine specimens may be obtained from one-time "straight" catheterizations or from indwelling Foley catheters. "Straight" catheterization is indicated when the client is unable to void for a random or a clean-catch specimen without excessively contaminating the sample. It is also used for samples for microbiologic and cytologic studies.

Indwelling catheters may be placed for a variety of reasons. In some cases, they may be inserted when serial urine specimens are needed at exact time intervals. In other cases, the catheter is already in place and must be used for urine sampling.

When obtaining a sample from an indwelling catheter, be sure that the drainage tube is empty; then clamp the tube distal to the specimen collection port. The sample is obtained with a needle (25- to 21-gauge) and a 3- to 5-mL (larger if a greater amount is needed) syringe after the tubing has been clamped for approximately 15 minutes. The specimen port is cleansed with an antiseptic swab (e.g., alcohol sponge) and the sample is aspirated. The sample is then placed in a sterile container or rubber-stoppered test tube and sent promptly to the laboratory. Bedside screening tests (e.g., for glucose and ketones) may be performed by instilling the sample directly from the syringe to the reagent strip. Care must be taken to ensure that the catheter is unclamped after the sample is obtained.

TWENTY-FOUR-HOUR (TIMED) SPECIMENS

Twenty-four-hour specimens allow quantification of substances in urine. Methods of preserving the accumulating sample vary among laboratories and, therefore, the laboratory should be consulted for advice regarding the use of a preservative or the need for refrigeration, or both. It is critical that all urine excreted during the 24-hour period be collected.

When a 24-hour specimen is required, it is desirable to begin in the morning, usually sometime between 6 and 8 AM. First the client voids and discards the specimen. The collection begins when the discard sample is obtained. All urine voided thereafter is collected. The next day, at the same time the specimen collection began, the client is instructed to void again. This final voiding is added to the sample, and the collection ends. The dates and times of specimen collection should be noted on the laboratory slip. In the hospital setting, it is helpful if a reminder to collect all urine is posted in or near the client's bathroom so that neither the client nor the hospital personnel inadvertently discard any portion of the specimen. The client should be instructed not to place toilet paper in the specimen container (devices that fit into toilet seats are often used). Individuals who use a bedpan should be instructed not to void into a pan containing feces.

Sometimes it is necessary to insert a Foley catheter for 24-hour urine collections, especially if the client is unable to participate in specimen collection. Other times, a Foley catheter may already be in place. When a 24-hour urine collection is to be obtained via an indwelling catheter, the collection should begin by changing the tubing and drainage bag so that a clean, fresh system is in use. If a preservative is required, it can be obtained from the laboratory and placed directly into the drainage bag. Others advocate using a container with preservative and emptying the drainage bag contents into it at frequent intervals (e.g., every 2 hours). If refrigeration of the specimen is necessary, the drainage bag is placed in a basin filled with ice. The ice supply must be renewed frequently to ensure that the specimen is properly chilled. If the urine must be protected from light, the drainage bag may be covered with dark plastic or with aluminum foil. If the drainage tubing is positioned correctly for continuous drainage, it need not be covered.

When the collection is completed, the sample should be transported promptly to the laboratory.

Some urine tests require 2-hour samples. A 2-hour sample is collected in the same manner as a 24-hour sample, with the exact starting and stopping times noted.

SUPRAPUBIC ASPIRATION

Suprapubic aspiration involves inserting a needle directly into the bladder to obtain a urine sample. Because the bladder is normally sterile, this method allows collection of samples that are free of extraneous contamination. In this procedure, the skin over the suprapubic area is cleansed with antiseptic and draped with sterile drapes. A local anesthetic may then be injected. The needle is inserted and the sample is removed, after which a sterile dressing is applied. The site is observed for inflammation and abnormal drainage. Suprapubic aspiration may be used for samples for microbiologic and cytologic analysis. It may also be used to obtain samples in infants and young children.

PEDIATRIC SAMPLES

Pediatric urine collections can be performed for random, first voided, clean-catch, or timed specimens. For infants, this procedure involves the attachment of a plastic collection device to the male penis or to the female genitalia to collect the urine. A female infant is placed in a supine position with the hips rotated and abducted and the knees flexed. The perineal area is cleansed and dried, and the collection device is taped to the perineum at the point between the anus and the vagina. The adhesive edges of the device toward the front and over the pubic area are sealed to prevent leakage of urine. A male infant is placed in supine position, and the penis and scrotum are cleansed and dried. The device is applied over the penis and scrotum and the edges are sealed against the perineum to prevent leakage of urine. A diaper is placed over the collection device. The device is removed after the specimen is obtained to prevent loosening of a moist bag. The urine is placed in a clean container, labeled correctly, and sent to the laboratory. A clean-catch specimen is collected using the same appliances applied after cleansing with soap or an antiseptic pad and then with sterile water. The specimen should be tested immediately for accurate results, as the number of bacteria can double every 20 to 30 minutes. If the infant has not voided within 45 minutes, the bag is removed and the cleansing and application are repeated. A 24-hour specimen collection requires a special collection bag that contains a collection tube attached to a container device that can be emptied periodically. Testing with Tes-Tape can be accomplished by placing a cotton ball in the diaper to collect the urine and placing the tape on the wet cotton ball. The wet diaper can also be used for this type of testing. Urine specimens are obtained from toilet-trained children in the same manner as for adults. It is helpful to follow the child's usual urinary pattern when collecting the specimen. A potty chair or bedpan placed on the toilet and terminology familiar to the child should be used ("tinkle," "potty," and so on). A parent can assist and often has more success in collecting a specimen than does the nurse.

III

Guidelines for Isolation Precautions in Hospitals*

INTRODUCTION

In 1996, the Centers for Disease Control and Prevention (CDC) revised its *Guidelines for Isolation Precautions in Hospitals* to meet the following objectives: (1) to be epidemiologically sound; (2) to recognize the importance of all bodily fluids, secretions, and excretions in the transmission of nosocomial pathogens; (3) to contain adequate precautions for infections transmitted by the airborne, droplet, and contact routes of transmission; (4) to be as simple and user friendly as possible; and (5) to use new terms to avoid confusion with existing infection control and isolation systems.

The revised guidelines contain two tiers of precautions. The first and most important precautions are those designed for the care of *all* patients regardless of their diagnosis or presumed infection status. These Standard Precautions are designed to prevent the occurrence of nosocomial infections. The second tier is designed to implement isolation precautions for specific patients with certain diagnoses. Included are airborne, droplet, and contact modes of transmission.

STANDARD PRECAUTIONS (TIER ONE)

1. Standard Precautions apply to all blood, bodily fluids, secretions, excretions, nonintact skin, and mucous membranes.
2. Handwashing is to be done between all client contacts, and after contact with blood, bodily fluids, secretions, excretions, or contaminated equipment.
3. Gloves are worn at all times when in contact with blood, bodily fluids, secretions, excretions, nonintact skin, and mucous membranes. Handwashing is to be done after removal of gloves.
4. Masks and eye protection are worn if splashing of blood or bodily fluids is possible.
5. Gowns are worn if contact with blood, bodily fluids, secretions, or excretions is possible.
6. Proper disinfection of equipment is necessary, and single-use items should be used and properly disposed of after use.
7. Contaminated linens are to be placed in leakproof bags and appropriately tagged.

*Adapted from Centers for Disease Control and Prevention @ http://www.cdc.gov
Author's Note: This is an excellent web site for up-to-date information on precaution guidelines and statistical data on infectious diseases.

8. Sharp instruments and needles are to be disposed of in a puncture-resistant container. This container should be placed in every client room. The CDC recommends that needles be disposed of uncapped or that a mechanical device be used for recapping.
9. Private rooms are generally not necessary unless client hygiene practices are inadequate or in cases of specific Tier Two situations.

TRANSMISSION CATEGORIES (TIER TWO)
Airborne Precautions

1. Droplet nuclei smaller than 5 microns (measles, chickenpox, disseminated varicella zoster, pulmonary or laryngeal tuberculosis).
2. Clients require a private room, negative airflow with at least six changes per hour, and a mask or other respiratory protection for the nurse. The client may also require a mask if coughing is excessive.

Droplet Precautions

1. Droplets larger than 5 microns (diptheria, rubella, streptococcal pharyngitis, pneumonia, scarlet fever, pertussis, mumps, mycoplasma or meningococcal pneumonia, or sepsis).
2. Private room or cohort (isolated grouping) of clients and a mask for the nurse are required.

Contact Precautions

1. Direct client contact or environmental contact, colonization or infection with drug-resistant organisms, *Shigella* and other enteric pathogens, herpes simplex, scabies, varicella zoster.
2. Private room, cohort of clients, gloves, and gown for the nurse are required.

IV

Units of Measurement (Including SI Units)*

SCIENTIFIC NOTATION

Sometimes it is necessary to use very large and very small numbers. These can best be indicated and handled in calculations by use of scientific notation, which is to say by use of exponents. Use of scientific notation requires writing the number so that it is the result of multiplying some whole number power of 10 by a number between 1 and 10. Examples are:

$$1234 = 1.234 \times 10^3$$
$$0.01234 = 1.234 \times \frac{1}{100} = 1.234 \times 10^{-2}$$
$$0.001234 = 1.234 \times \frac{1}{1000} = 1.234 \times 10^{-3}$$

To convert a number to its equivalent in scientific notation:

Place the decimal point to the right of the first non-zero digit. This will now be a number between 1 and 9.

Multiply this number by a power of 10, the exponent of which is equal to the number of places the decimal point was moved. The exponent is positive if the decimal point was moved to the left, and negative if it was moved to the right. For example:

$$\frac{1,234,000.0 \times 0.000072}{6000.0} = \frac{1.234 \times 10^6 \times 7.2 \times 10^{-5}}{6.0 \times 10^3}$$

Now, by simply adding or subtracting the exponents of ten, and remembering that moving an exponent from the denominator of the fraction to the numerator changes its sign,

$$= \frac{1.234 \times 10^6 \times 10^{-5} \times 10^{-3} \times 7.2}{6} = \frac{1.234 \times 10^{-2} \times 7.2}{6}$$

Now, dividing by 6,

$$= 1.234 \times 10^{-2} \times 1.2 = 1.4808 \times 10^{-2} = \frac{1.4808}{100} = 0.014808$$

* Adapted from Thomas, CL (ed): Taber's Cyclopedic Medical Dictionary, ed 18. FA Davis, Philadelphia, 1997, pp 2227–2233. Used with permission.

The last operation changed 1.4808×10^{-2} into the final value, 0.014808, which is not expressed in scientific notation.

SI UNITS (SYSTÈME INTERNATIONAL D'UNITÉS OR INTERNATIONAL SYSTEM OF UNITS)

This system includes two types of units important in clinical medicine. The *base units* are shown in the first table, derived units in the second table, and derived units with special names in the third table.

SI BASE UNITS

Quantity	Name	Symbol
Length	meter	m
Mass	kilogram	kg
Time	second	s
Electric current	ampere	A
Temperature	kelvin	K
Luminous intensity	candela	cd
Amount of a substance	mole	mol

SOME SI DERIVED UNITS

Quantity	Name of Derived Unit	Symbol
Area	square meter	m^2
Volume	cubic meter	m^3
Speed, velocity	meter per second	m/s
Acceleration	meter per second squared	m/s^2
Mass density	kilogram per cubic meter	kg/m^3
Concentration of a substance	mole per cubic meter	mol/m^3
Specific volume	cubic meter per kilogram	m^3/kg
Luminescence	candela per square meter	cd/m^2

SI DERIVED UNITS WITH SPECIAL NAMES

Quantity	Name	Symbol	Expressed in Terms of Other Units
Frequency	hertz	Hz	s^{-1}
Force	newton	N	$kg \cdot m \cdot s^{-2}$ or $kg \cdot m/s^2$
Pressure	pascal	Pa	$N \cdot m^{-2}$ or N/m^2
Energy, work, amount of heat	joule	J	$kg \cdot m^2 \cdot s^{-2}$ or $N \cdot m$
Power	watt	W	$J \cdot s$ or J/s
Quantity of electricity	coulomb	C	$A \cdot s$
Electromotive force	volt	V	W/A
Capacitance	farad	F	C/V
Electrical resistance	ohm	Ω	V/a
Conductance	siemens	S	A/V
Inductance	henry	H	$W\phi/A$
Illuminance	lux	lx	ln/m^2
Absorbed (radiation) dose	gray	Gy	J/kg
Dose equivalent (radiation)	sievert	Sv	J/kg
Activity (radiation)	becquerel	Bq	s^{-1}

PREFIXES AND MULTIPLES USED IN SI

Prefix	Symbol	Power	Multiple or Portion of a Multiple
tera	T	10^{12}	1,000,000,000,000
giga	G	10^{9}	1,000,000,000
mega	M	10^{6}	1,000,000
kilo	k	10^{3}	1,000
hecto	h	10^{2}	100
deca	da	10^{1}	10
unity			1
deci	d	10^{-1}	0.1
centi	c	10^{-2}	0.01
milli	m	10^{-3}	0.001
micro	μ	10^{-6}	0.000001
nano	n	10^{-9}	0.000000001
pico	p	10^{-12}	0.000000000001
femto	f	10^{-15}	0.000000000000001
atto	a	10^{-18}	0.000000000000000001

METRIC SYSTEM

MASSES

Table		Grams		Grains
1 Kilogram	=	1000.0	=	15,432.35
1 Hectogram	=	100.0	=	1,543.23
1 Decagram	=	10.0	=	154.323
1 Gram	=	1.0	=	15.432
1 Decigram	=	0.1	=	1.5432
1 Centigram	=	0.01	=	0.15432
1 Milligram	=	0.001	=	0.01543
1 Microgram	=	10^{-6}	=	15.432×10^{-6}
1 Nanogram	=	10^{-9}	=	15.432×10^{-9}
1 Picogram	=	10^{-12}	=	15.432×10^{-12}
1 Femtogram	=	10^{-15}	=	15.432×10^{-15}
1 Attogram	=	10^{-18}	=	15.432×10^{-18}

Arabic numbers are used with masses and measures, as 10 g, or 3 ml, etc. Portions of masses and measures are usually expressed decimally. 10^{-1} indicates 0.1; $10^{-6} = 0.000001$; etc.

WEIGHTS AND MEASURES

Arabic numerals are used with masses and measures, as 10 g, or 3 ml, etc. Portions of masses and measures are usually expressed decimally. For practical purposes, 1 cm³ (cubic centimeter) is equivalent to 1 ml (milliliter) and 1 drop (gtt.) of water is equivalent to a minim (m).

LENGTH

Millimeters (mm)	Centimeters (cm)	Inches (in.)	Feet (ft)	Yards (yds)	Meters (m)
1.0	0.1	0.03937	0.00328	0.0011	0.001
10.0	1.0	0.3937	0.03281	0.0109	0.01
25.4	2.54	1.0	0.0833	0.0278	0.0254
304.8	30.48	12.0	1.0	0.333	0.3048
914.40	91.44	36.0	3.0	1.0	0.9144
1000.0	100.0	39.37	3.2808	1.0936	1.0

1 μm = 1 micrometer = 0.001 millimeter. 1 mm = 100 μm.
1 km = 1 kilometer = 1000 meters = 0.62137 statute mile.
1 statute mile = 5280 feet = 1.609 kilometers.
1 nautical mile = 6076.042 feet = 1852.276 meters.

VOLUME (FLUID)

Milliliters (ml)	U.S. Fluidrams (f$\mathfrak{z}$)	Cubic Inches (in.^{3})	U.S. Fluidounces (f$\mathfrak{z}$)	U.S. Fluid Quarts (qt)	Liters (L)
1.0	0.2705	0.061	0.03381	0.00106	0.001
3.697	1.0	0.226	0.125	0.00391	0.00369
16.3866	4.4329	1.0	0.5541	0.0173	0.01639
29.573	8.0	1.8047	1.0	0.03125	0.02957
946.332	256.0	57.75	32.0	1.0	0.9463
1000.0	270.52	61.025	33.815	1.0567	1.0

1 gallon = 4 quarts = 8 pints = 3.785 liters.
1 pint = 473.16 ml.

WEIGHT

Grains (gr)	Grams (g)	Apothecaries' Ounces ($\mathfrak{z}$)	Avoirdupois Pounds (lb)	Kilograms (kg)
1.0	0.0648	0.00208	0.0001429	0.000065
15.432	1.0	0.03215	0.002205	0.001
480.0	31.1	1.0	0.06855	0.0311
7000.0	453.5924	14.583	1.0	0.45359
15432.358	1000.0	32.15	2.2046	1.0

1 microgram (μm) = 0.001 milligram.
1 mg = 1 milligram = 0.001 g; 1000 mg = 1 g.

APOTHECARIES' WEIGHT

20 grains = 1 scruple 　　　　　3 scruples = 1 dram
8 drams = 1 ounce 　　　　　12 ounces = 1 pound

AVOIRDUPOIS WEIGHT

27.343 grains = 1 dram 　　　　　16 drams = 1 ounce
16 ounces = 1 pound 　　　　　100 pounds = 1 hundredweight
2000 pounds = 1 short ton 　　　　　2240 pounds = 1 long ton
1 oz troy = 480 grains 　　　　　1 oz avoirdupois = 437.5 grains
1 lb troy = 5760 grains 　　　　　1 lb avoirdupois = 7000 grains

CIRCULAR MEASURE

60 seconds = 1 minute   60 minutes = 1 degree
90 degrees = 1 quadrant   4 quadrants = 360 degrees = circle

CUBIC MEASURE

1728 cubic inches = 1 cubic foot   27 cubic feet = 1 cubic yard
2150.42 cubic inches = 1 standard bushel   268.8 cubic inches = 1 dry (U.S.) gallon
1 cubic foot = about four fifths of a bushel   128 cubic feet = 1 cord (wood)

DRY MEASURE

2 pints = 1 quart   8 quarts = 1 peck   4 pecks = 1 bushel

LIQUID MEASURE

16 ounces = 1 pint   4 quarts = 1 gallon   2 barrels = 1 hogshead (U.S.)
1000 milliliters = 1 liter 31.5 gallons = 1 barrel (U.S.) 1 quart = 946.35 milliliters
4 gills = 1 pint   2 pints = 1 quart   1 liter = 1.0566 quart

Barrels and hogsheads vary in size. A U.S. gallon is equal to 0.8327 British gallon; therefore, a British gallon is equal to 1.201 U.S. gallons. 1 liter is equal to 1.0567 quarts.

LINEAR MEASURE

1 inch = 2.54 centimeters   40 rods = 1 furlong   8 furlongs = 1 statute mile
12 inches = 1 foot   3 feet = 1 yard   5.5 yards = 1 rod
1 statute mile = 5280 feet   3 statute miles = 1 statute league   1 nautical mile = 6076.042 feet

TROY WEIGHT

24 grains = 1 pennyweight   20 pennyweights = 1 ounce   12 ounces = 1 pound
Used for weighing gold, silver, and jewels.

HOUSEHOLD MEASURES* AND WEIGHTS

Approximate Equivalents: 60 gtt. = 1 teaspoonful = 5 ml = 60 minims
= 60 grains = 1 dram = ⅛ ounce

1 teaspoon = ⅛ fl. oz; 1 dram   16 teaspoons (liquid) = 1 cup
3 teaspoons = 1 tablespoon   12 tablespoons (dry) = 1 cup
1 tablespoon = ½ fl. oz; 4 drams   1 cup = 8 fl. oz
1 tumbler or glass = 8 fl. oz; ½ pint

Conversion Rules and Factors

To convert units of one system into the other, multiply the number of units in column I by the equivalent factor opposite that unit in column II.

---

* Household measures are not precise. For instance, a household tsp will hold from 3 to 5 ml of liquid. Therefore, household equivalents should not be substituted for medication prescribed by the physician.

Note: Traditionally, the word "weights" is used in these tables, but "masses" is the correct term.

WEIGHT

1 attogram	=	15.432×10^{-18} grains
1 femtogram	=	15.432×10^{-15} grains
1 picogram	=	15.432×10^{-12} grains
1 nanogram	=	15.432×10^{-9} grains
1 microgram	=	15.432×10^{-6} grains
1 milligram	=	0.015432 grain
1 centigram	=	0.15432 grain
1 decigram	=	1.5432 grains
1 decagram	=	154.323 grains
1 hectogram	=	1543.23 grains
1 gram	=	15.432 grains
1 gram	=	0.25720 apothecaries' dram
1 gram	=	0.03527 avoirdupois ounce
1 gram	=	0.03215 apothecaries' or troy ounce
1 kilogram	=	35.274 avoirdupois ounces
1 kilogram	=	35.151 apothecaries' or troy ounces
1 kilogram	=	2.2046 avoirdupois pounds
1 grain	=	64.7989 milligrams
1 grain	=	0.0648 gram
1 apothecaries' dram	=	3.8879 gram
1 avoirdupois ounce	=	28.3495 grams
1 apothecaries' or troy ounce	=	31.1035 grams
1 avoirdupois pound	=	453.5924 grams

VOLUME (AIR OR GAS)

1 cubic centimeter (cm³)	=	0.06102 cubic inch
1 cubic meter (m³)	=	35.314 cubic feet
1 cubic meter	=	1.3079 cubic yard
1 cubic inch (in³)	=	16.3872 cubic centimeters
1 cubic foot (ft³)	=	0.02832 cubic meter

CAPACITY (FLUID OR LIQUID)

1 milliliter	=	16.23 minims
1 milliliter	=	0.2705 fluidram
1 milliliter	=	0.0338 fluidounce
1 liter	=	33.8148 fluidounces
1 liter	=	2.1134 pints
1 liter	=	1.0567 quart
1 liter	=	0.2642 gallon
1 fluidram	=	3.697 milliliters
1 fluidounce	=	29.573 milliliters
1 pint	=	473.1765 milliliters
1 quart	=	946.353 milliliters
1 gallon	=	3.785 liters

TIME

1 millisecond = one thousandth (0.001) of a second

1 second = $\frac{1}{60}$ of a minute

1 minute = $\frac{1}{60}$ of an hour

1 hour = $\frac{1}{24}$ of a day

TEMPERATURE

Given a temperature on the Fahrenheit scale; to convert it to degrees Celsius, subtract 32 and multiply by 5/9. Given a temperature on the Celsius scale; to convert it to degrees Fahrenheit, multiply by 9/5 and add 32. Degrees celsius are equivalent to degrees Centigrade.

PRESSURE

TO OBTAIN	MULTIPLY	BY
lb/sq in.	atmospheres	14.696
lb/sq in.	in. of water	0.03609
lb/sq in.	ft of water	0.4335
lb/sq in.	in. of mercury	0.4912
lb/sq in.	kg/sq meter	0.00142
lb/sq in.	kg/sq cm	14.22
lb/sq in.	cm of mercury	0.1934
lb/sq ft	atmospheres	2116.8
lb/sq ft	in. of water	5.204
lb/sq ft	ft of water	62.48
lb/sq ft	in. of mercury	70.727
lb/sq ft	cm of mercury	27.845
lb/sq ft	kg/sq meter	0.20482
lb/cu in.	gm/ml	0.03613
lb/cu ft	lb/cu in.	1728.0
lb/cu ft	gm/ml	62.428
lb/U.S. gal	gm/L	8.345
in. of water	in. of mercury	13.60
in. of water	cm of mercury	5.3543
ft of water	atmospheres	33.95
ft of water	lb/sq in.	2.307
ft of water	kg/sq meter	0.00328
ft of water	in. of mercury	1.133
ft of water	cm of mercury	0.4461
atmospheres	ft of water	0.02947
atmospheres	in. of mercury	0.03342
atmospheres	kg/sq cm	0.9678
bars	atmospheres	1.0133
in. of mercury	atmospheres	29.921
in. of mercury	lb/sq in.	2.036
mm of mercury	atmospheres	760.0
g/ml	lb/cu in.	27.68
g/sq cm	kg/sq meter	0.1
kg/sq meter	lb/sq in.	703.1
kg/sq meter	in. of water	25.40
kg/sq meter	in. of mercury	345.32
kg/sq meter	cm of mercury	135.95
kg/sq meter	atmospheres	10332.0
kg/sq cm	atmospheres	1.0332

FLOW RATE

TO OBTAIN	MULTIPLY	BY
cu ft/hr	cc/min	0.00212
cu ft/hr	L/min	2.12
L/min	cu ft/hr	0.472

PARTS PER MILLION

Conversion of parts per million (ppm) to percent:

1 ppm = 0.0001%, 10 ppm = 0.001%, 100 ppm = 0.01% 1000 ppm = 0.1%, 10,000 ppm = 1%, etc.

ENERGY

1 foot pound = 1.35582 joule

1 joule = 0.2389 Calorie (kilocalorie)

1 Calorie (kilocalorie) = 1000 calories = 4184 joules

A large Calorie, or kilocalorie, is always written with a capital C.

pH

The pH scale is simply a series of numbers stating where a given solution would stand in a series of solutions arranged according to acidity or alkalinity. At one extreme (high pH) lies a highly alkaline solution, which may be made by dissolving 4 g of sodium hydroxide in water to make a liter of solution; at the other extreme (low pH) is an acid solution containing 3.65 g of hydrogen chloride per liter of water. Halfway between lies purified water, which is neutral. All other solutions can be arranged on this scale, and their acidity or alkalinity can be stated by giving the numbers that indicate their relative positions. If the pH of a certain solution is 5.3, it falls between gastric juice and urine on the above scale, is moderately acid, and will turn litmus red.

Tenth-normal HCL	−1.00	⎫ Litmus is red in
Gastric juice	*1.4	⎬ this acid range.
Urine	*6.0	⎭
Water	7.00	—Neutral
Blood	7.35–7.45	⎫
Bile	*7.5	⎬ Litmus is blue in
Pancreatic juice	8.5	⎪ this alkaline range.
Tenth-normal NaOH	13.00	⎭

---

* These body fluids vary rather widely in pH; typical figures have been used for simplicity. Urine samples obtained from healthy individuals may have pH anywhere between 4.7 and 8.0.

V

Profile or Panel Groupings and Laboratory Tests

PROFILE OR PANEL GROUPINGS OF DIAGNOSTIC PROCEDURES

A profile or panel grouping refers to a measurement of multiple laboratory tests that reflects the function of several organ systems (health profile) or to a group of selected diagnostic tests and procedures that reflects the function or status of a specific organ or disease. In general, profiles or panels help to determine the client's state of health, support or rule out the presence of physiological abnormalities, determine the effectiveness of therapy, and provide preventive measures or teaching to reduce the progression of a disease. They are also used as screening tests for asymptomatic clients as a preventive measure, although it is generally felt that routine individual screening tests are all that are needed for those who are healthy.

The panel or profile consists of a battery or group of 4 to 12 biochemical tests performed on a few milliliters of serum with an instrument called the sequential multiple analyzer (SMA). The tests are ordered as a unit designated as SMA-4, SMA-6, or SMA-12. SMA-4 includes red blood cell (RBC) count, white blood cell (WBC) count, hemoglobin (Hgb), and hematocrit (Hct). SMA-6 includes sodium (Na), potassium (K), chloride (Cl), bicarbonate (HCO_3), glucose, and blood urea nitrogen (BUN). SMA-12 includes total protein, albumin, calcium (Ca), BUN, inorganic phosphorus, cholesterol, glucose, uric acid, creatinine, total bilirubin, alkaline phosphatase (ALP), and aspartate aminotransferase (SGOT [AST]). The electrolytes included in the SMA-6 can replace uric acid, creatinine, cholesterol, and phosphorus (P) to provide another variety of SMA-12. Another type of analyzer, known as SMAC, can accommodate a large profile of roughly 20 tests (CHEM 20), provide several tests from each of the panels, and analyze components of the blood singly or in combination to note organ or body system associations in a single procedure. Patterns of abnormalities can be recognized by the physician, and more conclusive diagnostic procedures can be ordered based on these profile results (Table A–2).

LABORATORY TESTS FOR DISEASES, ORGANS, OR ORGAN SYSTEMS

Cardiovascular System

➤ *Cardiac enzymes:* Aspartate aminotransferase (AST, SGOT), creatine phosphokinase (CPK), creatine kinase (CK) and isoenzyme (CK-MB), lactate dehydrogenase (LH, LDH) and isoenzyme (LD_1, LD_2), hydroxybutyrate dehydrogenase (HBDH)

Table A–2 ➤ CHEM-20 HEALTH PROFILE
WITH SOME
ORGAN ASSOCIATIONS
OF EACH ANALYTE

Glucose *F, R*	Bilirubin, direct *L*
BUN *K, L, F*	Bilirubin, total *L*
Creatinine *K, F*	LDH *L, M*
Uric acid *K*	SGOT (AST) *L, M*
Sodium *K, F*	SGPT (ALT) *L*
Potassium *K, F*	Alkaline phosphatase *L, B*
Chloride *K, F*	Albumin *N, L, K*
Bicarbonate *K, F*	Total protein *N, L*
Calcium *B, F*	Cholesterol *N, R*
Phosphorus *K, B*	Triglycerides *N, R*

K = kidneys, *L* = liver, *B* = bone, *N* = nutrition, *M* = muscle,
R = cardiac risk assessment, *F* = fluid and electrolyte balance.
Source: Sacher, RA, and McPherson, FA; Widmann's Clinical
Interpretation of Laboratory Tests, ed 10. FA Davis, Philadelphia,
1991, p 14. Used with permission.

➤ *Lipids:* Total lipids, lipoprotein electrophoresis (HDL, LDL, VLDL), cholesterol, triglycerides, phospholipids
➤ *Electrolytes:* Potassium (K), sodium (Na)
➤ *Coagulation:* Prothrombin time (PT), activated partial thromboplastin time (aPTT), coagulation time (CT), clotting time, Lee-White coagulation time(LWCT)
➤ *Pericardial fluid:* Cytologic examination; other tests to measure RBC count, WBC count, differential, and glucose; microbiologic examination if endocarditis is suspected (Gram stain, culture)
➤ *Drug levels:* Digoxin, digitoxin, diltiazem, nifedipine, propranolol, verapamil, others included in therapeutic regimen
➤ *Miscellaneous:* Erythrocyte sedimentation rate (ESR), WBC, glucose, blood gases (pH, pCO_2, pO_2)
➤ *Procedures:* Cardiac nuclear scanning, cardiac radiography, echocardiography, electrocardiography (ECG), phonocardiography, exercise ECG, cardiac catheterization and angiography, heart and chest magnetic resonance imaging (MRI), non-nuclear computed tomography (CT) of the chest

Pulmonary System

➤ *Arterial blood gases* (ABGs): pH, pCO_2, pO_2, HCO_3, BE
➤ *Sputum:* Microbiologic examination (Gram and other stains, acid-fast bacillus [AFB] smear and culture), culture and sensitivity (C&S), cytologic examination
➤ *Pleural fluid:* Microbiologic examination (C&S, Gram stain); cytologic examination; other tests to measure LDH, RBC, WBC, differential, eosinophils, pH, and immunoglobulins
➤ *Drug levels:* Theophylline therapeutic regimen
➤ *Miscellaneous:* Alpha$_1$-antitrypsin, WBC

➤ *Procedures:* Bronchoscopy, mediastinoscopy, thoracoscopy, chest radiography and tomography; bronchography; pulmonary angiography; thoracic ultrasonography; lung nuclear scanning; non-nuclear thoracic CT; chest MRI; pulmonary function studies; exercise pulmonary function; body plethysmography; sweat test; lung biopsy; thoracentesis; oximetry; skin tests for allergens and bacterial and fungal pulmonary diseases

Neurological System

➤ *Cerebrospinal fluid:* Routine analysis (cell count and differential, protein, glucose); other tests such as enzymes, electrolytes, urea, lactic acid, and glutamine; microbiologic examination (C&S, Gram and AFB stains); cytologic examination; serologic examination (neurosyphilis tests)
➤ *Drug levels:* Anticonvulsants (phenobarbital, phenytoin, primidone) and others included in therapeutic regimen or considered for overdose in the comatose client (prescribed and otherwise)
➤ *Miscellaneous:* Electrolytes (K, Na, Cl, CO_2), glucose, alcohol, ABGs, BUN, creatinine, toxicology screen (blood and urine)
➤ *Procedures:* Skull and spinal radiography; cerebral angiography; brain and cerebrospinal fluid (CSF) flow nuclear scanning; echoencephalography; non-nuclear head, intracranial, neck, and spinal CT scanning; head and intracranial MRI; electroneurography; evoked brain potentials; spinal nerve root thermography; oculoplethysmography; visual-auditory and optic-acoustic nerve tests

Hematologic System

➤ *Blood cell counts:* Complete blood count (CBC), including RBC, Hgb, Hct, RBC indices (MCV, MCH, MCHC), WBC, WBC differential, platelet, and reticulocyte
➤ *Blood cell types:* Hgb electrophoresis, blood typing and cross-matching, sickle cell screening
➤ *Coagulation:* Bleeding time, platelet aggregation, platelet survival, clot retraction time, capillary fragility, PT, PTT, aPTT, whole blood clotting time (CT), thrombin clotting time (TCT), prothombin consumption time (PCT), factor assays, plasma fibrinogen, fibrin split products (FSP), euglobulin lysis
➤ *Iron deficiency:* Iron, total iron-binding capacity (TIBC), folic acid, ferritin
➤ *Hemolysis:* RBC enzymes (glucose-6-phosphate dehydrogenase [G-6-PD]), haptoglobin, indirect Coombs', bilirubin
➤ *Miscellaneous:* Erythrocyte osmotic fragility, ESR, WBC enzymes, T- and B-lymphocyte assay, immunoglobulin assay
➤ *Procedures:* Schilling test, bone marrow aspiration, bone marrow nuclear scanning, RBC survival time study, platelet survival time study, lymph node biopsy

Endocrine System

➤ *Thyroid tests:* Calcitonin, thyroid-stimulating immunoglobulins (TSI), thyroxine-binding globulin (TBG), triiodothyronine (T_3), T_3 uptake, thyroxine (T_4), free T_4 index, thyroid antibodies, thyroid-stimulating hormone (TSH)

➤ *Thyroid procedures:* Thyroid nuclear scanning, radioactive iodine uptake study, thyroid-stimulating hormone (TSH) study, thyroid Cytomel and perchlorate suppression studies, ultrasonography, iodine 131 (^{131}I) scanning

➤ *Parathyroid tests:* Parathyroid hormone (PTH), calcium, phosphorus, prednisone-cortisone suppression

➤ *Parathyroid procedures:* Ultrasonography, nuclear scanning

➤ *Pituitary tests:* Growth hormone (GH), GH stimulation, growth suppression, prolactin (LTH), adrenocorticotropic hormone (ACTH), TSH and stimulation test, follicle-stimulating hormone (FSH), luteinizing hormone (LH), FSH-LH challenge, antidiuretic hormone (ADH)

➤ *Pituitary procedures:* Skull radiography, cerebral angiography, nuclear brain scanning, intracranial MRI scanning

➤ *Adrenal tests:* Cortisol, ACTH, cortisol-ACTH challenge, aldosterone, aldosterone challenge, catecholamines, urinary hormones (cortisol, aldosterone, 17-hydroxycorticosteroids [17-OHCS], 17-ketosteroids [17-KS], 17-ketogenic steroids [17-KGS], pregnanetriol, vanillylmandelic acid [VMA])

➤ *Adrenal procedures:* Non-nuclear CT scanning, adrenal nuclear scanning, ultrasonography, angiography, skull radiography

➤ *Pancreas tests:* Glucose, glucose tolerance (GT), 2-hour postprandial glucose, ketones, glycosylated hemoglobin, BUN, creatinine, tobutamide tolerance, insulin, amylase, lipase, aldolase, potassium (K), sodium (Na), glucagon, C-peptide

➤ *Pancrease procedures:* Endoscopic retrograde cholangiopancreatography (ERCP), ultrasonography, abdominal MRI scanning, pancreas nuclear scanning, non-nuclear CT scanning

Renal-Urologic Systems

➤ *Blood tests:* BUN, creatinine, electrolyte panel, osmolality, proteins, ammonia, uric acid, renin, aldosterone, γ-glutamyl transpeptidase (GGT)

➤ *Urine tests:* Routine analysis, creatinine clearance, insulin clearance, protein, complement C_3 and C_4, tubular function (phenolsulfonphthalein [PSP]), concentration (osmolality, specific gravity), electrolytes, C&S

➤ *Procedures:* Kidney and renography nuclear scanning; non-nuclear abdominal CT; ultrasonography; angiography; kidney, ureter, bladder (KUB) radiography; antegrade pyelography; retrograde urethrography, cystography, and ureteropyelography; excretory urography (IVP); voiding cystourethrography; pelvic floor sphincter electromyography (EMG); cystometry; uroflowmetry and urethral pressure profile; cystoscopy; renal biopsy

Musculoskeletal System

➤ *Muscle/bone enzymes:* Adolase; alkaline phosphatase (ALP); creatine phosphokinase (CPK); AST, SGOT

> *Electrolytes:* Calcium (Ca)
> *Joint tests:* Rheumatoid factor (RF), ESR, antistreptolysin O (ASO), immunoglobulins (IgG, IgM), C-reactive protein (CRP), complement C_3 and C_4
> *Synovial fluid:* Routine analysis (RBC, WBC, neutrophils, protein, glucose, crystals); other tests such as rheumatoid factor (RA), complements
> *Procedures:* Bone and joint radiography, arthrocentesis, arthroscopy, arthrography, myelography, musculoskeletal MRI scanning, bone and joint nuclear scanning, EMG, muscle biopsy

Hepatobiliary-Gastrointestinal Systems

> *Liver enzymes:* Alkaline phosphatase (ALP) and isoenzymes (ALP_1), alanine aminotransferase (ALT, SGPT), 5'-nucleotidase (5'-N), lactic dehydrogenase (LDH) and isoenzymes (LDH_5), leucine aminopeptidase (LAP), γ-glutamyl transpeptidase (GTT), creatine phosphokinase (CPK) and isoenzymes (CPK_3)
> *Liver blood tests:* Bilirubin, protein (albumin, globulin) and protein electrophoresis, PT, cholesterol, ammonia, hepatitis B–associated antigen and antibody tests
> *Liver procedures:* Abdominal radiography, liver nuclear scanning, non-nuclear CT scanning; abdominal MRI scanning, ultrasonography, hepatic and portal angiography, liver biopsy
> *Gallbladder procedures:* Abdominal radiography, oral cholecystography (OCG), intravenous cholangiography (IVC), percutaneous transhepatic cholangiography (PTC), operative cholangiography, T-tube cholangiography, biliary ultrasonography, non-nuclear CT scanning, gallbladder and biliary system nuclear scanning, endoscopic retrograde cholangiopancreatography (ERCP)
> *Esophageal and stomach tests:* Electrolyte panel, gastrin
> *Esophageal and stomach procedures:* Gastric analysis (macroscopic and microscopic), gastric acidity and acid stimulation, esophagogastroduodenoscopy (EGD), gastric emptying and gastrointestinal bleeding nuclear scanning, gastroesophageal reflux nuclear scanning, barium swallow, upper gastrointestinal (UGI) series, fluoroscopy, esophageal manometry and associated tests, mesenteric angiography, esophageal or stomach biopsy
> *Small and large intestine tests:* Electrolyte panel, carotene, carcinoembryonic antigen (CEA); D-xylose absorption; lactose intolerance; fecal analysis (occult blood, fat, culture)
> *Small and large intestine procedures:* Duodenal contents analysis (macroscopic and microscopic), duodenal stimulation for cholecystokinin-pancreozymin (CCK-PZ) and secretin, abdominal radiography, colonoscopy, proctosigmoidoscopy, barium enema, Meckel's diverticulum nuclear scanning, paracentesis, peritoneal fluid analysis, non-nuclear CT scanning, colon biopsy

Reproductive System

> *Female blood tests:* Prolactin, estrogen, follicle-stimulating hormone (FSH), luteinizing hormone (LH), progesterone

➤ *Female urine tests:* Pregnanediol, FSH, estrogen
➤ *Female procedures:* Colposcopy, culdoscopy, laparoscopy, hysterosalpingography, pelvic and breast ultrasonography, mammography, breast thermography, breast biopsy, cervical biopsy, Papanicolaou (Pap) smear, cytologic analysis (Barr chromatin body, chromosome analysis), non-nuclear CT pelvic scanning
➤ *Male blood tests:* Testosterone, semen analysis for fertility, cytology analysis for chromosomal and genetic abnormalities
➤ *Male urine tests:* 17-ketosteroids (17-KS)
➤ *Male procedures:* Scrotal nuclear scanning, scrotal-prostate ultrasonography, prostate biopsy
➤ *Pregnant female tests:* Complete blood count (CBC), ABO and Rh typing, albumin, syphilis serology (rapid plasmin reagin [RPR], Venereal Disease Research Laboratory [VDRL]), renin, TORCH screen (toxoplamosis, other infections, rubella, cytomegalovirus, and herpes simplex), human placental lactogen (hPL), creatine phosphokinase (CPK), human chorionic gonadotropin (hCG), progesterone and urinary pregnanediol, enzymes (heat-stable alkaline phosphatase [HSAP], diamine oxidase [DAO], oxytocinase), estriol (E_3) in blood and urine, endocrine panel for hormones, hematology panel for blood cells, coagulation, iron, folate, ESR, routine urinalysis (UA), cytology analysis for sex chromatin and chromosomal anomalies, amniotic fluid analysis for lecithin:sphingomyelin (L:S) ratio, genetic defects, creatinine, phosphatidylglycerol (PG), uric acid
➤ *Pregnant female procedures:* Amnioscopy, amniocentesis, pelvimetry, contraction stress tests, pelvic ultrasonography, fetal monitoring (internal and external), fetoscopy
➤ *Newborn tests:* TORCH, type and Rh, bilirubin, glucose, calcium, albumin, phenylketonuria (PKU)

Immune and Autoimmune Conditions

➤ *Immune and autoimmune tests:* T- and B-lymphocyte assay; immunoblast transformation; immunoglobulin assay (IgG, IgA, IgM, IgD, and IgE); antinuclear antibodies (ANA); antibody tests; uric acid; rheumatoid factor (RF); antistreptolysin O (ASO) titer; C-reactive protein (CRP); protein electrophoresis for cryoglobulins; lupus erythematosus (LE); anti-DNA, complement C_3 and C_4 assay; ESR; human immunodeficiency virus (HIV or AIDS) antibody tests

Infectious and Febrile Conditions

➤ *Infectious and febrile tests:* Heterophil, febrile agglutinins; blood culture analysis; culture of other body fluids; fungal antibody tests; antistreptococcal antibody tests; viral antibody tests; other antibody tests; differential WBC count, ESR
➤ *Infectious and febrile procedures:* Abscess-inflammatory nuclear scanning, gallium 67 (^{67}Ga) nuclear scanning, skin tests, chest x-ray

Tumors

➤ *Tumor marker tests:* Prostate (prostatic acid phosphatase [PAP], prostate-specific antigen [PSA]); thyroid (calcitonin); colon, lung, breast (carcinoembryonic antigen [CEA]); liver, testes (α-fetoprotein [AFP]); testes, trophoblastic (human chorionic gonadotropin [hCG]); ovary (CA 125); breast (CA 15-3); pancreas; colon (CA 19-9, CA 50); lymphoma, leukemia (lymphocyte B and T)

➤ *Other tumor tests:* Oncogenes (DNA sequences by polymerase chain reaction [PCR]), cytology examination for B- and T-cell gene rearrangement and DNA content of tumor cells, vasoactive intestinal peptide (VIP), squamous cell carcinoma (SCC) antigen, tissue polypeptide antigen (TPA), neuron-specific enolase (NSE), glycoprotein antigen (DU-PAN-2), metabolic tests (uric acid, albumin, cholesterol, triglycerides), hematologic tests (leukocytes, platelets), endocrine tests (ADH, cortisol, ACTH), isoenzymes (alkaline phosphatase [ALP], creatine kinase [CK-BB], galactosyltransferase [GT II], lactate dehydrogenase [LD_1]), electrolyte panel, and other tests based on suspected tumor location

➤ *Tumor procedures:* Radiography of suspected area, lymph node and retroperitoneal ultrasonography, mammography, bone marrow aspiration, nuclear body scanning (^{67}Ga), non-nuclear CT scanning of body and head, body and head/intracranial MRI scanning, endoscopy of area, lymphangiography, biopsy of affected organ

Chronic Disorders

➤ *Hypertension:* Lipid panel (total lipids, HDL, LDL, cholesterol, triglycerides, phospholipids), glucose, ABGs, electrolyte panel, BUN, creatinine, creatinine clearance, uric acid, lactate dehydrogenase (LDH), aldosterone (blood and urine), catecholamines, CBC, renin, angiotensin-converting enzyme, urinalysis

➤ *Diabetes:* Blood and urine glucose and ketones: 2-hour postprandial, glucose tolerance (GT), triglycerides, glucagon, CBC, glycosylated hemoglobin, urinalysis, insulin assay

➤ *Arthritis:* Antinuclear antibodies (ANA), rheumatoid factor (RF), antistreptolysin O (ASO) titer, C-reactive protein (CRP), protein electrophoresis, uric acid, C_4 and total complement, immune complex assay, synovial fluid analysis

➤ *Chronic obstructive pulmonary disease (COPD):* Spirometry, theophylline level, ABGs, electrolyte panel, sputum culture, chest x-ray, pulmonary function

➤ *Coronary artery disease (CAD):* Glucose, lipid panel (see Hypertension above), electrolyte panel

➤ *Chronic heart failure (CHF):* Digoxin and other cardiac drug levels, coagulation profile (bleeding and clotting time, PT, PTT, and thrombin time; factor analysis; platelets), cardiac enzymes and isoenzymes (CK, GGTP, SGOT, SGPT, LD), CBC, electrolyte panel, ESR, ECG, cardiac radiography, angiography, echocardiography

➤ *Anemia:* Schilling test, iron, total iron-binding capacity (TIBC), ferritin, folate, CBC, bone marrow analysis
➤ *Drug abuse:* Opiates (meperidine [Demerol], codeine), heroin, cocaine, amphetamines, barbiturates, methaqualone, cannabinoids (marijuana, hashish), phencyclidine ("angel dust"), phenothiazines, tricyclic antidepressants

VI

Nursing Care Plan for Individuals Experiencing Laboratory and Diagnostic Testing

Diagnosis. Anxiety related to insufficient knowledge of laboratory and diagnostic testing.

Goal. Individual will verbalize feelings regarding upcoming testing.

Interventions. Introduce yourself and other health-care team members to the individual and family.
Encourage individual to voice concerns and ask questions regarding the procedures.
Permit family members to be present for support as is possible.
Provide the following information:
  Description of the test
  Purpose of the test
  Pre-procedure routines
  Who will perform the procedure and where it will be conducted
  Expected sensations
  After-procedure routines
  When results will be available and who will discuss the implications

Diagnosis. Altered comfort: Pain, nausea, vomiting, diarrhea related to laboratory or diagnostic procedure.

Goal. Increased level of comfort after symptom or comfort relief measures are provided.

Interventions. Acknowledge the report of pain or discomfort.
Relate how long the discomfort will last, if known.
Provide optimal pain relief with prescribed analgesia.
Provide appropriate medications and other nonpharmacological interventions to manage other symptoms of discomfort.
Reduce unpleasant odors and sights as indicated.
Assess relief of pain or discomfort frequently and provide additional measures if relief is inadequate.

Diagnosis. Risk for infection caused by invasive procedure.

Goal. No infection.

Interventions. Use aseptic techniques as indicated.
Change dressings as indicated; note amount and type of drainage.
Take baseline temperature and monitor as needed.
Assess site for redness and inflammation.

Diagnosis. High risk for bleeding related to altered bleeding tendencies and invasive vascular procedures.

Goal. Prevent acute bleeding episode.

Interventions. Assess laboratory values (platelet count, PTT/aPTT) for bleeding tendencies.
Apply pressure to vascular site for 3 to 5 minutes routinely.
Assess site frequently to determine appropriate coagulation.
Apply pressure dressing as indicated.
Instruct individual and family to report continued bleeding.

Note: From Carpenito, L. Nursing Care Plans and Documentation: Nursing Diagnosis and Collaborative Problems, ed 2. Philadelphia, JB Lippincott, 1995.

VII

Discussion and Answers to Case Studies and Critical Thinking Exercises

CHAPTER 1

1. a. Pernicious anemia.
   b. Hct and MCV are increased to compensate for decreased Hgb content.
   c. A 24-hour urine test to determine the absorption of vitamin B_{12}. The individual is given oral vitamin B_{12} tagged with a radioisotope and amounts are measured in excreted urine. Less than 7 percent excretion is indicative of impaired absorption.
2. a. Acute lymphocytic leukemia.
   b. Hct, RBCs, Hgb, and platelets are all decreased as bone marrow activity is increased with WBC production. WBCs, lymphocytes, and blasts are all increased in leukemia.
   c. The individual starts a chemotherapy regimen, institutes bleeding precautions, controls for infection, and treats side effects of chemotherapy.

CHAPTER 2

1. a. Idiopathic thrombocytopenic purpura (ITP).
   b. Because of risk for bleeding, institute bleeding precautions: avoid trauma, use gentle oral care measures, no IM injections, instruct individual to report signs of bleeding immediately, MedicAlert bracelet.

CHAPTER 3

1. a. AIDS
   b. The following should be considered: age, positive lymph nodes, and hepatosplenomegaly.
   c. ELISA test is enzyme-linked immunosorbent assay to detect antigens or antibodies. It is the most widely used test to diagnose AIDS. The Western blot test may also be used. Both tests require patient consent.
   d. *Pneumocystis carinii* pneumonia (PCP) is considered an opportunistic infection that occurs in persons who are immunosuppressed.

CHAPTER 4

1. a. Erythroblastosis fetalis or hemolytic disease of the newborn. It results from blood incompatibility between mother and fetus. It is characterized by jaundice, anemia, hepatosplenomegaly, and generalized edema.
   b. No. Rh-positive mothers will not have antibodies against Rh factor, and the fetus has no Rh antigens.

CHAPTER 5

1. a. Thyroid storm.
   b. Thyroid levels will be evaluated; T_3 and T_4 levels will be elevated.
2. a. Tetany.
   b. Serum calcium levels should be checked and would be decreased in this case. Chvostek's sign (spasm of the facial muscles after stimulation of the facial nerve) may be positive as well as Trousseau's sign (muscle spasm of the upper extremity after applying pressure, usually by inflation of a blood pressure cuff).
3. a. Diabetic ketoacidosis (DKA).
   b. Formula is 2Na + Glu/18 + BUN/2.8. His serum osmolality is 328, indicating a hyperosmolar state.
   c. Increased serum glucose acts as an osmotic diuretic and results in increased urination. Osmoreceptors and increased urine output trigger the mechanism of thirst, thereby resulting in increased drinking. Although glucose levels are high, they are not used for energy sources and protein is substituted, resulting in relative "starvation" and increased eating.
   d. These are Kussmaul respirations (Kussmaul's breathing) and are the body's attempt to lower pH levels by blowing off CO_2.
4. a. Hypernatremia with hypertonic imbalance.
   b. Her clincal manifestations could include tachycardia, dry mucous membranes, postural hypotension, altered mental state, complaints of thirst, and a high urine specific gravity.
   c. She is in need of free water sources. If she is able to drink, provide water. If IV therapy is indicated, D_5W would be ordered.
5. a. Metabolic acidosis.
   b. The most probable cause is overdose of a drug, probably ASA, which increases acid elements, therefore lowering pH. If an anion gap is calculated ($[Na^+ + K^+] - [Cl^- + HCO_3^-]$), the value is 26.4, indicating that the source of acidosis is anions other than normal metabolites, in this case acetylsalicylic acid.

CHAPTER 6

1. a. His lab values reveal abnormal color, increased specific gravity, positive RBCs, and increased protein.
   b. Poststreptococcal acute glomerulonephritis.
   c. The differential diagnosis is made considering his recent sore throat and fever, and the values are not as elevated as they would be in nephrotic syndrome.

CHAPTER 7

1. a. The following tests should be ordered: chest x-ray and sputum cultures and sensitivity.
   b. If cultures are positive, then bacterial pneumonia is the most likely diagnosis.

CHAPTER 8

1. a. Meningitis.
   b. This diagnosis would be confirmed by the presence of bacteria or viruses, cell count of greater than 500 per cubic millimeter, protein greater than 300 mg/dL, and decreased glucose and chloride levels.

CHAPTER 9

1. a. Pleural effusion.
   b. A mediastinal shift occurs as a result of "collapsing" part of the affected lung, resulting in the stabilized lung pulling the trachea to the stable side.

CHAPTER 10

1. a. Hemolytic disease of the newborn.
   b. If there has been a been a slight placental tear, the mother's blood could be sensitized to the Rh factor and develop antibodies against Rh-positive blood of the fetus.
   c. If fetal maturity is adequate, the choice may be made to deliver by cesarean section now or to institute an intrauterine blood transfusion with O-negative blood.

CHAPTER 11

1. a. Jim has a borderline infertility problem. Although the quality of his sperm is good, there are insufficient numbers and poor motility.
   b. A pituitary tumor can result in hypofunction of an endocrine gland caused by the lack of stimulating hormone — in this case, LH, or luteinizing hormone, which affects sperm production.
   c. If the infertility is caused by hypofunction of the pituitary gland and if removal of the tumor restores function, Jim's infertility problem is reversible.

CHAPTER 12

1. a. Stomach cancer.
   b. A diagnosis of cancer requires a tissue biopsy. Additional tests may include a flat plate film of the abdomen as well as contrast dye studies to determine the presence of tumor.

CHAPTER 13

1. a. Gastric ulcer.
   b. The following may be contributing factors to this problem: stress, smoking, irregular eating patterns, and ASA ingestion.
   c. The significance of tarry stools is bleeding in the UGI tract.

CHAPTER 14

1. a. Cervical cancer.
   b. A tissue biopsy is indicated to confirm the diagnosis.

CHAPTER 15

1. a. Septicemia.
   b. If this episode of septicemia is not corrected, the patient could develop septic shock, a life-threatening condition with high mortality.

CHAPTER 16

1. a. You would explain to the patient that, although a tube will be placed down the trachea into the lungs, it is not wide enough to obstruct breathing.
   b. It is probable that a tissue biopsy may reveal cancer.

CHAPTER 17

1. a. Although rectal polyps can be palpated on physical exam, a barium enema will visualize the entire colon for masses.
   b. He should be informed that his stools will be clay colored from the barium and that he should report any problem with constipation.

CHAPTER 18

1. a. Secondary hypertension.
   b. In decreased perfusion to the kidneys, the angiotensin I and II, renin, and aldosterone cycle are activated to increase volume and vasoconstriction, thereby resulting in increased blood pressure.
   c. A renal angiogram is likely to reveal renal artery stenosis.

CHAPTER 19

1. a. Mr. Brown has some occlusion to the carotid artery. The significance is that he is at risk to develop transient ischemic attacks (TIAs) or cerebrovascular accident (CVA).
   b. Doppler carotid studies may be ordered.
   c. If the degree of stenosis is severe, surgical endarterectomy may be recommended. If the degree of stenosis is not major or if the patient is a poor surgical risk, anticoagulation therapy may be recommended.

CHAPTER 20

1. a. Pulmonary embolism.
   b. The associated risk factors for pulmonary embolism in this case are: overweight, sedentary lifestyle, dehydration.
   c. The treatment plan for this problem is: anticoagulation therapy, hydration, weight reduction, and exercise.

CHAPTER 21

1. a. Transient ischemic attack (TIA). If the condition does not resolve in 24 hours, the diagnosis of cerebrovascular accident (CVA) would be made.
   b. Cerebral angiography is a contrast dye invasive study. CT scans use radiographic beams to produce a three-dimensional image; it is a noninvasive test. MRI technique uses magnetic beams to produce an image; it is a noninvasive test.
   c. Heparin therapy is used in embolic and thrombotic cerebral events. Heparin is contraindicated in hemorrhagic events.

CHAPTER 22

1. a. Neurogenic bladder associated with spinal shock.
   b. A Foley catheter would be indicated because he has lost the reflex to void.

CHAPTER 23

1. a. Second-degree heart block.
   b. Second-degree heart block may compromise cardiac output and develop into third-degree heart block, which requires immediate intervention, usually the insertion of a pacemaker.

CHAPTER 24

1. a. Myasthenia gravis.
   b. An anticholinesterase medication (neostigmine or pyridostigmine) will be ordered and the patient will take it for the rest of her life.

CHAPTER 25

1. a. Sputum cultures should be performed, specifically for acid-fast bacilli indicating tuberculosis, and a chest x-ray should be performed. Also, a tuberculin skin test should be performed on all family members.
   b. Isoniazid (INH) and rifampin are the drugs most commonly used and are taken for up to 1 year.

General Index

Page numbers in italics indicate figures; those followed by "t" indicate tables. See also the Index of Tests and Procedures Covered, which begins on page 1029.

Abdomen
    computed tomography scanning of, 810–811
    magnetic resonance imaging of, 817–819
    plain films of, *596,* 596–599
        obstruction series of, 598–599
    ultrasonography of, 698–700
ABGs. *See* Arterial blood gases (ABGs)
ABO blood groups, antigens/antibodies in, 130t
ABO blood typing, 129–132
Abscess, radionuclide scanning of, 755–756
Acanthocytosis, significance of, 30t
Accelerator globulin, deficiency states involving, 73t
Acetylcholinesterase, 215–216
Acetylcholinesterase in neural tube defect detection, 425–426
Acid, gastric
    basal tests for, 450
        procedure for, 453
    stimulation tests for, 450–451
        procedure for, 453
Acid phosphatase (ACP), 204–206
Acid phosphatase test for semen, 439
Acid-base imbalances, blood gases in, 278t
Acid-fast bacillus smear and culture in sputum analysis, 385–386
Acoustic admittance tests, 919–922
Acoustic reflexes testing, 919, 920, 921–922
ACP. *See* Acid phosphatase (ACP)
Acquired immunodeficiency syndrome (AIDS), tests for, 117–119
ACTH. *See* Adrenocorticotropic hormone (ACTH)
Activated partial thromboplastin time (aPTT), 66–68
Addis count, 322
Addison's disease, cortisol deficiency in, 247–248
ADH. *See* Antidiuretic hormone (ADH)
Adrenal glands
    angiography of, 659–660
    radionuclide scanning of, 741–743
Adrenal hormone(s), 247–254
    aldosterone as, 250–252
    catecholamines as, 252–254
    cortisol as, 247–250
Adrenalin, 252
Adrenocorticotropic hormone (ACTH), 226–228
    blood glucose levels and, 143t
Alanine aminotransferase (ALT), 191–192

Alcohols, blood levels of, 301t
Aldolase (ALS), 207–208
Aldosterone, 250–252
    urinary, measurement of, 353–354
        factors interfering with, 360
        indications for, 362
        reference values for, 358t
Alkaline phosphatase (ALP), 194–196
    serum levels of, elevated, conditions causing, 195t
Alkaline phosphatase isoenzymes, 196–199
Alkaptonuria, 366
α_1-Antitrypsin, 160–161
α-fetoprotein
    maternal, increased levels of, conditions causing, 425t
    in neural tube defect detection, 425–426
α-Hydroxybutyric dehydrogenase (HBD), 214–215
ALT. *See* Alanine aminotransferase (ALT)
Ambulatory electrocardiography, 856–858
Amino acids, urinary, 365–366
Ammonia, 168–169
    blood levels of, altered, causes of, 168t
Amniocentesis for amniotic fluid tests, 424, 431–432
    for bilirubin measurement in hemolytic disease of newborn detection, 426–427
Amnioscopy, 567–569
Amniotic fluid
    analysis of, 423–433
        tests for fetal maturity in, 427–429
        tests for genetic defects in, 424–426
        tests for hemolytic disease of newborn in, 426–427
        tests for neural tube defects in, 424–426
    production of, 423
Amylase
    serum, 201–203
        elevated, causes of, 202t
    urinary, 349
        reference values for, 350t
        tests of
            factors interfering with, 350
            indications for, 350–351
            nursing care before, 351
            procedure for, 352
Anal cultures, 521–522
Anemias
    classification of, 28t
    hemolytic, classification of, 782t
Anergy panel, 84

Angiography, 651–681
  access for, 652
  adrenal, 659–660
  cardiac, 654–659
  catheters for, 651, *652*
  cerebral, 661–663
  contrast media for, 651–652
  conventional film, 653
  digital subtraction, 653
  fluorescein, 671–673
  hepatic, 665–667
  lower extremity, 677–679
  lymphatic, 673–674
  magnetic resonance imaging,
    816–817
  mesenteric, 669–671
  portal, 665–667
  procedures using, 654–679
  pulmonary, 663–665
  renal, 667–669
  risks in, 653–654
  upper extremity, 675–676
Anion gap, 277–278
Anisocytosis, significance of, 30t
Antegrade pyelography, 627–630
Antibiotics, blood levels of, 298t
Antibody screening test, 135–136
Antibody(ies)
  in ABO blood groups, 130t
  cell and tissue-specific, 101t
Anticonvulsants, blood levels of, 298t
Antidiuretic hormone (ADH), 235–237
Anti-DNA, disorders related to, 99t
Antigen(s), 81
  in ABO blood groups, 130t
  Australian, 115
  cancer, tests for, 123–124
  human leukocyte, 136–138
  mature lymphocyte responses to, 88f
  prostate-specific, 206–207
Antiglobulin tests, 133–136
  direct, 134–135
    positive, drugs causing, 134t
  indirect, 135–136
Antihemophilic factor, deficiency states
  involving, 73t
Antinuclear antibodies (ANA), disorders
  related to, 99t
Antistreptolysin O (ASO) titer, 106
Antithrombin system, 52
Aortic ultrasonography, 698–700
Arterial blood gases, definition of, 901
Arterial blood gases (ABGs), 288–292
Arterial Doppler studies
  carotid, 717–718
  extremity, 715–717
  transcranial, 719–720
Arterial plethysmography, 839–840
Arteriography. *See also* Angiography
  access for, 652

Artery(ies)
  carotid, Doppler studies of, 717–718
  coronary, *654*
  foot, *677*
  hand, *675*
  leg, *677*
  mesenteric, *669*
  pulmonary, catheterization of, 891–894
  wrist, *675*
Arthrocentesis, 419–420
Arthrography, 638–640
Arthroscopy, 576–579, *577*
Arylsulfatase A, urinary, 349
  reference values for, 350t
  tests of
    factors interfering with, 350
    indications for, 351
    nursing care before, 351
    procedure for, 352
Aspartate aminotransferase (AST), 192–194
Aspirin, hemostasis and, 50
AST. *See* Aspartate aminotransferase (AST)
Audiometry
  Békésy, 924–926
  hearing loss, 914–917
Auditory brainstem electric response test,
  924–926
Auditory evoked potentials, 873
Auditory system studies
  acoustic admittance tests as, 919–922
  hearing loss audiometry as, 914–917
  hearing loss tuning fork tests
    as, 917–919
  otoneural lesion site tests as, 922–924,
    924–926
  otoneurological tests as, 922–924
  spondee speech reception threshold test as,
    927–928
Australian antigen, 115
Autoantibodies
  disorders related to, tests in diagnosis of,
    99t
  reference values for, 100t
  tests of, 98–101

B lymphocytes
  altered levels of, causes of, 85t
  assays of, 84–87
  functions of, 39
  in humoral immunity, 83–84
Bacteria
  in duodenal secretions, 454, 455t
  in urine, 325
  nitrite testing for, 321
Bacterial infection antibody tests, 104–109
Bands, altered levels of, causes of, 43t
Barbiturates, blood levels of, 299t–300t
Barium enema, 614–617
Barium swallow, 609–612

Basophilic stippling, significance of, 31t
Basophils
    altered level of, causes of, 43t
    functions of, 39
Békésy audiometry, 924–926
Bence Jones protein, 366t, 367
Benzodiazepines, blood levels of, 298t
Bicarbonate
    in duodenal secretions, 454, 455t
    serum, 276, 278–279
        altered levels of, disorders/drugs associated with, 277t
Bile in feces, tests and reference values for, 470
Biliary system
    radionuclide scanning of, 768–769
    Ultrasonography of, 703–705
Bilirubin, 186–189
    in amniotic fluid in fetal maturity assessment, 429
    elevations in, causes of, 188t
    measurement of, amniocentesis for, in hemolytic disease of newborn detection, 426–427
    in urine, 319–321
Bilirubinuria, 320
Binaural loudness balance test, 924–926
Binaural midplane localization test, 924–926
Binding proteins, 161–164
Biomicroscopy, slit-lamp, 938–939
Biopsy
    bladder, 487–489
    bone, 482–483
    bone marrow, 10–11
    breast, 484–485
    cervical punch, 485–487
    chorionic villus, 492–494
    intestinal, 498–500
    liver, 494–496
    lung, 501–503
    lymph node, 497–498
    muscle, 496–497
    needles for, 479
    pleural, 503–505
    prostate gland, 505–507
    renal, 489–492
    skin, 481–482
    thyroid gland, 507–508
    ureter, 487–489
Bladder. See also Urinary tract
    biopsy of, 487–489
    function of, urodynamic studies of, 829–836. See also Urodynamic studies
    neurogenic, types and effects of, 831t
    ultrasonography of, 706–707
Bleeding, gastrointestinal, conditions associated with, 468t–469t
Bleeding time, 56–58
Blood
    ammonia levels in, altered, causes of, 168t
    complete count of, 18–22

culture of, 513–515
    in duodenal secretions, 454, 455t
    dyscrasias of, drugs causing, 20t–21t
    fecal, occult
        reference values for, 470t
        tests for, 467
    functions of, 3
    glucose levels in
        hormones influencing, 143t
        measurement methods for, 143
    in stomach contents, 447
    in urine, 318–319
Blood banking, 129–139
    ABO typing in, 129–132
    antiglobulin tests in, 133–136
    Rh typing in, 132–133
Blood chemistry, 141–306
    arterial blood gases in, 288–292
    bilirubin in, 186–189
    carbohydrates in, 142–155. See also Glucose
    drugs in, 297, 298t–300t, 300, 303
    electrolytes in, 268–288. See also Electrolytes
    enzymes in, 189–220. See also Enzymes
    hormones in, 220–268. See also Hormone(s)
    lipids in, 172–186. See also Lipids; Lipoproteins
    proteins in, 156–172. See also Protein(s)
    toxic substances in, 297, 300, 301t–303t, 303
    trace minerals in, 296–297
    vitamins in, 292–296
Blood gases
    in acid-base imbalances, 278t
    arterial, 288–292
        definition of, 901
Blood sugar, postprandial, 146–148
Blood typing
    ABO, 129–132
    Rh, 132–133
Blood vessels
    activity in, in hemostasis, 49
    activity of, in hemostasis, 49
    carotid, 661
    cerebral, 661
    hepatic arterial, 665
    large, 654
    lower extremity, 677
    vertebral, 661
Blood volume study, total, 778–780
Body plethysmography, 841–843
Body plethysmography, definition of, 901
Body scanning
    computed tomography in, 801–804
    gallium 67, 773–775
    iodine 131, 775–776
    magnetic resonance imaging in, 813–816

Bone(s)
  biopsy of, 482–483
  cranial/facial, 589
  of extremities, 602
  radionuclide scanning of, 738–740
Bone marrow
  biopsy of, 10–11
  examination of, 8–11
    contraindications to, 10
    indications for, 9–10
    reference values for, 9t
  radionuclide scanning of, 740–741
Brain
  electroencephalography of, 869–871
  evoked potentials of, 871–874
  positron emission tomography of, 777
  radionuclide scanning of, 733–735
Breast
  positron emission tomography of, 777–778
  ultrasonography of, 709–711
Bronchial provocation, definition of, 901
Bronchodilators, blood levels of, 298t
Bronchography, 640–642
Bronchoscopy, 533–540
  contraindications to, 536
  factors interfering with, 535
  fibroptic, 534, 534–535
  indications for, 535–536
  nursing alert on, 536
  nursing care after, 539–540
  nursing care before, 537–538
  procedure for, 538–539
  reference values for, 535
  rigid, 534

C3, altered levels of, causes of, 95t
C4, altered levels of, causes of, 95t
Cabot's rings, significance of, 31t
Calcitonin, 244–245
Calcium
  in coagulation, 52
  serum, 279–282
    altered levels of, disorders/drugs associated with, 280t
  urinary
    measurement of, 342
    reference values for, 343t
Cancer
  bladder, biopsy in diagnosis of, 487–489
  bone, biopsy in detection of, 482–483
  cervical
    cervical punch biopsy in diagnosis of, 485–487
    Papanicolaou smear in detection of, 478–481
  immunologic tests related to, 119–124
  renal, biopsy in diagnosis of, 489–492
  skin, biopsy for detection of, 481–482
  ureteral, biopsy in diagnosis of, 487–489

Cancer antigen tests, 123–124
Carbohydrates, 142–155. See also Glucose
  utilization of, fecal
    tests for, 469
Carboxyhemoglobin, 33
Carcinoembryonic antigen (CEA) test, 122–123
Cardiac cycle, 852–853
Cardiac drugs, blood levels of, 299t
Cardiovascular system studies, 885–898
  cardiac catheterization as, 886–891. See also Catheterization, cardiac
Carotid artery, Doppler studies of, 717–718
Carotid vessels, 661
Casts in urine, 323–324, 324t
Catecholamines, 252–254
  urinary, measurement of, 355–356
    factors interfering with, 361
    indications for, 362
    reference values for, 359t
Catheterization
  cardiac, 886–891
    contraindications to, 889
    factors interfering with, 888
    indications for, 888–889
    insertion sites/routes for, 886
    nursing alert on, 889
    nursing care after, 891
    nursing care before, 889–890
    procedure for, 890–891
    reference values for, 887–888
  pulmonary artery, 891–894
Catheters for angiography, 651, 652
CBC. See Complete blood count (CBC)
Cell analysis, 477–509
Cell-mediated immunity, 82
  response to antigens in, 88f
Central nervous system (CNS), syphilis involving, serologic tests for, 399–400
Cerebral angiography, 661–663
Cerebral vessels, 661
Cerebrospinal fluid (CSF)
  analysis of, 389–401
    cell count and differential in, 391
    factors interfering with, 393
    glucose in, 391
    indications for, 393–394
    nursing care after, 396
    nursing care before, 394
    proteins in, 391
    reference values for, 392t–393t
    sample collection procedure for, 394–396
  cytologic examination of, 398–399
  flow of, scanning of, 735–737
  formation of, 389
  functions of, 389
  microbiologic examination of, 396–398
  neurologic tests of, for neurosyphilis, 399–400

Ceruloplasmin, 162–164
    altered levels of, causes of, 163t
Cervical spine, *589*
Cervix
    cancer of
        cervical punch biopsy in diagnosis,
            485–487
        Papanicolaou smear in detection of,
            478–481
    punch biopsy of, 485–487
Chemistry, blood, 141–306. *See also* Blood
    chemistry
Chest
    magnetic resonance imaging of,
        820–822
    plain films of, *593*, 593–596, *594*
    tomography of, 605–606
Chief cells, 445
Chloride(s)
    serum, 274–276
        altered levels of, disorders/drugs associ-
            ated with, 275t
    urinary
        measurement of, 341–342
        reference values for, 343t
Cholangiography
    intravenous, 620–621
    operative, 623–624
    percutaneous transhepatic, 624–627
    T-tube, 621–623
Cholangiopancreatography, endoscopic retro-
    grade, 548–552, *549*
Cholecystography, oral, 617–619
Cholecystokinin-pancreozymin (CCK-PZ) test,
    457
Cholesterol
    fractions of, 181–183
    total, 177–179
        altered levels of, disorders/drugs associ-
            ated with, 178t
Cholinesterases, 215–216
Chorionic gonadotropin, human, 259–261
    in FSH/LH challenge tests, 232
Chorionic villus biopsy, 492–494
Choroid plexus, 389
Christmas factor, deficiency states
    involving, 73t
Chylomicrons, 173
Cineradiography, 587
CK. *See* Creatine kinase (CK)
Clomiphene in FSH/LH challenge tests, 232
Closing volume, definition of, 901
Clot retraction test, 60–61
Clotting factors, 50t
    assays of, 71–74
    deficiencies of, states associated with, 73t
    reference values for, 72t
CMG. *See* Cystometry (CMG)
Coagulation
    in hemostasis, 50–52

studies of, 63–77
    euglobulin lysis time in, 76–77
    factor assays in, 71–74
    fibrin split products in, 75–76
    partial thromboplastin time/activated
        partial thromboplastin time in, 66–68
    plasma fibrinogen in, 74–75
    prothrombin consumption time in,
        70–71
    prothrombin time in, 63–66
    thrombin clotting time in, 69–70
    whole blood clotting time in, 68–69
Coagulation factors, 50t, 71–74. *See also*
    Clotting factors
Coagulation time, 68–69
Cold agglutinin tests, 107–109
Cold agglutinins, disorders related to, 99t
Cold stimulation test, 897–898
Colloid, 237
Colonoscopy, 555–559, *556*
Color perception tests, 933–934
Color-flow Doppler imaging, 687
Colposcopy, 563–565
Complement system, tests of, 94–97
Complete blood count (CBC), 18–22
    indications for, 18, 21
    reference values for, 18, 19t
Computed tomography (CT), 799–812
    abdominal scanning by, 810–811
    body scanning by, 801–804
    emission, 730
    head scanning by, 804–806
    intracranial scanning by, 804–806
    neck scanning by, 806–808
    pelvic scanning by, 811–812
    single-photon emission, 731
    spinal scanning by, 806–808
    thoracic scanning by, 808–809
Confrontation test, 931–933
Contraction stress test, 845–847
Contrast media
    for angiography, 651–652
    iodinated, adverse reactions to, 588t
    radiologic studies using, 587–588
    reactions to, 653
Coombs' tests, 133–136
Corneal staining, 940–941
Coronary arteries, *654*
Cortisol, 247–250
    blood glucose levels and, 143t
    urinary, measurement of, 353
        factors interfering with, 360
        indications for, 361–362
        reference values for, 358t
Cortisone glucose tolerance test, 152–153
C-peptide, 264–265
CPK. *See* Creatine phosphokinase (CPK)
Cranial bones, *589*
C-reactive protein (CRP), disorders related
    to, 99t

Creatine, serum, 169–170
Creatine kinase (CK), 208
Creatine phosphokinase (CPK), 208–211
  elevated, causes of, 209t
Creatinine
  in amniotic fluid in fetal maturity assessment, 429
  serum, 166–167
Creatinine, renal clearance tests for, 333–334
Cryoglobulins
  disorders related to, 99t
  tests for, 90, 92
Crystals
  in synovial fluid, 415–416, 417t
  in urine, 325, 326t–327t
CSF. *See* Cerebrospinal fluid (CSF)
Culdoscopy, 565–567, *566*
Culture(s), 511–512
  anal, 521–522
  blood, 513–515
  ear, 515–516
  eye, 515–516
  genital, 521–522
  nose, 516–518
  skin, 519–521
  sputum, 383–385
    acid-fast bacillus, 385–386
  stool, 472–474
  throat, 516–518
  wound, 518–519
Culture and sensitivity (C&S) testing
  antimicrobial susceptibility and, 512
  specimen collection for, 512–522
  on sputum, 383–385
Cushing's syndrome, cortisol excess in, 247
Cyanocobalamin. *See* Vitamin B$_{12}$
Cystic fibrosis, sweat test for, 908–910
Cystography, retrograde, 631–633
Cystometry (CMG), 830–833
Cystoscopy, 559–563
Cystourethrography, voiding, 636–637
Cystourethroscopy, *560*
Cytologic examination, of cerebrospinal fluid, 398–399
Cytology, 477
Cytomel suppression study, 790

Deep vein scanning, 766–767
Dexamethasone in cortisol/ACTH challenge tests, 248
Diabetes mellitus, glycosuria in, 316
Diarrhea, types of, 473t
Differential white blood cell (WBC) count, 41–42
  altered, causes of, 43t–44t
Diffusing capacity of lungs, definition of, 901
Digital subtraction angiography, 653
Dipyridamole in cardiac scanning, 745
Diverticulum, Meckel's, scanning for, 761–762

Donor, blood, universal, 130
Doppler ultrasound, 686–687, *687*
  arterial
    carotid, 717–718
    extremity, 715–717
    transcranial, 719–720
  studies using, overview of, 715t
  venous, extremity, 720–721
Drug(s)
  altering cholesterol levels, 178t
  altering free fatty acid levels, 174t
  altering prothrombin time, 65
  altering triglyceride levels, 176t
  blood glucose alterations from, 144t
  blood levels of, 297, 298t–300t, 300, 303
  causing blood dyscrasias, 20t–21t
  causing extracellular fluid level alterations, 269t
  causing false-positive autoantibody test reactions, 102t
  causing false-positive glycosuria results, 317t
  causing glycosuria, 317t
  causing hypoalbuminemia, 158t
  causing positive direct antiglobulin tests, 134t
  causing serum bicarbonate level alterations, 277t
  causing serum calcium level alterations, 280t
  causing serum chloride level alterations, 275t
  causing serum magnesium level alterations, 285t
  causing serum phosphorus/phosphate level alterations, 283t
  causing serum potassium level alterations, 272t
  causing serum sodium level alterations, 269t
  impairing platelet aggregation, 59t
  prolonging bleeding time, 57t
  urine screening tests for, 371–373
Duodenum
  contents of, analysis of, 454–456
  secretions of, 446
    stimulation tests for, 457–458
    tests of, 454–458
Dyscrasias, blood, drugs causing, 20t–21t

Ear. *See also* Auditory system
  culture of, 515–516
ECD. *See* Esophagogastroduodenoscopy (EGD)
ECG. *See* Electrocardiography (ECG)
Echinocytosis, significance of, 30t
Echocardiography, 688–691
  transesophageal, 692–693

Echoencephalography, 691–692
EEG. *See* Electroencephalography (ECG)
Effusions
    analysis of, 403–421
    definition of, 403
    tests of, 405–420
    transudates differentiated from, 404
Ejaculation, 435–436
Electrocardiography (ECG), 852–858
    ambulatory, 856–858
    exercise, 860–862
    factors interfering with, 854
    Holter, 856–858
    indications for, 854–855
    nursing alert on, 855
    nursing care after, 856
    nursing care before, 855
    procedure for, 855–856
    reference values for, 853–854
    signal-averaged, 862–863
Electrodiagnostic studies, 851–879
    electrocardiography as, 852–858. *See also*
        Electrocardiography (ECG)
    electroencephalography as, 869–871
    electromyography as, 863–867
    electroneurography as, 867–868
    electronystagmography as, 874–876
    electro-oculography as, 878–879
    electroretinography as, 876–878
    evoked brain potentials as, 871–874
    phonocardiography as, 858–859
Electroencephalography (EEG), 869–871
Electrolytes
    anion gap and, 277–279
    blood, 268–288
    serum
        bicarbonate, 276, 277t
        calcium as, 279–282
        chloride as, 274–276
        magnesium as, 284–286
        phosphorus/phospshate as, 282–284
        potassium as, 271–274
        sodium as, 268–271
    serum osmolality and, 286–288
    urinary
        measurement of, 341–345
            factors interfering with, 343–344
            indications for, 344
            nursing care for, 344–345
            procedures for, 344
        reference values for, 343t
Electromyography (EMG), 865–867
    pelvic floor sphincter, 863–865
Electroneurography, 867–868
Electronystagmography (ENG), 874–876
Electro-oculography (EOG)
Electrophoresis
    hemoglobin, 29, 31–34
    serum protein, for immunoglobulin assays,
        90, 92f

Electrophysiologic studies, 851–881
Electroretinography (ERG), 876–878
Elliptocytosis, significance of, 30t
EMG. *See* Electromyography (EMG)
Emission tomography
    computed, 730
    positron, 730–731, 776–778
Endoscopes
    procedures using, 528–579
        amnioscopy as, 567–569
        arthroscopy as, 576–579, *577*
        bronchoscopy as, 533–540. *See also*
            Bronchoscopy
        colonoscopy as, 555–559, *556*
        colposcopy as, 563–565
        culdoscopy as, 565–567, *566*
        cystoscopy as, 559–563
        endoscopic retrograde cholangiopancre-
            atography as, 548–552, *549*
        esophagogastroduodenoscopy as,
            544–548
        laparoscopy as, 569–576. *See also*
            Laparoscopy
        laryngoscopy as, 529–533
        mediastinoscopy as, 540–542
        proctosigmoidoscopy as, 552–555
        thoracoscopy as, 542–544
    studies using, 527–581
    types of, 527, *528*
Endoscopic retrograde cholangiopancreatogra-
    phy (ERCP), 548–552, *549*
Enema, barium, 614–617
ENG. *See* Electronystagmography (ENG)
Enzymes
    in blood, 189–220
        acid phosphatase as, 204–206
        alanine aminotransferase as, 191–192
        aldolase as, 207–208
        alkaline phosphatase as, 194–196
        alkaline phosphatase isoenzymes as,
            196–199
        α-hydroxybutyric dehydrogenase as,
            214–215
        aspartate aminotransferase as, 192–194
        cholinesterases as, 215–216
        creatine phosphokinase, 208–211
        hexosaminidase as, 213–214
        isocitrate dehydrogenase as, 199–201
        lactic dehydrogenase as, 211–213
        ornithine carbamoyltransferase, 200–201
        prostate-specific antigen as, 206–207
        red blood cell, 35–37
        serum amylase as, 201–203
        serum lipase as, 203–204
        study of, 190
        white blood cell, 42, 44–46
    digestive, 445
    renin as, 217–220
    urinary, 349–352
        reference values for, 350t

Enzymology, 190
EOG. *See* Electro-oculography (EOG)
Eosinophils
    altered levels of, causes of, 43t–44t
    functions of, 39
Epinephrine, 252
    blood glucose levels and, 143t
    urinary, measurement of, 355–356
        reference values for, 359t
Epithelial cells
    in feces, 463
    in urine, 323
ERCP. *See* Endoscopic retrograde cholan-
    giopancreatography (ERCP)
ERG. *See* Electroretinography (ERG)
Erythrocyte(s), 3
    abnormalities of, 30t–31t
    count of, 22–24
    in duodenal secretions, 454, 455t
    production of, 5
    studies of, 22–39
        erythrocyte count in, 22–24
        erythrocyte sedimentation rate in, 37–39
        hematocrit in, 24–25
        hemoglobin in, 25–27
        osmotic fragility in, 34–35
        red blood cell indices in, 27–28
        red blood cell (RBC) enzymes in, 35–37
    in urine, 322
Erythrocyte sedimentation rate (ESR), 37–39
Erythropoiesis, 5
    inadequate, causes of, 5, 7
    iron in, 13
Erythropoietin
    in RBC production, 5
    release of, causes of tissue hypoxia stimu-
        lating, 7t
Esophageal manometry, 836–839
Esophagogastroduodenoscopy (EGD),
    544–548
Estrogens, 254–256
    urinary, measurement of, 356–357
        factors interfering with, 361
        indications for, 363
        reference values for, 359t
Euglobulin lysis time, 76–77
Evoked brain potentials, 871–874
Evoked potential, His bundle, study of,
    894–897
Exercise electrocardiography, 860–862
Expiratory reserve volume, definition of, 900
Extracellular fluid level, altered, disorders/drugs
    associated with, 269t
Extremity(ies)
    arterial Doppler studies of, 715–717
    bones of, *602*
    lower, angiography of, 677–679
    plain films of, 602–603
    upper, angiography of, 675–676
    venous Doppler studies of, 720–721

Exudates, pleural, transudates differentiated
    from, 409t
Eye
    culture of, 515–516
    electrophysiologic studies of, 874–879
        electronystagmography as, 874–876
        electro-oculography as, 878–879
        electroretinography as, 876–878
    plethysmography of, 843–845

Facial bones, *589*
Factor assays, 71–74
Falling test, 922–924
Fats, fecal, 463–464
    reference values for, 470t
Febrile agglutinin tests, 107–109, 108t
Feces
    analysis of, 461–475
        microbiologic, 472–474
        microscopic, 463–466
    characteristics of, normal/abnormal,
        462t–463t
    composition of, 461
    cultures of, 472–474
    occult blood in, tests for, 467
    quantitative fats in, tests for,
        467, 469
Ferritin, 14
    reference values for, 15t
Fertility tests, 437–439
Fetoplacental adequacy studies, 845–847
Fetoscopy, 569–570
    indications for, 572
    procedure for, 575
    reference values for, 570
Fetus
    abnormalities of, chorionic villus biopsy in
        detection of, 492–494
    maturity of, tests for, 427–429
Fibrin split products (FSP), 75–76
Fibrinogen, 50
    plasma, 74–75
Fibrinogen uptake study, 766–767
Fibrinolytic system, 52
Fibrin-stabilizing factor, deficiency states in-
    volving, 73t
Fibrin-stabilizing factor, deficiency states in-
    volving, 73t
Fishberg test, 337
    nursing care after, 341
    nursing care before, 339
    procedure for, 341
Flow-volume loop, definition of, 901
Fluid
    amniotic, 423–433. *See also* Amniotic
        fluid
    pericardial, analysis of, 405–407
    peritoneal, analysis of, 412–415
    pleural, analysis of, 408–412

Fluid *(Continued)*
  serous
    characteristics of, 404
    formation of, 403
  synovial
    analysis of, 415–420
    characteristics of, 404–405
    crystals in, 415–416, 417t
    formation of, 403–404
    white blood cells and inclusions in, 416t
Fluorescein angiography, 671–673
Fluorescent treponema antibody-absorption
  (FTA-ABS) test for syphilis, 109–110
Fluoroscopy, 586–587
Folate. *See* Folic acid
Folic acid
  in erythropoiesis, 7
  studies of, 16–18
Follicle-stimulating hormone (FSH), 231–234
Foot, blood vessels of, *677*
Forced expiratory volume in 1 second, definition
  of, 901
Forced inspiratory flow rate, definition of, 901
Forced vital capacity, definition of, 900
Forward grouping, 130
Free fatty acids (FFAs), 173–175
    altered levels of, factors associated with,
      174t
FSH. *See* Follicle-stimulating hormone (FSH)
Functional residual capacity, definition of, 900
Fungal infection antibody tests, 102–104

Gallbladder, radionuclide scanning of, 768–769
Gallium 67 body scanning, 773–775
Gamma-glutamyl transpeptidase, serum,
  198–199
Gammopathies, 92t
Gastric emptying scanning, 756–758
Gastric hormones, 266–268
Gastrin, 267–268
  secretion of, 445
Gastrointestinal tract
  bleeding in
    conditions associated with, 468t–469t
    scanning for, 760–761
  reflux in, scanning for, 758–759
Gated blood pool imaging, 745
Genetic disorders
  fetal, chorionic villus biopsy in detection
    of, 492–494
  tests for, 424–426
Genital cultures, 521–522
Genitalia, male, *436*
GH. *See* Growth hormone (GH)
Gland(s)
  adrenal, radionuclide scanning of,
    741–743
  parathyroid, radionuclide scanning of,
    754–755

parotid, radionuclide scanning of, 737–738
prostate
    biopsy of, 505–507
    ultrasonography of, 707–708
salivary, radionuclide scanning of, 737–738
thyroid
    biopsy of, 507–508
    function of, radioactive iodine uptake
      study of, 786–788
    radionuclide scanning of, 752–754
Glaucoma, tonometry in diagnosis of, 934–936
Globulin, serum levels of, altered, causes of,
  159t
Glomerulonephritis, laboratory correlations
  with, 328t
Glucagon, 265–266
  blood glucose levels and, 143t
Glucose
  blood levels of, 144–146
    altered, causes of, 144t
    hormones influencing, 143t
    measurement methods for, 143
    two-hour postprandial, 146–148
  in cerebrospinal fluid analysis, 391
  functions of, 142
  plasma, 144–146. *See also* Glucose, blood
    levels of
  serum, 144–146. *See also* Glucose, blood
    levels of
  in urine, 315–317
Glucose tolerance tests (GTTs), 148–153
  cortisone, 152–153
  intravenous, 151–152
  oral, 148–151
Glucose-6-phosphate dehydrogenase (G-6-PD),
  36
Glutamic-oxaloacetic transaminase, 192
Glutamic-pyruvic transaminase, 191
Glycosuria, 316
    disorders/drugs causing, 317t
    false-positive, drugs causing, 317t
Glycosylated hemoglobin, 153–154
Gonadal hormones, 254–259
    estrogens as, 254–256
    progesterone as, 256–258
    testosterone as, 258–259
Gonadotropin, human chorionic, 259–261
  in FSH/LH challenge tests, 232
Gout, 365
Gram staining in sputum analysis, 380–383
Growth hormone (GH), 221–225
    blood glucose levels and, 143t
    stimulation tests for, 223–224
    suppression tests for, 224–225
GTTs. *See* Glucose tolerance tests (GTTs)

Hageman factor, deficiency states involving, 73t
Hand, arteries of, *675*
Haptoglobin, 161–162

HBD. *See* α-Hydroxybutyric dehydrogenase (HBD)
hCG. *See* Human chorionic gonadotropin (hCG)
Head
    computed tomography scanning of, 804–806
    magnetic resonance imaging of, 819–820
Hearing loss audiometry, 914–917
Hearing loss tuning fork tests, 917–919
Hearing tests
    acoustic admittance tests as, 919–922
    hearing loss audiometry as, 914–917
    hearing loss tuning fork tests as, 917–919
    spondee speech reception threshold test as, 927–928
Heart
    angiography of, 654–659
    catheterization of, 886–891. *See also* Catheterization, cardiac
    electrocardiographic study of, 852–858, 860–863. *See also* Electrocardiography (ECG)
    magnetic resonance imaging of, 820–822
    phonocardiography and, 858–859
    plain films of, 603–605
    positron emission tomography of, 777–778
    radionuclide scanning of, 744–749
        contraindications to, 747
        factors interfering with, 746
        indications for, 746–747
        nursing alert on, 747
        nursing care after, 749
        nursing care before, 747–748
        procedure for, 748–749
        reference values for, 744–745
Heinz bodies, significance of, 31t
Hematocrit, 24–25
Hematology, 3–47
Hematopoiesis, 4–18
    evaluation of, 7–18
        bone marrow examination in, 8–11
        iron studies in, 13–16
        reticulocyte count in, 11–13
    folic acid studies in, 16–18
    theory of, 6f
    vitamin B_{12} studies in, 16–18
Hematopoietic function tests, 3–47
Hematuria, 318
Heme synthesis, 345, 346f
Hemoglobin, 25–27
    glycosylated, 153–154
    types of, 29, 31
Hemoglobin (Hgb) electrophoresis, 29, 31–34
Hemoglobinuria, 319
Hemolytic anemias, classification of, 782t
Hemolytic assay, 95
Hemolytic disease of newborn, tests for, 426–427
Hemophilia, prothrombin time in, 63

Hemostasis, 49–78
    antagonists to, 52
    coagulation in, 50–52
    coagulation studies on, 63–77
    platelet function in, 49–50
    platelet studies of, 53–63
    vascular activity in, 49
Hepatic angiography, 665–667
Hepatic arteries, *665*
Hepatitis, tests for, 115–117
Hexaminidase, 213–214
5-HIAA. *See* 5-Hydroxyindoleacetic acid (5-HIAA)
His bundle evoked potential study, 894–897
Histology, 477
    applications of, 478
    biopsy in, 478. *See also* Biopsy
HLAs. *See* Human leukocyte antigens (HLAs)
Hollander insulin test, 451
    procedure for, 453
Holter electrocardiography, 856–858
Homovanillic acid (HVA), urinary, measurement of, 356
    factors interfering with, 361
    indications for, 362–363
    reference values for, 359t
Hormone(s), 220–268
    adrenal, 247–254. *See also* Adrenal hormone(s)
    adrenocorticotropic, 226–228
    altering free fatty acid levels, 174t
    follicle-stimulating, 231–234
    gastric, 266–268
    gonadal, 254–259. *See also* Gonadal hormones
    growth, 221–225
    hypophyseal, 220–237. *See also* Hypophyseal hormones
    influencing blood glucose levels, 143t
    intestinal, 266–268
    luteinizing, 234–235
    pancreatic, 262–266
    parathyroid, 245–247
    placental, 259–262
    thyroid, 237–245. *See also* Thyroid hormone(s)
    thyroid-stimulating, 228–231
        radionuclide-mediated study of, 788–790
    urinary, 352–364
    urinary, measurement of
        factors interfering with, 360–361
        nursing care for, 363–364
        procedure for, 364
Howell-Jolly bodies, significance of, 31t
hPL. *See* Human placental lactogen (hPL)
hPRL. *See* Prolactin (hPRL)
Human chorionic gonadotropin (hCG), 259–261
    in FSH/LH challenge tests, 232

Human chorionic gonadotropin (hCG)
 (Continued)
  urinary, measurement of, 357–358
   factors interfering with, 361
   indications for, 363
   reference values for, 360t
Human leukocyte antigens (HLAs), 136–138
  diseases associated with, 137t
Human placental lactogen (hPL), 261–262
Humoral immunity, 83
  response to antigens in, 88f
HVA. *See* Homovanillic acid (HVA)
Hydantoins, blood levels of, 298t
Hydrochloric acid secretion, 445
17-Hydroxycorticosteroids, urinary, measurement of, 354
   factors interfering with, 360
   indications for, 362
   reference values for, 358t
5-Hydroxyindoleacetic acid (5-HIAA), urinary, measurement of, 356
   factors interfering with, 361
   indications for, 363
   reference values for, 359t
Hydroxyproline, urine, 366
Hyperchromia, significance of, 30t
Hypernatremia, disorders/drugs associated with, 269t
Hypersensitivity reactions, IgE antibodies in, 97–98
Hyperthyroidism, Cytomel suppression study for, 790
Hypoalbuminemia, causes of, 158t
Hypochromia, significance of, 30t
Hyponatremia, disorders/drugs associated with, 269t
Hypophyseal hormones, 220–237
   adrenocorticotropic hormone as, 226–228
   antidiuretic hormone as, 235–237
   follicle-stimulating, 231–234
   growth hormone as, 221–225
   luteinizing hormone as, 234–235
   prolactin as, 225–226
   thyroid-stimulating hormone as, 228–231
Hypothyroidism, perchlorate suppression study for, 790
Hypoxia, tissue, stimulating erythropoietin release, causes of, 7t
Hysterosalpingography, 642–644

ICD. *See* Isocitrate dehydrogenase (ICD)
Immune complex assays, 96–97
Immunity
  cell-mediated, 81
   response to antigens in, 88f
  humoral, 83
   response to antigens in, 88f
Immunoblast transformation tests, 88–90

Immunodeficiency diseases, lymphocyte maturation and, 87f
Immunoelectrophoresis for immunoglobulin assays, 90
Immunoglobulin E (IgE), radioallergosorbent test for, 97–98
Immunoglobulins, 83
  assays of, 90–94
  functions of, 91t
  levels of
   altered, causes of, 91t
   excessive, conditions causing, 92f
  reference values for, 93t
  thyroid-stimulating, 234–244
Immunohematology, 129–139
  antiglobulin tests in, 133–136
  blood typing in, 129–133
   ABO, 129–132
   Rh, 132–133
  human leukocyte antigens in, 136–138
Immunologic antibody tests, 101–119
  bacterial, 104–109
  fungal, 102–104
  syphilis, 109–112
  viral, 112–119
Immunology, 81–125
  autoantibody tests in, 98–101
  complement system tests in, 94–97
  immunologic antibody tests in, 101–119
  immunology antibody tests in, 101–119.
   See also Immunologic antibody tests
  lymphocyte function tests in, 82–94. *See also* Lymphocytes, functions of, tests in
  radioallergosorbest test for IgE in, 97–98
  tests of, related to cancer, 119–124
Infection(s)
  bacterial, antibody tests for, 104–109
  cultures in diagnosis of, 511–522. *See also* Culture(s)
  fungal, antibody tests for, 102–104
  parasitic, immunologic tests for, 103t
  urinary tract
   leukocyte esterase testing for, 321–322
   nitrite testing for, 321
  viral, antibody tests for, 112–119
Infectious mononucleosis tests, 113–115
Inflammatory radionuclide scanning, 755–756
Inspiratory capacity, definition of, 900
Insulin, 263–264
  blood glucose levels and, 143t
Intestinal hormones, 266–268
Intestine, biopsy of, 498–500
Intracranial scanning
   computed tomography in, 804–806
   magnetic resonance imaging in, 819–820
Intravenous cholangiography (IVC), 620–621
Intravenous glucose tolerance test (IVGTT), 151–152

Intravenous pyelogram (IVP), 635–636
Inulin, renal clearance tests for, 332
Iodine 131 body scanning, 775–776
Ionizing radiation, therapeutic use of, 728, 730
Iron
    in erythropoiesis, 7, 13
    reference values for, 14t–15t
    serum, 14
    studies of, 13–16
        indications for, 15–16
        nursing care before and after, 16
        procedure for, 16
Islets of Langerhans, hormones produced by, 262–266
Isocitrate dehydrogenase (ICD), 199–201
Isoenzymes
    alkaline phosphatase, 196
    creatine phosphokinase, 208–211
    lactic dehydrogenase, 211–213
        elevated, tissue sources and causes of, 212t
Isoflow volume, definition of, 901
IVC. *See* Intravenous cholangiography (IVC)
IVP. *See* Intravenous pyelogram (IVP)

Joints, radionuclide scanning of, 738–740

Karyotyping, 425
17-Ketogenic steroids, urinary, measurement of, 355
    factors interfering with, 361
    indications for, 362
    reference values for, 358t
Ketones in urine, 317–318
17-Ketosteroids, urinary, measurement of, 354
    factors interfering with, 361
    indications for, 362
    reference values for, 358t
Kidney(s)
    angiography of, 667–669
    biopsy of, 489–492
    disease of, laboratory correlations with, 328t
    function of, tests of, 332–341
        clearance, 332–334
        concentration/dilution, 336–341
        phenolsulfonphthalein test as, 334–336
        tubular function, 334–336
    radionuclide scanning of, 769–772
    ultrasonography of, 705–706
Knee, arthroscopy of, *577*

Lactic acid in cerebrospinal fluid, 392
Lactic dehydrogenase (LDH), 211–213
Lactogen, human placental, 261–262
LAP. *See* Leucine aminopeptidase; Leucine aminopeptidase (LAP)

Laparoscopy, 569–576
    contraindications to, 572
    factors interfering with, 570
    gastrointestinal, 569, *570*
    gynecologic, 569, *571*
    indications for, 571–572
    nursing alert for, 573
    nursing care after, 575–576
    nursing care before, 573–574
    procedure for, 574–575
    reference values for, 570
Laryngoscopy, 529–533
Lecithin:sphingomyelin (L:S) ratio in fetal lung maturity assessment, 428
Lee-White coagulation time, 68–69
Leg, blood vessels of, *677*
Leptocytosis, significance of, 30t
Leucine aminopeptidase (LAP)
    serum, 197–198
    urinary, 349
        reference values for, 350t
        tests of
            factors interfering with, 350
            indications for, 351
            nursing care before, 352
            procedure for, 352
Leukocyte(s), 3–4
    in duodenal secretions, 454, 455t
    in feces, 463
    production of, 5
    studies of, 39–46
        differential white blood cell (WBC) count in, 41–42
        white blood cell (WBC) count in, 40–41
        white blood cell (WBC) enzymes in, 42, 44–46
    in urine, 322–323
Leukocyte alkaline phosphatase (LAP), 44–45
Leukocyte esterase in urine, 321–322
Leukocytosis, 40
Leukopenia, 40
Leukopoiesis, 5, 7
    altered, causes of, 8t
Liley graph in hemolytic disease of newborn detection, 426–427, *427*
Lipase, serum, 203–204
Lipids, 172–186. *See also* Lipoproteins
    free fatty acids as, 173–175
    functions of, 172
    phospholipids as, 179–181
    total cholesterol as, 177–179
    triglycerides as, 175–177
Lipoproteins
    classification of, 173
    composition of, 173t
    fractions of, 181–183
        altered levels of, conditions associated with, 182t
    phenotypes of, 184–186
        clinicopathological significance of, 185t

Liver
angiography of, 665–667
biopsy of, 494–496
radionuclide scanning of, 763–765
ultrasonography of, 703–705
Lumbar puncture
nursing care after, 396
nursing care before, 394
procedure for, 394–396
Lumbosacral spine, *601*
Lung(s)
angiography of, 663–665
biopsy of, 501–503
fetal, maturity of, tests for, 427–429
positron emission tomography of, 777–778
radionuclide scanning of, 749–752
Lupus erythematosus (LE), disorders related to, 99t
Luteinizing hormone (LH), 234–235
Lymph nodes
biopsy of, 497–498
ultrasonography of, 697–698
Lymphangiography, 673–674
Lymphocytes
altered levels of, causes of, 44t
assays of, 84–87
functions of, 39
tests of, 82–94
assays in, 84–87
immunoblast transformation tests in, 88–90
immunoglobulin assays in, 90–94
Lysozyme, urinary, 349
reference values for, 350t
tests of
factors interfering with, 350
indications for, 351
nursing care before, 351–352
procedure for, 352

Macrocytosis, significance of, 30t
Magnesium
serum, 284–286
altered levels of, disorders/drugs associated with, 285t
urinary
measurement of, 343
reference values for, 343t
Magnetic resonance imaging (MRI), 800–801, 813–824
abdominal, 817–819
angiography, 816–817
body imaging by, 813–816
chest, 820–822
head, 819–820
heart, 820–822
intracranial, 819–820
musculoskeletal, 822–824
Malabsorption, excess fecal fat in, 464
Mammography, 607–609

Manometric studies, 829–849
esophageal, 836–839
fetoplacental adequacy, 845–847
urodynamic, 829–836. *See also*
Urodynamic studies
Masking level differences test, 924–926
Maximum inspiratory/expiratory pressures, definition of, 901
Maximum midexpiratory flow, definition of, 901
Maximum volume ventilation, definition of, 901
Mean corpuscular hemoglobin concentration (MCHC), 27
Mean corpuscular hemoglobin (MCH), 27
Mean corpuscular volume (MCV), 27
Meat fibers in feces, 464
Meckel's diverticulum scanning, 761–762
Mediastinoscopy, 540–542
Meningitis, CSF examination in diagnosis of, 397–398
Mesenteric angiography, 669–671
Methemoglobin, 32
Metyrapone in cortisol/ACTH challenge tests, 248
Microbiologic examination of cerebrospinal fluid, 396–398
Microcytosis, significance of, 30t
Minerals
trace, 296–297
in urine, 368–369
Mixed lymphocyte culture technique before transplantation, 89
Monocytes
altered levels of, causes of, 44t
functions of, 39
Mosenthal test, 337
nursing care before, 340
procedure for, 340
Mucus
in stomach contents, 447
in urine, 325
Muscles, biopsy of, 496–497
Musculoskeletal system, magnetic resonance imaging of, 822–824
Myasthenia gravis, Tensilon test for, 912–914
Mycoplasma pneumoniae infection, cold agglutinin test for, 107
Myelography, 644–646
Myopathy, muscle biopsy in diagnosis of, 496–497

Narcotics, blood levels of, 299t
Neck, computed tomography scanning of, 806–808
Needle(s), biopsy, *479*
Nephrotic syndrome, laboratory correlations with, 328t
Nephrotoxicity from contrast media, 653–654

Nerve conduction studies, 867–868
Neural tube defects, tests for, 424–426
Neurogenic bladder, types and effects of, 831t
Neurologic tests of cerebrospinal fluid for neurosyphilis, 399–400
Neurological system studies, 910–941
    acoustic admittance tests as, 919–922
    color perception tests as, 933–934
    corneal staining as, 940–941
    hearing loss audiometry as, 914–917
    hearing loss tuning fork tests as, 917–919
    otoneural lesion site tests as, 924–927
    otoneurological tests as, 922–924
    refraction as, 936–937
    Schirmer tearing test as, 939–940
    slit-lamp biomicroscopy as, 938–939
    spinal nerve root thermography as, 910–912
    spondee speech reception threshold test as, 927–928
    Tensilon test as, 912–914
    tonometry as, 934–936
    visual acuity tests as, 928–930
    visual field tests as, 930–933
Neuropathy, muscle biopsy in diagnosis of, 496–497
Neurosyphilis, neurologic tests for, 399–400
Neutrophils
    altered levels of, causes of, 43t
    functions of, 39
Newborn, hemolytic disease of, tests for, 426–427
Nitrite in urine, 320
Non-nuclear scan studies, 799–825
    computed tomography as, 799–812. *See also* Computed tomography (CT)
    magnetic resonance imaging as, 800–801, 813–824. *See also* Magnetic resonance imaging (MRI)
Norepinephrine, 252
    urinary, measurement of, 355–356
        reference values for, 359t
Nose, culture of, 516–518
Nuclear scanning, 727–797
    abscess, 755–756
    adrenal, 741–743
    biliary system, 768–769
    bone, 738–740
    bone marrow, 740–741
    brain, 733–735
    cardiac, 744–749. *See also* Heart, radionuclide scanning of
    cerebrospinal fluid flow, 735–737
    deep vein, 766–767
    gallbladder, 768–769
    gallium 67, 773–775
    gastric emptying, 756–758
    gastrointestinal bleeding, 760–761
    gastrointestinal reflux, 758–759
    inflammatory, 755–756
    iodine 131, 775–776
    joint, 738–740
    kidney, 769–772
    liver, 763–765
    lung, 749–752
    Meckel's diverticulum, 761–762
    methodology of, 728
    pancreas, 762–763
    parathyroid, 754–755
    parotid gland, 737–738
    pheochromocytoma, 743–744
    positron emission tomography as, 730–731, 776–778
    risks in, 732
    salivary gland, 737–738
    scrotal, 772–773
    single-photon emission computed tomography as, 731
    spleen, 765–766
    thyroid, 752–754
    ventilation-perfusion, 749–752
5'-Nucleotidase, 196–197
Null cells, 82
Nystagmus, electrophysiologic study of, 874–876

Obstetric ultrasonography, 712–714
OCG. *See* Oral cholecystography (OCG)
OCT. *See* Ornithine carbamoyltransferase (OCT)
Ocular ultrasonography, 693–695
Oculoplethysmography, 843–845
Operative cholangiography, 623–624
Oral cholecystography (OCG), 617–619
Oral glucose tolerance test (OGTT), 148–151
Orbit, plain films of, 591–592
Ornithine carbamoyltransferase (OCT), 200–201
Osmolality, serum, 286–288
Osmotic fragility, erythrocyte, 34–35
Otoneural lesion site tests, 924–927
Otoneurological tests, 922–924
Oval fat bodies, 323
Oximetry, 906–908

P waves, 852
Pancreas
    radionuclide scanning of, 762–763
    ultrasonography of, 702–703
Pancreatic hormones, 262–266
    C-peptide as, 264–265
    glucagon as, 265–266
    insulin as, 263–264
Papanicolaou (Pap) smear, 478–481
Paracentesis, 414
Paranasal sinuses
    plain films of, 592–593
    tomography of, 606–607

Parasites
  in duodenal secretions, 454, 455t
  in feces, 464
  in urine, 325
Parasitic immunologic tests, 103t
Parathyroid gland, radionuclide scanning of,
  754–755
Parathyroid hormone (PTH), 245–247
Parathyroid ultrasonography, 695–696
Parotid gland, radionuclide scanning of,
  737–738
Partial thromboplastin time (PTT), 66–68
Past-pointing test, 922–924
Peak expiratory flow rate, definition of, 901
Peak inspiratory flow rate, definition of, 901
Pelvic floor sphincter electromyography,
  863–865
Pelvimetry, 599–600
Pelvis
    computed tomography scanning of,
      811–812
    ultrasonography of, 711–712
Pepsinogen secretion, 445
Perchlorate suppression study, 790
Percutaneous transhepatic cholangiography
  (PTHC), 624–627
Pericardial fluid analysis, 405–407
Pericardiocentesis, 406–407
Perimetric test, 931–933
Periodic acid-Schiff (PAS) stain, 45
Peritoneal fluid analysis, 412–415
Persantine in cardiac scanning, 745
PET. See Positron emission tomography (PET)
pH
    of duodenal secretions, 454, 455t
    of urine, 313–314
Phenolsulfonphthalein (PSP) test, 334–336
Phenylketonuria (PKU), 365
Pheochromocytoma, catecholamine excess in, 252
Pheochromocytoma scanning, 743–744
Phonocardiography, 858–859
Phosphate, serum, 282–284
    altered levels of, disorders/drugs associated
      with, 283t
Phosphatidyl glycerol in fetal lung maturity
  assessment, 428–429
Phospholipids, 179–181
Phosphorus
    serum, 282–284
      altered levels of, disorders/drugs associ-
        ated with, 283t
    urinary
      measurement of, 342–343
      reference values for, 343t
Pigments, urinary, 345–349
Pilocarpine iontophoresis sweat test, 908–910
Pituitary gland
    hormones secreted by, 220–237. See also
      Hypophyseal hormones
PKU. See Phenylketonuria (PKU)

Placental hormones, 259–262
Placental lactogen, human, 261–262
Plasma, glucose in, 144–146. See also Glucose,
  blood levels of
Plasma fibrinogen, 74–75
Plasma thrombin time, 69–70
Plasma thromboplastic antecedent (PTA), defi-
  ciency states involving, 73t
Plasmin, 52
Plasminogen, 52
Platelet(s), 3, 4
    count of, 54–56
    deficiency of, prolonged bleeding time in, 56
    functions of
      altered, causes of, 53t
      in hemostasis, 49–50
    levels of, altered, causes of, 54t
    studies of, 53–63
      bleeding time in, 56–58
      clot retraction test in, 60–61
      platelet aggregation test in, 59–60
      platelet count in, 54–56
      Rumple-Leeds capillary fragility test in,
        61–63
Platelet aggregation test, 59–60
Platelet survival time study, 784–786, *786*
Plethysmography, 829, 839–845
    arterial, 839–840
    body, 841–843
    body, definition of, 901
    ocular, 843–845
    venous, 840–841
Pleura, biopsy of, 503–505
Pleural fluid analysis, 408–412
Pleural transudates, exudates differentiated
  from, 409t
Pluripotential stem cells in hematopoiesis, 5
Poikilocytosis, significance of, 30t
Polychromase chain reaction in sputum analysis,
  380–383
Polychromatophilia, significance of, 30t
Polyhydramnios, 423
Porphyrins, urinary, 345–349
Portal angiography, 665–667
Positron emission tomography (PET), 730–731,
  776–778
Postprandial blood sugar, 146–148
Potassium
    serum, 271–274
      altered levels of, disorders/drugs associ-
        ated with, 272t
    urinary
      measurement of, 342
      reference values for, 343t
PR interval, 853
PR segment, 853
Pregnanediol, urinary, measurement of, 357
    factors interfering with, 361
    indications for, 363
    reference values for, 360t

Pregnanetriol, urinary, measurement of, 355
   factors interfering with, 361
   indications for, 362
   reference values for, 358t
Proconvertin, deficiency states involving, 73t
Proctosigmoidoscopy, 552–555
Progesterone, 256–258
   in FSH/LH challenge tests, 232
Prolactin (hPRL), 225–226
Prostaglandins in hemostasis, 50
Prostate gland
   biopsy of, 505–507
   in semen production, 435
   ultrasonography of, 707–708
Prostate-specific antigen (PSA), 206–207
Protein(s)
   in blood, 156–172
      binding, 161–164
      C-reactive, disorders related to, 99t
      metabolites of, 164–172
         ammonia as, 168–169
         serum creatine as, 169–170
         serum creatinine as, 166–167
         urea nitrogen as, 164–166
         uric acid as, 170–172
      serum, 156–160
         altered levels of, causes of, 157t
   in cerebrospinal fluid analysis, 391
   in urine, 314–315, 364–368
Proteinuria, 314–315
Prothrombin, deficiency states involving, 73t
Prothrombin consumption time (PCT), 70–71
Prothrombin time (PT), 63–66
Pseudocholinesterase, 215–216
Psychiatric drugs, blood levels of, 301t
Pteroylglutamic acid. See Folic acid
PTHC. See Percutaneous transhepatic cholangiography (PTHC)
Pulmonary angiography, 663–665
Pulmonary artery catheterization, 891–894
Pulmonary function study, 899–906
   contraindications to, 903
   exercise, 905–906
   factors interfering with, 902
   indications for, 902–903
   nursing care after, 904–905
   nursing care before, 903–904
   procedure for, 904
   reference values for, 901–902
   volumes/capacities measured in,
      900–901
Pulmonary system studies, 898–910
   oximetry as, 906–908
   pulmonary function study as, 899–906.
      See also Pulmonary function study
   sweat test as, 908–910
Pulse oximetry, 906–908
Pyelography
   antegrade, 627–630
   intravenous, 635–636

Pyelonephritis, laboratory correlations with,
   328t
Pyroglobulin, testing for, 92
Pyruvate kinase (PK), 36

QRS complex, 852–853
QRS interval, 853
QT interval, 853
Queckenstedt's test, 395

Radial immunodiffusion for immunoglobulin
   assays, 90
Radiation
   exposure risks for, 588
   therapeutic use of, 728, 730
Radioactive iodine uptake study, 786–788
Radioallergosorbent test (RAST) for IgE,
   97–98
Radioimmunoassays of immunoglobulins, 90
Radiologic studies, 585–647
   angiographic, 651–681. See also
      Angiography
   cineradiography as, 587
   contrast-mediated, 587–588, 609–646
      antegrade pyelography as, 627–630
      arthrography as, 638–640
      barium enema as, 614–617
      barium swallow as, 609–612
      bronchography as, 640–642
      hysterosalpingography as, 642–644
      intravenous cholangiography as, 620–621
      intravenous pyelogram as, 635–636
      myelography as, 644–646
      operative cholangiography as, 623–624
      oral cholecystography as, 617–619
      percutaneous transhepatic cholangiogra-
         phy as, 624–627
      retrograde cystography as, 631–633
      retrograde ureteropyelography as,
         633–635
      retrograde urethrography as, 630–631
      sialography as, 638
      T-tube cholangiography as, 621–623
      upper gastrointestinal series as, 612–614
      voiding cystourethrography as, 636–637
   film cassettes for, 585–586
   film for, 585
   fluoroscopy as, 586–587
   invasive, 586
   noninvasive, 586
   plain film, 589–605
      abdominal, 596, 596–599
      cardiac, 603–605
      chest, 593, 593–596, 594
      extremity, 602, 602–603
      orbital, 591–592
      paranasal sinus, 592–593
      pelvimetry as, 599–600

Radiologic studies *(Continued)*
　　plain film *(Continued)*
　　　skull, 589–591
　　　spinal, 600–601
　　tomography as, 586, 605–607
　　xeroradiography as, 587, 607–609
Radionuclide scanning, 727–795. *See also*
　　Nuclear scanning
Radionuclides
　　diagnostic scanning uses of, 729t–730t
　　laboratory studies using, 731–732,
　　　778–794
　　　of perchlorate suppression, 790–792
　　　of platelet survival time, 784–786, *786*
　　　of radioactive iodine uptake, 786–788
　　　of red blood cell survival time, 781–784
　　　Shilling test as, 792–794
　　　of thyroid cytomel suppression,
　　　　790–792
　　　of thyroid-stimulating hormone,
　　　　788–790
　　　of total blood volume, 778–780
Radiopharmaceuticals, diagnostic scanning uses
　　of, 729t–730t
Rapid plasma reagin (RPR) test for syphilis,
　　110–112
Raynaud's syndrome, cold stimulation test for,
　　897–898
Red blood cell (RBC) enzymes, 35–37
Red blood cell (RBC) indices, 27–28
Red blood cell survival time study, 781–784
Red blood cells, 3. *See also* Erythrocyte(s)
Reflexes, acoustic, testing of, 919, 920,
　　921–922
Refraction, 936–937
Renal angiography, 667–669
Renin, 217–220
Renography, 769–772
Respiration, process and control of, 899–900
Reticulocyte count, 11–13
Retina, electrophysiologic study of, 876–878
Retrograde cystography, 631–633
Retrograde ureteropyelography, 633–635
Retrograde urethrography, 630–631
Retroperitoneal ultrasonography, 697–698
Reverse grouping, 130
Rh typing, 132–133
Rheumatoid factor (RF), disorders related to,
　　99t
Rib cage, *601*
Rinne test, 917–919
Romberg test, 922–924
Rouleaux, 37
Rumple-Leeds capillary fragility test, 61–63

Salicylates, blood levels of, 299t
Salivary gland, radionuclide scanning of,
　　737–738
Schilling test, 792–794

Schirmer tearing test, 939–940
Schistocytosis, significance of, 30t
Schistosoma haematobium in urine, 325
Schwabach test, 917–919
Scrotum
　　radionuclide scanning of, 772–773
　　ultrasonography of, 708–709
Secretin test, 457
Semen
　　analysis of, 435–443
　　　factors interfering with, 440
　　　for fertility, 437–439
　　　indications for, 440
　　　nursing care after, 441
　　　nursing care before, 440–441
　　　procedure for, 441
　　　reference values for, 440t
　　formation of, 435
　　tests for presence of, 439
Seminal vesicles, 435
Sensitivity tests, on sputum, 383–385
Serous fluid
　　characteristics of, 404
　　formation of, 403
Serum
　　alkaline phosphatase levels in, elevated,
　　　conditions causing, 195t
　　amylase in, 201–203
　　bicarbonate in, 276, 278–279
　　　altered levels of, disorders/drugs associ-
　　　　ated with, 277t
　　creatine in, 169–170
　　creatinine in, 166–167
　　globulin in, altered levels of, causes of, 159t
　　glucose in, 144–146. *See also* Glucose,
　　　blood levels of
　　lipase in, 203–204
　　proteins in, 156–160
　　　altered levels of, causes of, 157t
Serum α-fetoprotein (AFP) test, 120–122
Serum complement assays, 95–96
Serum glutamic-oxaloacetic transaminase, 192
Serum glutamic-pyruvic transaminase, 191
Serum osmolality, 286–288
Serum protein electrophoresis for immunoglob-
　　ulin assays, 90, 92f
Serum prothrombin time, 70–71
Shake test in fetal lung maturity assessment, 429
Shift to the left/right, 41
Sialography, 638
Sickle cell disorders, hemoglobin abnormalities
　　in, 31–32
Siderotic granules, significance of, 31t
Signal-averaged electrocardiography, 862–863
Single-photon emission computed tomography
　　(SPECT), 731
Sinus, paranasal
　　plain films of, 592–593
　　tomography of, 606–607
Skin, culture of, 519–521

Skull, plain films of, 589–591
Slit-lamp biomicroscopy, 938–939
Small intestine, biopsy of, 498–500
Smear
    acid-fast bacillus, in sputum analysis,
        385–386
    Papanicolaou, 478–481
Sodium
    serum, 268–271
        altered levels of, disorders/drugs associ-
          ated with, 269t
    urinary
        measurement of, 341
        reference values for, 343t
Somatosensory evoked potentials, 873
Somatostatin, blood glucose levels and, 143t
Somatotropin, human chorionic, 261
Specific gravity of urine, 313
Sperm
    antibodies to, 438
    count of, 437
    morphology of, 438, *438*
    motility of, grades of, 437t
    production of, 435
Sperm penetration assay, 439
Spermatozoa, in urine, 325
Spherocytosis, significance of, 30t
Spinal nerve root thermography, 910–912
Spine
    cervical, *589*
    computed tomography scanning of,
        806–808
    lumbosacral, *601*
    thoracic, *601*
Spleen
    radionuclide scanning of, 765–766
    ultrasonography of, 700–702
Spondee speech reception threshold test,
    927–928
Sputum
    analysis of, 379–387
        acid-fast bacillus smear and culture in,
          385–386
        culture and sensitivity tests in,
          383–385
        staining in, 380–383
    color of, significance of, 380
    mucoid, significance of, 379
    mucopurulent, significance of, 380
    production of, 379
    purulent, significance of, 380
ST segment, 853
Stained red blood cell (RBC) examination,
    28–29
    red blood cell abnormalities seen on,
        30t–31t
Staining, corneal, 940–941
Staphylococcal tests, 104–106
Steatorrhea, 463
Stem cells in hematopoiesis, 5

Stomach
    acidity in, tests of, 450–453
    contents of
        analysis of
          factors interfering with, 449
          indications for, 449
          macroscopic, 447–448
          microscopic, 448–450
          nursing for, 449–450
          procedure for, 450
          reference values for, 448t–449t
        bacteria in, 448
        blood in, 447
        color of, 447
        epithelial cells in, 448
        mucus in, 447
        parasites in, 448
        pH of, 447–448
        red blood cells in, 448
        white blood cells in, 448
        yeasts in, 448
    secretions of, 445–453
        inhibition of, 446
        stimulation of, 445, 446
        tests of, 447–453
          gastric content analysis as, 447–450
Stomatocytosis, significance of, 30t
Stool, cultures of, 472–474
Streptococcal tests, 106–107
Stress test, 860–862
    contraction, 845–847
Stuart factor, deficiency states involving, 73t
Succinimides, blood levels of, 298t
Sulfhemoglobin, 33
Sulkowitch's test, 344
Sweat test, 908–910
Synovial fluid
    analysis of, 415–420
        arthrocentesis for, 419–420
        factors interfering with, 418
        indications for, 418–419
        reference values for, 417t
    characteristics of, 404–405
    crystals in, 417t
    formation of, 403–404
    white blood cells and inclusions in, 416t
Syphilis tests, 109–112

T lymphocytes
    altered levels of, causes of, 85t
    assays of, 84–87
    in cell-mediated immunity, 82
    development of, 82
    functions of, 39
    subsets of, 83
    subsets of, abnormal, disorders associated
        with, 85t
T waves, 853
Tangent screen test, 931–933

Tay-Sachs disease, hexosaminidase in, 213–214
TBG. *See* Thyroxine-binding globulin (TBG)
Technetium Tc 99m pyrophosphate in cardiac
    scanning, 745
Tensilon test for myasthenia gravis, 912–914
Testosterone, 258–259
Thalassemias, hemoglobin abnormalities in, 31,
    33f
Thallium chloride rest/stress studies, 744–745
Thermography, spinal nerve root, 910–912
Thoracentesis, 411
Thoracic spine, *601*
Thoracic ultrasonography, 696–697
Thoracoscopy, 542–544
Thorax, computed tomography scanning of,
    808–809
Throat, culture of, 516–518
Thrombin clotting time (TCT), 69–70
Thrombin in hemostasis, 50
Thrombocytes, 3. *See also* Platelets
Thrombocythemia, 54
Thrombocytopenia, causes of, 54t
Thrombocytosis, causes of, 54t
Thrombopoietin, 53
Thyrocalcitonin, 244–245
Thyroid gland
    biopsy of, 507–508
    function of, radioactive iodine uptake study
        of, 786–788
    radionuclide scanning of, 752–754
Thyroid hormone(s), 237–245
    calcitonin as, 244–245
    thyroid-stimulating immunoglobulins as,
        243–244
    thyroxine as, 238–240
    thyroxine-binding globulin as, 243
    triiodothyronine as, 240–242
Thyroid ultrasonography, 695–696
Thyroid-stimulating hormone (TSH), 228–231
    radionuclide-mediated study of, 788–790
Thyroid-stimulating immunoglobulins (TSI),
    243–244
Thyroxine (T₄), 238–240
    blood glucose levels and, 143t
Thyroxine-binding globulin (TBG), 243
TIBC. *See* Total iron-binding capacity (TIBC)
Tidal volume, definition of, 900
Tissue analysis, 477–509
Tolbutamide tolerance test, 154–155
Tomography, 586
    chest, 605–606
    computed, 799–812. *See also* Computed
        tomography (CT)
    emission, 730
        single-photon, 731
    paranasal sinus, 606–607
    positron emission, 730–731, 776–778
Tone decay test, 924–926
Tonometry, 934–936
Total blood volume study, 778–780

Total iron-binding capacity (TIBC), 14
    reference values for, 15t
Total lung capacity, definition of, 900
Tourniquet test, 61–63
Toxic substances, industrial/household, in blood,
    297, 300, 301t–303t, 303
Trace minerals, 296–297
Tracheal suctioning in sputum collection, 382
Transcranial ultrasound, arterial Doppler,
    719–720
Transesophageal echocardiography, 692–693
Transferrin, 14
Transudates
    effusions differentiated from, 404
    pleural, exudates differentiated from, 409t
Triglycerides, 175–177
    altered levels of, disorders/drugs associated
        with, 176t
    in feces, 464
Triiodothyronine (T₃), 240–242
Trypsin, fecal
    reference values for, 470t
    tests for, 469
TSI. *See* Thyroid-stimulating immunoglobulins
    (TSI)
T-tube cholangiography, 621–623
Tubular function tests, 334–336
Tumor markers, tests for, 119–124, 120t
Tympanometry, 919–921
Tyrosyluria, 365

Ultrasound, 685–724
    abdominal, 698–700
    aortic, 698–700
    biliary system, 703–705
    bladder, 706–707
    breast, 709–711
    diagnostic value of, 686
    display modes for, 685–686
    Doppler, 686–687, 687, 715–721. *See*
        also Doppler ultrasound
    echocardiography as, 688–691
    echoencephalography as, 691–692
    kidney, 705–706
    liver, 703–705
    lymph node, 697–698
    obstetric, 712–714
    ocular, 693–695
    pancreatic, 702–703
    parathyroid, 695–696
    pelvic, 711–712
    prostate, 707–708
    retroperitoneal, 697–698
    risks of, 687–688
    scrotal, 708–709
    spleen, 700–702
    thoracic, 696–697
    thyroid, 695–696
    transesophageal echocardiography as,
        692–693

Universal donor, 130
Universal recipient, 130
Upper gastrointestinal (UGI) series, 612–614
Urea
    in cerebrospinal fluid, 392
    renal clearance tests for, 332–333
Urea nitrogen, 164–166
    altered levels of, causes of, 165t
Ureter, biopsy of, 487–489
Ureteropyelography, retrograde, 633–635
Urethral pressure profile, 835–836
Urethrography, retrograde, 630–631
Uric acid, 170–172
    altered levels of, causes of, 171t
    urinary, 365
Urinalysis, 310–332
    appearance in, 311
    bilirubin in, 319–321
    blood in, 318–319
    clarity in, 311
    color in, 310–311, 312t–313t
    factors interfering with, 329
    glucose in, 315–317
    indications for, 330
    ketones in, 317–318
    leukocyte esterase in, 321–322
    macroscopic analysis in, 310–322
    microsopic analysis in, 322–325,
        326t–328t, 329–332
    nitrite in, 320
    nursing alert for, 330
    nursing care after, 331–332
    nursing care before, 331
    odor in, 311
    pH in, 313–314
    protein in, 314–315
    reference values for, 329t
    specific gravity in, 313
    urobilinogen in, 319–321
Urinary tract. *See also* Bladder
    infection of
        leukocyte esterase testing for,
            321–322
        nitrite testing for, 321
Urine
    amino acids in, 365–366
    amylase in, 349
    appearance of, 311
    arylsulfatase A in, 349
    bilirubin in, 319–321
    blood in, 318–319
    calcium in, measurement of, 342
    casts in, 323–324, 324t
    chlorides in, measurement of,
        341–342
    clarity of, 311
    color of, 310–311
        factors affecting, 312t–313t
    concentration of, in renal function testing,
        336–341

crystals in, 325, 326t–327t
cytologic examination of, 370–371
dilution tests on
    nursing care after, 341
    nursing care before, 340
    procedure for, 340
    in renal function testing, 338
drug screening tests of, 371–373
electrolytes in
    measurement of, 341–345
    reference values for, 343t
enzymes in, 349–352
epithelial cells in, 323
formation of, 309
glucose in, 315–317
hormones in, 352–364. *See also*
        Hormone(s) in urine
hydroxyproline in, 366
ketones in, 317–318
leucine aminopeptidase in, 349
leukocyte esterase in, 321–322
lysozyme in, 349
magnesium in, measurement of, 343
microbiologic examination of, 369–370
minerals in, 368–369
nitrite in, 320
odor of, 311
pH of, 313–314
phosphorus in, measurement of, 342–343
pigments in, 345–349
porphyrins in, 345–349
potassium in, measurement of, 342
protein in, 314–315
proteins in, 364–368
red blood cells in, 322
sodium in, measurement of, 341
specific gravity of, 313
studies of, 309–375. *See also* Urinalysis
    in renal function evaluation, 332–341
uric acid in, 365
urobilinogen in, 319–321
vitamins in, 368–369
white blood cells in, 322–323
Urobilinogen
    in feces, tests for, 469–470
    in urine, 319–321
Urodynamic studies, 829–836
    cystometry as, 830–833
    urethral pressure profile as, 835–836
    uroflometry as, 833–834
Uroflometry, 833–834

Vanillylmandelic acid (VMA), urinary, measure-
        ment of, 356
    factors interfering with, 361
    indications for, 362
    reference values for, 359t
Vascular activity in hemostasis, 49
Veins, deep, scanning of, 766–767

Venereal disease research laboratory (VDRL)
    test for syphilis, 110–112
Venography. *See also* Angiography
    access for, 652
Venous Doppler extremity studies, 720–721
Venous plethysmography, 840–841
Ventilation, maximum volume, definition of, 901
Ventilation-perfusion scanning, 749–752
Ventricular punctures, 395–396
Vertebral vessels, *661*
Viral infection antibody tests, 112–119
Visual evoked potentials, 873
Visual field tests, 930–933
Visual system studies, 928–941
    color perception tests as, 933–934
    corneal staining as, 940–941
    refraction as, 936–937
    Schirmer tearing test as, 939–940
    slit-lamp biomicroscopy as, 938–939
    tonometry as, 934–936
    visual acuity tests as, 928–930
    visual field tests as, 930–933
Vital capacity
    definition of, 900
    forced, definition of, 900
Vitamin A, 292–293
Vitamin B$_{12}$
    in erythropoiesis, 7
    studies of, 16–18

Vitamin B$_{12}$ deficiency, Schilling test for,
    792–794
Vitamin B$_{12}$ in erythropoiesis, 7
Vitamin C, 293–294
Vitamin D, 295–296
Vitamins, 292–296
    in urine, 368–369
VMA. *See* Vanillylmandelic acid (VMA)
Voiding cystourethrography, 636–637
von Willebrand's factor, 50

Weber test, 917–918
White blood cell (WBC) count, 40–41
White blood cell (WBC) enzymes, 42,
    44–46
White blood cells, 3. *See also* Leukocyte
Whole blood clotting time, 68–69
Wound culture, 518–519
Wright's stain in sputum analysis, indications
    for, 381
Wrist, arteries of, *675*

Xeroradiography, 587
    for mammography, 607–609

Yeast in urine, 325

Index of Tests and Procedures Covered

The tests and procedures in this index are grouped according to the substance or organ being examined, or the type of study, and are listed alphabetically.

Laboratory Tests

Amniotic Fluid

Tests for fetal maturity, 427
Tests for genetic and neural tube defects, 424
Tests for hemolytic disease of the newborn, 426

Blood

ABO blood typing, 129
Acid phosphatase (ACP), 204
Acquired immunodeficiency syndrome (AIDS) tests, 117
Adrenocorticotropic hormone (ACTH), 226
Alanine aminotransferase (ALT, SGPT), 191
Aldolase (ALS), 207
Aldosterone, 250
Aldosterone challenge tests, 250
Alkaline phosphatase (ALP), 194
α-hydroxybutyric dehydrogenase (α-HBD, HBD), 214
α₁-antitrypsin, 160
Ammonia, 168
Amylase, serum, 201
Anion gap calculation, 277
Antibody screening tests, 101, 135
Antidiuretic hormone (ADH), 235
Antiglobulin test, direct (DAT), 134
Antiglobulin test, indirect (IAT), 135
Arterial blood gases (ABGs), 288
Aspartate aminotransferase (AST, SGOT), 192
Autoantibody tests, 98
Bicarbonate (HCO₃), serum, 276
Bilirubin, 186
Bleeding time, 56
Blood urea nitrogen (BUN), 164
Ca 15-3, CA 19-9, Ca 50, CA 125 antigen tests, 123
Calcitonin, 244
Calcium (Ca), serum, 279
Capillary fragility test, Rumple-Leeds, 61
Carcinoembryonic antigen (CEA) test, 122
Catecholamines, 252
Ceruloplasmin (Cp), 162
Chloride (Cl), serum, 274
Cholesterol, total, 177
Cholesterol fractionation, 181
Cholinesterases, 215
Clot retraction test, 60
Complete blood count (CBC), 18

Coombs test, direct, 134
Coombs test, indirect, 135
Cortisol, 247
Cortisol/adrenocorticotropic hormone (ACTH) challenge tests, 248
C-peptide, 264
Creatine, serum, 169
Creatine phosphokinase (CPK) and isoenzymes, 208
Creatinine, serum, 166
Differential white blood cell count, 41
Drugs and toxic substances, 297
Enzyme-linked immunoabsorbent assay (ELISA), 117
Erythrocyte (RBC) count, 22
Erythrocyte sedimentation rate (ESR, Sed Rate), 37
Estrogens, 254
Euglobulin lysis time, 76
Factor assays, 71
Febrile/Cold agglutinin tests, 107
Fibrin split products (FSP), 75
5′-nucleotidase (5′-N), 196
Fluorescent treponemal antibody-absorption test (FTA-ABS), 109
Follicle-stimulating hormone (FSH), 231
Follicle-stimulating hormone (FSH)/Luteinizing hormone (LH) challenge tests, 232
Free fatty acids (FFA), 193
Fungal antibody tests, 102
Gamma glutamyl transpeptidase (GTT), 198
Gastrin, 267
Glucagon, 265
Glucose, 144
Glucose, two-hour postprandial, 146
Glucose tolerance test, cortisone, 152
Glucose tolerance test, intravenous, 151
Glucose tolerance test, oral, 148
Glycosylated hemoglobin, 153
Growth hormone (GH, STH, SH), 221
Growth hormone stimulation tests, 223
Growth hormone suppression test, 224
Haptoglobin, 161
Hematocrit (Hct), 24
Hemoglobin (Hgb), 25
Hemoglobin electrophoresis, 29
Hepatitis tests, 115
Hexosaminidase, 213
Human chorionic gonadotropin (hCG), 259
Human leukocyte antigens (HLA), 136
Human placental lactogen (hPL), 261

Blood — *Continued*

Immune complex assays, 96
Immunoblast transformation tests, 88
Immunoglobulin assays, 90
Infectious mononucleosis tests, 113
Insulin, 263
Iron studies, 13
Isocitrate dehydrogenase (ICD), 199
Lactic dehydrogenase (LDH) and isoenzymes, 211
Leucine aminopeptidase (LAP), 197
Lipase, serum, 203
Lipoprotein and cholesterol fractionation, 181
Lipoprotein phenotyping, 184
Luteinizing hormone (LH, ICSH), 234
Magnesium (Mg^{++}), serum, 284
Minerals, trace, 256
Ornithine carbamoyl transferase (OCT), 200
Osmotic fragility, 34
Parathyroid hormone (PTH), 245
Partial thromboplastin time/Activated partial thromboplastin time (PTT/aPTT), 66
Phospholipids, 179
Phosphorus and phosphate (P), serum, 282
Plasma fibrinogen, 74
Platelet aggregation test, 59
Platelet count, 54
Platelet survival time study, 784
Potassium (K), serum, 271
Progesterone, 256
Prolactin (hPRL, LTH), 225
Prostate-specific antigen (PSA), 206
Proteins, serum, 156
Prothrombin consumption time (PCT, Serum prothrombin time), 70
Prothrombin time (PT, Pro Time), 63
Radioactive iodine uptake (RAIU Study), 786
Radioallergosorbent test for IgE (RAST), 97
Red blood cell enzymes, 35
Red blood cell indices, 27
Red blood cell (RBC) survival time, 781
Renin, 217
Reticulocyte count, 11
Rh typing, 132
Rumple-Leeds capillary fragility test (tourniquet test), 61
Sed rate, 37
Serum α-fetoprotein test, 120
Serum complement assays, 95
Serum osmolality, 286
SGOT, 192
SGPT, 191
Sodium (Na), serum, 268
Stained red blood cell examination, 28
Staphylococcal tests, 104
Streptococcal tests, 106
T- and B-lymphocyte assays, 84
Testosterone, 258

Thrombin clotting time (TCT, Plasma thrombin time), 69
Thyroid cytomel/perchlorate suppression studies, 790
Thyroid-stimulating hormone (TSH), 228
Thyroid-stimulating hormone (TSH) stimulation test, 230
Thyroid-stimulating immunoglobulins (TSI, TSIg), 243
Thyroxine (T$_4$), 238
Thyroxine-binding globulin (TBG), 243
Tolbutamide tolerance test, 154
Total blood volume study, 770
Tourniquet test, 61
Transferrin, 13
Triglycerides, 175
Triiodothyronine (T$_3$), 240
Triiodothyronine uptake (RT$_3$U), 241
Uric acid, 170
Venereal disease research laboratory (VDRL) and Rapid plasma reagin (RPR) tests, 110
Viral infection antibody tests, 112
Vitamin A, 292
Vitamin B$_{12}$ and folic acid studies, 16
Vitamin C, 293
Vitamin D, 295
Western immunoblot assay (WIB), 117
White blood cell (WBC) count, 40
White blood cell enzymes, 42
Whole blood clotting time (Coagulation CT, Lee-White coagulation time), 68

Cells/Tissues

Bladder and ureter biopsy, 487
Bone biopsy, 482
Bone marrow examination, 8
Breast biopsy, 484
Cervical punch biopsy, 485
Chorionic villus biopsy (CVB), 492
Intestinal biopsy (small intestine), 498
Liver biopsy, 494
Lung biopsy, 501
Lymph node biopsy, 497
Mammotest, 484
Muscle biopsy, 496
Papanicolaou smear (Pap smear), 478
Pleural biopsy, 503
Prostate gland biopsy, 505
Renal biopsy, 489
Skin biopsy, 481
Thyroid gland biopsy, 507

Cerebrospinal Fluid

Cytologic examination, 398
Microbiologic examination, 396
Routine analysis, 391
Serologic tests for neurosyphilis, 399

Cultures

Blood, 513
Cerebrospinal fluid, 396
Effusions, 405
Eye/Ear, 515
Feces, 466
Gastrointestinal contents, 447
Genital and anal, 521
Nose and throat, 516
Skin, 519
Sputum, 386
Urine, 369
Wound, 518

Duodenal Contents/ Secretions

Analysis of duodenal contents, 454
Duodenal stimulation tests, 457

Effusions

Pericardial fluid analysis, 405
Peritoneal fluid analysis, 412
Pleural fluid analysis, 408
Synovial fluid analysis, 415

Feces

Microbiologic tests, 466
Microscopic analysis, 463
Tests for specific substances, 466

Gastric Contents/Secretions

Analysis of gastric contents, 447
Tests of gastric acidity, 450

Semen

Tests for fertility, 437
Tests for the presence of semen, 439

Sputum

Acid-fast bacillus (AFB) smear and culture, 385
Culture and sensitivity (C&S), 383
Cytologic examination, 386
Gram stain and other stains, 380

Urine

Clearance tests and creatinine clearance, 332
Concentration tests and dilution tests, 336
Cytologic examination, 370
Drug screening tests, 371
Electrolytes, 341
Enzymes, 349
Glucose tolerance test, cortisone, 152
Glucose tolerance test, intravenous, 151
Glucose tolerance test, oral, 148

Hormones and their metabolites, 352
Microbiologic examination, 369
Osmolality, 336
Pigments, 345
Proteins, 364
Routine urinalysis, 310
Schilling test, 792
Tubular function tests and phenolsulfonphthalein (PSP) test, 334
Vitamins and minerals, 368

Diagnostic Procedures

Angiography

Adrenal, 659
Bronchial and intercostal, 663
Cardiac, 654
Cerebral, 661
Fluorescein, 671
Hepatic and portal, 665
Lower extremity, 677
Lymphangiography, 673
Mesenteric, 669
Pulmonary, 663
Renal, 667
Upper extremity, 675

Electrophysiology

Apexcardiography, 853
Auditory evoked potential, 871
Brain mapping, 869
Electrocardiography (ECG), 852
Electroencephalography (EEG), 869
Electromyography (EMG), 865
Electroneurography, 867
Electronystagmography (ENG), 874
Electro-oculography (EOG), 878
Electroretinography (ERG), 876
Evoked brain potentials, 871
Exercise electrocardiography, 860
Holter electrocardiography, 856
Pelvic floor sphincter electromyography, 863
Phonocardiography, 858
Signal-averaged electrocardiography (SAE), 862
Somatosensory evoked potential, 871
Vectocardiography, 853
Visual-evoked potential, 846, 863

Endoscopy

Amnioscopy, 567
Anoscopy, 552
Arthroscopy, 576
Bronchoscopy, 533
Colonoscopy, 555
Colposcopy, 563
Culdoscopy, 565

Endoscopy — *Continued*

Cystoscopy, 559
Endoscopic retrograde
  cholangiopancreatography (ERCP), 548
Esophagogastroduodenoscopy (EGD), 544
Fetoscopy, 569
Laparoscopy, gastrointestinal, 569
Laparoscopy, gynecologic, 560
Laryngoscopy, direct, 529
Laryngoscopy, indirect, 529
Mediastinoscopy, 540
Proctosigmoidoscopy, 552
Thoracoscopy, 542

Manometry

Arterial plethysmography, 839
Body plethysmography, 841
Contraction stress test, 845
Cystometry (CMG), 830
Esophageal acid clearing and perfusion tests,
  836
Esophageal manometry, 836
Nonstress test, 845
Oculoplethysmography, 843
Urethral pressure profile, 835
Uroflowmetry, 833
Venous plethysmography, 840

Non-Nuclear Scanning

Abdominal scanning, 810
Abdominal magnetic resonance imaging (MRI),
  817
Angiography magnetic resonance imaging, 816
Body scanning (CT, CAT, CTT), 801
Body magnetic resonance imaging (MRI,
  NMR), 816
Head and intracranial scanning, 804
Head and intracranial magnetic resonance
  imaging, 819
Heart and chest magnetic resonance imaging,
  820
Musculoskeletal magnetic resonance imaging,
  822
Neck and spinal computerized tomography
  scanning, 806
Pelvic computerized tomography scanning, 806
Thoracic scanning, 808
Abscess/inflammatory, 755
Adrenal, 741
Bone and joint, 738
Bone marrow, 740
Brain, 733
Cardiac, 744
Cardiac multigated pool (MUGA), 745
Cardiac myocardial, 745
Cardiac stress or rest, 745
Cerebrospinal fluid flow, 735
Deep vein, 766

Fibrinogen uptake, 766
Gallbladder/biliary system, 768
Gallium 67, 773
Gastric emptying, 756
Gastroesophageal reflux, 758
Gastrointestinal bleeding, 760
Iodine-131, 775
Kidney and renography, 769
Liver, 763
Lung perfusion, 749
Lung ventilation, 749
Meckel's diverticulum, 761
Pancreas, 762
Parathyroid, 754
Parotid/salivary gland, 737
Pheochromocytoma, 743
Positron emission tomography (PET), 776
Schilling test, 792
Scrotal, 772
Spleen, 765
Thyroid-stimulating hormone (TSH) study,
  788
Thyroid Cytomel/perchlorate suppression
  studies, 790

Radiography

Abdominal films (KUB), 596
Antegrade pyelography, 627
Arthrography, 638
Barium enema (LGI), 614
Barium swallow, 609
Bronchography, 640
Cardiac films, 603
Chest films (CXR), 593
Chest tomography, 665
Excretory urography (EOG), 635
Extremity films, 602
Flat plate, 596
Hysterosalpingography, 642
Intravenous cholangiography (IVC), 620
Mammography, 607
Myelography, 644
Obstruction series, 598
Operative cholangiography, 623
Oral cholecystography (OCG), 617
Orbital films, 591
Paranasal sinus films, 592
Paranasal sinus tomography, 606
Pelvimetry, 599
Percutaneous transhepatic cholangiography
  (PTHC), 624
Retrograde cystography, 631
Retrograde ureteropyelography, 633
Retrograde urethrography, 630
Sialography, 638
Skull films, 589
Spinal films, 600
Transillumination, breast, 607
T-tube cholangiography, 621

Radiography — *Continued*

Upper gastrointestinal (UGI) series, 612
Voiding cystourethrography, 636

Ultrasound

Abdominal/aortic, 698
Arterial Doppler carotid studies, 717
Arterial Doppler extremity studies, 715
Arterial Doppler transcranial studies, 719
Bladder, 706
Breast, 709
Echocardiography, 688
Echoencephalography, 691
Kidney, 705
Liver/biliary system, 703
Lymph nodes/retroperitoneal, 697
Obstetric, 712
Ocular, 693
Pancreatic, 702
Pelvic, 711
Prostate, 707
Scrotal, 708
Spleen, 700
Thoracic, 696
Thyroid/parathyroid, 695
Transesophageal echocardiography, 692
Venous Doppler extremity studies, 720

Organ/System Specific Diagnostics

Ear

Acoustic admittance tests, 919
Air conduction and bone conduction tests, 914
Auditory brainstem electric response test, 924
Bekesy audiometry, 924
Binaural loudness balance, 924
Falling test, 923
Hearing loss audiometry tests, 924
Hearing loss tuning fork tests, 917
Otoneural lesion site tests, 924
Otoneurological tests, 922
Past-pointing test, 924
Romberg test, 924
Schwaback test, 918

Speech discrimination test, 924
Spondee speech reception threshold (SRT) test, 927
Tone decay test, 902
Tympanometry, 919

Eye

Color perception tests, 933
Confrontation test, 930
Corneal staining, 940
Jaeger visual acuity test, 928
Perimetry test, 930
Refraction, 936
Schirmer tearing test, 939
Slit lamp biomicroscopy, 938
Snellen visual acuity test, 928
Tangent screen test, 930
Tonometry, 934
Visual acuity tests, 928
Visual field tests, 930

Heart

Cardiac catheterization study, 886
His bundle (EP) study, 894
Pulmonary artery catheterization study, 891

Lung

Exercise pulmonary function study, 905
Oximetry, 906
Pulmonary function study, 899
Sweat test, 908

Miscellaneous

Cold stimulation test, 897
Spinal nerve root thermography, 910
Tensilon test, 912

Skin

Coccidioidomycosis/histoplasmosis/blastomycosis tests, 958
Intradermal tests for allergens, 951
Mumps test, 957
Patch tests for allergens, 949
Scratch tests for allergens, 948
Tests for immune competence, 952
Trichinosis/toxoplasmosis tests, 960
Tuberculin tests, 954